Kewal K. Jain

Textbook of Hyperbaric Medicine

Sixth Edition

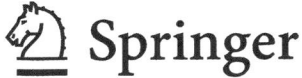 Springer

Kewal K. Jain, MD
Basel, Switzerland

ISBN 978-3-319-83664-5   ISBN 978-3-319-47140-2   (eBook)
DOI 10.1007/978-3-319-47140-2

This Springer imprint is published by Springer Nature
The registered company is Springer International Publishing AG
The registered company address is: Gewerbestrasse 11, 6330 Cham, Switzerland

Slowly but surely, hyperbaric medicine is becoming an established treatment modality for a variety of medical disorders, despite the rocky road that it has sometimes had to travel over the years. In some ways, I feel that the need for oxygen in medical treatments is akin to man's basic requirement for water and food, and I also think it is fair to say that the logic and utility of hyperbaric oxygen treatment now seem to be almost as undeniable as these basic requirements are.

It is certainly the case that, from time immemorial, remedies learned by trial and error have been handed down through the generations—with the result that many roots, berries, fruits, and leaves, as well as special waters containing minerals have been advocated throughout history for their curative powers. More recently, however, evidence-based medicine has come to the fore, demanding higher standards of evidence from basic and clinical/research trials and objective statistical results. One of the first instances of such objective studies in my lifetime was when Austin Bradford Hill and Richard Doll (Doll 2003) convinced colleagues to allocate patients with pulmonary tuberculosis randomly to prove the efficacy of streptomycin, although their trial followed a tradition started 200 years earlier by Linde, who provided citrus fruits aboard some, but not all ships in the British Navy to test whether they would prevent scurvy (Moberg and Chon 2000).

By means of prospective trials, it has been found that various "established" therapies can be detrimental for some diseases, while being clearly beneficial for others. This is precisely the case with hyperbaric medicine now: while a hyperoxic environment for newborn babies can lead to retrolental fibroplasia with blindness, there is also convincing evidence that hyperbaric treatments provide clear benefits in diseases such as various neurological disorders, stroke, cerebral ischemia, and wound healing. And, of course, those of us who have worked in high-altitude environments know the very short time window during which the human brain can function in hypoxic conditions. It never ceases to astonish me what a wide range of effects (beneficial or toxic) a seemingly innocuous substance such as oxygen can have in various circumstances.

By and large, the experts who have made such superb contributions to the *Textbook of Hyperbaric Medicine* are the world leaders in their fields. With their help, Dr. Jain has expanded his already outstanding book into a compendium of multiauthored chapters (containing over 2000 references) covering areas of medicine as disparate as wound healing, gastrointestinal disorders, trauma, and obstetrics. Of particular interest in this edition are the extensive discussions of cerebral circulation and its disorders, as well as of stroke, diving accidents, and neurosurgery.

For an earlier edition, Dr. Jain enlisted a remarkable Foreword by Professor Edward Teller (see next page), who began by stating "Hyperbaric medicine is new and controversial" and that we live "in an age that has the habit of treating progress with suspicion," and then went on to pose the question, "But what is the innovator to do?" He also raised the age-old problem of the ethics of the double-blind trial and cautioned us to be aware of the potential danger of high-pressure treatment for too long a period, in the same way that drug treatments at too high dosages bear clear risks. The field of hyperbaric medicine has indeed been subject to an at times intense debate, but much progress has been made since Professor Teller originally wrote his words (and will, I am sure, continue to be made in the future), on the basis of mutual respect, understanding, and cooperation, while also submitting beliefs to randomized trials.

Professor Teller wrote then: "It is not entirely impossible that, perhaps sometime in the next decade, professors of medicine will have difficulty in explaining why treatment with oxygen was not widely adopted much earlier." Reflecting today on these words by an elder statesman whose scientific observations went unheeded early on, we can safely conclude that the uphill battle for acceptance of hyperbaric oxygen as therapy now rests on a solid foundation. This solid foundation is described comprehensively and clearly within this outstanding text, in which the assembled experts provide a fair and balanced summary of the literature and evidence. And it also means that the "decade of HBO" to which Professor Teller indirectly referred has now come.

James F. Toole, MD
Teagle Professor of Neurology
Director, Cerebrovascular Research Center
Wake Forest University School of Medicine
Winston-Salem, NC, USA

References

Doll R. The evolution of the controlled trial. The Eighteenth John P. McGovern Award Lecture, delivered at the Thirty-third meeting of the American Osler Society, Edinburgh, Scotland; 23 May 2003.
Moberg CL, Chon ZA, editors. Launching the antibiotic era. Personal accounts of the discovery and use of the first antibiotics. New York: Rockefeller University Press; 1990.

Foreword to the First Edition

Hyperbaric medicine is new and controversial. Indeed, since it is new, it must be controversial in an age that has the habit of treating progress with suspicion. But what is the innovator to do? If he applies a new and safe procedure to patients, and the procedure appears to be successful, his success might well be denigrated as anecdotal. Will he be allowed to run a double-blind experiment in which half of the patients are denied the benefits of what appears to be a cure? It is an age-old problem that has grown sharper in the course of time.

Hyperbaric medicine grew out of the problems encountered by divers exposed to high pressures. The treatment of disturbances due to bubbles which develop during rapid decompression was the natural connection between high pressure and medicine. This limited application of a medical procedure is, of course, widely accepted. But its extension to counteract the damage due to the air bubbles resulting from other causes, such as those accidentally introduced during medical treatment, is less generally recognized.

What is attempted in this book is a detailed and critical treatment of a large subject. If thorough discussion will lead to some consensus, the subject could grow very much larger. Indeed, oxygen, which in the form of hyperbaric oxygen (HBO) is called a drug, is the most natural of all drugs.

The first problem we must face is the danger of high-pressure treatment used at excess pressure for too long a period, or in conjunction with the wrong kind of drug. Oxygen indeed has toxic effects. Furthermore, the delivery of the pressurized gas to the patient may be mishandled. A properly extensive discussion is devoted to such dangers, which are completely avoidable.

Perhaps the most natural use of HBO is to counteract carbon monoxide poisoning. The best known effect of carbon monoxide is to replace oxygen by being more firmly bound to hemoglobin. But, of course, high-pressure oxygen can drive out the carbon monoxide and produce a cure in an understandable fashion.

A little harder to grasp is why pure oxygen at two atmospheres of pressure (which is ten times as concentrated as the natural occurrence) should have any general uses. Indeed, under normal circumstances, the hemoglobin in arterial blood is 97% saturated with oxygen. Are we exerting ourselves to supply the remaining 3%? The answer, of course, is no. Oxygen is also soluble in blood. At two atmospheres of pressure, oxygen can be dissolved into the plasma at several times normal levels and can significantly improve tissue oxygenation. This is important because hemoglobin, while more eager to take up oxygen, is also more reluctant to part with it. The oxygen dissolved in the plasma, having a higher chemical potential, is pushed out from the capillaries and into the surrounding tissue. From there, it can spread small distances by diffusion.

Even in the blood itself, the dissolved oxygen may help the white blood cells in their phagocytic activity. Bacteria themselves may react in a variety of ways. It appears that many can use oxygen at normal pressures, but are damaged by oxygen at higher pressures. In the case of anaerobic bacteria, oxygen can act in a powerful way to stop the infection. In combination with other methods, HBO clearly appears effective in cases of gangrene.

But more is involved than the straightforward destruction of the pathogen. The natural healing process may also be assisted by the presence of oxygen. This obviously should be the case when hyperbaric treatment counteracts on oxygen deficiency. Many injuries involve the destruction of capillaries, the means of delivering oxygen. Under such circumstances, healing is itself tied to revascularization of the damaged tissue. But growth of the requisite capillaries is in turn tied to the oxygen supply. This relationship can explain why in the case of many slow healing wounds, HBO seems to have a strong positive effect. Very much more can and should be done to extend the study of the speed of healing to the more normal cases.

In the human body, 20 % of the oxygen consumption occurs in 3 % of the body mass: the brain. This is also the region most sensitive to a deficiency of oxygen, which can produce dramatic results. Indeed, surgical methods on the carotid artery are often used to relieve oxygen deficiency to the brain. It seems logical that in HBO we have a tool that can serve a similar purpose. This might be particularly important in the case of stroke, a high-ranking cause of death and disability. It is clearly worthwhile to explore whether and to what extent disability can be reduced or avoided by prompt use of hyperbaric treatment. If the blood supply to a small region of the brain is reduced, relief might come from the diffusion of oxygen into the ischemic region from neighboring capillaries.

For all new medical techniques, scientific evidence is demanded. Yet medicine is still partly an art, as well as a dramatically advancing science. Therefore in the complicated questions of life, disease, and recovery, it is sometimes hard to distinguish between the fight against the causes of a disease and our efforts to aid toward the reassertion of overall health. There are good indications that HBO is helpful in many diseases, such as multiple sclerosis and osteomyelitis. One may mention these two applications because, in the former, earlier recognition of the disease made possible by the use of magnetic resonance imaging has made early treatment a better possibility and seems to have given a real chance for help from HBO. In the latter case, osteomyelitis, the location of the disease is the bone, where oxygen is usually not amply available.

As members of the scientific community we are all naturally tempted to theorize, as long as a glimmer of a theory might be perceived. This book proceeds, however, along strictly step by step empirical lines. Case after case, the various pathologies are reviewed. In each situation, it is carefully stated to what extent the evidence merely indicates a conclusion and to what extent the conclusion can be proved. In the present stage of HBO, it is a certainty that there will be considerable criticism. On the other hand, those who disagree are likely at the same time to disagree among themselves. I believe that the result will be not only critical reflection, but also more experimentation, more reviews, more understanding, and more progress. It is not entirely impossible that, perhaps sometimes in the next decade, professors of medicine will have difficulty in explaining why the treatment with oxygen was not widely adopted much earlier.

Edward Teller[†]
Formerly Director Emeritus Lawrence
Livermore National Laboratories
California & Senior Research Fellow Hoover Institution
Stanford University, Stanford, CA, USA

Preface to the Sixth Edition

A quarter of a century has passed since the first edition of the book was published. Apart from incorporating new advances since the fifth edition, there was a major reorganization of the book for the new publisher, Springer. Of the more than 2500 publications relevant to hyperbaric medicine published during 2009–2015 that were reviewed, approximately 1300 have been selected and added to the bibliography which has been divided and appended at the end of each chapter. Several older references have been deleted, whereas others have been retained either for their historical interest or for research that has not been repeated. As in previous editions, proportionately more space has been devoted to disorders of the nervous system than other therapeutic areas. Nine chapters on new topics have been added to this edition, and two chapters from the first edition were deleted with incorporation of essential information into other chapters. With increasing application of biotechnologies to clinical medicine, applications in combination with hyperbaric oxygen have been explored, including a new chapter on personalized hyperbaric medicine. There is an increasing integration of multidisciplinary approaches in management of complex disorders, and the role of hyperbaric oxygen in these has been defined. Other new chapters include "Nursing in a Hyperbaric Medical Facility," "Hyperbaric Oxygen Therapy in Military Medicine," and "Ethics, Standards and Quality Control in Practice of Hyperbaric Medicine."

Finally, I would like to thank Gregory Sutorius, senior editor in Clinical Medicine at Springer, for his encouragement and oversight of this project. Diane Lamsback, developmental editor for Springer, has provided invaluable assistance in editing and managing this project.

Basel, Switzerland   K. K. Jain

Preface to the Fifth Edition

Almost 20 years have passed since the first edition of the *Textbook of Hyperbaric Medicine* was written, and since the publication of the fourth revised edition in 2004, there has been a considerable increase of research and development in applications of hyperbaric oxygen. Of the more than 1200 publications relevant to hyperbaric medicine during 2004–2008, approximately 300 have been selected and added to the list in this book, whilst a corresponding number of older references have been deleted to maintain the bibliography at 2000 entries. Several older publications have been retained for their historical interest, and some of these have indeed become classics.

There is an ever increasing use of hyperbaric oxygen for neurological disorders. Other areas of expansion include applications in ophthalmology, and the chapter on this has been rewritten and expanded by Frank Butler and Heather Murphy-Lavoie. A new chapter by Alan Wyatt on the role of hyperbaric oxygen in organ transplantation has been added as well as a chapter on the treatment of chronic Lyme disease by William Fife and Caroline Fife.

Multimodality treatment is required in some complex disorders, and hyperbaric oxygen has been combined with new advances in drug treatment and surgical procedures as well as with complementary medicine techniques such as acupuncture. As other new technologies such as those for manipulating stem cells develop, their interaction with hyperbaric oxygen is being studied. Hyperbaric oxygen may prove to be a useful adjunct to stem cell-based therapeutics and regenerative medicine.

I would like to thank the editorial staff at Hogrefe & Huber Publishers, particularly the Publishing Manager, Robert Dimbleby, for their help and encouragement during this revision.

Basel, Switzerland   K. K. Jain

Preface to the Fourth Edition

The textbook has been revised in accordance with the progress made in hyperbaric medicine during the past 4 years. There were over 1000 publications relevant to hyperbaric medicine during 1999–2002. Approximately 200 of these were selected and a corresponding number of older references were deleted to keep the total number of references in the bibliography to 2000. The number of clinical trials for various applications in hyperbaric oxygen therapy has increased. These are included wherever the published results are available. As personalized medicine is developing, it will be applied to hyperbaric oxygenation as well. It is already obvious that patients require an individualized approach in hyperbaric therapy protocols. The dose of oxygen, pressure, and duration of treatment need to be determined for each patient individually. It is difficult to reach any conclusions from clinical trials about a particular pressure of oxygen or even a range for a broad diagnostic category with many variants among patients that determine the response.

Applications in neurological disorders are developing further and space devoted to this area has been increased. A new chapter by Neubauer and Harch has been added on the treatment of cerebral palsy with hyperbaric oxygenation.

I wish to thank the publishing directors of Hogrefe Publishers and their Editor, Mr. Robert Dimbleby, for their help and encouragement throughout the period of revision.

Basel, Switzerland   K. K. Jain

Hyperbaric medicine continues to make progress. The textbook has been revised and expanded with inclusion of new contributors. We are fortunate to have an article from Prof. Hideyo Takahashi of Japan describing the state of development of hyperbaric oxygen therapy in Japan.

As in the previous edition, objective judgment has been exercised in deciding to include various reports and studies on this subject. There are more than 200 publications every year on hyperbaric medicine, and all the publications cannot be included in references. The bibliography already contains more than 2000 entries. Most of the older references have been retained because of their historical value.

Much of the original material still holds its value and has also been retained. Simply because no new work has been done in some areas does not mean that these indications for HBO are no longer valid. Research in hyperbaric medicine continues to be limited by lack of funding. However, the technique is available for clinical application in certain cases when the need arises and often a precedence in that area helps. Well-documented anecdotal reports have a teaching value, and this has been utilized in the textbook. This is particularly so in the case of emergency medicine and treatment of hypoxemic/ischemic encephalopathies, where it would be practically impossible to conduct controlled studies.

Much of the expansion of hyperbaric oxygen therapy is in the area of neurological disorders, which is reflected in the increased number of chapters devoted to this area. This application of hyperbaric oxygen holds the greatest promise for the future for diseases of the nervous system.

I wish to thank the publishing directors of Hogrefe & Huber and their Editor, Mr. Robert Dimbleby, for their help and encouragement throughout the period of preparation.

Basel, Switzerland   K. K. Jain

Preface to the Second Edition

A great deal of progress has taken place in Hyperbaric Medicine since the publication of the first edition. This has necessitated a thorough revision of the book and inclusion of new contributors. Some of the outdated references were removed and new ones have been added, bringing the total about 1800 entries. I have tried to keep my judgment objective, and this is helped by the fact that I have no involvement in the political and financial aspects of hyperbaric medicine.

In spite of this critical revision and corrections, I am pleased to state that a great deal of the old stuff still holds its value. Use of hyperbaric oxygen therapy in neurological disorders continues to expand and required a chapter on neurosurgery, for which I was fortunate to have the collaboration of Dr. Michael Sukoff of the United States, who has done much of the pioneer work in this field. The chapter on pediatric surgery by Prof. Baydin from Russia is a useful new addition. With the inclusion of unpublished work on the role of neuropeptides in oxygen therapy (Prof. G.T. Ni) from China, the book is now truly international.

I wish to thank the publishing directors of Hogrefe & Huber Publishers for their help and encouragement throughout the period of revision. Countless other colleagues also helped and their names are too numerous to list here.

Basel, Switzerland   K. K. Jain

This book goes considerably beyond the scope of the *Handbook of Hyperbaric Oxygen Therapy,* which was written by me and published by Springer Verlag in 1988. In addition, with the many rapid developments in this field, the *Handbook* has already become remarkably outdated. Our use of the word "textbook" in the title of the present work is in keeping with the increasing worldwide recognition of this branch of medicine and the need for a definite and inclusive source covering this body of knowledge, as it exists today.

In practice hyperbaric medicine of course involves mostly the use of hyperbaric oxygen, i.e., oxygen under pressure greater than atmospheric. As a result, this field overlaps with diving medicine in the areas of

The effect of high pressure on the human body

Physical exercise under hyperbaric environments

Air embolism

Decompression sickness

I have made no attempt to intrude any further into diving medicine, as there are several excellent textbooks on that subject. In addition, the use of normobaric oxygen has been discussed elsewhere in a 1989 title by K. K. Jain, *Oxygen in Physiology and Medicine.*

I have written this current work in a textbook style, and there is more discussion on the pathophysiology of diseases and the rational basis of hyperbaric oxygen than in the *Handbook.* Extensive and up-to-date references have been assembled as an integral part of this project, and these total about 1500.

The highlights of this present effort are the newly documented effectiveness of hyperbaric oxygen therapy in the rehabilitation of stroke patients and the validation of these gains via the iofetamine scan technique. This same method has also been used to document the improvement in multiple sclerosis patients undergoing hyperbaric oxygen therapy.

In the preparation of this work, I was considerably aided by the capable and cooperative management effort provided by the two directors of the Hogrefe & Huber publishing company. The execution of a project involving this degree of both scope and detail is certainly an exercise in teamwork between author and publisher, and it was a pleasure to have shaped the production in a creative and timely manner.

Basel, Switzerland   K. K. Jain

Contents

Part I Basic Aspects

1 The History of Hyperbaric Medicine 3
K. K. Jain
Hyperbaric Therapy and Diving Medicine 3
The Development of Hyperbaric Air Therapy 4
The Development of Hyperbaric Oxygen Therapy 7
References 9

**2 Physical, Physiological, and Biochemical Aspects
of Hyperbaric Oxygenation** 11
K. K. Jain
Introduction 11
Physical Basics 11
Physiology of Oxygenation 12
    The Oxygen Pathway 12
    Ventilation Phase 12
    Transport Phase 12
    Shift of the Oxygen-Hemoglobin Dissociation Curve 13
    Delivery of Oxygen to the Tissues 14
    Oxygen Transfer at the Capillary Level 14
    Relation Between the Oxygen Transport and Utilization 14
    Oxygen Utilization in the Cell 15
    Effect of Blood Flow 15
    Effect of Oxygen-Hemoglobin Reaction on Transport of CO_2 15
    Autoregulation of the Intracellular pO_2 16
Hyperbaric Oxygenation 16
    Theoretical Considerations 16
    General Effects of HBO on the Healthy Human Body 19
    Biochemical Effects of HBO 20
    Effect of HBO on Enzymes 20
    Effect of HBO on the Nervous System 20
    Effect of HBO at Molecular Level 21
Conclusion 21
References 21

3 Effects of Diving and High Pressure on the Human Body 23
K. K. Jain
Physical Effects of Pressure 23
Effects of Pressure on Various Systems of the Body 23
    Hematological and Biochemical Effects 23
    Effect on Ammonia Metabolism 24
    Effect on Blood Cells and Platelets 24

Changes in the Respiratory System and Blood Gases 24

Effects on the Cardiovascular System.. 25

Changes in the Endocrine System... 25

Effect on the Skeletal System 25

Effects of High-Pressure Environments on the Nervous System.......... 25

Damage to the Middle Ear and Inner Ear in Diving 29

Vertigo and Diving.. 30

Taste Sensation Under High Pressure 30

Effect of High Pressure on Effect of Drugs 30

Conclusion 31

References.. 31

4   Physical Exercise under Hyperbaric Conditions 33
K. K. Jain

Introduction.. 33

Exercise and Hypoxia 34

Exercise in Hyperbaric Environments 34

Exercise Under Hyperoxia 35

Physical Exercise Under Hyperbaric Conditions.............................. 35

General Effects.. 35

Effect on Lactate Production and Clearance................................ 36

Effect of Exercise on Ammonia Metabolism................................ 37

Effect of HBO on Antioxidant Enzymes in Skeletal Muscle............... 37

Effect of HBO on Blood Flow to the Muscles During Exercise.......... 37

Physical Exercise in Relation to Toxic Effects of HBO 38

Conclusion 38

References.. 38

5   Hypoxia.. 39
K. K. Jain

Introduction.. 39

Pathophysiology of Hypoxia.. 39

Hypoxia-Inducible Factor 40

Hypoxia and Heat Shock Proteins 40

Effect of Hypoxia on Cellular Metabolism................................. 40

Impact of Hypoxia on Various Body Systems 41

Respiratory Function.. 41

Cardiovascular System... 41

General Metabolic Effects 41

Effects of Hypoxia on the Brain 42

Role of HBO in the Treatment of Hypoxic States 46

The Role of Nitric Oxide Synthase in the Effect of HBO in Hypoxia.... 47

Possible Dangers of HBO in Hypoxic States............................... 47

References.. 48

6   Oxygen Toxicity.. 49
K. K. Jain

Introduction.. 49

Pathophysiology of Oxygen Toxicity 50

Free Radical Mechanisms 50

Pathology of Oxygen Toxicity 50

Pulmonary Oxygen Toxicity 52

Normobaric vs. Hyperbaric Oxygen in Induction of Pulmonary
Oxygen Toxicity.. 53

Oxygen-Induced Retinopathy 53
Factors That Enhance Oxygen Toxicity 53
Central Nervous System Oxygen Toxicity 54
Ammonia and Amino Acids 56
Biomarkers of Oxygen Neurotoxicity 56
Neuropathology of Oxygen Toxicity 56
Manifestations of CNS Oxygen Toxicity 57
Clinical Monitoring for Oxygen Toxicity 57
Protection Against Oxygen Toxicity 57
Extension of Oxygen Tolerance 59
Conclusion and Directions for Future Research 59
References 60

7 **Hyperbaric Chambers: Equipment, Technique, and Safety** 61
K. K. Jain
Introduction 61
Monoplace Chambers 61
Multiplace Chambers 62
Multiplace Chambers for the Critical Care Department 64
Surgery in the Multiplace Chamber 65
Mobile Multiplace Hyperbaric Chambers 65
Hyperbaric Chambers for Diving Medicine 66
Hyperbaric Chambers for Animal Research 66
Selection of a Hyperbaric Chamber 68
Technique of Hyperbaric Oxygenation 68
Ancillary Equipment 70
Oxygen Masks and Hoods 70
Respirators and Ventilators 70
Diagnostic Equipment 71
ECG and EEG 71
Transcutaneous Oxygen Tension 71
Glucose-Monitoring Devices 71
Use of Miscellaneous Medical Devices in the Hyperbaric Chamber 72
Cardiopulmonary Resuscitation 72
Use of Defibrillators in Hyperbaric Chambers 72
Pleural Suction Drainage 72
Endotracheal Tubes 72
Care of Tracheotomy 72
Continuous Bladder Irrigation and HBO 72
Transdermal Patches for Drug Delivery and Hyperbaric Chamber 73
Implanted Devices in Patients 73
Monitoring of Patients in the Hyperbaric Chamber 73
Safety in the Hyperbaric Chamber 74
Operational Safety 74
Masks and Breathing Control System 74
Fire Safety in the Chamber 74
Use of Portable Hyperbaric Chambers in Patient's Rooms 76
Regulatory Issues Relevant to Hyperbaric Medicine 76
Staffing of Hyperbaric Facilities 77
Conclusion 77
References 77

8   Indications, Contraindications, and Complications of HBO Therapy............... 79
      K. K. Jain
      Indications... 79
      Contraindications.. 79
      Complications of Hyperbaric Oxygenation 81
          Middle Ear Barotrauma.. 81
          Ophthalmological Complications of HBO.. 82
          Pulmonary Complications of HBO.. 82
          Oxygen Seizures 82
          Decompression Sickness.. 83
          Genetic Effects.. 83
          Claustrophobia.. 83
          Anxiety Reactions.. 83
          Coincidental Medical Events in the Hyperbaric Chamber................................ 84
      Precautions in Selection of Patients for HBO Treatment...................................... 84
      Conclusion 84
      References 84

9   Drug Interactions with Hyperbaric Oxygenation.. 85
      K. K. Jain
      Oxygen as a Drug.. 85
          Drug–Drug Interactions 85
          Interactions of HBO with Other Drugs... 85
      Interaction of HBO with Antimicrobials 86
          Carbapenem Antibiotics... 86
          Aminoglycoside Antibiotics 86
          Sulfonamides... 86
      Interaction of HBO with Anticancer Agents 86
      Interaction of HBO with Cardiovascular Drugs 86
          Adrenomimetic, Adrenolytic, and Ganglion-Blocking Agents 86
          Digitalis/Digoxin... 87
          Antianginal Drugs 87
          Heparin... 87
      Interaction of HBO with Drugs Acting on the CNS 87
          Anesthetics... 87
          CNS Stimulants... 87
          Ethanol 87
          Narcotic Analgesics... 87
          Pentobarbital 87
          Scopolamine.. 87
      Interaction of HBO with Miscellaneous Drugs 88
      Practical Considerations of Drug Administration During HBO Therapy................. 88
      Drugs that Enhance Oxygen Toxicity 88
      Drugs that Protect Against Oxygen Toxicity 88
      Conclusion 89
      References 89

**10   Neurophysiologic SPECT Brain Function Imaging and Hyperbaric
      Oxygen Therapy**.. 91
      J. Michael Uszler
      Introduction... 91
      Case Studies 93
      Conclusion 94
      Suggested Reading.. 96

Part II Clinical Applications

11 Decompression Sickness 101

Philip B. James and K. K. Jain

Introduction 101

Pathophysiology 102

    Gas Formation 102

    Pulmonary Changes 104

    Bubble-Induced CNS Injury 104

    Changes in Blood 105

    Dysbaric Osteonecrosis 106

    Role of Free Radicals 106

Clinical Features 106

    Decompression Sickness in Diving 106

    Altitude Decompression Sickness 107

    Ocular Complications of DCS 108

    Ultrasonic Detection of Bubbles 109

Diagnosis 109

    Blood Examination 109

    Ultrasound Monitoring of Bubbles 110

    Bone Scanning 110

    X-Rays 110

    Retinal Angiography 110

Imaging 110

Electrophysiological Studies 110

Neuropsychological Assessment 110

Treatment 110

    Emergency Management and Evaluation 110

    Recompression and HBO Treatment 111

    Management of Altitude Decompression Sickness 111

    Management of Neurological Manifestations of Decompression Sickness 114

Monoplace vs. Multiplace Chambers 115

Use of Oxygen vs. Other Gas Mixtures 115

Drugs 116

Importance of Early Treatment 117

Delayed Treatment 117

Treatment of Residual Neurological Injury and SPECT Brain
Imaging in Type II DCS 117

Risk Factors for DCS 117

Preventive Measures for DCS 118

Prognosis of DCS 118

Conclusion 118

References 119

12 Cerebral Air Embolism 121

K. K. Jain

Introduction 121

Causes 121

Mechanisms 122

Pathophysiology of Cerebral air Embolism 122

Clinical Features 123

Diagnosis 123

Treatment 123

Clinical Applications of HBO for Air Embolism 124
Ancillary Treatments 126
    Antiplatelet Drugs 126
    Steroids 126
    Hemodilution 126
    Control of Seizures 126
    Measures to Improve Cerebral Metabolism 126
Hyperbaric Treatment in Special Situations 126
    Cerebral Edema 126
    Cardiovascular Surgery 126
    Neurosurgery 127
    Pulmonary Barotrauma 127
    Air Embolism During Invasive Medical Procedures 127
    Cerebral Air Embolism During Obstetrical Procedures 127
    Cerebral Air Embolism in Endoscopic Retrograde
    Cholangiopancreatography 128
    Cerebral Embolism Due to Hydrogen Peroxide Poisoning 128
    Relapse Following Spontaneous Recovery 128
    Delayed Treatment 129
Conclusion 129
References 129

13   Carbon Monoxide and Other Tissue Poisons 131
     K. K. Jain
     Classification of Tissue Poisons 131
     Carbon Monoxide Poisoning 131
         Historical Aspects of CO Poisoning 131
         Biochemical and Physical Aspects of CO 131
         CO Body Stores 132
         Biochemical Effects of CO on Living Organisms 132
         Inhibition of the Utilization of Oxygen by CO 132
     Epidemiology of CO Poisoning 133
         Causes of CO Poisoning 134
         Sources of CO Poisoning 134
     Pathophysiology of CO Poisoning 134
         CO Binding to Myoglobin 134
         CO-Induced Hypoxia 135
     Effects of CO on Various Systems of the Body 135
         Cardiovascular System 135
         Hemorheological Effects of CO 136
         Effect of CO on Blood Lactate 136
         Effect of CO on the Lungs 136
         Exercise Capacity 136
         Sleep 136
         Effect on Pregnancy 136
         Musculoskeletal System 136
         Skin 136
         Gastrointestinal System 137
         Effects on the Peripheral Nervous System 137
         Effects on the Visual System 137
         Effect on the Auditory System 137
         Effect on the Central Nervous System 137
     Clinical Features of CO Poisoning 138
         Neuropsychological Sequelae of CO Poisoning 138

Clinical Diagnosis of CO Poisoning 140
   Pitfalls in the Clinical Diagnosis of CO Poisoning.. 140
   Occult CO Poisoning 140
Laboratory Diagnosis of CO Poisoning 140
   Brain Imaging Studies.. 141
General Management of CO Poisoning 142
   Rationale for Oxygen Therapy (NBO or HBO) for CO Poisoning 143
   Experimental Evidence 144
   Clinical Use of HBO in CO Poisoning 144
   Clinical Trials of HBO in CO Poisoning 145
   HBO for CO Intoxication Secondary to Methylene Chloride Poisoning 148
   Treatment of CO Poisoning in Pregnancy 148
   Treatment of Smoke Inhalation... 149
   Prevention and Treatment of Late Sequelae of CO Poisoning............................... 149
   Controversies in the Use of HBO for CO Poisoning 149
Cyanide Poisoning 150
   Pathophysiology... 150
   Clinical Features of Cyanide Poisoning.. 150
   Laboratory Diagnosis 150
   Treatment 150
   Rationale for Use of HBO in Cyanide Poisoning 150
Hydrogen Sulfide Poisoning 150
Carbon Tetrachloride Poisoning 151
Methemoglobinemias.. 151
   Treatment 151
Miscellaneous Poisons 152
   Organophosphorus Compounds.. 152
   Conclusions: Poisoning Other Than with CO.. 152
References.. 152

14 HBO Therapy in Infections... 155
K. K. Jain
Introduction.. 155
   Host Defense Mechanisms Against Infection... 155
   Impairment by Anoxia 155
   Oxygen as an Antibiotic... 155
HBO as an Adjuvant to Antibiotics 157
HBO in the Treatment of Infections 157
   HBO in the Treatment of Soft Tissue Infections 158
   Crepitant Anaerobic Cellulitis 158
   Progressive Bacterial Gangrene 158
   Necrotizing Fasciitis 158
   Nonclostridial Myonecrosis 159
   Fournier's Gangrene... 159
   Gas Gangrene 160
   Fungal Infection 163
   HBO in the Management of AIDS.. 164
   Miscellaneous Infections 164
Osteomyelitis 165
   Management of Osteomyelitis 166
   HBO Treatment of Osteomyelitis 167
   Clinical Results of HBO Treatment in Osteomyelitis... 168
   Osteomyelitis of the Jaw 168
   Osteomyelitis of the Sternum.. 168

Malignant Otitis Externa 168
References 169

15 Hyperbaric Oxygen Therapy and Chronic Lyme Disease:
The Controversy and the Evidence 171
Caroline E. Fife and Kristen A. Eckert
Introduction to Lyme Disease vs. Chronic Lyme Disease: A Brief Overview 171
Chronic Lyme Disease 173
HBOT for Lyme Disease and CLD 174
Rationale for Using HBOT 174
The Need for a HBOT Medical Registry 179
Conclusion 179
References 180

16 HBO Therapy in Wound Healing, Plastic Surgery, and Dermatology 183
K. K. Jain
Introduction 183
Wound Healing 184
Role of Oxygen in Wound Healing 184
Pathophysiology of Nonhealing Wounds 184
Wound Healing Enhancement by Oxygen 185
Clinical Applications 187
Role of HBO in Nonhealing Wounds and Ulcers 189
Ulcers Due to Arterial Insufficiency 189
Diabetic Ulcers 190
Clinical Use of HBO in Diabetic Foot 191
Guideline for the Use of HBO in the Treatment of Diabetic Foot Ulcers 192
Venous Ulcers 193
Decubitus Ulcers 195
Infected Wounds 195
Frostbite 195
Spider Bite 196
HBO for Inflammatory Bowel Disease 197
HBO as an Aid to the Survival of Skin Flaps and Free Skin Grafts 197
Basic Considerations 197
Animal Experimental Studies 198
Comparison and Combination of HBO with Other Methods
for Enhancing Flap Survival 199
Clinical Applications 199
Conclusion 200
HBO as an Adjunct in the Treatment of Thermal Burns 200
Basic Considerations 200
Experimental Studies 201
Clinical Applications 201
Conclusion 202
Applications of HBO in Dermatology 202
Necrobiosis Lipoidica Diabeticorum 202
Pyoderma Gangrenosum 202
Purpura Fulminans 203
Toxic Epidermal Necrolysis 203
Psoriasis 203
Scleroderma 203
References 204

17   HBO Therapy in the Management of Radionecrosis 207
K. K. Jain
Intoduction 207
   Radiation Physics 207
   Unit of Radiation 207
Radiation Biology 208
Radiation Pathology 208
   Clinicopathological Correlations 208
   Effect of Radiation on Blood Vessels 208
   Effect on Soft Tissues 208
   Radiation Effects on the Nervous System 208
   Radiation Effects on the Bone 209
HBO Therapy for Radionecrosis 209
   Effect of HBO on Radiation Damage to Skin and Mucous Membranes 209
   Rationale for Clinical Application 209
Management of Osteoradionecrosis 210
   Basic Studies 210
   Osteoradionecrosis of the Mandible 211
   Osteonecrosis of the Temporal Bone 212
   Osteoradionecrosis of the Chest Wall 212
   Osteoradionecrosis of the Vertebrae 212
   Management of Radionecrosis of CNS 212
   Management of Radionecrosis of Soft Tissues 214
   Effect of HBO on Cancer Recurrence 216
Conclusion 217
References 217

18   The Use of HBO in Treating Neurological Disorders 221
K. K. Jain
Introduction 221
   Effect of HBO on Cerebral Metabolism 221
   Effect of HBO on Cerebral Blood Flow 222
   Effect of HBO on the Blood–Brain Barrier 224
   Effect of HBO on Oxygen Tension in the Cerebrospinal fluid 224
Rationale for the Use of HBO in Neurological Disorders 225
   Cerebral Hypoxia 225
   Cerebral Edema 225
Role of HBO in Neuroprotection 226
Indications for the Use of HBO in Neurological Disorders 228
Clinical Neurological Assessment of Response to HBO 229
   Comatose Patients 229
   Paraplegics 229
   Hemiplegics (Stroke Patients) 230
Diagnostic Procedures Used for Assessing the Effect of HBO 230
   Electrophysiological Studies 230
   Cerebral Blood Flow 231
   Computerized Tomography 232
   Magnetic Resonance Imaging 232
   Positron Emission Tomography 233
   Single Photon Emission Computed Tomography 233
References 234

19 Role of Hyperbaric Oxygenation in the Management of Stroke 237
K. K. Jain
Introduction.. 237
    Epidemiology of Stroke 238
Risk Factors for Stroke 238
    Pathophysiology of Stroke 239
    Causes of Stroke 239
    Changes in the Brain During Ischemic Stroke.. 240
    Clinicopathological Correlations 240
    Structure of a Cerebral Infarct 240
    Cerebral Metabolism in Ischemia 242
Molecular Mechanism in the Pathogenesis of Stroke.................................... 244
    Gene Expression in Response to Cerebral Ischemia............................... 244
    Induction of Heat Shock Proteins 244
    Role of Cytokines and Adhesion Molecules in Stroke 244
    DNA Damage and Repair in Cerebral Ischemia..................................... 244
    Role of Neurotrophic Factors 244
Classification of Ischemic Cerebrovascular Disease 245
Recovery from Stroke 245
Complications of Stroke 246
Sequelae of Stroke 246
    Vascular Dementia 247
Diagnosis of Stroke 247
Stroke Scales 248
    Barthel Index 248
    Rankin Scale 248
    National Institutes of Health Stroke Scale 248
    Unified Neurological Stroke Scale.. 248
    Canadian Neurological Scale 249
    Evaluation of Various Scales... 249
An Overview of the Conventional Management of Stroke.............................. 249
    Acute Ischemic Stroke 249
    Neuroprotectives 250
Management of the Chronic Poststroke Stage 252
    Management of Spasticity.. 252
Role of HBO in the Management of Acute Stroke 253
    HBO in Relation to Cerebral Ischemia and Free Radicals 254
    Animal Experiments 254
    Neuroprotective Effect of HBO Preconditioning.................................... 257
    Review of Clinical Studies... 258
    HBO as a Supplement to Rehabilitation of Stroke Patients.................... 262
Conclusions of the Effects of HBO in Stroke Patients 265
Future Prospects.. 266
References.. 266

20 HBO Therapy in Global Cerebral Ischemia/Anoxia and Coma........................ 269
Paul G. Harch
Introduction... 269
Pathophysiology... 270
Rational Basis of HBO Therapy 271
Review of Animal Experimental Studies... 298
Review of Human Clinical Studies.. 300
Case Studies 304

Patient 1: HBO Treatment for Coma Due to Traumatic Brain Injury.................. 304

Patient 2: Near Drowning, Chronic Phase 307

Patient 3: Near Drowning, Chronic Phase 308

Patient 4: Battered Child Syndrome 309

Conclusion 311

References... 314

21   HBO Therapy in Neurosurgery 321

K. K. Jain

Introduction.. 321

Role of HBO in the Management of Traumatic Brain Injury: TBI 321

Mechanism of Action of HBO in TBI 322

Effect of HBO on ICP in Acute TBI 322

Effect of HBO Therapy in Chronic Sequelae of TBI............................... 323

Experimental and Clinical Studies of HBO in TBI 323

Controlled Clinical Trials of HBO for TBI... 325

Use of HBO for TBI in Clinical Practice... 326

Conclusions 326

Role of HBO in the Management of Spinal Cord Injury 326

Effects of Spinal Cord Injury 327

Rationale of the Use of HBO in SCI... 327

Animal Experimental Studies of HBO in SCI 327

Clinical Studies of HBO in SCI 328

Role of HBO in Rehabilitation of SCI Patients 329

Role of HBO in Compressive and Ischemic Lesions of the Spinal Cord 329

Conclusions About Use of HBO in SCI 330

HBO as an Adjunct to Radiotherapy of Brain Tumors............................. 330

Role of HBO in the Management of CNS Infections 331

Role of HBO in Cerebrovascular Surgery 332

Neuroprotection During Neurosurgery 337

Conclusion 337

References... 338

22   Oxygen Treatment for Multiple Sclerosis Patients 341

Philip B. James

Introduction.. 341

Pathophysiology.. 342

Rationale for Hyperbaric Oxygen Treatment.. 342

Clinical Trials of HBO in Multiple Sclerosis.. 345

Conclusion 349

References... 349

23   HBO in the Management of Cerebral Palsy 351

Paul G. Harch

Introduction: Causes of Cerebral Palsy... 351

Oxygen Therapy in the Neonatal Period.. 351

Treatment of Cerebral Palsy with HBO 353

Published Clinical Trials... 354

The United States Army Study on Adjunctive HBO Treatment of Children

with Cerebral Anoxic Injury 355

The New Delhi Study of HBOT in CP... 356

Unpublished Studies 356

The Cornell Study 356

Comparative Effectiveness Studies... 356

Recent Studies (Since 2007) 357
Side Effects 357
Case Reports 358
  Patient 1: Cerebral Palsy 358
  Patient 2: Cerebral Palsy 359
Conclusions 361
References 363

24 HBO Therapy in Miscellaneous Neurological Disorders 365
K. K. Jain
Introduction 365
HBO in the Treatment of Benign Intracranial Hypertension 365
Peripheral Neuropathy 366
  HBO for the Treatment of Peripheral Neuropathic Pain 366
  HBO for Treatment of Drug-Induced Neuropathy 366
HBO for the Treatment of Trigeminal Neuralgia 367
HBO in Susac's Syndrome 367
Cerebral Malaria 367
Vascular Headaches 367
  Rationale for the Use of HBO in Vascular Headaches 367
  Current Status of Use of HBO in Vascular Headaches 368
HBO for Autism Spectrum Disorder 368
Neurological Disorders in Which HBO Has Not Been Found to Be Useful ... 368
  Dementia Due to Degenerative Disorders of the Brain 368
  HBO in the Management of Neuromuscular Disorders 369
References 370

25 HBO Therapy in Cardiovascular Diseases 371
K. K. Jain
Introduction 371
Pathophysiology 371
  Risk Factors 371
  Hypoxia, Hyperoxia, and Atherosclerosis 371
Hyperbaric Oxygenation in Cardiology 372
  Effect of Hypoxia, Hyperoxia, and Hyperbaric Environments
  on Cardiovascular Function 372
  Metabolic Effects of HBO on the Heart 372
  Role of HBO in Experimental Myocardial Infarction 373
Clinical Applications of HBO in Cardiology 373
  Acute Myocardial Infarction 373
  Combination of HBO and Thrombolysis 376
  Chronic Ischemic Heart Disease (Angina Pectoris) 376
  Cardiac Arrhythmias 377
  Heart Failure 377
  Cardiac Resuscitation 377
HBO as an Adjunct to Cardiac Surgery 377
  Experimental Studies 377
  Human Cardiac Surgery 378
  Protective Effect of HBO Preconditioning in Cardiac Surgery 379
  CNS Complications of Cardiac Surgery 379
HBO in Preventive Cardiology 380
  Prevention and Rehabilitation of Coronary Artery Disease 380
  Physical Training of Patients with Chronic Myocardial Insufficiency 380
  Conclusion and Comments 380

HBO in Shock 380
   Pathophysiology of Shock 380
   Oxygen Delivery by Blood 380
   Traumatic and Hypovolemic Shock 381
   Cardiogenic Shock 381
Peripheral Vascular Disease 381
   Causes 381
   Symptoms and Signs 382
   Pathophysiology of Limb Ischemia 382
   Biochemical Changes in Skeletal Muscle in Ischemia
   and Response to Exercise 382
   Clinical and Laboratory Assessment of Patients with Peripheral
   Vascular Disease 383
   General Management of PVD Patients 384
   Drug Therapy 384
   Exercise Therapy 384
   Surgery 384
   Role of HBO in the Management of Peripheral Vascular Disease 385
   Role of HBO in Miscellaneous Arteriopathies 389
   HBO as an Adjunct to Peripheral Vascular Surgery 389
   Conclusions Regarding the Role of HBO in Peripheral Vascular Disease 390
References 390

26 HBO Therapy in Hematology and Immunology 393
K. K. Jain
Introduction 393
Effect of HBO on Red Blood Cells 393
   Deformability 393
   Oxygen Exchange 394
   Structure and Biochemistry 395
   Effect of HBO on Stored Blood 395
   Hemoglobin 395
   Erythropoiesis 396
   Effect of HBO on Hemorheology in Human Patients 396
Effect of HBO on Leukocytes 396
Effect of HBO on Platelets and Coagulation 396
Effect of HBO on Stem Cells 396
Effect of HBO Treatment on the Immune System 397
Effect of HBO Treatment on Plasma and Blood Volume 398
The Use of HBO in Conjunction with Oxygen Carriers 399
Clinical Applications of HBO in Disorders of the Blood 399
   Hypovolemia and Acute Anemia Due to Blood Loss 399
   Hemolytic Anemia 400
   Potential Benefits of HBO in Cerebrovascular Diseases
   Due to Blood Disorders 400
   Contraindication: Congenital Spherocytosis 400
References 401

27 HBO Therapy in Gastroenterology 403
K. K. Jain
Introduction 403
HBO in Peptic Ulceration 403
   Pathophysiology and Rationale of HBO Therapy 403
   Experimental Studies in Animals 404

Clinical Assessment of HBO in Gastric and Duodenal Ulcer Patients.................. 404
HBO in the Treatment of Intestinal Obstruction... 404
Basic Considerations and Rationale of HBO Therapy 404
Experimental Studies in Animals... 405
HBO Therapy in Adynamic Ileus 406
HBO in Adhesive Intestinal Obstruction 406
Methods... 407
HBO in Chronic Idiopathic Intestinal Pseudo-obstruction 407
HBO in Inflammatory Bowel Disease 407
Ulcerative Colitis and Crohn's Disease 407
Mechanism of Effectiveness of HBO in Ulcerative Colitis 408
HBO in Infections of the Gastrointestinal Tract 408
Toxic Megacolon.. 408
Pseudomembranous Colitis.. 409
Necrotizing Enterocolitis 409
Radiation Enterocolitis.. 409
HBO in Pneumatosis Intestinalis 409
Pathophysiology of Pneumatosis Cystoides Intestinalis........................ 409
Rationale for HBO Therapy... 410
Clinical Experience 410
HBO in Ischemic Disorders of the Intestine.. 410
Use of Hyperbaric Therapy in Removal of Entrapped Intestinal Balloons 411
HBO in Acute Pancreatitis.. 411
Animal Experimental Studies of HBO in Acute Pancreatitis 411
Clinical Applications of HBO in Acute Pancreatitis 411
HBO in Diseases of the Liver 412
Effect of HBO on the Normal Liver 412
Effect of HBO on Experimentally Induced Hepatic Disorders in Animals.......... 412
Clinical Applications 412
Conclusions Regarding the Use of HBO in Gastroenterology 413
References.. 414

28 HBO and Endocrinology 417
K. K. Jain
Introduction.. 417
Thyroid Glands 417
Glucocorticoid Receptors... 417
Adrenocortical Function.. 417
Epinephrine/Norepinephrine... 418
Prostaglandins.. 418
Testosterone 418
Clinical Applications 419
Thyroid Disease 419
Diabetes Mellitus 419
Conclusion 420
References.. 420

29 HBO and Pulmonary Disorders 423
K. K. Jain
Introduction.. 423
Effects of HBO on Lungs.. 423
Arterial and Pulmonary Arterial Hemodynamics 423
Lung Mechanics and Pulmonary Gas Exchange 424
Pulmonary Oxygen Toxicity 424

Clinical Applications 425
    Respiratory Insufficiency 425
    Bronchial Asthma 426
    Bronchitis 426
    Inflammatory Processes of the Lungs 426
    Pulmonary Embolism.. 426
    Pulmonary Edema 426
    Mechanism of Action of HBO in Type II Decompression Syndrome................... 427
Contraindications for the Use of HBO.. 427
    Nitrogen Dioxide Poisoning 427
    Paraquat Poisoning.. 427
    Emphysema.. 427
    Shock Lung 427
    Pneumothorax 427
Conclusion 428
References.. 428

30 Hyperbaric Oxygenation in Traumatology and Orthopedics 429
K. K. Jain
Introduction... 429
Crush Injuries.. 429
    Pathophysiology... 430
    Diagnosis.. 430
    Treatment 430
    Role of HBO in Treatment.. 430
    Traumatic Ischemia... 431
    Compartment Syndromes.. 433
HBO for High Pressure Water Gun Injection Injury... 433
Peripheral Nerve Injuries 433
    Rationale for the Use of HBO 434
    Experimental Studies 434
    Clinical Applications 435
    Concluding Remarks 435
Fractures... 435
    Basic and Experimental Considerations 435
    Clinical Experience 436
    Bone Fractures with Arterial Injuries 436
Traumatic Amputations and Reimplantations of Body Parts.. 436
    Reimplantation of Limbs 436
    Reimplantation of Other Body Parts... 437
Role of HBO in Battle Casualties 437
Effect of HBO on Osteogenesis 437
    HBO for Treatment of Osteonecrosis (Aseptic Necrosis) 437
    HBO Therapy of Osteonecrosis 438
Rheumatoid Arthritis 440
    Basic Considerations.. 440
    Rationale of Use of HBO in Rheumatoid Arthritis... 440
    Clinical Applications 441
Conclusion 441
References.. 441

31 HBO Therapy in Otolaryngology 443
K. K. Jain
Introduction.. 443
Tinnitus 443
Sudden Deafness... 445
    Role of HBO in the Management of Sudden Deafness 445
    Rationale for HBO Therapy in Sudden Deafness 445
    Acute Acoustic Trauma 446
    Concluding Remarks About the Use of HBO in Hearing Loss ... 449
Effect of HBO in Preventing Hearing Impairment from Chronic
Noise Exposure 451
Miscellaneous Disturbances of the Inner Ear 451
Neuro-otological Vascular Disturbances.. 451
    Meniere's Disease 452
    Facial Palsy 453
Otological Complications of HBO Therapy 453
Miscellaneous Conditions in Head and Neck Area 453
    Malignant Otitis Externa 453
    Aphonia Due to Chronic Laryngitis... 454
Conclusion 454
References 454

32 HBO Therapy and Ophthalmology 457
Heather Murphy-Lavoie, Tracy LeGros, Frank K. Butler Jr., and K. K. Jain
Introduction.. 457
Review of Pertinent Anatomy and Physiology of the Eye.............. 458
    The Process of Vision 458
    Factors Affecting Vision 458
    Retinal Blood Supply 458
    Ocular Oxygen Tension 458
    Physiology of the Eye in Hyperoxic Conditions....................... 458
Adverse Effects of Hyperoxia... 459
    Retinal Oxygen Toxicity 459
    Lenticular Oxygen Toxicity 460
Ocular Contraindications to Hyperbaric Oxygen Therapy 461
Pre-HBOT Ocular Examination.. 461
HBO in the Treatment of Diseases of the Eye 461
    Recommended Indications... 461
    Potential Indications for HBOT in Ophthalmology.................. 468
    Other Reported Uses 474
    Emergency HBO in Patients with Acute Vision Loss................. 477
Conclusion 478
References 478

33 Hyperbaric Oxygenation in Obstetrics and Gynecology 485
K. K. Jain
Introduction.. 485
HBO and Risk of Congenital Malformations 485
Role of HBO in Obstetrics 486
    Experimental Studies 486
    Clinical Applications 486
Use of HBO for Medical Conditions in Pregnancy 487
    Acute Carbon Monoxide Poisoning During Pregnancy............. 487
    Diabetes.. 487

Management of Pregnancy and Delivery in Women with Heart Disease 487
Applications of HBO in Neonatology.. 487
HBO in Gynecology 488
Animal Experimental Studies 488
Clinical Applications in Gynecology... 488
Conclusion 488
References 489

34   Use of Hyperbaric Oxygenation (HBO) in Neonatal Patients 491
E. Cuauhtémoc Sánchez-Rodríguez
Introduction.. 491
Hypoxic–Ischemic Encephalopathy of the Newborn.. 492
Uses of Hyperbaric Oxygenation in Hypoxic–Ischemic Encephalopathy
and Necrotizing Enterocolitis of the Neonate.. 492
Use of Hyperbaric Oxygenation in Neonates 493
Results... 494
Discussion 495
References 495

35   Hyperbaric Oxygenation in Geriatrics 499
K. K. Jain
Introduction.. 499
Physiology of Aging 499
Theories of Aging 499
Changes in the Brain with Aging... 501
Applications of HBO in Geriatrics 502
Rationale 502
Safety of HBO Treatments in the Elderly 504
Conclusion 504
References 504

36   HBO as an Adjuvant in Rehabilitation and Sports Medicine 505
K. K. Jain
Introduction.. 505
Role of HBO in Rehabilitation 505
Indications... 505
Advantages.. 506
Applications of HBO in Rehabilitation of Neurological Disorders...................... 506
Rehabilitation of patients with CNS injuries 506
Role of HBO in Rehabilitation after Myocardial Infarction............................. 506
HBO as an Adjunct to Rehabilitation in Peripheral Vascular Disease................. 506
HBO as an Adjunct to Rehabilitation of Limb Amputees 507
HBO for Treatment of Sports Injuries 507
HBO as an Adjunct to Sports Training 508
Future Prospects.. 509
References.. 509

37   Nursing and Hyperbaric Medicine.. 511
Valerie A. Larson-Lohr
History... 511
The Nursing Process 513
Hyperbaric Patient Education 513
Hyperbaric Nursing Research 521
References.. 521

38   Role of HBO in Enhancing Cancer Radiosensitivity 523
K. K. Jain
Introduction... 523
Role of Hypoxia in Tumors.. 523
Rationale of Use of HBO as Adjunct to Radiotherapy 524
Experimental Studies of the Radiosensitizing Effect of HBO.............................. 524
Clinical Studies of HBO as Radiation Sensitizer... 525
    Carcinoma of the Cervix 525
    Head and Neck Cancer.. 525
    Carcinoma of the Lung 526
    Carcinoma of the Bladder 526
    Malignant Melanoma 526
    Malignant Glioma 526
Advantages of HBO as an Adjunct to Radiotherapy 528
Limitations of HBO as Adjunct to Radiotherapy of Cancer................................. 528
    Drawbacks of HBO as Adjunct to Radiotherapy of Cancer 528
Alternative Methods for Enhancing Radiosensitivity of Cancer 528
Combination of Other Methods with HBO and Irradiation for Cancer 529
    Hyperthermia 529
    Hypothermia 529
    Vasodilators 529
    Induced Anemia and Red Cell Infusion.. 529
    Radiation Sensitizing Agents 529
    Use of Perfluorochemicals as Oxygen Carriers 529
HBO and Antineoplastic Agents... 529
HBO and Photodynamic Therapy 530
Conclusion 530
References.. 530

39   HBO Therapy and Organ Transplants 533
H. Alan Wyatt
Background 533
Role of HBO 534
Ischemia-Reperfusion Injury 534
Inflammation 534
Lung Transplants.. 535
Pancreas Transplants 535
Renal Transplants... 536
Liver Transplants.. 536
Face Transplants... 537
Hand Transplants 537
Miscellaneous Organs and Tissues 537
Clinical Applications 538
Conclusion 538
References.. 538

40   Hyperbaric Oxygen Pretreatment and Preconditioning 541
Gerardo Bosco and Enrico M. Camporesi
Introduction... 541
Hyperbaric Medicine Perspective 541
Diving Medicine 542
References.. 543

41 Anesthesia in the Hyperbaric Environment 545
Enrico M. Camporesi
Historical Perspective 545
Current Indications.. 546
Physical Considerations Concerning Anesthetic 546
Physiological Considerations.. 546
   Cardiovascular Effects 547
   Central Nervous System... 547
   Nitrous Oxide Anesthesia 547
   Intravenous Anesthesia 548
   Pharmacokinetics in the Hyperbaric Environment 548
Practical Aspects of Anesthesia in the Pressure Chamber.................. 548
   Noise 548
   Airway Equipment 548
   Ventilators 548
   Monitoring 549
   Prophylactic Myringotomy to Prevent Middle Ear Barotrauma 549
Conclusion 550
References.. 550

42 Hyperbaric Oxygen in Resuscitation 551
Keith Van Meter
Introduction.. 551
Indications.. 553
Cardiopulmonary Resuscitation 553
Case Studies 554
   Case 1 554
   Case 2 558
Discussion 562
Future Applications... 563
Conclusion 564
References.. 565

43 HBO in Military Medicine 567
Fabio Faralli, Alberto Fiorito, and Gerardo Bosco
Hyperbaric Oxygen Therapy and Combat Medicine 567
   Gas Gangrene: Crush Injuries and Traumatic Wounds................ 568
   Exceptional Loss of Blood... 568
   Burns 568
   Postconcussion Syndrome, Traumatic Brain Injuries,
   Posttraumatic Stress Disorders 569
   Hearing Loss and Tinnitus 570
   Spinal Cord Injury.. 570
   Hyperbaric Oxygen Therapy and Military Response
   to Natural Catastrophes.. 570
Hyperbaric Activities in Military Environment 571
   Offensive Activities or Activities Carried out During Wartime...... 571
   Defensive Activities or Activities Carried out During Peacetime ... 572
Field of HBO Application in Military Diving Medicine 573
   Military Diving Operations.. 573
   Diving Methods... 573
   Employee's Safety 573
   Personnel Training 573
   Personnel Recruitment 573

Submarine Medicine 573
   Submarines' Rescue 573
   Technical Aspects of Rescue Operations 573
   Transfer Under Pressure 574
References 574

Part III   Hyperbaric Medicine as a Specialty

44   Training and Practice of Hyperbaric Medicine 579
K. K. Jain
Introduction 579
Relation of Hyperbaric Medicine to Other Medical Specialties 580
   Hyperbaric Medicine and Diving Medicine 580
Training in Hyperbaric Medicine 580
   Admission Requirements 580
   Training Program 580
   Examinations 580
Proposal for a Curriculum for a Diploma Course in Hyperbaric
and Diving Medicine 581
Training of Nonphysician Healthcare Personnel for Hyperbaric Medicine.............. 581
Practice of Hyperbaric Medicine 581
Economic Aspects 582
Conclusion 582

45   Research in Hyperbaric Medicine 583
K. K. Jain
Introduction 583
Basic Research in HBO 583
Animal Experimental Studies 584
Application of Biotechnologies in Hyperbaric Medicine 584
   Biomarkers of Effect of HBO 584
   Action of HBO on Gene Expression 585
   HBO as Adjunct to Cell therapy and Regenerative Medicine 586
   Nanobiotechnology and HBO 586
Clinical Trials of HBO Therapy 587
   Problems with Clinical Trials of HBO 587
   Ethical Aspects of Clinical Trials with HBO 588
Conclusion 588
References 588

46   Personalized Hyperbaric Medicine 589
K. K. Jain
Introduction 589
Molecular Diagnostics as Guide to HBO Therapy 590
   Role of Sequencing in Personalized Medicine 590
   Biomarkers for Personalized HBO Therapy 591
   Imaging for Personalized HBO Therapy 591
   Brain Imaging as Guide to Therapy of Multiple Sclerosis 591
   Imaging Tumor Hypoxia for Personalized Cancer Therapy 591
Pharmacogenomics and Pharmacogenetics of HBO 592
   Oxygen Toxicity and Genes 592
   Susceptibility to HBO-Induced Cataract Formation 592
Economical Aspects of Personalized HBO Therapy 592
Conclusion 592
References 592

47 The Future of Hyperbaric Medicine 593
K. K. Jain
Introduction to Future Medicine 593
Important Medical Advances in the Next Decade 593
Advances in Surgery 594
Important Areas for Future Development 594
Role of HBO in Future Medicine 595
Role of Hyperbaric Oxygen in the Multidisciplinary Healthcare
Systems of the Future 595
Future Needs in Hyperbaric Medicine 595
References 596

**48 Ethical Issues, Standards, and Quality Control
in the Practice of Hyperbaric Medicine** 597
Caroline E. Fife, Kristen A. Eckert, and Wilbur Thomas Workman
Alternative Medical Treatments and Off-Label Use of Hyperbaric Oxygen 598
The Risks of the Public Information Gap 598
Is There an Alternative to HBOT? 599
Safety and Fire Hazard Issues from Misuse of Hyperbaric Chambers 599
The Controversy of Low Pressure Oxygen 602
The "Chamber" Effect 602
Ethical Challenges with HBOT Clinical Trial Design 603
Informed Consent 604
Desperate Measures 604
HBOT Fraud 605
HBOT Market Regulations 605
Food, Drug, and Cosmetic Act (FDC) 510(k) Clearance 605
National Hyperbaric Oxygen Therapy Registry 606
Conclusion 606
References 607

49 Worldwide Overview of Hyperbaric Medicine 609
K. K. Jain
Introduction 609
Hyperbaric Medicine in China 609
Hyperbaric Medicine in Japan 610
Hyperbaric Medicine in Russia 611
Hyperbaric Medicine in Germany 612
World Distribution of Hyperbaric Facilities 613
Conclusion 614
Reference 614

50 Hyperbaric Medicine in the United States 615
Thomas M. Bozzuto
Introduction 615
American College of Hyperbaric Medicine 617
National Board of Diving and Hyperbaric Medical Technology 619
Baromedical Nurses Association 619
Indications for Use of Hyperbaric Oxygen 620
Resources 620
Organizations for Subspecialty Certification 621
Currently Offered Fellowship Training Locations in Undersea
and Hyperbaric Medicine 621

51   Hyperbaric Medicine in Latin America.. 623
Cuauhtémoc Sánchez-Rodríguez

History... 623
Introduction... 623
Existing General Standards... 624
Responsible Existing Authorities.. 624
    Industry 624
    Labor 624
    Health 624
    Insurance 624
Latin American Consensus 624
Implementation of Minimum Standards and Regulations 625

Index... 627

Abbreviations

ADMA	Asymmetric dimethylarginine
ADP	Adenosine diphosphate
ASD	Autism spectrum disorders
AST	Aspartate aminotransferase
ATA	Atmospheres absolute
ATP	Adenosine triphosphate
BIH	Benign intracranial hypertension
BIS	Bispectral index monitor
CAAE	Cerebral artery air embolism
CABG	Coronary artery bypass graft
CAT	Catalase
CBF	Cerebral blood flow
CD	Crohn's disease
CLD	Chronic Lyme disease
CRT	Chemoradiotherapy
CT	Computed tomography
CTA	CT angiography
CVI	Chronic venous insufficiency
DCD	Donations after cardiac death
DCI	Decompression illness
DCS	Decompression sickness
DNS	Delayed neuropsychiatric sequelae
ECD	Expanded criteria donors
EfHBOT	Efficacy of HBOT
eNOS	Endothelial cell nitric oxide synthase
EVA	Extravehicular activities
FAD	Flavin adenine dinucleotide
FMS	Fibromyalgia syndrome
GOQ	Glucose oxidation quotient
GPx	Glutathione peroxidase
H_2O_2	Hydrogen peroxide
HBD	Donors who have a heartbeat
HBO	Hyperbaric oxygen
HBO-PC	HBO preconditioning
HBOT	Hyperbaric oxygen therapy
HIE	Hypoxic-ischemic encephalopathy
HIF	Hypoxia-inducible factor
HSP	Heat shock protein
ICH	Intracerebral hemorrhage
iNOS	Inducible nitric oxide synthase
I/R	Ischemia-reperfusion
IRI	Ischemia-reperfusion injury

LDF	Laser Doppler flowmetry
MCANS	Neurological Scale for Middle Cerebral Artery Infarction
MCAO	Middle cerebral artery occlusion
MDA	Malondialdehyde
MMPs	Matrix metalloproteinases
NBO	Normobaric oxygen
NHBD	Non-heart beating donors
NICE	National Institute for Health and Care Excellence
NO	Nitric oxide
NOS	NO synthase
NSE	Neuron-specific enolase
PAF	Platelet activation factor
PCS	Post-concussion syndrome
PDD	Pervasive developmental disorders
PET	Positron emission tomography
PFC	Perfluorocarbon
PTCI	Percutaneous transluminal coronary intervention
PLDS	Post-Lyme disease syndrome
PTLD	Posttreatment Lyme disease
PSTD	Post-traumatic stress disorders
rCBF	Regional cerebral blood flow
RCT	Randomized controlled trial
RION	Radiation-induced optic neuropathy
rTPA	Recombinant tissue plasminogen activator
SCUBA	Self-contained breathing apparatus
SIRS	Systemic inflammatory response syndrome
SNSS	Scandinavian Neurological Stroke Scale
SOD	Superoxide dismutase
TBI	Traumatic brain injuries
TCOM	Transcutaneous oxygen monitor
UC	Ulcerative colitis
UHMS	Undersea and Hyperbaric Medical Society
UNSS	Unified Neurological Stroke Scale
UPTD	Unit pulmonary toxic dose
VEGF	Vascular endothelial growth factor

About the Author

K. K. Jain is a retired neurosurgeon who has held fellowships and teaching positions at Harvard, UCLA, and the University of Toronto. He has been a visiting professor in Germany, Iran, and India and has served in the U.S. Army with the rank of lieutenant colonel. He trained in microsurgery with Prof. Yasargil at the University of Zurich, Switzerland. After devising new techniques in laser microvascular surgery, he wrote the pioneering *Handbook of Laser Neurosurgery*. Since 1976, he has been active in the field of hyperbaric medicine, beginning with the application of this technique to stroke patients. His 464 publications include 27 books such as *Oxygen in Physiology and Medicine*, *Textbook of Gene Therapy*, *The Handbook of Nanomedicine*, and *Textbook of Personalized Medicine*. Prof. Jain, in addition to his activities in biotechnology, serves as a consultant in hyperbaric medicine and neurology.

Contributors

Gerardo Bosco, MD, PhD Department of Biomedical Sciences, University of Padova, Padova, Italy

Thomas M. Bozzuto, DO, FACEP, FFACHM, UHM/ABEM Phoebe Putney Memorial Hospital, Wound Care and Hyperbaric Center, Albany, GA, USA

Frank K. Butler, MD, CAPT MC USN (Ret) Committee on Tactical Combat Casualty Care, Joint Trauma System, Pensacola, FL, USA

Enrico M. Camporesi, MD University of South Florida, Tampa, FL, USA

TEAMHealth Anesthesia Research Institute, Tampa General Hospital, Tampa, FL, USA

Kristen A. Eckert, MPhil Strategic Solutions, Inc., Cody, WY, USA

Fabio Faralli, MD, Surgeon Rear Admiral (Ret.) Italian Navy, Arcola, Italy

Caroline E. Fife, MD CHI St. Luke's Wound Clinic, The Woodlands, TX, USA

Baylor College of Medicine, Houston, Texas, USA

Intellicure, Inc., The Woodlands, TX, USA

Alberto Fiorito, MD, LtC (Ret.) Department of Biomedical Sciences, University of Padova, Lerici, Italy

Paul G. Harch, MD Section of Emergency and Hyperbaric Medicine, Louisiana State University School of Medicine, New Orleans, Louisiana University Medical Center, Louisiana Children's Medical Center, New Orleans, LA, USA

K. K. Jain, MD, FRACS, FFPM Basel, Switzerland

Philip B. James, MB, ChB, DIH, PhD, FFOM Department of Surgery, Ninewells Hospital and Medical School, Dundee, Angus, UK

Valerie A. Larson-Lohr, MSN, APRN Wound Healing Associates, San Antonio, TX, USA

Tracy LeGros, MD, PhD Department of Emergency Medicine, University Medical Center, Undersea and Hyperbaric Medicine, New Orleans, LA, USA

Keith Van Meter, MD Section of Emergency Medicine, LSU Health Sciences Center, University Medical Center, LCMC Health, New Orleans, LA, USA

Tulane School of Medicine, New Orleans, LA, USA

Heather Murphy-Lavoie, MD Department of Emergency Medicine, University Medical Center, Undersea and Hyperbaric Medicine, New Orleans, LA, USA

E. Cuauhtémoc Sánchez-Rodríguez, MD, MSc, MPH Department of Hyperbaric Medicine, Agustín O´Horan, SSY, Mérida, Yucatán, Mexico

J. Michael Uszler, MD, MS Department of Nuclear Medicine, Providence St. Johns Health Center, Santa Monica, CA, USA

Wilbur Thomas Workman, BS, MS Quality Assurance and Regulatory Affairs, Undersea and Hyperbaric Medical Society, San Antonio, TX, USA

H. Alan Wyatt, MD, PhD, CHT Department of Hyperbaric Medicine, West Jefferson Medical Center, Marrero, LA, USA

K.K. Jain

Abstract

This chapter reviews the historical relationship between hyperbaric therapy and diving medicine, recounting the important stages in the development of compressed-gas technology and a few of the more interesting early attempts to utilize it for medical purposes.

Keywords

Compressed air • Diving medicine • History • Hyperbaric chambers • Hyperbaric medicine • Oxygen

Hyperbaric Therapy and Diving Medicine

As is well known, the origins and development of hyperbaric medicine are closely tied to the history of diving medicine. While the attractions of the deep are easily understood, it was the various unpleasant physical consequences of venturing beneath the surface of the world's oceans that led directly to the many applications of compressed-gas therapy in modern medicine. Although scientifically based applications of hyperbaric technology are a relatively recent development, the use of compressed gas in medicine actually has ancient roots.

The origin of diving is not known, but it was recognized as a distinct occupation as far back as 4500 BC. However, since humans can only hold their breath for a few minutes, unaided dives are limited to depths of less than about 30 m. The first use of actual diving equipment to extend the limits of underwater activity is attributed in legend to none other than Alexander the Great, who, in 320 BC, is said to have been lowered into the Bosphorus Straits in a glass barrel (Fig. 1.1), which purportedly gave him a secret weapon in the siege of Tyre.

K.K. Jain, MD, FRACS, FFPM (✉)
1 Blaesiring 7, Basel 4057, Switzerland
e-mail: jain@pharmabiotech.ch

Around the year 1500, Leonardo Da Vinci made sketches of a variety of diving appliances, without developing any for practical use. It was not until 1620 that the Dutch inventor Cornelius Drebbel developed the first true diving bell. His device was extremely limited, especially by its simple air supply that delivered air pressurized at only one atmosphere, but it was certainly the forerunner of all submersible vehicles.

In 1691 Edmund Halley, after whom the comet is named, advanced diving bell technology by devising a method of replenishing the air supply using weighted barrels (Smith 1986). This was followed in the next two centuries by the development of compressed-air diving helmets and suits, which made it possible to remain under water for an hour or more.

Even though the duration of dives had been extended, divers were still limited to the same shallow waters as before. Undersea pioneers had quickly discovered the eardrum-rupturing effects of increasing water pressure. Those attempting to venture even deeper in diving bells also quickly learned about the best-known medical problem associated with diving: decompression sickness. It was not until the middle of the nineteenth century that the effectiveness of countering decompression sickness with hyperbaric recompression was finally discovered (Table 1.1). Although recompression in air was utilized first, hyperbaric oxygen (HBO) is now used, and this is the principal connection between diving medicine and the other forms of HBO therapy.

© Springer International Publishing AG 2017
K.K. Jain, *Textbook of Hyperbaric Medicine*, DOI 10.1007/978-3-319-47140-2_1

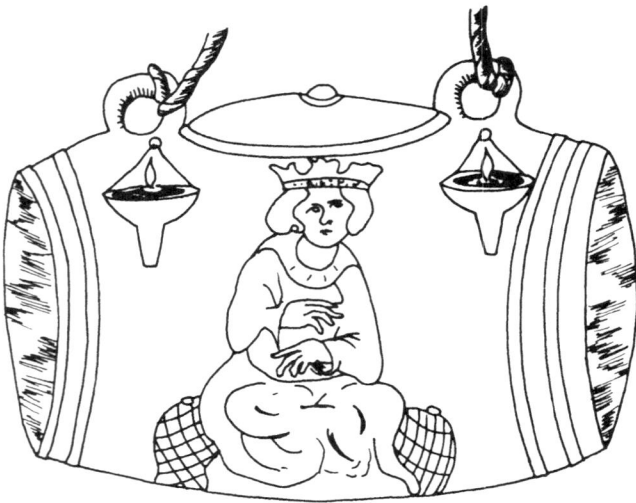

Fig. 1.1 Alexander the Great was said to have been lowered into the Bosphorus Straits in a glass barrel. Note that the candles are lighted and if, indeed, Alexander went into this barrel, he was lucky to survive. The illustration is redrawn from a thirteenth century manuscript in the Burgundy Library in Brussels and is reproduced courtesy of Dr. E. B. Smith

Table 1.1 Some important benchmarks in the history of diving medicine in relation to hyperbaric medicine

4500 BC	Earliest records of breath-holding dives for mother-of-pearl
400 BC	Xerxes used divers for work on ships and for salvaging sunken goods. Dives were for 2–4 min and to a depth of 20–30 m
320 BC	First diving bell used by Alexander the Great
300 BC	Aristotle described the rupture of the eardrum in divers
1670	Boyle gave the first description of the decompression phenomenon as "bubble in the eye of a snake in vacuum"
1620	Cornelius Drebbel developed a one-atmosphere diving bell, basically the forerunner of all modern submarines
1691	Edmund Halley improved bell technology by devising a method to replenish air supply in the diving bell
1774	Freminet, a French scientist, reached a depth of 50 ft (2.5 ATA) and stayed there for 1 h using a helmet with compressed air pumped through a pipe from the surface
1830	Cochrane patented the concept and technique of using compressed air in tunnels and caissons to balance the pressure of water in soil
1841	Pol and Watelle of France observed that recompression relieved the symptoms of decompression sickness
1869	Publication of *Twenty Thousand Leagues under the Sea*, a science fiction novel by Jules Verne, contains a description of diving gears with air reserves
1871	Paul Bert showed that bubbles in the tissues during decompression consist mainly of nitrogen
1920	Use of gas mixtures for diving (heliox); diving depth extended to 200 m
1935	Behnke showed that nitrogen is the cause of narcosis in humans subjected to compressed air above 4 ATA
1943	Construction of aqua lung by Cousteau; diving at 200 bar possible
1967	Founding of Undersea Medical Society, USA

The Development of Hyperbaric Air Therapy

The first documented use of hyperbaric therapy actually precedes the discovery of oxygen. Landmarks in the history of hyperbaric (compressed) air therapy are shown in Table 1.2. The British physician Henshaw seems to have used compressed air for medical purposes in 1662. The chamber he developed was an airtight room called a "domicilium," in which variable climatic and pressure conditions could be produced, with pressure provided by a large pair of bellows. According to Henshaw, "In times of good health this domicilium is proposed as a good expedient to help digestion, to promote insensible respiration, to facilitate breathing and expectoration, and consequently, of excellent use for the prevention of most afflictions of the lungs." There is, however, no account of any application of Henshaw's proposed treatment, and there were no further developments in the field of hyperbaric therapy for nearly two centuries.

In the nineteenth century, there was a rebirth of interest in hyperbaric therapy in France. In 1834 Junod built a hyperbaric chamber to treat pulmonary afflictions using pressures of two to four absolute atmospheres (ATA). In 1837 Pravaz built the largest hyperbaric chamber of that time and treated patients with a variety of ailments. Fontaine developed the first mobile hyperbaric operating theater in 1877 (Fig. 1.2), and by this time hyperbaric chambers were available in all major European cities. Interestingly, there was no general rationale for hyperbaric treatments, and prescriptions therefore varied from one

Table 1.2 Landmarks in the history of hyperbaric (compressed) air therapy

1662	Henshaw used compressed air for the treatment of a variety of diseases
1834	Junod of France constructed a hyperbaric chamber and used pressures of 2–4 ATA to treat pulmonary disease
1837	Pravaz of France constructed the largest hyperbaric chamber of that time and used it to treat a variety of ailments
1837–1877	Construction of pneumatic centers in various European cities, e.g., Berlin, Amsterdam, Brussels, London, Vienna, and Milan
1860	First hyperbaric chamber on the North American continent in Oshawa, Canada
1870	Fontaine of France used the first mobile hyperbaric operating theater
1891	Corning used the first hyperbaric chamber in the USA to treat nervous disorders
1921	Cunningham (USA) used hyperbaric air to treat a variety of ailments
1925	Cunningham tank was the only functional hyperbaric chamber in the world
1928	Cunningham constructs the largest hyperbaric chamber in the world; American Medical Association condemns Cunningham's hyperbaric therapy
1937	The Cunningham chamber is dismantled for scrap metal

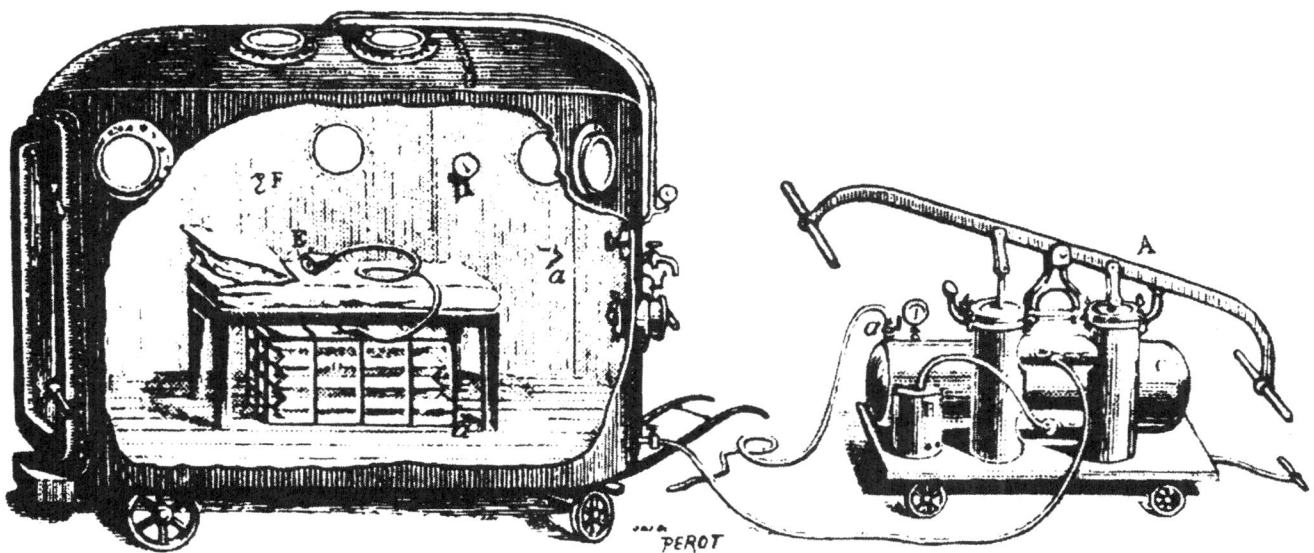

Fig. 1.2 Fontaine's mobile operating room of 1877. Note the manual nature of the compressor apparatus and the anesthesia gas container and mask in the chamber. Photo courtesy of Dr. Baixe, Toulon, France

physician to another. (In those days no methods were available to estimate the partial pressure of oxygen in blood, which at 2 ATA of air is about double that at sea level. In comparison, if pure oxygen is breathed at 2 ATA, the partial pressure of oxygen in the arterial blood is 12 times higher than normal.)

During the second half of the nineteenth century, hyperbaric centers were advertised as being comparable to health spas. Junod referred to his treatment as "le bain d'air comprimé" (the compressed-air bath). In 1855 Bertin wrote a book on this topic (the title page is shown in Fig. 1.3) and constructed his own hyperbaric chamber (Fig. 1.4).

The literature on hyperbaric medicine up to 1887 reviewed by Arntzenius contains 300 references, which is a remarkably large number for that period when publications on this topic were scarce.

The first hyperbaric chamber on the North American continent was constructed in 1860 in Oshawa, Ontario, Canada, just east of Toronto. The first such chamber in the United States was built by Corning a year later in New York to treat nervous disorders. The chamber that received the most publicity, however, and was the most actively used was that of Cunningham in Kansas City in the 1920s (Sellers 1965). He first used his chamber to treat the victims of the Spanish influenza epidemic that swept the USA during the closing days of the First World War. Cunningham had observed that mortality from this disease was higher in areas of higher elevation, and he reasoned that a barometric factor was therefore involved. Cunningham claimed to have achieved remarkable improvement in patients who were cyanotic and comatose. In 1923, the first recorded hyperbaric chamber fire occurred at Cunningham's sanatorium. He had installed open gas burners under the tank to keep it warm in winter, and someone turned the flame too high so

that it scorched the interior insulation. The patients were evacuated safely. However, one night a mechanical failure resulted in a complete loss of compression and all his patients died. This tragedy was a sobering lesson but ultimately did not deter Dr. Cunningham. His enthusiasm for hyperbaric air continued, and he started to treat diseases such as syphilis, hypertension, diabetes mellitus, and cancer. His reasoning was based on the assumption that anaerobic infections play a role in the etiology of all such diseases. In 1928, in Cleveland, Cunningham constructed the largest chamber ever built—five stories high and 64 ft in diameter (Fig. 1.5). Each floor had 12 bedrooms with all the amenities of a good hotel. At that time, it was the only functioning hyperbaric chamber in the world.

As the publicity surrounding his treatments grew, Dr. Cunningham was repeatedly requested by the Bureau of Investigations of the American Medical Association (AMA) to document his claims regarding the effectiveness of hyperbaric therapy. Apart from a short article in 1927, however, Cunningham made no efforts to describe or discuss his technique in the medical literature. He was eventually censured by the AMA in 1928, in a report that stated: "Under the circumstances, it is not to be wondered that the Medical Profession looks askance at the 'tank treatment' and intimates that it seems tinctured much more strongly with economics than with scientific medicine. It is the mark of the scientist that he is ready to make available the evidence on which his claims are based."

Dr. Cunningham was given repeated opportunities to present such evidence but never did so. A more detailed account of Cunningham's story and the history of hyperbaric medicine is recorded elsewhere (Trimble 1974). The Cunningham chamber was dismantled for scrap in 1937, which brought to a temporary end the era of hyperbaric air therapy for medical disorders.

ÉTUDE CLINIQUE

DE L'EMPLOI ET DES EFFETS

DU

BAIN D'AIR COMPRIMÉ

dans le

TRAITEMENT DES MALADIES DE POITRINE

notamment dans

LE CATARRHE CHRONIQUE, L'ASTHME ET LA PHTHISIE PULMONAIRE

SELON LES PROCÉDÉS

MÉDICO-PNEUMATIQUES OU D'ATMOSPHÉRIE DE M. ÉMILE TABARIÉ

PAR

EUGÈNE BERTIN

Directeur de l'Établissement medico-pneumatique de Montpellier; Professeur-Agrégé de la
Faculté de médecine; Membre titulaire de l'Académie des sciences et lettres et Médecin des
Prisons de la même ville; Correspondant de la Société d'hydrologie médicale de Paris, de la
Société médicale du canton de Genève, de la Société impériale de médecine de Marseille, de
la Société de médecine de Nimes, etc., etc

Deuxième Édition, avec une Planche.

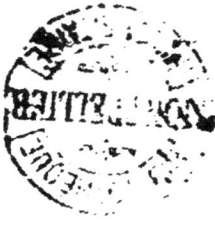

PARIS   MONTPELLIER

Adrien DELAHAYE, Libr.-Édit.   C. COULET, Libraire - Éditeur
Place de l'École-de-Médecine   Grand'rue, 5

1868

Fig. 1.3 Title page of the second edition (1868) of the book by Bertin on the treatment of diseases by compressed air

Fig. 1.4 Hyperbaric chamber constructed by Bertin in 1874

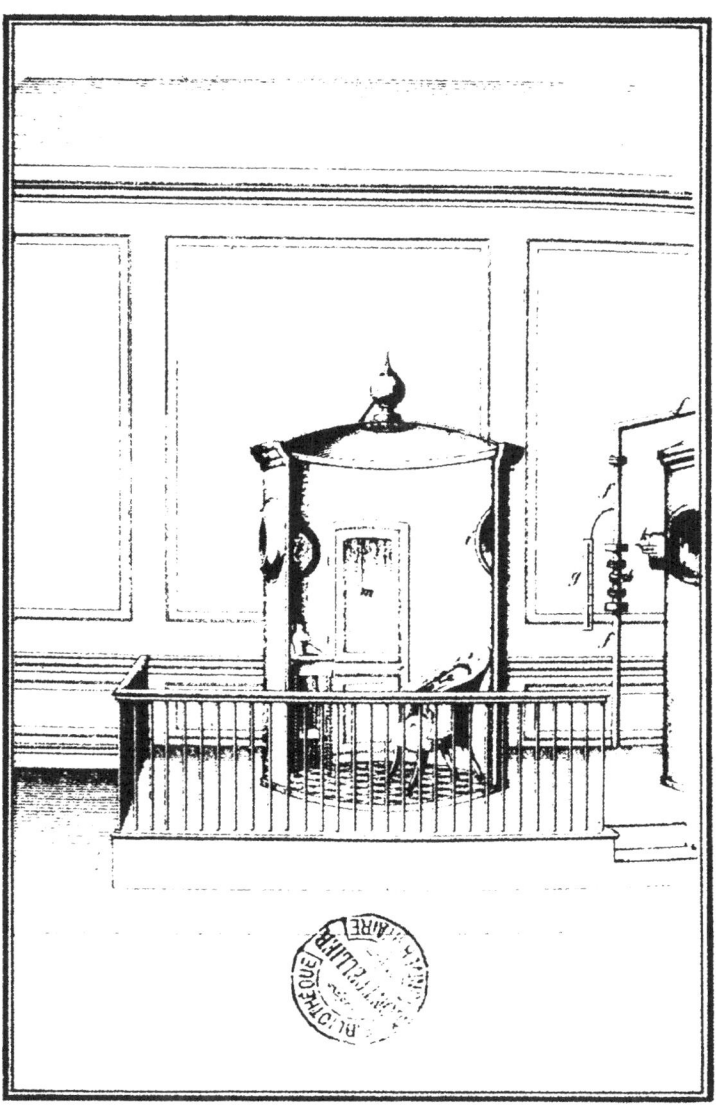

The Development of Hyperbaric Oxygen Therapy

Oxygen was not "discovered" until 1775, when the English scientist Joseph Priestley isolated what he called "dephlogisticated air." A more detailed history of the applications of oxygen since that time can be found in a book on oxygen (Jain 1989). Although hyperbaric air had been used as early as 1662, oxygen was not specifically added to early hyperbaric chambers. Landmarks in the development of hyperbaric oxygen therapy are shown in Table 1.3.

The toxic effects of concentrated oxygen reported by Lavoisier and Seguin in 1789 were reason enough for hesitation to use it under pressure. Beddoes and Watt, who wrote the first book on oxygen therapy in 1796, completely refrained from mentioning the use of oxygen under pressure.

Paul Bert, the father of pressure physiology, discovered the scientific basis of oxygen toxicity in 1878 and recommended normobaric, but not hyperbaric, oxygen for decompression sickness.

The history of hyperbaric chambers is covered in two books (Haux 2000; Stewart 2011). The potential benefits of using oxygen under pressure for the treatment of decompression sickness were first realized by Dräger, who in 1917 devised a system for treating diving accidents (Fig. 1.6). For some unknown reason, however, Dräger's system never went into production. It was not until 1937—the very year that Cunningham's "air chamber" hotel was demolished—that Behnke and Shaw actually used hyperbaric oxygen for the treatment of decompression sickness. The age of hyperbaric oxygen therapy had finally arrived.

Fig. 1.5 Cunningham's giant steel ball hyperbaric chamber built in 1928 in Cleveland, Ohio. It was six stories high and contained 72 rooms. Photo courtesy of Dr. K. P. Fasecke

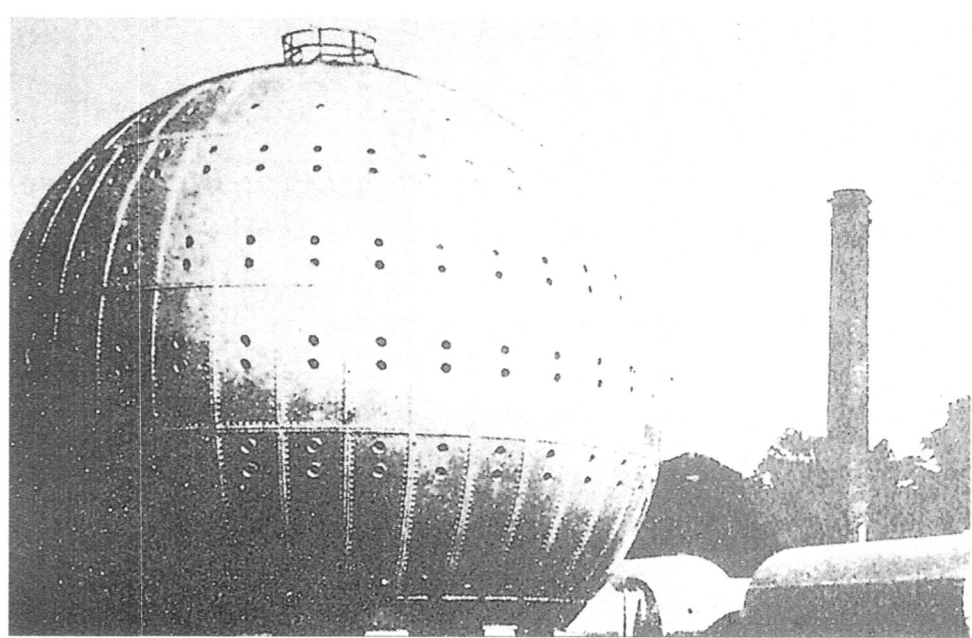

Table 1.3 Landmarks in the development of hyperbaric oxygen (HBO) therapy

1775	Discovery of oxygen by Priestley
1789	Toxic effects of oxygen reported by Lavoisier and Seguin: use of HBO discouraged
1796	Beddoes and Watt wrote the first book on medical applications of oxygen
1878	Bert (father of pressure physiology) placed oxygen toxicity on a scientific basis and recommended normobaric but not hyperbaric oxygen for decompression sickness
1895	Haldane showed that a mouse placed in a jar containing oxygen at 2 ATA failed to develop signs of carbon monoxide intoxication
1937	Behnke and Shaw first used HBO for treatment of decompression sickness
1938	Ozorio de Almeida and Costa (Brazil) used HBO for treatment of leprosy
1942	End and Long (USA) used HBO for treating experimental carbon monoxide poisoning in animals.
1954	Churchill-Davidson (UK) used HBO to enhance radiosensitivity of tumors
1956	Boerema (the Netherlands), father of modern hyperbaric medicine, performed cardiac surgery in a hyperbaric chamber
1960	Boerema showed life can be maintained in pigs in the absence of blood by using HBO
1960	Sharp and Smith become the first to treat human carbon monoxide poisoning by HBO
1961	Boerema and Brummelkamp used hyperbaric oxygen for treatment of gas gangrene; Smith et al. (UK) showed the protective effect of HBO in cerebral ischemia
1962	Illingworth (UK) showed the effectiveness of HBO in arterial occlusion in limbs
1963	First International Congress on Hyperbaric Medicine in Amsterdam
1965	Perrins (UK) showed the effectiveness of HBO in osteomyelitis
1966	Saltzman et al. (USA) showed the effectiveness of HBO in stroke patients
1970	Boschetty and Cernoch (Czechoslovakia) used HBO for multiple sclerosis
1971	Lamm (FRG) used HBO for treatment of sudden deafness
1973	Thurston showed that HBO reduces mortality in myocardial infarction
1970s	Extensive expansion of hyperbaric facilities in Japan and the USSR
1980s	Development of hyperbaric medicine in China
1983	Formation of the American College of Hyperbaric Medicine (founder/president, Dr. Neubauer of Florida)
1986	Undersea Medical Society (USA) adds the word hyperbaric to its name and is called UHMS. Reached a membership of 2000 in 60 countries
1987	Jain (Switzerland) demonstrated the relief of spasticity in hemiplegia due to stroke under HBO and integrated it with physical therapy
1988	Formation of the International Society of Hyperbaric Medicine

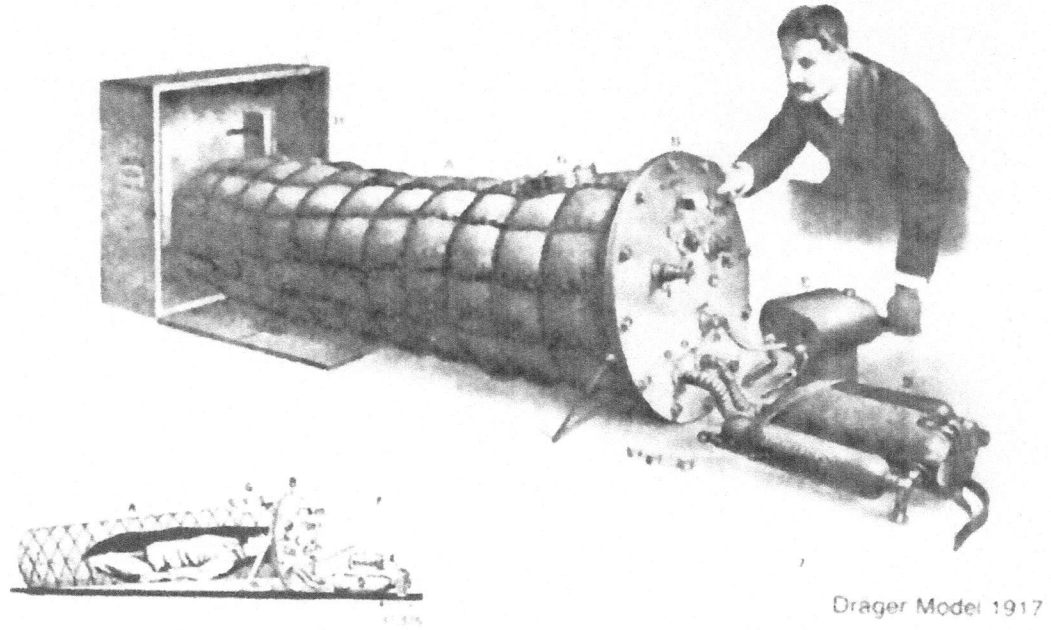

Fig. 1.6 Sketch of the 1917 Dräger 2 ATA system for diving accidents, including oxygen breathing system. Photo courtesy of Dr. Baixe, Toulon, France

References

Haux GF. History of hyperbaric chambers. Flagstaff: Best Publishing; 2000.

Jain KK. Oxygen in physiology and medicine. Springfield: Charles C. Thomas; 1989.

Sellers LM. The fallibility of Forrestian principle. Anesth Analg. 1965;44:9.

Smith EB. Priestley lecture: on the science of deep sea diving—observations of the respiration of different kinds of air. Chem Soc Rev. 1986;15:503–22.

Stewart J. Exploring the history of hyperbaric chambers, atmospheric diving suits and manned submersibles: the scientists and machinery. Bloomington: Xlibris Corporation; 2011. p. 151.

Trimble VH. The uncertain miracle—hyperbaric oxygen. New York: Doubleday; 1974.

Physical, Physiological, and Biochemical
Aspects of Hyperbaric Oxygenation

2

K.K. Jain

Abstract

This chapter presents a basic scientific foundation detailing the important and interesting properties of oxygen and then surveys how these realities come into play under hyperbaric conditions. Starting with physiology of oxygenation, general effects of hyperbaric oxygenation (HBO) are described on the healthy human body. There is a specific focus on the biochemical effects of HBO and effect of HBO at molecular level. Tissue oxygen tension and biomarkers of HBO are also described. More detailed effects of HBO on various systems of the body will be described along with clinical applications in various therapeutic areas in part II of this book.

Keywords

Oxygen • Hyperbaric oxygen (HBO) • Biochemical effects of HBO • Effect of DNA on DNA • Oxygen pathway • HBO biomarker • Glucose metabolism • Ammonia metabolism • Oxygen transport • Tissue oxygen tension

Introduction

Oxygen is the most prevalent and most important element on earth. A complete and in-depth discussion of the biochemical and physiological aspects of oxygen was described in a book on oxygen (Jain 1989), and an updated brief description of how oxygen is transported and the basic physical laws governing its behavior will be useful for discussion of clinical applications of hyperbaric oxygen in the following chapters of this book. The various terms frequently encountered in relation to oxygen include:

Partial pressure of a gas	p
Partial pressure of oxygen	pO_2
Partial pressure of oxygen in alveoli	pAO_2
Partial pressure of oxygen in arterial blood	paO_2
Partial pressure of oxygen in venous blood	pvO_2

K.K. Jain, MD, FRACS, FFPM (✉)
1 Blaesiring 7, Basel 4057, Switzerland
e-mail: jain@pharmabiotech.ch

Physical Basics

The atmosphere is a gas mixture containing by volume 20.94 % oxygen, 78.08 % nitrogen, 0.04 % CO_2, and traces of other gases. For practical purposes air is considered to be a mixture of 21 % oxygen and 79 % nitrogen. The total pressure of this mixture at sea level is 760 millimeters of mercury (mmHg). Dalton's law states that in a gas mixture, each gas exerts its pressure according to its proportion of the total volume:

$$\text{Partial pressure of a gas} = (\text{absolute pressure}) \times (\text{proportion of total volume of gas})$$

Thus, the partial pressure of oxygen (pO_2) in air is $(760) \times (21/100) = 160$ mmHg.

Pressures exerted by gases dissolved in water or body fluids are certainly different from those produced in the gaseous phase. The concentration of a gas in a fluid is determined not only by the pressure but also by the "solubility coefficient" of the gas. Henry's law formulates this as follows:

Concentration of a dissolved gas

$$= (\text{pressure}) \times (\text{solubility coefficient})$$

The solubility coefficient varies for different fluids, and it is temperature dependent, with solubility being inversely proportional to temperature. When concentration is expressed as volume of gas dissolved in each unit volume of water, and pressure is expressed in atmospheres, the solubility coefficients of the important respiratory gases at body temperature are as follows:

Oxygen: 0.024 mL O_2/mL blood atm pO_2 CO_2: 0.5 mL plasma/atm pCO_2
Nitrogen: 0.067 mL/mL plasma/atm pN_2

From this one can see that CO_2 is, remarkably, 20 times more soluble than oxygen.

Physiology of Oxygenation

The Oxygen Pathway

The oxygen pathway is shown in Fig. 2.1. It passes from the ambient air to the alveolar air and continues through the pulmonary, capillary, and venous blood to the systemic arterial and capillary blood. It then moves through the interstitial and intracellular fluids to the microscopic points of oxygen consumption in the peroxisomes, endoplasmic reticulum, and mitochondria.

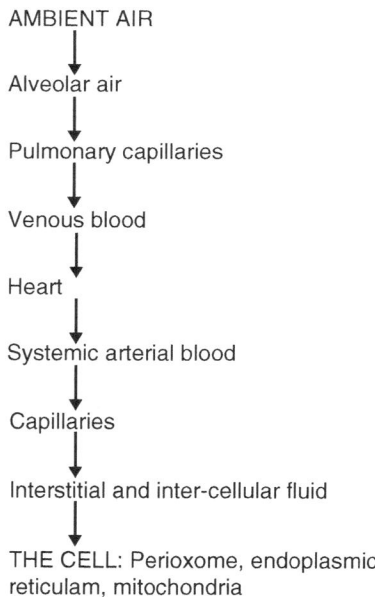

AMBIENT AIR

Alveolar air

Pulmonary capillaries

Venous blood

Heart

Systemic arterial blood

Capillaries

Interstitial and inter-cellular fluid

THE CELL: Perioxome, endoplasmic reticulam, mitochondria

Fig. 2.1 The oxygen pathway

Ventilation Phase

Respiration, the primary goal of the lungs, is inhalation of air with uptake of O_2 contained in it, and exhalation with removal of CO_2 from the body. At rest, a normal human breathing rate is 12–15 times a minute. With each breath containing ~500 mL of air, this amounts to 6–8 L of air that is inspired and expired every minute. Once the air reaches the depths of the lung in the alveoli, simple diffusion allows O_2 to enter the blood in the pulmonary capillaries and CO_2 to enter the alveoli, from where it can be expired. On average, 250 mL of O_2 enters the body per minute, and 200 mL of CO_2 is excreted.

Oxygen is continuously absorbed into the blood as it circulates through the lungs and enters the systemic circulation. The effect of alveolar ventilation and the rate of oxygen absorption from the alveoli on the pAO_2 are both shown in Fig. 2.2. At a ventilation rate of 5 L/min and oxygen consumption of 250 mL/min, the normal operating point is at A in Fig. 2.2. The alveolar oxygen tension is maintained at 104 mmHg. During moderate exercise, the rate of alveolar ventilation increases fourfold to maintain this tension and ~1000 mL of oxygen is absorbed per minute.

Carbon dioxide is being constantly formed in the body and discharged into the alveoli by secretion is 40 mmHg. It is well known that the partial pressure of alveolar CO_2 (pCO_2) increases directly in proportion to the rate of CO_2 excretion and decreases in inverse proportion to alveolar ventilation.

Transport Phase

The difference between pAO_2 (104 mmHg) and pvO_2 (40 mmHg), which amounts to 64 mmHg, causes oxygen to diffuse into the pulmonary blood. It is then transported, mostly in combination with hemoglobin, to the tissue capillaries, where it is released for use by the cells. There the oxygen reacts with various other nutrients to form CO_2, which enters the capillaries to be transported back to the lungs.

During strenuous exercise, the body oxygen requirement may be as much as 20 times normal, yet oxygenation of the blood does not suffer, because the diffusion capacity for oxygen increases fourfold during exercise. This rise results in part from the increased number of capillaries participating, as well as dilatation of both the capillaries and the alveoli. Another factor here is that the blood normally stays in the lung capillaries about three times as long as is necessary to cause full oxygenation. Therefore, even during the shortened time of exposure on exercise, the blood can still become nearly fully saturated with oxygen.

Fig. 2.2 Effect of alveolar ventilation and rate on oxygen absorption from the alveoli on the alveolar pO_2

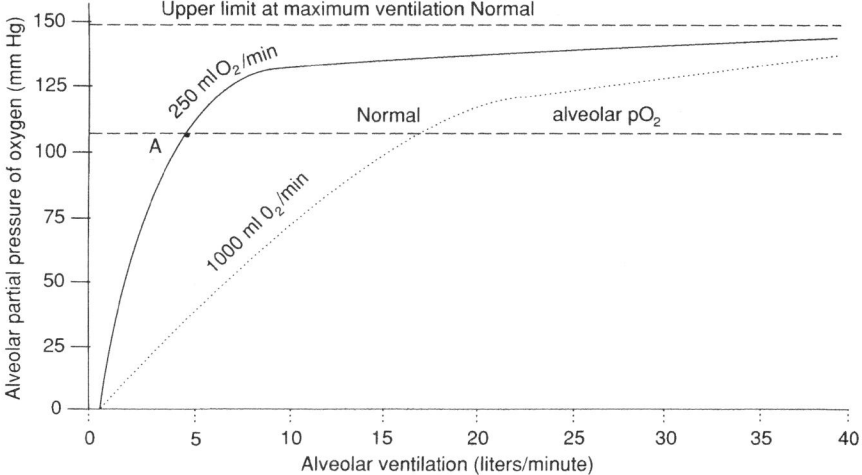

Normally 97 % of the oxygen transported from the lungs to the tissues is carried in chemical combination with hemoglobin of red blood cells and the remaining 3 % in a dissolved state in plasma. It turns out that 1 g of hemoglobin can combine with 1.34 mL oxygen from where it is removed continuously by ventilation. The normal concentration of hemoglobin is 15 g/100 mL blood. Thus, when hemoglobin is 100 % saturated with oxygen, 100 mL blood can transport about 20 (i.e., 15×1.34) mL oxygen in combination with hemoglobin. Since the hemoglobin is usually only 97.5 % saturated, the oxygen carried by 100 mL blood is actually 19.5 mL. However, in passing through tissue capillaries, this amount is reduced by 14.5 mL (paO_2 40 mmHg and 75 % oxygen saturation). Thus, under normal conditions, 5 (i.e., 19.5–14.5) mL of O_2 is transported to the tissues by 100 mL blood. On strenuous exercise, which causes the interstitial fluid pO_2 to fall as low as 15 mmHg, only 4.5 mL oxygen remains bound with hemoglobin in each 100 mL blood. Thus 15 (i.e., 19.5–4.5) mL oxygen is transferred by each 100 mL blood—three times the amount transferred under normal conditions. Since cardiac output can also increase up to six or seven times, for instance, in well-trained marathon runners, the end result is a remarkable 20-fold (i.e., 15×6.6=approximately 100; 100/5=20) increase in oxygen transport to the tissues. This is about the top limit that can be achieved.

Hemoglobin has a role in maintaining a constant pO_2 in the tissues and sets an upper limit of 40 mmHg. It usually delivers oxygen to the tissues at a rate to maintain a pO_2 of between 20 and 40 mmHg. In a pressurized chamber, pO_2 may rise tenfold, but the tissue pO_2 changes very little. The saturation of hemoglobin can rise by only 3 %, as 97 % of it is already combined with oxygen. This 3 % can be achieved at pO_2 levels of between 100 and 200 mmHg. Increasing the inspired oxygen concentration or the total pressure of inspired oxygen does not increase the hemoglobin-transported oxygen content of the blood. Thus, hemoglobin has an interesting tissue oxygen buffer function.

Shift of the Oxygen-Hemoglobin Dissociation Curve

Hemoglobin actively regulates oxygen transport through the oxygen-hemoglobin (oxyhemoglobin) dissociation curve, which describes the relation between oxygen saturation or content of hemoglobin and oxygen tension at equilibrium. There is a progressive increase in the percentage of hemoglobin that is bound with oxygen as pO_2 increases. It was first shown more than a century ago that that the dissociation curve was sigmoid-shaped (Bohr et al. 1904). This led Hill to postulate that there were multiple oxygen binding sites on the hemoglobin and to derive the following equation:

$$\left(\frac{\text{Oxygen tension}}{\text{P50}}\right)^2 = \frac{\text{Oxygen saturation}}{1 - \text{Oxygen saturation}}$$

where P50 is the oxygen tension (in mmHg) when the binding sites are 50 % saturated.

Within the range of saturation between 15 and 95 %, the sigmoid shape of the curve can be described in the Hill coefficient, and its position along the oxygen tension axis can be described by P50 which is inversely related to the binding affinity of the hemoglobin for oxygen. The P50 can be estimated by measuring the oxygen saturation of blood equilibrated to different levels of oxygen tension according to standard conditions and fitting the results to a straight line in logarithmic form to solve for P50. The resulting standard P50 is normally 26.3 mmHg in adults at sea level. It is useful for detecting abnormalities in the affinity of hemoglobin for oxygen resulting from hemoglobin variants or from disease. P50 is increased to enhance oxygen unloading when the primary limitation to oxygen transport is peripheral, e.g., anemia. P50 is reduced to enhance loading when the primary limitation is in

Fig. 2.3 Shift of the oxygen-hemoglobin dissociation curve. *DPG* diphosphoglycerate

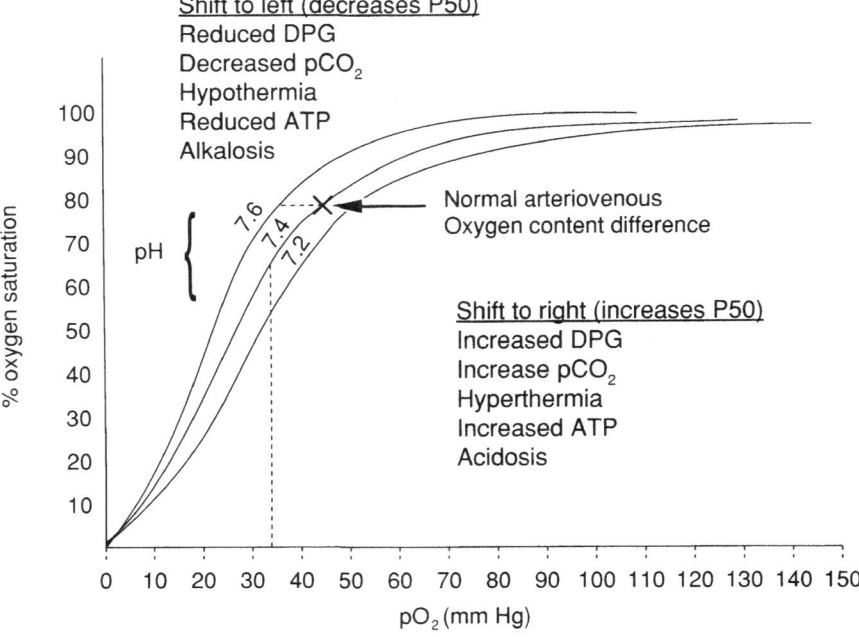

the lungs, e.g., lung disease. The balance between loading and unloading is regulated by allosteric control of the P50 and chemoreceptor control of ventilation which is matched to diffusing capacities of the lungs and the tissues. Optimal P50 supports the highest rate of oxygen transport in health and disease.

A number of conditions can displace the oxyhemoglobin dissociation curve to the right or the left, as indicated in Fig. 2.3.

Delivery of Oxygen to the Tissues

During transit from the ambient air to the cellular structures, the pO_2 of oxygen drops from 160 mmHg to a few mmHg in the mitochondria. This gradual drop is described as the "oxygen cascade" and is shown in Fig. 2.4.

Oxygen Transfer at the Capillary Level

There is considerable resistance to oxygen transfer in the capillaries, and this is as significant as the resistance in the surrounding tissues.

Microvascular geometry and capillary blood flow are the most important factors responsible for regulating the oxygen supply to the tissues to meet the specific oxygen demands of organs such as the heart and brain. The tissues, of course, form the end point of the oxygen pathway. The task of the active transport system is to ensure an adequate end-capillary pO_2 so that passive diffusion of oxygen to the mitochondria is maintained.

Relation Between the Oxygen Transport and Utilization

The relationship between the transportation of oxygen and its utilization was first described long ago by Fick (1870). According to the Fick principle, oxygen consumption of the tissues (pO_2) is equal to the blood flow to the tissues (Q), multiplied by the amount of oxygen extracted by the tissue, which is the difference between the arterial and the mixed venous oxygen contents, $C(a-v)O_2$:

$$\text{Oxygen Consumption}\left(VO_2\right) = (Q) \times \left(C\left(a-v\right)O_2\right)$$

As the VO_2 of a given tissue increases, the normal response in the human body is to increase the local blood flow to the area, to maintain the local $(a-v)O_2$ content difference close to the normal range. A marked increase of $(a-v)O_2$, above 4–5 vol.%, is observed during physical exercise, as discussed further in Chap. 5. An increase of this magnitude in non-exercising individuals usually means an impaired circulation, inadequate to meet the increased demand of the tissues in some disease states, or it means that the oxygen content of the arterial blood is very low. The increased extraction of oxygen from the blood leads to a lower pO_2 compared to the normal level of 35–40 mmHg with O_2 saturation at 75 %. Naturally the regional flow throughout the body is variable, and organs such as the heart and brain extract much more oxygen from the blood than do other organs. The brain makes up 2–3 % of body weight but receives 15 % of the cardiac output and 20 % of the oxygen

Fig. 2.4 The oxygen cascade

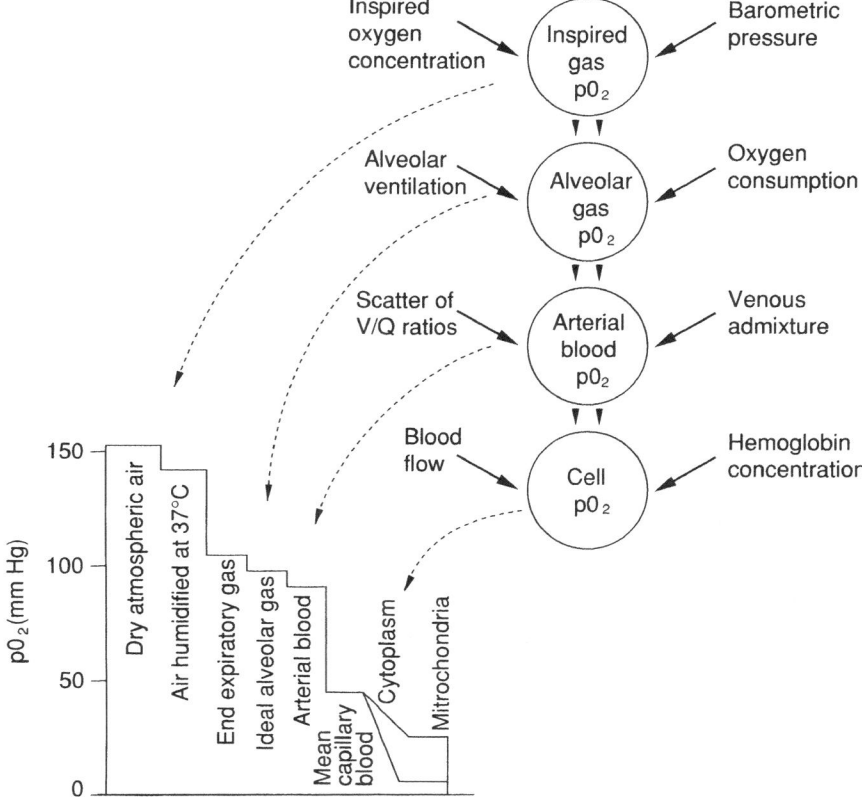

uptake of the entire body. Within the brain, cerebral blood flow and oxygen uptake vary according to the level of cerebral activity.

Oxygen Utilization in the Cell

The major site of utilization of molecular oxygen within the average cell is the mitochondria, which account for about 80%, while 20% is used by other subcellular organs, such as the microsomes, nucleus, plasma membrane, etc. Oxygen combines with electrons derived from various substrates to release free energy. This energy is used to pump H+ ions from the inside to the outside of the mitochondria against an electrochemical gradient. As H+ ions diffuse back, free energy is made available to phosphorylate adenosine diphosphate (ADP), and adenosine triphosphate (ATP) is generated.

Only a minute amount of oxygen is required for the normal intracellular chemical reactions to take place. The respiratory enzyme system is so geared that when tissue pO_2 is more than 1–3 mmHg, oxygen availability is no longer a limiting factor in the rate of chemical reactions. Under normal conditions, the rate of oxygen utilization by cells is controlled by the rate of energy expenditure within the cells, i.e., by the rate at which ADP is formed from ATP.

The diffusion distance from the capillary wall to the cell is rarely more than 50 µm, and normally oxygen can reach the cell quite readily. But, if pO_2 falls below the critical value of 1–3 mmHg, and if the cells are located farther away from the capillaries, the oxygen utilization is diffusion limited and not determined by ADP. This is particularly true for cerebral white matter, which is very sensitive to hypoxia as well as hyperoxia.

Effect of Blood Flow

Since oxygen is transported to the tissues in the bloodstream, interruption of blood flow means that the amount of available oxygen to the cells also falls to zero. Under these conditions, the rate of tissue utilization of oxygen is limited by blood flow.

Effect of Oxygen-Hemoglobin Reaction on Transport of CO_2

This response, known as the Haldane effect, results from the fact that combination of oxygen with hemoglobin causes it to become a stronger acid. This displaces CO_2 from the blood in two ways:

1. When there is more acid, hemoglobin has less of a tendency to combine with CO_2 to form carbhemoglobin. Much of the CO_2 present in this form in the blood is thus displaced.
2. The increased acidity of the hemoglobin causes it to release an excess of H+ ions, and these, in turn, bind with bicarbonate ions to form carbonic acid which then dissociates into water and CO_2, which is released from the blood into the alveoli.

Thus in the presence of oxygen, much less CO_2 can bind. The Haldane effect is far more important in promoting CO_2 transport than the Bohr effect on the transport of oxygen. The combined Bohr-Haldane effect on oxygen transport is more important than on pH or CO_2 transport. Equations have been described for predicting the limits of the rates of oxygen supply to the cells of living tissues and organs. It is possible to delineate the mechanisms by which molecular oxygen is transported from the red cells while being carried in the bloodstream longitudinally through capillaries into the moving plasma and thence radically out and through the capillary wall into the surrounding tissues for tissue cell respiration.

Autoregulation of the Intracellular pO$_2$

Intracellular pO_2 has not as yet been measured in humans, simply due to the lack of a suitable device for doing so. Such studies have been carried out in experimentally using microelectrodes implanted in the giant neurons of *Aplysia* (500 μm–1 mm) and comparing it with the extracellular pO_2 (EpO_2). At an EpO_2 value of +20 mmHg, the IpO_2 showed a stable value of between 4.5 and 8 mmHg. At between 10 and 50 mmHg EpO_2, IpO_2 is kept fairly constant by "autoregulation." A simple, minimally invasive method for the analysis of intracellular oxygen in live mammalian cells is available. Loading of the cells with the phosphorescent oxygen-sensing probe, MitoXpress (Luxcel Biosciences Ltd, Cork, Ireland), is achieved by passive liposomal transfer or facilitated endocytosis, followed by monitoring in standard microwell plates on a time-resolved fluorescent reader (O'Riordan et al. 2007). Phosphorescence lifetime measurements provide accurate, real-time, quantitative assessment of average oxygen levels in resting cells and their alterations in response to stimulation. MitoXpress® Xtra assay enables measurement of extracellular oxygen consumption rates with whole cell populations, isolated mitochondria, permeabilized cells, and a wide range of 3D cultures including: tissues, small organisms, spheroids, scaffolds, and matrixes.

The protoporphyrin IX-triplet state lifetime technique (PpIX-TSLT) was the first method to measure mitochondrial oxygen tension (mitoPO$_2$) in living cells and can be used in humans (Mik 2013). The technique is based on oxygen-dependent quenching of the delayed fluorescence lifetime of 5-aminolevulinic-acid-enhanced mitochondrial PpIX and enables comprehensive measurement of tissue oxygenation. MitoPO$_2$ in intact tissues reflects the balance between oxygen supply and demand at the cellular level. Clinical measurements of mitoPO$_2$ are possible as demonstrated by cutaneous measurements in healthy volunteers. Applications of PpIX-TSLT can be used in anesthesiology and intensive care for monitoring mitoPO$_2$ as a resuscitation end point, targeting oxygen homeostasis in the critically ill, and assessing mitochondrial function at the bedside.

Hyperbaric Oxygenation

Theoretical Considerations

Hyperbaric oxygenation (HBO) involves the use of oxygen under pressure greater than that found on earth's surface at sea level. Units commonly used to denote barometric pressure include:

mmHg	millimeters of mercury
in Hg	inches of mercury
psi	pounds per square inch
kg/cm^2	kilograms per square centimeter
bar	bar
fsw, msw	feet or meters of sea water
atm	atmospheres
ATA	atmospheres absolute

The standard atmosphere (symbol: atm) is a unit of pressure equal to 101,325 Pa or 1013.25 hectopascals or millibars, equivalent to 760 mmHg (torr), 29.92 in Hg, and 14.696 psi. (The pascal is a newton per square meter or in terms of SI base units kilogram per meter per second squared.)

$$Mpa\,(megapascal) = 9\ atm\,(1\ million\ force\ of\ Newton\,/\,sq\ meter)$$

Pressure at sea level = 0.1 Mpa or 101.325 kPa (1013.25 hPa or mbar) or 29.92 in. (inHg) or 760 millimeters of mercury (mmHg)

The only absolute pressures are those measured by a mercury barometer. In contrast, gauge pressures are a measure of difference between the pressure in a chamber and the surrounding atmospheric pressure. To convert pressure as measured by a gauge to absolute pressure (ATA) requires addition of the barometric pressure. A guide to these conversions is shown in Table 2.1. The range of partial pressures of oxygen under HBO is shown in Table 2.2, and the ideal alveolar oxygen pressures are shown in Table 2.3.

Boyle's well-known law states that if the temperature remains constant, the volume of a gas is inversely proportional to its pressure. Therefore, normal or abnormal gas-containing cavities in the body will have volume changes as HBO therapy is applied.

Table 2.1 Comparison of pressure units in range encountered in hyperbaric therapy

| ATA | Absolute pressures (bar) | | | | Gauge pressures | | |
	mmHg (torr)		Pa	fsw	msw	psi	atm
1	760	1.013	101.3	0	0	0	0
1.5	1140	1.519	151.9	16	5.16	7.35	0.5
2	1520	2.026	202.6	33	10.32	14.7	1
2.5	1900	2.532	253.2	50	15.48	21.05	1.5
3	2280	3.039	303.9	66	20.64	29.4	2
4	3040	4.052	405.2	99	30.97	44.0	3
5	3800	5.065	506.5	132	41.29	58.7	4
6	4560	6.078	607.8	165	51.61	73.3	5

Pa kilo pascal, pascal (newton per square meter) is the SI unit of choice

Table 2.2 Range of partial pressures in hyperbaric therapy

| Total pressure | | Oxygen pressure | |
ATA	mmHg	ATA	mmHg
1	760	0.21	159.7
1.5	1140	0.31	239.4
2	1520	0.42	319.2
2.5	1900	0.53	394.0
3	2280	0.63	478.8
4	3040	0.84	638.4
5	3800	1.05	798.0
6	4560	1.26	957.6

Table 2.3 Ideal alveolar oxygen pressures

| Total pressure | | pAO_2 breathing air | pAO_2 breathing 100% O_2 |
ATA	mmHg	mmHg	mmHg
1	760	102	673
1.5	1140	182	1053
2	1520	262	1433
2.5	1900	342	1813
3	2280	422	2193
4	3040	582	O_2 not administered at pressures >3 ATA
5	3800	742	
6	4560	902	

Density

As barometric pressure rises there is an increase in the density of the gas breathed. The effect of increased density on resting ventilation is negligible within the range of the 1.5–2.5 ATA usually used in HBO. However, with physical exertion in patients with decreased respiratory reserves or respiratory obstruction, increased density may cause gas flow problems.

Temperature

The temperature of a gas rises during compression and falls during decompression. According to Charles' law, if the volume remains constant, there is a direct relationship between absolute pressure and temperature.

Effect of Pressure on Oxygen Solubility in Blood

Only a limited amount of oxygen is dissolved in blood at normal atmospheric pressure. But, under hyperbaric conditions, as seen in Table 2.4, it is possible to dissolve sufficient oxygen, i.e., 6 vol.% in plasma, to meet the usual requirements of the body. In this case oxyhemoglobin will pass unchanged from the arterial to the venous side because the oxygen physically dissolved in solution will be utilized more readily than that bound to hemoglobin. The typical arterial oxygen uptake under HBO is shown in Fig. 2.5. Here the usual oxygen dissociation curve has been extended to include increases in oxygen content as a result of inspiring oxygen up to 3 ATA. The pO_2 simply rises linearly with rise of pressure.

Table 2.4 Effect of pressure on arterial O_2

Total pressure		Ideal dissolved oxygen content (vol%)	
ATA	mmHg	Breathing air	Breathing 100 % O_2
1	760	0.32	2.09
1.5	1140	0.61	3.26
2	1520	0.81	4.44
2.5	1900	1.06	5.62
3	2280	1.31	6.80
4	3040	1.80	O_2 not administered at pressures >3 ATA
5	3800	2.30	
6	4560	2.80	

Values assume arterial pO_2 = alveolar pO_2 and that hemoglobin oxygen capacity of blood is 20 vol.%

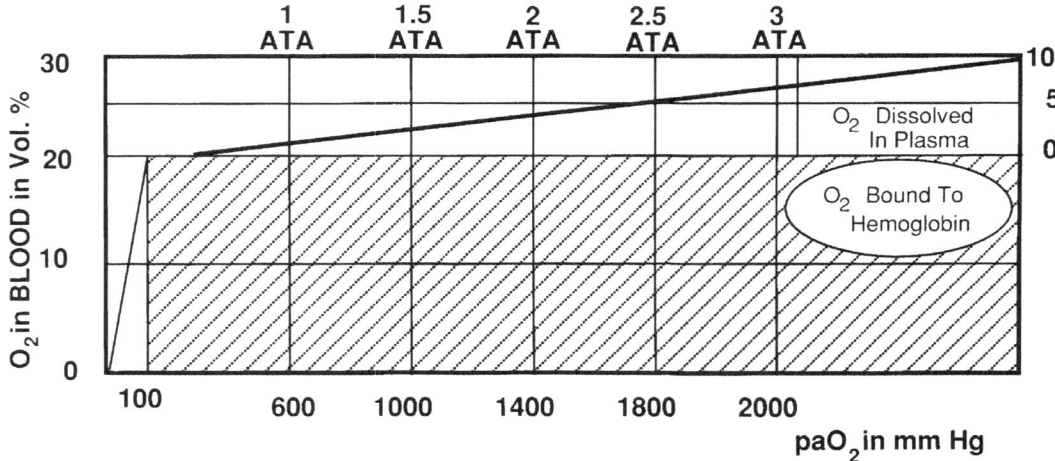

Fig. 2.5 Oxygen uptake curve under HBO in humans

Effect of HBO on Capillary Oxygen Pressure Drop

The oxygen extraction by average tissues of 5 vol.% results in a remarkable pressure drop of 60 (100 down to 40) mmHg from the arterial end to the venous end of the capillary. At 2000 mmHg the oxygen content is approximately 25 (20 + 5) vol%. The extraction of 5 vol.% in this case causes a pressure drop of about 1900 mmHg. Each of the differences in pO_2 represents the same number of oxygen molecules, in the first case carried by the hemoglobin and in the second case by the plasma. The metabolic requirement of the cells can ultimately be expressed as a certain number of molecules of oxygen per minute.

HBO and Retention of CO_2

When HBO results in venous blood being 100 % saturated with oxygen, there is a rise in blood pCO_2 and a shift of pH to the acid side. This is due to loss of hemoglobin available to transport CO_2. This affects only the 20 % of the venous content of CO_2 which is transported by hemoglobin. Excess CO_2 is transported by the H_2CO_3/HCO_3 mechanism, as well as by entering into physical solution in plasma. The eleva-tion of cerebral venous pCO_2 is of the order of 5–6 mmHg when venous hemoglobin is 100 % saturated with oxygen. CO_2 does not continue to rise in venous blood and the tissues as long as the blood flow remains constant, and presents no major problems.

Tissue Oxygen Tension Under HBO

Various factors relating to tissue oxygen tension under HBO are:

- Arterial pO_2 is the maximum pO_2 to which any tissue will be exposed and plays a major part in determining the pO_2 diffusion gradient driving oxygen into the tissues. Arterial pO_2 depends on the inspired pO_2.
- Arterial pO_2 content is the total amount of oxygen available. It depends on the inspired oxygen and the blood hemoglobin level.
- Tissue blood flow regulates the delivery of oxygen to the tissues.
- Tissue oxygen levels vary according to utilization of the available oxygen.

In a *typical* tissue, arteriovenous oxygen difference rises to 350 mmHg when 100 % oxygen is breathed at 3 ATA. If the blood flow to the tissues is reduced by half, the corresponding values of capillary pO_2 will be 288 and 50 mmHg. But, of course, the oxygen requirement of different tissues varies. For example, the needs of cardiac muscle are ten times that of the skin.

Another factor is the vasoconstricting effect of HBO, which reduces the blood flow. Effective cellular oxygenation can be accomplished at very low rates of blood flow when arterial pO_2 is very high.

General Effects of HBO on the Healthy Human Body

The important general effects of hyperoxia on a healthy human body are listed in Table 2.5. The effects vary according to the pressures used, the duration of exposure, and health of the subject. Unless otherwise stated, HBO refers to the use of 100 % oxygen. The effects of HBO on each system, both in health and in disease, will be discussed in chapters dealing with disorders of those systems. As an introduction, some important effects are described here briefly.

Cardiovascular System

The cardiovascular system responds to HBO with vasoconstriction, hypertension, bradycardia, and reduced cardiac output (CO). Experimental studies at 2.5 ATA in conscious rats and at 3 ATA for anesthetized rats have shown that hypertension, bradycardia, and reduced CO—the initial cardiovascular responses to moderate levels of HBO—are coordinated through a baroreflex-mediated mechanism initiated by HBO-induced vasoconstriction (Demchenko et al. 2013). Furthermore, this study showed that baroreceptor activation

Table 2.5 Effects of hyperoxia

I. Oxygen transport and metabolism
1. Inactivation of the hemoglobin role in oxygen and CO_2 transport
2. The biological burning of normal oxygen metabolism
II. Respiratory system
1. Suppression of carotid and aortic bodies with depression of ventilation
2. Washout of N_2 with increased susceptibility to lung collapse
III. Cardiovascular system
1. Bradycardia
2. Decreased cardiac output and decreased cerebral blood flow
IV. Peripheral vessels
1. Vasoconstriction of peripheral blood vessels: brain, kidney, eye
2. Increased peripheral resistance
V. Metabolic and biochemical

in HBO inhibits sympathetic outflow and can partially reverse an O_2-dependent increase in arterial pressure.

In human patients, HBO results in a decrease in CO due to bradycardia, rather than a reduction in stroke volume. Blood pressure remains essentially unchanged. Blood flow to most organs falls in proportion to the fall of CO except to the right and the left ventricles of the heart. There is no impairment of the function of any of these organs because the raised pO_2 more than compensates for the reduction of the blood flow. Vasoconstriction may be viewed as a regulatory mechanism to protect the healthy organs from exposure to excessive pO_2. Usually the vasoconstrictor response does not take place in the hypoxic tissues.

Dermal blood flow has been shown to decrease as a response to hyperoxia; it has been measured by laser Doppler flowmeter. It was also demonstrated that the reduction of blood flow does not occur in the vicinity of a chronic skin ulcer and that the vasoconstrictor response is restored after the ulcer had healed.

A study examined the effect of hyperbaric air and HBO on arterial and pulmonary arterial hemodynamics and blood gas measures (Weaver et al. 2009). The data presented are in agreement with that of others that heart rate and Q' fall with HBO_2 exposure. The PaO_2, Pv O_2, Sv O_2, and $PaCO_2$ values were within expected ranges during hyperbaric air and HBO exposures. PVR and Pv CO_2 decreased during HBO exposure. Finally, $Q's/Q't$ was higher than expected with subjects breathing air at atmospheric pressure and fell to 0 during HBO exposure.

HBO modifies fibrinolytic activity in the blood. To clarify the stage of fibrinolytic activation by HBO exposure, the activities and antigens have been estimated during and after the HBO exposure. The plasminogen activator inhibitor-1 (PAI-1) activity and PAI-1 antigen show significant decrease after compression to a pressure 284 kPa (2.8 ATA), before the start of decompression, and after decompression. The euglobulin fibrinolytic activity (EFA) level and tissue-type plasminogen activator (t-PA) activity rise significantly shortly after decompression, and 3 h later return to baseline. These findings suggest that fibrinolytic activity is elicited after HBO rather than during HBO.

Effect of HBO on Microcirculation

HBO improves the elasticity of the red blood cells and reduces platelet aggregation. This, combined with the ability of the plasma to carry dissolved oxygen to areas where RBCs cannot reach, has a beneficial effect on the oxygenation of many hypoxic tissues in various circulatory disorders.

Effect of HBO on Respiratory System

Hyperoxia suppresses the respiratory reactivity to CO_2. After an initial depression of respiration, there is hyperventilation. HBO reversibly depresses the hypoxic ventilatory drive, most probably by a direct effect on the carotid CO_2 chemoreceptors.

Usually there are no differences between forced vital capacities (FVC) and maximal expiratory flows before and after HBO exposure while breathing dry or humidified oxygen. However, decreases in mean expiratory flow with steady FVC have been reported after 14 days of daily HBOc therapy (0.24 MPa) with although 80 % of the patients are symptom free and remain so afterwards. This toxicity is clinically insignificant in subjects free of inflammatory lung diseases. HBO therapy, though safe, is not entirely without effect on the lungs.

Biochemical Effects of HBO

Biomarkers of HBO

Urine methylguanidine (MG) which is known as a uremic toxin is synthesized from creatinine. Urine MG/urine creatinine/serum creatinine ratio is used as an index of MG synthesis rate which has been shown to increase during HBO therapy in human subjects and can be used as a biomarker of active oxygen products in vivo.

Magnetic resonance imaging (MRI) is useful for evaluating oxygenation in several types of tissue and blood. A study has evaluated brain tissue oxygenation changes between normoxia and hyperoxia in healthy subjects using dynamic T1- and T2*-weighted imaging sequences (Haddock et al. 2013). This study concluded that T1 and T2* responses to FiO_2 serve as independent biomarkers of oxygen physiology in the brain with a potential to provide quantitative information on tissue oxygenation.

Effect of HBO on the Acid-Base Balance

Increased partial pressure of oxygen in the blood disturbs the reduction of oxyhemoglobin to hemoglobin. Of the alkali that neutralizes the transported CO_2, 70 % originates from the hemoglobin. As a result of HBO and due to increased solubility of CO_2, there is retention of CO_2 leading to a slight rise of H+ ions in the tissues. HBO reduces excess lactate production in hypoxic states, as well as during exercise. This important subject is discussed in detail in Chap. 5.

Effect of HBO on Enzymes

Cyclooxygenase inactivation. This results in decreased production of prostacyclin by hyperoxic tissues. In experimental studies, brief exposure of human umbilical arteries to hyperoxia results in a 30 % decrease in activity of cyclooxygenase, in contrast to a 49 % increase in its activity throughout the hypoxic arterial segments.

Heme oxygenase (HO). This enzyme catalyzes the rate-limiting step in the oxidative degradation of heme to biliverdin. The isoform HO-1 is inducible by a variety of agents causing oxidative stress and has been suggested to play an important role in cellular protection against oxidant-mediated cell damage. A low-level overexpression of HO-1 induced by HBO exposure provides protection against oxidative DNA damage by further exposures to HBO.

Tyrosine hydroxylase. Increased oxygen saturation of this enzyme leads to increased turnover of catecholamines. Hyperoxia inhibits phenylalanine and tyrosine hydroxylase.

Succinic Dehydrogenase (SDH) and Cytochrome Oxidase (CCO). These enzymes are activated by HBO. Their levels decline in the liver and kidneys of patients with intestinal obstruction. HBO after surgery led to the normalization of the levels of these enzymes.

Effect of HBO on Oxidative Stress

The role of hyperbaric oxygen (HBO) therapy in free radical-mediated tissue injury is not clear. HBO has been shown to enhance the antioxidative defense mechanisms in some animal studies, but HBO has also been reported to increase the production of oxygen free radicals. Hyperoxia causes an increase in nitric oxide (NO) synthesis as part of a response to oxidative stress. Mechanisms for neuronal nitric oxide synthase (nNOS) activation include augmentation in the association with Hsp90 and intracellular entry of calcium. In animal experimental studies, tissue oxygenation and cellular defenses have been shown to effectively limit damage from chronic oxidative stress more effectively than chemical antioxidants (Verma et al. 2015).

Effect of HBO on the Nervous System

Vasoconstriction and reduced cerebral blood flow do not produce any clinically observable effects in a healthy adult when pressures of 1.5–2.5 ATA are used. Pressures higher than 3 ATA for prolonged periods can lead to oxygen convulsions as a result of oxygen toxicity. The effects of HBO are more pronounced in hypoxic/ischemic states of the brain. HBO reduces cerebral edema and improves the function of neurons rendered inactive by ischemia/hypoxia. The improvement of brain function is reflected by the improved electrical activity of the brain. The effect of HBO on cerebral blood flow is discussed in Chap. 18.

Effect of HBO on Cerebral Metabolism

The most important metabolic effects of HBO are on the brain. Most of the investigations of this topic have been prompted by the problem of oxygen toxicity. It is believed that the preconvulsive period of oxygen toxicity is characterized by alterations in several interrelated physiological functions of the brain, such as electrical activity, blood flow, tissue pO$_2$, and metabolic activity. The relation of these changes to the development of oxygen-induced convulsions has not yet been clarified. Nonetheless, several interesting observations have been made as a result of these studies which throw some light on the effect of HBO on cerebral metabolism in the absence of clinical signs of oxygen toxicity. Most of the cerebral metabolic studies are now done on human patients with various CNS disorders. Use of brain imaging in metabolic studies is described in Chaps. 10, 18, and 20.

Effect of HBO on Glucose Metabolism

Studies on regional cerebral glucose metabolic rate (rCMRgl) in rats after exposure to pressures of 1, 2, and 3 ATA show that the degree of central nervous system effects of HBO depends upon the pressure as well as the duration of exposure. Increased utilization of glucose in some neuronal structures precedes the onset of central nervous system manifestations of oxygen toxicity. Exposure of rats to 100 % oxygen at 3 ATA causes an increase in rCMRgl, and this is related to the oxygen-induced preconvulsive pattern of the electrocorticogram.

In cats HBO (3 ATA for 60 min) has a definite effect on the glycerophosphate shuttle mechanism following acute blood loss. HBO stimulates the mitochondrial glycerol-3-phosphate dehydrogenase in the sensorimotor cortex and the medulla oblongata, providing glycerol-3-phosphate dehydrogenation. There is activation of the cytoplasm hydrogen delivery to the mitochondrial respiratory chain. In addition, there is prevention of a rise in glycerol-3-phosphate and NADH levels, as well as inhibition of glycerol-3-phosphate dehydrogenase, which limits lactate production. Energy metabolism has also been found to be highly sensitive to raised pressures of oxygen, which can reduce the formation of ATP molecules considerably.

Effect of HBO on Ammonia Metabolism

Following injury to the brain, the activity of glutaminase increases sharply, providing a release of ammonia from glutamine and a rise in transcapillary transfer of ammonia into the brain tissue from the blood. At the same time, there is activation of glutamate formation pathways under the effect of glutamine dehydrogenase and decrease of glutamine formation due to inhibition of glutamine synthase. This also leads to a decrease in the amount of α-ketoglutarate. HBO at 3 ATA for 60 min prevents ammonia toxicity from increasing in the dehematized brain. The toxic effects of ammonia ions on the brain are eliminated via:

- Stimulation of the activity of the mitochondrial GDG providing glutamate formation from α-ketoglutarate
- Binding of ammonia with glutamate resulting in glutamine formation
- A decrease of glutaminase activity inhibiting the process of deaminization of glutamine—a potential source of ammonia
- Transcapillary discharge of ammonia in the form of glutamine from the brain to the blood

Effect of HBO at Molecular Level

Effect on DNA

HBO treatment under therapeutic conditions induces DNA damage in leukocytes in various studies on human subjects. However, there is no indication of induced chromosomal breakage in cultivated leukocytes. Increased DNA damage is usually found immediately at the end of the treatment, whereas it is not detectable 24 h later. DNA damage is detected only after the first treatment and not after further treatments under the same conditions, indicating an increase in antioxidant defenses. DNA damage does not occur when the HBO treatment is started with a reduced treatment time which is then increased stepwise. HBO-induced DNA strand breaks and oxidative base modifications are rapidly repaired, leading to a reduction in induced DNA effects of >50 % during the first hour. A similar decrease is found in blood taken immediately after exposure and 2 h after exposure.

Conclusion

The practical significance of many of the general effects of HBO is not clear. The study of the effects on cerebral metabolism was motivated by a search for the mechanism of oxygen-induced seizures. High pressures such as 6 ATA have been used which have no clinical relevance; the pressures for treatment of cerebral disorders usually do not exceed 2 ATA. The starting optimal pressure for treating patients with brain injury is 1.5 ATA. The cerebral glucose metabolism is balanced at this pressure. Raising the pressure even only to 2 ATA may have unfavorable effects on the human brain.

Generally HBO therapy is safe and well tolerated by humans at 1.5–2 ATA. The duration of exposure and the percentage of oxygen also have a bearing. No adverse effects are seen at 1.5 ATA for exposures up to 40–60 min.

References

Bohr C, Hasselbalch K, Krogh A. Concerning a biologically important relationship—the influence of the carbon dioxide content of blood on its oxygen binding. Translation of: Über einen in biologischer Beziehung wichtigen Einfluss, den die Kohlensäurespannung des Blutes auf dessen Sauerstoffbindung übt. Skand Arch Physiol. 1904;16:401–12.

Demchenko IT, Zhilyaev SY, Moskvin AN, Krivchenko AI, Piantadosi CA, Allen BW. Baroreflex-mediated cardiovascular responses to hyperbaric oxygen. J Appl Physiol. 2013;115:819–28.

Fick A. Über die Messung des Blutquantums in den Herzventrikeln. S.B. Phys-Med Ges, Würzburg, v. 16., 1870.

Haddock B, Larsson HB, Hansen AE, Rostrup E. Measurement of brain oxygenation changes using dynamic T(1)-weighted imaging. Neuroimage. 2013;78:7–15.

Jain KK. Oxygen in physiology and medicine. Springfield: Charles C. Thomas; 1989.

Mik EG. Special article: measuring mitochondrial oxygen tension: from basic principles to application in humans. Anesth Analg. 2013;117:834–46.

O'Riordan TC, Zhdanov AV, Ponomarev GV, Papkovsky DB. Analysis of intracellular oxygen and metabolic responses of mammalian cells by time-resolved fluorometry. Anal Chem. 2007;79:9414–9.

Verma R, Chopra A, Giardina C, Sabbisetti V, Smyth JA, Hightower LE, et al. Hyperbaric oxygen therapy (HBOT) suppresses biomarkers of cell stress and kidney injury in diabetic mice. Cell Stress Chaperones. 2015;20:495–505.

Weaver LK, Howe S, Snow GL, Deru K. Arterial and pulmonary arterial hemodynamics and oxygen delivery/extraction in normal humans exposed to hyperbaric air and oxygen. J Appl Physiol. 2009;107:336–45.

Effects of Diving and High Pressure on the Human Body

3

K.K. Jain

Abstract

This chapter examines physiological responses to variations in environmental pressure and physical effects of pressure. High pressure also has an effect on action of drugs on the human body. Effects of high-pressure environments are described on various systems of the body, particularly the nervous system. Hearing and vestibular functions, as well as taste sensation, are impaired under high pressure. In addition to detailing effects on specific body systems, the symptoms and treatments related to a variety of pressure-induced medical conditions are presented.

Keywords

Complications of diving • Decompression sickness • Diver's headache • Diver's vertigo • Diving medicine • Environmental pressure • High-pressure neurological syndrome • Middle ear damage in diving • Nitrogen narcosis • Pressure and action of drugs

Physical Effects of Pressure

When human beings descend beneath the surface of the sea, they are subjected to tremendous pressure increases. To keep the thorax from collapsing, air must be supplied under high pressure, which exposes the blood in the lungs to extremely high alveolar gas pressures. This is known as hyperbarism. Workers in caissons, for example, must work in pressurized areas.

Relation of Sea Depth to Pressure. A vertical column of sea water 33 ft (~10 m) high exerts the same absolute pressure as that of the atmosphere at sea level (760 mmHg, as measured by a mercury barometer) and referred to as 1 ATA or 1.013 bar. Therefore, a person 33 ft beneath the surface of the sea is exposed to a pressure of 2 ATA (1 ATA caused by the weight of the water and 1 ATA by the air above the water) and a dive to 66 ft involves exposure to pressure of 3 ATA. Studies in diving medicine may refer to a dive to so many feet or the diver being subjected to so many ATA or bar. Similar terms are used to describe simulations in hyperbaric chambers.

K.K. Jain, MD, FRACS, FFPM (✉)
1 Blaesiring 7, Basel 4057, Switzerland
e-mail: jain@pharmabiotech.ch

Effect of Depth on Volume of Gases. Boyle's law states that the volume to which a given quantity of gas is compressed is inversely proportional to the pressure. Thus, 1.0 L of air at sea level is compressed to 0.5 L at 10 m (33 ft).

The effects of pressure on the human body vary according to the following factors:

- Total pressure
- Duration of exposure to pressure
- State of activity of the diver resting or exercising
- Temperature
- Drugs in the body
- Gas mixtures used
- Rate of descent

Effects of Pressure on Various Systems of the Body

Hematological and Biochemical Effects

A 14-day exposure to 5.2 % oxygen and nitrogen at pressure of 4 ATA has been shown to cause hemoconcentration with slight elevation of Hb, Hct, RBC, plasma proteins, and cholesterol because of a decrease of plasma volume with diuresis. Loss of intracellular fluid has been observed, but this reverses partially during the postexposure period. Weight loss has been observed in divers compressed to 49.5 ATA (488 msw) in He-oxygen environments. This loss was shown to be 3.7–10.2 kg in 14 days of hyperbaric exposure.

Diuresis occurs in practically all saturation dives and is associated with natriuresis at pressures greater than 31 ATA. Three mechanisms may be involved in the development of this diuresis:

1. Inhibition of ADH release
2. Inhibition of tubular reabsorption of NA+ (pressure inhibits active transcapillary transport of NA+)
3. Inhibition of hydrostatic action of ADH on the tubules

Fluid loss induced by diving and/or weightlessness might also add substantially to the pressure-induced diuresis. Because the sense of thirst is impaired in hyperbaric environments, and the resultant fluid imbalance reduces performance of divers, countermeasures against fluid loss should be taken during operational saturation diving.

Effect on Ammonia Metabolism

Long-term exposure to hyperbaric conditions has been shown to increase blood urea in US Navy divers. This is interpreted as evidence of hyperammonemia because urea is formed with ammonia buffering.

Effect on Blood Cells and Platelets

Increase of neutrophils, blood platelets, and fibrinogen concentration in the blood plasma immediately after diving is of temporary character, being a typical reaction observed during diving. The values usually return to normal spontaneously. Environmental stress such as cold water may contribute to platelet activation, which plays an important role in the pathogenesis of prethrombotic states and thus may be responsible for decompression illness during compressed air diving.

Changes in the Respiratory System and Blood Gases

Breathing mixtures with normal oxygen content at pressures up to 60 bar produces moderate changes in respiration, compared with the pattern of respiration at normal ambient pres-

sure. At pressures from 80 to 100 bar, oxygen transport is likely to be compromised by changes in hemoglobin affinity. Breathing of high concentrations of oxygen (pO_2 over 500 mbar) causes retention of CO_2 in the tissues, which leads to hyperventilation. However, if the subject is exercising, reduced chemoreceptor activity leads to impaired alveolar ventilation.

Rapid changes in environmental pressure produce an inequality between inspiratory and expiratory volumes; compression causes hypercapnia while decompression causes hypocapnia. The following influence the respiratory effects of pressure:

Position of the diver. The upright position causes less dyspnea than the prone position.
Physical activity, which increases the tendency for CO_2 accumulation.
Gas density. The higher the density of the gas mixture breathed, the greater the airway resistance is; it therefore requires more energy to breathe denser mixtures.
If the diver uses a face mask, the breathing gas should provide a static lung load of approximately 0 to +10 cm of water (0–0.01 ATA) regardless of the diver's orientation in the water.

The increased ventilation observed in experimental animals breathing He-oxygen mixtures at extremely high pressures (up to 10 MPa) is responsible for fatigue of the respiratory muscles and may lead to ventilatory failure.

Adaptation has been shown to occur during a 14-day exposure to a high nitrogen pressure environment of 4 ATA with naturally inspired oxygen tensions. This modification of respiratory control is exemplified by a diminished ventilatory response to CO_2. The diminished response is more likely related to the density of respiratory gas than to the narcotic influence of the respired nitrogen.

Multiple diving exposures affect both the vital capacity and the forced rotatory flow rate of smaller lung volumes. This is evidence for the narrowing of the airways that may be secondary to diving-induced loss of elasticity of the lung tissue. Longitudinal studies of lung function in oxygen divers have shown that substantial exposure to elevated oxygen partial pressure while diving is not associated with an accelerated decline in lung function. Factors other than hyperoxia (e.g., venous gas microemboli and altered breathing gas characteristics) may account for the long-term effects that have been found in professional divers.

Hypoxic states usually do not occur in divers, but the response of divers to hypoxia is the same as that of nondivers. The effects of repeated acute exposures to breathing 100% oxygen at pressure—such as those encountered during oxygen diving—may affect the peripheral oxygen chemosensors.

Effects on the Cardiovascular System

Exposure to hyperbaric environments has been shown to cause a variety of disturbances in the electrical activity of the mammalian heart. Arrhythmias under these conditions are considered to be the result of an increase in parasympathetic tone. Increased hydrostatic pressure also decreases excitability and conduction through direct effects on the myocardial cell membrane. Hyperbaric exposure alters cardiac excitation–contraction coupling in anesthetized cats during He-oxygen dives to 305 msw. Some conclusions of the studies of the effects of moderate hyperbaric exposure on the rat heart are as follows:

• Cardiac contractility is increased during hyperbaric exposures despite administration of calcium and sodium channel blockers, thus reducing the possibility of involvement of these channels in the mechanism of this effect. Starling's mechanism or neurotransmitter involvement was also excluded.

• Repeated hyperbaric exposures causes hypertrophy of the heart.
• Left ventricular pressure increased at 5 bar and the degree of rise varied with the breathing gases used.
• Heart rate remained unchanged in all normoxic experiments.

Doppler-echocardiographic studies in healthy divers indicate that circulating gas bubbles are associated with cardiac changes, suggesting a right ventricular overload and an impairment of ventricular diastolic performance. Postdive humoral and hematologic changes are consistent with the hypothesis that "silent" gas bubbles may damage pulmonary endothelium and activate the reactive systems of the human body.

The increased environmental pressure seems responsible for the hemodynamic rearrangement causing reduction of cardiac output seen in diving humans because most of the changes are observed during diving (Marabotti et al. 2009). Left ventricular diastolic function changes suggest a constrictive effect on the heart possibly accounting for cardiac output reduction. Breath holding (BH) induces progressive left ventricular (LV) enlargement both in air and whole-body immersion, associated with reduced LV ejection fraction and progressive hindrance to diastolic filling (Marabotti et al. 2013). For a similar apnea duration, SaO_2 decreased less during immersed BH, indicating an O_2-sparing effect of diving, suggesting that interruption of apnea was not triggered by a threshold critical value of blood O_2 desaturation.

Changes in the Endocrine System

The following changes in the endocrine function can occur as a result of hyperbaric exposures exceeding 4 ATA (30 msw) while breathing 6.2 % nitrogen in oxygen:

• Increase in the circulating levels of epinephrine, norepinephrine, and dopamine.
• Decrease in ADH secretion without a change in aldosterone excretion.
• Severe hyperbaric conditions associated with deep dives have a profound effect on male reproductive function due to fall in the quality of semen and oligozoospermia.
• Decrease of thyroxine levels in the blood.
• Increase in the insulin and angiotensin I level in plasma.
• Increase in the circulating concentration of atrial naturetic factor (ANF, a diuretic hormone). This may explain the diuresis observed in divers.

The endocrine reactions as well as the accompanying reductions in cognitive performance in divers, however, may be the result of emotional reactions to the dive rather than the direct effect of nitrogen narcosis.

Effect on the Skeletal System

Dysbaric osteonecrosis is a type of avascular necrosis caused by ischemia and subsequent infarction of bone. This usually involves the head of the femur. The disruption of blood flow in bone has been attributed to the formation of nitrogen bubbles as a result of diving, but blood pressure at the femoral head has been shown to be reduced by prolonged exposure to compressed air. Dysbaric osteonecrosis has been reported in 25 % of workers who perform in high-pressure environments (Cimsit et al. 2007).

Effects of High-Pressure Environments on the Nervous System

Neuropsychological Effects
Scuba diving was shown to have adverse long-term neuropsychological effects only when performed in extreme conditions, i.e., cold water, with >100 dives per year, and maximal depth <40 m. Deterioration of both mental and motor function has been reported in dives to 10 and 13 ATA—while breathing air and at rest. Hyperbaric air at 7 ATA does not impair short-term or long-term memory in test subjects, but, long-term memory is impaired at 10 ATA although it recovers on switching to an 80/20 He-oxygen mixture.

Non-saturation construction divers may not reveal clear evidence of neuropsychological deficit due to repeated diving but the prolonged reaction time can be ascribed to extensive non-saturation diving. Middle-aged divers who are exposed to critical depths of >60 msw have navigational problems and the number of brain lesions detected on MRI can be related to the number of hyperbaric exposures. There is a belief among occupational divers that a "punch drunk" effect is produced by prolonged compressed air diving. Most of the studies on this topic have serious limitations in statistical analysis and use of control groups. Dementia is recognized as a complication of severe hypoxia, cerebral embolism, or cerebral decompression sickness, but temporary neurological insults experienced by divers breathing compressed air cannot be translated into hard evidence of brain damage.

Nitrogen Narcosis

Behnke noted in 1935 that humans subjected to compressed air >5 ATA exhibited symptoms similar to alcohol intoxication. As the symptoms were immediate in onset and did not occur when He-oxygen mixtures were used, Behnke concluded that nitrogen was the causal agent. Since then many investigators have studied this phenomenon which Cousteau calls "l'ivresse des grandes profondeurs" or "rapture of the depths." The symptoms of nitrogen narcosis are euphoria, dulled mental ability, difficulty in assimilating facts, and quick decision-making.

Many suggestions have been made to explain the narcotic effects of inert gases, but the most satisfactory explanation seems to be the degree of lipid solubility. Auditory evoked potential studies have been used to assess the degree of narcosis induced by diving and indicate that nitrogen is the major cause of compressed air narcosis and that oxygen does not have a synergistic effect with nitrogen. Some of the noble gases, which have been substituted for nitrogen, also tend to cause some narcosis, but to a much lesser degree. Nitrogen and a raised CO_2 tension in the tissues as a result of hypoventilation and impaired CO_2 elimination are the causes of narcosis, but they can also cause a deterioration in the performance of the affected diver. Increasing the oxygen partial pressure and the density of the breathing mixture causes retention of the carbon dioxide in the cerebral tissues and synergistically potentiates the nitrogen narcosis.

Most of these studies were carried out under hyperbaric conditions although nitrous oxide is known to be an inducer of narcosis at atmospheric pressure as well. Animal experimental studies indicate that nitrous oxide could be considered as a normobaric model of hyperbaric narcosis.

Effects of anesthetics and high-pressure nitrogen can be compared. Conventional anesthetics, including inhalational agents and inert gases, such as xenon and nitrous oxide, interact directly with ion channel neurotransmitter receptors. However, there is no evidence that nitrogen, which only exhibits narcotic potency at increased pressure, may act by a similar mechanism; rather nitrogen at increased pressure might interact directly with the GABAA receptor. Repetitive exposures to nitrogen narcosis produce a sensitization of postsynaptic N-methyl D-aspartate receptors on dopaminergic cells, related to a decreased glutamatergic input in substantia nigra pars compacta (Lavoute et al. 2008). Consequently, suc-cessive nitrogen narcosis exposures disrupt ion channel receptor activity revealing a persistent nitrogen-induced neurochemical change underlying the pathologic process.

Diving deeper than 100 m cannot be done breathing air, as the nitrogen contained in such a mixture becomes narcotic at pressures greater than 6 ATA. In order to avoid nitrogen narcosis, mixtures of helium and oxygen (heliox) are used, and this permits dives beyond 100 m.

High-Pressure Neurological Syndrome

This subject has been reviewed in detail elsewhere (Jain 1994, 2016). High-pressure neurological syndrome (HPNS) is a condition encountered in deep diving beyond a depth of 100 m which is made possible by breathing of special gas mixtures such as helium and oxygen (heliox). It is characterized by neurological, psychological, and electroencephalographic abnormalities. Clinical features of HPNS have been reviewed by several authors and can be summarized as follows:

Symptoms
- Headache
- Vertigo
- Nausea
- Fatigue
- Euphoria

Neurological signs
- Tremors
- Postural sway
- Opsoclonus
- Myoclonus
- Dysmetria
- Hyperreflexia
- Sleep disorders
- Drowsiness
- Convulsions (only in experimental animals)

Neuropsychiatric
- Memory impairment
- Cognitive deficits
- Psychoses

Pathophysiology of HPNS

HPNS is primarily a result of excessive atmospheric pressure on different structures in the central nervous system (CNS). The rate of compression influences the manifestations of HPNS; a faster rate of compression increases the intensity of HPNS and decreases the pressure threshold for the onset of symptoms. The manifestations persist during a stay at a constant depth and decrease during decompression. The symptoms usually subside after the pressure is normalized, but some of these, such as lethargy, may linger on for days. In some cases, complaints such as memory disturbances take several months to resolve. Eventually, all of the divers who experience only HPNS recover. There is no evidence of permanent neurological sequelae or histopathological changes in the brain resulting from HPNS.

Intraspecies and interspecies variations of high-pressure neurological syndrome exist. There appears to be a genetic basis for adaptation to high-pressure neurological syndrome. Some individuals are more susceptible than others to development of the syndrome as a whole, or manifest various symptoms at different pressures. A single mutation in 3'UTR (untranslated region) of vacuolar protein sorting gene 52 (Vps52) is associated with greater than 60 % of the seizure risk difference between the high- and low-risk seizure susceptibility strains of mice (McCall 2011). By gene homology with human VPS52, this mutation may be considered a risk factor for seizures on exposure to high pressure.

High pressure differentially affects ionic currents of eight specific N-methyl-D-aspartate receptor subtypes generated by the co-expression of GluN1-1a or GluN1-1b with 1 of the 4 GluN2(A–D) subunits. A further study reports that eight GluN1 splice variants, when co-expressed with GluN2A, mediate different ionic currents at normal and high pressure of 45 atm, indicating that both GluN1 and GluN2 subunits play a critical role in determining N-methyl-D-aspartate receptor currents under normal and high-pressure conditions (Bliznyuk et al. 2015). Because of the differential spatial distribution of various N-methyl-D-aspartate receptor subtypes in the CNS, these data offer an explanation for the mechanism governing the complex signs and symptoms of high-pressure neurological syndrome as well as for the long-term health sequelae of repetitive deep dives by professional divers.

Sensitivity of the nervous system to high pressures may be compensated by a physiological adaptive response. Synaptic depression that requires less transmitter turnover may serve as an energy-saving mechanism when enzymes and membrane pumps activity are slowed down at pressure. Lethargy and fatigue, as well as reduction in cognitive and memory functions, are compatible with this state. Maladaptation to high pressure may lead to a pathophysiological response, i.e., HPNS. Some of the neurological signs may be an unmasking of previously silent brain lesions as a result of DCS. Various neurological manifestations appear at different depths. Tremor is seen at 200–300 m, myoclonus at 300–500 m, and EEG abnormalities are noted at 200–400 m.

Psychotic-like episodes in divers exposed to high pressure have been attributed to either the HPNS, confinement in pressure chamber, the subject's personality, or the addition of nitrogen or hydrogen to the basic helium-oxygen breathing mixture used for deep diving. Alternatively, it is suggested that these disorders are in fact paroxysmal narcotic symptoms that result from the sum of the individual narcotic potencies of each inert gas in the breathing mixture. This hypothesis has been tested against a variety of lipid solubility theories of narcosis and the results clearly support the hypothesis that there are cellular interactions between inert gases at raised pressure and pressure itself.

Role of Neurotransmitters in the Pathogenesis of HPNS

Various neurotransmitters and amino acids have been implicated in the pathogenesis of HPNS: GABA, dopamine, serotonin (5-HT), acetylcholine, and glutamate. Conclusions from various studies on this subject are:

- Various neurological and behavioral disturbances of HPNS are regulated by different mechanisms in the same areas of the brain.
- Neurotransmitter interactions in HPNS differ in various parts of the brain.
- The biochemical substrates for epileptic and HPNS-associated convulsions are different, for example, adenosine compounds protect against epilepsy but not against HPNS seizures.

The motor symptoms of HPNS are attributed to changes in neural excitability at spinal and midbrain levels. Serotonin may be implicated in hyperbaric spinal cord hyperexcitability. Quinolinic acid and kynurenine are metabolites of 5-HT that have been proposed as endogenous convulsants. The precise balance between these two may be an important determinant of onset of HPNS.

The clinical features of serotonin syndrome are changes in mental status, restlessness, myoclonus, hyperreflexia, shivering, and tremor. Behavioral changes in rats exposed to pressure resemble serotonin syndrome and are consistent with the activation of 5-HT receptor subtype 1A.

Prevention and Management of HPNS

Measures for the prevention and management of HPNS are as follows:

- Reduction of the speed of compression
- Modifications and additions to breathing gas mixtures: addition of nitrogen or hydrogen to heliox
- Anesthetics
- Barbiturates
- Anticonvulsant drugs
- Non-anesthetic compounds

A promising pharmacological approach is based on the resemblance of HPNS to serotonin syndrome. 5-HT1A receptor antagonists may provide a promising approach to prevent HPNS.

Headaches in Divers

Headaches in divers are uncommon include benign causes such as exertion, cold stimulus, migraine, and tension as well as serious causes such as decompression sickness, air embolism, and otic or paranasal sinus barotrauma. Inadequate ventilation of compressed gases can lead to carbon dioxide accumulation, cerebral vasodilatation, and headache. Rarely cerebral aneurysm rupture is associated with barotrauma. It is unclear whether volume expansion of trapped air, the blood pressure increase associated with barotrauma, or systemic vasodilation causes an aneurysm to rupture in this situation. Correct diagnosis and appropriate treatment require a careful history and neurologic examination as well as an understanding of the unique physiologic stresses of the subaquatic environment.

Central Nervous System Lesions in Divers

Decompression sickness is described in Chap. 10. Hyperintense lesions of the subcortical white matter seen on MRI are more common in amateur divers than in normal controls. These results differ from studies on saturation divers who have fewer such lesions than control subjects, even though neurological manifestations are more common among divers. Professional saturation diving involves breathing of helium/oxygen mixtures rather than compressed air as in the case of amateur divers. It is possible that MRI lesions in amateur divers are due to intravascular gas microbubbles. The only direct evidence for this is the demonstration by fluorescein angiography of pathological changes in the retinal microvasculature of divers even when they have not experienced decompression sickness.

Microbubble Damage to the Blood–Brain Barrier

Myelin damage has been discovered at the autopsy of divers with no recorded incidence of neurological decompression syndrome during life. Hyalinization of cerebral vessels has also been described in divers. Subtle neuropsychological changes in divers have not always been correlated with any pathology in the brain.

It has been proposed that as divers undergo decompression, microbubbles (15 ± 5 mm) pass the pulmonary filter into the cerebral arterial circulation and impair the blood–brain barrier, leading to extravasation of protein and focal cerebral edema (James and Hills 1988). This can account for the myelin damage and cerebral vascular pathology in divers.

Effect of Pressure on the Peripheral Nerve Conduction Velocity

Moderate pressure has been shown to increase nerve conduction velocity and amplitude in experimental animals, whereas high pressures depress these parameters. Various studies of nerve conduction velocities of divers at depth have concluded:

- There is no significant correlation between slow sensory conduction and hyperbaric pressure.
- Distal motor latencies increase with increases in hyperbaric pressure as well as with decreases in ambient temperature.
- The effect of pressure is independent of the temperature.
- No significant changes were detected in the main nerve trunk proximal to the wrist, or in the F-wave response.
- The effect on peripheral nerves may contribute to the reduced work capacity of divers at depth.
- Effect of hyperbaric pressure on autonomic nerve functions.

Autonomic nerve functions under severe hyperbaric pressure has been evaluated by measuring heart rate variability (HRV) and catecholamine excretion rate to assess sympathetic and parasympathetic tone in normal volunteers in submarine experimental facilities simulating conditions 330 m below sea level. There was significant negative correlation between HRV and urinary catecholamine levels. Evaluation of autonomic nerve functions under hyperbaric conditions by measuring HRV was shown to be a useful method. Thus, the present results indicate that the autonomic nerve functions of people who work under deep-sea conditions can be evaluated adequately by measuring HRV.

Hearing and Vestibular Impairment in Hyperbaric Environments

Hearing loss in professional divers is well known. A general etiological classification of hearing loss that is associated with hyperbaric environments is shown in Table 3.1. The hearing threshold in water appears to be 20–60 dB higher than in air. In the hyperbaric chamber, application of pressure on the middle ear or the external ear causes temporary impairment of hearing—especially in the low frequency range. At 4–11 ATA in hyperbaric air, the threshold of hearing is raised to 30–40 dB—proportional to the

Table 3.1 Hearing loss related to hyperbaric environments: an etiological classification

Conductive
Hearing acuity under hyperbaric conditions
Under water
Hyperbaric chamber
Obstruction to the external ear tympanic membrane perforation
Middle ear barotrauma of descent shock wave
Forceful autoinflation
Middle ear cleft
Middle ear barotrauma of descent otitis media
Sensorineural
Inner ear barotrauma
Otologic problems occurring at depths
Otologic decompression sickness
Noise-induced deafness

pressure. In a heliox environment at 31 ATA, the hearing loss does not exceed 30–40 dB. Conclusions of studies on this subject are:

- Humans with patent Eustachian tubes, exposed to hyperbaric heliox conditions, develop a conductive hearing loss related to depth.
- After exposure at a depth of 600 ft for several days, there is less variation in the hearing levels and a greater loss in the lower frequencies.
- Sensory-neural auditory functions, as measured by sensory acuity levels and frequency differences, are not altered by hyperbaric heliox exposures up to 19.2 ATA.
- The conductive hearing loss is assumed to be the result of an increased impedance of the middle ear transformer in the denser atmosphere plus an upward shift in resonance frequency of the ear in a helium atmosphere.

Damage to the Middle Ear and Inner Ear in Diving

The pressure changes that are encountered in diving can cause damage to the ear in at least three distinctly different ways:

1. Middle ear barotrauma of descent
2. Middle ear barotrauma as a manifestation of pulmonary barotrauma during ascent
3. Inner ear barotrauma

Middle ear barotrauma occurs during descent when there is a failure to equalize the middle ear and the ambient pressures by means of the Eustachian tube. When this occurs, there may be bleeding in the middle ear and even rupture of the ear drum.

Forceful autoinflation of the middle ear (Valsalva maneuver) during descent may cause rupture of the round window membrane and leakage of perilymph into the middle ear. Damage to the inner ear may occur by decompression sickness, that is, release of dissolved nitrogen bubbles during ascent from a deep dive. It can lead to hearing loss and dizziness. This damage is usually unilateral and can be reversed with prompt recompression procedure, including HBO therapy. Barotrauma of the ear has been shown to be preventable by myringotomy (puncture of the tympanic membrane) before the dive.

Temporal bones of divers who died of unrelated causes, but had a history of barotrauma of the ears have been examined the. The classical findings, shown in Figs. 3.1 and 3.2, are very similar to experimental findings in monkeys subjected to barotrauma. New bone formation in the inner ear

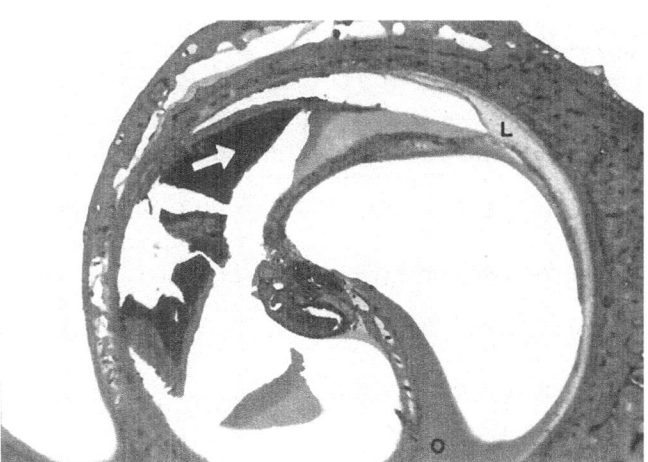

Fig. 3.1 Blood in the middle turn of the cochlea (*white arrow*) in a diver following decompression sickness. Postmortem examination. *L* spiral ligament, *O* osseous spiral lamina

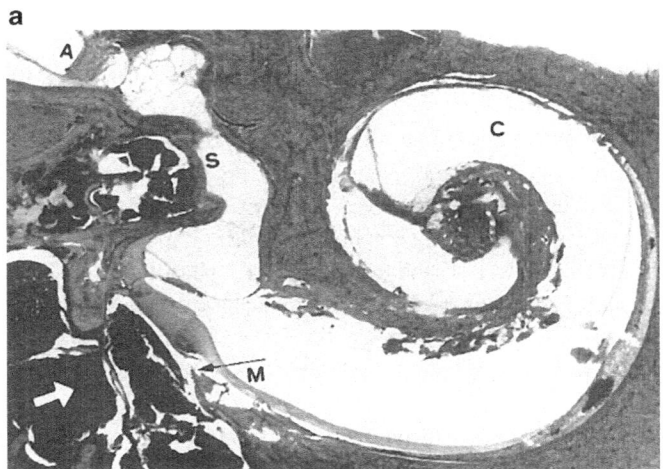
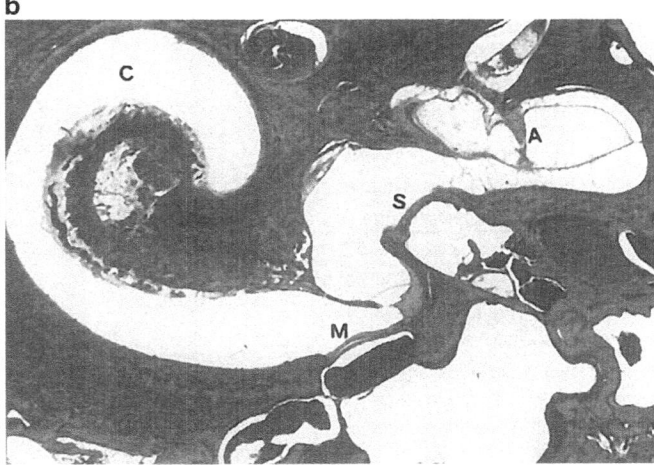

Fig. 3.2 (**a**, **b**) Middle and inner ears, left (*top*) and right (*bottom*) of a diver who died underwater from unknown causes. Left ear has the round window membrane (*M*) ripped (*black arrow*) and the middle ear is filled with blood (*white arrow*). *C* cochlea, *A* lateral ampullary crista, *S* footplate of stapes. Photos courtesy of Dr. K.E. Money, reproduced from Money et al. (1985)

following decompression sickness may have been responsible for the late onset of hearing deficits.

Professional diving may cause a more rapid deterioration of high frequency hearing loss than is seen in the general population. An audiometric survey of abalone divers has shown that >60 % of them suffered from high frequency deafness unacceptable by the Australian standards. The hearing loss was unilateral in one-half of the cases and bilateral in the rest.

In experimental studies, minipigs subjected to a compression/decompression profile that was considered to be safe for compressed air workers showed that there was loss of hearing as well as loss of hair cells in the cochlea of all the compressed animals.

Vertigo and Diving

Because of the close anatomical relationship between the hearing organ and the vestibular apparatus, vestibular disorders like dizziness and vertigo are frequently associated with barotrauma of the ear. Inner ear barotraumas and decompression sickness may cause acute vestibular symptoms in divers. The result may be irreversible damage to the vestibular end organs or their central connections. An etiological classification of vertigo in divers is shown in Table 3.2.

Table 3.2 Vertigo in diving: an etiological classification

Due to unequal vestibular stimulation
1. Caloric; unilateral external auditory canal obstruction
(a) Cerumen
(b) Otitis externa
(c) Miscellaneous causes tympanic membrane perforation
(a) Shock wave
(b) Middle ear barotrauma of descent
(c) Forceful autoinflation
2. Barotrauma external and/or middle ear
(a) External ear barotrauma of descent
(b) Middle ear barotrauma of descent
(c) Middle ear barotrauma of ascent
(d) Forceful inflation
3. Inner ear barotrauma
(a) Fistulas of the round window
(b) Fistulas of the oval window
4. Decompression sickness
(a) Peripheral decompression sickness
(b) Central decompression sickness
5. Air embolism
6. Miscellaneous causes
Due to unequal vestibular responses
1. Caloric
2. Barotrauma
3. Abnormal gas pressures
4. Sensory deprivation

In a survey of divers and nondiver controls, the prevalence of dizziness (28 %), spinning vertigo (14 %), and unsteady gait (25 %) was significantly higher in divers than controls (Goplen et al. 2007). These symptoms were strongly associated with a previous history of DCS, particularly Type I, which was reported by 61 % of the divers. Symptoms were less strongly associated with the number of dives. In divers with dizziness, the prevalence of abnormal postural sway, nystagmus, canal paresis, or pathological smooth pursuit was 32 %,9 %, 7 %, and 11 %, respectively. Among the reasons for the high prevalence of vestibular symptoms among the divers, the high exposure to DCS is probably an important factor.

Inert gas narcosis may lead to balance disturbances and nystagmus. Velocity of the slow component of the vestibular ocular reflex, as determined by electronystagmography (ENG) increases by 50 % after inhalation of 25 % nitrous oxide. Caloric tests conducted during saturation dives to 450 msw (4.6 mPa) while breathing trimix do not show any significant nystagmus upon ENG.

Taste Sensation Under High Pressure

Significant changes in taste sensation have been shown to occur on exposure to heliox at 18.6 ATA. These changes include:

* Increased sensitivity to sweetness
* Increased sensitivity to bitter taste
* Decline of sour sensitivity
* Decrease of salt sensitivity

Effect of High Pressure on Effect of Drugs

The efficiency of a number of drugs is affected by pressure—usually manifested as a decrease in activity—but the results may be unpredictable. High pressure has been reported to reduce the efficiency of drugs which act on cell membranes, such as anesthetics, tranquilizers, and narcotics. This effect is ascribed to the pressure changes affecting the cell membrane itself. The major enzyme involved in drug metabolism is cytochrome P-450 which is bound to the cell membrane. The effect of pressure on the membrane may be differential. The so-called pressure of anesthesia may be due to an antagonism, not only on a pharmacological level, but also on a physiological level via increased sensory feedback under high pressure.

Dimenhydrinate, an antihistamine, often is used by divers to control seasickness. Its effects in the hyperbaric environment have been poorly studied although decrements in learning were reported. Dimenhydrinate adversely affects mental flexibility and depth can impair memory. It is likely that these effects in combination increase the risk to scuba divers. Divers who suffer from severe seasickness may have to take dimenhydrinate to avoid the miseries of this condition, but they would be wise to incorporate extra margins of safety into planning dives.

Information on the manner in which high pressure affects the drug disposition in the body is scarce.

Conclusion

Important effects of pressure on the human body were reviewed in this chapter. This may be of interest to physicians who treat complications of diving with HBO. For those interested in diving medicine, several excellent texts are available including that by (Edmonds et al. 2015). The most important effect of high pressure is on the nervous system. This should be distinguished from oxygen toxicity. The major complication of diving and decompression sickness are discussed in Chap. 12; cerebral air embolization is described in Chap. 13.

References

Bliznyuk A, Aviner B, Golan H, Hollmann M, Grossman Y. The N-methyl-D-aspartate receptor's neglected subunit—GluN1 matters under normal and hyperbaric conditions. Eur J Neurosci. 2015;42:2577–84.

Cimsit M, Ilgezdi S, Cimsit C, Uzun G. Dysbaric osteonecrosis in experienced dive masters and instructors. Aviat Space Environ Med. 2007;78:1150–4.

Edmonds C, Bennett M, Lippmann J, Mitchell S. Diving and subaquatic medicine. 5th ed. Boca Raton: CRC Press; 2015.

Goplen FK, Grønning M, Irgens A, Sundal E, Nordahl SH. Vestibular symptoms and otoneurological findings in retired offshore divers. Aviat Space Environ Med. 2007;78:414–9.

Jain KK. High pressure neurological syndrome (HPNS). Acta Neurol Scand. 1994;90:45–50.

Jain KK. High pressure neurological syndrome. In: Greenamyre JT, editor. Medlink Neurology; 2016 (online).

James PB, Hills BA. Microbubbles damage the blood-brain barrier. Abstract 21. In: Proceedings of the XIV Annual meeting of the EUBS, Aberdeen, Scotland; 1988.

Lavoute C, Weiss M, Sainty JM, Risso JJ, Rostain JC. Post effect of repetitive exposures to pressure nitrogen-induced narcosis on the dopaminergic activity at atmospheric pressure. Undersea Hyperb Med. 2008;35:21–5.

Marabotti C, Scalzini A, Cialoni D, Passera M, L'Abbate A, Bedini R. Cardiac changes induced by immersion and breath-hold diving in humans. J Appl Physiol. 2009;106:293–7.

Marabotti C, Piaggi P, Menicucci D, Passera M, Benassi A, Bedini R, et al. Cardiac function and oxygen saturation during maximal breath-holding in air and during whole-body surface immersion. Diving Hyperb Med. 2013;43:131–7.

McCall RD. HPNS seizure risk: a role for the Golgi-associated retrograde protein complex. Undersea Hyperb Med. 2011;38 (1):3–9.

Money KE, Buckingham IP, Calder IM, Johnson WH, King JD, Landolt JP, et al. Damage to the middle ear and the inner ear in underwater divers. Undersea Biomed Res. 1985;12:77–84.

Physical Exercise under Hyperbaric Conditions

4

K.K. Jain

Abstract

This chapter discusses the role of physical exercise under normoxic and hyperoxic conditions, as well as the impact of greatly reduced supplies of oxygen. Experimental studies of effect of HBO on hypoxia associated with exercise will also be described. The results of these studies help set the stage for later detailed analyses of the strengths and limits of HBO therapy itself.

Keywords

Exercise in hyperbaric environments • Exercise under hyperoxia • Exercise and hypoxia

Introduction

Oxygen plays an important role in exercise physiology, and this subject was discussed extensively in an earlier book (Jain 1989). The following brief account of what happens during exercise under normoxic conditions serves as an important introduction to the effects of hyperbaric conditions on physical exercise.

The dynamic transition among different metabolic rates of VO_2 (VO_2 kinetics) that are initiated, e.g., at the onset of exercise, provides a unique window into understanding metabolic control. Because of the differences in O_2 supply relative to VO_2 among various types of fibers, the presence of much lower O_2 levels in the microcirculation supplying fast-twitch muscle fibers, and the demonstrated metabolic sensitivity of muscle to O_2, it is possible that fiber type recruitment profiles might help explain the slowing of VO_2 kinetics at higher work rates and in chronic diseases (Poole et al. 2008).

Oxygen demands of the body can of course increase dramatically during exercise. Our normal oxygen consumption of about 150 mL/min might rise to 1000 mL/min during moderate exercise, even though alveolar pO_2 is maintained at 104 mmHg. This situation is achieved by a fourfold increase of alveolar ventilation. During strenuous physical activity, such as a marathon race, the body's oxygen requirements may be 20 times normal, yet oxygenation of the blood does not suffer. There is, however, tissue hypoxia in some of the working muscles and strenuous exercise may be considered as a hypoxic episode. The response to physical exercise is outlined in Table 4.1.

Mild physical exercise improves the efficiency of the oxygen delivery as demonstrated in a study on patients suffering from metabolic syndrome (Passoni et al. 2015). Prescription of exercise (40 min/session, 3 times/week) was tailored at workload corresponding to $\sim$90 % individual anaerobic threshold. Exercise significantly improved peak values of oxygen consumption (VO_2) by $\sim$10 %. This study supports a positive effect of a mild exercise for the adaptive response of the oxygen chain to face metabolic needs compatible with daily life in patients affected by metabolic syndrome.

Physical activity, in the form of voluntary wheel running, induces gene expression changes in the brain. Animals that exercise show an increase in brain-derived neurotrophic factor (BDNF), a molecule that increases neuronal survival, enhances learning, and protects against cognitive decline. Microarray analysis of gene expression provides further support that exercise enhances and supports brain function.

K.K. Jain, MD, FRACS, FFPM (✉)
1 Blaesiring 7, Basel 4057, Switzerland
e-mail: jain@pharmabiotech.ch

© Springer International Publishing AG 2017
K.K. Jain, *Textbook of Hyperbaric Medicine*, DOI 10.1007/978-3-319-47140-2_4

Table 4.1 Effect of physical exercise on the human body

System	Acute effects (in untrained subjects)	Effects of chronic dynamic exercise
Cardiovascular	Tachycardia	Bradycardia
	Rise of cardiac output from 5 to 30 L/min	Increase of stroke volume of the heart
		Increase of heart size
		Increase of myocardial capillary to fiber ratio
Respiratory	Rise of alveolar ventilation linearly with rise of O_2 uptake	Increase of number of alveoli available for O_2 exchange
	Increased work of respiratory muscles, using up 10 % of total O_2 uptake	Increase of extraction fraction of $(a–v)$ O_2 difference
Blood	Hemoconcentration due to fluid loss	Increase of hemoglobin
	Reduction of O_2 saturation (5 %)	Increase of 2,3-diphosphoglycerate
	Rise of ammonia and lactate	Less accumulation of ammonia and lactate
Metabolism		Raised anaerobic thresholds
		Increased utilization of FFA
		Increased intracellular pools of ATP and phosphocreatine
Skeletal muscle		Increase of maximal blood flow rate
		Increase of mitochondrial volume and oxidative enzymes
		Increase of capillary density
Brain		Increase of cerebral blood flow
		Increase in brain-derived neurotrophic factor
		Enhances leaning and prevents cognitive decline

Exercise and Hypoxia

Some decline in pO_2 may occur during intensive exercise, particularly in individuals with high VO_2 max. Whether this can be termed "hypoxia" or not is controversial. Exercise is not considered to be hypoxia unless the pO_2 falls below the critical level of 40 mmHg. Exercise is hypoxic under the following circumstances:

- Exhausting exercise by normal individuals in normoxic environments
- Exercise at high altitudes
- Exposure to carbon monoxide in the atmosphere
- In patients with chronic obstructive pulmonary disease.

The effects of physical exercise under hypoxic conditions are shown in Table 4.2. The main changes in chronic hypoxia in relation to exercise are:

1. Decrease in arterial saturation (due to a fall of inspired oxygen pressure)
2. Decrease in maximal cardiac output (due to a fall of maximal heart rate)
3. Increase in hemoglobin concentration
4. Decrease in the maximal oxygen flow through muscle capillaries
5. Change in respiratory potential of the muscles due to loss of oxidative enzymes.

Table 4.2 Effects on the human body of exercise under hypoxic conditions

Cardiovascular system
– Increase of cardiac output and muscle blood flow compared with normoxic conditions
Respiratory system
– Increase of ventilation
– Increase in oxygen consumption
– No appreciable change in alveolar and arterial CO_2 transport
Metabolic

Hypoxia is a rationale for use of HBO in medical conditions where physical activity is limited due to a disease condition associated with hypoxia and normobaric oxygen is not sufficient. It may be used in complications caused by physical activity under hypoxic conditions at high altitude. Use of HBO to improve physical performance in competitive sports would be considered a form of doping and is forbidden.

Exercise in Hyperbaric Environments

The study of human work performance in hyperbaric environments is important for evaluating the effects of diving on the human body. The effects of physical exercise while diving depend upon the following key factors:

1. Pressure to which the diver is subjected
2. Composition of the breathing mixture

3. Type of activity, e.g., swimming, walking underwater, or operating a machine
4. Body posture, e.g., vertical or prone
5. Ambient temperature.

The increase of VO_2 under hyperbaric conditions corresponds to the rise in oxygen needs. The oxygen consumption during a standard exercise at 5 ATA of air is higher than at 1 ATA. The main reason for this is the increase of respiratory resistance due to a rise of gas density. Whereas the total oxygen consumption at 1 ATA is 81.5% of the total oxygen needs, this value decreases to 73.9% at 5 ATA. Factors that limit work capacity at depth include:

1. Increased respiratory resistance to breathing dense gases
2. Increased energy cost of ventilation
3. Carbon dioxide retention
4. Dyspnea
5. Adverse cardiovascular changes.

Exercise in hyperbaric environments depresses the heart rate. Part of this depression is due to the effects on the heart of a rise in the partial pressure of oxygen, both directly and via the parasympathetic efferents. In addition, other factors such as gas density, high inert gas pressure, or hydrostatic pressure may interfere with sympathetic stimulation of the heart.

A reduction of ventilation and bradycardia during exercise under 2 ATA in air has been attributed to the increase in gas density.

Hyperbaric conditions are known to increase the subjective feeling of fatigue in divers. There is a decrease of vigilance and a subjective feeling of change in the body functions of divers who undergo saturation dives to simulated pressures of 40 ATA. This feeling is more pronounced during compression and saturation and decreased during compression.

Exercise Under Hyperoxia

Hyperoxia here refers to the use of raised oxygen fractions in the inspired air, but at a pressure not higher than 1 ATA. The results may vary according to the method used to achieve hyperoxia, i.e., whether the hyperoxia is achieved by breathing a gas with high fractional concentration of oxygen at sea level, or by the study being carried out in a pressure chamber. The response to exercise at a given arterial pO_2 is not the same under these two conditions. Performance increases with increasing pO_2 under both conditions, but in hyperbaric studies performance levels were somewhere between 200 and 400 mmHg. In hyperoxia at 1 ATA, performance increases continuously as pO_2 increases. Increased gas density in the hyperbaric environment increases the work of breathing and

Table 4.3 Effect on the human body of physical exercise under hyperoxic conditions

Cardiovascular response
– Variable decrease of heart rate
– Decrease of blood flow to the exercising limb to offset the raised O_2 tension
Pulmonary function
– Reduction of pulmonary ventilation
– Decrease of oxygen consumption compared with exercise under normoxia
Biochemical
– H+ ion concentration is higher than during exercise under normoxia
– Reduction of excess lactate
Energy metabolism
– Decreased rate of glucose utilization and lactate production
– Shift of respiratory quotient (RQ) toward fat metabolism, thus lowering RQ

compromises performance at high pressures. The effects of hyperoxia on exercise and the possible mechanisms involved are listed in Table 4.3. Cardiovascular function during exercise under hypoxia is described in Chap. 24.

Exercise studies on healthy volunteers have shown that leg VO_2 max is limited by oxygen supply during normoxia, but it does not increase during hyperoxia in proportion to either the femoral venous pO_2 or mean leg capillary pO_2.

Physical Exercise Under Hyperbaric Conditions

General Effects

The effects of physical exercise under hyperbaric oxygenation (HBO) are often quite difficult to evaluate, due to the variable interaction of three factors: oxygen, pressure, and exercise. The effects of these factors are better known when applied individually. HBO at 1.5 ATA accentuates some of the effects of normobaric hyperoxia, but higher pressures may cancel some of the advantages of HBO such as reduction of the metabolic complications of exhausting physical exercise. Most of the studies on this topic have concentrated on the metabolic aspects, particularly the lactate accumulation in the blood, which can be easily measured.

A decrease of ventilation and some bradycardia is usually observed while exercising under HBO conditions. VO_2 max increases by 3% during exercise while breathing 100% O_2 at 1 ATA, but does not increase further when the pressure is raised to 3 ATA. There are no changes in oxygen consumption or oxygen extraction during exercise under HBO at 2 ATA, as compared with exercise while breathing normobaric air.

The $(a-v)O_2$ difference is the same in healthy young volunteers whether they exercise breathing normal air or under HBO at 3 ATA (pAO$_2$ 1877 mmHg). It appears probable, therefore, that the maximum oxygen uptake in active muscles does not increase when the arterial oxygen content is increased. Thus, the maximum oxygen uptake in an active muscle seems not to be limited by the blood flow to the muscle or the oxygen diffusion from the blood to the interior of the muscle cell, but rather by the oxygen utilization system inside the cell.

Effect on Lactate Production and Clearance

Studies of the effect of HBO (3 ATA) on excess lactate production during exercise in dogs show that the values of excess lactate are much lower than those observed during previous exercise by the same animals at 1 ATA while breathing air. If exercise is conducted under HBO first, not only is the excess lactate low, but it remains so during subsequent exercise at 1 ATA breathing air 45 min later. Three mechanisms for this effect are:

- Oxygen provided to the exercising muscles during hyperoxia is sufficient to lower the excess lactate formation. It counteracts the hypoxia that usually results while exercising at atmospheric pressure and is responsible for the production of lactic acid.
- There is increased removal of excess lactate as a result of stimulation of the oxidative enzymatic process.
- HBO produces inhibition of glycolytic sulfhydryl enzymes. This results in an improvement of glycolysis, and therefore, in lowered lactate formation. Such an inhibitory effect could well persist for up to 45 min and explain the continual decrease of excess lactate after HBO exposure when exercise under atmospheric air followed.

The myocardium and liver of dogs exercised under 3 ATA HBO can eliminate the increased amount of lactate at the expense of glucose consumption. Studies of the blood chemistry parameters in healthy adult volunteers who exercised while breathing air, normobaric oxygen, and oxygen at 1.5 ATA revealed that in the rest period following exercise, uric acid, lactate, and pyruvate decreased significantly compared with the levels after exercise without HBO. The drop in the level of ammonia was less. However, the ammonia levels 1 and 15 min after exercise under HBO were much lower than the corresponding values during exercise while breathing normobaric oxygen (see Fig. 4.1).

Lactate levels immediately after exercise (1–20 min) were lower during exercise while breathing oxygen than during exercise in room air. Lactate levels were lower during exercise under HBO than they had been 1, 5, 10, and 15 min previously after exercise, breathing normobaric oxygen. The rise of excess lactate was less after exercise under HBO than after exercise under oxygen breathing. The excess lactate (XL) was calculated according to the formula:

$$XL = (Ln - Lo) - (Pn - Po)\frac{Lo}{Po}$$

where Lo is the resting and Ln the exercise blood lactate, and Po and Pn are the resting and exercise blood pyruvate values, respectively.

There was a fall of glucose during exercise under HBO, suggesting inhibition of glycolysis, which is a contributory factor to the rise in the level of ammonia. Inhibition of glycolysis should lead to diminution of uremia. Whether there is stimulation or depression of the Krebs cycle at 1.5 ATA HBO remains to be determined. But in any case, the tendency of ammonia levels to fall is striking. These findings tend to support the hypothesis that more glycogenic amino acids than α-ketoglutaric acid go into the citric acid cycle.

Fig. 4.1 Effect of physical exercise on lactate levels under normobaric oxygenation (- - - O$_2$) and hyperbaric oxygenation (—HBO). Arterial blood lactate levels were determined before treadmill exertion as well as 1 and 15 min following the completion of exercise

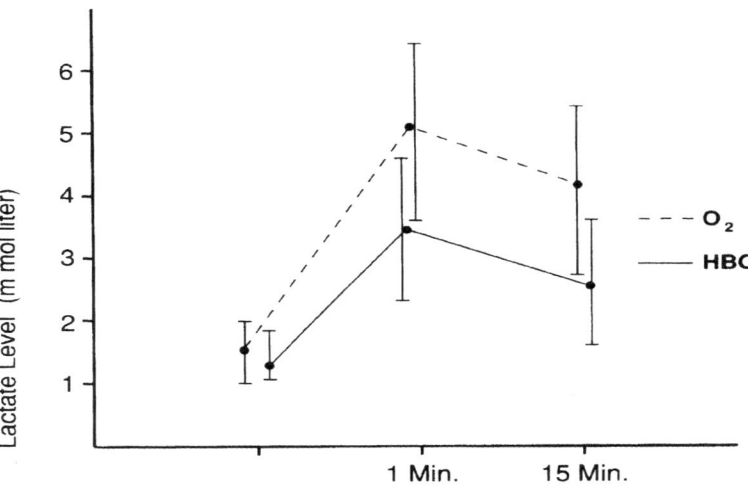

Physical exercise in sports is associated with muscle injury that can cause ischemia. Usually, it is accompanied by anaerobic glycolysis, the formation of lactate, and depletion of high-energy phosphates within the extracellular fluid of the affected skeletal muscle tissue. In experimental animals, HBO treatment has been shown to attenuate significantly the increase of lactate and glycerol levels caused by ischemia, without affecting glucose concentration and modulating antioxidant enzyme activity in the postischemic skeletal muscle (Bosco et al. 2007). The clinical use of HBO in sports injuries is discussed in Chap. 36.

Effect of Exercise on Ammonia Metabolism

Lactate accumulation is well-known as a factor in causing fatigue and limiting the capacity for physical exertion. However, the role of ammonia in causing fatigue is not quite so clear.

At rest, skeletal muscle is consistently an ammonia consumer with a clearance of ~0.3 mmol/kg wet wt/min by resting muscle. Assuming that the body is 40% muscle, there is 8 mmol/min uptake of ammonia by the resting muscle. Ammonia levels are known to rise steeply following muscular exertion, but they decline spontaneously in a short time in healthy adults. Hyperammonemia of exercise is due mainly to a release of ammonia from muscles during the recovery phase. As muscle pH returns to the resting level, more ammonia diffuses from the muscle into the blood. If the ammonia levels do not subside promptly, untoward effects may be experienced by a person doing exhaustive physical exercise. This is likely to happen in untrained persons with neurological disorders. Healthy young athletes usually do not suffer from "ammonia hangover."

Ammonia levels are lower in those exercising under HBO compared with those exercising under normobaric conditions. The mechanism by which HBO lowers ammonia levels in the blood is not clear. Ammonia is formed in the body by deamination of amino acids where the amino group is transferred to α-ketoglutaric acid, which becomes glutamic acid and may release ammonia again. Most of the ammonia is removed from the blood by conversion to urea in the liver. HBO has been shown to lower blood ammonia in hepatic encephalopathy (see Chap. 26). Blood urea can be lowered in volunteers exercising under HBO, an effect attributed to inhibition of glycolysis.

Effect of HBO on Antioxidant Enzymes in Skeletal Muscle

In skeletal muscle, the activity of the enzymatic antioxidants superoxide dismutase (SOD), glutathione peroxidase (GPx), and catalase (CAT) is regulated in response to generation of reactive oxygen species (ROS). Increased activity of these enzymes is observed after repeated bouts of aerobic exercise, a potent stimulus for intracellular ROS production. Although ROS formation in response to vigorous physical exertion can result in oxidative stress, ROS also play an important role as signaling molecules (Niess and Simon 2007). ROS modulate contractile function in unfatigued and fatigued skeletal muscle. Furthermore, involvement of ROS in the modulation of gene expression via redox-sensitive transcription pathways represents an important regulatory mechanism, which may be involved in the process of adaptation through training.

HBO inhalation also stimulates intracellular ROS production, but the effects of HBO on skeletal muscle SOD, GPx, and CAT activity have not been studied. In adult male rats, acute HBO inhalation at 3 ATA reduced catalase activity by ~51% in slow-twitch soleus muscles (Gregorevic et al. 2001). Additionally, repeated HBO inhalation (twice daily for 28 days at a pressure of 2 ATA) increased Mn-superoxide dismutase activity by ~ 241% in fast-twitch extensor digitorum longus muscles. Thus, both acute and repeated HBO inhalation can alter enzymatic antioxidant activity in skeletal muscles.

At rest, skeletal muscle is consistently an ammonia consumer with a clearance of ~0.3 mmol/kg wet wt/min by resting muscle. Assuming that the body is 40% muscle, there is 8 mmol/min uptake of ammonia by the resting muscle. Ammonia levels are known to rise steeply following muscular exertion, but they decline spontaneously in a short time in healthy adults. Hyperammonemia of exercise is due mainly to a release of ammonia from muscles during the recovery phase. As muscle pH returns to the resting level, more ammonia diffuses from the muscle into the blood. If the ammonia levels do not subside promptly, untoward effects may be experienced by a person doing exhaustive physical exercise. This is likely to happen in untrained persons with neurological disorders. Healthy young athletes usually do not suffer from "ammonia hangover."

Ammonia levels are lower in those exercising under HBO compared with those exercising under normobaric conditions. The mechanism by which HBO lowers ammonia levels in the blood is not clear. Ammonia is formed in the body by deamination of amino acids where the amino group is transferred to α-ketoglutaric acid, which becomes glutamic acid and may release ammonia again. Both acute and repeated HBO inhalation can alter enzymatic antioxidant activity in skeletal muscles.

Effect of HBO on Blood Flow to the Muscles During Exercise

Large increases in systemic oxygen content resulting from exercise under HBO produce substantial reductions in limb blood flow due to increased vascular resistance as oxygen is a vasoconstrictor. In a study on young healthy male volunteers, forearm exercise (20 % of maximum) was performed in a hyperbaric chamber at 1 ATA while breathing 21 % O_2 and at 2.82 ATA while breathing 100 % O_2 with estimated change in arterial O_2 content ~6 mL O_2/100 mL (Casey et al. 2013). Forearm blood flow (FBF ml/min) was measured using Doppler ultrasound. During exercise, vasoconstrictor responsiveness was slightly greater during hyperoxia than normoxia. However, during α-adrenergic blockade, hyperoxic exercise FBF and vascular resistance remained lower than during normoxia. Although the vasoconstrictor responsiveness during hyperoxic exercise was slightly greater, it likely does not explain the majority of the large reductions in FBF and vascular resistance during exercise under HBO.

Physical Exercise in Relation to Toxic Effects of HBO

The toxic effects of oxygen are not usually seen during HBO below pressures of 3 ATA. Concern has been expressed that physical exercise may predispose patients to oxygen toxicity.

Breathing oxygen at 2 ATA during exercise lowered ventilation and restores arterial pH and pCO_2 toward resting levels. There is either a slight elevation of cerebral blood flow or a diminished rate of cerebral oxygen consumption during exercise while breathing oxygen at 2 ATA, without gross elevation of cerebral venous pO_2. Physical exercise overrules the decrease in cerebral blood flow velocity (CBFV) during hyperoxia and leads to even higher CBFV-increases with increasing pO_2 (Koch et al. 2013). A tendency towards CO_2 retention with elevated end-tidal CO_2 may have a vasodilator effect and thus heighten the risk of oxygen neurotoxicity due to increased blood flow.

Physical exercise is accompanied by a rise in body temperature that may increase the possibility of oxygen toxicity. In the hyperbaric chamber, the temperature is usually controlled and this factor is eliminated. Peripheral vasoconstriction usually limits blood flow and oxygen delivery under hyperoxia, but exercise may have a vasodilating effect, which might allow exposure of the tissues to high oxygen concentrations.

Conclusion

Although HBO reduces the biochemical disturbances resulting from physical exertion, it has not been shown that HBO extends human physical performance. The duration of time to physical exhaustion does not decrease in the hyperbaric chamber. Unlike other methods that elevate oxygen content of the blood, acute HBO exposure appears to have no significant effect on subsequent high-intensity running or lifting performance (Rozenek et al. 2007). However, HBO, by facilitating biochemical recovery after exhaustive exercise, may shorten the recovery time from exhaustion. Further studies need to be done on this topic to determine the role of HBO in the training of athletes. The current knowledge may also help in using HBO for the rehabilitation of patients with neurological disability, such as hemiplegia and paraplegia, as HBO may enable these patients to undertake more strenuous exercise than possible for them under normobaric conditions.

References

Bosco G, Yang ZJ, Nandi J, Wang J, Chen C, Camporesi EM. Effects of hyperbaric oxygen on glucose, lactate, glycerol and anti-oxidant enzymes in the skeletal muscle of rats during ischaemia and reperfusion. Clin Exp Pharmacol Physiol. 2007;34:70–6.
Casey DP, Joyner MJ, Claus PL, Curry TB. Vasoconstrictor responsiveness during hyperbaric hyperoxia in contracting human muscle. J Appl Physiol. 2013;114:217–24.
Gregorevic P, Lynch GS, Williams DA. Hyperbaric oxygen modulates antioxidant enzyme activity in rat skeletal muscles. Eur J Appl Physiol. 2001;86:24–7.
Jain KK. Oxygen in physiology and medicine. Springfield: Charles C. Thomas; 1989.
Koch AE, Koch I, Kowalski J, Schipke JD, Winkler BE, Deuschl G, et al. Physical exercise might influence the risk of oxygen-induced acute neurotoxicity. Undersea Hyperb Med. 2013;40:155–63.
Niess AM, Simon P. Response and adaptation of skeletal muscle to exercise— the role of reactive oxygen species. Front Biosci. 2007;12:4826–38.
Passoni E, Lania A, Adamo S, Grasso GS, Noè D, Miserocchi G, et al. Mild training program in metabolic syndrome improves the efficiency of the oxygen pathway. Respir Physiol Neurobiol. 2015;208:8–14.
Poole DC, Barstow TJ, McDonough P, Jones AM. Control of oxygen uptake during exercise. Med Sci Sports Exerc. 2008;40:462–74.
Rozenek R, Fobel BF, Banks JC, Russo AC, Lacourse MG, Strauss MB. Does hyperbaric oxygen exposure affect high-intensity, short-duration exercise performance? J Strength Cond Res. 2007;21:1037–41.

K.K. Jain

Abstract

Tissue hypoxia plays an important role in the pathogenesis of many disorders, particularly those of the brain. Correction of hypoxia by hyperbaric oxygenation is, therefore, an important adjunct in the treatment of those disorders. This chapter describes pathophysiology of hypoxia with general impact on the functions of various systems of the body and particularly the brain. Role of HBO in the treatment of hypoxic states is discussed as well as possible adverse effects of HBO.

Keywords

Hypoxia • Tissue hypoxia • Cerebral hypoxia

Introduction

The term "hypoxia" generally means a reduced supply of oxygen in the living organism. Hypoxia may be either generalized, affecting the whole body, or local, affecting a region of the body. It is difficult to define hypoxia precisely, but it may be described as a state in which aerobic metabolism is reduced by a fall of pO_2 within the mitochondria. In this situation, the partial pressure of oxygen, which in dry air is 160 mmHg, drops to about 1 mmHg, by the time it reaches the mitochondria of the cell. Below this value aerobic metabolism is not possible. Hypoxia is not always a pathological condition as variations in arterial oxygen concentrations can be physiological, e.g., during strenuous physical exercise. In contrast, "anoxia" implies a total lack of oxygen, although the word is sometimes used as a synonym for hypoxia.

The subject of hypoxia was dealt with in detail in a book on oxygen (Jain 1989). Recent developments and a few important aspects should be discussed here because relative tissue hypoxia is frequently the common denominator of many diseases that are amenable to HBO therapy.

Pathophysiology of Hypoxia

Within the cell, 80 % of the total oxygen consumption is by mitochondria, and 20 % by a variety of other subcellular organs. The biochemical reactions in these locations serve a variety of biosynthetic, biodegradative, and detoxificatory oxidations. Some of the enzymes involved in the synthesis of neurotransmitters have low affinities for oxygen and are impaired by moderate depletions of oxygen. Some of the manifestations of oxygen depletion are related to "transmitter failure" (decreased availability of transmitter), rather than bioenergetic failure. The disturbances that lead to decreased oxygen supply could operate at any of the three phases mentioned in Chap. 2, i.e.:

- The respiratory phase
- The phase of oxygen transport
- The phase of oxygen use by the tissues

Hypoxia can potentiate injury due to oxidative stress. The proposed sequences are shown in Fig. 5.1.

K.K. Jain, MD, FRACS, FFPM (✉)
1 Blaesiring 7, Basel 4057, Switzerland
e-mail: jain@pharmabiotech.ch

© Springer International Publishing AG 2017
K.K. Jain, *Textbook of Hyperbaric Medicine*, DOI 10.1007/978-3-319-47140-2_5

Fig. 5.1 Proposed sequence in which hypoxia potentiates injury due to oxidative stress. *ROS* reactive oxygen species, *HIF* hypoxia-inducible factor, *ATP* adenosine triphosphate

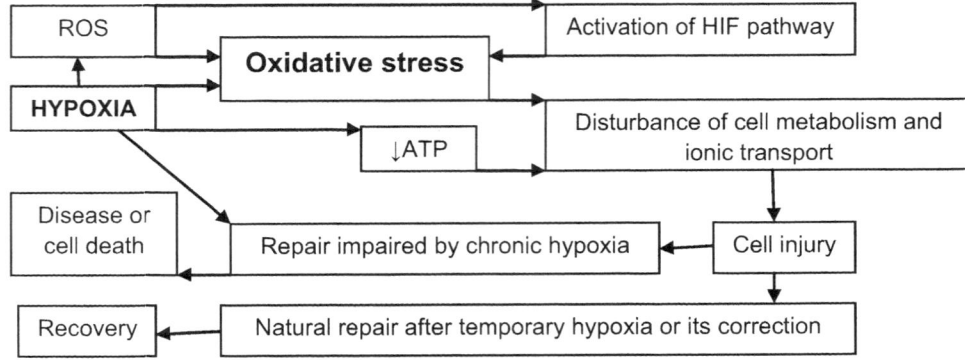

Hypoxia-Inducible Factor

Hypoxia-inducible factor (HIF) senses and coordinates cellular responses to hypoxia. HIFs mediate the ability of the cell to cope with decreased oxygen tension. These transcription factors regulate cellular adaptation to hypoxia and protect cells by responding acutely and inducing production of endogenous metabolites and proteins to promptly regulate metabolic pathways. HIF pathway plays an important role in physiological adaptation, cell survival, pH regulation, and adaptation during exercise (Kumar and Choi 2015). HIF-1α, the most well-established member of the HIF family, is a master regulator for the expression of genes involved in the response to hypoxia in most mammalian cells.

HIF-1α plays a role in the pathogenesis of several diseases and can be modulated by HBO. Interaction of HBO with HIF is variable according to whether the disease is characterized by upregulation or downregulation of HIF-1α. For example, the ability to downregulate the expression of HIF-1α may partially explain the therapeutic effect of HBO on taurocholate-induced acute pancreatitis in Wistar rats (Bai et al. 2009). Another study has shown that induction of fibroblast proliferation in HBO disappears when HIF-1α is knocked down (Sunkari et al. 2015). Furthermore, the local transfer of stable HIF-1α-expressing adenovirus into experimental wounds in diabetic animals has an additive effect on HBO-mediated improvements in wound healing. In conclusion, HBO stabilizes and activates HIF-1, which contributes to increased cellular proliferation. In diabetic animals, the local transfer of active HIF further improves the effects of HBO on wound healing.

Hypoxia and Heat Shock Proteins

Heat shock proteins (Hsps) is the term used for a family of proteins that are produced by cells in response to exposure to stressful conditions. Originally described as a response to heat shock or rise in temperature, they are now known to

be induced by other stressful situations such as hypoxia. Hsps are named according to their molecular weight, e.g., Hsp60, Hsp70, and Hsp90. A study on healthy volunteers subjected to transient normobaric hypoxia has shown that hypoxic conditions can trigger the release of Hsp70 (Lichtenauer et al. 2014).

A study has shown that HBO treatment prevents nitric oxide (NO)-induced apoptosis in articular cartilage injury via enhancement of the expression of Hsp70 (Ueng et al. 2013). The histological scores showed that HBO markedly enhanced cartilage repair. Immunostaining showed that HBO enhanced HSP70 expression and suppressed iNOS and caspase 3 expressions in chondrocytes.

Effect of Hypoxia on Cellular Metabolism

Hypoxia depresses mitochondrial oxidative phosphorylation. Creatine phosphorylase is released, as evidenced by sarcolemmal damage during hypoxia. This process is considered to be calcium mediated, because calcium channel blockers protect the cell from hypoxic damage.

A rapid decline in ATP levels under hypoxic conditions may cause an increase in calcium flux into the cytosol because of inhibition of the calcium pump in the plasma membrane, mitochondria, and endoplasmic reticulum. Alternatively, ATP may be metabolized to hypoxanthine, a substrate for superoxide anion formation. Barcroft's classification of hypoxia is as follows (Barcroft 1920):

- Hypoxic: includes all types of hypoxia in which not enough oxygen reaches the alveoli.
- Anemic: caused by inadequate hemoglobin or abnormal hemoglobin, so that not enough oxygen can be transported to the tissues.
- Stagnant or circulatory: blood flow is inadequate to carry the oxygen to the tissues.
- Histotoxic: the tissues cannot use the oxygen even though it reaches the tissues in adequate quantities.

Table 5.1 Causes of hypoxia

I. Inadequate oxygenation in the lungs
   1. Deficient oxygen in the atmosphere: high altitudes (mountain sickness), closed spaces
   2. Hypoventilation
      (a) Respiratory muscle paralysis or weakness due to neuromuscular or neurological diseases
      (b) Extreme obesity
      (c) Central depression of respiration due to the effect of sedatives, narcotics, or anesthetics
   3. Pulmonary disorders
      (a) Chronic obstructive pulmonary disease, such as chronic bronchitis and emphysema, hypoxic cor pulmonale
      (b) Restrictive lung disease: adult respiratory distress syndrome, chest injuries, deformities of the chest and the thoracic spine
      (c) Pulmonary infections: pneumonia, diphtheria, whooping cough
   4. Sleep-disordered breathing: sleep apnea, snoring, nocturnal hypoxia
II. Inadequate transport and delivery of oxygen
   1. Carriage of oxygen combined with hemoglobin
      (a) Anemia, reduced RBC
      (b) Reduced effective hemoglobin concentration: COHb, MetHb, etc.
   2. Increased affinity of hemoglobin for oxygen
      (a) Reduced DPG in RBC
      (b) Reduced temperature
      (c) Increased pH of blood
   3. Circulatory disorders
      (a) Global decrease of cardiac output
      (b) Systemic arteriovenous shunts, right to left cardiac shunts
      (c) Maldistribution of cardiac output, regional circulatory disturbances
   4. Disturbances of hemorheology and microcirculation
      (a) Increased viscosity
      (b) RBC disease: decreased surface, stiff cell membrane, etc.
III. Increased demand of tissues beyond normal supply (relative hypoxia)
   1. Inflammation
   2. Hyperthermia
   3. Strenuous physical exercise
IV. Capability of the tissue to use oxygen is inadequate
   1. Cellular enzyme poisoning: cytochrome P-450 and a3 cytochrome oxidase
   2. Reduced cellular enzymes because of vitamin deficiency

The causes of hypoxia are shown in Table 5.1.

Impact of Hypoxia on Various Body Systems

The effects of hypoxia vary in accordance with its cause, whether the situation is acute or chronic, and also with the overall state of health of the individual in question.

Cellular hypoxia may develop in multiple organ failure syndrome because of the increased oxygen demand at the tissue level and/or because the ability to extract oxygen at the cellular level is decreased. Restoration of oxygen transport and metabolic support are important components of treatment.

Respiratory Function

Hypoxia initially leads to an increase in the respiratory rate, but later the rate is decreased. It remains controversial whether there is depression of the respiratory center, decreased central chemoreceptor pCO_2, or both. Respiratory depression is likely due to a fall in tissue pCO_2 resulting from an increase in blood flow caused by hypoxia.

In hypoxia caused by hypoventilation, CO_2 transfer between alveoli and the atmosphere is affected as much as oxygen transfer, and hypercapnia results, i.e., excess CO_2 accumulates in the body fluids. When alveolar pCO_2 rises above 60–75 mmHg, dyspnea becomes severe, and at 80–100 mmHg stupor results. Death can result if pCO_2 rises to 100–150 mmHg.

Cardiovascular System

Circulatory responses to hypoxia have been studied mainly in the laboratory animals and a few conclusions that can be drawn are as follows:

- The local vascular effect of hypoxic vasodilation is probably common to all but the pulmonary vessels. It is strongest in active tissues (heart, brain, working skeletal muscle) that are dependent on oxygen for their metabolism.
- A chemoreceptor reflex produces an increase in cardiac contractility and selective vasoconstriction that support arterial pressure and some redistribution of cardiac output.
- The overall response to hypoxia involves an increase in cardiac output and selective vasodilation and vasoconstriction in an attempt to maintain oxygen delivery and perfusion pressure to all organs.

General Metabolic Effects

The following disturbances have been observed as a result of experimental hypoxia produced in animals:

- Appearance of excess lactate in the blood
- Appearance of 2,3-DPG in the blood of animals exposed to hypoxia of high altitudes

- Higher plasma levels of corticosterone, leading to neo-glucogenesis
- Decrease of long-chain unsaturated fatty acids in the blood sera of rats adapted to hypoxia

Effects of Hypoxia on the Brain

Although any part of the body can be affected by hypoxia, the effects are most marked on the cells of the central nervous system, for the following key reasons:

- The brain has unusually high resting energy requirements, which can only be met by oxidative breakdown of the exogenous substrate. Anaerobic production of energy by glycolysis is not adequate to maintain normal brain function.
- The brain cannot store oxygen. Its energy reserves are low and usually it cannot tolerate anoxia (due to lack of circulation) for more than 3 min.
- The brain, unlike muscle tissue, is incapable of increasing the number of capillaries per unit of volume.
- Neurons have a poor capacity to recover or regenerate after dysoxia.

Cerebral Metabolism

Cerebral metabolism, particularly that of oxygen, is closely tied in with cerebral blood flow (CBF). The brain, although it makes up only 2 % of the body weight, consumes 20 % of the oxygen taken in by the body and receives 15 % of the cardiac output. This is remarkably high oxygen consumption, considering that the brain, unlike the heart muscle, does not perform any physical work. Cerebral metabolism is depicted by another term, glucose oxidation quotient (GOQ). It denotes the ratio

$$\text{AVD of Glucose} - \text{AVD of Lactate} (\text{in mg}/\text{dL}):$$
$$\text{AVD Oxygen} (\text{in vol\%})$$

where AVD is the arteriovenous difference. Normally this value is 1.34, because 1.0 mL of oxygen oxidizes 1.34 mg of glucose.

Cell energy metabolism is simply a balance between use of adenosine triphosphate (ATP) during the performance of work and its resynthesis in anabolic sequence, which provides the energy required to rephosphorylate adenosine diphosphate (ADP). The resulting energy metabolism is depicted by the following equations:

$$\text{Energy utilization}: \text{ATP} + \text{H}_2\text{O} > \text{ADP} + \text{Phosphate} + \text{energy}$$

$$\text{Energy production}: \text{ADP} + \text{Phosphate} + \text{energy} \rightarrow \text{ATP} + \text{H}_2\text{O}$$

The brain produces about as much CO_2 as it consumes in oxygen; i.e., the respiratory quotient is close to 1.0. On a molar basis, the brain uses a remarkable six times as much oxygen as glucose. Glucose is normally the sole substrate and is completely utilized.

The rate of electron transport, and thereby of oxygen use, is determined by the rate of consumption of ATP and the rate of accumulation of ADP and Pi. Most studies in humans have shown that oxygen consumed accounts for only 90–95 % of the glucose extracted, leading to the view that 5–10 % of the glucose extracted by the brain is metabolized to lactic acid. The cause of this is not known, but it may be an "emergency metabolic exercise" by the brain.

Pathways of cerebral metabolism (glycolysis, the citrus cycle, and the GABA pathway) are shown in Fig. 5.2. Glycolysis includes a series of enzymatic reactions by which the cytoplasmic glucose is built into two molecules of lactate. Thus no oxygen is necessary, but nicotinamide adenine dinucleotide (NAD+) is required. In all, glycolysis produces two molecules of NADH and ATP from each molecule of glucose. Under aerobic conditions, pyruvate is decarboxylated oxidatively:

$$\text{pyruvate} + \text{CoA} + \text{NAD+} \rightarrow \text{acetyl CoA} + \text{NADH} + \text{CO}_2$$

Acetyl CoA is transported in the mitochondria and goes into the citrus cycle; NADH is oxidized through mitochondrial electron transfer. Pyruvate and several other products of intermediate metabolism are oxidized through the citrate cycle, whereby the hydrogen of NAD+ and flavine adenine dinucleotide (FAD) is carried over by substrate-specific dehydrogenases. In summary, the balance of the cycle is

$$\text{acetyl CoA} + \text{NAD} + +\text{FAD} + \text{GDP} + \text{Pi} + 2\text{H}_2\text{O} \rightarrow 3\text{NADH}$$
$$+ \text{FADH2} + \text{GTP} + 2\text{CO}_2 + 2\text{H} + \text{CoA}$$

where lactate is the end product of the glycolytic reaction, and we obtain

$$\text{glucose} + 2\text{ADP} + 2P_i \rightarrow 2\text{ATP} + 2\text{lactate}$$

If we add up all ATP formed from the oxidation of one molecule of glucose, we find the following balance:

$$\text{glucose} + 6\text{CO}_2 + 38\text{ADP} + 38P_i > 6\text{CO}_2 + 44\text{H}_2\text{O} + 38\text{ATP}$$

Thus the complete oxidation of a glucose molecule provides 19 times as much ATP as anaerobic glycolysis.

The key enzyme for the regulation of the rate of glycolysis is phosphofructokinase, which is activated by P_i, adenosine monophosphate (AMP), cyclicAMP (cAMP), ADP, and ammonia. It is inhibited by ATP and citrate. Glucose degradation is partly regulated by glucose availability.

In the presence of glucose, norepinephrine-induced glycogenolysis is blocked despite elevations in cAMP. On the whole, the brain energy turnover is 7 molecules/min. One molecule of ATP contains 29.7 kJ of energy. It is postulated

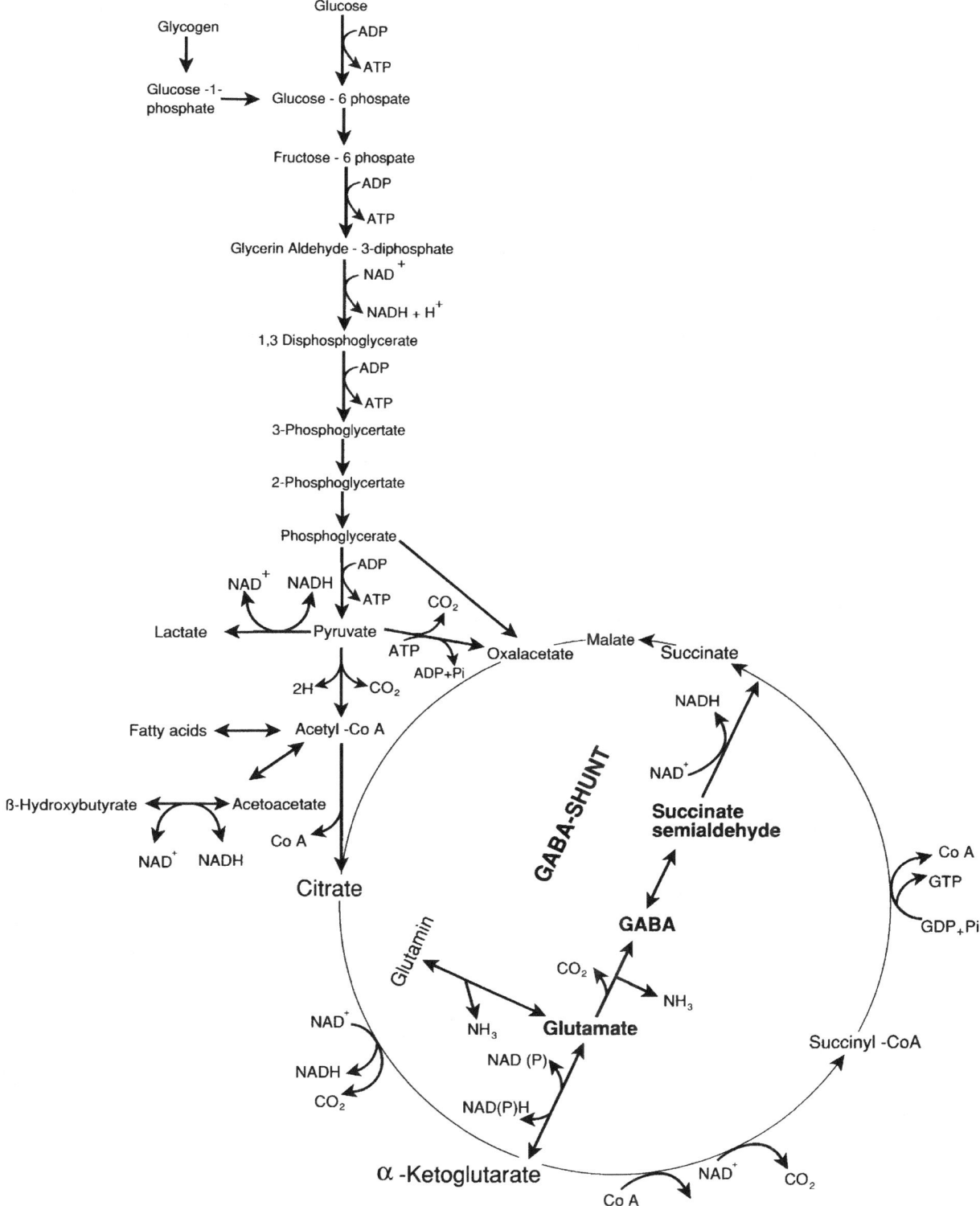

Fig. 5.2 Glycolytic pathway, critic acid cycle, and GABA shunt

that the relative concentration of adenine nucleotide, also expressed as energy charge (EC), has the most important metabolic regulatory effect:

$$\frac{EC + ATP + \frac{1}{2}ADP}{AMP + ADP + ATP}$$

Under physiological conditions this quotient generally has a value between 0.85 and 0.95, and this value falls significantly in cerebral ischemia.

The GABA Shunt

It has been shown that 10% of the carbon atoms from pyruvate molecules are metabolized via the GABA shunt. When coupled with the aspartate aminotransferase (AST) reaction, aspartate formation results:

$$glutamate + oxaloacetate > aspartate + \alpha \ ketoglutarate$$

Two associated reactions give rise to the formation of glutamine and alanine:

$$glutamate + NH_3 + ATP \rightarrow glutamine + ADP + P_i$$

$$pyruvate + glutamate \rightarrow \alpha \ ketoglutarate + alanine$$

The GABA shunt pathway and its associated reactions allow the synthesis of glutamate, GABA, aspartate, alanine, and glutamine from ammonia and carbohydrate precursors. They have two main functions: detoxification of ammonia and resynthesis of amino acid transmitters that are lost from neurons during functional activity.

Pyruvate and the Citric Acid Cycle

Under some conditions pyruvate can be introduced into the citric acid cycle via pyruvate decarboxylase or malate dehydrogenase. Pyruvate dehydrogenase is an intramitochondrial enzyme complex that catalyzes the conversion of pyruvate into acetyl CoA and CO_2. The proportion of pyruvate dehydrogenase in active form in the brain intramitochondrial enzyme complex that catalyzes the conversion of pyruvate into acetyl CoA and CO_2 changes inversely with changes in mitochondrial energy charge. Normally there is a slight excess of pyruvate dehydrogenase in comparison with pyruvate flux, as the brain usually depends on carbohydrate utilization.

Cerebral Metabolism During Hypoxia

During tissue hypoxia, molecular oxygen or the final receptor of hydrogen is reduced. This results in diminution in the amount of hydrogen which can reach the molecular oxygen via the respiratory chain. As a sequel, not only is the oxidative energy production reduced, but the redox systems are shifted to the reduced side with ensuing tissue acidosis.

The reduction of oxidative ATP formation leads to an increase of nonoxidative energy production, i.e., by glycolysis due to decrease of the ATP/AMP quotient. The increased glycolysis results in an accumulation of pyruvate and NADH within the cytoplasm of the cell.

Since triose phosphate dehydrogenase is an enzyme of glycolysis dependent on NAD, the activity of this enzyme, and thus of the glycolytic pathways, requires NAD within the cytoplasm for maintenance of the cell function. Under hypoxic conditions NAD is provided within the cytoplasm by means of the following reaction catalyzed by lactate dehydrogenase:

$$pyruvate + NADH \rightarrow lactate + NAD$$

This causes a reduction of intracellular pyruvate and NADH concentration, and a supply of NAD and lactate. Whereas lactate, the final product of glycolysis, is bound, NAD is made available as hydrogen receptor to the triose phosphate dehydrogenase. This is how glycolysis, with its relatively low energy production, may be maintained even under hypoxic conditions. This biochemical process is extremely valuable for the structural conservation of the neurons under hypoxic conditions.

Hypoxia also disturbs the acid–base balance of the tissues by an increase of H+ ion concentration and an excess of lactate as a result of intensified glycolysis. It affects the cytoplasmic NADH/NAD as well as lactate/pyruvate ratios, as expressed in the following equation:

$$\frac{lactate}{pyruvate} \times \frac{K}{H} = \frac{NADH}{NAD}$$

where K is an equilibrium constant. The redox system is shifted to the reduced side. There is increased pyruvate concentration, which, however, falls short of the increase in lactate.

In total anoxia the glycolysis increases four to seven times. There is a decrease of glucose, glucose-6-phosphate, and fructose–hexose phosphate and an increase of all substrates from fructose diphosphate to lactate. These changes can be interpreted as resulting from facilitation of phosphorylation of glucose to fructose–hexose phosphate.

Studies with labeled glucose uptake in the brain under hypoxic conditions show that the hippocampus, the white matter, the superior colliculi, and the geniculate bodies are the areas most sensitive to the effects of hypoxia. The relatively greater sensitivity of the white matter to hypoxia may lead to an understanding of the white matter damage in postanoxic leukoencephalopathy and its possible prevention with HBO. The relative paucity of capillaries in white matter may predispose them to compression by edema.

Anoxia and hypoxia have different effects on the brain. In hypoxia, the oxidative metabolism of the brain is impaired but not abolished. A three-stage model of ischemic–hypoxic disturbances of the brain is shown in Fig. 5.3.

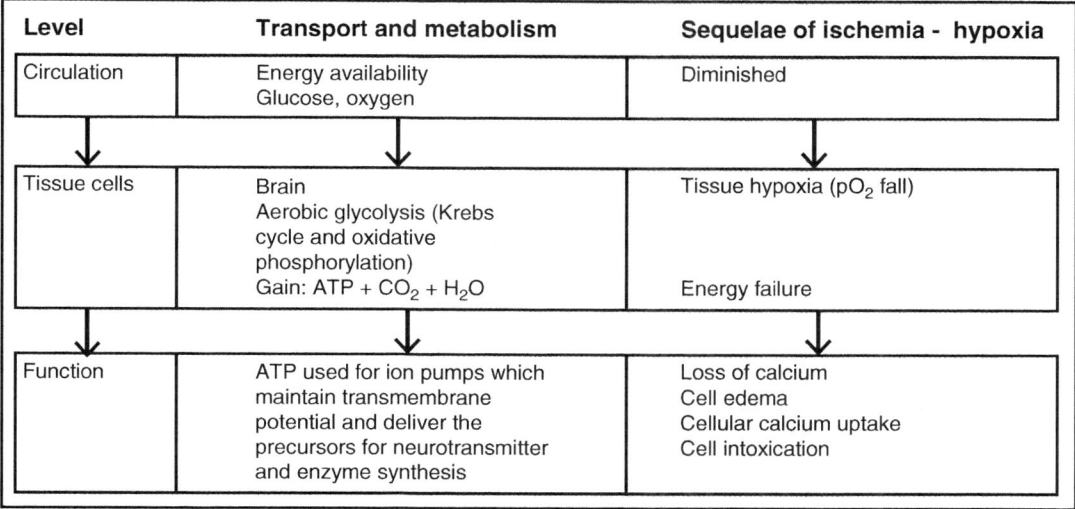

Level	Transport and metabolism	Sequelae of ischemia - hypoxia
Circulation	Energy availability Glucose, oxygen	Diminished
Tissue cells	Brain Aerobic glycolysis (Krebs cycle and oxidative phosphorylation) Gain: ATP + CO_2 + H_2O	Tissue hypoxia (pO_2 fall) Energy failure
Function	ATP used for ion pumps which maintain transmembrane potential and deliver the precursors for neurotransmitter and enzyme synthesis	Loss of calcium Cell edema Cellular calcium uptake Cell intoxication

Fig. 5.3 A three-stage model of ischemic–hypoxic disturbances of the brain

Changes in Neurotransmitter Metabolism

The following changes in neurotransmitter metabolism during hypoxia are particularly significant:

Synthesis of Acetylcholine Is Impaired by Hypoxia. Decrease of acetylcholine following cerebral hypoxia correlates with impairment of memory and learning processes. Indirect evidence for this includes the ameliorating effect of cholinergic drugs in cerebral insufficiency due to hypoxia.

Reduction of Brain Catecholamines. Norepinephrine, epinephrine, and dopamine are synthesized by a combination of tyrosine and oxygen. Hypoxia limits this biosynthesis; the turnover of 5-HT is reduced. A reduction has also been observed in the synthesis of glucose-derived amino acids.

Disturbances of CBF Regulation

In the normal person, CBF remains constant in spite of variations in blood pressure up to a certain extent by virtue of autoregulation. This reflects an inherent capacity of the brain to regulate the circulation according to its requirements. The arteries and arterioles contract when the blood pressure rises and dilate when the blood pressure falls. Hypoxia impairs and blocks this critical mechanism; indeed, there may be marked vasodilatation in the hypoxic brain. Thus, the blood supply of the affected brain region is dependent upon the prevailing blood pressure. The disruption of autoregulation accompanied by focal ischemia and peripheral hyperemia is called the "luxury perfusion syndrome." Following hypoxia, CBF increases as much as twofold initially, but the blood flow increase is blunted somewhat by a decreasing arterial pCO_2 as a result of the hypoxia-induced hyperventilatory response. After a few days, however, CBF begins to fall back toward baseline levels as the blood oxygen-carrying capacity is increasing due to increasing hemoglobin concentration and packed red cell volume as a result of erythropoietin upregulation. By the end of 2 weeks of hypoxic exposure, brain capillary density is increased with resultant decreased intercapillary distances. The relative time courses of these changes suggest that they are adjusted by different control signals and mechanisms.

Disturbances of Microcirculation

In the hypoxic brain, there is aggregation of thrombocytes regardless of the etiology of hypoxia. This is followed by aggregation of red cells, and the phenomenon of "sludging" in the blood. This is aggravated by a reduction of velocity in the blood flow and can result in stasis with its sequelae, such as extension of the area of infarction.

Disturbances of the Blood–Brain Barrier

The hypoxic brain tissue is readily affected by disturbances of the permeability of the blood–brain barrier (BBB) and the cell membranes, because the energy-using mechanisms are dependent upon the integrity of these membranes. Disturbances of the BBB impair the active transport of substances in and out of the brain tissues. This may particularly affect glucose transport to the neurons during its metabolism. The oxygen deficiency can also result in a secondary disturbance of the utilization of the substrate.

Cerebral Edema

A further sequel of BBB damage is cerebral edema. Although injury to the brain contributes to the edema, the loss of autoregulation is also an important factor. The rise of intracapillary pressure leads to seepage of fluid into the extracellular

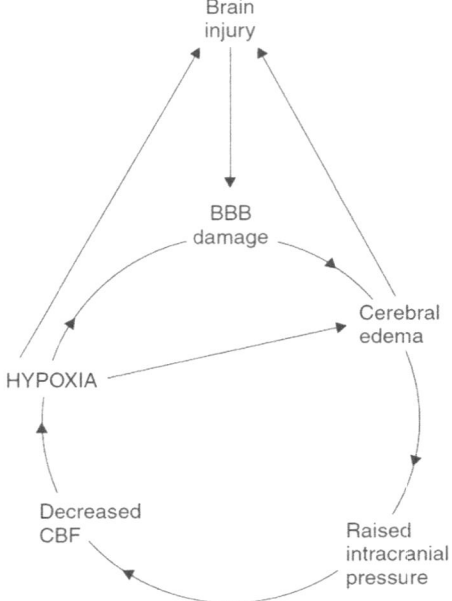

Fig. 5.4 Hypoxia as a central factor in edema due to brain injury

space. The edema impairs the oxygen supply to the brain and leads to an increase of intracranial pressure and a decrease of CBF. Hypoxia which complicates a brain injury is a dreaded phenomenon and represents a decisive factor in the outcome of the illness. Hypoxia is the central factor in the vicious circle shown in Fig. 5.4.

Effect of Hypoxia on the Electrical Activity of the Brain

The electrical activity of the neurons in the human CNS is remarkably sensitive to hypoxia. EEG activity is attenuated after 10–30 s, and evoked potentials are depressed within 1–3 min of hypoxia. Little is known of the important mechanisms underlying these effects.

Disappearance of EEG activity with hypoxia and reappearance on oxygenation are related to the creatine phosphate (CrP)/creatine (Cr) quotient, pointing to a close functional relationship between brain energy potentials and EEG activity. Computer analysis of EEG in induced hypoxia in human subjects shows that both the mean frequency and the mean amplitude closely reflect the degree of hypoxia.

Electrocerebral silence occurs when cerebral venous pO_2 reaches 20 mmHg or after only 6 s of total anoxia.

Disturbances of Mental Function in Cerebral Hypoxia

McFarland et al. (1944) demonstrated that oxygen deprivation, whether induced by high altitude or CO poisoning, leads to loss of capacity of sensory perception and judgment. The subjects recovered when oxygen supply was resumed.

Some important causes of hypoxia that lead to impairment of mental function are:

- Chronic carbon monoxide poisoning
- High altitudes, climbing peaks over 8000 m without supplemental oxygen
- Sleep-disordered breathing
- Chronic obstructive pulmonary disease

Hypoxia has been considered a causal factor in the decline of intellectual function in the elderly. Cerebral symptoms appear at even a moderate degree of hypoxic hypoxia, demonstrating that certain higher functions are very sensitive to restriction of the oxygen supply, as suggested in Fig. 5.5. Delayed dark adaptation has been reported at alveolar oxygen tensions of 80 mmHg, but abnormalities in psychological tests do not occur until alveolar pO_2 is reduced below 50 mmHg, and gross deterioration of mental functions appears only below alveolar pO_2 values of 40 mmHg.

A mild and rapid hypoxic challenge, by breathing 14.5 % oxygen or rapid ascent by helicopter to a mountain peak 3450 m high, may improve a simple measure of cognitive performance (Schlaepfer et al. 1992). Effects of hypoxia vary according to the mode of induction, severity, and duration.

Structural Changes in the Brain After Hypoxia

Patients who recover following resuscitation for cardiopulmonary arrest may not show any structural changes demonstrable by imaging studies. Patients with a residual vegetative state usually develop cerebral atrophy with decrease of rCBF and oxygen consumption. In the subacute phase, these patients may show white matter lucencies on CT scan. PET findings (decrease of rCBF and rCMRO), weeks after the ischemic–hypoxic insult, correlate with the neuropsychiatric deficits due to cardiopulmonary arrest.

Conditions Associated with Cerebral Hypoxia

Various conditions associated with cerebral hypoxia are shown in Table 5.2. Pathophysiology and management of these are discussed in various chapters of this book.

Assessment of Hypoxic Brain Damage

Various abnormalities demonstrated on brain imaging are described in Chaps. 18 and 19. Delayed hypoxic changes are likely to manifest by changes in basal ganglia. The classical example of hypoxic brain damage is that after cardiac arrest. Hypoxic brain damage after cardiac arrest can be estimated by measurements of concentrations of serum S protein which is an established biomarker of central nervous system injury. It is a reliable marker of prediction of survival as well as of outcome.

Fig. 5.5 Influence of inspired oxygen concentration on alveolar pO_2 in man, with symptoms of and physiological responses to hypoxia. Reproduced from Siesjö et al. (1974)

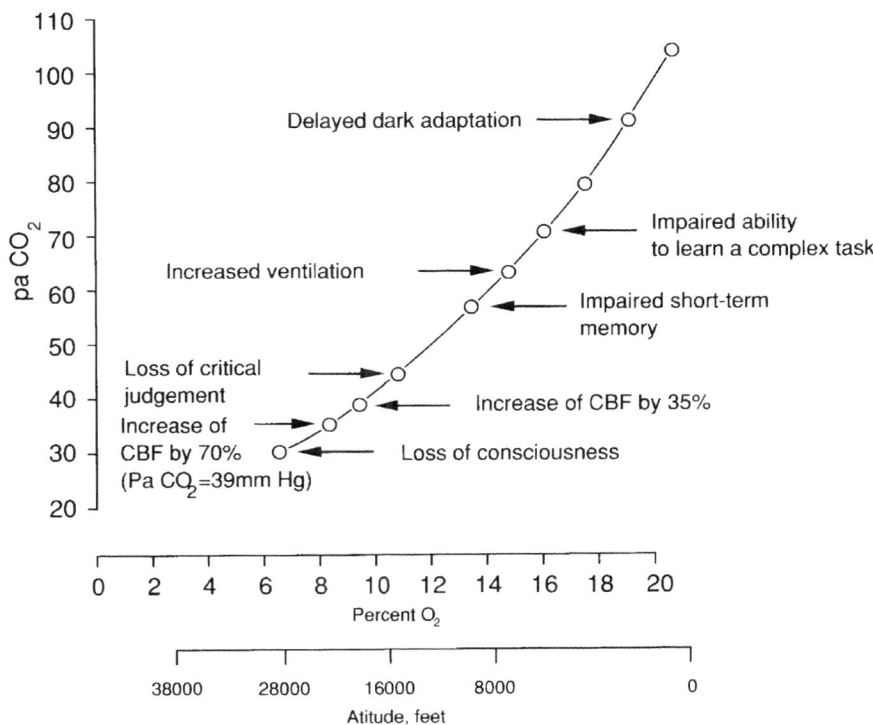

Table 5.2 Conditions associated with cerebral hypoxia

- Air embolism
- Carbon monoxide poisoning
- Cardiac arrest
- Cardiac arrhythmia
- Complications of general anesthesia
- Cyanide poisoning
- Decompression sickness involving the brain
- Drowning
- Drug overdose
- Fat embolism
- Malignant brain tumors, e.g., glioblastoma multiforme
- Severe head injury
- Strangulation
- Stroke
- Very low blood pressure

in other chapters: myocardial ischemia in Chap. 25, CO poisoning in Chap. 13, stroke in Chap. 19, and global ischemia/anoxia and coma in Chap. 20.

Neurons can tolerate between 20 and 60 min of complete anoxia without irreversible changes. Following these severe insults, neurons regain the ability to synthesize protein, produce ATP, and generate action potentials. HBO can facilitate this recovery process. The most significant effects of hypoxia are on the brain, and a review of the metabolic effects leads to the rationale of HBO therapy in hypoxic conditions of the brain, particularly those due to cerebrovascular ischemia.

Hypoxia is also a common feature of the tumor microenvironment and a major cause of clinical radioresistance. Role of HBO in enhancing cancer radiosensitivity is discussed in Chap. 38.

Role of HBO in the Treatment of Hypoxic States

Hypoxia due to inadequate oxygenation in the lungs, either from extrinsic factors or owing to pulmonary disease, can usually be corrected by oxygen. The role of HBO in pulmonary disorders is discussed in Chap. 29. The major applications of HBO are in conditions with inadequate transport and delivery of oxygen to the tissues or inadequate capacity of the tissues to use oxygen. The uses of HBO in the treatment of circulatory disturbances and tissue edema are discussed

The Role of Nitric Oxide Synthase in the Effect of HBO in Hypoxia

The adhesion of polymorphonuclear leukocytes to endothelial cells is increased following hypoxic exposure and is reduced to control levels following exposure to HBO. In experimental studies, HBO exposure induced the synthesis of endothelial cell nitric oxide synthase (eNOS). The NOS inhibitor nitro-L-arginine methyl ester attenuated HBO-mediated inhibition of intercellular adhesion molecule-1 (ICAM-1) expression. These findings suggest that the beneficial effects of HBO in treating hypoxic injury may be mediated in part by inhibition of ICAM-1 expression through the induction of eNOS.

Possible Dangers of HBO in Hypoxic States

Although it appears logical that HBO would be useful in hypoxic states, some concern has been expressed about the free radical damage and damage to the carotid bodies which impairs hypoxic ventilatory drive.

Free Radicals

Hypoxia can potentiate tissue injury due to oxidative stress and free radicals and there is theoretical concern that oxygen given in hypoxia may cause further cell damage. The counterargument is that correction of hypoxia by HBO would reduce the free radical formation resulting from hypoxia. Although the concept of oxygen toxicity at reduced oxygen tensions is a paradox, it cannot be dismissed. It is conceivable that partial lack of oxygen, by impeding electron acceptance at the cytochrome oxidase step, increases the "leak current," i.e., free radical formation. This subject is discussed further in Chap. 6 (oxygen toxicity).

Damage to Carotid Bodies

The carotid body chemosensory response to hypoxia is attenuated following prolonged exposure to normobaric hypoxia in the cat and is attributed to generation of free radicals in the carotid bodies. Further studies on the cat using exposure to 5 ATA showed diminution of chemosensory responsiveness to hypoxia within 2 h which was not considered to be due to lack of neurotransmitters (Torbati et al. 1993). Ultrastructural changes in the carotid bodies (increased number of mitochondria in the glomus cells) after HBO exposure could be explained by the oxidative stress.

Besides their role in ventilation, carotid bodies also regulate peripheral insulin sensitivity. Based on the knowledge that carotid bodies are functionally blocked by hyperoxia and that HBO therapy improves fasting blood glucose in diabetes patients, a study has investigated the effect of HBOT on glucose tolerance in type 2 diabetes patients (Vera-Cruz et al. 2015). The results show that HBO ameliorates glucose tolerance and can be used as a therapeutic intervention in type 2 diabetes.

References

Bai X, Sun B, Pan S, Jiang H, Wang F, Krissansen GW, et al. Down-regulation of hypoxia-inducible factor-1alpha by hyperbaric oxygen attenuates the severity of acute pancreatitis in rats. Pancreas. 2009;38:515–22.

Barcroft J. Anoxemia. Lancet. 1920;11:485.

Jain KK. Oxygen in physiology and medicine. Springfield: Charles C. Thomas; 1989.

Kumar H, Choi DK. Hypoxia inducible factor pathway and physiological adaptation: a cell survival pathway? Mediators Inflamm. 2015;2015:584758.

Lichtenauer M, Zimmermann M, Nickl S, Lauten A, Goebel B, Pistulli R, et al. Transient hypoxia leads to increased serum levels of heat shock protein-27, -70 and caspase-cleaved cytokeratin 18. Clin Lab. 2014;60:323–8.

McFarland RA, Roughton FJ, Halperin MH, et al. The effects of carbon monoxide and altitude on visual thresholds. J Aviat Med. 1944;15:381–94.

Schlaepfer TE, Bärtsch P, Fisch HU. Paradoxical effect of mild hypoxia and moderate altitude on human visual perception. Clin Sci. 1992;83:633–6.

Siesjö BK, Johannson H, Ljunggren B, Norberg K. Brain dysfunction in cerebral hypoxia and ischemia. Nerv Ment Dis. 1974;53:75–105.

Sunkari VG, Lind F, Botusan IR, Kashif A, Liu ZJ, Ylä-Herttuala S, et al. Hyperbaric oxygen therapy activates hypoxia-inducible factor 1 (HIF-1), which contributes to improved wound healing in diabetic mice. Wound Repair Regen. 2015;23:98–103.

Torbati D, Sherpa AK, Lahiri S, Mokashi A, Albertine KH, DiGiulio C. Hyperbaric oxygenation alters carotid body ultrastructure and function. Respir Physiol. 1993;92:183–96.

Ueng SW, Yuan LJ, Lin SS, Niu CC, Chan YS, Wang IC, et al. Hyperbaric oxygen treatment prevents nitric oxide-induced apoptosis in articular cartilage injury via enhancement of the expression of heat shock protein 70. J Orthop Res. 2013;31:376–84.

Vera-Cruz P, Guerreiro F, Ribeiro MJ, Guarino MP, Conde SV. Hyperbaric oxygen therapy improves glucose homeostasis in type 2 diabetes patients: a likely involvement of the carotid bodies. Adv Exp Med Biol. 2015;860:221–5.

K.K. Jain

Abstract

Prolonged exposure to oxygen at high pressure can have toxic effects, particularly on the central nervous system (CNS), but at pressures used clinically it does not pose a problem. The main topics discussed in this chapter are pathophysiology of CNS oxygen toxicity, pulmonary oxygen toxicity, and oxygen-induced retinopathy. Various factors that enhance oxygen toxicity, as well as protection against oxygen toxicity, are discussed. Directions are given for future research.

Keywords

Cerebral metabolism • Free radicals • Hyperbaric oxygen • Neurotoxicity of oxygen • Normobaric oxygen • Oxygen at high pressure • Oxygen toxicity • Pulmonary oxygen toxicity • Retinal oxygen toxicity • Tolerance to oxygen

Introduction

Priestley (see Chap. 1), the discoverer of oxygen in 1775, theorized about the effects of hyperoxia in this charming passage:

> We may also infer from these experiments, that though pure dephlogisticated air might be very useful as a medicine, it might not be so proper for use in the healthy state of the body: for, as a candle burns out much faster in dephlogisticated than in common air, so we might, as might be said, live out too fast, and the animal powers be too soon exhausted in this pure kind of air. A moralist, at least, may say that the air which nature has provided for us is as good as we deserve (Priestley 1973).

Paul Bert (see Chap. 1) was the first to actually document the toxicity of oxygen a century later by conducting experiments to test the effects of hyperbaric oxygen (HBO), not only on himself but also on other life forms (Bert 1878). Indeed, seizures resulting from the toxicity of oxygen to the central nervous system (CNS) are still referred to as the "Paul Bert effect." Although his work is a classic, Bert completely missed pulmonary toxicity as an effect of normobaric oxygen. This was later discovered two decades later by Lorraine Smith and is fittingly referred to as the "Lorraine Smith effect" (Smith 1899). In the twentieth century, several experiments were carried out in human subjects to show the effects of oxygen toxicity (Behnke et al. 1936). Toxic effects of continuous exposure to HBO beyond the point of seizures to irreversible neurological damage and eventual death were discovered half a century later and are now referred to as the "John Bean effect" (Bean et al. 1945).

As a result of these earlier studies it became generally accepted that a 3-h exposure at 3 ATA and a 30- to 40-min exposure at 4 ATA were the limits of safe tolerance by healthy human adults. It is now generally accepted that HBO at 3 ATA affects primarily the nervous system, while the respiratory system is affected independently at 2 ATA. There is a vast amount of literature on basic mechanism of oxygen toxicity. This chapter describes mainly the toxic effects of HBO. Normobaric hyperoxia, which usually leads to pulmonary oxygen poisoning, has been dealt with in detail elsewhere (Jain 1989).

K.K. Jain, MD, FRACS, FFPM (✉)
1 Blaesiring 7, Basel 4057, Switzerland
e-mail: jain@pharmabiotech.ch

© Springer International Publishing AG 2017
K.K. Jain, *Textbook of Hyperbaric Medicine*, DOI 10.1007/978-3-319-47140-2_6

Pathophysiology of Oxygen Toxicity

The molecular basis of CNS, as well as pulmonary oxygen poisoning, involves generation of reactive oxygen species (ROS). This has been known as the free radical theory of oxygen poisoning. The basis of this theory, for the CNS oxygen toxicity, is that an increased generation of ROS during HBO may ultimately lead to alterations in cerebral energy metabolism and electrical activity due to membranes lipid peroxidation, enzyme inhibition, and/or enzyme modulation. Although HBO-induced generation of ROS could directly alter the functions of various SH-containing enzymes, membrane-bound enzymes and structures as well as the nucleus, the physiological effects of HBO may also indirectly cause hypoxic-ischemia, acidosis, anemia, and hyperbilirubinemia.

At higher pressures of oxygen, events in the brain are a prelude to distinct lung pathology. The experimental observation that CNS-mediated component of lung injury can be attenuated by selective inhibition of neuronal nitric oxide synthase (nNOS) or by unilateral transection of the vagus nerve has led to the hypothesis that non-pulmonary neurogenic events predominate in the pathogenesis of acute pulmonary oxygen toxicity in HBO, as nNOS activity drives lung injury by modulating the output of central autonomic pathways (Demchenko et al. 2007).

Free Radical Mechanisms

Oxygen free radicals are products of normal cellular oxidation reduction processes. Under conditions of hyperoxia, their production increases markedly. The nature of the oxygen molecule makes it susceptible to univalent reduction reactions in the cells to form superoxide anion (O_2^-) a highly reactive, cytotoxic free radical. In turn, other reaction products of oxygen metabolism, including hydrogen peroxide (H_2O_2), hydroxyl radicals (OH·), and singlet oxygen ($^1O_2$), can be formed. These short-lived forms are capable of oxidizing the sulfhydryl (SH) groups of enzymes, interact with DNA, and promote lipoperoxidation of cellular membranes.

Boveris and Chance presented an excellent unifying concept of the mechanism of oxygen toxicity in 1978, which is a classic now. H_2O_2 generation as a physiological event has been documented in a variety of isolated mitochondria and is rapidly enhanced by hyperoxia. Superoxide ions, generated submitochondrial fractions, are the source of H_2O_2 (Boveris and Chance 1978). This hypothesis is shown in Fig. 6.1. As a primary event, the free radical chain reactions produce lipoperoxidation. Lipoperoxides, in turn, will have disruptive effects on the structure of the biomembranes, inhibit enzymes with SH groups, and shift the cellular redox state of

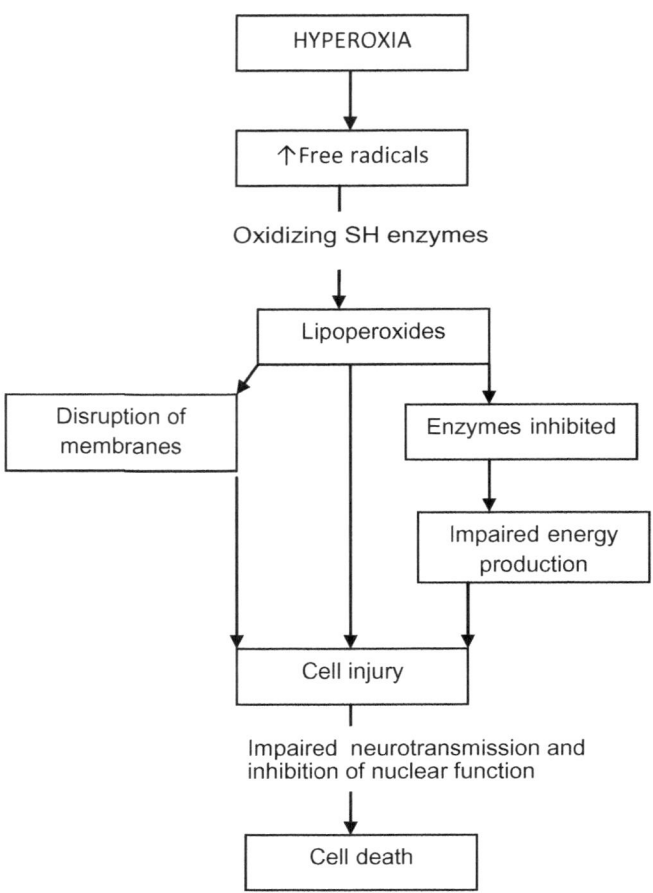

Fig. 6.1 Summary of the hypothesis of oxygen toxicity. *SH* sulfhydryl. Updated and modified from Boveris and Chance (1978)

glutathione toward oxidation. This will be transmitted through the secondary events to pyridine nucleotides, with the mitochondrial NADH oxidation resulting in impaired energy production. Enzyme inhibition, altered energy production, and decrease or loss of function may be consequences of either increased peroxides or a decline in the antioxidant defense.

Although increased generation of ROS before the onset of HBO-induced convulsions has been demonstrated in conscious rats, their production in association with oxygen toxicity has not been demonstrated satisfactorily in human subjects. There are increased electron spin resonance signals from blood of persons exposed to HBO but these return to normal within 10 min of cessation of exposure to HBO.

Pathology of Oxygen Toxicity

The pathology of oxygen toxicity has been documented comprehensively in a classical work on this topic (Balentine 1982). The various manifestations of oxygen poisoning are summarized in Table 6.1. It is well known that the development of pulmonary and CNS toxicity depends upon the partial pressure and the duration of exposure, as shown in Fig. 6.2. Fortunately, the early effects of poisoning are completely reversible, but prolonged exposure first lengthens the recovery period and then eventually produces irreversible changes. Many organs have been affected in experimental oxygen toxicity studies of long exposure to high pressures — a situation that is not seen in clinical practice.

High-pressure oxygen leads to increased pyruvate/lactate and pyruvate malate redox couples, as well as to a decrease in the incorporation of phospholipid long-chain fatty acid and pyruvate into the tissue lipid. During recovery from the effects of high-pressure oxygen these changes are reversed. These data indicate that oxygen poisoning of tissues is not the result of an inhibition of carbohydrate metabolism, but instead may result from the formation of toxic lipoperoxides.

The power expression for cumulative oxygen toxicity and the exponential recovery were successfully applied to various features of oxygen toxicity at the Israel Naval Medical Institute in Israel (Arieli et al. 2002). From the basic equation, the authors derived expressions for a protocol in which PO_2 changes with time. The parameters of the power equation were solved by using nonlinear regression for the reduction in vital capacity (DeltaVC) in humans:

$$\text{Delta } VC = 0.0082 \times t2 \left(PO_2 / 101.3 \right) \left(4.57 \right)$$

where t is the time in hours and PO_2 is expressed in kPa.

The recovery of lung volume is:

$$\text{Delta } VC(t) = \text{Delta } VC(e) \times e\left(-\left(-0.42 + 0.00379 \ PO_2\right)t\right),$$

where DeltaVC(t) is the value at time t of the recovery, DeltaVC(e) is the value at the end of the hyperoxic exposure, and PO_2 is the prerecovery oxygen pressure.

Data from different experiments on CNS oxygen toxicity in humans in the hyperbaric chamber were analyzed along with data from actual closed-circuit oxygen diving by using a maximum likelihood method. The parameters of the model were solved for the combined data, yielding the power equation for active diving:

Table 6.1 Manifestations of oxygen toxicity

Effects on the central nervous system (see Table 6.4)
Retinal toxicity
Effects on the respiratory system
Chemical toxicity: tracheobronchial tree, capillary endothelium, alveolar epithelium
Pulmonary damage: atelectasis
Hypoxemia → acidosis → death
Cardiovascular system
Hemolysis of erythrocytes
Myocardial damage
Endocrine system
Adrenals
Gonads
Thyroid
Hepatotoxicity
Renal damage

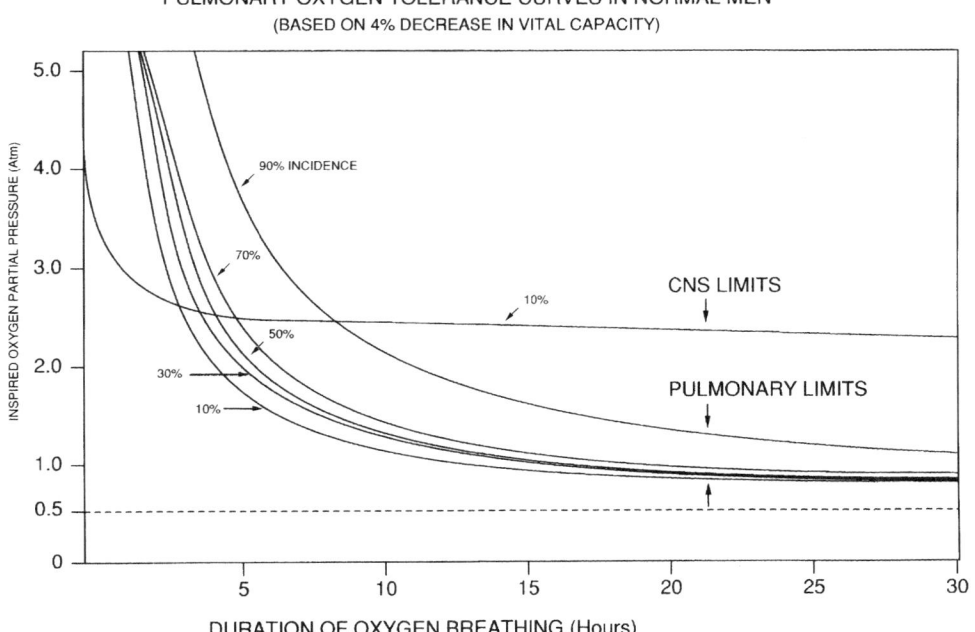

Fig. 6.2 Individual variation in susceptibility to oxygen poisoning. *Curves* designated as pulmonary limits are inspired pO$_2$ exposure duration relationships for occurrence of one or more neurological signs and symptoms listed in Table 6.5. From Clark JM, Fischer AB: Oxygen toxicity and extension of tolerance in oxygen therapy. In: Davis JC, Hunt TK (Eds.): Hyperbaric oxygen therapy, Bethesda, MD, Undersea and Hyperbaric Medical Society 1977. By permission

PULMONARY OXYGEN TOLERANCE CURVES IN NORMAL MEN
(BASED ON 4% DECREASE IN VITAL CAPACITY)

$$K = t2\left(PO_2 / 101.3\right)\left(6.8\right),$$

where t is in minutes.

It was suggested that the risk of CNS oxygen toxicity in diving can be derived from the calculated parameter of the normal distribution:

$$Z = \left[\ln\left(t\right) - 9.63 + 3.38 \times \ln\left(PO_2 / 101.3\right)\right] / 2.02.$$

The recovery time constant for CNS oxygen toxicity was calculated from the value obtained for the rat, taking into account the effect of body mass, and yielded the recovery equation:

$$K\left(t\right) = K\left(e\right) \times e\left(-0.079t\right),$$

where $K(t)$ and $K(e)$ are the values of K at time t of the recovery process and at the end of the hyperbaric oxygen exposure, respectively, and t is in minutes.

Pulmonary Oxygen Toxicity

This is usually a manifestation of prolonged exposure (more than 24 h) to normobaric 100 % oxygen, as well as during exposure to HBO from 2 to 3 ATA O_2 in human and experimental animals. The pathology and pathophysiology of pulmonary oxygen toxicity are described in more detail elsewhere (Jain 1989). The major mechanism by which HBO produces lung injury in rabbits is by stimulating thromboxane synthesis. Lung injury induced by free radicals has been demonstrated in an animal model of smoke inhalation, and the free radicals clear up after about an hour. Normobaric 100 % oxygen given for 1 h does not increase the level of free radicals in this model, but HBO at 2.5 ATA does so.

Breathing HBO at pressures >3 ATA can cause acute pulmonary injury that is more severe if there are concomitant signs of CNS toxicity and indicates activation of an autonomic link between the brain and the lung. Findings of an experimental study indicate that pulmonary damage in HBO is caused by an abrupt and significant increase in pulmonary vascular pressure that is sufficient to produce barotrauma in capillaries (Demchenko et al. 2011). According to the authors, extreme HBO exposures specifically produce massive sympathetic outflow from the CNS that depresses left ventricular function, resulting in acute left atrial and pulmonary hypertension. These effects on the heart and on the pulmonary vasculature are attributed to HBO-mediated central sympathetic excitation and catecholamine release that disturbs the normal equilibrium between excitatory and inhibitory activity in the autonomic nervous system.

The role of GDF15 (growth and differentiation factor 15), a secreted cytokine induced by oxidative stress in vitro, in a model of pulmonary oxygen toxicity, is expected to play a critical role in decreasing cell death and oxidative stress. Knockdown of p53, a direct target of p53, significantly decreases the induction of GDF15 by hyperoxia (Tiwari et al. 2015). This study shows that GDF15 has a pro-survival and anti-oxidant role in hyperoxia and that p53 plays a key role in its induction.

Acute changes in the lungs resulting from oxygen toxicity consist of alveolar and interstitial edema, alveolar hemorrhages, and proteinaceous exudates. This is followed by an inflammatory reaction. Further prolonged exposure to oxygen leads to a proliferative phase, which includes proliferation of type II epithelial cells and fibroblasts, followed by collagen deposits. Healing may occur after discontinuance of oxygen exposure, but areas of fibrosis and emphysema may remain. In patients with heart failure or in patients with reduced cardiac ejection fractions, HBO may contribute to pulmonary edema by increasing left ventricular afterload, increasing oxidative myocardial stress, decreasing left ventricular compliance by oxygen radical-mediated reduction in NO, increasing pulmonary capillary permeability, or by causing pulmonary oxygen toxicity.

Repeated exposure to HBO at intervals insufficient to allow total recovery from pulmonary oxygen toxicity may lead to cumulative effects. The progression of toxicity can be monitored by serial pulmonary function studies. The concept of a "unit pulmonary toxic dose" (UPTD) was developed to enable comparison of the pulmonary effects of various treatment schedules of HBO (Bardin and Lambertsen 1970). The UPTD was designed to express any pulmonary toxic dose in terms of an equivalent exposure to oxygen at 1 ATA. It is only an arbitrary measure and did not allow for the recovery between HBO exposures. For example, 10 HBO treatments at 2.4 ATA for 90 min each would give the patient a UPTD of >200 and would indicate significant pulmonary toxicity with a 20 % reduction in vital capacity. In practice, however, no clinical evidence of pulmonary toxicity is seen with this schedule. There is no significant impairment of pulmonary diffusing capacity in divers who have been intermittently exposed to HBO at 4 ATA for years. The term "UPTD" is now hardly used in clinical practice of HBO therapy.

Prolonged exposure to elevated oxygen levels is a frequent and important clinical problem. Superoxide dismutase (SOD) and catalase, the major intracellular antioxidant enzymes, cooperate in the detoxification of free oxygen radicals produced during normal aerobic respiration. Therapeutic approaches designed to deliver SOD or catalase to these intracellular sites would be useful in mitigating the pulmonary oxygen toxicity. A number of approaches to deliver these enzymes have not been successful. Adenovirus-mediated transfer to lungs of both catalase and SOD cDNA has been shown to protect against pulmonary oxygen toxicity. Distal airway epithelial cells, including type II alveolar and non-ciliated bronchiolar epithelial cells, are important targets for oxygen radicals under the hyperoxic condition. The accessibility of these distal airway epithelial cells to in vivo gene transfer through the tracheal route of administration suggests the potential for in vivo transfer of MnSOD and extracellular SOD genes as an approach for the prevention of pulmonary oxygen toxicity.

Normobaric vs. Hyperbaric Oxygen in Induction of Pulmonary Oxygen Toxicity

Some studies had found that different pathology may exist in normobaric vs. hyperbaric oxygen-induced pulmonary oxygen toxicity, and that nitric oxide synthase (NOS) may play a role. One study has investigated changes of NOS in normobaric and hyperbaric pulmonary oxygen toxicity in rats (Liu et al. 2014). Various groups were exposed to 100 % oxygen at 1 ATA, 1.5 ATA, 2 ATA, 2.5 ATA, and 3 ATA for 56, 20, 10, 8, and 6 h, respectively. There was a control group exposed to normobaric air. After exposure, expression of eNOS and nNOS was measured in bronchoalveolar lavage fluid and was found to be elevated in1 ATA group as compared to the air group, whereas these changes were not so obviously in the other groups. The expression of nNOS was not changed in normobaric and hyperbaric pulmonary oxygen toxicity, while the expression of eNOS was significantly decreased in 2 ATA group, and significantly elevated in 2.5 ATA and 3 ATA group. The conclusion was that the expression of eNOS can change when exposed to different pressures of oxygen.

Oxygen-Induced Retinopathy

Retrolental fibroplasia is considered to be an oxygen-induced obliteration of the immature retinal vessels when 100 % oxygen is given to premature infants. A study showed that oxygen therapy for more than 3 days, in infants delivered following 32–36 weeks of gestation, was not associated with an increased risk of retinopathy of prematurity (Gleissner et al. 2003). HBO (2.8 ATA, 80 % oxygen) given to premature rats does not result in retinopathy, whereas control animals given normobaric 80 % oxygen developed retinopathy. This topic is discussed further in Chap. 32.

Factors That Enhance Oxygen Toxicity

Various factors which enhance oxygen toxicity are listed in Table 6.2. Combining HBO with the substances listed, together with morbid conditions such as fever, should definitely be avoided.

Table 6.2 Enhancers of oxygen toxicity

Gases
Carbon dioxide
Nitrous oxide
Hormones
Insulin
Thyroid hormones
Adrenocortical hormones
Neurotransmitters
Epinephrine and norepinephrine
Drugs and chemicals
Acetazolamide
Aspirin
Dextroamphetamine
Disulfiram
Guanethidine
NH_4Cl
Paraquat
Perfluorocarbon
Trace metals
Iron
Copper
Morbid conditions
Congenital spherocytosis
Fever
Vitamin E deficiency convulsions
Physiological states of increased metabolism
Diving
Hyperthermia
Physical exercise

Intravenous perfluorocarbon emulsions, administered with supplemental inspired oxygen, are being evaluated for their ability to eliminate nitrogen from blood and tissue prior to submarine escape. These agents can increase the incidence of CNS oxygen toxicity by enhancing oxygen delivery to the brain. In an experimental study, conscious rats that were pretreated with perfluorocarbon emulsion at 3 or 6 mL/kg intravenously and exposed to 100 % oxygen at 5 ATA (Demchenko et al. 2012). At the lower dose, 80 % of the animals experienced seizures after 33 min of exposure compared with 50 % of the control animals. At the higher dose, seizures occurred in all rats within 25 min. At these doses, administration of perfluorocarbon emulsion poses a clear risk of CNS oxygen toxicity in conscious rats exposed to HBO at 5 ATA.

Trimix SCUBA diving involves regulating mixtures of nitrogen, oxygen, and helium in an attempt to overcome the risks of narcosis and decompression sickness during deep dives, but introduces other potential hazards such as hypoxia and convulsions due to oxygen toxicity (Farmery and Sykes 2012).

The best known effect of increasing CO_2 concentration is global warming, but large increases in CO_2 concentration (to 1 or 10 %) are also known to affect cellular biochemical reactions. Increased CO_2 concentration is a risk factor for oxygen toxicity as it exacerbates ROS generation, which increases oxidative cellular lesions. CO_2 probably also reacts with ROS in vivo, such as H_2O_2, to exacerbate oxidative stress (Ezraty et al. 2011).

Mild hyperthermia (38.5 °C) has been used therapeutically for a number of conditions. An increase of temperature increases oxygen uptake by body tissues. Hyperthermia may thus be expected to enhance oxygen toxicity. Transient biochemical side effects of mild hypothermia such as hyperammonemia can be inhibited by HBO, but this combination should be used cautiously to avoid oxygen toxicity.

It is generally believed that high humidity enhances oxygen toxicity as manifested by lung damage and convulsions. This has been experimentally verified in rodents exposed to HBO (515–585 kPa) under conditions of low humidity as well as 60 % relative humidity.

Physical exercise definitely lowers the threshold for CNS oxygen toxicity in the rat over the entire range of pressures from 2 to 6 ATA. This observation should be kept in mind in planning physical exercise in hyperbaric environments (see Chap. 4). Various enzymes inhibited by hyperoxia are shown in Table 6.3. This may explain how hyperoxia leads to oxygen toxicity. Glutathione reductase is an integral component of the antioxidant defense mechanism. Inhibition of brain glutathione reductase by carmustine lowers the threshold for seizures in rats exposed to HBO.

Central Nervous System Oxygen Toxicity

Effect on Cerebral Metabolism

Disturbances of cerebral metabolism resulting from hyperoxia have been described in Chap. 2. HBO at 2 ATA has been shown to stimulate cerebral metabolic rate of glucose lightly, but does not result in any toxic manifestations. Oxidative metabolism of the brain is usually not affected by pressures up to 6 ATA. In the rat cortical neuron culture, HBO exposure to 6 ATA for 30, 60, and 90 min increases the lactate dehydrogenase activity in the culture medium in a time-dependent manner. Accordingly, the cell survival is decreased after HBO exposure. Pretreatment with the NMDA antagonist MK-801 or L-N(G)-nitro-arginine methyl ester, an NOS inhibitor, protects the cells against the HBO-induced damage suggesting that activation of NMDA receptors and production of NO play a role in the neurotoxicity produced by HBO exposure.

There is no evidence that seizures are related to oxidative metabolic changes. However, increase of glucose utilization precedes the onset of electrophysiological manifestations of CNS oxygen toxicity. Increased NO production during pro-

Table 6.3 Enzymes Inhibited by Hyperoxia at 1–5 ATA

1. Embden-Meyerhof pathway
   Phosphoglucokinase
   Phosphoglucomutase
   Glyceraldehyde-phosphate-dehydrogenase[a]
2. Conversion of pyruvate to acetyl-CoA
   Pyruvate oxidase
3. Tricarboxylic acid cycle
   Succinate dehydrogenase[a]
   α-ketoglutarate dehydrogenase[a]
   Malate dehydrogenase[a]
4. Electron transport
   Succinate dehydrogenase[a]
   Malate dehydrogenase[a]
   Glyceraldehyde-phosphate dehydrogenase[a]
   DPNH dehydrogenase[a]
   Lactate dehydrogenase[a]
   Xanthine oxidase
   D-Amino acid oxidase
5. Neurotransmitter synthetic enzymes
   Glutamic acid decarboxylase
   Choline acetylase
   Dopa decarboxylase
   5-HTP decarboxylase
   Phenylalanine hydroxylase
   Tyrosine hydroxylase
6. Proteolysis and hydrolysis
   Cathepsin
   Papain
   Unspecified proteases and peptidases
   Unspecified in autolysis
   Arginase
   Urease
   Ribonuclease
7. Membrane transport
   NA+, K+-ATPase+
8. Molecular oxygen reduction pathway
   Catalase
9. Other enzymes
   Acetate kinase
   Cerebrosedase
   Choline oxidase
   Fatty acid dehydrogenase
   Formic acid dehydrogenase
   Glutamic dehydrogenase
   Glutamic synthetase
   Glyoxylase
   Hydrogenase
   Isocitrate lyase
   Malate syntase
   Myo kinase (adenylate kinase)
   Phosphate transacetylase
   Transaminase
   Zymohexase (aldolase)

[a]Indicate enzymes containing essential sulfhydryl (SH) groups, emphasized as being inactivated by oxidation of these groups

longed HBO exposure is responsible for escape from hyperoxic vasoconstriction in cerebral blood arterioles suggesting that NO overproduction initiates CNS oxygen toxicity by increasing regional cerebral blood flow (rCBF), which allows excessive oxygen to be delivered to the brain. The hypothetical pathophysiological pathways leading to acute and chronic oxygen neurotoxicity are illustrated in Fig. 6.3.

Effect on Neurotransmitters

Neurotransmitters are downregulated under hyperbaric hyperoxia. With the recognition of NO as a neurotransmitter, its relationship to hyperoxia has been studied. Experimental studies in rats have shown that they can be protected against oxygen neurotoxicity by a combination of

Fig. 6.3 Basic mechanisms of CNS oxygen toxicity. *ROS* reactive oxygen species, *NO* nitric oxide. Image by D. Torbati, Ph.D.

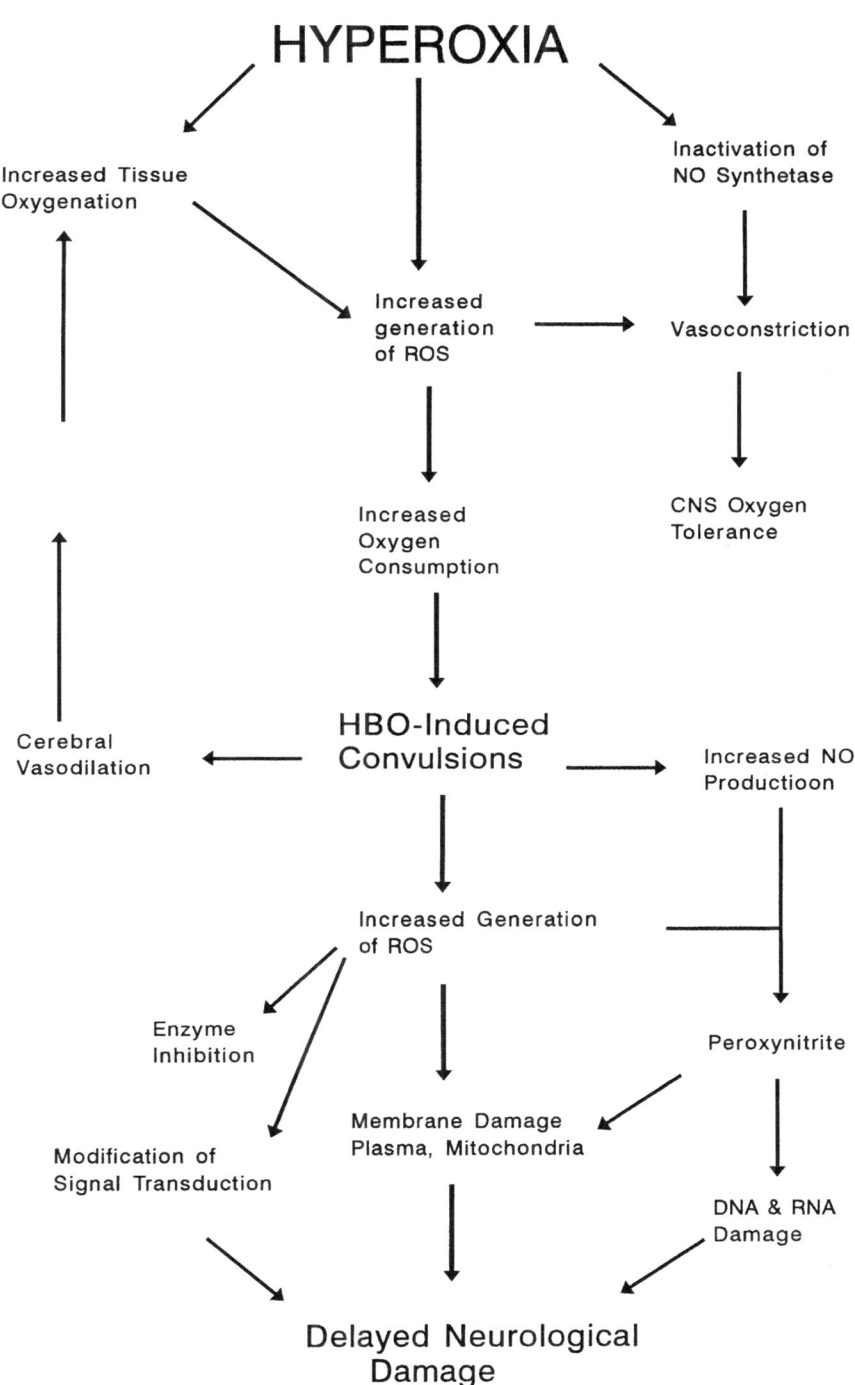

a monoamine oxidase inhibitor and a NOS inhibitor. Protection against oxygen toxicity by these agents is not related to the preservation of the GABA pool. Oxygen-dependent norepinephrine metabolism and NO synthesis are inactive during oxygen neurotoxicity. These findings indicate that NO is an important mediator in oxygen neurotoxicity and suggest that extracellular SOD increases oxygen neurotoxicity by inactivation of NO.

Exposures to HBO at 2–3 ATA stimulate neuronal NOS (nNOS) and at both pressures, elevations in NO concentration are inhibited by the nNOS inhibitor 7-nitroindazole and the calcium channel blocker nimodipine. Infusion of SOD inhibits NO elevation at 3, but not 2 ATA HBO. Hyperoxia increased the concentration of NO associated with hemoglobin. These findings highlight the complexity of oxidative stress responses and may help explain some of the dose responses associated with therapeutic applications of HBO.

Ammonia and Amino Acids

Single seizures induced in rats subjected to HBO at 6 ATA have been shown to be associated with accumulation of ammonia and alterations in amino acids in the brain. These changes are considered to be caused by an increase in oxidative deamination or possibly the result of glial failure to capture released amino acids. The subsequent imbalance between the excitatory and inhibitory mediators in the striatum has been offered as an explanation of the recurrence of seizures in animals maintained on HBO.

Biomarkers of Oxygen Neurotoxicity

Changes in the Electrical Activity of the Brain and Seizures

Conscious rats and rabbits exposed to HBO usually demonstrate an increased EEG slow wave activity which eventually develops into bursts of paroxysmal electrical discharges. These electrical events precede the onset of visible HBO-induced convulsions, and therefore were suggested as early biomarkers of CNS oxygen toxicity in experimental animals. In vitro studies with HBO also show changes in neuronal electrical activity, which may be associated with seizures.

The seizure associated with HBO usually occurs toward the end of the oxygen exposure while the patient is being decompressed. It is a violent motor discharge with a brief period of breath holding. In such cases, therefore, decompression should be temporarily halted until the seizure is over; otherwise, there could be rupture of lung alveoli.

Oxygen-induced seizures are not a contraindication for further HBO therapy. Further HBO treatments may be carried out at lower pressures and shorter exposures. Anticonvulsant medications are usually not indicated, but may be used. Carbamazepine and vigabatrin are effective in preventing HBO-induced convulsions in patients under high ATA HBO. Acupuncture has been claimed to protect against oxygen-induced convulsions by increasing GABA in the brain levels but there is no experimental evidence to confirm it.

Epilepsy has been listed as a contraindication for using HBO therapy. This is based on the assumption that oxygen is liable to precipitate a seizure in an epileptic patient and such an event in a chamber might be detrimental to the patient. Seizures in epileptic patients are rare during HBO therapy where pressures less than 2 ATA are used. There is no published study that reexamines this issue. The question therefore still arises: is HBO really dangerous for an epileptic? If epilepsy is included in the contraindications for HBO, patients with head injuries and strokes who happen to have seizures would be deprived of the benefit of HBO therapy. The mechanism of epilepsy in such patients is different from that of an oxygen-induced convulsion. It has even been shown that EEG abnormalities in stroke patients improve with HBO treatment. It is possible that HBO may abort a seizure from a focus with circulatory and metabolic disturbances by correcting these abnormalities. Seizures are extremely rare and no more than a chance occurrence during HBO sessions at pressures between 1.5 and 2 ATA even in patients with a history of epilepsy.

Hyperoxic Hyperpnea as a Biomarker of HBO Neurotoxicity

HBO stimulates central CO_2-chemoreceptor neurons, increases minute ventilation (V_{min}), decreases heart rate and, if breathed for sufficiently long periods, produces CNS oxygen toxicity, i.e., seizures, which are variable between individuals and their onset is difficult to predict. In an experimental study, breathing HBO in Dawley rats induced an early transient increase in V_{min} and heart rate during pressurization, followed by a second significant increase of V_{min} several minutes prior to seizure (Pilla et al. 2013). The study showed that hyperoxic hyperpnea is an early biomarker that predicts an impending seizure while breathing HBO.

Neuropathology of Oxygen Toxicity

In experimental studies, there is no damage to the CNS of rats exposed to HBO until the pressure exceeds 4 ATA. The brain damage is increased by CNS-depressant drugs, increase of pCO_2, acetazolamide, and NH_4Cl. Permanent spastic limb paralysis has been observed in rats (the John Bean effect) after repeated exposure to high oxygen pressures (over 5 ATA). There is selective necrosis of white matter both in the spinal cord and the brain, and this is considered to be the effect of hyperoxia. HBO-induced rat brain lesions, examined by electron microscopy, show two types of nerve cell alterations: (1) type A lesions characterized by pyknosis and hyperchromatosis of the nerve cells, vacuolization of the cytoplasm, and simultaneous swelling of the perineural glial processes; (2) type B lesions are characterized by lysis in the cytoplasm and karyorrhexis.

Manifestations of CNS Oxygen Toxicity

Signs and symptoms of CNS oxygen toxicity are listed in Table 6.4.

Clinical Monitoring for Oxygen Toxicity

The most important factor in early detection of oxygen toxicity is the observation of signs and symptoms. For monitoring pulmonary function, determination of vital capacity is the easiest and most reliable parameter, as it is reduced before any irreversible changes occur in the lungs. EEG tracings do not show any consistent alterations before the onset of seizures and are not a reliable method of early detection of oxygen toxicity.

Decrease in [9,10–3H] oleic acid incorporation by human erythrocytes that is detected in vitro after HBO exposure in vivo may reflect an early event in the pathogenesis of oxygen-induced cellular injury and may be a useful monitoring procedure. An increase in CBF velocity (BCFV) precedes onset of symptoms of oxygen toxicity during exposure to 280 kPa oxygen, which may be followed by seizure (Koch et al. 2008). At rest a delay of ~20 min precedes the onset of CNS oxygen toxicity and seizure can be aborted with timely oxygen reduction.

Protection Against Oxygen Toxicity

Various agents and measures for prevention or treatment of oxygen toxicity are listed in Table 6.5; these are mostly experimental. The most promising agents are the antioxidants. The use of vitamin E (tocopherol) is based on the free-radical theory of oxygen toxicity. It has been used to protect premature infants (who lack vitamin E) against oxygen toxicity. Dietary supplementation with selenium and vitamin E, which increase the cerebral as well as extra-cerebral GSH content, does not protect rats against the effect of HBO by delaying the onset of first electrical discharge. However, such diets may still be advantageous in promoting recovery and reversal of toxic process, as occurs between consecutive HBO exposures or during intermittent oxygen exposure. Not all of the dietary free-radical scavengers are effective in counteracting oxygen toxicity. In ani-

Table 6.4 Signs and symptoms of CNS toxicity

Visual disturbances
Loss of visual acuity
Constriction of visual field
Disturbances of alertness and consciousness
Sleepiness
Syncope
Behavior and mood disorders
Apprehension
Changes of behavior
Clumsiness
Dazzle
Depression
Disinterest
Euphoria
Fidgeting
Abnormal perception
Acoustic perception of music, bell ringing, knocking, etc.
Unpleasant olfactory sensations
Unpleasant gustatory sensations
Movement disorders
Decrease of intensity of movement
Fibrillation of lips
Lateral movements
Lip twitching
Twitching of cheek and nose
Cardiovascular
Bradycardia
Palpitations
Respiratory
Choking sensation
Changes in breathing patterns
Diaphragmatic spasms
Grunting
Hiccoughs
Inspiratory predominance
Panting
Gastrointestinal
Epigastric tensions
Severe nausea
Spasmodic vomiting
Miscellaneous neurological manifestations
Convulsions
Vertigo
Miscellaneous general symptoms
Facial pallor
Sweating

mal experiments, no correlation was found between in vitro inhibition of lipid peroxidation and in vivo protection against oxygen toxicity. Hypothermia has been considered to be a protector against oxygen toxicity, but HBO at 5 ATA induces hypothermia in mice, and this has little protective effect against convulsions.

Table 6.5 Factors protecting against generalized oxygen toxicity

Antioxidants, free radical scavengers, and trace minerals
Allopurinol
Ascorbic acid
Edaravone
Glycine
Magnesium
Selenium
Superoxide dismutase, SOD
Tyloxapol
Vitamin E
Chemicals and enzymes modifying cerebral metabolism
Arginine
Coenzyme Q10 and carnitine
Gamma-aminobutyric acid, GABA
Glutathionehemocarnisine
Interleukin-6
Leukotriene B4 antagonist SC-41930
Paraglycine and succinic acid
Sodium succinate and glutamate
Drugs
Adrenergic-blocking and ganglion-blocking drugs
Barbiturates
BCNU
Chlorazepate
Diazepam
Ergot derivatives: lisuride and quinpirole
Isonicotinic acid hydrazide
Levodopa
Lithium
Milecide
MK-801 (a competitive NMDA receptor antagonist)
Neuroleptics: chlorpromazine, thorazine
Propranolol
Intermittent exposure to HBO
Acclimatization to hypoxia
Interposition of air-breathing periods
Endocrine factors
Adrenalectomy
Hypophysectomy
Thyroidectomy
Gene therapy

One approach to prevent pulmonary oxygen toxicity is to augment antioxidant enzyme activity in the respiratory system. A study investigated the ability of aerosolized extracellular SOD (EC-SOD) to protect the lungs from hyperoxic injury (Yen et al. 2011). Treatment with aerosolized EC-SOD increased the survival rate of mice with hyperoxia-induced pulmonary oxygen toxicity. The protective effects of EC-SOD against hyperoxia were further confirmed by reduced lung edema and systemic oxidative stress. The results indicate the potential of an aerosol therapy with recombinant human EC-SOD for reducing oxidative injury

in patients with severe hypoxemic respiratory failure, including acute respiratory distress syndrome.

The detoxifying function of cytochrome c to scavenge ROS in mitochondria has been confirmed experimentally (Min and Jian-Xing 2007). A concept of mitochondrial radical metabolism is suggested based on the two electron leak pathways mediated by cytochrome c that are metabolic routes of oxygen free radicals. The main portion of oxygen consumed in the electron transfer of respiratory chain is used in ATP synthesis, while a subordinate part of oxygen consumed by the leaked electrons contributes to ROS generation. The models of respiratory chain operating with two cytochrome c-mediated electron-leak pathways and a radical metabolism of mitochondria accompanied with energy metabolism are helpful in understanding the pathological problems caused by oxygen toxicity. Animal experimental studies show that perfluorocarbon increases the risk of CNS neurotoxicity under HBO and edaravone (marketed as a neuroprotective agent for acute ischemic stroke in Japan) could serve as a promising chemoprophylactic agent to prevent it (Liu et al. 2012).

Distal airway epithelial cells, including type II alveolar and non-ciliated bronchiolar epithelial cells, are important targets for O_2 radicals under the hyperoxic condition. The accessibility of these distal airway epithelial cells to in vivo gene transfer through the tracheal route of administration, suggests the potential for in vivo transfer of MnSOD and extracellular SOD genes as an approach in the prevention of pulmonary O_2 toxicity.

Every clinician who treats patients should be aware of oxygen toxicity, although it is rare. At pressures of 1.5 ATA, even prolonged use in patients with cerebrovascular disease has not led to any reported case of oxygen toxicity. It should not be assumed that experimental observations regarding oxygen toxicity under hyperbaric conditions are applicable to normobaric conditions. Whereas disulfiram protects against HBO, it potentiates the toxicity of normobaric oxygen in rats. Ascorbic acid is also a free radical scavenger and protects against oxygen toxicity, but large doses of this vitamin may prove counterproductive in treating oxygen toxicity if the reducing enzymes are overloaded. An oxidized ascorbate might actually potentiate oxygen toxicity through lipoperoxide formation. Mg^{2+} has a double action against the undesirable effects of oxygen. It is a vasodilator and also a calcium blocker and protects against cellular injury. Magnesium sulfate suppresses the electroencephalographic manifestations of CNS oxygen toxicity and an anticonvulsant effect has been demonstrated in rats exposed to HBO at 6 ATA. A prophylactic regimen of 10 mmol Mg^{2+} 3 h before a session of HBO and 400 mg of vitamin E daily, starting a couple of days before the HBO treatment, is useful in preventing oxygen toxicity, but no controlled study has been done to verify the efficacy of this regime.

Extension of Oxygen Tolerance

Tolerance to oxygen primarily means tolerance to the toxic effects, because the physiological effects have no prolonged consequences. Various approaches to extend tolerance to hyperoxia are discussed in the following sections.

Tolerance Extension by Adaptation

At low levels of atmospheric hyperoxia, some forms of true protective adaptation appear to occur, such as that related to changing antioxidant defenses in some tissues. At higher oxygen pressures, some adaptation could conceivably occur in some cells of the intact human being with progressive and severe poisoning in other cells. At very high oxygen pressure, rapid onset of poisoning would make adaptation inadequate and too late.

Tolerance Extension by Drugs

A pharmacological approach, such as that of providing free radical scavengers, will attain broad usefulness only if the drug can attain the free permeability of the oxygen molecule. The drug should reach the right location at the right time, and remain effective there in the face of continuous hyperoxia, without itself inducing any toxic effects. There is no such ideal drug available at present.

Tolerance Extension by Interrupted Exposure to Oxygen

Interruption of exposure to HBO is known to extend the safe exposure time. In experimental animals, intermittent exposure to HBO postpones the gross symptoms of oxygen toxicity along with changes in enzymes, such as SOD, in the lungs. There is no accepted procedure for quantifying the recovery during normoxia. A cumulative oxygen toxicity index—K, when K reaches a critical value (K_c) and the toxic effect is manifested, can be calculated using the following equation:

$$K = t2e \times PO_2 c,$$

where $t(e)$ is hyperoxic exposure time and PO_2 is oxygen pressure and c is a power parameter.

Recovery during normoxia (reducing K) is calculated by the following equation

$$K2 = K1 \times e\left[-rt(r) \right],$$

where $t(r)$ is recovery time, r being the recovery time constant.

A combination of accumulation of oxygen toxicity and its recovery can be used to calculate CNS oxygen toxicity. Predicted latency to the appearance of the first electrical discharge in the electroencephalogram, which precedes clinical convulsions, can be compared to measured latency for different exposures to HBO, followed by a period of normoxia and further HBO exposure. Recovery follows an exponential path, with $r = 0.31$ (SD 0.12) min (-1).

Calculation of the recovery of the CNS oxygen toxicity is in accordance with exponential recovery of the hypoxic ventilatory response and is probably a general recovery process. The recovery can be applied to the design of various hyperoxic exposures. Inclusion of air breaks in prolonged HBO treatment schedules is a recognized practice. The return to normobaric air between HBO sessions may lead to low pO_2 seizures, which are also described as a "switch off" phenomenon. However, much research still needs to be done to find the ideal schedules to extend oxygen tolerance.

Effect of HBO on the CNS of Newborn Mammals

Newborn mammals are extremely resistant to the CNS effects of HBO compared to adults. Indirect evidence indicates that HBO in newborn rats induces a persistent cerebral vasoconstriction concurrently with a severe and maintained reduction in ventilation. The outcome of these exposures may be as follows:

- Extension of tolerance to both CNS and pulmonary oxygen toxicity,
- Creation of a hypoxic–ischemic condition in vulnerable neuronal structures, and
- Impairment of circulatory and ventilatory responses to hypoxic stimuli on return to air breathing, with subsequent development of a hypoxic–ischemic condition.

These events may set the stage for development of delayed neurological disorders.

Conclusion and Directions for Future Research

The exact mechanism underlying oxygen toxicity to the CNS is not known, but the free radical theory appears to be the most likely explanation. The role of nitric oxide in the effect of HBO has also been established. Fortunately, CNS oxygen toxicity is rare because most HBO treatments are carried out at pressures below 2.5 ATA, and the duration of treatment does not exceed 90 min. Nevertheless, a physician treating patients with HBO must be aware of oxygen toxicity. There is no rational prevention or treatment, but free radical scavengers are used in practice to prevent the toxic effects of oxygen. Until a better understanding of the mechanism of oxygen toxicity and better methods of treatment are available, use of the free radical scavengers that are available appears to be a reasonable practice, particularly when these are relatively nontoxic. In situations where prolonged exposures to HBO are required, the benefits of treatment vs. the risks of oxygen toxicity should be carefully weighed.

The chemiluminescence index, which is a measure of tissue lipid peroxidation, indicates individual sensitivity of the body to HBO. Such a technique would enable the prediction of the effectiveness of HBO treatment as well as control its duration. Oxygen toxicity can also be exploited for therapeutic purposes. One example of this is the use of HBO as an antibiotic. Induced oxygen toxicity by HBO with protection of the patient by free radical scavengers should be investigated as an adjunctive treatment for AIDS, because the virus responsible for this condition has no protective mechanisms against free radicals. Since induction of antioxidative defense mechanisms has been determined after HBO exposure, a modified treatment regimen of HBO therapy may avoid genotoxic effects.

The methods for estimating free radicals are still cumbersome and not in routine use. More practical methods should be developed as a guide to the safe limits of HBO therapy.

The molecular basis of oxygen toxicity should be sought at the cellular and organelle levels. Simultaneous monitoring of cerebral, electrical, circulatory, and energy-producing functions is a useful tool for determining the safety margins of HBO, as well as for tracing the primary mechanisms of oxygen toxicity in the CNS.

Mammalian cell lines have been shown to develop tolerance to oxygen by repetitive exposure to HBO at 6–10 ATA for periods up to 3 h. Repeated screening of various cell lines may lead to the discovery of oxygen-resistant cell types, which might provide an insight into the factors inherent in the development of oxygen tolerance.

The latest approach to counteract pulmonary oxygen toxicity is gene therapy by viral-mediated transfer SOD and catalase to the pulmonary epithelium. This appears to be the most promising method of delivery of these enzymes.

References

Arieli R, Yalov A, Goldenshluger A. Modeling pulmonary and CNS O(2) toxicity and estimation of parameters for humans. J Appl Physiol. 2002;92:248–56.

Balentine JD. Pathology of oxygen toxicity. New York: Academic; 1982.

Bardin H, Lambertsen CJ. A quantitative method for calculating pulmonary toxicity. Use of "unit pulmonary toxicity dose" (UPTD). Institute for Environmental Medicine Report. Philadelphia: University of Pennsylvania; 1970.

Bean JE, Lingnell J, Coulson J. Effects of oxygen at increased pressure. Physiol Rev. 1945;25:1–147.

Behnke AR, Forbes HS, Motley EP. Circulatory and visual effects of oxygen at 3 atmospheres pressure. Am J Physiol. 1936;114:436–42.

Bert P. La pression barométrique. Recherches de physiologie expérimentelle. Paris, G Masson, 1878. Translated by Hitchcock MA and Hitchcock FA and published as Barometric pressure: Researches in Experimental Physiology, College Book Company, Columbus, Ohio, 1943. Reprinted by the Undersea Medical Society, Bethesda, Maryland; 1978.

Boveris A, Chance B. The mitochondrial generation of hydrogen peroxide. Biochem J. 1978;134:707–16.

Demchenko IT, Welty-Wolf KE, Allen BW, Piantadosi CA. Similar but not the same: normobaric and hyperbaric pulmonary oxygen toxicity, the role of nitric oxide. Am J Physiol Lung Cell Mol Physiol. 2007;293:L229–38.

Demchenko IT, Zhilyaev SY, Moskvin AN, Piantadosi CA, Allen BW. Autonomic activation links CNS oxygen toxicity to acute cardiogenic pulmonary injury. Am J Physiol Lung Cell Mol Physiol. 2011;300:L102–11.

Demchenko IT, Mahon RT, Allen BW, Piantadosi CA. Brain oxygenation and CNS oxygen toxicity after infusion of perfluorocarbon emulsion. J Appl Physiol. 2012;113:224–31.

Ezraty B, Chabalier M, Ducret A, Maisonneuve E, Dukan S. CO_2 exacerbates oxygen toxicity. EMBO Rep. 2011;12:321–6.

Farmery S, Sykes O. Neurological oxygen toxicity. Emerg Med J. 2012;29:851–2.

Gleissner MW, Spantzel T, Bucker-Nott HJ, Jorch G. Risk factors of retinopathy of prematurity in infants 32 to 36 weeks gestational age. Z Geburtshilfe Neonatol. 2003;207:24–8.

Jain KK. Oxygen in physiology and medicine. Springfield: Charles C. Thomas; 1989.

Koch AE, Kähler W, Wegner-Bröse H, Weyer D, Kuhtz-Buschbeck J, Deuschl G, et al. Monitoring of CBFV and time characteristics of oxygen-induced acute CNS toxicity in humans. Eur J Neurol. 2008;15:746–8.

Liu S, Li R, Ni X, Cai Z, Zhang R, Sun X, et al. Perfluorocarbon-facilitated CNS oxygen toxicity in rats: reversal by edaravone. Brain Res. 2012;1471:56–65.

Liu AZ, Bao XC, Fang YQ, Sang ZN, Li HJ, Zhang WQ. The change of NOS in pulmonary oxygen toxicity induced by different oxygen pressure. Zhongguo Ying Yong Sheng Li Xue Za Zhi. 2014;30:227–9.

Min L, Jian-Xing X. Detoxifying function of cytochrome c against oxygen toxicity. Mitochondrion. 2007;7:13–6.

Pilla R, Landon CS, Dean JB. A potential early physiological marker for CNS oxygen toxicity: hyperoxic hyperpnea precedes seizure in unanesthetized rats breathing hyperbaric oxygen. J Appl Physiol. 2013;114:1009–20.

Priestley J. The discovery of oxygen (1775), part 1. In: Faulconer A, Keys TC, editors. Foundations of anesthesiology, vol. 1. Springfield: Charles C. Thomas; 1965. p. 39–70.

Smith JL. The Pathological effects due to increase of oxygen tension in air breathed. J Physiol. 1899;24:19–35.

Tiwari KK, Moorthy B, Lingappan K. Role of GDF15 (growth and differentiation factor 15) in pulmonary oxygen toxicity. Toxicol In Vitro. 2015;29:1369–76.

Yen CC, Lai YW, Chen HL, Lai CW, Lin CY, Chen W, et al. Aerosolized human extracellular superoxide dismutase prevents hyperoxia-induced lung injury. PLoS One. 2011;6, e26870.

K.K. Jain

Abstract

This chapter deals with the equipment used in hyperbaric medicine. Main components are hyperbaric chambers of various types, e.g., monoplace, multiplace, and mobile as well as those used for diving medicine. Advantages and limitations of each type of chamber are given. Various techniques of hyperbaric oxygenation (HBO) are described. A wide variety of ancillary equipment is used for monitoring of patients in the hyperbaric chamber. Safety in the hyperbaric chamber is an important consideration and regulatory issues relevant to hyperbaric medicine should be taken into consideration. Finally, there is discussion of staffing of hyperbaric facilities.

Keywords

Compressed air • Diving chambers • Fire safety in chambers • HBO • Hyperbaric chamber • Hyperbaric oxygen • Mobile chambers • Monoplace chambers • Multiplace chambers • Oxygen masks • Patient monitoring devices • Ventilators for hyperbaric environments

Introduction

The main facility required for hyperbaric medicine is of course the hyperbaric chamber itself. This is essentially a chamber constructed to withstand pressurization, so that oxygen can be administered inside at pressures greater than at sea level. Mostly the chambers are hard shell constructed from metal, but soft shell mobile monoplace chambers are also available. Essential parts of a hard shell chamber are view ports (windows) made of acrylic and control panel for monitoring pressure and gas content as well as the patient's condition and two-way communication from outside to inside of the chamber. The size, shape, and pressure capabilities of the designs chambers vary considerably. The technical details of each model now available are provided by the manufacturers, and a classification of various types of chambers is shown in Table 7.1.

K.K. Jain, MD, FRACS, FFPM (✉)
1 Blaesiring 7, Basel 4057, Switzerland
e-mail: jain@pharmabiotech.ch

Monoplace Chambers

Monoplace chambers are the most commonly used; in most of them the pressure cannot be raised over 3 ATA. The patient can be transferred into this chamber on a gurney, and the chamber is filled with oxygen under pressure. There are two types of oxygen flow mechanisms:

- Constant purging: This type has a fixed rate of oxygen flow through the chamber and out again to the external environment.
- Recycling: This type recycles all or a portion of the gases, which are used again after they are properly cleaned and unwanted CO_2 and water vapor are absorbed. Communication with the patient is through an intercom.

Advantages of monoplace chambers are:

1. Handling of patients individually; privacy and, in case of infection, isolation.
2. Ideal for recovery room and transfer within hospital departments by a chamber with storable gurney

Table 7.1 Types of hyperbaric chambers

1. Monoplace
2. Multiplace or "walk-in" chambers
3. Mobile or portable
– Monoplace: transportable by air, sea, or land
– Multiplace: chamber can be driven from place to place
4. Chambers for testing and training divers
5. Small hyperbaric chambers
– For neonates
– For animal experiments

(OxyHeal 1000 series). There is no interruption of medical treatment as the patient can stay in the chamber during transfer.

3. It is comfortable. Face mask not required and there is no danger of oxygen leak.
4. Ideal for patients confined to bed in acute stage of illness or injury, e.g., paraplegics.
5. Easy to observe patient inside the chamber.
6. No special decompression procedures required.
7. Economy of space and cost; can be easily moved and placed anywhere in hospital.
8. Fewer operators required.

The disadvantages of monoplace chambers are:

- There is a potential fire hazard in an oxygen-filled environment.
- Direct access to the patient is very limited, except in the case of modified chambers with a side room for the attendant (Reneau dual compartment).
- Monoplace ventilators are less advanced and require the use of muscle relaxants and excessive sedation.
- Intravenous lines must be changed to specially designed IV pumps located outside the chamber with chamber pass-through and risk of inaccurate drug delivery (Lind 2015).
- Physical therapy cannot be carried out in the limited space.
- It is difficult to provide an "air brake" for a patient with decompression sickness unless the patient is conscious, cooperative, and able to put on a mask himself.

This design is ideal for the care of a patient who does not require the presence of medical personnel in the chamber. Most of the essential body functions can be monitored externally, and even the respirator can be controlled from outside the chamber.

A Sechrist monoplace chamber, in common use in the USA, is shown in Fig. 7.1. The design of a monoplace chamber for an acute care facility or an intensive care unit is shown in Fig. 7.2. An example of a small 1-man portable chamber is the Hyperlite folding hyperbaric chamber (SOS Ltd, London, UK) shown in Fig. 7.3. It is made of modern lightweight material and can be easily pressurized on site and then transferred under pressure to and into virtually any therapeutic facility. It is suitable for diving complications, trauma, and other emergency indications for HBO. It may be useful for the emergency treatment of acute stroke.

Another transportable chamber which is in development is the Gamow bag, which can be carried as a back pack and pressurized when required. It has been found to be useful for treating high altitude illness. The pressure limit of the original bag is set at 2 psi because of the fragility of the fabric. However, improvement of the hardware to make the bag capable of withstanding higher pressures has made it possible to perform standard HBO therapy with the newly devised portable chamber, the Chamberlite 15. In this study, the safety of the new bag was examined using healthy human volunteers, and the bag was shown to be usable in clinical emergency cases, such as CO intoxication and decompression sickness (Shimada et al. 1996). The effectiveness of emergency hyperbaric oxygen therapy was also examined using the CO intoxication model of the rat. Evidence suggested that HBO was especially beneficial if applied during the first 30 min of rescue work. It was concluded that the transportable chamber was a promising emergency tool for CO intoxication. This bag can be considered for HBO treatment of acute stroke patients during transport to a medical center.

Multiplace Chambers

Multiplace chambers are used for simultaneous treatment of a number of patients. The capacity varies from a few to as many as 20 patients. The chamber is filled with air and breathing is done via a mask covering the mouth and nose. Modern chambers of this type are fitted with a comprehensive gas supply and monitoring systems; the gas composition in the chamber is monitored and corrected, particularly if there are oxygen leaks from the masks. The atmosphere is air-conditioned for humidity as well as temperature. Examples of multiplace hyperbaric chambers manufactured in the USA are:

- Dual OxyHeal 2000 Hyperbaric chamber (OxyHeal Health Group). A pair of Class A multiplace hyperbaric chambers accommodate 4 occupants (Fig. 7.4).
- OxyHeal 4000 Multiplace hyperbaric chamber (OxyHeal Health Group). A 3-lock, 6 ATA, 18-patient horizontal cylinder Class A hyperbaric chamber system is used for critical care treatments (Fig. 7.5).
- OxyHeal 5000 Rectangular Chamber (OxyHeal Health Group). The 3 ATA hyperbaric chamber complex Class A hyperbaric chamber is designed to accommodate 12 patients and to perform critical care (Fig. 7.6).

Uses and advantages of multiplace chambers are as follows:

Fig. 7.1 The Sechrist monoplace hyperbaric chamber

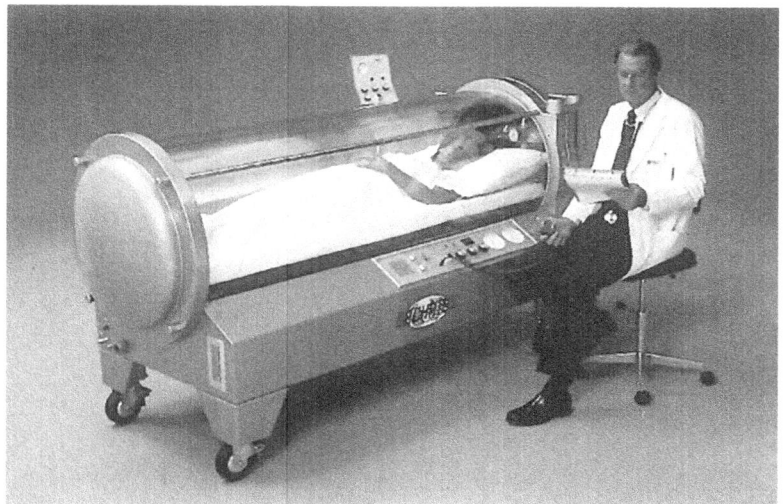

Fig. 7.2 Monitoring and routine care functions for acute medical care in a monoplace chamber

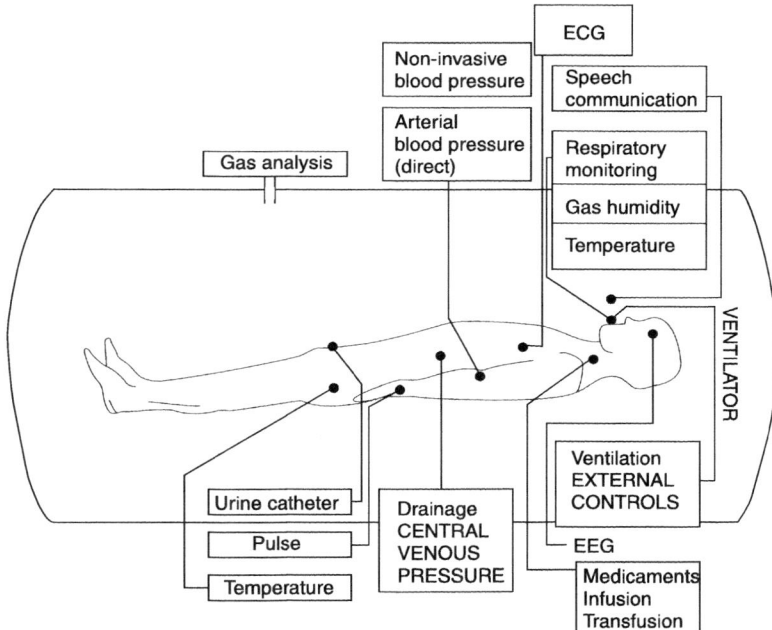

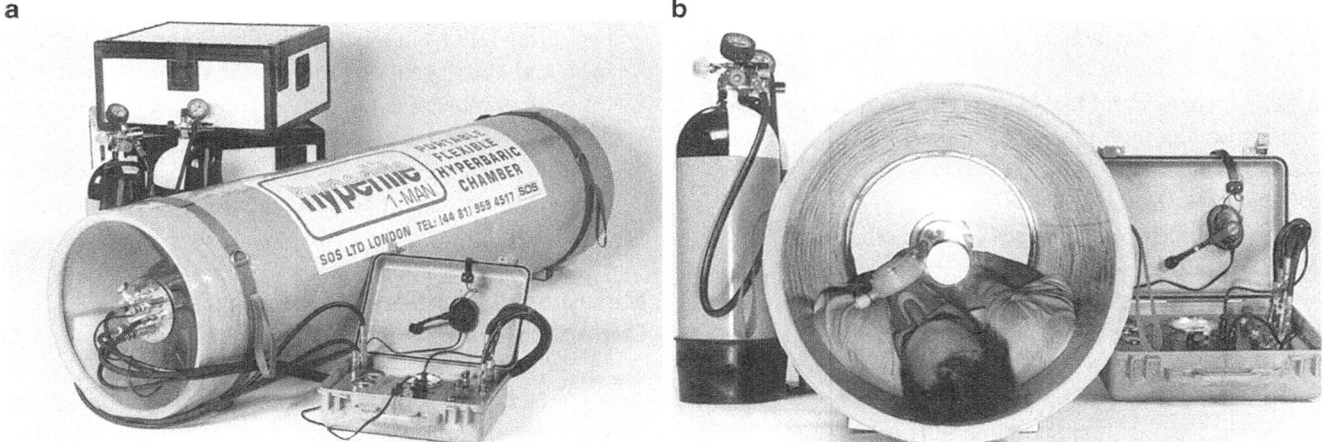

Fig. 7.3 (**a**, **b**) The Hyperlite 1-man portable hyperbaric chamber. Photos courtesy of SOS Ltd, London, UK

Fig. 7.4 A pair of OxyHeal 2000 Class A multiplace hyperbaric chambers. These 3 ATA chambers accommodate four occupants. All BIBS gases can be controlled internally or externally. An extension tube permits the introduction of supine patients. Low-voltage automated devices with manual back-ups control treatments. Photo courtesy of OxyHeal Health Group, La Jolla, CA 92038, USA

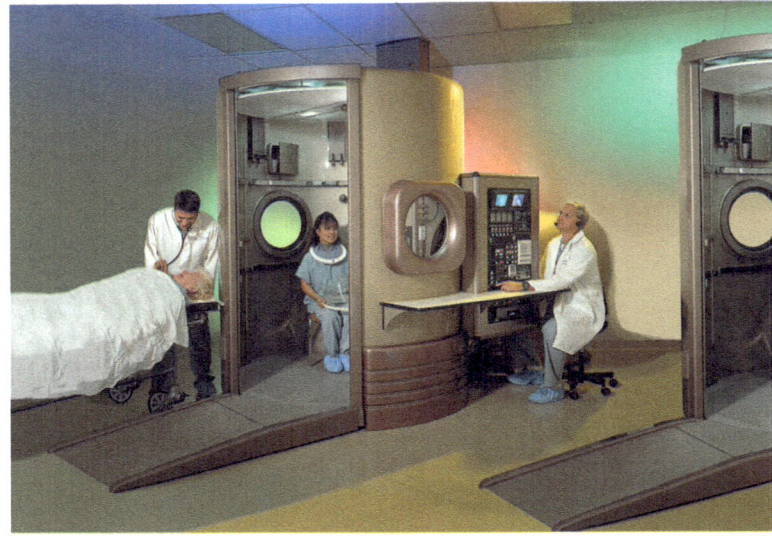

Fig. 7.5 OxyHeal 4000 Class A Multiplace hyperbaric chamber. A 3-lock, 6 ATA, 18-patient horizontal cylinder hyperbaric chamber system at Presbyterian/St. Luke's Hospital in Denver, Colorado, USA. This chamber performs a significant number of critical care treatments annually. Photo courtesy of OxyHeal Health Group, La Jolla, CA 92038, USA

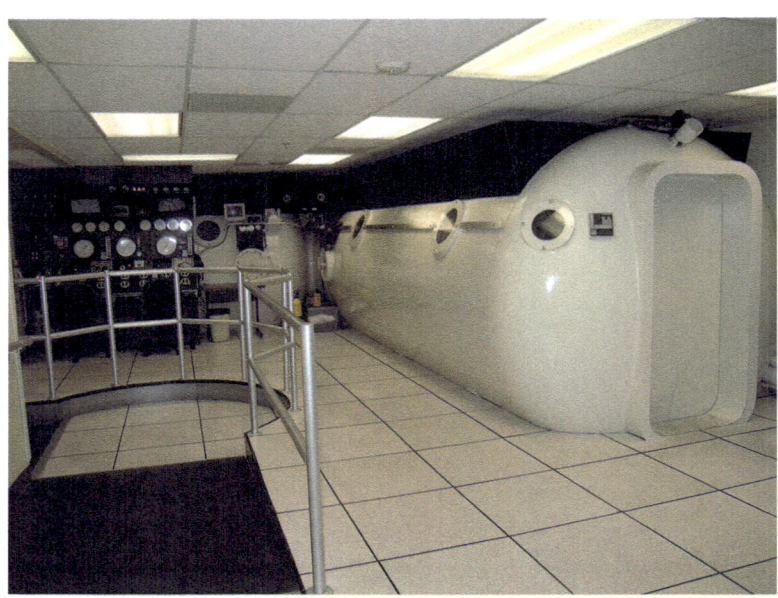

1. Simultaneous treatment of a large number of patients is possible.
2. They are essential for treatment that requires presence of a physician and special equipment, as in an operating room.
3. There is reduced fire hazard.
4. Physical therapy can be performed in the chamber.
5. Sports physiology and physical therapy research. A treadmill is placed in the chamber and all the necessary investigations can be done while the patient exercises in the chamber particularly for patients with stroke, peripheral vascular disease, and myocardial ischemia.
6. "Brain jogging" using computer-based mental exercises and psychological testing can be performed in the chamber during HBO administration. This is useful in the treatment and assessment of patients with cognitive deficits.
7. Pressure can be raised to 6 ATA for special situations in air embolism and decompression sickness.
8. Multiplace chamber is better suited for HBO therapy in the critical care department and intensive care units (ICU).

Multiplace Chambers for the Critical Care Department

A multiplace chamber is better suited for HBO therapy of critically ill patients with failing vital functions and organ systems, primarily because it permits appropriate ICU

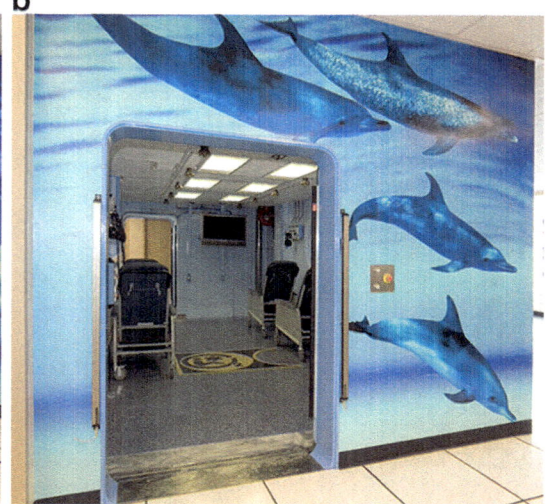

Fig. 7.6 (**a**) OxyHeal 5000 Rectangular Chamber. The 3 ATA hyperbaric chamber complex adjoining the Regional Burn Center at the University Medical Center, Las Vegas, Nevada, USA. The complex consists of a large two-lock rectangular geometry Class A hyperbaric chamber designed to accommodate 12-patients and to perform critical care. The OxyHeal 2000, shown in the foreground, is used to enable routine hyperbaric treatments when the larger chamber is performing critical care treatments. The chamber complex Control Console operates both hyperbaric systems. (**b**) OxyHeal 5000 Rectangular Chamber Interior. The view shows non-dedicated seating, large entertainment screen, and floor level doors large enough to roll a hospital bed into. Underwater scene murals are applied in order to reduce patient anxiety. Photo courtesy of OxyHeal Health Group, La Jolla, CA 92038, USA

equipment to be used inside the chamber by accompanying staff. Normal "hands-on" intensive care continues during HBO therapy with close attention to all aspects of critical patient care (Lind 2015). Multiplace hyperbaric chambers can be used to deliver patient care with enormous flexibility. Standard critical care techniques, such as mechanical ventilation, endotracheal suctioning, hemodynamic monitoring, blood gas measurement, and emergency therapy such as cardiopulmonary resuscitation can be performed inside a multiplace chamber. The multiplace chamber can be considered an extension of the ICU. This flexibility is accompanied by increased complexity of chamber operation. Defibrillation plays a crucial role in the resuscitation of patients from acute life-threatening cardiac dysrhythmias causing cardiac arrest. Concerns over safety and function of defibrillators under pressure have so far prevented their routine use in clinical hyperbaric chambers. Now increasing numbers of unstable and critically ill patients are being treated in such facilities.

Surgery in the Multiplace Chamber

Minor surgical procedures can be performed in the usual multiplace hyperbaric chamber, but major surgery such as heart surgery requires a specially designed chamber. There are many such chambers in existence in the USSR and Japan, but few in Europe (Graz and Amsterdam). The hyperbaric chamber with an operating room located at the University of Nagoya, Japan, is shown in Fig. 7.7. There are some technical problems of surgery in a hyperbaric chamber as some types of equipment cannot be operated in a chamber, e.g., electrocoagulation for hemostasis.

Mobile Multiplace Hyperbaric Chambers

The first mobile multiplace chamber was constructed in the form of a bus in Nagoya, Japan, but it is no longer in use. Other mobile chambers are now available, in various locations throughout the world. An OxyHeal 4000 triple lock, 6 ATA, 18-patient mobile hyperbaric chamber (OxyHeal-HealthGroup) resides within the over-the-road trailer. This chamber complex is now permanently installed on a roof of the Hermann Hospital in Houston, Texas, USA, where it has been in continuous operation since 1990. OxyHeal 4000 dual lock, 6 ATA, 12-patient hyperbaric chamber (OxyHeal Health Group), shown in Fig. 7.8 is placed next to the emergency department of Advocate/Lutheran General Hospital in Park Ridge, Illinois, USA. This was one of the first American hospitals to perform hyperbaric surgeries and the hyperbaric center there has been in continuous operation since the early 1960s.

The advantages of a mobile chamber are:

- It can be moved where needed. It can function, for instance, in the parking lot of a hospital.
- It is comfortable and safe.
- It is ideal for clinical use as well as for research.

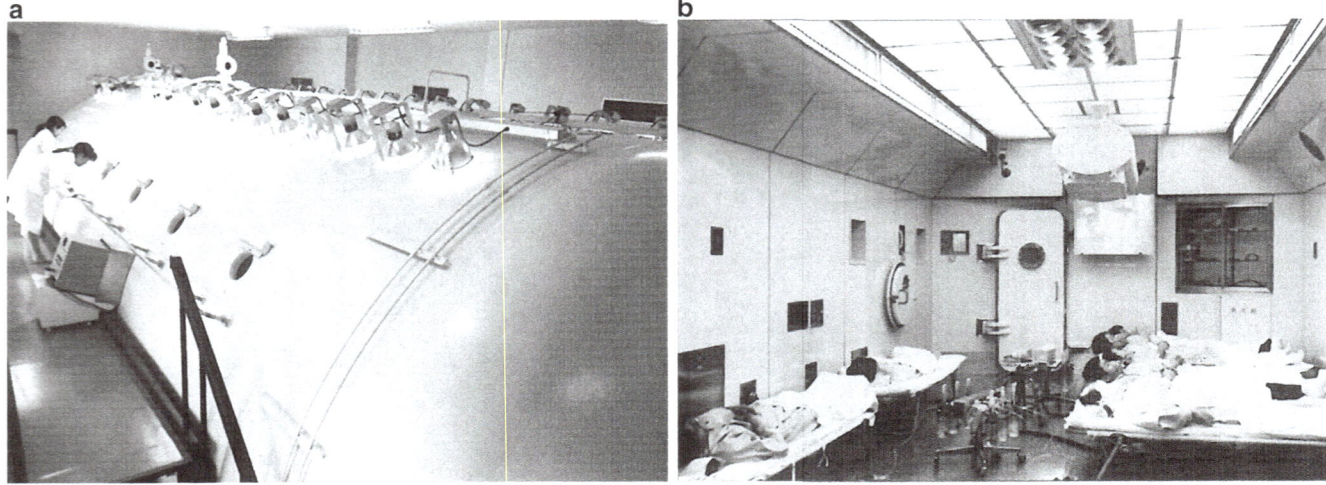

Fig. 7.7 (**a**) Large hyperbaric chamber at the University of Nagoya, Japan, outside view. (**b**) Inside view. Operations can be carried out in this chamber

Fig. 7.8 Mobile hyperbaric system interior. An OxyHeal 4000 dual lock, 6 ATA, 12-patient hyperbaric chamber inside a 52′ over-the-road trailer, installed adjoining the Emergency Room at Advocate/Lutheran General Hospital in Park Ridge, Illinois, USA. Photo courtesy of OxyHeal Health Group, La Jolla, CA 92038, USA

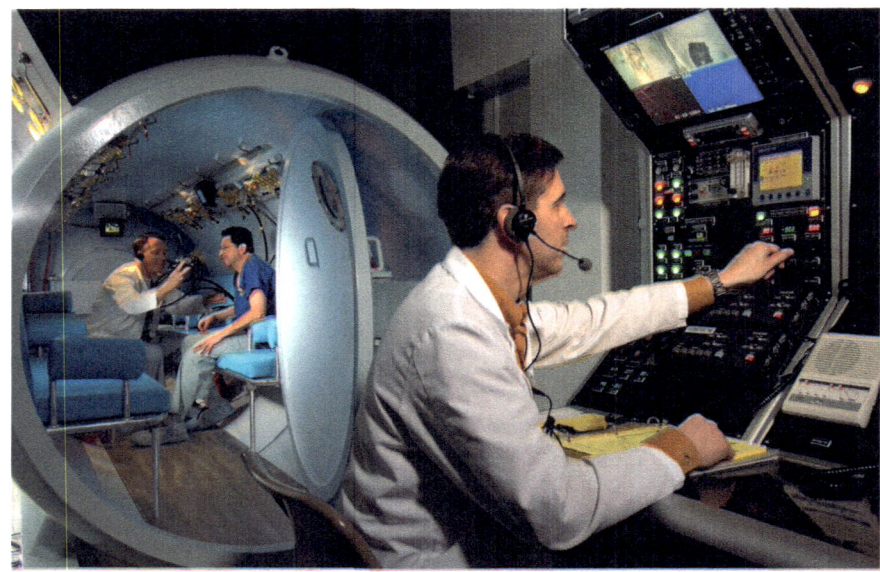

- It is suitable for use in military medicine. It can be moved to the base hospital in case of war. It can also be transported by air and sea.
- Emergency treatment of the patient with stroke, myocardial infarction and CNS injuries can be carried out during long-distance transport in the chamber.

Hyperbaric Chambers for Diving Medicine

Diving chambers are used for testing and training divers with simulated depths. These facilities can be combined with hyperbaric chambers for patient treatment in a hyperbaric center. An example of this is shown in Fig. 7.9.

Hyperbaric Chambers for Animal Research

Hyperbaric chambers have been constructed for use in experiments with small animals. Small portable chambers are available for resuscitation of newborns. A specially designed chamber for animal experiments is shown in Fig. 7.10. OxyCure 3000 Hyperbaric Cellular Incubator (OxyHeal Health Group) is a class C chamber with controls for the pressure, gases, temperature, and humidity shown in Fig. 7.11. It is used in cellular studies and to induce autologous stem cell replication.

A novel preclinical rodent-sized pressure chamber system has been developed that is compatible with computed tomography (CT), positron emission tomography (PET), and magnetic resonance imaging (MRI) and enables continuous uncompromised and minimally invasive data acquisition throughout hyperbaric exposures (Hansen et al. 2015). This pressure chamber system is compatible with CT, PET, and MRI. No correction in image intensity was required with pressurization up to 1.013 mPa for any of the imaging modalities. However, CT demonstrated an increase in

Hounsfield units in proportion to the pressure. Pressurization induced no effect on the longitudinal relaxation rate (R_1) for MRI, whereas the transversal relaxation rate (R_2) changed slightly. The R_2 data further revealed an association between pressure and the concentration of the paramagnetic nuclei gadolinium, the contrast agent used to mimic different tissues in the MRI phantoms.

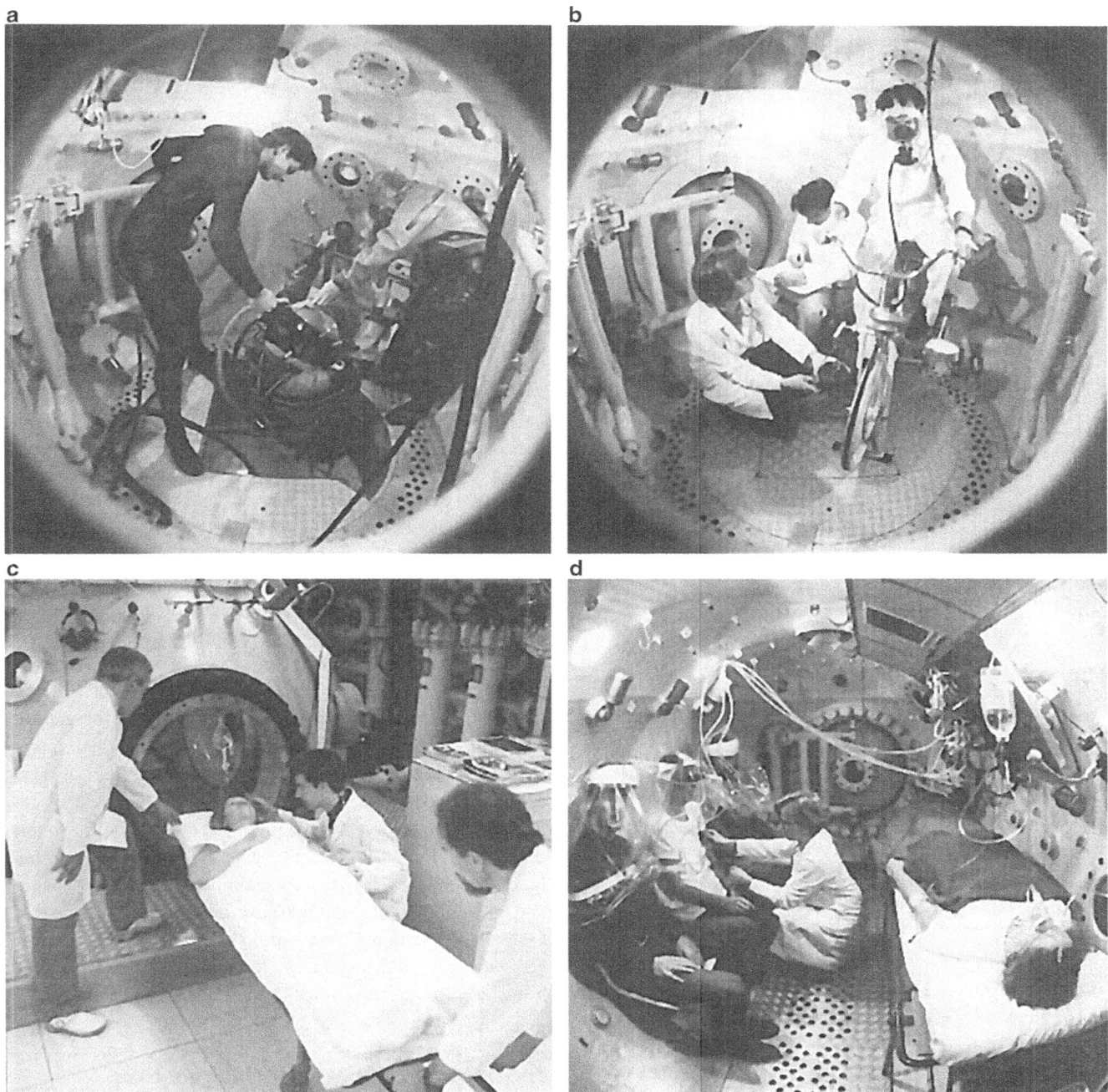

Fig. 7.9 Combined treatment and diver testing hyperbaric chamber at the University Hospital, Zurich, Switzerland. (**a**) Diving testing; (**b**) exercise testing; (**c**) a patient being transferred into the chamber on a special device; (**d**) patients being treated inside the chamber—note the oxygen tents used by the patients; (**e**) overall view. This chamber can be used for simulating dives to depths of 1000 m and high altitude simulation up to 10,000 m

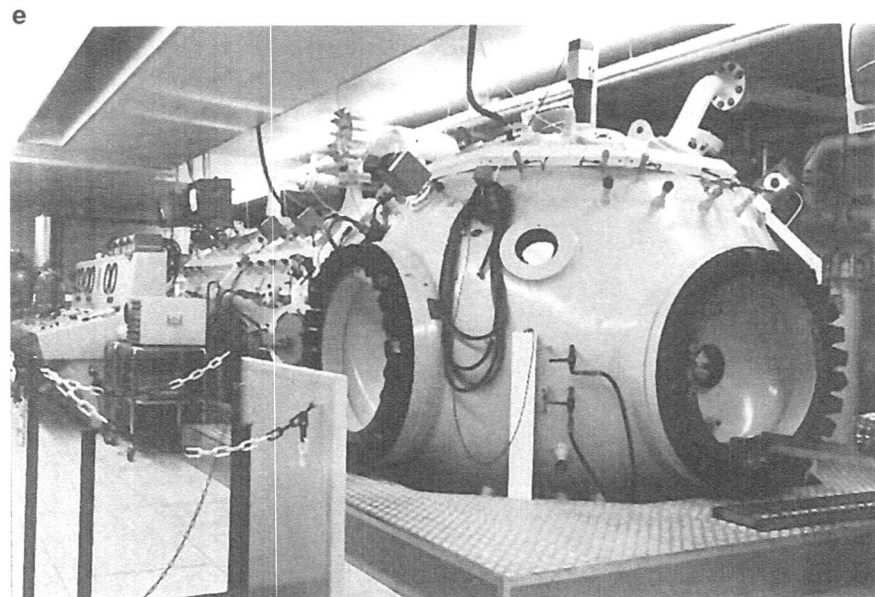

Fig. 7.9 (continued)

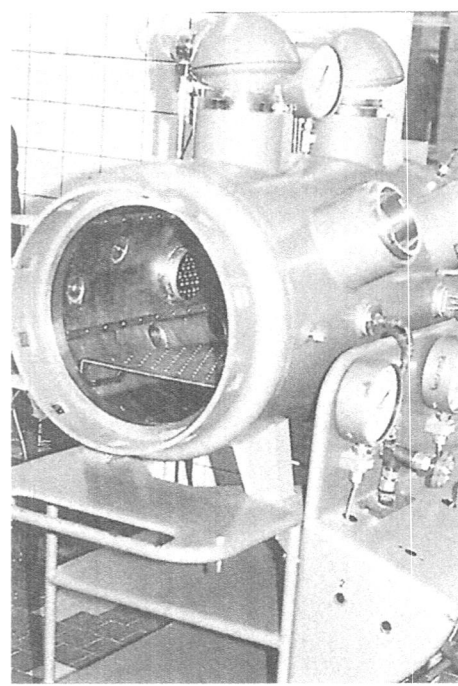

Fig. 7.10 A hyperbaric chamber for animal experiments at the All Union Center for Surgical Research, Moscow

Selection of a Hyperbaric Chamber

A classification of hyperbaric chambers according to pressure, size, and uses is shown in Table 7.2. Most of the indications (90 %) can be covered by chambers of types I and II. Pressure up to 2.5 ATA is not only the upper limit for most applications, it is also the starting point for compulsory inspection by the technical inspection agency (TÜV) in Germany. This classification may help the manufacturer as well as the consumer to choose a chamber within a certain category. It would be uneconomical to make all the chambers capable of withstanding a pressure of 6 ATA. Two indications for which pressures of 6 ATA have been used in the past, i.e., decompression sickness and air embolism, are being reassessed. For both these conditions, the highest pressures required may not exceed 3 ATA, as discussed in Chaps. 11 and 12.

The hyperbaric chamber is a durable piece of equipment and many old chambers are still performing well. The safety record has been good. However, as in any other technology, there is constant evolution and improvement. The latest addition to the hyperbaric chamber family is the mobile multiplace chamber. This chamber gives us an ideal opportunity to conduct further investigations in the field of rehabilitation and sports medicine. Another advantage of the mobile chamber is that the equipment can be moved to any desired location at short notice with no necessity for installation procedures. Hyperbaric chambers are still expensive, and the number of chambers available is not adequate to treat all the patients who would potentially benefit from HBO therapy. In this situation, the mobile hyperbaric chamber is an economical proposition.

Technique of Hyperbaric Oxygenation

The schedules of pressure for different diseases are listed in the appropriate chapters. We restrict ourselves here to some general comments about technique.

Fig. 7.11 OxyCure 3000 Hyperbaric Cellular Incubator for cellular studies. Photo courtesy of OxyHeal Health Group, La Jolla, CA 92038, USA

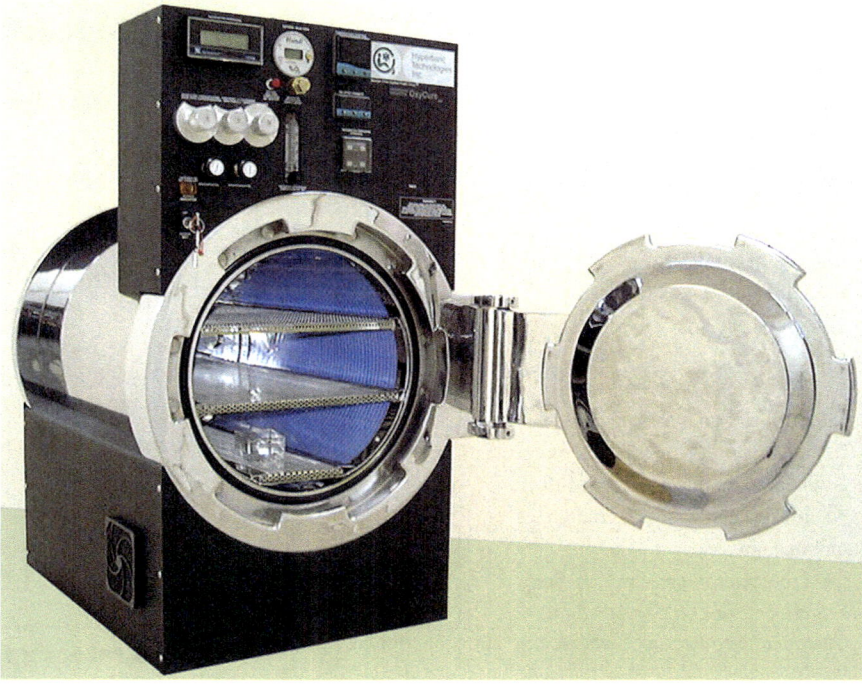

Table 7.2 Classification of hyperbaric chambers according to use and pressure

Type	Pressure	Type	Typical indications
I	Up to 1.5 ATA	Mobile and multiplace	Ischemic disorders: cerebral, cardiac, peripheral-vascular: adjuvant to physical therapy and sports medicine; adjuvant to survival of skin flaps; acoustic trauma
II	Up to 2.5 ATA	Monoplace and portable	Gas gangrene
	Up to 3.0 ATA		Burns
			Crush injuries of extremities
			Emergency treatment of decompression sickness
III	Up to 6.0 ATA	Multiplace	Air embolism
			Decompression sickness

The hyperbaric technician follows the prescribed instructions from the hyperbaric physician about the pressure, duration, and frequency of treatment. Most of the treatments at our hyperbaric center are given at pressures between 1.5 and 2.5 ATA, and the usual duration of a hyperbaric session is 45 min. Of this, 10 min are required for compression and 5 min for decompression if pressures of 1.5 ATA are used. Thus, the maximal oxygen saturation is maintained for about 0.5 h. In the case of infections, the treatment duration is doubled. The treatment sessions for most chronic conditions are given daily, including weekends. For the multiplace chamber, patients are grouped according to indications. For example, all stroke patients are grouped to go in the same session and are accompanied by a physiotherapist or a physician if a research project is involved. The technician keeps a complete log of the session and the data can be recorded and reproduced by com-

puter. Compression and decompression are quite smooth, and if the patient complains of any discomfort such as ear pain, the procedure can be halted. In case of a more severe problem, the affected patient can be moved to the anteroom of the multiplace chamber and decompression started while the treatment of the remaining patients is continued in the main chamber with the door between the two chambers locked.

In the case of a monoplace chamber, oxygen is introduced into the chamber at the start while pressure is raised. In the multiplace chamber, oxygen masks are used and oxygen inhalation is started only when the chamber has been pressurized to the desired level.

Oxygen partial pressures are not measured routinely, but only for research purposes or in some special cases. Most of the measured values of paO_2 are around 1000 mmHg at 1.5 ATA.

Table 7.3 Ancillary equipment for the hyperbaric chamber

1. Oxygen masks and hoods
2. Respirators and ventilators
3. Miscellaneous equipment for treatment
Cardiopulmonary resuscitation apparatus
Endotracheal tubes
Suction equipment
Intravenous infusions
4. Equipment for diagnosis
Basic medical examination tray
Transcutaneous oxygen measurement
EEG
ECG
Blood gases and hemorrheology equipment
Intracranial pressure and CSF oxygen tension monitors
Blood pressure measurement cuff
5. Neurological assessment equipment
Ophthalmoscope
Dynamometer to measure spasticity
6. Equipment for exercise: treadmill
7. Therapeutic equipment such as cervical traction for cervical spine injuries

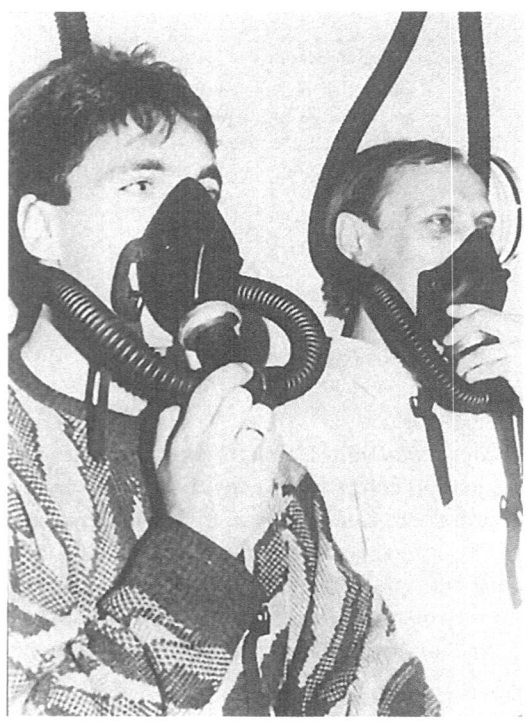

Fig. 7.12 Oxygen masks for use in hyperbaric chambers

Ancillary Equipment

Various types of ancillary equipment are listed in Table 7.3.

Oxygen Masks and Hoods

Oxygen masks are required only in the multiplace hyperbaric chambers. The mask should fit tightly and not allow any leakage of oxygen. The US Air Force aviator's mask, when properly fitted, has end-inspired oxygen levels of 96.9–99 %, and paO_2 of 1640 mmHg is reached at 2.4 ATA. One type of mask in common use is shown in Fig. 7.12. The masks are made of rubber or silicon and can be cleaned and disinfected easily. Headbands of the masks can be placed easily. Oxygen hoods and oxygen tents have been used as an alternative to the masks and are particularly useful in patients with head and neck lesions.

Respirators and Ventilators

Various ventilators found to be effective in hyperbaric environments at pressures up to 6 ATA are:

- The Sechrist model 500A mechanical ventilator, shown in Fig. 7.13, for use with the Sechrist monoplace chamber. Patients with respiratory failure can be placed in it and it will compensate for changes in pressure inside the chamber. Its specifications are shown in Table 7.4.
- The Penlon Oxford ventilator: this is a bellows type, volume-set, timed-cycle device and is used at some medical facilities.
- The Siemens Servo ventilators—sophisticated, volume-set, timed-cycle devices used in intensive care units.
- The Monaghan 225 ventilator is driven by compressed air rather than oxygen. At 1 ATA, this ventilator delivers between 35 and 40 L of the gas/min to the patient. Although this ventilator functions satisfactorily, gas delivery drops to 18 L/min, still adequate for the majority of patients.

The desirable features of a ventilator for hyperbaric environments are:

- No electrically driven components.
- Volume and rate remain stable with all changes in pressure.
- Low oxygen bleeds into the chamber to prevent contamination of the air inside.

Table 7.4 Specifications of the hyperbaric ventilator, Model 500A (Sechrist)

Principals of function	Automatic adjustment of delivery pressure of ventilation to variations of pressure in the hyperbaric chamber
Regulating system	Two components: breathing circuit in the chamber and control module outside the chamber
Respiratory frequency	8–30 breaths/min
Respiratory minute volume	0–15 L/min at 3 ATA
Tidal volume range	0–1.5 L at 3 ATA
Breathing time relationship (inspiration: expiration)	1:5–3.5:1
Respiratory flow range	0–100 L/min at ambient
	0–60 L/min at 3 ATA
Inspiratory pressure	20–80 cm water limit

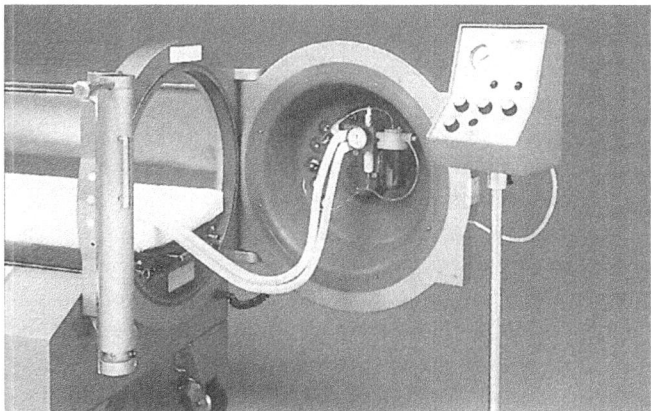

Fig. 7.13 Sechrist Model 500A Mechanical Ventilator for the Sechrist monoplace hyperbaric system. Photo courtesy of Sechrist Industries Inc., Anaheim, CA

- Continuous flow in intermittent mandatory ventilation is superior to a demand valve, as it minimizes the inspiratory work and maintains a constant airway pressure.

Diagnostic Equipment

Basic medical diagnostic equipment such as reflex hammers, stethoscope, and ophthalmoscope should be available in the chamber.

ECG and EEG

ECG and EEG pose no special problems and should be standard in chambers for treating patients with cardiovascular and cerebrovascular disorders. Changes in the signal quality of ECG can occur with high pressures. EEG power spectrum recording can be performed quite satisfactorily in the hyperbaric chamber. Somatosensory-evoked potential studies can also be conducted.

Transcutaneous Oxygen Tension

Transcutaneous oxygen tension ($tcpO_2$) measurement is a noninvasive technique for measuring oxygen tension of the tissues by means of an electrode taped on the skin. It cannot be used in the monoplace chamber, as the electrodes are electrically heated and constitute a fire hazard. The results of measurements of $tcpO_2$ in volunteers breathing air and HBO up to 4 ATA show close correlation with pO_2 values measured directly in blood from arterial puncture inside the hyperbaric chamber. In patients with various degrees of peripheral vascular occlusive disease, the $tcpO_2$ are significantly lower than in control subjects.

Blood gases should ideally be determined inside the chamber due to the problem of release of gases if the sample is brought outside to sea-level pressure. Several blood gas analysis systems have been modified to function inside the hyperbaric chamber. Blood samples of gases can also be analyzed at the pressure of measurement with specially calibrated equipment. The ratio of arterial to alveolar pO_2 (*a/A* ratio) is a constant, independent of the inspired oxygen concentration. This is also true at elevated atmospheric pressure, in healthy volunteers as well as patients. It is possible to predict the paO_2 at 3 ATA from the values obtained at 1 ATA.

Glucose-Monitoring Devices

Diabetic patients may experience fluctuations in blood glucose levels during HBO treatment for ischemic non-healing wounds. Therefore, whole blood glucose levels should be monitored during treatment. Most of the currently marketed glucose monitoring devices (glucometers) measure glucose with glucose oxidase or glucose dehydrogenase-based methods. Glucose dehydrogenase methods do not utilize oxygen, but inaccuracies have been reported between measurements at ground level and at 2.36 ATA. Glucose oxidase-impregnated reagent strips are affected because both high and low pressures of oxygen interfere with enzymatic reactions involved which utilize oxygen.

Use of Miscellaneous Medical Devices in the Hyperbaric Chamber

Cardiopulmonary Resuscitation

Basic cardiopulmonary resuscitation equipment should be available in the chamber. Endotracheal tubes and Foley catheter cuffs should be inflated with water or saline instead of air. Suction can be generated in the chamber by compressed air or made available from outside through a pressure reduction regulator. Special injection kits for intravenous infusion are available from the manufacturers for use in their chambers. In the case of monoplace chambers, special precautions are necessary when running an intravenous infusion because of the difference between chamber pressure and external pressure. A treadmill motor can be placed under the hyperbaric chamber and the motion transmitted by a shaft through the floor of the chamber (see Fig. 7.10).

Use of Defibrillators in Hyperbaric Chambers

Electrical defibrillation is the only effective therapy for cardiac arrest caused by ventricular fibrillation or pulseless ventricular tachycardia. Defibrillation under hyperbaric conditions is inherently dangerous owing to the risk of fire, but it can be conducted safely if certain precautions are taken. New defibrillators have been introduced for hyperbaric medicine, which makes the procedure easier technically, nevertheless sparks and fire have been observed during defibrillation, even under normobaric conditions. Therefore, delivery of defibrillation shock in a hyperbaric environment is still considered to be a hazardous procedure (Kot 2014).

Pleural Suction Drainage

Pleural suction drainage systems can be dramatically affected by pressure change, but can be used safely in a hyperbaric environment provided that the following precautions are taken (Walker et al. 2006):

- Suction should not be applied during pressurization.
- Pressurization needs to be slow, 10 kPa/min or less.
- Suction must be applied during depressurization if there is an air leak of 5/min or greater coming from the patient, otherwise suction is not essential.
- Hyperbaric compatibility should be tested before use.

Endotracheal Tubes

Humidification of inspired gas is critical in ventilated patients who are treated in hyperbaric chambers. This is usually achieved by heat and moisture exchange devices and the endotracheal tube adds airflow resistance. Increased gas density may increase total airway resistance, peak pressures, and mechanical work of breathing under hyperbaric conditions, particularly if the endotracheal tubes are <8 mm (Arieli et al. 2011). Use of the largest possible endotracheal tube is recommended to reduce work of breathing in the chamber.

Care of Tracheotomy

HBO therapy has been in patients with anastomotic complications after tracheal repair and shown to promote healing. Patients with tracheostomy experience increased respiratory distress inside the chamber due to increased density of the respired gases and the narrowing of the airway lumen by the tracheostomy. Because patients with tracheostomy cannot breathe through a facemask, two other options remain to deliver oxygen to patients treated in a multiplace chamber. The first option is to use a hood; however, most of the hoods will not be suitable for these patients because the neck seal of the hood corresponds to the tracheostomy opening. The second option is to attach a T-tube to the tracheostomy, which separately provides inspiration and expiration from the two limbs. However, this technique dramatically increases the respiratory resistance and makes breathing extremely hard for the patient. Therefore, monoplace chambers, which are compressed with oxygen and in which the patients breathe directly from the surroundings without the need for accessories, will be more suitable and comfortable for these patients (Uzun and Mutluoglu 2015). Patients with tracheostomy might require myringotomy or tympanostomy tube placement to avoid middle ear barotrauma, because they will not be able to efficiently autoinflate their middle ear compartment. Finally, the tracheostomy tube cuff in patients undergoing HBO treatment should, preferably, be inflated with water rather than air. Air-filled cuffs will shrink at high pressure and cause the tracheostomy tube to be displaced.

Continuous Bladder Irrigation and HBO

Radiation-induced hemorrhagic cystitis is complication of radiation therapy and HBO is used to support the healing process (see Chap. 17). Continuous bladder irrigation (CBI) is often required to prevent further clot formation, accumulation, and obstruction. This should not be stopped during

HBO treatment and a method of providing CBI in a monoplace hyperbaric chamber has been described as used in patients (Cooper et al. 2015). An IV to catheter adapter is used to enable an IV pump to control CBI flow into the chamber. Drainage is collected in an extra-large (2–5 L) bag. The rate is set, so the volume does not exceed the bag's capacity. The bag is placed in a manner that avoids spilling and allows monitoring of outflow.

Transdermal Patches for Drug Delivery and Hyperbaric Chamber

Transdermal patches are commonly used for drug delivery. HBO safety protocols usually require all transdermal products to be removed prior to entrance into the hyperbaric chamber, and many institutional policies state that removed patches are not to be reapplied. For patients with painful conditions who are undergoing HBO for conditions such as osteomyelitis and non-healing wounds due to diabetes mellitus, fentanyl patches would need to be changed on a daily basis. Although the recommended dosing interval is 72 h, shorter intervals have been considered in selected patients. Pain was shown to be successfully managed with daily application of fentanyl transdermal patch while receiving HBO (Pawasauskas and Perdrizet 2014).

Implanted Devices in Patients

These devices create a risk of malfunction when exposed to hyperbaric conditions. For example, deep brain stimulators should not be subjected to pressures >203 kPa as they get deformed. There are no standard guidelines for use of various devices in a hyperbaric chamber. Some manufacturers support patients and medical practitioners with information on how their devices behave under increased pressure, and they should be contacted for confirmation that their device can be safely exposed to the treatment pressure and time. In some cases, an individual risk-benefit analysis should be conducted on the patient and the specific implanted device, taking into consideration the patient's clinical condition, the indication for HBO therapy, and the capability of the hyperbaric facility for monitoring and intervention in the chamber (Kot 2014).

Monitoring of Patients in the Hyperbaric Chamber

Patients and attendants in the chamber can be monitored by any of the following means:

- Visual. Direct view into a monoplace chamber; closed circuit TV in the multi-place chamber.

- Auditory. For both monoplace and multiplace chambers, several 2-way communication systems are available for this purpose.
- Use of diagnostic and monitoring equipment both inside and outside the chamber; direct observation by the accompanying attendants in case of multiplace chambers.

The level of monitoring depends on the severity and type of illness. With critically ill patients, the routine monitoring in the ICU can be continued into the chamber. In patients not requiring medical attention by contact, most of the essential monitoring can be done in a suitably equipped hyperbaric chamber, such as the Dräger HTK 1200 monoplace chamber. Some of the problems of monitoring head-injured patients in the monoplace chamber are:

1. If the arterial blood pressure is monitored by an indwelling radial artery catheter, a pressure infuser should be used to keep the line flushed open with a heparinized solution. Any obstruction of the catheter during pressure changes may dampen the wave form or flatten it.
2. Central venous pressure can be measured by connecting the line to a transducer and a monitoring module.
3. Swan-Ganz catheter. Pulmonary artery pressures can be monitored during HBO therapy; satisfactory wave forms are obtained without significant changes in the pulmonary artery pressure.
4. For EEG monitoring, the electrodes should be attached prior to entry to the chamber, and the collodion should be allowed to dry because when wet, it is flammable. Properly placed electrodes can stay in position for up to 5 days.
5. The cuffs of the endotracheal tubes should be filled with sterile normal saline during HBO. After the treatment, the saline is removed and replaced by air.
6. Arterial blood gas analysis. Arterial blood gas samples can be aspirated from the arterial line for analysis during HBO treatment. Transcutaneous oxygen monitoring cannot be done in a monoplace chamber because the electrode presents a fire hazard.
7. Intracranial pressure monitoring is important in patients with head injuries and cerebral edema. The Richmond subarachnoid bolt system connected to a standard arterial pressure transducer located inside the chamber with electrical leads passing through the walls is satisfactory. Intracellular current passage and recording inside a hyperbaric chamber can be carried out without danger of fire by using glass microelectrodes and micromanipulators. The cerebrospinal fluid (CSF) reflects the oxygen tension of the brain. CSF examination by cistern puncture or after removal from an Ommaya CSF reservoir may give an idea of the state of oxygenation of the brain tissues. This is important, as there is no satisfactory practical method of measuring cerebral blood flow in the hyperbaric chamber.

Safety in the Hyperbaric Chamber

Operational Safety

Safety is a very important consideration in the construction of hyperbaric chambers. Loss of chamber structural integrity can result in rapid decompression and decompression sickness. Most chambers in the United States are constructed according to the requirements of the ASME Boiler and Pressure Vessels Code, as amplified by ANSI-ASME PUHO (Sect. VIII, Div. 1, American Society of Mechanical Engineers, New York). A chamber built according to these standards can be expected to give years of reliable service, if it is properly maintained.

The windows of a hyperbaric chamber are usually made of acrylic plastic because it is easily formed and gives ample warning of impending failure. These materials are subject to corrosion and alcohol-based solutions should not be used for cleaning windows. Acrylic is subject to damage by heat and nuclear radiation.

Essential controls and monitors for a hyperbaric chamber should be provided with an emergency power source in the event of loss of power, and the transfer from normal to emergency power should be automatic.

Atmospheric Control

This refers to maintenance of a safe atmosphere inside the chamber. Contamination of the atmosphere is possible by products carried into the chamber. The hyperbaric chamber is pressurized by one of three methods:

- Compressed gas directly from a compressor,
- Compressed gas from a pressurized accumulator,
- Gas from a cryogenic supply system through a suitable vaporizer.

Large multiplace chambers are pressurized by compressed air from an accumulator that acts as a buffer in the event of compressor failure or loss of electric power. Pressurized air, regardless of the source, should be checked periodically for composition and purity. Sufficiently clean air can be provided by locating the air intake away from sources of pollution and providing suitable absorbers for pollutants. Safety standards for the composition of chamber air are given in Table 7.5.

Masks and Breathing Control System

The breathing control system is also referred to as BIBS (built in breathing system) in a multiplace chamber. It provides a safe and secure source of breathing gas in case of contamination of the chamber atmosphere. The masks for supplying oxygen are supplied by an overhead dumping system where the exhaled breath is directed out of the chamber. The masks should fit well. Oxygen leaking from the masks not only reduces the effectiveness of the treatment, but also raises the oxygen concentration of the chamber air above accepted levels and should not exceed 23 vol.%. The expired gases are removed directly by a so-called "overboard dumping system." In the case of hoods, special attention is required to CO_2 removal and prevention of excessive humidity. The oxygen supply to the mask should be humidified to prevent the irritating effect of oxygen.

Fire Safety in the Chamber

Prior to 1970, there were no national fire safety standards for clinical hyperbaric chambers in the United States. Fire prevention was a matter left to common sense of the operators. Considering the widespread use of hyperbaric oxygen therapy, the record of fire safety in hyperbaric chambers has been good. The first hyperbaric chamber fire occurred in 1923 in Cunningham's chamber in the United States (see Chap. 1). There were 25 fires in clinical hyperbaric chambers worldwide from 1923 to 1996 (Sheffield and Desautels 1997, 1998). The review by these authors was based on reports in the literature as well as the Chambers Experience and Mishap Database of the Undersea and

Table 7.5 Recommended maximum values for contaminants in hyperbaric chamber

Contaminant	Maximum value
Carbon dioxide	1000 ppm by volume (0.1 %) in hyperbaric air
	5000 ppm by volume (0.5 %) in HBO at 1 ATA
Carbon monoxide	5 ppm in hyperbaric air
Gaseous hydrocarbons (methane, ethane, etc.)	25 ppm by volume (0.0025 %)
Halogenated solvents	0.2 ppm by volume (0.00002 %)
Particulate matter	0.005 mg/L, weight/volume
Total water	0.3 mg/L, weight/volume
Odor	None objectionable or unusual

Hyperbaric Medical Society. During the 73-year period reviewed, there were 91 human fatalities associated with 40 fires in pressure-related chambers of all types including diving bells, decompression chambers, and pressurized Apollo Command Module. There were 60 deaths in 21 clinical hyperbaric chamber fires. No death occurred in clinical hyperbaric chambers in the United States. Most of the deaths prior to 1980 were associated with electrical ignition inside the chamber, but after this period the reported source of ignition has usually been a prohibited source of ignition carried by an occupant inside the chamber. All fatal fires occurred in enriched oxygen environments and only reported survivors were in chambers pressurized with air.

The first fire in a clinical monoplace chamber was reported in Japan in 1967 and three more occurred in the following years; all were initiated by hand warmers. An explosion due to static electricity was reported while a patient was having cobalt irradiation under HBO at 3 ATA in a monoplace chamber (Tobin 1978). The patient developed a lung rupture due to explosive decompression, but survived. From 1976 to 1989, static electricity was considered to be the cause of seven fires resulting in five deaths in monoplace chambers filled with pure oxygen. Static charge stored in the fiberglass tray was considered to be the initiating factors and these trays were replaced with stainless steel trays. Strict guidelines to this effect as well as for grounding were laid down by the National Fire Protection Association of the United States and no such incidents have been reported since then.

Another accident occurred in 1987 in Naples, when a child died in a fire in a monoplace chamber. The child was playing with a toy pistol that may have caused the ignition. The accident was attributed to the laxity of the attendant in allowing the child to take a toy into the chamber. No prompt measures were taken to rescue the child, who was practically incinerated.

The first occurrence of a fire in a multiplace chamber was precipitated by an externally heated microwave blanket introduced through the safety lock (Youn et al. 1989). The fire was rapidly extinguished with a central deluge system. A second mishap occurred in Milan, Italy, in 1997 when a fatal explosion occurred in a multiplace chamber with 11 deaths. A gas-operated hand warmer was the likely trigger and it is likely that the chamber was pressurized with oxygen rather than air as explosive fire would not occur in a chamber pressurized with air. There have been no fires reported in hyperbaric chambers during the past 5 years.

Fatal hyperbaric fires are usually caused by a combination of factors: abundance of combustible materials, high oxygen levels, faulty electrical components, inadequate fire extinguishing equipment, and lack of vigilance for carriage of prohibited items into the chamber. Emphasis should be placed on the prevention, detection, and elimination of known and suspected fire hazards in a hyperbaric chamber. Fire is more of a hazard in a monoplace chamber because it is filled with 100% oxygen.

The following measures should be taken to prevent fire in a monoplace chamber:

- There should be no electrical equipment inside the chamber. All leads for diagnostic equipment should be connected to instruments outside the chamber. All ignition sources inside the chamber should be eliminated.
- There should be no nylon garments inside the chamber.
- The patient should not use an oil-based or volatile cosmetic (facial cream, body oil, or hair spray) before a hyperbaric session.
- In case of fire, prompt decompression should be performed and the chamber opened. Fire precautions should be continued outside the chamber until the oxygen soaked into the garment or the mattress under the patient has dissipated.

For multiplace hyperbaric chambers, guidelines of the U. S. National Fire Protection Association should be followed: NFPA-56D dealing with hyperbaric facilities, and NFPA53M dealing with fire hazards in oxygen-enriched environments. Although there might be some flammability-inhibiting effect of the increased nitrogen present in compressed air, this effect is more than offset by the increased partial pressure of the oxygen present (up to 5 ATA). The standards include the following basic points:

- All equipment should be designed and tested to be intrinsically safe for hyperbaric conditions, i.e., it must be pressure-tested and spark proof.
- All wiring and fixed electrical equipment must comply with NFPA-70, National Electrical Code, Article 500, Class I, Division I.
- All equipment, circuits included, must be waterproof and explosion-proof.

The following additional measures should be taken in multiplace chambers:

1. No volatile or flammable liquid should be allowed inside the chamber.
2. Lubricants for mechanical devices inside the chamber should be of the halogenated polymer hydrocarbon type. All combustible lubricants should be avoided.
3. Electric motors should be replaced by air-driven or hydraulic motors.
4. Oxygen concentration in the chamber must be kept below 23%. If it goes over 25%, the oxygen supply should be shut off until the source of the leak is found.

5. Fire-detecting systems, manual or automatic, should be installed. The latter should have a safeguard for false alarms.
6. A fire extinguishing system should be provided. Pressurized water should be supplied by a built-in flooding system with additional hand-held hoses. Fire drill and escape procedures should be practiced periodically.

NFPA 99, Chap. 19, has specific guidance for fire extinguishing systems in class A (multiplace) chambers (National Fire Protection Association 2013). The important points are:

• Fire extinguishing systems must be capable of activation from inside or outside of chambers.
• Water is the extinguishing element of choice.
• Each member of the hyperbaric team should be trained in activating the chamber fire extinguishing system.
• NFPA has no guidelines on extinguishing fires in monoplace pure oxygen chambers as fires in this atmosphere are not survivable.

Use of Portable Hyperbaric Chambers in Patient's Rooms

It is safe to use a portable hyperbaric chamber in a patient's room in a hospital provided all the precautions for an oxygen-rich environment are observed and adequate technical supervision is provided. Particular measures to be taken are:

1. All combustible material should be removed from the room
2. Electrical appliances should be placed at least 5 ft (1.5 m) away from areas where the oxygen concentration is greater than 23.5 %.
3. All personal items likely to produce static discharges should be removed from the patient.

Regulatory Issues Relevant to Hyperbaric Medicine

There does not appear to be a clear-cut single authority for regulating hyperbaric medicine in any country. In the United States, the local fire marshal's office enforces the safety regulations of the National Fire Protection Association. The Food and Drug Administration (FDA), which is the main regulatory authority for pharmaceuticals and medical devices, had a rather background role in clinical hyperbaric medicine in the past, but it is becoming more significant now. Oxygen is classified as a drug by the FDA. Therefore, both its application and the devices used to administer it fall under FDA's jurisdiction. Hyperbaric chambers are medical devices

used for the administration of oxygen and are subject to FDA control, which applies to all medical devices which entered into use since 1976. Hyperbaric chambers constructed prior to 1976 are not subject to FDA control. Medical devices are divided by the FDA into three classes with differing levels of FDA involvement according to the class:

Class I: General controls. These are simple devices where performance is not much of a concern, such as tongue depressors. Notification of intention to market the device is required under Section 510 (k) of the Safe Medical Device Amendments enacted in 1976. FDA clearance of the Premarket Notification (hence the term 510K) is required prior to marketing the device or placing it for commercial distribution.

Class II: Special controls. These are complex devices where performance is a concern, but at a somewhat general level. Class II devices must comply with general controls and the requirement of some applicable standards. A 510K Premarket Notification to the FDA is required. FDA clearance of the Pre-market Notification is required prior to marketing the device or placing it in commercial distribution.

Class III: Pre-market approval. These are generally devices that are directly related to patient life support with a substantial risk of injury in the event of malfunction. An example is a cardiac pacemaker. Pre-market approval by the FDA is required. The resulting design and manufacturing controls are very strict.

Hyperbaric chambers are considered to be class II devices and the applicable industry standard is NFPA 99, Chap. 19 and "Safety Standard for Pressure Vessels for Human Occupancy (PVHO-1)" issued by the Safety Code Committee of the ASME.

All classes of medical devices are subject to the FDA's Good Manufacturing Practice (GMP) regulations. These are similar to the international quality assurance regulations (ISO 9000, ISO 9001, etc.) that have come into widespread use in recent years. The main requirements are:

• As established design for the product (e.g., drawings) approved by some reasonable person.
• Production in accordance with the design
• Testing to confirm performance in accordance with design requirements
• Receipt control and inspections of incoming materials
• Established procedures for resolving problems and customer complaints
• Production documentation sufficient to maintain accountability and to confirm that the above requirements are being met.
• The manufacturing establishment and the product must be registered annually with the FDA.

Conformance with the FDA's rules as they apply to the manufacture of hyperbaric chambers is usually not difficult in a technical sense. However, it does require a commitment to procedural controls that can be difficult to maintain.

"Labeling" is interpreted by the FDA to mean just about everything the manufacturer says about what the device can be used for and how it can be used. In case of oxygen, the recognized claims are the indications recommended by the Undersea and Hyperbaric Medical Society.

Adultered devices are prohibited by the FDA. This term applies to devices that are:

- Built in an unregistered establishment
- Built without a cleared 510K Premarket Notification
- Altered or otherwise not built in accordance with the approved design

Avoidance of appearance of endorsement of products. Manufacturers are not permitted to refer to their FDA 510K Premarket notification, nor resulting FDA clearance in advertising in any published literature. However, a manufacturer can respond to a request from a potential customer regarding whether or not a manufacturer has a cleared 510K Pre-market Notification for a specific device. Regulation of hyperbaric chambers varies in other countries. A European code of good practice for hyperbaric oxygen therapy represents the harmonized European view on safety in therapeutic hyperbaric facilities and can be used as a reference document for European countries for guidelines, regulations, and standards in hyperbaric medicine. One of the countries with very strict technical regulations is Germany where a certificate from an organization called TÜV (Technischer Überwachungsverein) is required before a hyperbaric chamber can be approved for use. Guidelines for quality control have been laid down by GTÜM (Gesellschaft für Tauchund Überdruckmedizin e.V.), which is an organization for diving and hyperbaric medicine. Germany has an excellent record of safety in hyperbaric medicine and no mishaps have occurred in recent years. Currently, all the hyperbaric chambers approved for use in Germany are multiplace and monoplace chambers are not allowed because of the fire hazard.

Staffing of Hyperbaric Facilities

All personnel employed in hyperbaric facilities should be properly trained and familiar with all relevant safety precautions and decompression procedures. Paramedical personnel are hyperbaric technicians and nurses. The technicians are mostly concerned with the operation and safety of the chamber, but they should also have an elementary knowledge of hyperbaric medicine. In "round-the-clock" emergency services, the attending nurse and critical care specialist should understand the physics and physiology of HBO for safe treatment and compression/decompression procedures. Nurses are concerned mostly with the care of the patients before, during, and after HBO treatments. Although they are expected to have a fair medical knowledge of conditions treated by HBO, they should also be familiar with the operation of the hyperbaric chambers. The role of nurses in hyperbaric medicine is described in Chap. 37.

The occupational health and safety of hyperbaric attendants is an important issue for staff of hyperbaric medicine units. The reported incidence of DCI in attendants ranges from 0.01 to 1.3%. This is mostly related to depth of pressure exposure. DCI can be prevented by oxygen breathing and rotation of attendants. Ear trauma is a frequent complaint. No complaints have been reported from physical therapists carrying out treatments on patients at 1.5 ATA on a daily basis for several weeks. The health and safety record of hyperbaric chamber attendants has been very good with only one death reported.

Conclusion

There is a great variety of hyperbaric chambers available and the hyperbaric physician has to choose the equipment best suited to the needs of his unit and according to the financial resources. The choice of ancillary equipment also depends upon the requirements. In general, the operation of hyperbaric chambers is safe if the safety precautions are followed. There is still room for improvement in the technical devices for monitoring the patients during hyperbaric treatment.

The basic technology for hyperbaric chambers is well established, though innovations continue to be made according to requirements. Gas supplies, the chamber hulls, control systems, monitoring equipment, and safety devices are constantly being adapted according to the most recent technical developments. Subtypes of hyperbaric chambers such as those for treatment or training or experimental use require different technical devices. Alarm as well as technical monitoring systems, fire-fighting equipment, and pressure locks are absolute requirements for any hyperbaric chamber. In chambers used for therapeutic purposes, facilities for invasive as well as noninvasive patient monitoring need to be ensured.

References

Arieli R, Daskalovic Y, Ertracht O, Arieli Y, Adir Y, Abramovich A, et al. Flow resistance, work of breathing of humidifiers, and endotracheal tubes in the hyperbaric chamber. Am J Emerg Med. 2011;29:725–30.

Cooper JS, Allinson P, Winn D, Keim L, Sippel J, Shalberg P, et al. Continuous bladder irrigation in the monoplace hyperbaric chamber: two case reports. Undersea Hyperb Med. 2015;42: 419–23.

Hansen K, Hansen ES, Tolbod LP, Kristensen MC, Ringgaard S, Brubakk AO, et al. A CT-, PET- and MR-imaging-compatible hyperbaric pressure chamber for baromedical research. Diving Hyperb Med. 2015;45:247–54.

Kot J. Medical devices and procedures in the hyperbaric chamber. Diving Hyperb Med. 2014;44:223–7.

Lind F. A pro/con review comparing the use of mono- and multiplace hyperbaric chambers for critical care. Diving Hyperb Med. 2015;45:56–60.

National Fire Protection Association. Standard for health care facilities. NFPA 99, Chapter 19, Hyperbaric facilities. Boston: National Fire Protection Association; 2013.

Pawasauskas J, Perdrizet G. Daily application of transdermal fentanyl patches in patients receiving hyperbaric oxygen therapy. J Pain Palliat Care Pharmacother. 2014;28:226–32.

Sheffield PJ, Desautels DA. Hyperbaric and hypobaric chamber fires: a 73-year analysis. Undersea Hyperbaric Med. 1997;24:153–64.

Sheffield PJ, Desautels DA. Hyperbaric chamber fires: an up-date. Undersea Hyperb Med. 1998;25:26 (abstract).

Shimada H, Morita T, Kunimoto F, et al. Immediate application of hyperbaric oxygen therapy using a newly devised transportable chamber. Am J Emerg Med. 1996;14:412–5.

Tobin DA. Explosive decompression in a hyperbaric oxygen chamber. AJR. 1978;111:622–4.

Uzun G, Mutluoglu M. Clinical challenges in the treatment of patients with tracheostomy in a hyperbaric chamber. J Thorac Cardiovasc Surg. 2015;149:646–7.

Walker KJ, Millar IL, Fock A. The performance and safety of a pleural drainage unit under hyperbaric conditions. Anaesth Intensive Care. 2006;34:61–7.

Youn BA, Kozikowski RJ, Myers RAM. The development of treatment algorithm in methylene chloride poisoning based on a multi-case experience. Undersea Biomed Res. 1989;12(Suppl):20 Abstract #16.

Indications, Contraindications, and Complications of HBO Therapy

8

8

K.K. Jain

Abstract

This chapter lists indications for the use of hyperbaric oxygen therapy (HBO) in different parts of the world including approved as well as those that are not approved. Various contraindications are also described.

Complications of HBO are discussed, particularly middle ear barotrauma, and their management is described. Precautions in selection of patients for HBO therapy are also mentioned.

Keywords

Anxiety reactions • Chamber claustrophobia • Complications of HBO • Contraindications for HBO • Decompression sickness • Hyperbaric oxygen (HBO) • HBO-induced DNA damage • Indication for HBO • Middle ear barotrauma • Ophthalmic complications • Otological complications • Oxygen seizures • Pulmonary barotrauma • Pulmonary oxygen toxicity

Indications

Indications for hyperbaric oxygen (HBO) therapy vary in different countries. The indications approved by the Undersea and Hyperbaric Medical Society (Table 8.1) are very limited and rely on the proof of efficacy of HBO by controlled studies. A summary of indications is shown in Table 8.2. The table lists all the conditions where HBO has been shown to be useful, although, to date, few of these have been proven by controlled studies.

Contraindications

Contraindications for HBO therapy are shown in Table 8.3.

Pneumothorax. The only absolute contraindication for HBO is untreated pneumothorax. Surgical relief of the pneumothorax before the HBO session, if possible, removes the obstacle to treatment.

K.K. Jain, MD, FRACS, FFPM (✉)
1 Blaesiring 7, Basel 4057, Switzerland
e-mail: jain@pharmabiotech.ch

The contraindications listed below are not absolute but relative. The potential benefits should be weighed against the condition of the patient and any ill effects that may occur.

Upper Respiratory Infections. These predispose to otic barotrauma and sinus squeeze.

Emphysema with CO2 Retention. Patients with this problem may develop pneumothorax due to rupture of an emphysematous bulla during HBO. Pretreatment X-rays of the chest should be taken to rule this out.

Air Cysts or Blebs in the Lungs Seen on Chest X-Ray. These may predispose to pulmonary barotrauma by causing air trapping during HBO treatment. A survey was conducted to determine how patients were evaluated for pulmonary blebs or bullae in different hyperbaric centers (Toklu et al. 2008). Of the 98 centers that responded to questionnaires, 65 (66.3%) reported that they applied HBO to the patients with air cysts in their lungs. X-ray was the most widely used screening method for patients with a history of a lung disease. The prevalence of pulmonary barotrauma in these centers was quite low at 0.00045%.

History of Thoracic Surgery or Ear Surgery. The patient should be thoroughly evaluated before HBO therapy is considered.

© Springer International Publishing AG 2017
K.K. Jain, *Textbook of Hyperbaric Medicine*, DOI 10.1007/978-3-319-47140-2_8

Table 8.1 Uses of HBO approved by the Undersea and Hyperbaric Medical Society, USA

Air or gas embolism
Carbon monoxide poisoning and carbon monoxide poisoning complicated by cyanide poisoning
Clostridial myonecrosis (gas gangrene)
Compromised skin grafts and flaps
Crush injury, compartment syndrome, and other acute traumatic ischemias
Decompression sickness
Enhancement of healing in selected problem wounds
Exceptional anemia resulting from blood loss
Intracranial abscess
Necrotizing soft tissue infections (of subcutaneous tissue, muscle, or fascia)
Radiation tissue damage (osteoradionecrosis)
Refractory osteomyelitis
Sensory neural hearing loss
Skin grafts and flaps (compromised)
Thermal burns

Table 8.2 Summary of international indications for HBO

Aid to rehabilitation: spastic hemiplegia of stroke, paraplegia, chronic myocardial insufficiency, peripheral vascular disease
Air embolism
Asphyxiation: drowning, near hanging, smoke inhalation
Cardiovascular diseases: shock, myocardial ischemia, aid to cardiac surgery
Decompression sickness
Dentistry: refractory periodontitis, adjunctive therapy for the implants in irradiated jaws
Endocrines: diabetes
For enhancement of radiosensitivity of malignant tumors
Gastrointestinal: gastric ulcer, necrotizing enterocolitis, paralytic ileus, pneumatosis cystoides intestinalis, hepatitis
Head and neck surgery: osteoradionecrosis and osteomyelitis of jaws
Hematology: sickle cell crises, severe blood loss anemia
Lung diseases: lung abscess, pulmonary embolism (adjunct to surgery)
Neurological: stroke, multiple sclerosis, migraine, cerebral edema, multi-infarct dementia, spinal cord injury and vascular diseases of the spinal cord, brain abscess, peripheral neuropathy, radiation myelitis, vegetative coma
Obstetrics: complicated pregnancy—diabetes, eclampsia, heart disease, placental hypoxia, fetal hypoxia, congenital heart disease of the neonate
Ophthalmology: occlusion of central artery of retina
Orthopedics: nonunion of fractures, bone grafts, osteoradionecrosis
Otorhinolaryngology: sudden deafness, acute acoustic trauma, labyrinthitis, Meniere's disease, malignant otitis externa (chronic infection)
Peripheral vascular disease: ischemic gangrene, ischemic leg pain
Plastic and reconstructive surgery: for nonhealing wounds as an aid to the survival of skin flaps with marginal circulation, as an aid to reimplantation surgery, and as an adjunct to the treatment of burns
Poisoning: carbon monoxide, cyanide, hydrogen sulfide, carbon tetrachloride
Traumatology: crush injuries, compartment syndrome, soft tissue sport injuries
Treatment of certain infections: gas gangrene, acute necrotizing fasciitis, refractory mycoses, leprosy, osteomyelitis

Table 8.3 Contraindications for HBO therapy

Absolute
Untreated tension pneumothorax
Relative
Upper respiratory infections
Emphysema with CO_2 retention
Asymptomatic air cysts or blebs in the lungs seen on chest X-ray
History of thoracic or ear surgery
Uncontrolled high fever
Pregnancy
Claustrophobia (see complications of HBO)

Uncontrolled High Fever. Fever predisposes to seizures. If HBO therapy is indicated for an infection with fever, the temperature should be lowered before therapy is commenced.

Pregnancy. There is animal experimental evidence that exposure to HBO during early pregnancy increases the incidence of congenital malformations. However, if a pregnant woman is poisoned with CO_2, the primary consideration is to save the mother's life. Exposure to HBO later in pregnancy appears to have no adverse effects. If the mother's life is threatened, for example, in CO poisoning, she should receive HBO therapy, as this has priority over consideration for the fetus. Many successful HBO treatments have been carried out during pregnancy without any danger to the fetus (see Chap. 33).

The following conditions have been considered to be contraindications previously but are not supported by evidence. Several patients have been treated by the use of HBO without aggravation of these conditions.

Seizure Disorders. Patients with CNS disorders such as stroke may suffer seizures as a manifestation of their primary disorder. However, seizures are rare during HBO sessions for neurological indications where the pressures do not exceed 1.5 ATA. If the disorder is due to a focal cerebral circulatory disorder or hypoxia, HBO should help to reduce the tendency toward seizures. Improvement in control of seizures and reduction in the dosage of antiepileptic drugs have been reported in epileptic children treated with HBO.

Malignant Disease. There is some concern regarding the effect of HBO on tumor growth because HBO is used as an adjunct to radiotherapy and also for the treatment of radiation necrosis in patients who may have residual cancer. This topic is discussed in Chap. 38 where it is concluded that malignant disease is generally not considered to be a contraindication for HBO therapy.

Optic Neuritis. A history of optic neuritis was previously considered a relative contraindication to HBO therapy. However, a large number of patients with multiple sclerosis, some of whom have optic neuritis, have been treated with HBO, but no aggravation of vision has been reported. A case report of a patient with a history of optic neuritis, who underwent comprehensive ophthalmologic evaluation before and after 40 treatments with HBO therapy, showed no detectable ophthalmologic deficit (Register et al. 2011).

Complications of Hyperbaric Oxygenation

Some of the complications of HBO therapy are listed in Table 8.4.

Middle Ear Barotrauma

This is the commonest reported complication of HBO, but the incidence varies in different series. Patients may have to be removed from the hyperbaric chamber during HBO treatment because of an inability to equalize middle ear pressure; the sessions can be resumed after treatment and training. In large series of HBO therapy sessions, as many as 17 % of all patients have been reported to experience ear pain. Most episodes are not related to a persistent Eustachian tube dysfunction. Barotraumatic lesions on visual otological examinations (ear microscopy) can be verified in a small percentage of these patients.

A Japanese study of otological complications for HBO therapy and the risk factors for these complications enrolled 1115 patients (Yamamoto et al. 2015). Otological symptoms were experienced by 165 (14.8 %) of the patients of which nearly half reported them at the first HBO therapy session. Some of these required myringotomy or tube insertion, and HBO therapy was stopped in only four patients because of these symptoms. Risk factors for otological complications of HBO include the following:

1. Unconscious patients are more likely to show barotrauma in the middle ear due to obvious inability to equalize pressure changes.
2. Elderly patients >60 years are more susceptible.
3. Patients with history of cardiovascular disease.
4. Patients with sensory deficits involving the ear region need special attention, because they seem to be at risk for rupture of the tympanic membrane.

Table 8.4 Complications of hyperbaric oxygen therapy

Middle ear barotrauma
Sinus pain
Ophthalmological complications (see Table 8.5)
Pulmonary barotrauma
Oxygen seizures
Decompression sickness
Genetic effects
Claustrophobia

Although some significant risk factors for middle ear barotrauma have been identified, a 1-year prospective study using multivariate logistic regression to analyze the data was unable to predict accurately enough which patients needed tympanostomy tubes during their HBO therapy to recommend the prophylactic procedure in selected patients (Commons et al. 2013).

The Eustachian tube openings in the nasopharynx are slit-like, and the patient may have difficulty in equalizing the middle ear pressure with that of outside air during compression. Most patients can learn to remedy this by Frenzel's maneuver which consists of pinching the nose, closing the mouth, and pushing the tongue against the soft palate to force air through the Eustachian tubes into the middle ears. This complication can lead to permanent hearing loss and vertigo. Unconscious patients and infants present a special diagnostic challenge because of difficulties in communicating pain and equalizing pressure across the ears. The slow compression method of HBO has proved to be safer as well as better than the standard compression technique and reduces the incidence of middle ear barotrauma (Vahidova et al. 2006).

Clinical practice with regard to middle ear barotrauma prophylaxis varies in US HBO centers. The use of nasal decongestants is considered to be helpful. Topical nasal decongestants, particularly oxymetazoline, are preferred over systemic oral medications. However, some controlled studies found no significant difference in the occurrence of ear discomfort in those receiving the decongestant oxymetazoline from those receiving spray of distilled water. Only a third of centers routinely administer prophylactic drugs before HBO treatment. Some centers perform routine prophylactic myringotomies on intubated patients. Less than half of centers never performed the procedure as routine prophylaxis.

Some complications such as otorrhea and persistent tympanic membrane perforations occur after conclusion of HBO therapy. Coexisting illness, such as diabetes mellitus, may contribute to the development of complications in patients undergoing HBO therapy. Alternative methods of tympanostomy, with emphasis on shorter duration of intubation, should be considered in this patient population. Patients with history of Eustachian tube dysfunction after first HBO treatment were found to be at greater risk of developing serous otitis media with subsequent treatments. Unconscious patients are more likely to show barotrauma in the middle ear due to obvious inability to equalize pressure changes.

A modified 24-gauge intravenous cannula has been used as a tool for tympanostomy tube placement as prophylactic for middle ear barotrauma and found to be effective in 99 % cases and enable removal without anesthesia and spontaneous healing of tympanic membrane in 99.6 % of cases (Zhang et al. 2013). Given the safety, effectiveness, and low risk of complications associated with this novel tympanostomy technique, it provided a simple yet effective therapeutic option for the management of otic barotrauma.

Table 8.5 Ophthalmological complications of HBO therapy

Aggravation of pre-existing ocular diseases
Keratoconus
Age-related macular degeneration
Cataract
Myopia
Retinal oxygen toxicity
Retrolental fibroplasia

Sinus Pain. Sinus block during pressurization may produce severe pain, particularly in the frontal sinuses. If a patient has upper respiratory infection, the HBO treatment should be postponed, or, if it is urgently required, the patient should be given decongestant medication and the compression performed slowly.

Ophthalmological Complications of HBO

Ophthalmological complications of HBO are listed in Table 8.5 and are discussed in detail in Chap. 32. Myopia is a reversible complication of acute exposure to HBO, and cataract is a complication of chronic long-term exposure. Increase in free radicals may play a role in pathogenesis of these complications, and prophylactic use of free radial scavengers during HBO therapy is one of the strategies for prevention of these complications.

Pulmonary Complications of HBO

Oxygen is rarely used for pulmonary disorders. Most of the pulmonary adverse effects are related to breathing under pressure and are considered under the headings of acute pulmonary oxygen toxicity and pulmonary barotrauma.

Acute Pulmonary Oxygen Toxicity

Breathing of HBO at pressures above 3 ATA can cause acute pulmonary injury that is more severe if signs of central nervous system (CNS) toxicity occur. This is consistent with the activation of an autonomic link between the brain and the lung, leading to acute pulmonary oxygen toxicity. This pulmonary damage is characterized by leakage of fluid, protein, and red blood cells into the alveoli, compatible with hydrostatic injury due to pulmonary hypertension, left atrial hypertension, or both. To prove this hypothetical connection, experiments were performed on rats in which cerebral blood flow, electroencephalographic activity, cardiopulmonary hemodynamics, and autonomic traffic were measured during exposure to HBO at 5 and 6 ATA (Demchenko et al. 2011). In some animals, autonomic pathways were disrupted pharmacologically or surgically. The findings indicate that

pulmonary damage in HBO is caused by an abrupt and significant increase in pulmonary vascular pressure, sufficient to produce barotrauma in capillaries. Specifically, extreme HBO exposures produce massive sympathetic outflow from the CNS that depresses left ventricular function, resulting in acute left atrial and pulmonary hypertension. The authors of this study attribute these effects on the heart and on the pulmonary vasculature to HBO-mediated central sympathetic excitation and catecholamine release that disturbs the normal equilibrium between excitatory and inhibitory activity in the autonomic nervous system.

Pulmonary Barotrauma

Incidence of pulmonary barotrauma is quite low and most series with treatments under 2 ATA do not report any cases. However, overinflation with pressure may lead to lung rupture, which may present as an air embolus, mediastinal emphysema, or tension pneumothorax.

Pneumothorax in a patient under HBO treatment is a serious complication. In a multiplace chamber, the physician should auscultate the patient, although the lung sounds are difficult to hear. Lung rupture may be suspected from the symptoms—sudden stabbing chest pain and respiratory distress. Tracheal shift and asymmetrical movements of the chest may be the only signs on physical examination. Decompression should be halted and thoracentesis performed. Plainly, this complication is more difficult to detect and to treat if it happens in a monoplace chamber.

Rarely comatose patients develop tension pneumothorax while receiving HBO therapy for CO poisoning. Serial physical examinations, arterial blood gas determinations, and chest X-rays are recommended in patients with a high index of suspicion of this complication in the setting of emergency HBO therapy.

Oxygen Seizures

Seizures as a manifestation of oxygen are described in Chap. 6. In a series of 80,000 patient treatments with HBO, only two seizures were documented, yielding an incidence of 2.4 per 100,000 patient treatments, and both cases occurred in a multiplace chamber pressurized to 2.4 ATA with O_2 delivered by mask for three times 30 min with 5-min air breaks (Yildiz et al. 2004). Use of pressure at 1.5 ATA does not lead to any oxygen-induced seizures when the duration of treatment was kept below 1 h. If a seizure occurs in a multiplace chamber, the oxygen mask should be removed; this will invariably stop the seizure. If not, 60–120 mg of phenobarbital should be given. The chamber pressure should not be changed: sudden decompression of the chamber during a seizure can cause lung rupture. Decompression can be carried out after the seizure stops.

Decompression Sickness

Decompression sickness (DCS) associated with diving is described in Chap. 11. DCS may occur during HBO therapy only if very high pressures are used and decompression is sudden. It is more likely to occur in the attendants in the hyperbaric chamber who breathe air. DCS occurs rarely during therapeutic compression to 6 ATA in air embolism cases. The first report of fatal accident involving DCS in a hyperbaric chamber occurred in Hanover, Germany (Richter et al. 1978). Twenty elderly patients were receiving HBO in a multiplace chamber at 4 ATA. One patient developed air embolism after 1 h when decompression was started during the first dive. During the second dive, at about 5 h, the chamber door was opened with a sudden explosive reduction of pressure. Five patients died of DCS. There are no reports of such a complication in recent years.

Genetic Effects

In vitro studies of HBO therapy suggest that HBO may cause DNA damage as shown by comet assay. However, a single HBO exposure causes limited DNA damage to human umbilical cord endothelial cells, which repairs quickly (Yuan et al. 2011). HBO protects against H_2O_2-induced DNA damage and involves rise of cellular glutathione levels. These findings imply that endothelial cells are unlikely to be compromised during HBO therapy.

Treatment of cells with HBO can result in generation of reactive oxygen species and induction of DNA strand breakages especially in lymphocytes. In one study, blood samples were drawn by venipuncture before and immediately after the first session of HBO treatment in 100 voluntary patients, and DNA-damaging effect of HBO was evaluated (Üstündağ et al. 2012). DNA strand breakages were significantly increased in lymphocytes after the first session of HBO treatment, but returned to their normal levels after 2 h of in vitro incubation. The elevated DNA strand breaks consistently decreased and reached to the baseline levels after the fifth session of HBO therapy. The results of this study support the existence of the previously reported cellular adaptive response against HBO-mediated oxidative DNA damage in experimental studies.

Cytogenetic data obtained from peripheral blood of patients who were treated with HBO at 1.5–2 ATA for 40 min daily for 10 days have shown significant increase of chromosome aberrations. These are considered to be mainly caused by chromatid and chromosome breaks and showed individual variations. These results indicate that HBO may have an indirect effect on the genetic apparatus of the human somatic cells. High quantity of chromosome breaks in cells of somatic tissues is an adaptive reaction of the organism to HBO.

Exposure to 100 % oxygen at a pressure of 1.5 ATA for a total of 1 h has been shown to induce DNA damage in the alkaline comet assay with leukocytes from test subjects. Under these conditions, HBO does not lead to an induction of gene and chromosome mutations. Because of known toxic effects, exposure of humans to HBO is limited, and possible genetic consequences of HBO cannot be completely evaluated in vivo. HBO treatment of cell cultures is a suitable model for investigating the relationship between oxygen-induced DNA lesions and the formation of gene and chromosome mutations. The results of one study indicate that HBO induces sister chromatid exchange and that lymphocytes retain increased sensitivity to the genotoxicity of mitomycin C 1 day after completing the HBO (Duydu et al. 2006).

In another study, peripheral blood mononuclear cells (PBMCs), freshly isolated from non-divers and pure oxygen divers, were exposed to ambient air (21 kPa) and hyperoxia at different levels, 100, 240, 400, and 600 kPa, for up to 6.5 h in an experimental pressure chamber (Witte et al. 2014). The conclusion is that visible DNA damage increases with pO_2 and exposure time dose-dependently and that PBMCs of oxygen divers seem to be more resistant to HBO.

Claustrophobia

This is often referred to as a complication of or contraindication for hyperbaric therapy, and some patients decline or discontinue treatment for this reason. Claustrophobia is relatively common in the general population, and some of the claustrophobic individuals may require HBO treatments. Claustrophobia can be a manifestation of anxiety due to confinement in a closed space and unfamiliar surroundings. It is more likely to be experienced in a small monoplace or portable chamber and less likely in a large multiplace chamber with easy communication to the outside. Claustrophobia should be treated prior to elective HBO treatments in a monoplace chamber.

Anxiety Reactions

There are several reports in the literature of anxiety reactions in patients undergoing HBO treatment. Anxiety levels of patients undergoing HBO treatments can be assessed by Spielberger State-Trait inventory Questionnaire. There is an increase in magnitude of anxiety with a new treatment, which decreases after the treatment. It is important to communicate with the patient and explain the procedure with reassurance. Larger studies on this topic would be useful.

Coincidental Medical Events in the Hyperbaric Chamber

A medical event may take place in the hyperbaric chamber and may not have any relation to the HBO therapy. Often such events are mistakenly attributed to HBO therapy. Reported coincidental events include the following:

1. Stroke
2. Myocardial infarction patients with known atherosclerotic disease and other risk factors for heart disease
3. Focal seizures in patients with a history of epilepsy or intracranial lesions

Precautions in Selection of Patients for HBO Treatment

In emergency situations, it is not possible to select patients and sometimes a risk has to be taken. For elective treatments, the patients should be screened carefully. History taking should include information of any chest or ear operations.

Examination of the patient should include the following:

- Chest X-ray
- Pulmonary function testing
- Examination of the eardrums

In many other conditions, the decision should be made on an individual basis. Particular attention should be paid to the following two situations:

1. Large skull defects. In a patient with a large skull defect following surgery, HBO treatments should be avoided if the scalp flap is caved in.
2. Implanted devices that are affected by increased pressure.

Cardiac Pacemakers. If the patient is wearing a cardiac pacemaker, it should be ascertained that it is one of the newer models that are pressure proof. Failure of temporary cardiac pacemakers has been reported under HBO. They recommended the use of permanent hermetically sealed pacemakers, which function quite well under hyperbaric conditions. Currently most of the pacemakers are unaffected by treatment depths below 3 ATA.

Intrathecal pumps are used for administration of drugs directly into the intrathecal space of the spinal canal for relief of spasticity or pain. Baclofen infusion pump is used in paraplegic patients with spinal cord spasticity. There may be retrograde leakage of CSF into the pump reservoir while undergoing HBO treatment at 2 ATA. There is no adverse effect of this except for the dilution of the medication in the pump. Tests by the manufacturers of these pumps have not shown any collapse of the pump although the pumps do not function during the exposure to high atmospheric pressure. This information may be important if spasticity is to be treated with HBO.

Conclusion

Generally speaking, no serious complications are associated with moderate pressure HBO treatment, but some complications may be related to the primary disease treated. Contraindications should be noted and precautions taken during treatment of those with risk factors for complications. Some implanted devices used in treatment of patients may not function properly in hyperbaric chambers.

References

Commons KH, Blake DF, Brown LH. A prospective analysis of independent patient risk factors for middle ear barotrauma in a multiplace hyperbaric chamber. Diving Hyperb Med. 2013;43:143–7.

Demchenko IT, Zhilyaev SY, Moskvin AN, Piantadosi CA, Allen BW. Autonomic activation links CNS oxygen toxicity to acute cardiogenic pulmonary injury. Am J Physiol Lung Cell Mol Physiol. 2011;300:L102–11.

Duydu Y, Ustündag A, Aydin A, Eken A, Dündar K, Uzun G. Increased sensitivity to mitomycin C-induced sister chromatid exchange in lymphocytes from patients undergoing hyperbaric oxygen therapy. Environ Mol Mutagen. 2006;47:185–91.

Register SD, Aaron ME, Gelly HB. Hyperbaric oxygen therapy and optic neuritis: case report and literature review. Undersea Hyperb Med. 2011;38:557–9.

Richter K, Löblich HJ, Wyllie JW. Ultrastructural aspects of bubble formation in human fatal accidents after exposure to compressed air. Virchows Arch. 1978;380:261–72.

Toklu AS, Korpinar S, Erelel M, Uzun G, Yildiz S. Are pulmonary bleb and bullae a contraindication for hyperbaric oxygen treatment? Respir Med. 2008;102:1145–7.

Üstündağ A, Şimşek K, Ay H, Dündar K, Süzen S, Aydın A, et al. DNA integrity in patients undergoing hyperbaric oxygen (HBO) therapy. Toxicol In Vitro. 2012;26:1209–15.

Vahidova D, Sen P, Papesch M, Zein-Sanchez MP, Mueller PH. Does the slow compression technique of hyperbaric oxygen therapy decrease the incidence of middle-ear barotrauma? J Laryngol Otol. 2006;120:446–9.

Witte J, Kähler W, Wunderlich T, Radermacher P, Wohlrab C, Koch A. Dose-time dependency of hyperbaric hyperoxia-induced DNA strand breaks in human immune cells visualized with the comet assay. Undersea Hyperb Med. 2014;41:171–81.

Yamamoto Y, Noguchi Y, Enomoto M, Yagishita K, Kitamura K. Otological complications associated with hyperbaric oxygen therapy. Eur Arch Otorhinolaryngol. 2015;273(9):2487–93.

Yildiz S, Aktas S, Cimsit M, Ay H, Toğrol E. Seizure incidence in 80,000 patient treatments with hyperbaric oxygen. Aviat Space Environ Med. 2004;75:992–4.

Yuan J, Handy RD, Moody AJ, Smerdon G, Bryson P. Limited DNA damage in human endothelial cells after hyperbaric oxygen treatment and protection from subsequent hydrogen peroxide exposure. Biochim Biophys Acta. 2011;1810:526–31.

Zhang Q, Banks C, Choroomi S, Kertesz T. A novel technique of otic barotrauma management using modified intravenous cannulae. Eur Arch Otorhinolaryngol. 2013;270:2627–30.

Drug Interactions with Hyperbaric Oxygenation

9

K.K. Jain

Abstract

Interactions of HBO with other drugs should be recognized for prevention of adverse reactions as well as for enhancement of therapeutic effects. This chapter looks at oxygen as a drug and its interactions with commonly used drugs. Particular attention is paid to drugs affecting the central nervous system (CNS). Practical points of drug administration during HBO therapy are described. Drugs that enhance oxygen toxicity as well as those that protect against oxygen toxicity are also described.

Keywords

Drug interactions • CNS drugs • Oxygen toxicity • Free radical scavengers • Antioxidants

Oxygen as a Drug

When oxygen is breathed in concentrations higher than those found in the atmospheric air, it is considered to be a drug. By this definition, hyperbaric oxygen (HBO) is definitely a drug and it can interact with other drugs.

Drug–Drug Interactions

A drug–drug interaction occurs when pharmacologic action of a drug is altered by coadministration of second drug. This may result in an increase or decrease of the known effect of either drug or a new effect which is seen with neither of the drugs. Drug–drug interactions are classified on the basis of mechanism that is involved primarily. These are as follows:

- *Pharmacokinetic interactions* occur as the drug is transported to and from its site of action, and the result is a change in plasma level or tissue distribution of the drug.

- *Pharmacodynamic interactions* occur at biologically active (receptor) sites and result in a change in the pharmacologic effect of a given plasma level of the drug.

- *Idiosyncratic interactions* occur unpredictably in a small number of patients and are unexpected from known pharmacologic actions of individual drugs. Their mechanisms are generally unclear but may be based on genetic susceptibility.

Interactions of HBO with Other Drugs

It is important to be aware of these interactions in patients who are receiving other drugs, for HBO can either potentiate or reduce the effects of other drugs. Conversely, there are also drugs that reduce or potentiate the effects of HBO. These correspond to protectors against and enhancers of oxygen toxicity, respectively, as discussed in Chap. 6.

Many drugs, including nonprescription drugs, have undesirable side effects that may be modified in the hyperbaric environment. Some drug effects are potentiated and some are antagonized; some agents produce entirely different effects than those observed in normobaric environments. A review has documented interactions with HBO involving 38 of the 69 commonly prescribed drugs (Smith 2011).

K.K. Jain, MD, FRACS, FFPM (✉)
1 Blaesiring 7, Basel 4057, Switzerland
e-mail: jain@pharmabiotech.ch

© Springer International Publishing AG 2017
K.K. Jain, *Textbook of Hyperbaric Medicine*, DOI 10.1007/978-3-319-47140-2_9

Interaction of HBO with Antimicrobials

HBO enhances the effects of antibiotics as it has an antimicrobial effect of its own. HBO-induced free radicals may be toxic for the microorganisms. HBO may be considered to have synergistic effects with antibiotics. This topic will be discussed further in Chap. 14 dealing with infections.

Carbapenem Antibiotics

Imipenem (Primaxin), an intravenous β-lactam antibiotic, is a member of the carbapenem class of antibiotics. Burn wounds are infected with *Pseudomonas aeruginosa*, which is sensitive to imipenem. Because such wounds are treated with HBO, its possible interaction with imipenem has been studied. The effects of HBO (100 % O_2, 3 ATA, 5 h) in combination with imipenem tested on bacterial counts of six isolates of *P. aeruginosa* and bacterial ultrastructure were investigated (Lima et al. 2015). Infected macrophages were exposed to HBO and the production of reactive oxygen species (ROS) was monitored. Results showed that HBO enhanced the effects of imipenem and increased superoxide anion production by macrophages, which likely kills bacteria by oxidative mechanisms. Therefore, HBO in combination with imipenem can be used to kill *P. aeruginosa* in vitro, and such treatment may be beneficial for the patients with injuries containing *P. aeruginosa*.

Aminoglycoside Antibiotics

CSF transfer of the aminoglycoside antibiotic tobramycin is not altered under HBO in rabbits, and HBO has no significant effect on the CSF concentration of this agent. CO_2, which is known to damage BBB, more than doubles the CSF/blood ratio for tobramycin. Pharmacokinetics of gentamicin does not change in healthy volunteers exposed to HBO.

Sulfonamides

Increase of oxygen tension has a synergistic bactericidal effect with sulfonamides rather than the usual bacteriostatic action. HBO and antibiotic synergism are discussed in Chap. 14.

Mafenide acetate (Sulfamylon), an antibacterial agent used in burn patients, is a carbonic anhydrase inhibitor and tends to promote CO_2 retention and vasodilatation. This drug must be discontinued before patients are placed in a hyperbaric chamber for HBO treatment.

Interaction of HBO with Anticancer Agents

The role of HBO in enhancing cancer radiosensitivity is discussed in Chap. 38. Hypoxia is a common phenomenon in solid tumors, associated with chemotherapy and radiotherapy resistance, recurrence, and metastasis. HBO therapy can increase tissue oxygen content to counteract hypoxia and enhance the effect of anticancer therapy. Interaction of HBO with some anticancer agents will be described here.

Exposure of cancer cells to HBO at 3 ATA for 2 h has been shown to produce inhibition of DNA synthesis or mitosis. Simultaneous exposure to HBO and adriamycin results in decreased cytotoxicity. However, exposure to adriamycin 2–8 h before or after HBO produces an increase in the drug effect. Cytotoxicity increases when cells were exposed to HBO before, during, or after nitrogen mustard administration.

HBO enhances the chemotherapeutic effect of doxorubicin both in cell culture and in animal models. HBO reduces the rate of misonidazole metabolism, thus increasing the concentration of this substance in tumors, which enhances radiosensitivity. However, doxorubicin is regarded as a contraindication for concomitant use with HBO therapy because of the increased risk of cardiotoxicity. An experimental study has shown that HBO exposure does not potentiate doxorubicin-induced cardiotoxicity in rats but confers cardioprotection against doxorubicin, which warrants further investigation (Karagoz et al. 2008).

Sorafenib is a first-line drug for hepatocellular carcinoma (HCC) but effective in only a small portion of patients and can induce tumor hypoxia. A study has investigated the effect of HBO in combination with sorafenib on hepatoma cell lines, which were exposed to HBO at 2 ATA pressure for 80 min per day or combined with sorafenib or cisplatin (Peng et al. 2014). HBO combined with sorafenib results in synergistic growth inhibition and apoptosis in hepatoma cells, suggesting a potential application of HBO combined with sorafenib in HCC patients. It was also shown that HBO significantly altered microRNA expression in hepatoma cells.

Interaction of HBO with Cardiovascular Drugs

Adrenomimetic, Adrenolytic, and Ganglion-Blocking Agents

Under HBO, there is a considerable reduction of hypotensive effect of α- and β-blockers, ganglion blockers, and β-adrenomimetics and elimination of the effects of central adrenomimetics. The pressor effects of the directly and particularly of the indirectly acting α-adrenomimetics, as well as the cardiotropic effects of β-adrenoblockers, are potentiated. Therefore, these drugs should be given after but not before the HBO session.

Digitalis/Digoxin

HBO has been reported to decrease the effectiveness of cardiac glycosides. There is some evidence that HBO may reduce the toxic effects of digitalis.

Antianginal Drugs

The effect of a single HBO session (1.5 ATA, duration 40 min), in combination with antianginal drugs, has been investigated in patients with ischemic heart disease and angina pectoris of effort, NYHA functional classes II–III. HBO reduces the degree of indirect hemodynamic effect of nifedipine and potentiates negative chronotropic and inotropic effects of propranolol—but has no impact on the degree of hemodynamic effect of depot–glycerol trinitrate.

Heparin

Heparin-treated animals exposed to HBO develop pulmonary hemorrhages as a result of interactions of the anticoagulant effect of heparin- and oxygen-induced pulmonary lesions. The pressures and exposure times in experimental studies are much longer than those used clinically and these observations are not applicable to humans. However, since heparin has been used as an adjunctive measure in patients undergoing HBO treatments, this potential complication should be kept in mind, although none has been reported in patients on heparin undergoing HBO treatments.

Interaction of HBO with Drugs Acting on the CNS

Anesthetics

The interactions of anesthetics with HBO are discussed in Chap. 41, but some of the drugs used are reviewed briefly here, due to their importance in many aspects of the current topic.

CNS Stimulants

CNS stimulants such as amphetamines interact unfavorably with HBO. And, notably, excessive coffee drinking in those who are susceptible to caffeine may also predispose to oxygen toxicity.

Ethanol

Hyperbaric air has a synergistic effect with ethanol and increases the sleeping time in mice. This may explain the increased susceptibility to the effects of compression and decompression of those who have imbibed alcohol. There are no special ill effects of HBO on patients who suffer carbon monoxide poisoning while they are inebriated. There is no evidence that HBO accelerates the metabolism of "sobering up" in alcoholics.

Narcotic Analgesics

Narcotic drugs generally depress respiration by reducing the reactivity of medullary centers to CO_2. This, combined with the depressing effect of HBO on respiration, can lead to a rise in $paCO_2$, which causes vasodilatation and enhances oxygen toxicity.

Pharmacokinetics of meperidine in dogs breathing air at 1 ATA is not altered under HBO at 2.8 ATA or breathing air at 6 ATA. The findings in dogs cannot, of course, be extrapolated to humans, as the two species handle drugs very differently. The action of morphine also is unchanged by HBO.

Pentobarbital

It has been mentioned in Chap. 3 that pentobarbital anesthesia can be reversed in rats under atmospheric pressure. Attempts to distinguish between the two possible causes of this reversal—changes in the drug disposition and changes in drug–receptor interaction—by studying the pharmacokinetics of pentobarbital in dogs exposed to HBO show no significant effect of HBO on total plasma clearance, volume of distribution, or elimination half-life of pentobarbital, thus ruling out changes in drug disposition as a cause of reversal of CNS depression by pentobarbital.

Scopolamine

This is an anticholinergic compound used widely for management of motion sickness and may be used concomitantly with HBO, particularly in divers. Interaction of scopolamine with HBO at 5 ATA has been tested in rats. The duration of the latent period preceding the onset of hyperoxic convulsions was not altered. However, the visual and cardiovascular side effects of the drug should be taken into consideration when scopolamine is used in combination with HBO. Scopolamine is also used as a transdermal patch, and no changes in its action were observed in divers exposed to pressures of over 2 ATA.

Interaction of HBO with Miscellaneous Drugs

Insulin. The dosages of insulin required in diabetes are decreased during HBO therapy and should be readjusted.

Losartan. Addition of HBO therapy to losartan, an angiotensin receptor blocker, increases the drug efficacy and has significant benefits in the management of proteinuria (Yilmaz et al. 2006).

Reserpine and guanethidine. Reserpine and guanethidine have been shown to interact unfavorably with HBO.

Salicylates. There is a significant increase in salicylate clearance in dogs at 2.8 ATA. There are no studies in humans.

Theophylline. There are no effects of HBO (2.8 ATA) on the pharmacokinetics of theophylline in the dog. There are no studies in humans.

Practical Considerations of Drug Administration During HBO Therapy

The mechanical effect of the pressure on the drug containers should be taken into consideration. Drugs stocked in a multiplace chamber and subjected to repeated compression and decompression should be put into pressure-proof containers. There are no problems of explosion with small vials when pressures are below 3 ATA. Multidose rubber top vials should be used only once in a hyperbaric chamber because of possible contamination while withdrawing a drug. Precautions for drug delivery devices are discussed in Chap. 7.

Elastomeric drug delivery devices are commonly used for long-term IV therapy in the outpatient setting. Patients receiving HBO therapy occasionally need these devices. A study compared the performance of the Baxter infusor LV10 elastomeric device in repetitive conditions at pressures of 243 kPa (Lewis et al. 2015). The fluid delivered by each device was measured and the device weighed at the end of each pressurization. No significant differences in delivery rate of the devices were observed between hyperbaric and control conditions.

Drugs that Enhance Oxygen Toxicity

Acetazolamide. Acetazolamide is a carbonic anhydrase inhibitor that prevents oxygen-induced vasoconstriction and increases blood flow under HBO. This predisposes the brain to the toxic action of oxygen. Acetazolamide should not be used at pressures greater than 2 ATA.

CNS stimulants. See section "CNS Stimulants."

Disulfiram. This drug is used in alcohol aversion therapy. It may potentiate oxygen toxicity via in vivo reduction to diethyldithiocarbamate and subsequent inhibition of superoxide dismutase.

Perfluorocarbon (PFC). Treatment of decompression sickness may involve the use of PFC and these patients may also receive HBO. It has been hypothesized that PFC can potentially increase the risk of CNS oxygen toxicity under HBO conditions. A rat model was used to evaluate the effects of intravenously administered PFC emulsion and was recorded during treatment with HBO at 6 ATA in the presence and absence of PFC (Liu et al. 2012). Concentrations of malondialdehyde (MDA), nitric oxide (NO), and hydrogen peroxide (H_2O_2) in the brain cortex and hippocampus were quantified. Changes in the activities of superoxide dismutase (SOD), glutathione peroxidase (GPx), catalase (CAT), and NO synthase (NOS) in the brain cortex and hippocampus were also determined. Edaravone, a potent antioxidant, was used to prevent PFC-induced CNS oxygen toxicity. The results showed that after PFC administration, the latency to first electrical discharge in EEG was significantly shortened; MDA, H_2O_2, and NO levels and NOS activity increased; and SOD, GPx, and CAT activities decreased. Edaravone effectively protected against CNS oxygen toxicity and the adverse effects of PFC. Results demonstrate that PFC administered before HBO would promote the occurrence of CNS oxygen toxicity, and edaravone could serve as a promising chemoprophylactic agent to prevent this.

Thyroid extract. Thyroid or thyroid extract given to experimental animals under HBO enhances the toxic effects of oxygen. The increase of metabolic rate is thought to predispose to oxygen-induced convulsions. It is a reasonable assumption that this would also occur in humans).

Drugs that Protect Against Oxygen Toxicity

This topic has been discussed in Chap. 6 and a list of drugs that protect against oxygen toxicity is given in Table 6.5.

Anticonvulsants. Phenytoin (Dilantin) and diazepam (Valium) are used to prevent seizures and do not have any protective effect against oxygen toxicity as such. Barbiturates are also used as antiepileptics and may have a protective effect against oxygen toxicity. But the disadvantage of using barbiturates is that they are respiratory depressants. Diazepam (Valium) is used to prevent and control seizures of nonhyperbaric origin. The dosage is 5–50 mg given slowly by intravenous injection. It may also lead to respiratory depression. Lorazepam is similar in action to diazepam but requires one-fifth the dose. If phenytoin is used, care should be taken not to use high pressures of oxygen for long periods: CNS toxicity may occur without the warning signs of seizures. Carbamazepine has been found to be useful for the prevention of CNS toxicity during HBO therapy of epilepsy-prone patients.

Ergot derivatives. Two ergot derivatives lisuride and quinpirole have been shown to antagonize convulsions in mice induced by HBO at 5 ATA. This protection was found to about 50 % of that obtained by diazepam. There is no report of use of any ergot derivatives in patients for this purpose.

Lidocaine. In subconvulsant doses, the local anesthetic, lidocaine, has a neuroprotective effect against CNS toxicity during exposure to HBO; the mechanism of this protection is unknown, but it may involve changes in the brain monoamine systems or changes in the excitability of neuronal membranes.

Magnesium. Mg ion compounds are substances with antioxidant and vasodilating effects and therefore reduce oxygen toxicity. A single dose of 10 mmol of magnesium sulfate can be given 3 h before a HBO session.

Phenothiazines. Chlorpromazine is considered to be protective against oxygen toxicity.

Propranolol. L-Propranolol has been shown to protect mice against HBO-induced seizures. There have been no reports of clinical application of this effect.

Vitamin E. Vitamin E is believed to protect against oxygen toxicity by counteracting the oxygen free radicals. A dose of 400 mg daily should be given to patients scheduled for HBO therapy starting 2 days before the therapy.

Conclusion

Drug interactions with HBO represent an important subject, but there is a lack of studies for many of the commonly used medications. Animal studies cannot always be applied to humans. Therefore, studies of the pharmacokinetics of commonly used drugs in patients receiving HBO should be carried out and an authoritative drug incompatibility list compiled; such a list would be incorporated in various pharmacopoeias and displayed in hyperbaric treatment facilities. A careful history should be taken on drug use by patients, and caution should be exercised in the use of drugs known to interact with oxygen.

References

Karagoz B, Suleymanoglu S, Uzun G, Bilgi O, Aydinoz S, Haholu A, et al. Hyperbaric oxygen therapy does not potentiate doxorubicin-induced cardiotoxicity in rats. Basic Clin Pharmacol Toxicol. 2008;102:287–92.

Lewis I, Smart D, Brown B, Baines C. Performance of the Baxter Infusor LV10 under hyperbaric conditions. Diving Hyperb Med. 2015;45:37–41.

Lima FL, Joazeiro PP, Lancellotti M, de Hollanda LM, de Araújo LB, Linares E, et al. Effects of hyperbaric oxygen on Pseudomonas aeruginosa susceptibility to imipenem and macrophages. Future Microbiol. 2015;10:179–89.

Liu S, Li R, Ni X, Cai Z, Zhang R, Sun X, et al. Perfluorocarbon-facilitated CNS oxygen toxicity in rats: reversal by edaravone. Brain Res. 2012;1471:56–65.

Peng HS, Liao MB, Zhang MY, Xie Y, Xu L, Zhang YJ, et al. Synergistic inhibitory effect of hyperbaric oxygen combined with sorafenib on hepatoma cells. PLoS One. 2014;9, e100814.

Smith RG. An appraisal of potential drug interactions regarding hyperbaric oxygen therapy and frequently prescribed medications. Wounds. 2011;23:147–59.

Yilmaz MI, Korkmaz A, Kaya A, Sonmez A, Caglar K, Topal T, et al. Hyperbaric oxygen treatment augments the efficacy of a losartan regime in an experimental nephrotic syndrome model. Nephron Exp Nephrol. 2006;104:e15–22.

J. Michael Uszler

Abstract

Modern medical date diagnostic imaging includes a variety of technologies, with the most prominent being SPECT (and PET) for function imaging and CT and MRI for anatomic, nonfunctional imaging. SPECT brain function imaging is the prominent technology that has been used for more than 25 years to evaluate brain function in relation to changes and functional characteristics of an individual's brain before and after any type of therapy; in this case, the effects of hyperbaric oxygen (HBO) therapy (HBOT). This chapter indicates some roles of brain SPECT function imaging in the evaluation of different types of brain dysfunctional states, before and after treatment, including the utilization of HBO therapy regarding any one of these conditions discovered by imaging and their comorbidities.

Keywords

Brain imaging • Single photon emission computed tomography (SPECT) • Computed tomography (CT) • Hyperperfusion • Hypoperfusion • Radioisotope • Radiopharmaceutical • Positron emission tomography (PET) • Magnetic resonance imaging (MRI) • Hyperbaric oxygen therapy (HBOT)

Introduction

Nuclear medicine imaging involves the use of intravenously injected radiopharmaceuticals, with a radiopharmaceutical selected for the particular organ system of interest that for the diagnostic and functional study is to be performed. The radiopharmaceutical substance distributes to the organ system of interest in accordance with the "tracer" principle, namely, that only a trace quantity of the tracer is injected such that it does not disturb the function of the organ system to be evaluated. Because only a "trace" quantity of radiopharmaceutical is used, for example, the radiation dose for a representative 10 year old is approximately 1/30th that of a CT scan for that same 10-year-old person.

The modern-day technology record for this process requires three factors: the first one is the radio tracer itself; second is the imaging hardware, in this case the SPECT scanner which gathers the radiopharmaceutical emission information from the body organ system that is being imaged. Finally, proprietary software is utilized to process the three-dimensional (3-D) data that is gathered from any one study, such that the imaging data can be presented in both 2-D and 3-D image formats, as well as to provide the semi-quantitative functional information.

A key point to note is that the purpose of any functional imaging study is actually not to make one clinical diagnosis. Rather it is for the purpose of gathering organ function information and then analyzing that functional information to determine the clinical single or multiple comorbidities that may be represented by that functional information. For instance, a common factor is that brain SPECT imaging may be clinically intended to evaluate for mild traumatic brain injury, but the scan functional information may also indicate

J.M. Uszler, MD, MS (✉)
Department of Nuclear Medicine, Providence St. Johns Health Center, 2121 Santa Monica Blvd., Santa Monica, CA 90404, USA
e-mail: uszler58@gmail.com

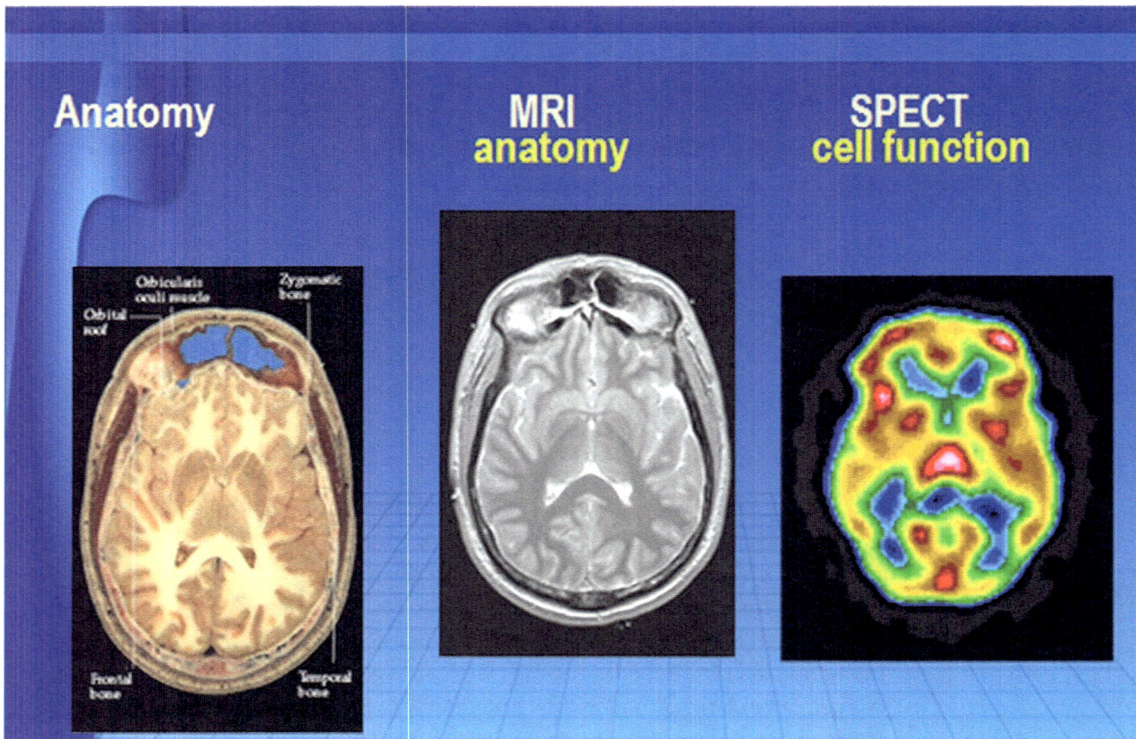

Fig. 10.1 Transverse post-mortem image along with another living state individual's transverse MRI and SPECT tomographic images showing anatomic correspondence at the mid-brain level

concomitant occurrence of (PTSD) post-traumatic stress disorder or neurotoxic substance exposure.

So the main reasons for getting a SPECT brain function scan are: (1) visual documentation of the presence and the extent of neurological disorder and regional dysfunction; (2) documenting possible multi-focal dysfunction secondary to disease etiologies that may be vascular, inflammatory, traumatic, or neurotoxic; and (3) uncovering comorbidities not considered in the initial clinical diagnosis.

Figure 10.1, a 3-image comparison, shows representative mid-brain anatomy in terms of the postmortem state compared with the living state images of MRI (anatomy) and the SPECT (actual neuronal function). Figure 10.2 is an example of SPECT brain imaging device with three imaging "heads" that slowly revolve around the patient's head during the 20-min scan.

The clinical utilization of brain SPECT function imaging requires the radiopharmaceutical being taken up only by functioning neurons; this is not a process simply of blood vessel flow, such as angiography. If the intravenously injected radiopharmaceutical is not taken up by neurons, i.e., the neurons are non-functioning, this indicates that these regions of the brain are actually not working adequately. Because of "injury" they may be functioning at only a low level, the so-called "idling neurons," and are not actually non-viable. It has been shown that "idling neurons" can have their functional level increased,

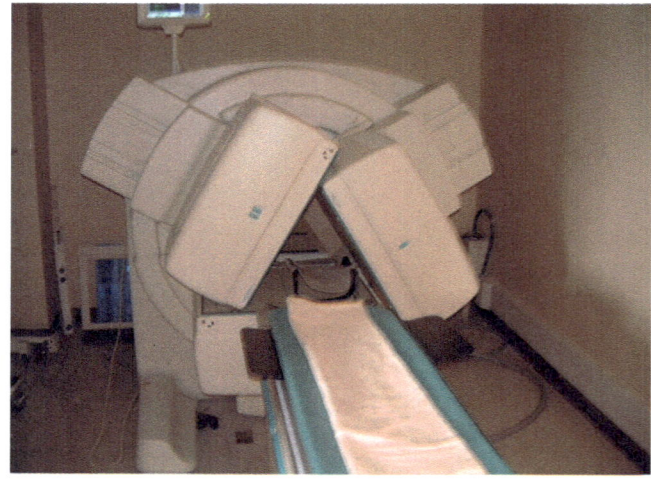

Fig. 10.2 Example of SPECT brain imaging device with three imaging "heads" that slowly revolve around the patient's head during the 20-min scan

possibly back to full normal function. This improved functional state is what is exemplified by increased, improved radiopharmaceutical uptake on SPECT brain imaging.

Remember that the way the brain cells work is that the brain cells do not store their own metabolites and thus need a continuous, variable supply of both the glucose and oxygen in order to maintain their ongoing function.

Basically, all disease processes start at the cellular level. And given that CT and MRI anatomic imaging is at a macroscopic level, CT and MRI are not effective at evaluating or diagnosing a dysfunctional or disease process, that is, unless a sufficient number of millions of cells are involved with the process so as to produce a macroscopic-sized lesion, whether that be mass lesion or distortion of anatomy.

Case Studies

The clinical applications for the utilization of brain SPECT function imaging in patients who are being evaluated for hyperbaric oxygen therapy include: cerebral palsy, CVA/stroke, concussion and traumatic brain injury, exposure to neurotoxic substances, be they environmental, therapeutic, or recreational, and for the evaluation of atypical brain function and clinical entities included in so-called Autism Spectrum Disorders (ASD) and Pervasive Developmental Disorders (PDD). In virtually all of these conditions, patients present with a cluster of dysfunctional symptoms and signs, and SPECT brain function imaging clarifies via regional brain function information that there are multiple comorbidities present. Based upon the brain SPECT imaging of atypical brain region function, rather than clinical diagnostic labeling, triaging of the patient's actual therapeutic indicators can be decided.

A clinical example of a "stroke" is represented in the following case. The patient was a 20-year-old female who had suffered a traumatic laceration of her right middle cerebral artery approximately 2 years prior to presenting for brain SPECT function imaging in relation to her start of hyperbaric oxygen therapy. As is frequently and unfortunately typical in cases such as this, it's important to notice that more than 2 years had elapsed from the time the patient actually suffered the brain injury and has undergone all different forms of rehabilitation therapy before finally presenting for actual medical imaging of the brain function injury along with the onset of hyperbaric oxygen therapy.

Figure 10.3 shows brain SPECT 3-D brain images before and after the performance of 40 h of hyperbaric oxygen therapy. The image on the left indicates that there are a variety of different degrees of brain function, including one focal area (black area) of virtually absent function in the right middle cerebral artery territory. This area clinically corresponds to the clinically observable left hemiparesis. The image on the left shows that while clinically all the therapy has been focused on the person's left hemiparesis, the SPECT function imaging shows that there is bilateral functional impairment in this person's brain, especially with significantly altered function in the frontal and temporal lobes bilaterally. These visualized function imaging

findings made other clinicians finally aware of frontal lobe dysfunctions in this person, which had not been attended to; frontal lobe dysfunctions corresponded to this person's inability to drive, not able to express emotions, not able to continue with her college studies, and not able to hold a job. Thus, she had a significant loss of overall quality of life, not just being functionally neurologically impaired. The brain SPECT function imaging made that overtly apparent. The image on the right shows one corresponding view of brain 3-D brain function after 40 hyperbaric treatments. The therapeutic regimen was 1.75–2.0 ATA in a 100 % oxygen flow through chamber, with the therapy sessions being 3–5 per week, such that the 40 hyperbaric treatments were accomplished in approximately 8 weeks. The brain SPECT function image (on the right side of the image) indicates two important facts. Firstly, there was no improvement of the focal markedly decreased perfusion in the right motor cortex area that was non-viable. Secondly, the scan indicated that multiple areas in the bilateral areas of the cerebral cortex showed improved functioning. And clinically corresponding to this was the observation that she could now engage more effectively in executive functions such as concentration, decision-making, and a better awareness of her emotional state. And yes, corresponding to the focal defect pattern in the right motor cortex, there was unfortunately no improvement in her left hemiparesis.

The longer term (beyond her initial 40 HBOT course and follow-up SPECT brain scan) showed that the patient subsequently had a total of at least 100 hyperbaric oxygen therapy treatments (before being lost to clinical follow-up). Over the ensuing 4–5 months, there was significant clinical improvement, she regained executive function, was able to drive a motor vehicle, able to return to her college studies and get her college degree. In essence, she regained much of her normal life, albeit with a residual left-sided hemiparesis. Thus, the take-home message from this case is that brain SPECT function imaging portrayed the bilateral brain dysfunction that was occurring in the patient and which had been clinically unrecognized and untreated. The subsequent hyperbaric oxygen therapy resulted in a marked bilateral cerebral improvement such that the patient regained much of her normal life.

The SPECT scan observation of multiple comorbidities also includes hyperperfused focal cortical areas that are SPECT evidence of possible epileptogenic foci (Figs. 10.4a, b). Clinical communications with practitioners treating pediatric and young adult age individuals seems to indicate that individuals with these hyperperfused "hyperactive" areas may get temporarily worse during the mid-course of a 40 dive HBOT course, resulting in temporary clinically increased hyperactive behavior. This reportedly clinically .subsides by the completion of a 40 sessions of HBOT therapy. However, the presence

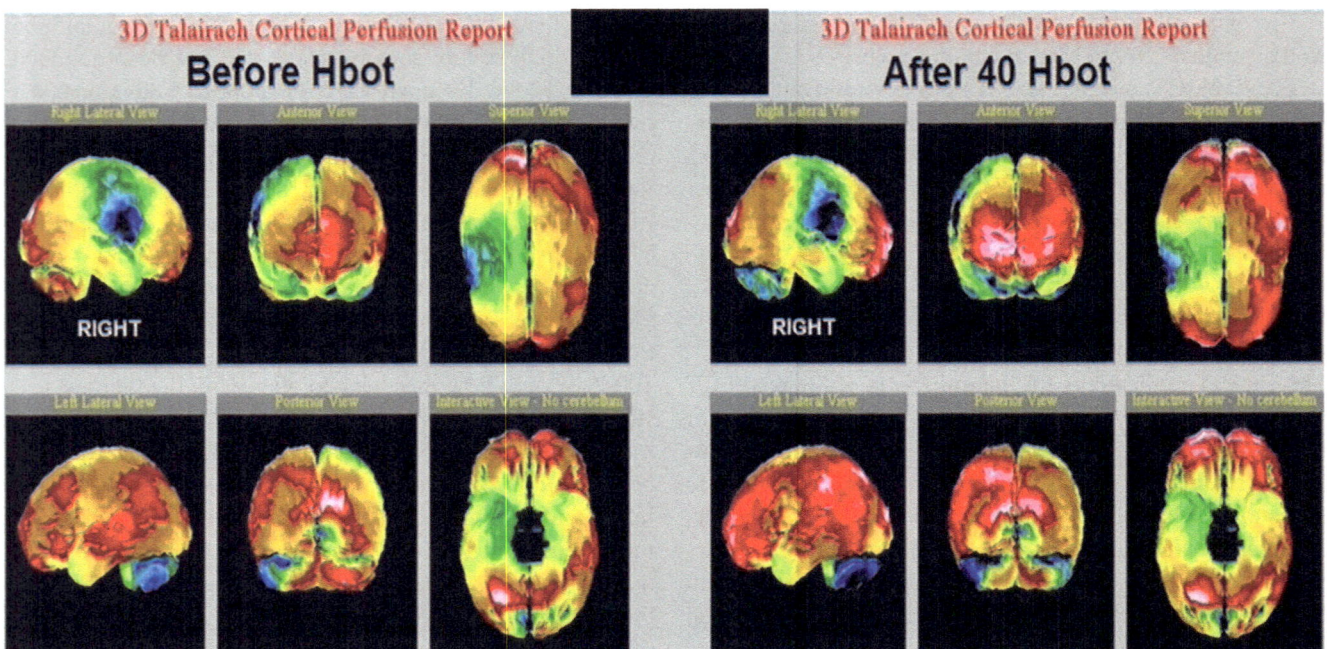

Fig. 10.3 3D semi-quantitative SPECT brain functions images before (*left*) and after (*right*) 40 HBO treatments (HBOT) using 100% O$_2$ at 1.75–2.0 ATA over 6- to 8-week period

of this brain cortically extensive hyperperfusion has led some practitioners to treat hyperactivity with anticonvulsants before initiating HBOT.

How often one uses SPECT brain function scanning is related to the clinical context of neurologic symptoms and the absence of abnormality on anatomic CT or MRI imaging. Remember that SPECT is much more sensitive for atypical, abnormal neuronal function because it represents what is occurring at a cellular, not macroscopic, level. After the SPECT documentation of traumatic brain injury, stoke or neurotoxic injury, the SPECT scan also serves as the baseline documentation prior to the onset of any therapy. If there is clinical improvement, then no follow-up SPECT scan is necessary. However, if one is considering an additional course of HBOT or any other type of therapy even with the occurrence of clinical improvement, then a follow-up scan can be performed to serve as a new baseline at the onset of any new therapy. Generally, no more than three SPECT brain function scans are done per year.

Conclusion

1. Brain SPECT function imaging is utilization of radioisotope imaging to evaluate organ system function on a regional (fundamentally a cellular) level. In this way, the focus is on making decisions based upon the physiologic basis of the patient's problem, thereby leading to appropriate targeted therapies. Brain SPECT functional imaging has been in clinical use for almost 30 years and is neither investigational nor experimental.

2. SPECT brain function imaging at a cellular level actually represents in vivo imaging of biochemistry and cellular function or dysfunction. The interpretation of brain SPECT imaging 30 years ago was based on anatomic distortion rather than the cellular dysfunction. It's only with the recent utilization of more sophisticated software, including semi-quantitative analysis and three-dimensional imaging, that one can observe cellular dysfunction before any anatomic changes have happened. This is the fundamental reason why SPECT brain function imaging is significantly more sensitive for the detection of regional cellular dysfunction or disease processes than macroscopic anatomic imaging with CT or MRI.

3. Brain SPECT function imaging can be used before and after courses of therapy to uncover a seizure disorder that is not clinically manifest, uncover traumatic brain injury or post-traumatic stress disorder, uncover temporal lobe dysfunction (which may subsequently improve with HBOT leading to improved languaging in ASD), uncover cerebellar dysfunction (that could be improved with HBOT thereby leading to improved sensory integration), and uncover brain dysfunction that has not been responding to present therapy (of any type).

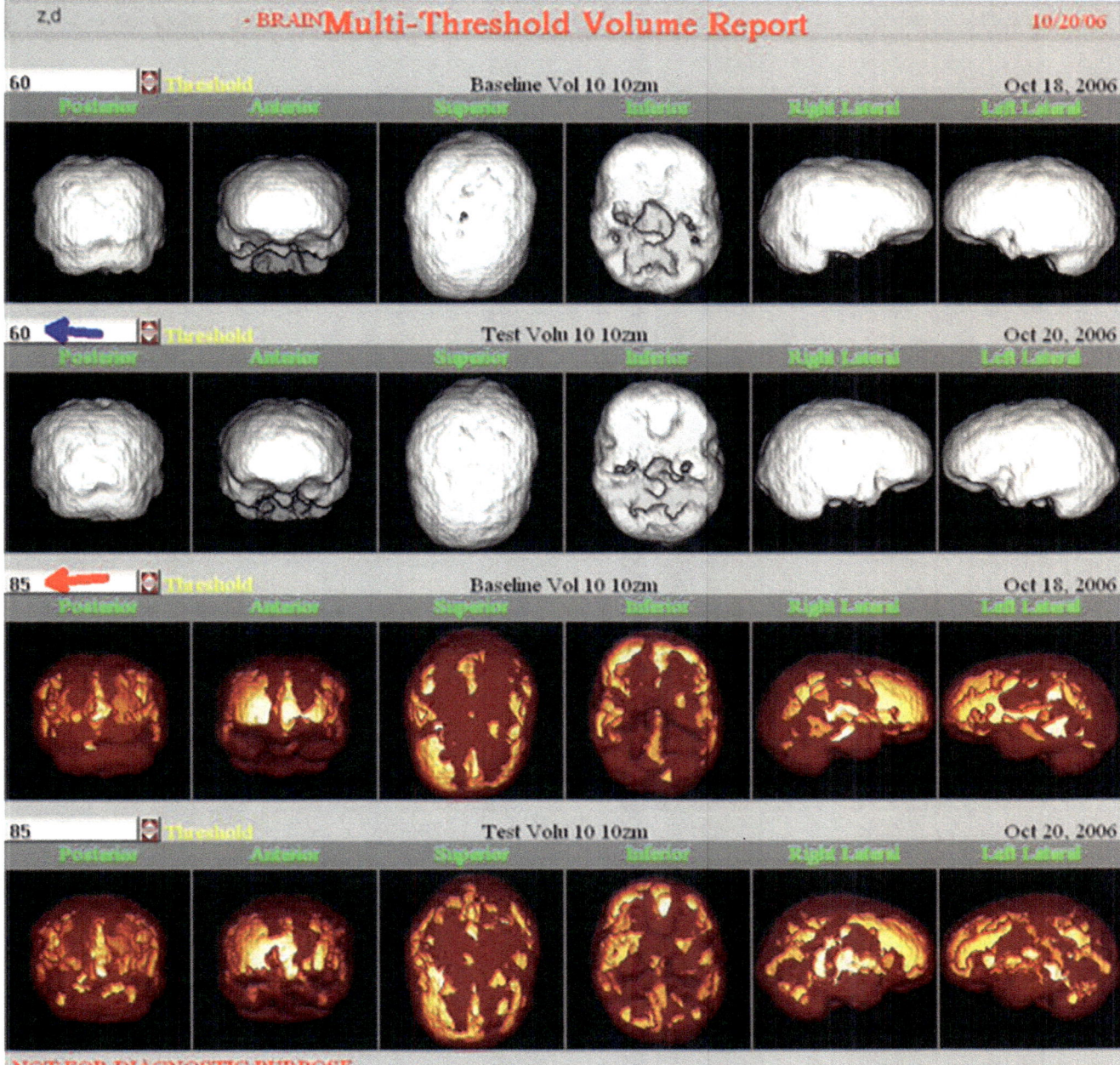

Fig. 10.4 (**a**) 3D SPECT brain function images indicating grayscale findings of temporal lobe decreased function and color scale findings of multiple cortical areas of hyperfunctioning areas. This combination is seen in autism spectrum disorder (ASD) and was evidence against the original clinical diagnosis of attention deficit hyperactivity disorder (ADHD), for which the patient was treated for 4 years. (**b**) Tomographic cross-sectional images also showing focal areas (*red* and *white*) of hyperperfusion, consistent with epileptogenic (seizure) foci

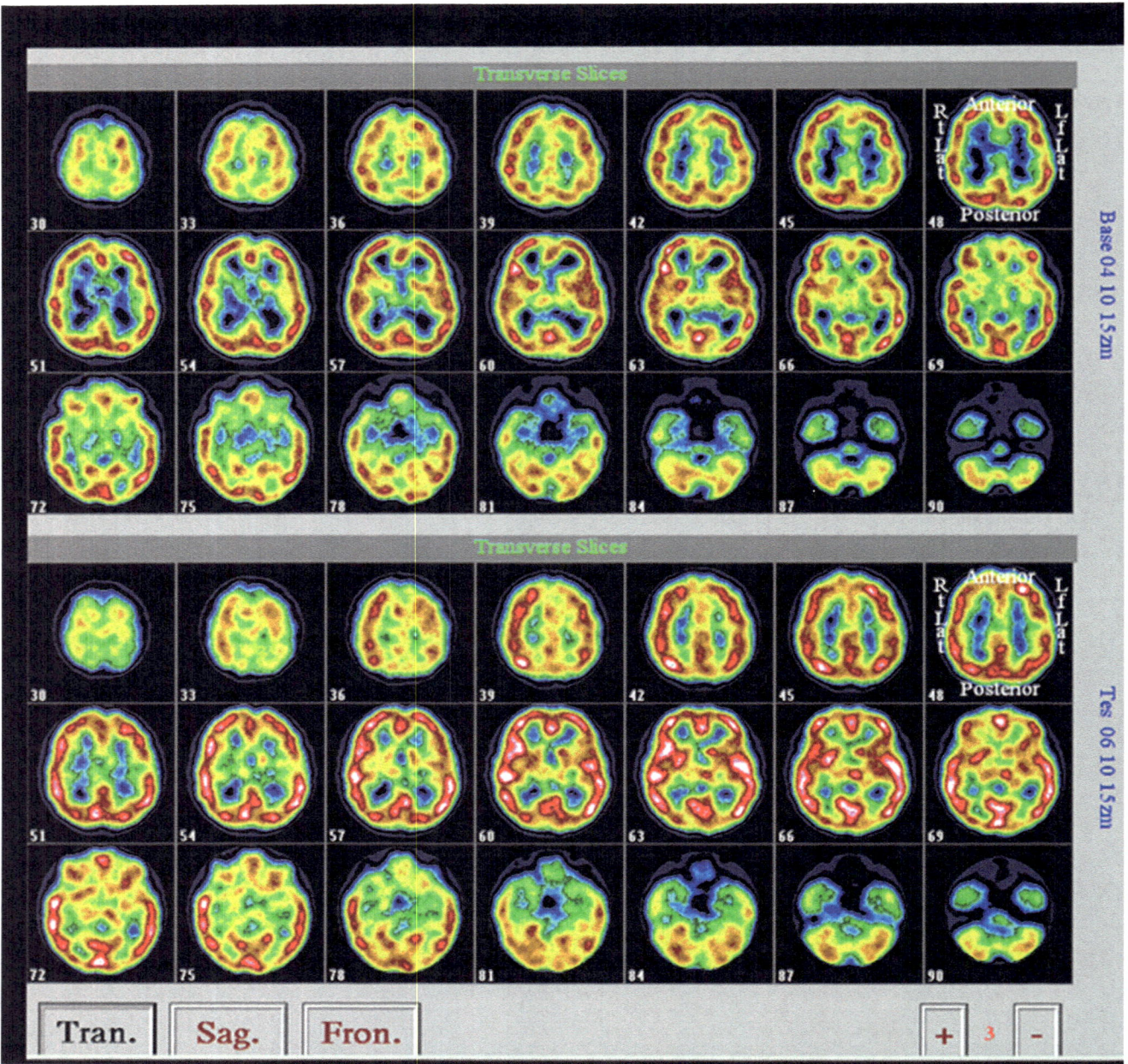

Fig. 10.4 (continued)

4. Because brain SPECT function imaging reveals dysfunction or disease processes at a cellular level, it is not necessarily focused on any one diagnostic entity, and thus represents functional information secondary to any cause of physiologic disturbance. Because of this, although there is usually one clinical diagnostic consideration, SPECT brain function imaging reveals the presence of multiple comorbidity factors in literally every patient. In this way, it serves a clinically very useful purpose by providing a much more profound insight into multiple factors that may be causing the clinically apparent dysfunction, be it behavioral, anatomic, or physiologic.

Suggested Reading

Boussi-Gross R, Golan H, Fishlev G, Bechor Y, Volkov O, Bergan J, et al. Hyperbaric oxygen therapy can improve post concussion syndrome years after mild traumatic brain injury—randomized prospective trial. PLoS One. 2013;8, e79995.

Chang DC, Lee JT, Lo CP, Fan YM, Huang KL, Kang BH, et al. Hyperbaric oxygen ameliorates delayed neuropsychiatric syndrome of carbon monoxide poisoning. Undersea Hyperb Med. 2010;37:23–33.

Efrati S, Fishlev G, Bechor Y, Volkov O, Bergan J, Kliakhandler K, et al. Hyperbaric oxygen induces late neuroplasticity in post stroke patients—randomized, prospective trial. PLoS One. 2013;8, e53716.

Harch PG, Fogarty EF, Staab PK, Van Meter K. Low pressure hyperbaric oxygen therapy and SPECT brain imaging in the treatment of blast-induced chronic traumatic brain injury (post-concussion syndrome) and post traumatic stress disorder: a case report. Cases J. 2009;2:6538.

Lin YT, Chen SY, Lo CP, Lee JT, Tsai CF, Yip PK, et al. Utilizing cerebral perfusion scan and diffusion-tensor MR imaging to evaluate the effect of hyperbaric oxygen therapy in carbon monoxide-induced delayed neuropsychiatric seqeulae—a case report and literature review. Acta Neurol Taiwan. 2015;24:57–62.

Neubauer RA, James P. Cerebral oxygenation and the recoverable brain. Neurol Res. 1998;20 Suppl 1:S33–6.

Raji CA, Tarzwell R, Pavel D, Schneider H, Uszler M, Thornton J, et al. Clinical utility of SPECT neuroimaging in the diagnosis and treatment of traumatic brain injury: a systematic review. PLoS One. 2014;9, e91088.

Rossignol DA, Bradstreet JJ, Van Dyke K, Schneider C, Freedenfeld SH, O'Hara N, et al. Hyperbaric oxygen treatment in autism spectrum disorders. Med Gas Res. 2012;2:16.

Shi XY, Tang ZQ, Sun D, He XJ. Evaluation of hyperbaric oxygen treatment of neuropsychiatric disorders following traumatic brain injury. Chin Med J (Engl). 2006;119:1978–82.

Decompression Sickness

Philip B. James and K.K. Jain

Abstract

Decompression sickness (DCS) is a form of dysbarism, which is the general term applied to all changes, pathophysiological changes secondary to altered environmental pressure. This chapter looks at risk factors, pathophysiology, clinical features, diagnosis, and the treatment of DCS. Early recompression is the only effective treatment for DCS, the increase in pressure redissolving the gas phase and oxygen restoring endothelial disruption and downregulating neutrophil interactions. For air diving recompression with oxygen or helium and oxygen mixtures is preferred to recompression breathing air. Helium and oxygen divers should not be recompressed breathing air. The management of neurological manifestations of DCS is given special attention to avoid late sequelae.

Keywords

Dysbarism • Altitude sickness • Decompression sickness (DCS) • Dysbaric osteonecrosis • Recompression • Hyperbaric chamber • Hyperbaric oxygenation (HBO) • Helium-oxygen mixtures • Comex 30 • Microembolism • Perivenous syndrome (PS) • Neutrophils

Introduction

Decompression sickness (DCS) is one form of dysbarism, which is a general term applied to all pathological changes secondary to altered environmental pressure. Other forms are pulmonary barotrauma and also aseptic bone necrosis, which is likely to be a form of decompression sickness. DCS is caused by gas phase formed by a sufficiently rapid reduction of environmental pressure to cause supersaturation of the gases dissolved in the tissues. The principle component is most usually nitrogen, but when helium and oxygen mixtures are used it is helium. DCS is also described by the terms, cais-

son disease, "the bends" (joint pains), "the chokes" (pulmonary symptoms), the "staggers" (vestibular symptoms), and "hits" (spinal cord symptoms). DCS occurs most commonly in divers usually within 24 h of a reduction in ambient pressure on ascent from a minimum depth of 6 m of sea water. DCS also occurs in those who work in compressed air as in caissons and tunnels. It can also result from a reduction of normal barometric pressure, such as in a hypobaric chamber or ascent in aircraft to altitudes in excess of 5000 m even when oxygen is breathed. It complicates flight in some high altitude military aircraft and may occur when astronauts don suits for undertaking extravehicular activity. Bubble formation may also be a component of altitude sickness in climbers making a rapid ascent. At sea level, 1 ATA almost 1 L of nitrogen is dissolved in the body. A little less than one-half of this is dissolved in water and a little more than one-half in the fat, which constitutes only 15 % of the normal male body—nitrogen is five times more soluble in fat than in water. In diving the additional amount of nitrogen that dissolves in the body depends upon the depth and the duration of a dive. For steady-state conditions, the volume of nitrogen that is liberated returning

P.B. James, MB, ChB, DIH, PhD, FFOM (✉)
Department of Surgery, Ninewells Hospital and Medical School, Ninewells Avenue, Dundee, Angus DD1 9SY, UK
e-mail: pbjames@talktalk.net

K.K. Jain, MD, FRACS, FFPM
1 Blaesiring 7, Basel 4057, Switzerland
e-mail: jain@pharmabiotech.ch

from 10 msw (2 ATA) to normal barometric pressure is 2 L. However, an exposure to 80% helium and 20% oxygen at 2 ATA would result in only 1 L of gas being dissolved, the difference being mainly due to the lower solubility of the gas in fat. However on resumption of air breathing at 1 ATA, the elimination of helium is very rapid. To achieve steady state at a particular pressure—often known as saturation—requires many hours and the time required in greater for nitrogen than for helium. The formulation of decompression tables is generally based on methods introduced by Haldane from his observation that decompression sickness is rare when the absolute pressure is halved as, for example, from 2 ATA to 1 ATA. However, he warned against the extrapolation of this principle to pressures above 6 ATA but erred in stating that the 2 to 1 decompression ratio was not associated with gas formation (Haldane 1922). Figure 11.1 shows the approximate half-lives of nitrogen in various tissues. However, the demonstration of gas formation in tissues after a decompression halving the absolute pressure on the Haldanian principle indicates that this method is empirical and should only be used to guide decompression table formulation.

After achieving steady-state conditions in air diving the central nervous system has a high concentration of nitrogen because of the high solubility of the gas in lipids. Using helium the amount dissolved under equivalent steady-state conditions is much less because of the lower solubility of the gas in fat. Consequently, neurological DCS is rare in helium and oxygen diving. Commercial diving expanded dramatically with the exploration for offshore oil and gas, and the experience gained has influenced practice in both military and amateur diving. For depths in excess of 50 msw, "saturation" techniques have been developed where divers live at constant pressure in a helium and oxygen environment (heliox), using a bell to transfer to the water. Attempts to use nitrox for saturation dives have not been successful. Operational dives have been undertaken to 450 msw using

heliox and experimental dives to 523 msw, using mixtures of hydrogen, helium, and oxygen. The inclusion of hydrogen reduces gas density and the work of breathing and also ameliorates the effects of the high pressure on nervous system function. These symptoms are known as the high pressure nervous syndrome (see Chap. 3).

Decompression illness (DCI) has been proposed to encompass both DCS and AGE (arterial gas embolism) because the neurological presentations of DCS and AGE may be difficult to distinguish may coexist. However, the proposal has not widely accepted the traditional terms: DCS and arterial gas embolism (see Chap. 12).

Pathophysiology

Gas Formation

The elimination of the excess "inert" gas taken up during a dive ultimately depends upon the transfer of gas from blood to the respired gas in the lungs. All decompression tables assume that blood passing through the lungs is equilibrated with the partial pressure of the gas being respired, but because of ventilation/perfusion mismatch in the lung this cannot be the case and some supersaturated blood must achieve the systemic circulation on decompression. Decompression sickness can follow repeated breath-hold dives because the elevation of the partial pressure of the nitrogen in the air compressed in the lungs is reflected in an increase in the plasma and tissue nitrogen content. Cerebral symptoms have been described following multiple breath-hold dives and decompression beyond the unsaturation associated with the metabolic use of oxygen (the oxygen window) produces supersaturation and risks the emergence of dissolved gas from solution. The formation of gas phase can be imaged in tissue fascia, for example, in muscle, using ultrasound. The principle component is the diluent gas present, but oxygen, carbon dioxide, and water vapor also contribute to the gas volume. Gas formation is believed to depend on the presence of gas nanobubbles (Weijs 2012) which are very small quantities of undissolved gas and the enlargement of such bubbles may occur very rapidly. It is universally agreed that the formation of gas is the initial event in the etiology of DCS. The principles underlying bubble formation are shown in Fig. 11.2.

There is considerable evidence that gas formation in the tight connective tissue of tendon is responsible for the classical joint pain of the "bends." Investigations using radiographs in aviators decompressed to altitude has demonstrated gas phase in the ligaments and tendons of the knee, and these observations are relevant to those seen in decompression after exposure to hyperbaric environments. Sequential perfusion has been observed in connective tissue, and this intermittent perfusion is probably a major factor in gas formation

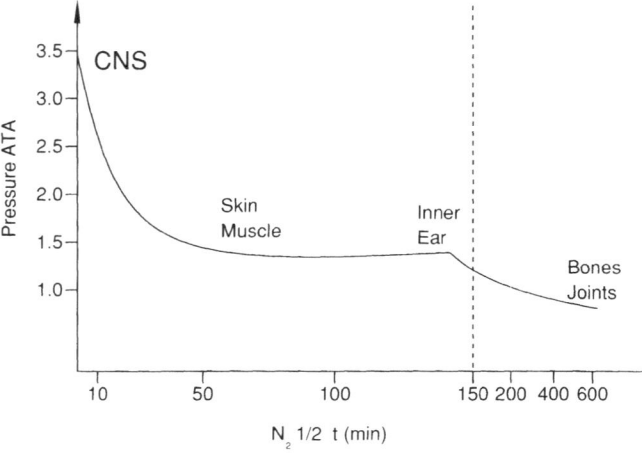

Fig. 11.1 Half-life of nitrogen in various tissues

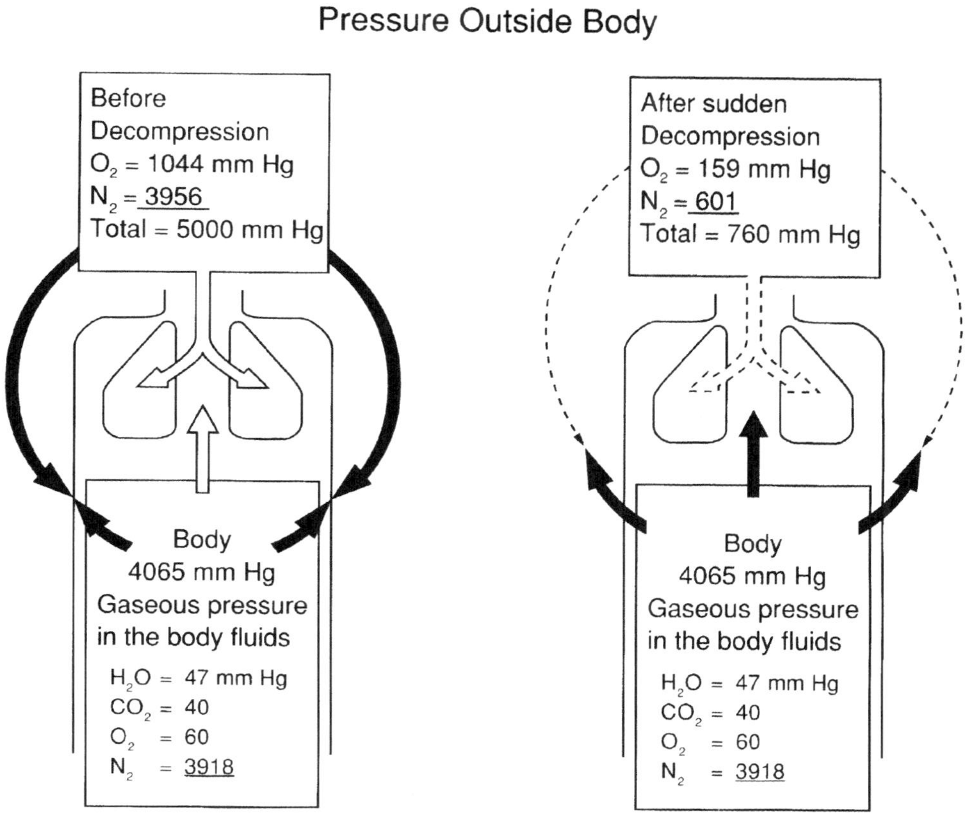

Fig. 11.2 Bubble formation after decompression due to great excess of intrabody pressure shown at *right*

Pressure Outside Body

Before Decompression
O_2 = 1044 mm Hg
N_2 = 3956
Total = 5000 mm Hg

Body
4065 mm Hg
Gaseous pressure in the body fluids
H_2O = 47 mm Hg
CO_2 = 40
O_2 = 60
N_2 = 3918

After sudden Decompression
O_2 = 159 mm Hg
N_2 = 601
Total = 760 mm Hg

Body
4065 mm Hg
Gaseous pressure in the body fluids
H_2O = 47 mm Hg
CO_2 = 40
O_2 = 60
N_2 = 3918

in this and other tissues because a tissue will take up gas when it is perfused, but release of gas will be limited if the microcirculation closes during decompression. The gas exchange will then be diffusion, not perfusion limited. Also, because the oxygen contained in the area of tissue will be metabolized, there may be a reduction in the inherent unsaturation as more nitrogen is absorbed. Intravascular bubbles are often detectable in the pulmonary artery during or after decompression. The timing is dependent on the nature of the dive. For example, circulating bubbles may be detected during the decompression from heliox saturation dives, but in air diving they are generally only detectable after decompression has been completed.

Electron microscopy studies of human tissues from fatal cases of DCS have shown that each bubble is covered with an osmiophilic, nonhomogeneous coat of a flocculent material that is associated with an electrokinetic zonal activity. This surface coat reduces the rate of nitrogen elimination via the blood–lung barrier when bubbles are trapped in the pulmonary capillaries. Bubbles induce changes in vascular permeability, and in severe decompression sickness this may precipitate hypovolemic shock and a reversible blood sludging. In addition to formation of bubbles in tissues, humoral agents may be released from tissues secondary to trauma caused by expanding gas. Intra-arterial bubble formation occurs only if there is a very sudden decompression from a

high pressure exposure. DCS generally increases in severity as the free gas in the body becomes more abundant. Exercise increases the elimination of gas but may also increase the release of gas in tissues and bubbles into the circulation. Following rapid decompression bubbles first form on the venous side of the circulation and then, if they exceed a certain number, move through the pulmonary circulation into the systemic circulation.

It is generally accepted that there is a threshold for the transpulmonary passage of emboli, and the transfer of bubbles into the systemic circulation may also occur through an atrial septal defect. The location and extent of bubble formation depends upon the severity of the supersaturation and the solubility of the diluent gas. Only in very severe experimental situations have bubbles been found intracellularly, in the anterior chamber of the eye, or in the cerebrospinal fluid. Diving using only oxygen as the respired gas is employed in the armed forces and although it is not associated with bubble formation, it carries the risk of acute oxygen toxicity manifest by convulsions which may lead to drowning. Oxygen-enriched air mixtures are used to reduce the risk of decompression sickness and/or extend bottom time and are becoming popular in amateur diving. They reduce but do not eliminate the risk of DCS and because there is a very real risk of convulsions from oxygen toxicity, divers should use a full face mask or helmet.

Pulmonary Changes

The first attempt to detect bubbles using ultrasound found them present in the inferior vena cava in a pig during decompression at 4 ATA after an exposure to compressed air at a pressure of 6 ATA for an hour (Gillis et al. 1968). Human studies have used transcutaneous ultrasonic detectors which are much less sensitive than implanted devices. Bubbles can be detected in the pulmonary artery in the majority of divers after significant dives, but they generally do not produce symptoms. Experimental studies have shown that venous bubbles can cross the lungs of anesthetized dogs when driving pressures are high enough to overcome the normal filtering function of the lungs. Bubbles trapped in the lung may also cross the pulmonary circulation as a result of the reduction in their size on compression. Before decompression tables were formulated, pulmonary decompression sickness—the "chokes"—often proved fatal and the events have been followed in experimental animals. The pulmonary changes are accompanied by hypoxemia, pulmonary hypertension, and respiratory distress. These features are shared by other microembolic syndromes as, for example, fat embolism, and are examples of the (adult) respiratory distress syndrome. Noncardiac pulmonary edema has been found to be the principal response of the lung to decompression stress, and the precipitating event is a large number of microbubbles arriving in the lung. Peribronchial edema has also been described.

Pulmonary barotrauma may occur in divers because an increase in the volume of gas entrapped in the lungs during ascent, leading to alveolar rupture, entry of the gas into systemic circulation via the pulmonary veins, and systemic air embolism (see Chap. 12). The gas may track around the vessels, leading to mediastinal emphysema. Rupture of peripheral alveoli may lead to pneumothorax. Pulmonary barotrauma is much more common in amateur divers using self-contained breathing apparatus (SCUBA) than professional divers, because of panic, or the exhaustion of their gas supply. When arterial gas embolism occurs as a result of a rapid ascent at the end of a dive, it is complicated by the excess of nitrogen in the tissues.

Bubble-Induced CNS Injury

Large and numerous bubbles may enter the cerebral circulation in arterial gas embolism associated with pulmonary barotrauma and cause gross obstruction to flow and ischemia. However, in contrast, bubbles formed on decompression are small, generally measuring about 25 μm on the surface (Haldane 1922). As with solid microemboli, the diameter of microbubbles is a critical factor in their behavior in the circulation and the size of such gaseous emboli depends on the absolute pressure. Ischemic hypoxia is a major factor in bub-

ble-induced CNS injury in decompression sickness. In experiments using labeled neutrophils (granulocytes), hypoxia signaling as a chemotaxic process occurs at an early stage and neutrophils may be involved in the typical perivenular neurological lesions. They can be visualized on MRI as white matter hyperintensities. Ischemia is conventionally associated with vascular occlusion, but gas embolism also causes endothelial damage and in the CNS this involves opening of the blood–brain barrier and edema. This has also been produced by the transit of microbubbles without being associated with ischemia (Hills and James 1991). Opening the blood–brain barrier causes the extravasation of plasma proteins which triggers the complement cascade. This induces inflammation with ischemia only developing when focal edema causes compression of the microcirculation. In animal experimental models, bubbles have been observed in the cerebral circulation, which precede changes in evoked potentials. Blood complement may also induce erythrocyte clumping in shock associated with omitted decompression. The result of these interactions between blood and the damaged tissues may well be a major determinant of the extent of neuronal recovery following focal blood–brain barrier disturbance and ischemia in the CNS. Fat embolism may also occur on decompression and even cause death from an acute disseminated encephalitis. Fat emboli, being fluid, also cross the lung filter and cause cerebral edema because of damage to the blood–brain barrier. The protein leakage and edema leads to focal demyelination with relative preservation of axons. The nutrition of areas of the white matter of both the cerebral medulla and the spinal cord depends on long draining veins which have been shown to have surrounding capillary free zones. Because of the high oxygen extraction in the microcirculation of the gray matter of the central nervous system, the venous blood has low oxygen content. When this is reduced further by embolic events, tissue oxygenation may fall to critically low levels, leading to blood–brain barrier dysfunction, inflammation, demyelination and eventually, axonal damage. These are the hallmarks of the early lesions of multiple sclerosis, where MR spectroscopy has also shown the presence of lactic acid. Significant elevation of the venous oxygen tension requires oxygen to be provided under hyperbaric conditions. Arterial tension is typically increased tenfold breathing oxygen at 2 ATA, but this results in only a 1.5-fold increase in the cerebral venous oxygen tension. The treatment of DCS, and both animal and clinical studies, have confirmed the value of oxygen provided under hyperbaric conditions in the restoration and preservation of neurological function in the "perivenous" syndrome (James 2007).

An additional mechanism by which bubbles may generate CNS injury is their nucleation within the white matter. Bubbles are seen in the myelin sheaths on the rapid decompression of experimental animals from high pressures and decompression from normal atmospheric pressure to altitude. Autochthonous (formed in situ) bubbles have been shown to traumatize neurons at the site of nucleation and compress adjacent ones, and this is one mechanism which can explain the abrupt onset of symptoms. However, the conditions used in these experiments are much more extreme than in most cases of human DCS. Because of the need for a reliable animal model and to avoid the unpredictability of decompression sickness which characterizes human dives very extreme conditions and often double exposures have been used.

The most obvious disability from neurological (Type II) DCS in diving is paraplegia due to the involvement of the spinal cord, but this rarely occurs as a complication of hypobaric decompression, indicating the importance of bubble size and tissue gas loading. Most divers with spinal cord symptoms when questioned actually admit to symptoms which indicate disturbed brain function. Three mechanisms have been postulated to explain the pathophysiology of spinal cord lesion:

- Arterial bubble embolism
- Epidural venous obstruction leading to infarction
- Autochthonous bubbles

The paramount difficulty is the attribution of spinal cord decompression sickness to arterial embolism has been the failure to recognize a natural disease of the spinal cord due to arterial microembolism. However, this has been answered by the recognition that multiple sclerosis (MS) may be due to subacute fat embolism (James 1982) and, notably, retinal changes occur in both decompression sickness and MS. In MS as in decompression sickness, the clinical presentation is dominated by symptoms affecting the spinal cord. decompression sickness being one cause of transverse myelitis. It may become progressive with late deterioration been described 13 years after acute spinal cord decompression sickness. In MS and DCS, focal cranial nerve problems, such as optic neuritis and oculomotor palsies, have been described and vestibular damage may leave permanent nystagmus. The pathology of epidural venous obstruction is central infarction of the cord and not the characteristic focal changes seen in the decompression sickness. Gas or edema may cause ischemia in the cord because of an increase in the internal pressure due to non-elasticity of the pia mater (Hills and James 1982).

It is unfortunate that fibrocartilaginous embolism has been overlooked in the debate about the mechanism of neurological decompression sickness. Material from the nucleus pulposus of spinal discs can cause microembolic damage to the nervous system, and the first human case was described over 50 years ago (Naiman et al. 1961). Again retrograde venous flow has been suggested as the mechanism but the postmortem finding of a 200 μm fibrocartilage embolus in the middle cerebral artery of a 17-year-old girl (Toro-

Gonzalez et al. 1993) demonstrated beyond doubt that system embolization does occur. As in decompression sickness, material may gain access to the systemic circulation by transpulmonary passage, or through an atrial septal defect. The girl, who had collapsed while playing basketball, died of myocardial infarction, and emboli were found in the coronary arteries. The size of the emboli, ranging from 20 to 200 μm, indicates that the microcirculation of the lung sizes the material. The mechanism has been described in other mammals and even in birds and is regarded as a relatively common cause of acute neurological symptoms in veterinary medicine.

Changes visible with both light and electron microscopes are seen in the spinal cords of animals subjected to severe experimental DCS. The finding of widened myelin sheaths showing a banded pattern of myelin disruption may be compatible with autochthonous gas, but similar patterns are seen in experimental allergic encephalomyelitis due to edema. Divers, compressed air workers and even U2 pilots, may be at risk of long-term CNS damage from non-symptomatic hyperbaric exposure. The effect of severe, controlled hyperbaric exposure was investigated on goats exposed to various dive profiles over a period of 5 years, with some experiencing DCS (Blogg et al. 2004). MRI was done and the animals were then sacrificed for neuropathological examination the brain and spinal cord. No significant correlation was found between age, years diving, DCS, or exposure to pressure with MRI-detectable lesions in the brain, or with neuropathological lesions in the brain or spinal cord. However, spinal scarring was noted in animals that had suffered from spinal cord DCS.

Changes in Blood

Even asymptomatic decompression of sufficient severity can be associated with a reduction of the number of circulating platelets by one-third during a 24-h period following a severe dive. A smooth muscle-activating factor released during decompression may potentiate other bioactive amines, such as bradykinin, serotonin, and histamine, which are known to be involved in shock caused by rapid decompression. Hyperagglutinability of the platelets may be a factor in the pathogenesis of severe neurological DCS. This phenomenon may be based on production of metabolites of arachidonic acid and prostaglandin-like compounds.

Adhesion of platelets to the surfaces of bubbles and formation of platelet aggregates have been shown by scanning electron microscopy. Other platelet agonists like ADP, epinephrine, and serotonin, which may be present in vivo, accelerate this interaction, and the platelet antagonists have been shown to depress platelet aggregation. These factors may delay gas resolution on recompression.

Dysbaric Osteonecrosis

Dysbaric osteonecrosis (DON) has been reported in humans and experimental animals after a single hyperbaric air exposure with inadequate decompression. It is usually considered to be the result of gas bubbles entering the end arteries in the bone and is seen most commonly in compressed air workers. According to one hypothesis, DON does not result from primary embolic or compressive effects of the nitrogen bubbles on the osseous vasculature (Jones et al. 1993). These authors report the presence of gas bubbles in the fatty marrow of the femoral and humeral heads and lipid and platelet aggregates were found on the surface of marrow bubbles. Fibrin platelet thrombi were found in systemic vessels, suggesting that injured marrow adipocytes can release liquid fat, and this fat embolism causes the release of thromboplastin, and other vasoactive substances that can trigger systemic intravascular coagulation and DON.

Role of Free Radicals

There is increasing awareness of the role of oxygen-derived free radicals in reperfusion injury but occlusion of flow is more a feature of air embolism rather than decompression sickness, the latter being associated with increased vascular permeability and inflammation in perivenous syndrome (James 1982). After the first phase of neurological DCS caused by the mechanical action of bubbles on endothelium, the symptoms in the second phase may result from oxygen-free radicals released by neutrophil invasion signaled by developing hypoxia (Martin and Thom 2002). It has been recognized since the introduction of the minimal recompression tables using 100% oxygen at 2.8 ATA (US Navy Manual 1970) that these procedures could be associated with worsening and convulsions from cerebral oxygen toxicity. However, convulsions have not been associated with any residual problems and are probably due to hypoglycemia as in some cases exposure to 2.8 ATA may be associated with intense vasoconstriction (James 2014). However, it is universally recognized that recompression treatment should be carried out as quickly as possible and that recompression with the additional use of heparin, superoxide dismutase, and catalase does not improve the outcome of severe DCS in experimental animals. A schematic of the pathogenesis of the forms of DCS is shown in Fig. 11.3.

Clinical Features

Decompression Sickness in Diving

Haldane (1907) classified DCS into three categories: Type I, joint pain; Type II, systemic symptoms or signs, caused by the involvement of the CNS or the cardiopulmonary systems;

and Type III characterized by convulsions and death. The first two parts of the classification are still the accepted standard internationally.

Clinical features of DCS are shown in Table 11.1. DCS is a disease that manifests itself in a variety of organ systems. However, studies of both compressed air workers and divers have shown that Type I DCS is the most common presentation, but the nature of the dive is important. For example, mild joint pains are not unusual during heliox saturation decompressions but Type II symptoms are extremely rare. In surface decompression procedures, Type II DCS is more common and on deep dives presents more frequently than Type I symptoms. It is obvious that joint pain is easier for a diver to recognize than symptoms affecting the nervous system. Cutis marmorata (Fig. 11.4), a rare cutaneous manifestation of decompression sickness with rash and pruritus, may precede illness involving the central nervous system (Kalentzos 2010). Occasionally, cutis marmorata is accompanied by other symptoms such as visual distortions, vertigo, or mild cerebral dysfunction. According to one hypothesis, the pathogenesis of these neurological manifestations is embolization of the brain stem with gas bubbles resulting in disturbance of regulation of skin blood vessel dilation and constriction by the of autonomic nervous system (Germonpre et al. 2015). However, gas bubbles have been observed in the skin after decompression in experimental animals suggesting systemic microbubbles are involved, and vigilance is needed to exclude the presence of neurological symptoms. The skin manifestations show only a modest response to recompression breathing oxygen.

The majority of divers who have undertaken surface-orientated dives experience symptoms within 3 h of surfacing although the onset of symptoms may be delayed for as long as 35 h and even longer if air travel is undertaken. In air diving, nearly one-half of the cerebral cases become apparent within 3 min of surfacing, and a similar proportion of spinal cases also become apparent within 3 min of surfacing. The most serious sequelae are those involving the CNS: neurologic manifestations of DCS comprise symptoms from the cerebral hemispheres, the spinal cord, as well as vestibular disturbances (Jain 2016). Inner ear decompression sickness has been reported to manifest as vertigo and additional hearing loss (Klingmann 2012). The distribution of the areas varies: in diving spinal cord symptoms dominate whereas in aviators cerebral symptoms are by far the most common (Fryer 1967; McGuire et al. 2013).

The most common area involved is the lower thoracic spinal cord, but the level can vary from C4 to L1. In air diving with in-water decompression CNS involvement occurs in approximately 25% of DCS cases. Late deterioration of spinal cord function has been reported several years after initial episodes of DCS, and other neurologic syndromes may also occur. Some divers develop evidence of acute cerebral hemisphere dysfunction, such as hemiparesis, aphasia, or hemianopsia, memory loss, and seizures.

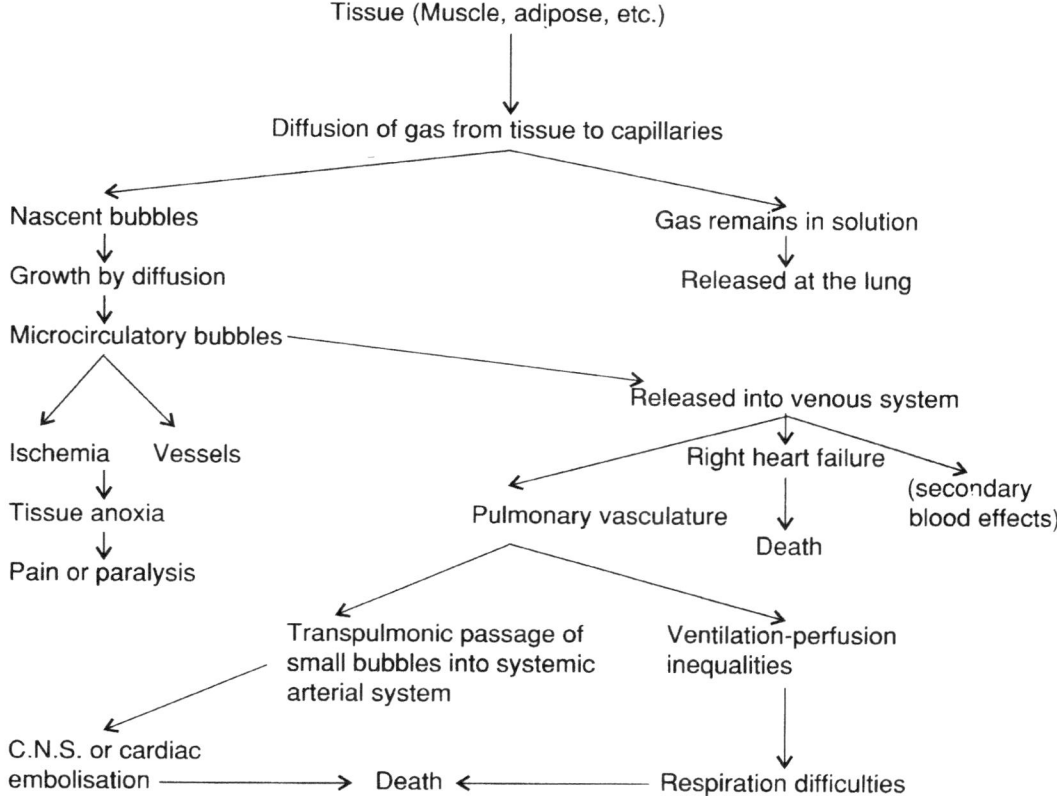

Fig. 11.3 Physiological sequelae in decompression sickness

Repetitive breath-hold diving can lead to accumulation of nitrogen in blood and tissues, which may give rise to DCS. MRI in four professional Japanese breath-hold divers (Ama) with histories of diving accidents showed cerebral infarcts localized in the watershed areas of the brain (Kohshi et al. 2005). A survey conducted on their island revealed that many Ama divers had experienced stroke-like events. A clinical feature of DCS in breath-hold diving is that the damage is limited to the brain. Although the mechanisms of brain damage in breath-hold diving are unclear, nitrogen bubbles passing through the lungs or the heart so as to become arterialized are most likely to be the causative factor.

Cardiac arrhythmias, usually supraventricular tachycardia, have been reported in DCS and pulmonary symptoms occur in about 2% of severe cases. Noncardiogenic pulmonary edema is an uncommon manifestation of Type II DCS. It usually occurs within 6 h of a dive and is believed to be caused by microbubbles in the pulmonary circulation. Shock is rare in DCS but may follow severe dives.

Altitude Decompression Sickness

Altitude DCS is usually seen in aviators at an altitude of 6098 m (20,000 ft), but it may occur at lower altitudes in those with risk factors for DCS. A case of DCS with rapid decompression at 2439 m (8000 ft) and a good response to recompression therapy has been reported by Rudge (1990). A review of 133 cases from the US Air Force by Wirjosemito et al. (1989) showed that the most common manifestations were joint pain (43.6%), headaches (42.1%), visual disturbances (30.1%), limb paresthesias (27.8%), and mental confusion (24.8%). Spinal cord involvement, chokes, and unconsciousness were rare. HBO treatment was successful in 97.7% of the cases, and residual deficits were noted in only 2.3% of the cases. Altitude-related DCS can present with a wide variety of symptoms in the same patients, such as nausea, headache, fatigue, and respiratory difficulty, which can be misdiagnosed as viral illness. Rudge (1991) reported two such patients in whom the symptoms resolved following recompression with HBO, thus confirming the diagnosis of DCS.

Cerebral hypoxia is usually not a feature of diving-related DCS, but explains the greater severity of the cerebral presentations at altitude. HBO was used in the treatment of a pilot who underwent rapid decompression from 753 hPa (2348 m altitude) to 148 hPa (Sheffield and Davis 1976). The pilot lost consciousness in 5–8 s. Supplemental oxygen was given after a delay of 6–8 min. On the ground, the pilot was blind and disoriented and remained so for the next 6.5 h until HBO therapy was started. The pilot eventually recovered with no neurological deficits. Davis et al. (1977) reviewed 145 cases

Table 11.1 Signs and symptoms of decompression sickness (DCS)

Type I DCS
Limb and joint pains (bends)
Skin rash (cutis marmorata)
Type II DCS
Neurological
1. Cerebral
– Visual disturbances
– Aphasia
– Hemiplegia
– Memory loss
– Convulsions
– Coma
2. Spinal ("hit")
– Sensory disturbances of extremities: paresthesias, numbness
– Weakness, difficulty in walking
– Bladder dysfunction
– Paraplegia or quadriplegia
3. Vestibular disturbances ("staggers")
– Nystagmus
– Vertigo
Pulmonary ("chokes")
1. Dyspnea
2. Hyperventilation
3. Chest pain
4. Acute respiratory distress syndrome (ARDS)
Cardiac
1. Tachycardia
2. Cardiac arrhythmias

of altitude DCS and recommended immediate compression to 2.8 ATA and a series of intermittent oxygen-breathing and air-breathing periods during the subsequent slow decompression. The US Air Force has modified the US Navy procedure Table 6. A degree of optic atrophy has been reported in a parachutist after repeated hypobaric exposures (Butler 1991) and vision improved with recompression and HBO therapy.

A review of 233 cases treated at the USAF School of Aerospace Medicine concluded that, as in diving, the treatment of altitude DCS with compression therapy is most useful when it is begun as early as possible (Rudge and Shafer 1991). The greater the delay in treatment, the longer the symptoms of DCS persist and the greater the rate of residual symptoms.

Another manifestation at altitude is acute mountain sickness (AMS), which usually occurs in individuals ascending above 3000 m without adequate acclimatization. The clinical signs and symptoms of AMS include headache, nausea, irritability, insomnia, dizziness, and vomiting. In some individuals, AMS may proceed to cerebral edema and/or pulmonary edema. Cerebral edema is considered to be secondary to hypoxic cerebral vasodilation and elevated capillary hydrostatic pressure, but it cannot be ruled out that bubbles may be a contributing factor. These events elevate peripheral sympathetic activity that may act in concert with pulmonary capillary stress failure to cause pulmonary edema but again pulmonary entrapment of bubbles offers an alternative explanation. Oxygen breathing and descent from altitude are proven effective measures for AMS, and a portable hyperbaric chamber has been found to be useful. During acute ascent in the Alps, an early 3-h pressurization of unacclimatized subjects using air was shown to slightly delay the onset of AMS, but did not prevent it or attenuate its severity on presentation (Kayser et al. 1993).

Extravehicular activity during missions on space stations and possibly to establish a permanent presence on the Moon or Mars carry a risk of DCS because of the reduction of pressure to one-third of normal atmospheric pressure required to use space suits. Loss of pressure from a space suit requires urgent recompression, and the International Space Station has a hyperbaric treatment capability.

Ocular Complications of DCS

Ocular complications of DCS are very rare. Nitrogen bubble formation may have contributed to vitreal separation from the retina in an otherwise healthy leisure diver who presented with simultaneous unilateral posterior vitreal detachment and DCS (Dan-Goor et al. 2012). Retinal vein occlusion with visual impairment has also been reported.

There are some reports of visual impairment in DCS that improved with recompression breathing oxygen. Optic disc swelling occurs when there is an obstruction to axonal transport at the level of the lamina cribrosa. A case has been reported of a high-performance fighter pilot who presented with unilateral optic disc swelling 2 days after an F-16 flight, where altitude decompression sickness was suspected (Pokroy et al. 2009). Visual acuity of the affected eye was decreased to 20/25, with enlarged blind spot and shallow arcuate scotomata on visual field testing. Marked swelling of the entire optic disc, retinal flame-shaped hemorrhages, and engorgement of the retinal veins were seen. Obstruction of the optic nerve head vasculature by microbubbles was suspected, and a course of hyperbaric oxygen treatment led to recovery of full visual function within a week.

A case of choroidal ischemia with DCS has been described that resulted from decompression-induced intravascular gaseous microemboli (Iordanidou et al. 2010). Central serous chorioretinopathy, an idiopathic condition associated with hypoxia and medications, has been reported in an aviator following a simulated flight in a hypobaric chamber (Ide 2014). This raises the possibility of similar problems in altitude decompression illness and needs further investigation.

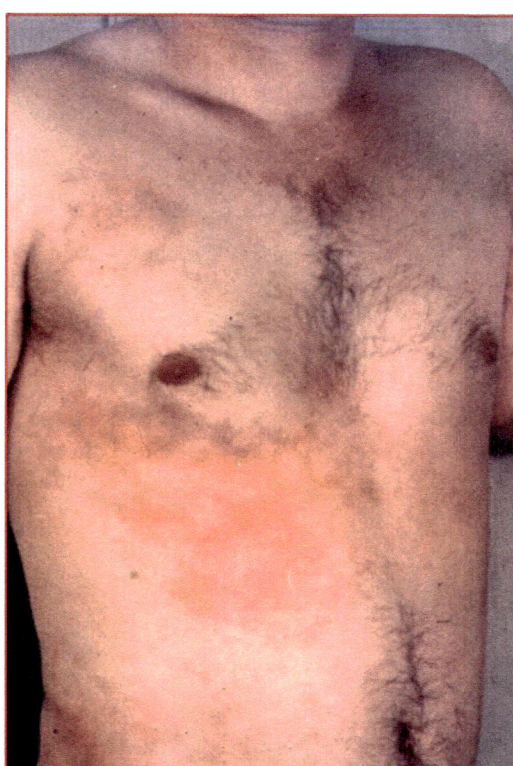

Fig. 11.4 Cutis marmorata, a skin manifestation of decompression sickness, has a mottled appearance with areas of pallor surrounded by cyanotic patches. It resolved with recompression therapy

Ultrasonic Detection of Bubbles

It is of course not possible in conventional diving to use ultrasonic monitoring, but it has been used to develop and monitor decompression procedures. Ultrasound has been used to detect venous gas emboli in divers and no bends developed prior to detection of bubbles over the precordium (Spencer 1976). However, during decompression with elevated oxygen, precordially determined bubbles at depth are predictive of limb pain in only 50% of cases; 70% of the divers were reported to develop bends without detectable bubbles (Powell et al. 1983). The amplitude of the Doppler-detected pulmonary artery flow sound, however, increased, and it was suggested that this may have indicated the presence of numerous microbubbles.

Pulse-echo ultrasound imaging techniques have been used to study the formation of bubbles. These can monitor the extent of bubble formation during decompression with a view to predicting symptoms. The results of such studies confirm that:

- A threshold of supersaturation for bubble formation exists
- The earliest bubbles are intravascular
- There is usually an accumulation of stationary bubbles before precordial bubbles are detected and symptoms of Type II DCS develop.

Diagnosis

DCS is rare in divers and compressed air workers unless pressure is greater than 2 ATA although cases have been described from long exposures to lesser pressures. The diagnosis can be made on the basis of history and clinical features, and it is essential to stress that if a significant dive has been undertaken then the presumption must be made that the symptoms are due to DCS and not natural disease. The differential diagnosis of neurological DCS, particularly in atypical cases, should include multiple sclerosis.

Recompression has been advocated as a definitive test for DCS, and providing it is undertaken immediately it is a valuable guide. However, immediate recompression is usually only possible in commercial diving operations where in most cases a chamber is on site. In Type I DCS, a small increase in pressure may resolve the pain, and on decompression it may recur in the same site suggesting a mechanical origin. In general, the higher the pressure of the onset of pain, the greater the pressure increase that is required for its resolution indicating a relationship to gas volume. With CNS symptoms, as bubbles may induce tissue hypoxia by interfering with blood flow it may be difficult to determine if improvement is due to a reduction in gas volume with pressure, or the resolution of edema and hypoxia from the use of a high partial pressure of oxygen. In general, laboratory tests are not helpful in DCS, but several have been used in experimental animal studies and some in human laboratory dives.

Blood Examination

Blood examination may include serum albumin measurement. Hypoalbuminemia at initial presentation due to capillary leak, although rare, accurately predicts the neurologic manifestations of DCS in scuba divers (Gempp et al. 2014). However, serum albumin as a biomarker of Type II decompression syndrome has not been validated yet for prognosis or as a guide to albumin infusion as treatment.

The fibrinogen degradation products test reflects disseminated intravascular coagulation or agglutination. The diagnostic value of this test in the absence of clinical information is questionable.

Ultrasound Monitoring of Bubbles

Ultrasonic monitoring of bubbles during experimental decompression has not been shown to be helpful in prediction of neurologic involvement in DCS (Kayar 2008). Detection of marrow bubbles with MRI after musculoskeletal decompression sickness, however, can be predictive of subsequent dysbaric osteonecrosis (Stéphant et al. 2008).

Bone Scanning

A Tc 99 bone scan has been shown to be positive as early as 72 h after the traumatic insult in a patient with joint pain Type I DCS. This test, however, like epidemiological studies, has not shown a relationship between symptoms of DCS and the sites of bone lesions.

X-Rays

Bone necrosis due to decompression may be detectable by X-rays after a delay of months because the radiological changes take time to appear. More than 10 % of men who have been deep air diving for 12 or more years have some bone necrosis, and the proportion is much higher in compressed air workers. The most frequent sites are the head of the humerus, the lower part of the shaft of the femur, and the upper end of the tibia.

Retinal Angiography

Bubbles in arteries of the retinal circulation have been visualized through a fundus camera in 25 % of sheep that were air compressed to 6 ATA and then rapidly decompressed to the surface (Parsons et al. 2009). This study demonstrates that retinal angiography is a practical experimental tool for real-time, noninvasive detection of bubbles in the retinal circulation, a visible window to the cerebral circulation. Fluorescein angiography demonstrated occluded blood flow caused by arterial gas emboli and may prove invaluable in the early detection of arterial gas emboli in the cerebral circulation in animal models.

Imaging

CT is a method of densitometry; it is not surprising that it has failed to reveal useful information, and it has been superseded by magnetic resonance imaging (MRI), which has much greater soft tissue resolution. Lesions in the spinal cord and cerebral have been detected after scuba diving have also been demonstrated using MRI. MRI can be useful in follow-up studies and in early diagnosis of DCS when symptoms do not fit the classic picture or loss of consciousness occurs during surfacing. MRI has revealed acute subcortical lesions and hyperintense white matter lesions in U-2 pilots with neurologic DCS and others who have not (McGuire et al. 2013; Jersey et al. 2013). As usual clinical correlations have proven difficult to establish as in other conditions such as compressed air workers (Fuerecdi et al. 1991). The unusual presentation of a case with mixed signs and symptoms of cervical myelopathy and Type II neurologic DCS presented a diagnostic dilemma that required the use of cervical spine MRI, which revealed the presence of tiny hypointensities (possibly bubbles) and edema within the spinal cord corresponded to the clinical findings (Liow et al. 2014). Some recovery was obtained using hyperbaric oxygen therapy but with residual neurologic deficits.

Electrophysiological Studies

EEG has been a useful technique to monitor the effect of recompression in cerebral disturbance in experimental animals and somatosensory evoked potentials have also shown abnormalities when the spinal cord is involved in DCS.

Neuropsychological Assessment

Neuropsychological assessment cannot be used as a test in acute decompression sickness because it requires considerable time and expertise. However, cognitive impairment may be detected by neuropsychological testing, even in the absence of neurological signs. Monitoring of the recovery of neurological deficits following HBO therapy can be demonstrated by using this method.

Treatment

Emergency Management and Evaluation

In amateur divers, there may be problems in the differentiation of air embolism and decompression sickness on the history because they may run out of gas and make a rapid ascent. Barotrauma is exceptionally rare in altitude excursions and also in commercial divers who usually have an unlimited supply of gas provided from the surface. It is also less likely to occur at the greater depths achieved in bell diving because the volumetric change is less for a given pressure change with increasing depth. It is important to recognize that barotrauma can occur on rapid ascent from a depth of a few meters. However, the essentials of therapy are the same for both air embolism and decompression sickness, that is, after ensuring a clear airway and using cardiopulmonary resuscitation when necessary, a diver must be given 100% oxygen as soon as possible and transferred to a chamber. The treatment of air embolism is described in Chap. 12. The Diver Alert Network (DAN) provides a 24 h hotline in the USA and internationally for advice regarding the management of diving accidents.

Recompression and HBO Treatment

The objectives of recompression are:

- To reduce bubble volume
- To redistribute and redissolve gas
- To reduce tissue edema and hypoxia

The joint pain of Type I DCS resulting from in surface-orientated diving generally resolves rapidly with prompt rapid recompression. In very rare cases, there may be an initial increase in the pain which is thought to be due to a "squeeze." Many cases will improve breathing oxygen at the surface, and it is important to note that no sequelae have been described from this presentation of DCS. It is important to ensure that the patient does not have neurological symptoms and as a neurological examination is difficult and unreliable in the presence of pain and reliance must be placed on the patient's account of their symptoms. Even 100% oxygen at normal atmospheric pressure is also of value in Type II DCS, but it must be emphasized that a tight fitting mask must be used to ensure that there is minimal dilution of the oxygen by air. Fluids can be given by mouth if the patient is not nauseated; otherwise, intravenous fluid therapy should be used.

Recompression has been established as the definitive treatment for DCS and was first introduced in compressed-air working where traditionally air was used. However, recompression breathing air is accompanied by the respiration of additional nitrogen and problems with air recompression tables led to the development of recompression to 2.8 ATA breathing oxygen. This became standard practice following the development of Tables 5 and 6 by the US Navy in 1970. This pressure reduces the volume of any gas present by almost a third and has the advantage of counteracting the hypoxic/ischemic effects of DCS, particularly those on the CNS. The limitation of oxygen breathing is that it cannot be undertaken at pressures higher than 2.8 ATA because of oxygen toxicity. Although rare, convulsions do indeed occur at 2.8 ATA using US Navy procedures. The more complex procedures necessary in commercial diving are beyond the scope of this text, but recompression and increased partial pressures remain the cornerstones of therapy.

For Type I DCS (joint pain only), USN Table 5 may be used, as shown in Fig. 11.5. The schedule is 135 min in length and has 5-min breaks before beginning the ascent from 60 fsw (2.8 ATA). However, it must be emphasized that if pain does not resolve or Type II symptoms are present USN Table 6 must be used and many centers have ceased using Table 5 because of the relapse rate and failure to recognize underlying neurological problems. If symptoms of joint pain do not respond within 10 min of oxygen breathing at 2.8 ATA, USN Table 6, that is the schedule shown in Fig. 11.6, should be used. Three sessions of 20 min oxygen breathing are undertaken at 2.8 ATA interspersed by 5 min air breaks. The 150-min period at 30 fsw (1.9 ATA) is divided into alternating periods of 60-min of oxygen breathing with two 15 min periods of air breathing. The total length of this schedule is 285 min, and it may be extended by 100 min if necessary. The US Air Force has produced modifications of these tables for use in altitude decompression sickness.

As an alternative, the flow chart (Fig. 11.7) should be consulted. If a COMEX 30 schedule is to be followed, the information is given in Tables 11.2 and 11.3. The gas of preference for this schedule is 50/50 helium and oxygen as much less satisfactory results have been obtained using a 50/50 nitrogen/oxygen mixture. USN Table 6A (1979) is intended for use when it is unclear whether the symptoms are due to air embolism or decompression sickness. This table has been modified by adding three or more stops from 165 to 60 ft. With this approach, the total cure rate has can be substantially improved.

In a retrospective study, HBO therapy, administered within 24 h of onset of Type I decompression syndrome, was associated with rapid relief of symptoms after a single treatment (Lee et al. 2015). In this study, seasoned military divers showed a faster response after recompression with fewer residual symptoms in comparison with commercial and recreational divers. Microscopic and ultrastructural findings of an experimental study confirm that the lung is an important organ affected in rabbits with Type II DCS and that HBO can alleviate pulmonary damage affecting alveolar gas exchange (Geng et al. 2015).

Management of Altitude Decompression Sickness

Altitude decompression sickness is usually treated with hyperbaric therapy in the same manner as diving DCS. Expanding space operations and higher flying, more remotely placed military aircraft have stimulated a reexamination of this paradigm. A treatment table, USAF Treatment Table 8 (TT8) has been used, which consists of 100% oxygen delivered at 2 ATA for four 30-min periods with intervening 10-min air breaks (a total oxygen dose of 2 h). Treatment has

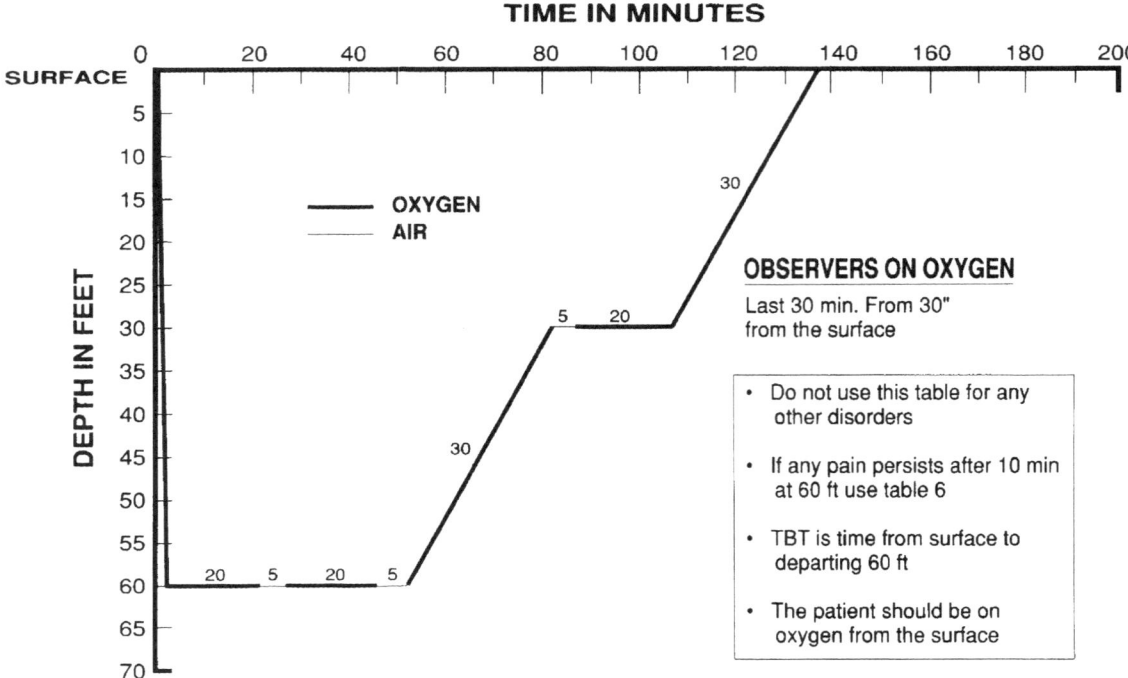

Fig. 11.5 The US Air Force modification of US Navy treatment Table 5

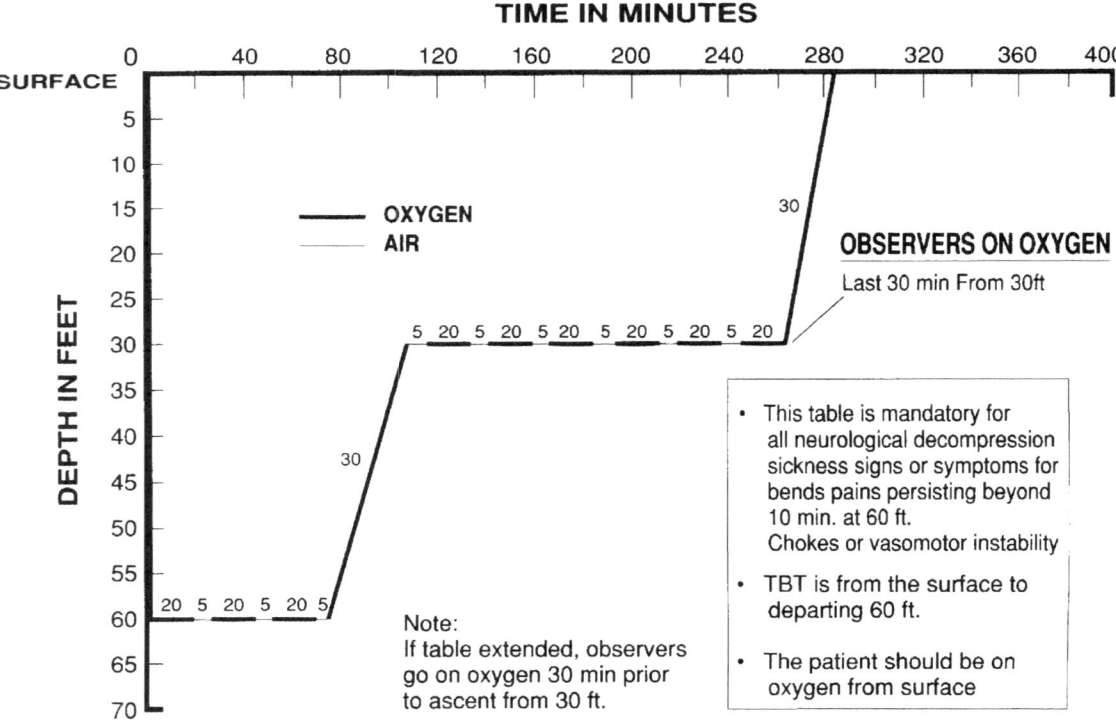

Fig. 11.6 The US Air Force modification of the US Navy treatment Table 6

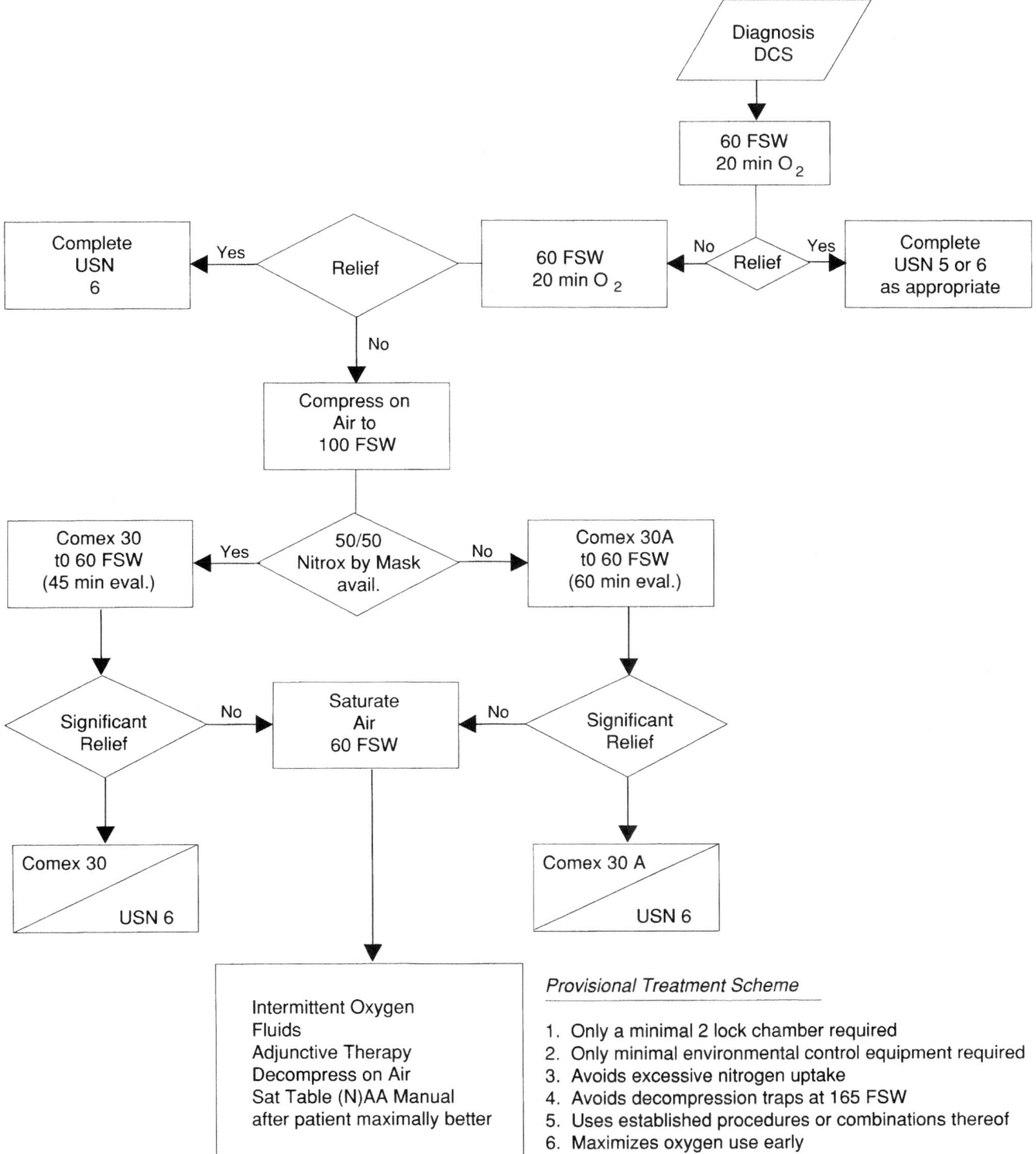

Fig. 11.7 Flow chart for decision-making in decompression sickness

Table 11.2 Therapeutic table: COMEX 30A

Depths (m)	Time (min)	Gas breathed patient attendant		Total time (min)
30	40	50/50	Air	40
30 to 24	5	Air	Air	45
(5 min/m)	25	50/50	Air	40
24	5	Air	Air	75
24	25	50/50	Air	100
24 to 18	5	Air	Air	105
(5 min/m)	25	50/50	Air	130
18	5	Air	Air	135
18	25	O_2	Air	160
18	5	Air	Air	165
18	25	O_2	Air	190
18 to 12	5	Air	Air	195
(5 min/m)	25	O_2	Air	220
12	10	Air	Air	230
12	45	O_2	Air	275
12	10	Air	Air	285
12	45	O_2	O_2	330
12	10	Air	Air	452
12	45	O_2	O_2	385
12	10	Air	Air	395
12 to surface	24	O_2	O_2	419
(Rate = 2 min/m)				

Table 11.3 Therapeutic table: COMEX 30A

Depths (m)	Time (min)	Gas breathed patient attendant		Total time (min)
30	30	Air	Air	60
30 to 24 (1 min/m)	6	Air	Air	66
24 to 21 (20 min/m)	60	Air	Air	126
21 to 18 (22 min/m)	66	Air	Air	192
18 to 15 (24 min/m)	72	Air	Air	264
15 to 12 (26 min/m)	78	Air	Air	342
(2 tablets 5 mg Valium on arrival at 12 m) 18				
12	10	Air	Air	352
12	40	O_2	O_2	392
12	10	Air	Air	402
12	40	O_2	O_2	442
12	10	Air	Air	452
12	40	O_2	O_2	492
12	5	Air	Air	497
12 to surface	24	O_2	O_2	521
(Rate = 2 min/m)				

been reported to be successful in 9 of 10 cases with Type I altitude DCS (Butler 2002). One failure with a recurrence of elbow pain required further therapy. Two patients were treated

for Type II altitude DCS with one failure (incomplete clearance of sensory deficits and weakness in the shoulder) requiring further therapy. Although TT8 had two failures, its successes suggest that a new protocol using TT8 for the treatment of altitude decompression sickness is viable but requires further clinical trials.

Management of Neurological Manifestations of Decompression Sickness

Spinal Cord DCS

The response of spinal cord DCS to HBO therapy depends upon the pathophysiology of the lesions. Magnetic resonance imaging (MRI) of the spinal cord may reveal demyelination and also show dorsal white matter lesions typical of venous infarction (Kei et al. 2007). Cases with short latency may have direct neuronal damage and hemorrhage present. In general such cases require more HBO treatments, and fare less well than those with DCS of late onset. In the latter case, ischemia contributes to neurological deficits and is responsive to HBO treatments. Improvement in MRI findings is not associated with improved clinical status, suggesting that delayed damage subsequent to initial spinal cord lesions may affect the clinical course (Yoshiyama et al. 2007). HBO therapy was shown by the US Navy to be more effective than the air recompression tables, and this has been confirmed in spinal cord DCS.

Helium and oxygen mixtures have been extensively used in recompression therapy in commercial diving (James 1981). The treatment of spinal cord DCS with helium saturation has significant advantages when there has been no clear improvement in neurological status after three 20 min sessions of 100 % oxygen at 2.8 ATA. Helium has the advantage of increasing the rate of nitrogen elimination from the tissues. Helium has been used in cases of spinal cord injury in DCS following air diving (Kol et al. 1993). This method of treatment was used in six cases following Comex-30 oxyhelium tables initially and some had additional HBO therapy. Five of these patients made full recoveries and 2 had mild residual neurological deficits. In one case a US Navy Table 6 had failed, but the patient recovered dramatically on recompression to 30 msw breathing a 50/50 helium and oxygen mixture 24 h later on Comex 30.

HBO at lower pressure (2 ATA) can be a useful tool in the treatment of acute and subacute phases of CNS ischemia and continued treatment is now recommended by the US Navy.

Experience in treating 68 sports divers with spinal cord DCS at the Israeli Naval Medical Institute over a period of 16 years was reviewed (Aharon-Peretz et al. 1993). Hydration and 100 % oxygen breathing were used until the patients reached the hyperbaric chamber. All patients received recompression therapy based on US Navy treatment tables using oxygen, except for six who were treated on Comex Treatment Table CX-30, which uses a 50/50 helium and oxygen mixture in addition to oxygen. Full recovery was achieved in 79% of these patients. In another review, cases of spinal DCS from a US naval station were classified according to severity and time to recompression with oxygen (Ball 1993). Delay in treatment was found to worsen the outcome for severely injured divers. Residual severity after all treatments was correlated with the severity after first treatment. Retreatment did not alter the outcome in these patients.

Spinal cord DCS presenting as complete Brown-Séquard syndrome with MRI signal abnormalities corresponding to an infarction in the posterior spinal artery territory has been reported to improve considerably following HBO therapy (Louge et al. 2012). Six further cases of this syndrome with DCS have been described in the literature, and the diagnosis is mainly based on clinical findings rather than MRI (Tseng et al. 2015).

Inner Ear Disturbances

Inner ear disturbances are unusual in air diving but may follow a switch from heliox to air in mixed gas diving. In this situation, the problem may reside in the inner ear, the brain stem, or the cerebellum. Hearing loss is also an unusual manifestation of decompression sickness and in the absence of other manifestations of DCS, it is difficult to distinguish it from middle and inner ear barotrauma. Once the diagnosis is established, immediate recompression with HBO may result in complete recovery of hearing. These disturbances can be treated with vasodilators, anti-inflammatory agents, and HBO. The last is a useful adjunct even if applied after a delay.

Facial Baroparesis

Ischemic neuropraxia of the facial nerve occurs during decompression if impaired Eustachian tube function causes the overpressure to persist in the middle ear in a person with a deficient facial canal; it is not a common event. The importance of recognition of this complication lies in differentiating it from DCS of the CNS and avoiding prolonged recompression therapy. There is no definite treatment, but HBO may be used, as this approach has been found useful in cases of Bell's palsy (see Chap. 18).

Late Sequelae of DCS

Divers who have had episodes of DCS are more liable to be hospitalized in the following years. These admissions may be due to late sequelae of DCS some of which are:

1. Persistent joint and limb pains.
2. Aseptic necrosis of bone. The cause of aseptic necrosis of bone, which is a late manifestation of DCS, is not known. It may be the result of damage to the endothelium or the capillaries supplying blood to the bone (see Chap. 30).

3. Motor disorders.
4. Peripheral neuropathy.
5. Patients who have suffered DCS have a higher incidence of vascular diseases.
6. Neuropsychological deficits

Monoplace vs. Multiplace Chambers

Most recompression facilities available to divers are two compartment multiplace chambers. The use of monoplace chambers for DCS has been controversial because examination of the casualty is not possible and most cannot be compressed beyond 3 ATA. However, compression to 6 ATA is unnecessary and even dangerous in DCS following surface-orientated diving, especially when treatment is delayed. Monoplace chambers can be used for the treatment of DCS under the following circumstances:

- Diving accident victims who arrive at a hyperbaric facility where only a monoplace chamber is available should be accepted for treatment.
- Monoplace chambers should be equipped to provide air breaks using a mask and an external source of compressed air to allow USN Tables 5 and 6 to be followed.

Air breaks are possible in a Sechrist model 2500-B monoplace chamber, and the equipment is easily fitted into other monoplace designs.

Use of Oxygen vs. Other Gas Mixtures

Oxygen treatment has disadvantages because it cannot be used at pressures greater than 2.8 ATA because of oxygen toxicity and air breaks are therefore used at this pressure. In fact, convulsions may occur after even 20 min at 2.8 ATA. It is likely that the convulsions are associated with the severe vasoconstriction which can be observed in the retina, and the same mechanism is likely to be responsible for the worsening recorded in successive US Navy Diving Manuals issued since the introduction of the minimal recompression oxygen breathing tables in 1970. Because of a perceived fire hazard raised by the use of oxygen, compressed air is still commonly used for the treatment of DCS in workers in compressed air working, but the results are inferior to those obtained using oxygen treatment. Oxygen treatment in recompression has the following advantages over air:

- A large gradient for nitrogen elimination
- No further addition of nitrogen
- Tissue oxygenation is improved even without full restoration of blood flow

- Reduced red blood cell aggregation
- Improved WBC filterability

In commercial diving, it is essential to avoid the use of compressed air in the recompression therapy of helium and oxygen mixture divers because the addition of nitrogen may cause dramatic worsening of symptoms and even death because of gas counter-transport (James 1981). For cases presenting after surfacing, the oxygen tables may be used but for deeper recompression therapy helium and oxygen mixtures must be used. This practice has now been incorporated into US Navy procedures (USN Manual 1993). Considerable commercial experience has been gained in the use of 50/50 heliox on the Comex 30 table for both air and heliox divers (see Table 11.2). In contrast to the use of oxygen at 2.8 ATA no cases of deterioration in divers have been recorded using heliox in recompression therapy. This is now fully supported by extensive animal experimentation with direct observation of bubbles in tissue. The only contrary experimental data has been from a severe experimental models where following the use of heliox a transient in pulmonary arterial pressure was seen. However, this has not been a problem in the therapy of human decompression sickness and the advice first given by the US Navy in 1959 to use helium-oxygen mixtures is still current in the US Navy (James 1988). Helium and oxygen mixtures can be used in place of air on any of the USN air recompression tables and are the preferred choice for recompression beyond 2.8 ATA.

Drugs

No drug treatment has been trialed for Type I pain only DCS. However, intravenous fluids are recommended in Type II DCS when the patient cannot take fluid orally. Isotonic, glucose-free fluids such as intravenous (IV) saline are recommended for prevention and treatment of hypovolemia as well as rehydration for reversal of the sludging of blood. Other plasma expanders are ineffective and dextrans may provoke allergic reactions.

Experimentally, the following interventions have been suggested but given the overall success of the current management of DCS are unlikely to be adopted:

1. IV perfluorocarbon emulsions, which are halogen substituted carbon nonpolar oils with resultant enhanced oxygen solubility, have been investigated as oxygen therapeutics as well for the enhancement of other gas movements within the body. One particularly promising area of research is the use of perfluorocarbon for the treatment of DCS (Spiess 2009). Improved oxygenation partly explains therapeutic effects of perfluorocarbons in decompression syndrome (Smith et al. 2012).

One concern is that perfluorocarbon may further decrease platelet count, which is already low in DCS because of platelet activation. In a swine model of decompression sickness, treatment with Oxycyte, a perfluorocarbon, did not impact platelet numbers and whole blood clotting by thromboelastometry, or result in bleeding (Cronin et al. 2016).

2. Steroids: As in spinal cord injury, there is some evidence that steroids may be beneficial when edema is present. However, the use of high-dose steroids has not been tested in DCS, and their use remains controversial (Jallul et al. 2007).

3. Intramuscular diclofenac sodium, a nonsteroidal anti-inflammatory agent, has been used to relieve the residual pain of DCS.

4. Lidocaine, a sodium-channel blocking agent used clinically as an antiarrhythmic and local anesthetic, can be used as a neuroprotective agent but clinical evidence of efficacy in DCS is limited to anecdotal reports. Expeditious administration of lidocaine may be justified in severe neurologic DCS after patient counseling and consent.

5. Nitric oxide (NO)-donating agents. This is based on the hypothesis that exogenous NO administration or pharmacological upregulation of NO may reduce DCS risk and severity by decreasing bubble formation, reduction of bubble-mediated inflammatory and coagulation cascades and protection of endothelial integrity (Duplessis and Fothergill 2008). Some of these effects can be achieved by statins, which are approved for the treatment of hypercholesterolemia. Statin-mediated lipid reduction may reduce bubble generation via alterations in plasma rheology and surface tension. Use of NO-donor medications such as isosorbide mononitrate and nitroglycerine should be investigated for the treatment of DCS.

6. Leukotrienes. Zafirlukast and zileuton, which are 5-lipoxygenase inhibitors, can reduce inflammatory responses to DCS in rats (Little and Butler 2008).

7. Fluoxetine, an antidepressant with anti-inflammatory properties, decreases the incidence of experimental decompression sickness in mice and improves motor recovery by limiting the inflammation process as evidenced by the reduction of circulating IL-6, a biomarker of systemic inflammation (Blatteau et al. 2012).

Platelet antagonists such as aspirin can reduce platelet aggregation surrounding microbubbles. Substances that increase the intracellular levels of cyclic AMP seem most promising in this respect. There has been no significant human experience with heparin which may promote hemorrhage. In experimental animals, perfluorocarbon emulsion (FC-43) combined with 100 % oxygen breathing has been shown to provide hemodynamic and neurological protection in DCS. On balance, it seems unlikely that pharmacological strategies will become available for the management of DCS and reliance must be placed on early recompression therapy with high partial pressures of oxygen and helium oxygen mixtures.

Importance of Early Treatment

The importance of early treatment has been established beyond dispute in military and commercial diving experience and a review of the treatment of DCS in US Navy divers indicated no mortality or obvious morbidity after recompression therapy. The common factors in these cases were as follows:

1. Medical screening and conditioning were strict.
2. Physicians and divers were acquainted with the signs and symptoms.
3. The interval between onset of symptoms and recompression was short.
4. There was aggressive diagnostic and therapeutic use of HBO.
5. There was judicious use of adjunctive measures such as intravenous fluids and dexamethasone.

Immediate hyperbaric treatment is the main factor in ensuring complete recovery from severe DCS. Following treatment, current guidelines recommend an observation period of at least 6 h for patients with neurological symptoms in case of relapse. Surveys have shown a symptom relapse rate as high as 38.5%, with half of those occurring in the first 24 h. A short-term observation unit is recommended for monitoring of these patients. A retrospective study of patients presenting with DCS at a major hyperbaric facility showed that of 102 consecutive patients with DCS who were receiving HBO, 42 (41.2%) had neurological sequelae, 10 required more than one treatment for refractory symptoms or relapse, 38 received up to three treatments, which can be done within the time requirements of short-term observation (Tempel and Severance 2006). Therefore, short-term observation units would provide a safe and efficient disposition for patients after receiving HBO.

Delayed Treatment

Patients with residual symptoms of DCS who present several days following the exposure may also benefit from HBO treatment, often with complete resolution. Therefore, DCS cases should be treated with HBO whenever they are seen, even as late as 2 weeks after the onset symptoms.

A transportable recompression rescue chamber (TRRC) has been suggested as an alternative to delayed treatment TRRC for one person can be used for the rapid initiation of treatment and evacuation in severe scuba-diving accidents.

This chamber has also been used for evacuation although a two-compartment chamber (one compartment for the victim and one for the attendant) is better.

There is some risk is involved in commercial air transport as gas bubbles may expand with increase in altitude in an aircraft and hypoxia will be worsened. However, some aircraft can maintain sea level conditions (1 ATA) at altitude and the Swiss air-rescue service can also transport a monoplace hyperbaric chamber in a helicopter. The ideal transportable hyperbaric chamber should be two compartment and fully equipped for ancillary treatment. Some chambers are available for surface transport and can be modified and fitted into a boat or a helicopter so that the patients can be treated while they are being transported to a regular medical facility for further care.

Treatment of Residual Neurological Injury and SPECT Brain Imaging in Type II DCS

The first DCS case where HMPAO–SPECT brain imaging was used to identify viable brain tissue and document the response to HBO at pressures lower than those used conventionally for the treatment of DCS was in 1993 (Harch et al. 1993). Following this a total of 13 divers who had Type II DCS or cerebral arterial gas embolism were managed by this approach (Harch et al. 1994). HMPAO–SPECT scans were done after test exposure to HBO at 1.5 or 1.7 ATA for 90 min. The initial scans were abnormal in all cases. "Tailing" HBO treatments at low pressures (1.5–2 ATA) were continued with primary HBO treatment for DCS in 9 of these and 4 with delays of 4–86 days. Neurological improvement was correlated with improvements shown on SPECT scans. This approach has now been adopted by the US Navy, and it is essential to recognize that this therapy is addressing hypoperfusion due to edema by utilizing the vasoconstrictive properties of oxygen at increased dosage and is not directed at persisting gas phase.

Risk Factors for DCS

The following risk factors for DCS have been recorded for air diving:

1. Obesity. Obesity increases the risk of DCS. Divers who are more than 20% in excess of ideal weight, according to standard tables, should be prohibited from diving until they have reduced their weight to acceptable levels.
2. Early, retrospective reports of the incidence of altitude DCS during altitude chamber training exposures indicated that women were more susceptible than men but in later studies, no differences in altitude DCS incidence were observed between the sexes. Women are at a higher

risk of developing altitude-related DCS during their menstrual periods.

3. Sensitivity to complement fixation. Individuals who are more sensitive to complement activation by alternate pathways are more susceptible to DCS.

4. High serum cholesterol levels and hemoconcentration predispose to bubble formation.

5. The presence of a foramen ovale is a risk factor for the development of DCS in divers because it allows the passage of venous emboli into the systemic circulation. The fetus may be at risk of DCS in a pregnant diver. The pulmonary filter is not functioning in the fetus, and the bubbles generated by either the fetal or the placental tissues will pass through the foramen ovale into the fetal arterial circulation, where they can proceed to embolize the brain, the spinal cord, and other organs.

6. A prolonged stay under pressure followed by rapid decompression.

7. Heavy exercise or other stress at depth.

8. Flying after diving and a rapid ascent to high altitude.

9. An experimental study in rats has shown that pretreatment with sildenafil, a phosphodiesterase-5 blocker used for the treatment of erectile dysfunction, promotes the onset and severity of neurologic DCS (Blatteau et al. 2013). This effect could be related to vasodilation with increased cerebral blood flow.

Shortness of breath after heavy exercise during the dive, dehydration, and dive depths exceeding 30 msw are relative risk factors for decompression sickness (Suzuki et al. 2014). Persons with a patent foramen ovale and a cardiac right-to-left shunt have an increased risk of developing neurologic complications even after recreational scuba diving in shallow water. Whether cigarette smoking increases the risk of developing DCS has not been established.

Preventive Measures for DCS

In 1908, Haldane devised the first set of validated schedules for diving exposures and decompression with the aim of preventing DCS, which he referred to as compressed air sickness (Boycott et al. 1908). DCS can be prevented when care is taken during ascent to normal pressure. Both navies and commercial diving companies have detailed decompression tables, including some that are computerized, which are available for the guidance of divers. Essentially, all calculations assume that the additional gas taken up remains in solution and gas equilibrates in the lung to ambient conditions. Both of these assumptions are now known to be untrue. In effect, decompression tables contrive to minimize bubble formation and allow the safe elimination of the bubbles formed.

The hypothesis that number of bubbles evolving during decompression from a dive, and therefore the incidence of DCS, might be reduced by pretreatment with HBO, has been tested in rats (Katsenelson et al. 2007). HBO pretreatment was shown to be equally effective at 304, 405, or 507 kPa, bringing about a significant reduction in the incidence of DCS in rats decompressed from 1013 kPa. This method has not yet been tested in humans.

Pre-dive conditioning measures such as endurance exercise in a warm environment, oral hydration, and normobaric oxygen breathing can reduce the risk of DCS in scuba divers by upregulation of cytoprotective proteins and reduction of bubbles formation (Gempp and Blatteau 2010).

In divers with a history of major neurologic decompression symptoms without evident cause, transesophageal echocardiography must be performed to exclude patent foramen ovale. Whether all divers should be screened for patent foramen ovale is an ongoing discussion. If a cardiac right-to-left shunt is present, divers with a history of decompression sickness should stop diving.

Prognosis of DCS

According to a study on military divers with DCS, the main independent risk factor associated with a poor outcome is the severity of neurologic manifestations at onset, and recovery is not significantly improved by prompt administration of recompression treatment (Blatteau et al. 2011). A prospective study on divers with neurologic DCS at a hyperbaric facility showed that those who presented more than 17 h after surfacing were likely to have more intense symptoms than those who presented earlier for treatment (Mutzbauer and Staps 2013). Neither had more HBO treatment or worse outcome related to the delay, but the amount of oxygen that had to be administered in total during the whole course of treatment was lower in cases that responded better.

In contrast to immediate treatment in commercial diving, therapeutic response in amateur divers with vestibular and inner ear decompression sickness remains poor, and incomplete recovery was found in 68 % of the patients that were followed (Gempp and Louge 2013). Time to recompression did not seem to influence the clinical outcome in these cases.

Conclusion

Air diving beyond 30 msw (4 ATA) is associated with a greatly increased risk of DCS. Decompressions and adherence to published "no-decompression" limits or decompression tables does not necessarily eliminate the risk of DCS. Early recognition and prompt management of a patient with DCS is essential and early recompression treatment reduces the incidence of late complications. Recompression with a high partial pressure of oxygen is recommended for the initial treatment and US Navy Tables 5 and 6 are the most widely used in surface-orientated diving. When required, further recompression should be undertaken using helium and oxygen mixtures which are preferred in the treatment of neurological DCS. Adherence to good diving practice and the recognition of risk factors for DCS are important to reduce the incidence of this disease.

References

Aharon-Peretz JS, Adir Y, Gordon CR, Kol S, Gal N, Melamed Y. Spinal cord decompression sickness in sport diving. Arch Neurol. 1993;50:753–6.

Ball R. Effect of severity, time to recompression with oxygen, and re-treatment on outcome in forty-nine cases of spinal cord decompression sickness. Undersea Hyperb Med. 1993;20:133–45.

Blatteau JE, Gempp E, Constantin P, Louge P. Risk factors and clinical outcome in military divers with neurological decompression sickness: influence of time to recompression. Diving Hyperb Med. 2011;41:129–34.

Blatteau JE, Barre S, Pascual A, Castagna O, Abraini JH, Risso JJ. Protective effects of fluoxetine on decompression sickness in mice. PLoS One. 2012;7, e49069.

Blatteau JE, Brubakk AO, Gempp E, Castagna O, Risso JJ, Vallée N. Sidenafil pre-treatment promotes decompression sickness in rats. PLoS One. 2013;8, e60639.

Blogg SL, Loveman GA, Seddon FM, Woodger N, Koch A, Reuter M, et al. Magnetic resonance imaging and neuropathology findings in the goat nervous system following hyperbaric exposures. Eur Neurol. 2004;52:18–28.

Boycott AE, Damant GC, Haldane JS. The prevention of compressed air illness. J Hyg (Lond). 1908;8:342–443.

Butler FK. Decompression sickness presenting as optic neuropathy. Aviat Space Environ Med. 1991;62:346–50.

Butler WP, Topper SM, Dart TS. USAF treatment table 8: treatment for altitude decompression sickness. Aviat Space Environ Med. 2002;73:46–9.

Cronin WA, Senese AL, Arnaud FG, Regis DP, Auker CR, Mahon RT. The effect of the perfluorocarbon emulsion Oxycyte on platelet count and function in the treatment of decompression sickness in a swine model. Blood Coagul Fibrinolysis. 2016;27:702–10.

Dan-Goor E, Asaria R, Borthwick B, Firth O, Hughes I, Sheather D, et al. Posterior vitreal detachment in decompression illness—case report and discussion. Am J Emerg Med. 2012;30:637.e5–6.

Davis JC, Sheffield PJ, Schuknecht L, et al. Altitude decompression sickness: hyperbaric therapy results in 145 cases. Aviat Space Environ Med. 1977;48:722–30.

Duplessis CA, Fothergill D. Investigating the potential of statin medications as a nitric oxide (NO) release agent to decrease decompression sickness: a review article. Med Hypotheses. 2008;70:560–6.

Fuerecdi GA, Czarnecki DJ, Kindwall EP. MR findings in the brains of compressed-air tunnel workers; relationship to psychometric results. Am J Roentgen. 1991;12:67–70.

Gempp E, Blatteau JE. Preconditioning methods and mechanisms for preventing the risk of decompression sickness in scuba divers: a review. Res Sports Med. 2010;18:205–18.

Gempp E, Louge P. Inner ear decompression sickness in scuba divers: a review of 115 cases. Eur Arch Otorhinolaryngol. 2013;270:1831–7.

Gempp E, De Maistre S, Louge P. Serum albumin as a biomarker of capillary leak in scuba divers with neurological decompression sickness. Aviat Space Environ Med. 2014;85:1049–52.

Geng M, Zhou L, Liu X, Li P. Hyperbaric oxygen treatment reduced the lung injury of type II decompression sickness. Int J Clin Exp Pathol. 2015;8:1797–803.

Germonpre P, Balestra C, Obeid G, Caers D. Cutis Marmorata skin decompression sickness is a manifestation of brainstem bubble embolization, not of local skin bubbles. Med Hypotheses. 2015;85:863–9.

Gillis MF, Peterson PL, Karagianes MT. In vivo detection of circulating gas emboli associated with decompression sickness using the Doppler blood flow detector. Nature. 1968;217:965–7.

Haldane JS. Admiralty report on deep water diving. London HMSO CN 1549; 1907.

Haldane JS. Respiration. New Haven: Yale University Press; 1922. p. 332–57.

Harch PG, Van Meter KW, Gottlieb SF, et al. Delayed treatment of type II DCS: the importance of low pressure HMPAO-SPECT brain imaging in its diagnosis and management. Undersea Hyperbaric Med. 1993;20(Suppl.):51 (abstract).

Harch PG, Van Meter KW, Gottlieb SF, et al. The effect of HBO tailing treatment on neurological residual and spect brain images in type II (cerebral) DCI/CAGE. Undersea Hyperbaric Med. 1994;21(Suppl):(abstract).

Hills BA, James PB. Microbubble damage to the blood-brain barrier. Undersea Biomed Res. 1991;18:111–6.

Ide WW. Central serous chorioretinopathy following hypobaric chamber exposure. Aviat Space Environ Med. 2014;85:1053–5.

Iordanidou V, Gendron G, Khammari C, Rodallec T, Baudouin C. Choroidal ischemia secondary to a diving injury. Retin Cases Brief Rep. 2010;4:262–5.

Jain KK. Decompression sickness: neurologic manifestations. In: Greenamyre T, editor. MedLink neurology. San Diego: Medlink Corporation; 2016.

Jallul S, Osman A, El-Masry W. Cerebro-spinal decompression sickness: report of two cases. Spinal Cord. 2007;45:116–20.

James PB. Evidence for subacute fat embolism as the cause of multiple sclerosis. Lancet. 1982;1:380–6.

James PB. Helium and oxygen mixtures in the treatment of compressed-air illness. Undersea Biomed Res. 1988;15:321.

James PB. Hyperbaric oxygenation in fluid microembolism. Neurol Res. 2007;29:156–61.

James PB. Oxygen and the brain: the journey of our lifetime. North Palm Beach: Best Publishing; 2014.

James PB. Problem areas in the therapy of neurological decompression sickness. In: James PB, editor. The size distribution of gas emboli arising during decompression: a review of the concept of critical diameter. Proceedings of XIII annual congress of EUBS, Dragerwerke, Travemunde; 1981. p. 481–6.

Jersey SL, Jesinger RA, Palka P. Brain magnetic resonance imaging anomalies in U-2 pilots with neurological decompression sickness. Aviat Space Environ Med. 2013;84:3–11.

Jones JP, Ramirez S, Doty SB. The pathophysiologic role of fat in dysbaric osteonecrosis. Clin Orthop. 1993;296:256–64.

Kalentzos VN. Images in clinical medicine. Cutis marmorata in decompression sickness. N Engl J Med. 2010;362(23), e67.

Katsenelson K, Arieli Y, Abramovich A, Feinsod M, Arieli R. Hyperbaric oxygen pretreatment reduces the incidence of de-compression sickness in rats. Eur J Appl Physiol. 2007;101:571–6.

Kayar SR. On beginning a second century of decompression sickness research: where are we and what comes next? Aviat Space Environ Med. 2008;79:1071–2.

Kayser B, Jean D, Herry JP, Bärtsch P. Pressurization and acute mountain illness. Aviat Space Environ Med. 1993;64:928–31.

Kei PL, Choong CT, Young T, Lee SH, Lim CC. Decompression sickness: MRI of the spinal cord. J Neuroimaging. 2007;17:378–80.

Klingmann C. Inner ear decompression sickness in compressed-air diving. Undersea Hyperb Med. 2012;39:589–94.

Kohshi K, Wong RM, Abe H, Katoh T, Okudera T, Mano Y. Neurological manifestations in Japanese Ama divers. Undersea Hyperb Med. 2005;32:11–20.

Kol S, Adir Y, Gordon CR, Melamed Y. Oxy-helium treatment of severe spinal cord decompression sickness after air diving. Undersea Hyperb Med. 1993;20:147–54.

Lee J, Kim K, Park S. Factors associated with residual symptoms after recompression in type I decompression sickness. Am J Emerg Med. 2015;33:363–6.

Liow MH, Ho BH, Kim SJ, Soh CR, Tang KC. MRI findings in cervical spinal cord type II neurological decompression sickness: a case report. Undersea Hyperb Med. 2014;41:599–603.

Little T, Butler BD. Pharmacological intervention to the inflammatory response from decompression sickness in rats. Aviat Space Environ Med. 2008;79:87–93.

Louge P, Gempp E, Hugon M. MRI features of spinal cord decompression sickness presenting as a Brown-Sequard syndrome. Diving Hyperb Med. 2012;42:88–91.

Martin JD, Thom SR. Vascular leukocyte sequestration in decompression sickness and prophylactic hyperbaric oxygen therapy in rats. Aviat Space Environ Med. 2002;73:565–9.

McGuire S, Sherman P, Profenna L, Grogan P, Sladky J, Brown A, et al. White matter hyperintensities on MRI in high altitude U2 pilots. Neurology. 2013;81:729–35.

Mutzbauer TS, Staps E. How delay to recompression influences treatment and outcome in recreational divers with mild to moderate neurological decompression sickness in a remote setting. Diving Hyperb Med. 2013;43:42–5.

Naiman JL, Donohue WL, Prichard JS. Fatal nucleus pulposus embolism of spinal cord after trauma. Neurology. 1961;11: 83–7.

Parsons JT, Smith CR, Zhu J, Spiess BD. Retinal angiography: noninvasive, real-time bubble assessment from the ocular fundus. Undersea Hyperb Med. 2009;36:169–81.

Pokroy R, Barenboim E, Carter D, Assa A, Alhalel A. Unilateral optic disc swelling in a fighter pilot. Aviat Space Environ Med. 2009; 80:894–7.

Powell MR, Thoma W, Fust HD, et al. Gas phase formation and Doppler monitoring during decompression with elevated oxygen. Undersea Biomed Res. 1983;10:217–24.

Rudge FW. A case of decompression sickness at 2,432 meters (8,000 feet). Aviat Space Environ Med. 1990;61:1026–7.

Rudge FW. Decompression sickness presenting as viral syndrome. Aviat Space Environ Med. 1991;62:60–1.

Rudge FW, Shafer MR. The effect of delay on treatment outcome in altitude-induced decompression sickness. Aviat Space Environ Med. 1991;62:687–90.

Sheffield PJ, Davis JC. Application of hyperbaric oxygen therapy in a case of prolonged cerebral hypoxia following rapid de-compression. Aviat Space Environ Med. 1976;47:759–62.

Smith CR, Parsons JT, Zhu J, Spiess BD. The effect of intravenous perfluorocarbon emulsions on whole-body oxygenation after severe decompression sickness. Diving Hyperb Med. 2012;42:10–7.

Spencer MP. Decompression limits for compressed air determined by ultrasonically detected blood bubbles. J Appl Physiol. 1976;40:229–35.

Spiess BD. Perfluorocarbon emulsions as a promising technology: a review of tissue and vascular gas dynamics. J Appl Physiol. 2009;106:1444–52.

Stéphant E, Gempp E, Blatteau JE. Role of MRI in the detection of marrow bubbles after musculoskeletal decompression sickness predictive of subsequent dysbaric osteonecrosis. Clin Radiol. 2008;63:1380–3, discussion 1384–5.

Suzuki N, Yagishita K, Togawa S, Okazaki F, Shibayama M, Yamamoto K, et al. A case-control study evaluating relative risk factors for decompression sickness: a research report. Undersea Hyperb Med. 2014;41:521–30.

Tempel R, Severance HW. Proposing short-term observation units for the management of decompression illness. Undersea Hyperb Med. 2006;33:89–94.

Toro-Gonzalez G, Navarro-Roman L, Roman GC, Cantillo J, Serrano B, Herrera M, et al. Acute ischemic stroke from fibrocartilagenous embolism to the middle cerebral artery. Stroke. 1993;24:730–40.

Tseng WS, Huang NC, Huang WS, Lee HC. Brown-Séquard syndrome: a rare manifestation of decompression sickness. Occup Med (Lond). 2015;65:758–60.

Weijs JH, Snoeijer JH, Lohse D. Formation of surface nanobubbles and the universality of their contact angles: a molecular dynamics approach. Phys Rev Lett. 2012;108:104501.

Wirjosemito SA, Touhey JE, Workman WT. Type II altitude decompression sickness (DCS): US Air Force experience with 133 cases. Aviat Space Environ Med. 1989;60:256–62.

Yoshiyama M, Asamoto S, Kobayashi N, Sugiyama H, Doi H, Sakagawa H, et al. Spinal cord decompression sickness associated with scuba diving: correlation of immediate and delayed magnetic resonance imaging findings with severity of neurologic impairment—a report on 3 cases. Surg Neurol. 2007;67:283–7.

Cerebral Air Embolism

K.K. Jain

Abstract

This chapter on air embolism examines the causes, mechanisms, and pathophysiology of air embolism with focus on cerebral air embolism. Clinical features, diagnosis, and treatment are described. The focus is on applications of HBO, but ancillary treatments are also mentioned. HBO is the most effective treatment of air embolism; it reduces the size of air bubbles and counteracts the secondary effects. Finally, hyperbaric treatment in special situations is considered. It is concluded that HBO plays an important role in the management of air embolism.

Keywords

Air bubbles • Air embolism • Arterial gas embolism (AGE) • Cerebral embolism • Decompression sickness • Hyperbaric oxygen (HBO) • Iatrogenic air embolism • Pulmonary barotrauma • Pulmonary embolism • Venous gas embolism (VGE)

Introduction

Gas can enter arteries (arterial gas embolism, AGE) due to alveolar-capillary disruption caused by pulmonary over-pressurization such as in breath-hold ascent by drivers or veins (venous gas embolism, VGE) as a result of tissue bubble formation due to decompression (diving, altitude exposure) or during certain surgical procedures where capillary hydrostatic pressure at the incision site is subatmospheric (Moon 2014). Both AGE and VGE can be caused by iatrogenic gas injection. The introduction of air into the venous or the arterial system can cause cerebral air embolism leading to severe neurological deficits. The first known recognition of arterial air embolism was reported by Morgagni in 1769, and later, in 1821, Magendie described the consequences of pulmonary overinflation leading to arterial gas embolism.

Causes

The most common causes reported in the literature are iatrogenic, the embolism occurring as a result of invasive medical procedures or surgery. Less commonly, air embolism occurs in divers undergoing rapid decompression and in submarine escape. Causes of air embolism are shown in Table 12.1. There are ~20,000 cases of air embolism per year in the USA. The exact incidence of various causes is difficult to determine, as not all cases are reported in the literature. Some victims recover spontaneously.

The incidence of air embolism during cardiopulmonary bypass operations is 0.1 %. The actual prevalence may be higher because several such complications are not recognized and reported.

Air enters the venous system in 30–40 % of the patients undergoing neurosurgical operations in the sitting position. A case of massive cerebral gas embolism has been reported during lumbar discectomy in the prone position resulting from hydrogen peroxide irrigation of the wound (Zhang et al. 2015). The patient developed severe neurological deficits including quadriplegia. In spite of supportive treatment and HBO therapy, the patient survived with significant neurological disability.

K.K. Jain, MD, FRACS, FFPM (✉)
Blaesiring 7, Basel 4057, Switzerland
e-mail: jain@pharmabiotech.ch

Table 12.1 Causes of air embolism

A. Diving-related: sudden decompression or ascent in diving and
   submarine escape
   – Breath-holding ascent in divers
   – Pulmonary barotrauma—"burst lung" in divers
   – Rapid decompression in an altitude chamber for flight training
B. Trauma
   – Cardiopulmonary resuscitation in patients with undetected lung injury
   – Head and neck injuries
   – High-altitude accidents
C. Iatrogenic
   1. Diagnostic and minor procedures
      – Air contrast salpingogram
      – Air insufflation with pneumatic otoscope
      – Angiography: diagnostic and therapeutic catheterization of blood
        vessels
      – Arterial lines for blood and medication infusion
      – Gastrointestinal endoscopy: endoscopic retrograde
        cholangiopancreatography
      – Hemodialysis
      – Intravenous fluids and central venous pressure (CVP) lines
      – Mechanical positive pressure ventilation
      – Needle biopsy of the lung
      – Pleural lavage
   2. Intraoperative complications
      – Cardiac surgery: open heart surgery with extracorporeal
        circulation
      – Cesarean section
      – Endobronchial resection of lung tumor using
        Neodymium-YAG laser
      – Neurosurgical operations in the sitting position: tear
        into veins in the posterior
      – Fossa or the cervical spinal canal
      – Pelvic surgery in Trendelenburg position. Operative
        hysteroscopy with laser
      – Pulmonary surgery: lung transplantation
      – Spinal surgery: wound irrigation with hydrogen peroxide
      – Thoracic surgery: opening of pulmonary veins at
        subatmospheric pressures
      – Vascular surgery: carotid endarterectomy with shunt
D. Miscellaneous and rare causes
   – Faulty abortion
   – Inhalation of helium directly from a pressurized helium tank
   – Ingestion of hydrogen peroxide solution
   – Orogenital sex during pregnancy

Air embolism can occur during neuro-angiographic interventional procedures such as aneurysm coiling embolization and carotid stent placement but overall incidence during diagnostic neuroangiographic procedure is very low in the order of 0.08 % (Gupta et al. 2007).

Mechanisms

In iatrogenic cases, the air is either sucked into the veins with negative pressure or introduced into the veins or arteries under pressure. Small amounts of gas introduced into the venous system are often tolerated. The lung is usually an effective filter for air bubbles greater than 22 μm in diameter when air is injected slowly. A bolus injection of air >1.5–3 mL/kg exceeds the filter capacity of the lungs and produces embolization through the left heart into the arterial circulation until it blocks arterioles 30–60 μm in diameter. Air has a large surface tension at the blood–air interface and the globules of air cannot be deformed enough to navigate the capillaries.

A patent foramen ovale occurs in 20–35 % of the normal adult population and in one out of ten of these is at risk of having arterial air embolism when air enters the venous system inadvertently. The exact prevalence rate of functional right to left atrial shunt in the healthy adult population, however, is unknown. In the absence of such a shunt, venous air must first traverse the pulmonary vasculature in order to enter the cerebral circulation.

In pulmonary barotrauma, lung volumes expand during rapid ascent. When alveolar pressure exceeds 80–100 mmHg, air can be forced into pulmonary capillaries. Alveoli may rupture into the pleural space, causing pneumothorax, or into the pulmonary veins, where the embolus may traverse the left side of the heart to enter the aorta and may ascend the carotid arteries to the cerebral circulation, as the diver is usually upright during ascent.

Pathophysiology of Cerebral air Embolism

Air emboli lodge distally in the smaller arteries and arterioles of the brain and obstruct the flow of blood. The result is ischemia, hypoxia, and cerebral edema. Even when the bubble is dissolved, a "no reflow" phenomenon may occur in the damaged tissues. The bubble acts as a foreign body and starts a number of biochemical reactions in the blood. Platelets are activated and release vasoactive substances including prostaglandins. The bubble may damage the endothelial cells of the vessel wall by direct contact. Margination and activation of leukocytes follows and may cause a secondary ischemia. If the bubble persists, it is surrounded by platelets and fibrin deposit, which may prevent dislodging of the bubble. Although the potential of large bubbles to cause cerebral injury is not disputed, there is controversy over the significance of exposure to small bubbles in cardiac surgery. It is known that postsurgical neuropsychological deficits do correlate positively with the number of emboli to which patients are exposed; to date, however, the technology for distinguishing between gaseous and particulate emboli or for sizing emboli accurately is not readily available.

Air bubbles injected directly into the cerebral circulation of experimental animals can open the blood–brain barrier (BBB). The barrier, however, repairs itself within a few hours. Ischemic hypoxia produced by air embolism is not severe enough to produce gross cerebral infarction, but produces necrosis of the deep cortical layers at the gray–white matter junction.

There may be segmental arterial vasospasm followed by dilatation, and some of the air may escape from the arteries into the veins via capillaries. As a result of arterial obstruction, regional cerebral blood flow (rCBF) declines, and EEG activity may cease in the affected region. The changes are typical of cerebral ischemia, but the BBB permeability increases immediately after air embolism, in contrast to vascular occlusion from other causes, where the onset is delayed. Focal ischemia of short duration does not lead to cell loss, and the processes causing deterioration are potentially reversible. The other potentially reversible process that occurs in the tissues is cerebral edema. Although the brain is the major concern in arterial embolism, the coronary arteries may occasionally be involved.

Animal brain models of cerebral arterial gas embolism are useful for neurophysiological investigations of pathophysiology of central nervous system (CNS) damage and for comparing the effectiveness of various recompression schedules. Most of such studies involve injection of air into cerebral vasculature. Secondary CNS deterioration may be due to endothelial damage or change in blood constituents rather than mechanical action of bubbles and may explain the failure of recompression therapy in such cases. The results of these animal studies cannot be extrapolated to humans.

Clinical Features

Clinical manifestations, essentially neurological or cardiovascular disorders vary greatly. The clinical features of air embolism depend on the patient's posture, the route of entry of air, the volume of air, the size of the bubbles, and the rate of entry of air. If the patient is reclining, air is more likely to enter the coronary arteries, whereas it is more likely to enter the cerebral arteries if the patient is upright. Neurological sequelae have been estimated to occur in 19–50 % of the patients with cerebral air embolism.

Signs and symptoms of air embolism in divers may not be clear-cut. In 50 % of such cases, dysbaric air embolism was found to be part of dysbarism syndrome including decompression sickness. A sudden change in sensorium is the most common symptom and ranges from disorientation to coma. Focal neurological deficits such as hemiplegia or monoplegia may occur, according to the location of the lesions. Respiratory arrest and seizures are less common. A shock-like state may occur with massive embolism. Associated symptoms may be those of pneumothorax (in pulmonary barotrauma) or myocardial ischemia. Liebermeister's sign, i.e., the presence of areas of pallor on the tongue after air embolism, may be observed in some cases.

Diagnosis

The diagnosis of air embolism is based on a careful consideration of the patient's history and neurological findings. In cases of sudden decompression with neurological deficit, the diagnosis is easier. During surgical procedures monitored by Doppler ultrasound, air embolization is detected at an early stage and appropriate measures can be taken to stop further air entering the blood vessels. Transcranial Doppler studies show that microscopic cerebral artery air emboli are present in virtually all patients undergoing cardiac surgery. Microbubbles can be detected with two-dimensional echocardiography, which is often used for this purpose during open heart and bypass surgeries. EEG monitoring is also useful for early detection of acute cerebral dysfunction.

Subtle changes in mental function may be a major manifestation even in the absence of other objective neurological signs. Air bubbles may also be seen on fundoscopic examination. Air may be seen in the cerebral arteries during a neurosurgical operation, or air can be demonstrated in a specimen of arterial blood. A high index of suspicion is very important in diagnosis. Under suspicious circumstances air embolism should be assumed present unless otherwise proven. In some cases, the diagnosis is proven only after successful response to hyperbaric therapy. In air embolism associated with diving, there is muscle injury and elevated serum creatine kinase which a biomarker of the severity of this complication.

CT and MRI offer a possibility of diagnosis of subclinical lesions of the brain. Cerebral air embolism can be easily identified on CT and MRI scans. However, intracranial air can be promptly absorbed and although cerebral infarcts due to air are clearly visualized on diffusion-weighted images, the air may rapidly disappear from images (Kaichi et al. 2015). CT may not be practical, especially if the cerebral air embolism occurs during an operation and cannot be relied on for exclusion of the diagnosis.

Treatment

Treatment of air embolism is similar to that of decompression sickness (see Chap. 11). Emergency measures include administration of 100 % oxygen, using a closely fitting mask, and transport of the patient to a hyperbaric facility. If transport by air is unavoidable, the patient should travel in a pressurized cabin, and the aircraft should stay at a low altitude. A bolus dose (10 mg) of dexamethasone may be given to prevent cerebral edema. Oxygen serves to reduce the size of the air bubble by depletion of nitrogen and also counteracts the hypoxia and ischemia of the surrounding brain tissue.

The important consideration in the treatment of cerebral air embolism is preparedness and anticipation. Procedures with a known risk of air embolism should not be performed far away from a hyperbaric facility, and a hyperbaric chamber should be available in institutions that conduct open heart surgery. Time is the more important element in management— the shorter the delay, the better the outcome. Emboli large enough to produce symptoms require immediate treatment because of the risk of "gas lock" in the right side of the heart and subsequent circulatory failure (Jorgensen et al. 2008).

The generally accepted treatment of air embolism is immediate compression to 6 ATA air for a period of not more than 30 min followed by ascent to 2.8 ATA with oxygen. The rationale of this approach is as follows:

1. Compression of the bubbles reduces their size. According to Boyle's law, the volume of a gas is inversely proportional to the pressure exerted on the gas. Compression to 6 ATA would reduce the size of a bubble to one-sixth, or ~17 %, of its original size (Table 12.2). The reduction of the surface area of the bubble to 30 % reduces the inflammatory effect of the bubble–blood interface.
2. Delivery of high levels of oxygen is important to counteract the ischemic and hypoxic effects of vascular obstruction. Breathing oxygen (100 %) at 2.8 ATA leads to an arterial pO_2 level of 1800 mmHg. At this pressure, 6 mL oxygen is dissolved in 100 mL plasma.
3. Fick's law can be applied to relate the rate of nitrogen diffusion to the concentration gradient between the bubble and the surrounding tissue. Oxygen at 100 % concentration improves the diffusion of nitrogen from the bubble.
4. Cerebral edema associated with cerebral air embolism leading to intracranial hypertension is decreased by HBO.
5. Vasoconstriction induced by HBO inhibits air embolus redistribution. This is possible because the reactivity of the cerebral arteries is not impaired in cerebral air embolism.

In the first experimental study employing hyperbaric therapy air was injected into the carotid arteries of rabbits, and there was a remarkable improvement in the survival rate of the animals treated with HBO (Meijne et al. 1963). Two decades later, a series of experimental studies were carried out to reassess the hyperbaric treatment of air embolism (Leitch et al. 1984a-d). They tested the question, "Is there a benefit in beginning treatment at 6 ATA?" in dog models of air embolism treated at various pressures. The effectiveness of the treatment was assessed by sensory-evoked potentials (SEP) and CBF. It was concluded that there was no advantage in

using air at 6 ATA prior to treatment with oxygen at 2.8 ATA. The data showed that clearance of air is probably independent of pressure past the threshold of 2 ATA and is certainly hastened by oxygen. Approximately 8 min were required to clear the embolism. A number of air-treated dogs had redistribution of air embolism after initial decompression and concomitant reduction of CBF. Later, a study of various pressure schedules in experimental feline arterial air embolism was carried out with assessment of severity by cortical SEP, and no additional benefits of initial treatment at 6 ATA were found as compared to 2.8 ATA (McDermott et al. 1992).

Transcranial Doppler studies show that microscopic cerebral artery air emboli (CAAE) are present in virtually all patients undergoing cardiac surgery, but massive cerebral arterial air embolism is rare. If it occurs, HBO is recommended as soon as surgery is completed. A mathematical model can be used to predict the absorption time of air embolus, assuming that the volumes of clinically relevant air emboli vary from 10^{-7} to at least 10^{-1} mL. Absorption times are predicted to be at least 40 h during oxygenation using breathing gas mixtures of fraction of inspired oxygen approximately equal to 40 %. When air emboli are large enough to be detected by CT, absorption times are calculated to be at least 15 h. Decreases in CBF caused by the air emboli would make the absorption even slower. If the diagnosis of massive CAAE is suspected, CT should be performed, and consideration should be given to HBO therapy if the emboli are large enough to be visualized, even if patient transfer to a HBO facility will require several hours.

Some authors recommend supportive care as the primary therapy for venous gas embolism, while HBO therapy in addition to supportive care is the first line of treatment for arterial gas embolism (Fukaya and Hopf 2007). The criterion for use of HBO is clinical manifestation, particularly neurological and not the source of air embolism.

Clinical Applications of HBO for Air Embolism

Clinical applications of HBO for air embolism during the past decade are shown in Table 12.3. If we consider the overall mortality of air embolism without hyperbaric treatment as 30 %, these results represent a remarkable improvement. Controlled prospective studies have shown that mortality can be reduced to <15 % if HBO therapy is given within 12 h of the accident. Treatment appears to be ineffective after irreversible damage has already been done. An experimental study on pigs failed to show an effect of HBO on cerebral function after a delay of 2 or 4 h following induction of cerebral air embolism (Weenink et al. 2013). The injury caused in this model may have been too severe for a single session of HBO to be effective. This study should not change current HBO strategies for

Table 12.2 Relative volume and surface area of a bubble with compression

Pressure (ATA)	Relative volume (%)	Relative surface area (%)
1	100	100
2.8	35	50
6	17	30

Table 12.3 Examples of applications of HBO for cerebral air embolism

Author and year	Number of cases	Cause	HBO/pressure used	Results and comments
Davis et al. (1990)	1	Cesarian section	US Navy (USN) Treatment 6 ATA	HBO treatment started 8 h after onset with impairment of consciousness and left hemiplegia. Recovered with minimal neurological deficits
Armon et al. (1991)	1	Open heart surgery	USN Treatment Table 6A	HBO started 30 h after the incident with coma, decerebrate rigidity and seizures. Recovered with residual deficits in 14 m
Kol et al. (1993)	6	Cardiopulmonary bypass	USN Treatment Table 6A	2 died
				2 partial recovery
				2 full recovery
Rios-Tejada et al. (1997)	1	Flight level 28,000 ft in an altitude chamber	Table 6A + 3 HBO sessions at 2 ATA/90 m	Complete recovery from left hemiplegia
Droghetti et al. (2002)	1	Percutaneous nephrolithotripsy in the prone position	USN Treatment Table 6	Patient presented neurological deficits 8 h later, when HBO treatment was started. Full recovery
Wherrett et al. (2002)	1	Diagnostic bronchoscopy	USN modified Table 6	Treated 52 h after the event. Discharged after fully recovery 1 w later
Rider et al. (2008)	1	Ingestion of H_2O_2	3 ATA/30 m + 2.5 ATA 60 m	Recovered
Tomabechi et al. (2008)	1	Needle biopsy of lung	HBO	Recovered
Guy et al. (2009)	1	During aortic valve replacement surgery	2.8 ATA/ 30 m, decompressed to 2 ATA/60 m	Cerebral perfusion during surgery and HBO day after surgery with full neurological recovery
Um et al. (2009)	4	Transthoracic lung biopsy	2.2 ATA/60 m	2 full recovery; 1 recovery but died of pneumonia; 1 HBO not available, died
Müller et al. (2010)	1	Intra-articular inject-ion of 20 mL of air for CT-arthrography	HBO given >6 h after episode	Full recovery/paradoxical embolism (migration of air from the venous to the arterial circulation via right-left shunt)
Le Guen et al. (2012)	1	During lung transplantation	HBO	Recovery
Bothma et al. (2012)	1	Retrograde cerebral venous gas embolism	HBO	Recovery
Janisch et al. (2013)	1	Pleural streptokinase instillation	HBO	Recovery
Byrne et al. (2014)	1	Hydrogen peroxide ingestion	HBO	Recovery
Lin et al. (2014)	1	Aspergillosis lung	USN Table 6	Significantly improvement in stroke resulting from cerebral embolism
Wilson and Sayer (2015)	1	Professional diving	Royal Navy Table 62	Complete resolution
Eoh et al. (2015)	1	Endoscopic balloon dilation for esophageal stricture	HBO	Improved
Park et al. (2016)	1	Esophageal ballooning	HBO	Recovered

cerebral AGE, but further research is necessary to elucidate the effectiveness of late initiation of HBO therapy. Whether less severe injury benefits from HBO should be investigated in models using smaller amounts of air and clinical outcome measures.

HBO has been used successfully in cases of air embolism as a complication of open heart surgery, endoscopy and transthoracic percutaneous thin-needle biopsy. The usual schedule of hyperbaric treatment is US Air Force Modification of US Navy Table 6 (Fig. 11.5; Chap. 11). The initial approach is to compress the patient to 6 ATA. After 30 min, decompression is carried out to 2.8 ATA.

Ancillary Treatments

The following treatments have been used in addition to hyperbaric therapy.

Antiplatelet Drugs

These have been used to counteract the platelet aggregation associated with air embolism. The use of heparin as anticoagulant is considered risky due to the danger of hemorrhage in infarcted areas. Patients who are already on heparin have a better prognosis after air embolism than those who are not anticoagulated. This is particularly noted during cardiopulmonary bypass for cardiac surgery. Oral aspirin is safer but takes about 30 min to act after ingestion.

Steroids

These have been used to prevent cerebral edema. Delayed cerebral edema can occur after initially good results from recompression following air embolism. Steroids should be administered cautiously during HBO as they may accelerate the development of oxygen toxicity.

Hemodilution

Hematocrit has been shown to have a relation to the infarct size in vascular occlusion, and many cases of air embolism display hemoconcentration. Hemodilution, e.g., by dextran-40, is indicated. Lowering of hematocrit also causes a reduction in oxygen-carrying capacity, but this is more than adequately compensated by HBO.

Control of Seizures

An anticonvulsant medication may be required for control of seizures. Prophylactic use of lidocaine not only controls seizures but also reduces infarct size and prevents cardiac arrhythmias associated with air embolism.

Measures to Improve Cerebral Metabolism

Loss of blood supply causes immediate reduction of neuronal pools and increased production of lactate. The total energy available is reduced. Increased blood glucose levels are associated with increased lactate production by the ischemic brain and increase in infarction. The control of blood glucose, therefore, is important after air embolism and routine use of intravenous dextrose should be avoided. There is evidence that HBO serves to normalize the cerebral metabolism (see Chap. 18) and also lowers blood glucose.

Hyperbaric Treatment in Special Situations

HBO has been used in for management of cerebral air embolism during several situations. Some examples are listed as case reports in Table 13.2. And others are listed in this section.

Cerebral Edema

The following example is given to illustrate the special use of HBO in cerebral edema. A patient with air embolism who responded to initial compression to 6 ATA but deteriorated into coma and decerebrate posturing during decompression at 1.9 ATA. There was increased intracranial pressure, indicating cerebral edema. The patient was given repeated HBO treatments twice daily at 2.8 ATA (100 % oxygen) and recovered completely. HBO in this case was doubly indicated— for air embolism as well as for cerebral edema.

Cardiovascular Surgery

Air embolism can occur during cardiac catheterization in infants with ventricular septal defect as air is inadvertently injected into the right ventricle. Anesthesia should be terminated and air compression should be done to 6 ATA as soon as possible after the episode and completed within a few hours. Oxygen need not be given. The infants make a good recovery with this approach, and the planned cardiac surgery can be carried out. If air embolism occurs during nitrous oxide anesthesia, nitrous oxide diffuses rapidly into enclosed pockets of gas, causing an increase in pressure (or an increase in volume if the surrounding tissues permit). Therefore, nitrous oxide anesthesia should be discontinued if air embolism occurs.

HBO has been used to treat patients with extensive neurological deficits from air emboli during open heart surgery. Treatment is usually not started until after completion of surgery, but is still effective. Some complicated operations in cardiac surgery and neurosurgery cannot be aborted because of air embolism. In such cases, compression treatment can be started after completion of the operation. Anecdotal successful cases of use of HBO for air embolism with delay of >20 h have been reported. HBO should be used as soon as feasible but within 48 h of massive air embolism.

Massive proven arterial air embolism during surgical closure of an atrial septal defect in infants can be successfully treated with intraoperative (retrograde cerebral perfusion) combined with postoperative procedures (deep barbiturate anesthesia and HBO).

Hypothermia has been used in cardiac surgery for cerebral protection. Patients who suffer massive air embolism during cardiopulmonary bypass can be treated by using a combination of hypothermia and HBO with good results. According to Charles' law, the volume of a gas varies according to temperature. Theoretically hypothermia is expected to decrease the size of the gas bubbles and should be beneficial in air embolism. Hypothermia has also a neuroprotective effect.

Neurosurgery

Air embolism following posterior fossa surgery in the sitting position can be promptly treated by recompression according to the standard schedule. The patients usually recover without neurological deficits. Nevertheless, occurrence of such an episode may lead to disruption of critical operation. Therefore, precautions should be taken to avoid such a complication. Sitting position for neurosurgical procedures may be a well-tolerated approach for the patient if neurosurgeons and neuroanesthesiologists meticulously follow a strict team protocol, including all necessary monitoring. Following suggestions have been made (Gracia and Fabregas 2014):

- A modified semisitting (lounging) position aiming to create a positive pressure in the transverse and sigmoid sinuses, with lower head and higher legs positioned above the top of the head, decreases the incidence and severity of venous air embolism.
- Hyperventilation, which compromises CBF, should be avoided during a sitting position.
- Precordial Doppler or transesophageal echocardiography monitoring improves the detection of small venous air embolism enabling early treatment to diminish its adverse effects.
- Patients with known patent foramen ovale can be operated on in a sitting position, under strict protocol, with few reported clinical venous air embolism and no paradoxical air embolism.

Pulmonary Barotrauma

A review of treatment of 89 cases of air embolism due to pulmonary barotrauma in divers showed a 65 % success rate with hyperbaric treatments (Leitch and Green 1986).

Although most cases would recover with oxygen at 2.8 ATA, there is no reason to alter the established technique of initial compression with air to 6 ATA prior to HBO at 2.8 ATA. Air embolism associated with pulmonary barotrauma during rapid decompression in an altitude chamber can be managed by the use of treatment Table 6A.

Pulmonary barotrauma with air embolism has been reported as a complication of HBO therapy for a nonhealing ulcer of the foot. Pneumothorax has been reported as a complication of recompression therapy for cerebral arterial gas embolism associated with diving.

Unusual presentations of cerebral air embolism include a patient who became unresponsive and developed subcutaneous emphysema during the direct insufflation of oxygen into the right middle lobe bronchus (Wherrett et al. 2002). An endotracheal tube and bilateral chest tubes were immediately placed with resultant improvement in the oxygen saturation. However, the patient remained unresponsive with extensor and flexor responses to pain. Later, there was seizure activity requiring anticonvulsant therapy. CT scans of the head and cerebral spinal fluid examination were negative though the electroencephalogram was abnormal. A CT of chest showed evidence of barotrauma. Fifty-two hours after the event, a presumed diagnosis of cerebral air embolism was made, and the patient was treated with HBO using a modified US Navy Table 6. Twelve hours later he had regained consciousness and was extubated. He underwent two more HBO and was then discharged from hospital 1 week after the event, fully recovered. Although HBO was started after significant delay, the patient made a good recovery.

Air Embolism During Invasive Medical Procedures

HBO has been used to treat patients with cerebral air embolism resulting from invasive medical procedures. Most of these patients recover without any evidence of damage on clinical examination and MRI if diagnosis is made early and treatment is started.

Cerebral Air Embolism During Obstetrical Procedures

Venous air embolism is likely during cesarean section as air enters uterine sinuses, particularly if the placenta separates before delivery as in the case of placenta previa. Cases of cerebral air embolism occurring during cesarean sections have been treated successfully with the use of HBO. Air embolism manifested by cortical blindness was reported in a patient following induced abortion by means of intra-amniotic hypertonic saline instillation and the patient made a complete recovery after treatment with HBO (Weissman et al. 1989).

Cerebral Air Embolism in Endoscopic Retrograde Cholangiopancreatography

Hepatic portal venous air embolism was considered to be a rare complication of endoscopic retrograde cholangiopancreatography and endoscopic biliary sphincterotomy and may be fatal. During endoscopy, the gastrointestinal tract is insufflated with airflows as high as 2000 mL/min. Normally, this air is able to escape via orifices, but if this does not occur, pressures up to 43 kPa may build up within the intestine and insufflated air can enter the portal venous system through duodenal vein radicles that may be torn during the procedure. Until 2009, 13 cases of air embolism after endoscopic retrograde cholangiopancreatography had been reported. Systemic spread in four of these cases proved fatal; pulmonary air embolism in two cases, and cerebral air embolism in another two. Regional or systemic air embolism to the heart or cerebrum during endoscopic retrograde cholangiopancreatography (ERCP) is now an increasingly recognized phenomenon. A Medline search in 2010 revealed that systemic air embolism after ERCP occurred in 14 cases with cerebral air embolism in 8 of these; 6 had fatal outcome, 1 survived with hemiplegia and only 1 survivor recovered completely (Finsterer et al. 2010). In only two of these cases, transgression of air from the venous to the arterial branch occurred through a patent foramen ovale. In none of the patients was transgression attributable to arteriovenous shunts within the lung or other tissues, or insertion of the caval veins directly into the left atrium. In five patients, systemic air embolism occurred in the absence of a foramen ovale. In all these cases, it was assumed that air entered the vasculature through the portal or hepatic veins. More cases of ERCP are being reported.

A fatal systemic air embolism occurred during endoscopic retrograde cholangiopancreatography, where immediate resuscitation attempts for cardiac arrest failed to revive the patient (Cha et al. 2010). An additional fatal case was reported of a patient, who several years previously had undergone gastroduodenal resection with cholecystectomy and papillotomy, and was admitted for recurrent ascending cholangitis secondary to bile duct stones (Bisceglia et al. 2009). During the third endoscopic cholangioscopic procedure for removal of bile duct stones, sudden cardiopulmonary arrest occurred. Death was due to massive pulmonary air embolism and cerebral air embolism. A spontaneous duodenobiliary fistula was found on autopsy, which was the pathway for entry of air insufflated during duodenal endoscopy. A case of a venous air embolism resulting in cardiorespiratory collapse was reported in a child with splenomesenteric portal shunt for portal cavernoma during endoscopic retrograde cholangiopancreatography under general inhalation anesthesia without using nitrous oxide (Di Pisa et al. 2011). Recovery fol-

lowed chest compressions, advanced life support measures and inhalation of 100 % oxygen.

Air embolism should be suspected if a patient does not wake up after ERCP. Cerebral and thoracic CT scans should be ordered, and appropriate measures should be taken, including aspiration of air from the right ventricle through an acutely floated pulmonary artery catheter or HBO should be initiated.

Cerebral Embolism Due to Hydrogen Peroxide Poisoning

Hydrogen peroxide can produce acute gas embolism. There is a case report of an adult who suffered an apparent stroke shortly after an accidental ingestion of concentrated hydrogen peroxide (Mullins and Beltran 1998). Complete neurologic recovery occurred quickly following HBO treatment. In another case report, a patient developed cerebral air embolism a short time after ingestion of a small amount of hydrogen peroxide manifested by hematemesis, left-sided hemiplegia, confusion, and left homonymous hemianopsia. Initial laboratory studies, chest X-ray, and brain CT were normal. MRI demonstrated areas of ischemia and 18 h after arrival, the patient underwent HBO treatment with complete resolution of symptoms (Rider et al. 2008). Of the seven reported cases of air embolism from hydrogen peroxide that did not undergo HBO, only in one patient was there a report of symptom resolution. HBO can be considered as the definitive treatment for gas embolism from hydrogen peroxide ingestion as with all other causes of acute gas embolism.

Relapse Following Spontaneous Recovery

In cases of spontaneous redistribution of air bubbles, a period of apparent recovery is frequently followed by relapse. The etiology of relapse appears to be multifactorial and is chiefly the consequence of a failure of reperfusion. Prediction of who will relapse is not possible, and any such relapse carries poor prognosis. It is advisable, therefore, that air embolism patients who undergo spontaneous recovery be promptly recompressed while breathing oxygen. Therapeutic compression serves to antagonize leukocyte-mediated ischemia-reperfusion injury; to limit potential re-embolization of brain blood flow, secondary to further leakage from the original pulmonary lesion or recirculation of gas from the initial occlusive event; to protect against embolic injury to other organs; to aid in the resolution of component cerebral edema; to reduce the likelihood of late brain infarction reported in patients who have undergone spontaneous clinical recovery; and to prevent decompression sickness in high gas loading dives that precede accelerated ascents and omitted stage decompression.

Delayed Treatment

Air embolism should be treated as quickly as possible after it is detected. This is not always possible and several cases receive delayed treatment. HBO treatments have led to recovery in cases of air embolism with severe neurological deficit where treatment was delayed for 24 h. In patients with air embolism secondary to cardiopulmonary bypass accidents, pulmonary barotrauma induced by mechanical ventilation and central vein catheterization, significant recovery has been noted even when treatment was started 15–60 h after the event.

Conclusion

Hyperbaric treatment has been proven to be unquestionably indicated for the treatment of air embolism with neurological deficits. The conventional methods of treatment, such as posturing the patient in certain ways, aspirating the air, providing normobaric oxygen, closed chest massage, and steroids, have not been adequate to manage this problem. The consensus concerning the pressure favors the retention of 6 ATA initial compression with air. If the patient's condition does not permit exposure to this high pressure or the chamber immediately available cannot provide this pressure, 100 % oxygen at 2.8 ATA would be acceptable as an alternative, particularly when only a monoplace chamber is available. The diagnosis of air embolism cannot always be made with certainty. There is need to improve technologies for early detection of air bubbles. It is acceptable to treat the patient with compression if air embolism is suspected, and the response to compression may be diagnostic in such cases. Early treatment provides better results than late treatment but HBO treatment should be considered at any stage the patient presents.

Considering that air embolism is a complication of medical and surgical procedures, it stands to reason that hyperbaric chambers should be available at clinics that perform such procedures. Although air embolism is extremely rare with modern bypass equipment, open heart surgery, preferably should be done in a hospital that has a hyperbaric chamber.

References

Armon C, Deschamps C, Adkinson C, Fealey RD, Orszulak TA. Hyperbaric treatment of cerebral air embolism sustained during an open-heart surgical procedure. Mayo Clin Proc. 1991;66:565–71.

Bisceglia M, Simeone A, Forlano R, Andriulli A, Pilotto A. Fatal systemic venous air embolism during endoscopic retrograde cholangiopancreatography. Adv Anat Pathol. 2009;16:255–62.

Bothma PA, Brodbeck AE, Smith BA. Cerebral venous air embolism treated with hyperbaric oxygen: a case report. Diving Hyperb Med. 2012;42:101–3.

Byrne B, Sherwin R, Courage C, Baylor A, Dolcourt B, Brudzewski JR, et al. Hyperbaric oxygen therapy for systemic gas embolism after hydrogen peroxide ingestion. J Emerg Med. 2014;46:171–5.

Cha ST, Kwon CI, Seon HG, Ko KH, Hong SP, Hwang SG, et al. Fatal biliary-systemic air embolism during endoscopic retrograde cholangiopancreatography: a case with multifocal liver abscesses and choledochoduodenostomy. Yonsei Med J. 2010;51:287–90.

Davis FM, Glover PW, Maycock E. Hyperbaric oxygen for cerebral air embolism occurring during cesarian section. Anesth Intensive Care. 1990;18:403–5.

Di Pisa M, Chiaramonte G, Arcadipane A, Burgio G, Traina M. Air embolism during endoscopic retrograde cholangiopancreatography in a pediatric patient. Minerva Anestesiol. 2011;77:90–2.

Droghetti L, Giganti M, Memmo A, Zatelli R. Air embolism: diagnosis with single-photon emission tomography and successful hyperbaric oxygen therapy. Br J Anaesth. 2002;89:775–8.

Eoh EJ, Derrick B, Moon R. Cerebral arterial gas embolism during upper endoscopy. A A Case Rep. 2015;5:93–4.

Finsterer J, Stöllberger C, Bastovansky A. Cardiac and cerebral air embolism from endoscopic retrograde cholangio-pancreatography. Eur J Gastroenterol Hepatol. 2010;22:1157–62.

Fukaya E, Hopf HW. HBO and gas embolism. Neurol Res. 2007;29:142–5.

Gracia I, Fabregas N. Craniotomy in sitting position: anesthesiology management. Curr Opin Anaesthesiol. 2014;27:474–83.

Gupta R, Vora N, Thomas A, Crammond D, Roth R, Jovin T, et al. Symptomatic cerebral air embolism during neuro-angiographic procedures: incidence and problem avoidance. Neurocrit Care. 2007;7:241–6.

Guy TS, Kelly MP, Cason B, Tseng E. Retrograde cerebral perfusion and delayed hyperbaric oxygen for massive air embolism during cardiac surgery. Interact Cardiovasc Thorac Surg. 2009;8:382–3.

Janisch T, Siekmann U, Kopp R. Cerebral air embolism after pleural streptokinase instillation. Diving Hyperb Med. 2013;43:237–8.

Jorgensen TB, Sorensen AM, Jansen EC. Iatrogenic systemic air embolism treated with hyperbaric oxygen therapy. Acta Anaesthesiol Scand. 2008;52:566–8.

Kaichi Y, Kakeda S, Korogi Y, Nezu T, Aoki S, Matsumoto M, et al. Changes over time in intracranial air in patients with cerebral air embolism: radiological study in two cases. Case Rep Neurol Med. 2015;2015:491017.

Kol S, Adir Y, Gordon CR, Melamed Y. Oxy-helium treatment of severe spinal cord decompression sickness after air diving. Undersea Hyperb Med. 1993;20:147–54.

Le Guen M, Trebbia G, Sage E, Cerf C, Fischler M. Intraoperative cerebral air embolism during lung transplantation: treatment with early hyperbaric oxygen therapy. J Cardiothorac Vasc Anesth. 2012;26:1077–9.

Leitch DR, Greenbaum LJJ, Hallenbeck JM. Cerebral arterial air embolism: 1. Is there benefit in beginning HBO treatment at 6 bar? Undersea Biomed Res. 1984a;11:221–35.

Leitch DR, Greenbaum LJJ, Hallenbeck JM. Cerebral arterial air embolism: II. Effect of pressure and time on cortical evoked potential recovery. Undersea Biomed Res. 1984b;11:237–48.

Leitch DR, Greenbaum LJJ, Hallenbeck JM. Cerebral arterial air embolism: III. Cerebral blood flow after decompression from various pressure treatments. Undersea Biomed Res. 1984c;11:249–63.

Leitch DR, Greenbaum LJJ, Hallenbeck JM. Cerebral arterial air embolism: IV. Failure to recover with treatment, and secondary deterioration. Undersea Biomed Res. 1984d;11:265–74.

Leitch DR, Green RD. Pulmonary barotrauma in divers and the treatment of cerebral arterial gas embolism. Aviat Space Environ Med. 1986;57:931–8.

Lin C, Barrio GA, Hurwitz LM, Kranz PG. Cerebral air embolism from angioinvasive cavitary aspergillosis. Case Rep Neurol Med. 2014;2014:406106.

McDermott JJ, Dutka AJ, Koller WA, Flynn ET. Effects of an increased PO2 during recompression therapy for the treatment of experimental cerebral arterial gas embolism. Undersea Biomed Res. 1992;19:403–13.

Meijne NG, Shoemaker G, Bulterijs AB. The treatment of cerebral gas embolism in a high pressure chamber. J Cardiovasc Surg. 1963;4:757.

Moon RE. Hyperbaric oxygen treatment for air or gas embolism. Undersea Hyperb Med. 2014;41:159–66.

Müller MC, Lagarde SM, Germans MR, Juffermans NP. Cerebral air embolism after arthrography of the ankle. Med Sci Monit. 2010;16:CS92–4.

Mullins ME, Beltran JT. Acute cerebral gas embolism from hydrogen peroxide ingestion successfully treated with hyperbaric oxygen. J Toxicol Clin Toxicol. 1998;36:253–6.

Park S, Ahn JY, Ahn YE, Jeon SB, Lee SS, Jung HY, et al. Two cases of cerebral air embolism that occurred during esophageal ballooning and endoscopic retrograde cholangiopancreatography. Clin Endosc. 2016;49(2):191–6. doi:10.5946/ce.2015.071.

Rider SP, Jackson SB, Rusyniak DE. Cerebral air gas embolism from concentrated hydrogen peroxide ingestion. Clin Toxicol (Phila). 2008;46:815–8.

Rios-Tejada F, Azofra-Garcia J, Valle-Garrido J. Neurological manifestation of arterial gas embolism following standard altitude chamber flight: a case report. Aviat Space Environ Med. 1997;68:1025–8.

Tomabechi M, Kato K, Sone M, Ehara S, Sekimura K, Kizawa T, et al. Cerebral air embolism treated with hyperbaric oxygen therapy following percutaneous transthoracic computed tomography-guided needle biopsy of the lung. Radiat Med. 2008;26:379–83.

Um SJ, Lee SK, Yang DK, Son C, Kim KN, Lee KN, et al. Four cases of a cerebral air embolism complicating a percutaneous transthoracic needle biopsy. Korean J Radiol. 2009;10:81–4.

Weenink RP, Hollmann MW, Vrijdag XC, Van Lienden KP, De Boo DW, Stevens MF, et al. Hyperbaric oxygen does not improve cerebral function when started 2 or 4 hours after cerebral arterial gas embolism in swine. Crit Care Med. 2013;41:1719–27.

Weissman A, Peretz BA, Michaelson M, Paldi E. Air embolism following intra-uterine hypertonic saline instillation: treatment in a high pressure chamber; a case report. Eur J Obstet Gynecol Reprod Biol. 1989;33:271–4.

Wherrett CG, Mehran RJ, Beaulieu MA. Cerebral arterial gas embolism following diagnostic bronchoscopy: delayed treatment with hyperbaric oxygen. Can J Anaesth. 2002;49:96–9.

Wilson CM, Sayer MD. Cerebral arterial gas embolism in a professional diver with a persistent foramen ovale. Diving Hyperb Med. 2015;45:124–6.

Zhang J, Zhang C, Yan J. Massive cerebral gas embolism under discectomy due to hydrogen peroxide irrigation. Case Rep Neurol Med. 2015;2015:497340.

Carbon Monoxide and Other Tissue Poisons

13

K.K. Jain

Abstract

Hyperbaric oxygenation (HBO) is a recognized treatment for carbon monoxide (CO) poisoning and has a supplemental role in the treatment of some other tissue poisons. Basic mechanisms, diagnosis, and management of carbon monoxide (CO) poisoning are discussed including controversies in the use of HBO for CO poisoning. Guidelines for the use of both normobaric oxygen (NBO) and HBO are discussed. HBO is more effective than NBO for the prevention of delayed neurological sequelae. HBO is also useful in the management of poisons other than CO: cyanide, hydrogen sulfide, carbon tetrachloride, and methemoglobinemias.

Keywords

Carbon monoxide poisoning • Carbon tetrachloride poisoning • Carboxyhemoglobin (COHb) • Carboxymyoglobin (COMb) • Cyanide poisoning • Hydrogen sulfide poisoning • Hyperbaric oxygen therapy (HBO) • Hypoxia • Methemoglobinemias • Normobaric oxygen (NBO) • Tissue poisons

Classification of Tissue Poisons

This chapter deals mainly with the role of hyperbaric oxygenation (HBO) in the treatment of carbon monoxide (CO) poisoning; several other tissue poisons that have been treated with HBO are also discussed. Classification of these poisons by their mode of action is presented in Table 13.1.

Carbon Monoxide Poisoning

Historical Aspects of CO Poisoning

Human beings have been exposed to CO ever since they have made fire inside sheltered caves. In 300 BC, Aristotle stated that "coal fumes lead to heavy head and death." Obviously, this was a reference to CO poisoning. Claude Bernard

showed in 1857 that CO produces hypoxia by reversible combination with hemoglobin (Bernard 1857); and in 1865, Klebs described clinical and pathologic findings in rats exposed to CO (Klebs 1865). The classical bilateral lesions of the globus pallidus and diffuse subcortical demyelination were described and correlated with psychic akinesia in 1924 (Pineas 1924). Connection of CO poisoning with parkinsonism was described a couple of years later (Grinker 1926).

In 1895, Haldane showed that rats survived CO poisoning when placed in oxygen at a pressure of 2 atm (Haldane 1895). The effectiveness of hyperbaric oxygen (HBO) in experimental CO poisoning in dogs and guinea pigs was demonstrated in 1942 (End and Long 1942). In 1960, HBO was first used successfully in treating human cases of CO poisoning (Smith and Sharp 1960).

Biochemical and Physical Aspects of CO

This subject has been dealt with in detail by Jain (1990), and it will be briefly reviewed here with more recent findings.

K.K. Jain, MD, FRACS, FFPM (✉)
Blaesiring 7, Basel 4057, Switzerland
e-mail: jain@pharmabiotech.ch

© Springer International Publishing AG 2017
K.K. Jain, *Textbook of Hyperbaric Medicine*, DOI 10.1007/978-3-319-47140-2_13

Table 13.1 Classification of tissue poisons where HBO has been used successfully

1. Action by combination with cytochrome α3 oxidase and P-450
   - Carbon monoxide
   - Hydrogen sulfide
2. Hepatotoxic free radical formation mediated by P-450
   - Carbon tetrachloride
3. Drug-induced methemoglobinemias
   - Nitrites
   - Nitrobenzene

Table 13.2 Biochemical effects of carbon monoxide

1. Effects on the blood
   - Increase of the carboxyhemoglobin level
   - Shift to the left of the oxygen dissociation curve
   - Rise of the lactate level
2. Action at the cellular level
   - Inhibition of cytochrome α3 oxidase and P-450

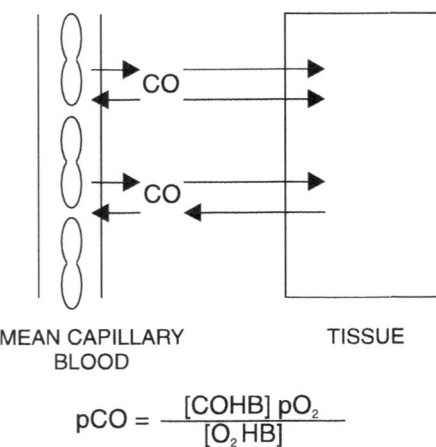

MEAN CAPILLARY BLOOD   TISSUE

$$pCO = \frac{[COHB]\ pO_2}{[O_2HB]}$$

Fig. 13.1 Mean tissue CO tension is equal to the mean CO tension in capillary blood. CO tension in mean capillary blood depends on the parameters listed in the Haldane equation depicted in this figure. Modified from Coburn 1970

CO Body Stores

Most of the body deposits of CO are found in the blood chemically bound to Hb. However, 10–15 % of the total body content of CO is located in extracellular space, probably in combination with myoglobin (Mb). The combination of Hb with CO is governed by Haldane's law. Accordingly, when a solution containing Hb is saturated with a gas mixture containing oxygen and CO_2, the relative proportions of the Hb that combine with the two gases are proportional to the relative partial pressures of the two gases (Fig. 13.1), allowing for the fact that the affinity of the CO for Hb is 240 times greater than that of O_2. This is expressed by the equation:

$$\frac{COHb}{O_2Hb} = K \times \frac{pC=_2}{pO_2}$$

where K is 240.

The rate of formation of COMb can also be expressed by the Haldane equation, except that the estimated value of the constant K is then 40. Apparently Mb is involved in the oxygen transport mechanism and is ready to deliver oxygen when needed. Examination of O_2Hb and O_2Mb dissociation curves reveals that, at pO_2 less than 60 mmHg, O_2 has greater affinity for Mb than for Hb.

Biochemical Effects of CO on Living Organisms

Carbon monoxide inhibits oxygen transport, availability, and utilization; its biochemical effects are summarized in Table 13.2. CO lowers the oxygen saturation in direct proportion to the COHb concentration, thus blocking oxygen transport from the lungs to the tissues. The binding of one or more CO molecules to Hb also induces an allosteric modification in the remaining heme group, distorting the oxygen dissociation curve and shifting it to the left. Tissue anoxia is thus far greater than would result from the loss of oxygen-carrying capacity alone. A concentration of 0.06 % of CO in the air is enough to block one-half of the Hb available for oxygen transport. The manner of CO combination with Hb differs appreciably from that of oxygen at high levels of CO saturation but is virtually the same at low levels of CO saturation.

Important factors that influence the accumulation of COHb are pH, pCO_2, temperature, and 2,3-DPG (diphosphoglycerate). The affinity of oxygen for the Hb is strongly influenced by 2,3-DPG, which is located inside the red blood cells (RBC). When 2,3-DPG levels rise, for example, in anaerobic glycolysis, hypoxia, anemia, and at high altitudes, affinity of the oxygen for Hb is reduced.

Inhibition of the Utilization of Oxygen by CO

Until recently it was believed that the sole effect of CO was to produce COHb, which blocks oxygen transfer to the cells. Warburg had already demonstrated in 1926 that CO competes with oxygen for the reduced form of cytochrome a3 oxidase, which is the terminal enzyme of the cellular respiratory chain. The possibility that CO is directly cytotoxic is borne out by in vitro demonstration of CO interactions with non-Hb hemoproteins. Reduced cytochrome a3 (cytochrome c oxidase) and cytochrome P-450 bind sufficient CO to inhibit their function in vitro. The possibility that CO inhibits mitochondrial electron transport in vivo is interesting because of the close relationship between the respiratory chain function and the

Fig. 13.2 The mitochondrial respiratory chain indicating sequence of electron transport, three sites of energy coupling (oxidative phosphorylation), and location of action of CO

Mitochondrial Respiratory Chain

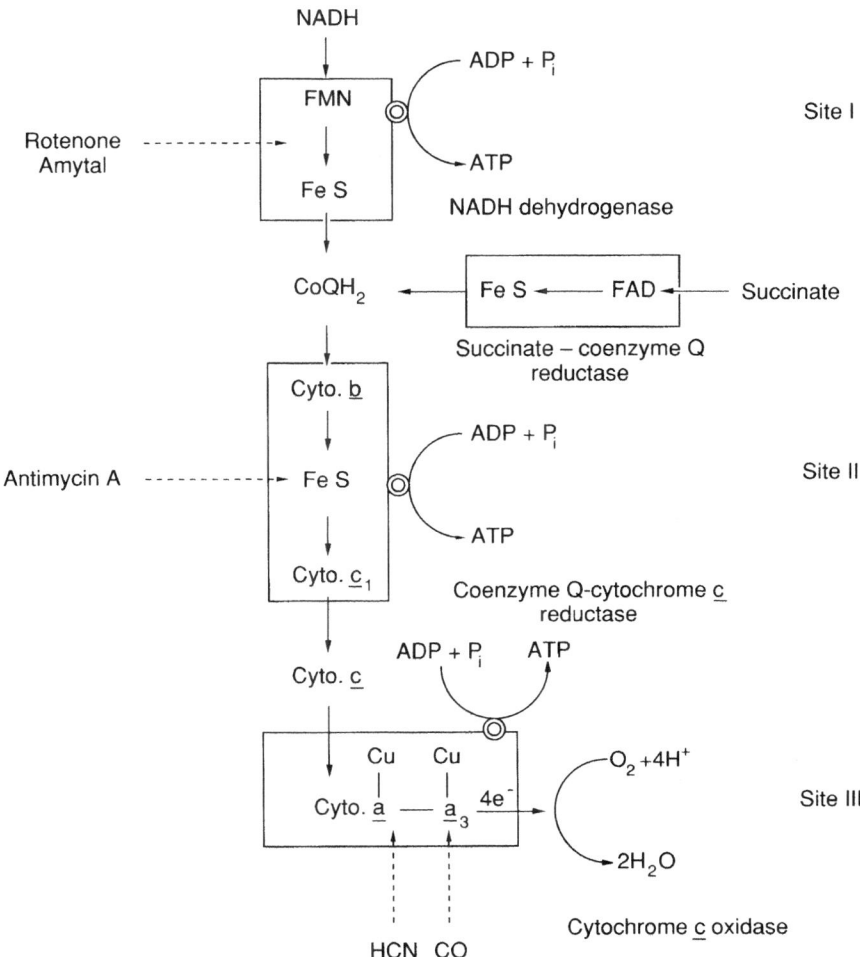

cellular energy metabolism (Fig. 13.2). These basic mechanisms have been confirmed (Chance et al. 1970).

CO combines with cytochrome a3 oxidase, and cytochrome P-450, thus blocking cellular oxidation and causing cellular hypoxia. Organs with high metabolic rate, such as the heart and brain, are particularly affected by CO. Cytochrome prefers oxygen to CO by a factor of 9:1, and this may explain the disparity between COHb levels and the clinical effects. This also explains the beneficial effect of HBO therapy. CO alters brain metabolism in vivo independently of the COHb-related decreases in oxygen delivery.

In conclusion, it can be stated that CO poisoning is highly complex, and a great deal more is involved than simple production of COHb. Formation of carboxycytochrome oxidase has been postulated to act as a toxin by blocking cellular use of oxygen. The half-life of CO bound with cytochrome a3 oxidase is not known. More research is needed to determine

this value, as it may be an important factor in the genesis of late sequelae of CO poisoning, and it may also provide a rational basis for determining the duration of treatment by oxygen therapy.

Epidemiology of CO Poisoning

Each year 50,000 persons visit emergency departments for CO poisoning in the United States. More than 4000 persons die annually from CO poisoning and in addition to this, CO accounts for more than half of the ~12,000 annual fire-associated deaths. In Korea, the incidence of CO poisoning in households using charcoal briquettes for heating and cooking was 5.4–8.4 % as shown in a survey of four major cities (Cho et al. 1986). There are no figures available for a much larger number of sufferers from occult CO poisoning.

Table 13.3 Causes of CO poisoning

1. Endogenous
Hemolytic anemias (rise of COHb to 4–6%)
2. Exogenous
A. Natural environments
– Microbial activity in plant life
B. Artificial
– Automobile exhaust
– Defective domestic appliances for heating and cooking
– Industrial plant exhausts
– Mining accidents
– Fires
C. Indirect
– Poisoning by methylene chloride (paint-stripping solvent) due to its conversion to CO in vivo
D. Cigarette smoking
– Active smoking
– Passive smoking

Causes of CO Poisoning

CO is present universally, but clinically manifest poisoning occurs only when critical levels are exceeded. Various causes for this are listed in Table 13.3. Endogenous CO is unimportant because the values seldom exceed 3% COHb. The most important sources of CO poisoning are exogenous.

Sources of CO Poisoning

The commonest source of CO poisoning in industrialized urban areas of Western countries is automobile exhausts. They contain 6–10% CO and are responsible for 90% of the CO content of the atmosphere of a city. Frequently such fatal poisoning occurs in a closed garage with the car engine running, a common method of suicide. There are ~2300 such suicides annually in the USA.

At busy city intersections, CO concentrations as high as 0.03% have been measured. A pedestrian on a street with heavy automobile traffic is exposed to CO. A concentration of 20–40 mg/mL can raise COHb 1.5–2-fold within 1 h. Jogging in this environment increases the CO intake and further raises the COHb. Persons doing manual work on streets with heavy automobile traffic can suffer a rise of COHb to toxic levels. Jogging in Central Park in New York City can be more dangerous than walking or just standing around. Smoking in such environments further aggravates CO intoxication and COHb levels of 13% can be reached.

After the garage, the kitchen is the most dangerous place and a frequent site of CO poisoning. Cooking gas usually contains 4–14% CO. If not burned properly (as in a defective oven or stove), CO can leak into the room. Other sources of

danger in the house are space-heating systems, such as a gas boiler. In Korea, household appliances are the commonest source of CO poisoning, open wood or coal-burning furnaces being the most frequent culprits.

Even though natural gas has been substituted for coal gas, 1000 persons still die annually in England and Wales as a result of CO poisoning from this source. Although natural gas burns more efficiently and cleanly than other forms of fuel, it is also the most potentially lethal if combustion is incomplete and is responsible for most of the deaths from domestic CO poisoning in the US. Incomplete combustion of other fuels such as charcoal and wood can also release CO, which can be trapped inside the building if the chimney is clogged. CO poisoning is more likely to occur in houses that are insulated and airtight to conserve energy.

Exhausts of many industrial plants, mills, and workshops contain CO. Risks are particularly high in blast furnaces and coal mines. Explosives can emit as much as 60% CO. Smoke contains CO, and smoke inhalation injury is usually associated with CO intoxication. Wood and paper fires contain 12% CO. Firefighters are particularly at risk from CO poisoning. COHb levels of 50% have been found in those dying within 12 h of receiving burns, implicating CO as the main culprit.

Pathophysiology of CO Poisoning

CO Binding to Myoglobin

It has been known for decades that death from CO poisoning is caused by hypoxia resulting from displacement of oxygen from the Hb. The mechanism of this, however, is not straightforward. Oxygen is stored in myoglobin and this is made possible by the crooked angle at which oxygen binds to the protein. CO, which prefers to sit upright, competes with for space with oxygen in this molecular shuttle. When myoglobin's structures forces CO to lie on its side, it is excluded. This classical view has been challenged by the use of spectroscopic techniques which provide evidence that a nearly perpendicular CO fits comfortably in myoglobin and that forced bending has little to do with CO exclusion. The reason is more likely that the unbound CO is pinned on its side near the binding site and little binding takes place.

Both CO and oxygen bind to an iron atom in the middle of the ring-shaped portion of myoglobin known as the heme group. Heme when isolated in experiments, binds to CO 10,000 times as strongly as it does to oxygen but when embedded in myoglobin, it binds only 20–30 times as strongly as oxygen. This led the belief that protein must be doing something to suppress CO relative to oxygen.

CO-Induced Hypoxia

Although the toxic effect of CO is postulated to be at the cellular level, by formation of carboxycytochrome oxidase, CO poisoning is primarily a hypoxic lesion caused by the replacement of OHb by COHb. Studies comparing the effect in dogs of anoxia induced by 0.5 % CO ventilation with that induced by breathing low oxygen mixtures found no significant differences in oxygen consumption or oxygen extraction in the two sets of animals who were subjected to equal reduction of arterial OHb, although the mode of desaturation was CO poisoning in one group.

The term CO-hypoxia implies that there is inhibition of oxygen transport from the blood to the tissues. Tissue oxygen tension may be decreased directly through a reduction in oxygen content by a lowered arterial oxygen tension, as well as through the presence of COHb. The oxygen dissociation curve is shifted to the left. The clinical effects of CO are usually attributed to tissue hypoxia, but they do not always correlate with COHb levels. Because CO combines with extravascular proteins such as myoglobin, its combination with cytochrome C-oxidase and cytochrome P-450 has been considered possibly to cause cellular hypoxia by inhibiting the mitochondrial respiratory chain.

Effects of CO on Various Systems of the Body

CO involves most parts of the body, but the areas most affected are those with high blood flow and high oxygen requirement, such as the brain and the heart. The effects of CO on various systems are presented in Table 13.4.

Cardiovascular System

The heart is particularly vulnerable to CO poisoning, because CO binds to cardiac muscle three times as much as to skeletal muscle. Studies on isolated animal hearts have shown that CO may have a direct toxic effect on the heart regardless of the formation of COHb. At levels of 1–4 % COHb, myocardial blood flow is higher, but no adverse effects are demonstrated. If the perfusion medium of an isolated rat heart muscle is gassed with 10 % CO, there is a 40 % increase in coronary blood flow, which is likely to be due to vasodilatation secondary to anoxia. Increase in myocardial blood flow occurs mostly without an increase in COHb levels.

Angina patients are particularly susceptible to CO exposure. The onset of angina during physical exertion can be accelerated by elevating COHb levels to the 5–9 % range.

Table 13.4 Effect of CO on various systems of the body

Cardiovascular system
- Precipitation of myocardial ischemia in patients with angina
- ECG abnormalities
- Cardiomyopathy as an acute effect and cardiomegaly as a chronic effect
- Hypertension and atherosclerosis as chronic effects

Elements of the blood and hemorrheology
- Increased platelet aggregation
- Lower RBC deformability
- Increased plasma viscosity and hematocrit
- Erythrocytosis as a chronic effect

Nervous system
- Brain: cerebral edema, focal necrosis
- Peripheral nerves: neuropathy and delayed motor conduction velocity

Special senses
- Visual system: retinopathy and visual impairment
- Auditory system: hearing loss due to hypoxia of the cochlear nerve

Lungs
- Pulmonary edema

Muscles
- Myonecrosis, compartment syndrome

Exercise physiology
- Decrease of physical work capacity and V2 max

Liver
- Impaired function due to inhibition of cytochrome P-450

Kidneys
- Impairment of renal function, renal shutdown
- Endocrines
- Impairment of hypophysis, hypothalamus, and suprarenals

Bone and joints
- Degenerative changes, hypertrophy of bone marrow
- Skin
- Erythema and blisters

Reproductive system
- Impaired menstruation and fertility in women
- Impotence in men
- Fetal toxicity with low conceptus weight and growth retardation

CO precipitates ischemia by reducing oxygen delivery to the myocardium. Changes in ECG have been shown to occur in workers chronically exposed to CO when COHb levels reach 20–30 %. These changes are reversible after withdrawal from exposure to CO. Various abnormalities in the ECG reported in CO poisoning are summarized in Table 13.5. Depression of the S-T segment is the most common ECG finding in these cases and may precede myocardial infarction resulting from exposure to CO. Conduction abnormalities may be the result of anoxia or a direct toxic effect of CO on hemorrhages into the conducting system of

Table 13.5 ECG abnormalities due to CO poisoning

1. Arrhythmias, extrasystoles, atrial fibrillation
2. Low voltage
3. Depression of S–T segment
4. Prolongation of ventricular complex, particularly the Q–T interval
5. Conduction defects
   - Increased P–R interval
   - A–V block
   - Branch bundle block

the heart. Abnormalities of the motion of the left ventricular wall, as shown by echocardiography, are frequently seen in CO poisoning, and these correlate with a high incidence of papillary muscle lesions in fatal cases.

In a study on 9046 patients with CO poisoning and 36,183 controls, the overall risks for developing peripheral arterial disease were 1.85-fold in the patients with CO poisoning compared with the comparison cohort after adjusting for age, sex, and comorbidities (Chen et al. 2015). Oxidative stress caused by toxicological free radicals results in endothelial cell damage, inflammatory reactions, and subsequent atherogenic processes in peripheral artery circulative systems.

Hemorheological Effects of CO

Viscosity of the whole blood as well as of the plasma increases after inhalation of 400 ppm of CO. An increase in COHb levels also decreases the deformability of erythrocytes, thus impairing the microcirculation.

Effect of CO on Blood Lactate

Levels of COHb over 5 % have been shown to raise blood lactate levels. This is presumed to be an effect of hypoxia. Severity of CO poisoning depends on the duration of exposure rather than on COHb levels alone. Severe poisoning associated with long exposure is accompanied by high blood lactate and pyruvate levels.

Effect of CO on the Lungs

Pulmonary edema is present in 36 % of patients with CO poisoning and is considered to be caused by hypoxia. X-rays of the lungs show a characteristic ground-glass appearance. Perihaler haze and intra-alveolar edema may also be present. Vomiting in an unconscious patient may lead to aspiration pneumonia.

Exercise Capacity

Endurance and VO_2 max decrease as the COHb levels rise. Fatigue and reduced exercise capacity may also be caused by the accumulation of lactate resulting from exposure to CO. Lactate levels over 4 mmol hinder physical training.

Sleep

Sleep is severely disturbed by CO, without a detectable effect on the respiratory frequency and pulmonary ventilation. The aortic body receptors mediating circulatory reflexes are more sensitive to CO than the carotid body receptors mediating respiratory reflexes. Disruption of sleep could result from afferent discharges from aortic receptors in response to CO or low oxygen content. Anoxia is known to abolish REM sleep.

Effect on Pregnancy

Studies of the effects of CO inhalation on the conceptus weight in gravid rats lead to the following conclusions:

- Continuous CO inhalation lowered the conceptus weight on days 14 and 20 of pregnancy.
- The effect was more pronounced in the group exposed to cigarette smoke (CO plus nicotine) than the group exposed to CO alone.
- CO affects the fetus more adversely during the last trimester of pregnancy, which is the phase of rapid growth.

Experimental studies in neonatal animals have shown that acute exposure to CO can alter neurotransmitter function in the brain and that some of the effects persist for several weeks. Exposure of neonatal rats to CO has also been shown to produce hyperactivity that persisted for up to 3 months of age.

Musculoskeletal System

Compartment syndromes of the lower extremities may be caused by necrosis and swelling of the muscles.

Skin

Cutaneous blisters occur in CO poisoning. It seems possible that necrobiosis in eccrine glands starts early, but that the epidermal basal cells, notably at the papillary apices, suffer the same change only after temporary pressure anoxia and reactive hyperemia.

Gastrointestinal System

Extensive bowel ischemia with infarction has been reported in fatal cases of CO poisoning.

Effects on the Peripheral Nervous System

Peripheral neuropathy can be caused by CO poisoning. Possible causes include anoxia, the toxic effect of CO on the nerves, and positional compression of the nerves during the comatose stage.

Effects on the Visual System

Measurable decreases in sensitivity to light and adaptation to darkness have been shown to result from low levels of CO exposure. These alterations persist even after elimination of COHb from the blood, indicating that a significant amount of CO may be retained in the tissues. Retinal hemorrhages have been observed on ophthalmoscopy of patients with acute CO poisoning. Retinal venous engorgement and peripupillary hemorrhages resemble those seen in hypoxia. CO retinopathy has been recorded as an acute effect of CO poisoning leading to visual impairment.

Effect on the Auditory System

Hearing loss of a central type caused by anoxia from CO poisoning is only partially reversible. The loss of auditory threshold activity is pronounced at the level of the auditory cortex; the relative vulnerability of the central auditory pathway has been demonstrated. Vestibular function is more frequently involved than the auditory function. Recovery from hearing loss is uncommon; this is the result of hypoxia of the cochlear nerve and the brain stem nuclei.

Effect on the Central Nervous System

The most important lesions of CO poisoning are in the central nervous system (CNS). This subject has been discussed in detail elsewhere (Jain 2016).

Neuropathology
Of the cells of the CNS, the astrocytes are more sensitive than neurons to the effects of CO. The critical lesions in CO poisoning are in the brain. There are three stages in the evolution of the brain lesions:

1. In immediate death after CO poisoning, there are petechial hemorrhages throughout the brain, but no cerebral edema
2. In patients who die within hours or days after poisoning, cerebral edema is present. There is necrosis of the globus pallidus and substantia nigra.
3. In patients who die days or weeks later from delayed sequelae of CO poisoning, edema has usually disappeared.

Degenerative and demyelinative changes are usually seen. Necrosis of the globus pallidus in a patient is revealed by CT scan as a low-density area. The corpus callosum, hippocampus, and substantia nigra may also be affected. In the late stages, there is cerebral atrophy, which is also demonstrated by CT scan; this usually correlates with poor neurological recovery. White matter damage is considered to be significant in the pathogenesis of parkinsonism in patients with CO poisoning.

Pathophysiology
The tendency for effects on certain areas of the brain such as the globus pallidus and substantia nigra has been considered to be caused by a hypoxic effect of CO. Clinical instances of "pure hypoxia" are rare, and many investigators consider CO intoxication to represent cerebral hypoxia aggravated by relative ischemia, as the lesions are similar to those induced by other forms of hypoxia and/or ischemia. It was shown 80 years ago that CO damages the blood–brain barrier, particularly in the cerebral white matter, where the venous drainage pattern predisposes to focal edema similar to that seen in multiple sclerosis (Putnam et al. 1931). This may lead to hypoxia and set up the cycle of hypoxia–edema–hypoxia. Delayed neurological deterioration can occur following anoxia from other causes and can explain similar deterioration after CO poisoning, in the absence of elevated levels of COHb.

The mechanism of delayed neurological toxicity is based on several reactions triggered by increased calcium concentrations in the cell, which persist long enough to produce alterations in cell function and delayed neurological damage. White matter demyelination is believed to be responsible for delayed neuropsychiatric syndrome.

Harmful effects of an acute nonlethal CO exposure do not cease with a decrease in COHb concentration. The decreased cytochrome oxidase activity may later on be mediated by a loss of mitochondria because of lipid peroxidation, rather than by specific inhibitory effects of CO. A similar mechanism would explain the acid proteinase activity in the glial cell fraction within 24 h of reoxygenation.

CO may alter the oxidative metabolism of the brain independently of a COHb-related decrease in oxygen delivery. Binding of CO to cytochrome oxidase in the brain cortex is a possible explanation of a nonhypoxic mechanism of CO toxicity. Mitochondria may contribute to CO-mediated neuronal damage during reoxygenation after severe CO intoxication. CO-mediated brain injury is a type of post-ischemic reperfusion phenomenon and xanthine-oxidase-derived reactive oxygen species may be responsible for lipid peroxidation. These explanations are offered for a number of poorly understood clinical observations regarding CO poisoning, particularly the neuropsychological effects at concentrations below 5%. Delayed amnesia induced by CO exposure in experimental animals may result from delayed neuronal death in the hippocampus and dysfunction of the acetylcholinergic neurons in the frontal cortex, the striatum, and/or the hippocampus. In animal studies it has been shown that N-methyl-D-aspartate (NMDA) receptor/ion channel complex is involved in the mechanism of CO-induced neurodegeneration, and that glycine binding site antagonists and NMDA-antagonists may have neuroprotective properties. In spite of various explanations that have been offered, nothing is known with certainty about the pathomechanism of CO poisoning. Recognition of CO a putative neural messenger that interacts with the enzyme guanylyl cyclase may provide an important clue to the pathomechanism of CO toxicity. Endogenously formed CO arises from the enzymatic degradation of heme oxygenase and acts as a neuromodulator. In addition to its physiological role, CO that arises subsequent to the appearance of heme oxygenase-1 may underlie various pathological states.

Relative cerebral hyperperfusion has been observed during CO-hypoxia and is considered to be due to a fall in the P50 (PO$_2$ at 50% saturation of non-CO bound sites on hemoglobin) rather than a direct tissue effect of CO. Cerebral blood flow has been shown to increase in anesthetized animals exposed to 1% CO, despite a fall of mean arterial blood pressure. In the presence of tissue hypoxia with undiminished plasma PO$_2$, the brain vasculature allows greater flow of blood while the microvasculature adjusts to reduce the diffusion distance for O$_2$.

Clinical Features of CO Poisoning

Signs and symptoms of CO poisoning are nonspecific and involve most of the body systems. They vary according to the COHb levels, as presented in Table 13.6. The clinical signs and symptoms depend on both the dose of CO and the duration of exposure. COHb levels do not necessarily correlate with the severity of clinical effects.

Neuropsychological Sequelae of CO Poisoning

The neurological sequelae of CO poisoning as reported in the literature are summarized in Table 13.7. There is some disparity in the results of the studies summarized here. However, psychological impairment can be detected at COHb levels between 2.5 and 5% by appropriate tests.

Higher levels of COHb during acute exposure may lead to impairment of consciousness, coma, and convulsions. Most of the neurological manifestations of CO poisoning

Table 13.6 Degree of severity of CO poisoning, COHb levels, and clinical features

Severity	COHb level	Clinical
Occult	>5%	No apparent symptoms
		Psychological deficits on testing
	5–10%	Decreased exercise tolerance in patients with chronic obstructive pulmonary disease
		Decreased threshold for angina and claudication in patients with atherosclerosis. Increased threshold for visual stimuli
Mild	10–20%	Dyspnea on vigorous exertion headaches, dizziness
		Impairment of higher cerebral function
		Decreased visual acuity
Moderate	20–30%	Severe headache, irritability, impaired judgment
		Visual disturbances, nausea, dizziness, increased respiratory rate
		Cardiac disturbances, muscle weakness
	30–40%	Vomiting, reduced awareness
		Fainting on exertion
		Mental confusion
Severe	40–50%	Collapse
		Convulsions
		Paralysis
	50–60%	Coma, frequently fatal within a few minutes
	Over	Immediately fatal

Table 13.7 Neuropsychological sequelae of CO poisoning

Authors and year	Subjects	COHb level or CO/ppm	Effects
Lilienthal and Fugitt (1946)	Humans	5–10 % COHb	Impairment in the FFT test
Trouton and Eysenck (1961)	Humans	5–10 % COHb	Impairment of the precision of control
			Multiple limb incoordination
Schulte (1963)	Humans	2–5 % COHb	Decrease in cognition and psychomotor ability
			Increase in the number of errors and the completion time in arithmetic tests, t-crossing test, and visual discrimination tests
Beard and Wertheim (1967)	Humans	90 min at 50 ppm shorter time at 250 ppm (=COHb of 4–5 %)	Impaired ability to discriminate short
	Rats	100 ppm for 11 min	Disruption of ability to judge time (assessed by differential reinforcement at a low rate of response)
Mikulka et al. (1973)	Humans	125–250 ppm briefly (COHb 6.6 %)	No effect on time estimation
			No disruption of tracking
Gliner et al. (1983)	Humans	100 ppm for 2.5 h controls (room air)	Decreased arousal and interest with fatigue resulting in decrease in performance
Schrot et al. (1984)	Rats	500 ppm—90 min (40 % COHb)	Disruption of the rate at which the rats acquired a chain of response
		850 ppm—90 min (50 % COHb)	
		1200 ppm—90 min (60 % COHb)	
Schaad et al. (1983)	Humans	COHb 20 %	No impairment on a tracking simulator device
Yastrebov et al. (1987)	Humans	900 ± 20 mg/m^3 for 10 min (COHb of 10 to +0.5 %)	Impairment in a two-dimensional compensatory tracking task combined with mental arithmetic. Symptoms of mild CO intoxication at COHb levels of 10 %

are late sequelae (listed in Table 13.8); these late sequelae are also referred to as "secondary syndromes." The complications may develop a few days to 3 weeks after exposure to CO, and as late as 2 years after apparently complete recovery from acute CO poisoning. Neuropsychiatric symptoms are prominent in the late sequelae. The incidence of secondary syndromes varies from 10 to 40 %. Patients poisoned by CO and treated by oxygen still developed late sequelae but such sequelae are rare in patients treated by HBO therapy.

In the largest reported series of 2360 victims of CO poisoning, delayed neurological sequelae were diagnosed in 11.8 % of those admitted to hospital and 2.75 % of the total group (Choi 1983). The lucid interval before appearance of neurological symptoms was 2–40 days (mean, 22.4 days). The most frequent symptoms were mental deterioration, urinary incontinence, gait disturbance, and mutism. The most frequent signs were masked face, glabellar sign, grasp reflex, increased muscle tone, short-step gait, and retropulsion. Most of these signs indicate parkinsonism. There were no important contributing factors except anoxia and age. Previous associated disease did not hasten the development of sequelae. Of the 36 patients followed for 2 years, 75 % recovered within 1 year.

Table 13.8 Delayed neuropsychological sequelae of CO poisoning

- Akinetic mutism
- Apallic syndrome
- Apraxia, ideomotor as well as constructional
- Ataxia
- Convulsive disorders
- Cortical blindness
- Deafness (neural)
- Delirium
- Dementia
- Depression
- Diminished IQ
- Dysgraphia
- Gilles de la Tourette syndrome
- Headaches
- Memory disturbances
- Movement disorders, parkinsonism, choreoathetosis
- Optic neuritis
- Peripheral neuropathy
- Personality change
- Psychoses
- Symptoms resembling those of multiple sclerosis
- Temporospatial disorientation
- Urinary incontinence
- Visual agnosia

Clinical Diagnosis of CO Poisoning

Few symptoms of CO poisoning occur at COHb concentrations of <10%. The presence of symptoms and history of exposure to CO and the circumstances in which the patient is found should lead to strong suspicion of CO poisoning. Therapy may be started before the laboratory investigations are completed.

Pitfalls in the Clinical Diagnosis of CO Poisoning

The following points should be taken into consideration in making a diagnosis of CO poisoning:

1. Clinical signs and symptoms of CO poisoning do not always correspond to COHb levels.
2. The cherry red color of the skin and the lips, usually considered to be a classical sign, is not present when the COHb levels are below 40% and there is cyanosis caused by respiratory depression. In practice this sign is rarely seen.
3. Some of the symptoms are aggravated by preexisting disease, such as intermittent claudication.
4. Tachypnea is frequently absent, because the carotid body is presumably responsive to the oxygen partial pressures rather than the oxygen content.
5. Examples of frequent misdiagnosis of CO poisoning are psychiatric illness, migraine headaches, stroke, acute alcohol intoxication or delirium tremens, heart disease, and food poisoning.
6. CO poisoning in infants is a frequently missed diagnosis. When unexplained neurological symptoms occur in an infant who has been a passenger in a car, COHb determinations should be made and CO poisoning should be considered in the differential diagnosis.
7. A bit of detective work may be required to locate the source of carbon monoxide poisoning. A simple tool based on the CH^2OPD^2 mnemonic (Community, Home, Hobbies, Occupation, Personal habits, Diet and Drugs) is helpful in obtaining an environmental exposure history.

Occult CO Poisoning

This is a syndrome of headache, fatigue, dizziness, paresthesias, chest pains, palpitation, and visual disturbances associated with chronic CO exposure. Headache and dizziness are early symptoms of CO poisoning and occur at COHb concentrations of 10% or more. Among patients taken to an emergency department during the winter heating season with complaints of headache or dizziness, 3–5% have COHb levels in excess of 10%. They are usually unaware of exposure to toxic levels of CO in their home prior to the visit to the emergency department. In patients who present with ill-defined symptoms and no history of CO exposure, CO poisoning must be considered when two or more patients are similarly or simultaneously sick.

Laboratory Diagnosis of CO Poisoning

Various laboratory procedures that may be used in the diagnosis of CO poisoning are as follows:

1. Determination of CO in the blood
   (a) Direct measurement of the COHb levels
   (b) Measurement of CO released from the blood
   (c) Measurement of CO content of the exhaled air
2. Arterial blood gases and lactic acid levels
3. Screening tests for drug intoxication and alcohol intoxication
4. Biochemistry
   (a) Enzymes: creatine kinase, lactate dehydrogenase, SGOT, SGPT
   (b) Serum glucose
5. Complete blood count
6. Electroencephalogram
7. Electrocardiogram
8. Brain imaging: CT scan, MRI, SPECT/PET
9. Magnetic resonance spectroscopy
10. Neuropsychological testing

COHb Measurement. This is the most commonly used investigation. Measurement is done spectrophotometrically, offering an accurate and rapid determination of the patient's COHb levels. An instrument like the CIBA Corning 2500-CO oximeter determines various selected wavelengths from 520 to 640 nm, and the following hemoglobin derivatives are measured: oxyhemoglobin (O_2Hb), deoxyhemoglobin (HHb), carboxyhemoglobin (COHb), and methemoglobin (MetHb).

Determination of CO Released from the Blood. Several methods are available for releasing CO from samples of blood. CO is then measured by gas chromatography. The amount of CO in the blood sample is calculated from the ratio of the CO content to the full CO capacity of the same sample.

CO Measurement in Exhaled Air. This can be measured by gas chromatography. A bag can be used to collect exhaled air and CO is determined by a flame ionization detector after catalytic hydration with methane. The values are given as parts per million (ppm) in the range of 0–500.

Clinical Significance of Monitoring Blood COHb. The following recommendations are based on various studies of monitoring of COHb in patients with acute CO poisoning:

1. Blood COHb greater than 10 % has diagnostic significance and, COHb > 30 % should be considered serious.
2. Clinical manifestations should be primary and COHb secondary when judging the degree of CO poisoning.
3. Treatment should be continued even when COHb levels have returned to normal, if the clinical symptoms are still present.
4. COHb sampling need not be continued when the patient has been away from the toxic environment for more than 8 h.
5. Monitoring of COHb is useful in making a differential diagnosis and in the event of death, a definitive diagnosis.

Pitfalls in the Diagnosis of CO Poisoning from COHb Level Determinations. COHb levels may be normal when first obtained and not reflect the true insult. This is likely to happen when:

- There is delay in obtaining samples following cessation of exposure to CO.
- Oxygen is administered before blood samples are withdrawn.
- COHb is calculated from oxygen partial pressures using a slide-rule nomogram.

Arterial pO_2 may be normal in the presence of CO if the patient is not dyspneic. The calculated oxyhemoglobin saturation may be grossly wrong in this case.

Changes in Blood Chemistry. Increased levels of lactate, pyruvate, and glucose are influenced by the duration of exposure to CO and are more pronounced after prolonged acute exposure than after a short exposure. Hyperglycemia may occur as a result of hormonal stress response. Blood lactate and COHb levels both correlate with the changes of consciousness in CO poisoning and are useful for defining indications for HBO treatment (Icme et al. 2014).

Electroencephalographic Changes. Various EEG abnormalities noticed in CO poisoning are diffuse abnormalities (continuous theta or delta activity) and low voltage activity accompanied by intervals of spiking or silence, as well as rhythmic bursts of slow waves. Topographic quantitative EEG methods may have promise in the study of acute and long-term effects of CO poisoning. Longitudinal and quantitative EEG recording after acute CO poisoning may show the following:

1. Elevated Absolute Power of all EEG frequencies with the most marked voltage increases occurring in the alpha-theta range.

2. Sharply defined regional increases in the absolute power of delta activity over the posterior temporal–parietal–occipital cortex bilaterally.
3. Increased relative power of the alpha wave that is most marked over the prefrontal cortex.
4. Decreased relative power of the alpha wave that is most marked over the prefrontal cortex.
5. Pronounced decreases in interhemispheric coherence for most frequency bands.

The multimodality evoked potentials have proved to be sensitive indicators in the evaluation of brain dysfunction and in the prognosis of acute CO poisoning and development of delayed encephalopathy. Pattern shift visual evoked potential (PSVEP) N75 and P100 latencies are not a sensitive screening tool for treatment decision making in a group of acutely CO poisoned patients.

Neuropsychological Testing. It has long been known that CO poisoning has a spectrum of effects on cognitive functioning. Neuropsychological impairments in CO-poisoned subjects include memory, intellectual, executive, and visuospatial defects. Various psychological tests have been designed for patients with CO poisoning. One neuropsychological screening battery for use in assessment of such patients consists of six tests: general orientation, digit span, trail making, digit symbols, aphasia, and block design (Messier and Myers 1991). These tests can be administered in an emergency by a nonpsychologist in 20 min. There is a strong correlation between abnormalities detected on psychometric testing and COHb levels. The former measures actual neurological disability and is a better index of severity of CO poisoning.

CO poisoning is significantly associated with impairment of context-aided memory, with the degree of pretreatment impairment predicting the number of HBO treatments judged to be necessary on the basis of clinical monitoring of the patient. In patients with poisoning of moderate severity, pretreatment performance in context-aided memory improved after the first HBO treatment. The memory measure used in this study appears to have considerable potential usefulness in the clinical assessment of the severity of CO poisoning in patients treated in an emergency setting.

Brain Imaging Studies

Various brain imaging studies have been found to be useful in assessing the brain involvement in CO poisoning. These are described in the following pages and a comparison of the value of various techniques is presented in Table 13.9.

CT Scan. The CT scan is the most widely used neuroimaging method for patients with CO poisoning. Common CT findings

Table 13.9 Comparative value of brain imaging studies in CO poisoning

	CT	MRI	SPECT/PET
Basal ganglia lesions	+	++	
White matter lesions	+	+++	
Both white and gray matter	+	++	+++
Cerebral edema	+	++	
Cerebral perfusion	+	+	+++
Predicting late sequelae	+	++	+++
Assessing response to HBO	+	++	+++

are symmetrical low-density abnormalities of the basal ganglia and diffuse low-density lesions of the white matter. The globus pallidus lucencies may be unilateral and white matter involvement may show marked asymmetry. Postcontrast CT offers an advantage when noncontrast CT is normal in CO poisoning. Acute transient hydrocephalus has been observed in acute CO poisoning but it may resolve in a few weeks. In the interval form of CO poisoning, low-density lesions bilaterally in the frontal regions, centrum semiovale, and pallidum have been correlated with demyelination of white matter of the corresponding parts at autopsy. An initial normal CT scan in a comatose patient does not rule out CO poisoning. Serial CT scanning showed no low-density lesions of the frontal lobes and basal ganglia until 3 days after exposure to CO.

Magnetic Resonance Imaging (MRI). Most of the knowledge of MRI findings in CO poisoning is based on case studies of patients in the subacute or chronic phase following exposure. MRI studies in the acute phase of CO poisoning show that, although the globus pallidus is the commonest site of abnormality in the brain, the effects are widespread.

In patients with CO poisoning, MRI can demonstrate bilateral edematous lesions in the globus pallidus and it is considered to be a more sensitive examination than serial CT in acute CO poisoning. Although the severity of white matter lesions correlates with the prognosis in acute CO poisoning, it does not always correspond to the neurological outcome in the subacute stage.

MRI has been used less often in cases of delayed encephalopathy after CO poisoning. The main finding in such cases is a reversible demyelinating process of the cerebral white matter. Lesions of the anterior thalami, which may be missed on CT scan, can be demonstrated by MRI. A spectrum of MRI changes has been seen even years after relatively mild CO poisoning. Patients with severe CO intoxication may develop persistent cerebral changes independently of their neuropsychiatric findings in the chronic stage, which may present with characteristic MRI findings. Diffusion tensor MRI is a promising technique to characterize and track delayed encephalopathy after acute carbon monoxide poisoning.

Positron Emission Tomography (PET). PET studies in acute CO poisoning show a severe decrease in rCBF, rOER, and rCMRO in the striatum and the thalamus, even in patients treated with HBO. These changes are temporary and the values return to normal in patients without clinical sequelae or only transient neurological disturbances. PET findings remain abnormal in patients with severe and permanent sequelae.

Single Photon Emission Computed Tomography (SPECT). This can provide imaging of cerebral perfusion. Diffuse hypoperfusion has been shown in both the gray and the white matter of the cerebral cortex in CO poisoning. SPECT is helpful in documenting the increase in cerebral perfusion along with clinical improvement as a result of HBO treatment. Cerebral vascular changes may be the possible cause of hypoperfusion in patients with CO poisoning and there is a good correlation between the clinical outcome and the findings of SPECT. SPECT can be used for predicting and evaluating the outcome of delayed neurological sequelae after CO poisoning. In comparison to traditional brain imaging techniques, 99 mTc-HMPAO brain imaging with fanbeam SPECT in combination with surface 3D display is a better tool for early detection of regional cerebral anomalies in acute CO poisoning. HMPAO-SPECT has been used in the management of patients with acute and delayed neurological sequelae of CO poisoning and found to be helpful in identifying potentially recoverable brain tissue and the response to HBO (see Chap. 20). The case history and SPECT scans of one of the patients are reproduced in Chap. 20.

Magnetic Resonance Spectroscopy (MRS). MRS is a noninvasive method that provides information about brain metabolites such as *N*-acetyl aspartate, choline, and creatine. MRS can reflect the severity of delayed sequelae of CO poisoning precisely. Increase in choline in the frontal lobes indicates progressive demyelination. Appearance of lactate and decrease in *N*-acetyl aspartate reflect the point at which neuron injury becomes irreversible. These findings have been correlated with those of MRI and SPECT. It may be a useful method to determine neuron viability and prognosis in CO poisoning. The combination of proton MRS and diffusion tensor imaging is useful for monitoring the changes in brain damage and the clinical symptoms of patients with delayed encephalopathy after CO poisoning and response to HBO treatment.

General Management of CO Poisoning

General guidelines for the management of CO poisoning are presented in Table 13.10. Once the patient is removed from CO environments, CO slowly dissociates from the Hb and is eliminated. The half-life of the COHb is presented in Table 13.11.

Table 13.10 Guidelines for the management of CO poisoning

1. Remove patient from the site of exposure
2. Immediately administer oxygen, if possible after taking a blood sample for COHb
3. Endotracheal intubation in comatose patients to facilitate ventilation
4. Removal of patient to HBO facility when indicated
5. General supportive treatment: for cerebral edema, acid–base imbalance, etc.
6. Keep patient calm and avoid physical exertion by the patient

Table 13.11 Half-life of COHb

	Pressure	Time
Air	1 ATA	5 h 20 min
100 % oxygen	1 ATA	1 h 20 min
100 % oxygen	3 ATA	23 min

At atmospheric pressure in fresh air, the circulating half-life of CO is 5 h 20 min. This time decreases to 23 min with HBO at 3 ATA. These half-lives are not constant, as they depend on a number of variable factors. They are particularly inaccurate when COHb levels are high. The objectives of treatment in CO poisoning are as follows:

- To hasten elimination of CO
- To counteract hypoxia
- To counteract direct tissue toxicity.

A flow chart as a guide for handling patients with CO poisoning is shown in Fig. 13.3. HBO therapy is the most important factor in treatment, but the following adjunctive measures should be considered:

- Treatment of cerebral edema. HBO therapy itself is effective against cerebral edema, but the use of steroids and mannitol may be helpful.
- Cellular protection. $Mg2+$ can be used; the usual dose is 20–30 mmol/day.
- Fluid and electrolyte balance should be carefully maintained and overhydration, which may aggravate cerebral edema and pulmonary complications, should be avoided. Acidosis should not be corrected pharmacologically, as slight acidosis aids in the delivery of oxygen to the tissues by shifting the oxygen dissociation curve to the right. HBO usually limits the metabolic acidosis associated with CO poisoning.
- Management of cardiac arrhythmias. Cardiac arrhythmias are a common complication of CO poisoning. They may subside with reversal of tissue hypoxia but may require pharmacological management.
- Preclinical studies show that the novel synergism of hydroxocobalamin (B12) with ascorbic acid has the potential to extract CO through conversion to CO_2, independently of high-flow or high-pressure O_2 (Roderique et al. 2015). This results in a clinically significant off-gassing of CO_2 at levels five to eight times greater than those of controls, a clinically significant reduction in COHgb half-life, and evidence of increased brain oxygenation. Reduced B12 has major potential as an injectable antidote for CO toxicity.

Rationale for Oxygen Therapy (NBO or HBO) for CO Poisoning

Hyperoxygenation enhances oxygen transfer into the anoxic tissues. At normal concentrations of tissue oxygen it should physically dilute the CO and possibly halt the movement of CO from Hb to Mb and cytochrome enzymes. Hyperoxygenation may be achieved by breathing 100 % oxygen either at atmospheric pressure (normobaric) or under hyperbaric conditions. HBO is more effective than NBO. HBO accomplishes the following therapeutic goals in CO poisoning:

- Immediate saturation of plasma with enough oxygen to sustain life and to counteract tissue hypoxia in spite of high levels of COHb.
- It causes a rapid reduction of CO in the blood by mass action of O_2. In the equation "$HbO2 + CO = HbCO + O_2$," an increase in either oxygen or CO results in a comparable increase in the corresponding compound with hemoglobin.
- It assists in driving CO away from cytochrome oxidase and in restoration of function. The increase in oxygen tension in plasma and not simply an increase in dissolved oxygen is responsible for the efficacy of HBO.
- HBO reduces cerebral edema.
- Brain lipid peroxidation caused by CO is prevented by 100 % oxygen at 3 ATA.
- HBO prevents immune-mediated delayed neurologic dysfunction following exposure.

Although breathing NBO hastens the removal of COHb, HBO hastens COHb elimination and favorably modulates inflammatory processes initiated by CO poisoning, an effect not observed with breathing NBO (Weaver 2014). HBO inhibits leukocyte adhesion to injured microvasculature, and reduces brain inflammation caused by the CO-induced adduct formation of myelin basic protein. Based upon three supportive randomized clinical trials in humans and considerable evidence from animal studies, HBO should be considered for all cases of acute symptomatic CO poisoning. HBO is indicated for CO poisoning complicated by concomitant cyanide poisoning, as happens often in smoke inhalation.

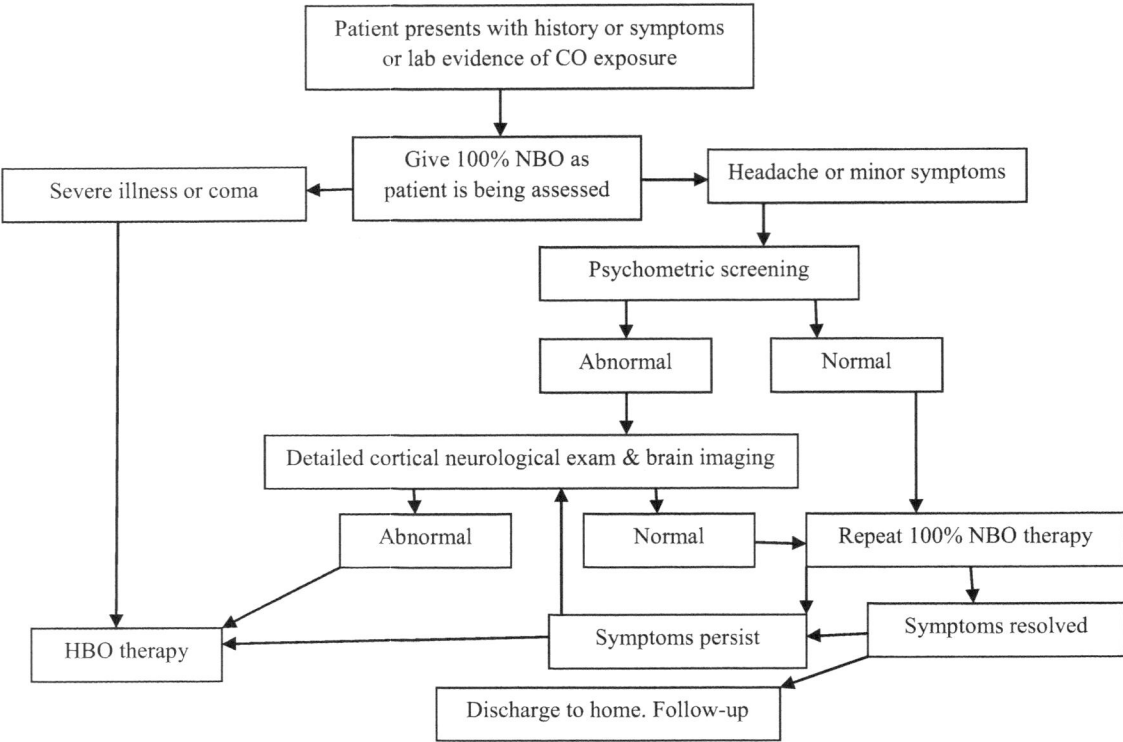

Fig. 13.3 Flow chart to guide treatment of carbon monoxide poisoning

HBO improves mitochondrial function. Mitochondrial complex IV (mtCIV) inhibition, along with COHb-induced hypoxia, may influence acute clinical symptoms and outcome in acute CO poisoning. To evaluate mitochondrial aspect of treatment efficacy, a study has correlated intoxication severity and symptoms with mitochondrial function and oxidative stress (lipid peroxidation) in 60 poisoned patients and determined recovery depending on either NBO or HBO therapy in a 3-month follow-up (Garrabou et al. 2011). Results show that mtCIV is a good biomarker of recovery from acute CO poisoning, efficacy of treatment, as well as development of delayed neurological sequelae, and favor HBO therapy as the treatment of choice.

Experimental Evidence

The results of some experimental studies of the use of HBO in CO poisoning are presented in Table 13.12.

Clinical Use of HBO in CO Poisoning

Guidelines for the use of HBO versus NBO are given in Table 13.13. Some open clinical studies of CO poisoning treated by HBO are presented in Table 13.14. HBO, if available, should be used at COHb levels of 25 % or above, but the clinical picture of the patient with a history of CO exposure is the deciding factor for the initiation of HBO therapy, and the COHb levels should be a secondary consideration. Because of the cost and limited availability of hyperbaric chambers, a decision regarding transfer of the patient to a hyperbaric facility is not always easy, particularly when the patient is critically ill. If possible, the patient should be transferred to a multiplace chamber with facilities for critical care and suitably qualified personnel. During transport to such a facility, the patient should receive 100 % oxygen, using a mask, and care should be taken that the patient does not rebreathe the exhaled air. The argument that NBO is always satisfactory for severe CO poisoning can no longer be sustained. A pO_2 of 1800 mmHg achieved by HBO is definitely more effective than the maximal pO_2 of 760 mmHg attainable by normobaric 100 % oxygen. In practice, it is much lower than this, since few oxygen masks exist that are suitable for administering oxygen to achieve a pO_2 above 600 mmHg.

The Undersea and Hyperbaric Medical Society of USA recommends HBO therapy for patients suffering from serious CO poisoning as manifested by transient or prolonged unconsciousness, abnormal neurologic signs, cardiovascular dysfunction, or severe acidosis or patients who are 36 years

Table 13.12 Experimental studies on the effect of HBO on carbon monoxide poisoning

Authors and year	Experimental subjects	Mode of oxygen therapy	Results
End and Long (1942)	Dogs and guinea pigs	HBO 3 ATA, 100% oxygen	HBO more effective than normobaric oxygen in eliminating CO from the body
Pace et al. (1950)	Human volunteers	HBO 2 ATA	Rate of diminution of CO accelerated
Ogawa et al. (1974)	Dogs	HBO	Hemoconcentration (20% decrease of blood volume reversed by HBO)
Koyama (1976)	Dogs	Half of the animals treated by conventional methods and the other half by HBO 2 ATA	COHb determination and biochemical studies showed that HBO was more effective than the conventional methods
Sasaki (1975)	Dogs	HBO	Acceleration of the half-clearance time of COHb
			Proposed procedure for HBO therapy based on it:
			1. For severe CO poisoning, HBO at 2.8 ATA for 20 min followed by 1.9 ATA for 57 min
			2. For moderate CO poisoning, 2.8 ATA oxygen for 20 min followed by 1.9 ATA for 46 min
			3. For light CO poisoning, 2.8 ATA oxygen for 20 min followed by 1.9 ATA for 30 min
Jiang and Tyssebotn (1997)	Rats with occluded left carotid artery	NBO in one group versus HBO in the other, normoxic animals as controls	1. Compared to the normoxic treatments, the HBO, but not the NBO, significantly reduced the mortality and the neurologic morbidity
			2. HBO was also significantly better than NBO in increasing surviving time and survival rate
			3. The results support the value of HBO in improving short-term outcome of acute CO poisoning in this rat model

Table 13.13 Hyperbaric oxygen (HBO) versus normobaric oxygen

Hyperbaric facilities available	COHb > 25%	HBO
	COHb < 25%	HBO if symptoms, NBO if none
No hyperbaric facilities	COHb > 40% no symptoms	NBO
	COHb < 40% with symptoms	Referral to HBO center

of age or older, were exposed for 24 h or more (including intermittent exposures), or have a carboxyhemoglobin level of 25% or more. Results of the latest study on this topic show that the indications of HBO therapy for CO poisoning are still not universally recognized (Mutluoglu et al. 2016). HBO therapy protocols used at European hyperbaric centers vary significantly, suggesting a need for more education regarding the published guidelines.

Clinical Trials of HBO in CO Poisoning

Clinical trials of HBO in CO poisoning are listed in Table 13.15. These are discussed in more detail later.

A trial of normobaric and hyperbaric oxygen for acute CO intoxication carried out in 629 adults who had been poisoned at home in the 13 h preceding admission to hospital (Raphael et al. 1989). It was a randomized study with grouping based on whether or not there was initial loss of consciousness. In those without any loss of consciousness HBO was compared with normobaric oxygen (NBO) treatments, with no difference being noticed in the recovery rate. Those who had an episode of loss of consciousness were treated either by a single session of 2 h of HBO at 2 ATA followed by 4 h of NBO, or by 4 h of NBO with two sessions of HBO 6–12 h apart. Two sessions of HBO were shown to have no advantage over a single session. The authors concluded that those who do not sustain initial loss of consciousness should be

Table 13.14 Open clinical studies of HBO in CO poisoning

Authors and year	No. of patients	Pressure	Results
Smith et al. (1962)	22	2 ATA	All recovered
Sluitjer (1963)	40	3 ATA	Group I: conscious or drowsy. 21 patients. Excellent results
			Group II: comatose with neurological abnormalities. 10 patients. Two died, 7 recovered fully and one had severe neurological sequelae
			Group III: Attempted suicide with combination of CO and barbiturates. Nine patients. Cardiorespiratory depression mainly with little localizing neurological signs. All recovered completely
Goulon et al. (1969)	302	2 ATA	Mortality when treatment started before 6 h was 13.5%, and when after 6 h 30.1%
Heyndrickx et al. (1970)	11	3 ATA	Clinical improvement more than in another 11 patients treated by NBO
Kienlen et al. (1974)	370	2–3 ATA	93.7% of the patients recovered
Adamiec et al. (1975)	44	2.5 ATA	80% showed good recovery
Yun and Cho (1983)	2242	?	98.2 recovered
Mathieu et al. (1985)	203	?	Mortality 1.7%; incidence of secondary syndromes, 4%: rest recovered
Norkool and Kirkpatrick (1985)	115	?	88% recovered fully
Colignon and Lamy (1986)	111	83 ATA	0.5% died in emergency room; 3.3% admitted to ICU; rest 96.2% had minor symptoms and recovered completely
Tirpitz and Bakyara (1988)	276	2–2.5 ATA	4 deaths. Rest recovered. Many treated and released to home the same day
Sloan et al. (1989)	297	3 ATA	Extremely ill patients with mortality of 6%. Rest recovered
Abramovich et al. (1997)	24	2.8 ATA	20 (84%) recovered consciousness during one treatment, 3 required a second treatment, and one who arrived in deep coma died

treated by NBO regardless of the COHb levels. The authors did not deny the usefulness of HBO in those with loss of consciousness, but stated that two sessions of HBO had no advantage over a single session. The methodology in the study is questionable.

A randomized study compared the effects of NBO versus HBO therapy in patients with moderate CO poisoning (Ducassé et al. 1995). In conscious patients without neurological impairment, one HBO treatment at 2.5 ATA for 0.5 h, within the first 2 h after admission, had the following advantages:

- Faster recuperation from symptoms such as headache and nausea.
- Quicker elimination of CO during the first 2 h. After 12 h, there was no difference in blood COHb levels between the two groups.
- Fewer EEG abnormalities after 3 weeks in the group treated with HBO.
- Recovery of the cerebral vasomotor response in the group treated with HBO, as shown using the acetazolamide test.

In a longitudinal study of 100 consecutive patients, the frequency of neuropsychiatric sequelae among patients who received oxygen at atmospheric pressure was 63%, among those who received one HBO treatment it was 46%, and in those who received two or more HBO treatments it was 13% (Gorman et al. 1992). The frequency of sequelae was greater if HBO treatment was delayed. In a prospective randomized clinical study, delayed neuropsychiatric sequelae were found to be less frequent with HBO treatment as compared with normobaric oxygen administration (Thom 1992). These authors recommend that HBO should be used in the initial treatment of all patients with CO poisoning, regardless of the severity of their initial clinical manifestations. It is difficult to compare the results of different reported studies, because the patient conditions differed widely and the HBO technique used also varied. The overall results of HBO therapy, however, were favorable. Some patients in critically ill condition died from other complications, and in some other cases the HBO therapy was instituted too late to be lifesaving.

Table 13.15 Clinical trials of HBO in CO poisoning

Authors and year	Study design	HBO pressure	Results
Annane et al. 2011	Randomized, not blinded 2 trials	Trial 1: 1 session HBO 2 ATA versus NBO if transient loss of consciousness	Trial 1: HBO was nonsuperior to NBO
		Trial 2: 2 sessions HBO versus 1 session HBO if initial coma	Trial 2: patients with 2 HBO sessions had worse outcomes than those with 1 HBO session
Weaver et al. (2002)	Double-blind, randomized trial to study the effect of HBO on cognitive sequelae of acute CO poisoning	HBO (2–3 ATA)	3 HBO treatments within a 24-h period reduced the risk of cognitive sequelae 6 weeks and 12 months after
	Control with normobaric oxygen + air		
Scheinkestel et al. (1999)	Randomized controlled double-blind trial and sham treatments in a multiplace hyperbaric chamber. Neuropsychological assessments	HBO (2.8 ATA/1 h) or 100 % oxygen	Both groups received high doses of oxygen but HBO therapy did not benefit
Thom et al. (1995)	Prospective, randomized study in patients with mild to moderate CO poisoning who presented within 6 h. Incidence of delayed neurological sequelae (DNS) compared between groups treated with oxygen or HBO	Normobaric 100 % oxygen or HBO (2.8 ATA for 30 min + 2 ATA for 90 min)	HBO treatment decreased the incidence of DNS after CO poisoning
Ducassé et al. (1995)	Randomized study in acute CO poisoning: normobaric oxygen (NBO) versus hyperbaric oxygen	2 h treatment with normobaric oxygen or HBO (2.5 ATA)	Patients treated with HBO had a significant clinical improvement compared with patients treated with NBO
Raphael et al. (1989)	Randomization of patients with acute CO intoxication to normobaric or hyperbaric oxygen. Grouping based on whether or not there was initial loss of consciousness	Single session of HBO (2 ATA/2 h) followed by 4 h of NBO, or by 4 h of NBO with 2 sessions of HBO, 6–12 h apart	Better recovery with HBO treatment in those with initial loss of consciousness. There was no advantage of 2 sessions of HBO over a single session

The treatments may be carried out in a monoplace or a multiplace hyperbaric chamber. A large chamber with intensive care facilities is preferable in case of a critically ill patient. Various regimens have been used for the treatment of CO poisoning. The pressures used vary between 2 and 3 ATA. The most commonly used protocol is an initial 45 min of 100 % oxygen at 3 ATA followed by further treatment at 2 ATA for 2 h or until the COHb is less than 10 %. HBO is the treatment of choice in patients who lost consciousness during toxic exposure, who are comatose on admission to hospital and who have persisting neurological abnormalities (Wattel et al. 1996). Complications of HBO in comatose patients include rupture of the eardrum in about 10 % of the patients. Seizures may occur in patients with brain injury who are subjected to high HBO pressures. In a series of 300 consecutive CO-poisoned patients, there was one seizure at 2.45 ATA (0.3 %), nine seizures at 2.80 ATA (2 %), and six seizures at 3 ATA (Hampson et al. 1996). This difference is statistically significant and should be considered when selecting the HBO treatment pressure for CO poisoning. Concern has been expressed that patients with severe CO poisoning, who are intubated and mechanically ventilated, may not achieve adequate hyperbaric oxygenation in a multiplace chamber. In a review of 85 such patients, pO_2 greater than 760 mmHg was documented in 95 % of the patients (Hampson 1998). Such patients should not be excluded from HBO treatment for fear that adequate oxygenation cannot be achieved.

North American HBO facilities were surveyed to assess selection criteria applied for treatment of acute CO poisoning (Hampson et al. 1995). Responses were received from 85 % of the 208 facilities in the United States and Canada which treated a total of 2636 patients in 1992. A majority of facilities treat CO-exposed patients in coma (98 %), transient loss of consciousness (77 %), focal neurologic deficits (94 %), or abnormal psychometric testing (91 %), regardless of carboxyhemoglobin (COHb) level. Although 92 % would use HBO for a patient presenting with headache, nausea, and a COHb value of 40 %, only 62 % of facilities utilized a specified minimum COHb level as the sole criterion for HBO therapy of an asymptomatic patient. It was concluded that when COHb is used as an independent criterion to determine HBO treatment, the level utilized varies widely between institutions. The limitations of some clinical trials were lack of long-term follow-up. Most of these studies comparing HBO with NBO had significant methodological limitations that make it difficult to draw any conclusions about the efficacy of HBO.

As of April 2016, only two clinical trials of use of HBO in CO poisoning that were initiated in 2007 were in progress. The first of these is investigating important clinical outcomes of patients with acute CO poisoning randomized to receive either one or three HBO treatments and is expected to be completed by 2019 (ClinicalTrials.gov Identifier: NCT00465855). HBO will be given 3 ATA for 25 min breathing oxygen, 5 min air breathing, 25 min oxygen breathing, 5 min air breathing, pressure reduced to 2 ATA for 30 min breathing oxygen, 5 min air breathing, and 30 min oxygen breathing. For the second and third HBO sessions, the subject will breathe 100 % oxygen delivered at 2 ATA for 90 min with two 5-min air breathing periods. The second clinical study is a retrospective review of the principal investigator's experience using SPECT brain imaging and HBO therapy in the diagnosis and treatment of nonacute phases of CO poisoning (ClinicalTrials.gov Identifier: NCT00596180). The purpose is to see if the SPECT brain imaging is consistent with the clinical condition and cognitive testing on the patients with neuropsychiatric sequelae. It is expected to be completed by end of 2016.

HBO for CO Intoxication Secondary to Methylene Chloride Poisoning

Methylene chloride (dichlormethane) is converted to CO by cytochrome P450 after it enters the human body. Occupational exposure to dichloromethane is frequent and can result in both acute and chronic toxicity, affecting mostly the central nervous system, directly or through its metabolite, CO. In 1 of the earliest series of 12 cases of methylene chloride poisoning from a single exposure, 9 required HBO treatment and made a good recovery (Youn et al. 1989). The authors observed that CO derived from methylene chloride has an effective half-life 2.5 times that of exogenously inhaled CO. In the case of methylene chloride poisoning, tissue levels of CO continue to rise after exposure, whereas in CO poisoning, the CO levels begin to fall after the exposure is terminated. The practical implication of this observation is that patients with methylene chloride poisoning should be treated adequately with HBO and observed for 12–24 h after exposure. Bilateral hypoacusis developing after accidental exposure to methylene chloride has been reported to improve following 25 days treatment with HBO (Bonfiglioli et al. 2014).

Treatment of CO Poisoning in Pregnancy

In the past, pregnancy was considered to be a relative contraindication for the use of HBO, because of the possible toxic effects of oxygen on the fetus. Dangers of hyperoxic exposure to the fetus have been demonstrated in animals.

However, these experimental exposures exceeded the time and pressures routinely used in clinical therapy. If 100 % oxygen given to pregnant women with CO intoxication, it should be prolonged to five times what the mother needs, because of the slow elimination of CO by the fetus. A 17-year-old pregnant woman with CO intoxication (COHb 47.2 %) at 37 weeks of gestation was treated by using HBO at 2.4 ATA for a 90-min treatment resulting in recovery and produced a healthy baby at full-term normal delivery (Van Hoesen et al. 1989). If the mother had been left untreated, considerable morbidity would have been anticipated for the mother as well as for the fetus. HBO treatment for acute CO poisoning in pregnant women is usually well tolerated without any hazards to the fetus or the mother. Results of the first prospective, multicenter study of acute CO poisoning in pregnancy showed that severe maternal CO toxicity was associated with significantly more adverse fetal cases when compared to mild maternal toxicity (Koren et al. 1991). Because fetal accumulation of CO is higher and its elimination slower than that in the maternal circulation, HBO decreases fetal hypoxia and improves outcome. Based on the available clinical evidence, the following recommendations are made for the treatment of CO poisoning during pregnancy:

- Administer HBO therapy if the maternal COHb level is above 20 % at any time during the exposure.
- Administer HBO therapy if the patient has suffered or demonstrated any neurological signs, regardless of the COHb level.
- Administer HBO therapy if signs of fetal distress are present, that is, fetal tachycardia, decreased beat-to-beat variability on the fetal monitor, or late decelerations, consistent with the COHb levels and exposure history.
- If the patient continues to demonstrate neurological signs or signs of fetal distress 12 h after initial treatment, additional HBO treatments may be indicated.
- Treatment requires HBO sessions of a longer duration for fetal CO elimination than in the nonpregnant patients (Friedman et al. 2015).

It is generally agreed that oxygen therapy should be offered in all cases of CO poisoning, especially if there are maternal symptoms during exposure (Bothuyne-Queste et al. 2014). In addition, a fetal echography directed on the cephalic pole and even a fetal MRI should also be done 3 weeks after exposure. A prospective single-center cohort study spanning 25 years (1983–2008) included all pregnant women living in the Nord-Pas-de-Calais region of France who received HBO for CO poisoning and who gave birth to a living child (Wattel et al. 2013). There were no significant psychomotor or height/weight sequelae in those exposed to HBO treatment. Therefore, no specific follow-up of the children is necessary if their neonatal status is normal.

Treatment of Smoke Inhalation

Smoke inhalation involves multiple toxicities and pulmonary insufficiency, as well as thermal and chemical injury. CO intoxication is the most immediate life-threatening disorder in such cases. As a practice guideline, the following patient groups in smoke inhalation injury should be directed by rescue personnel to an emergency service with a hyperbaric facility:

- Those who are unconscious
- Those who are responsive but combative
- Those not responding to verbal instructions or painful stimuli.

If the patient meets these criteria, 100 % oxygen is administered initially during transport to a hyperbaric emergency medical center. If the COHb is over 20 % and the surface burns are covered less than 20 % of the patient's body, the patient should be treated initially with HBO and then transferred to a burn center, unless the burn service is located in the hyperbaric facility itself. HBO is given at 2.8 ATA for 46 min using 100 % oxygen. Patients with surface burns more extensive than 10 % should be treated initially at a burn center.

Experimental pulmonary edema caused by smoke inhalation is lessened by HBO. This may be the explanation of benefit of HBO on respiratory insufficiency associated with smoke inhalation and CO poisoning. Administration of HBO 2.8 ATA for 45 min inhibits adhesion of circulating neutrophils subsequent to smoke inhalation in rats whether used in a prophylactic manner before smoke inhalation, or as treatment immediately after the smoke insult. However, the beneficial effect appears related to inhibition of neutrophil adhesion to the vasculature rather than prevention of CO poisoning.

Prevention and Treatment of Late Sequelae of CO Poisoning

Several reports indicate that the incidence of secondary syndromes is reduced by adequate treatment with HBO in the acute stage of CO poisoning. Empirical overtreatment has been used in the belief that it would prevent late sequelae. The half-life of CO bound with cytochrome a3 oxidase, which is the determining factor for late sequelae, is not known. Further research is required to evaluate the CO bound to cytochrome a3 oxidase, so that the necessary duration of HBO treatment can be determined more realistically. HBO has been used for the treatment of late sequelae of CO poisoning. Patients with severe CO poisoning who have abnormalities on brain imaging that persist after HBO treatment are more likely to develop neuropsychiatric sequelae. Cognitive deficits demonstrated at time of assessment have been successfully reversed by HBO, despite the delay between the exposure and treatment. Controlled clinical trials have shown that incidence of delayed neurologic sequelae (DNS) in a group of patients acutely poisoned with CO decreases with HBO but not NBO treatment. In patients with CO-induced akinetic mutism and cortical as well as subcortical lesions, improvement in rCBF correlated well with functional recovery after HBO treatment (Chen et al. 2016).

Controversies in the Use of HBO for CO Poisoning

Even those who recognize the value of HBO question its role in CO poisoning, because there are no definite correlations of clinical manifestations with COHb levels, and COHb levels are not a definite guide for therapy. There is a particularly poor correlation between carboxyhemoglobin levels and neurological presentation. Neurological effects are due to unmeasured tissue uptake of CO, which increases during hypoxia because of competition between CO and oxygen at the oxygen-binding sites on hemoproteins. The efficacy of HBO therapy cannot be ascribed to hastened dissociation of carboxyhemoglobin. Additional mechanisms of action of HBO found in studies in animals include:

- Improved mitochondrial oxidative metabolism
- Inhibition of lipid per oxidation
- Impairment of adherence of neutrophils to cerebral vasculature.

Randomized controlled trials have shown that HBO is the only effective therapy for acute CO poisoning if delayed neurologic sequelae are to be minimized. NBO should not be used between multiple HBO treatments, as this can contribute to oxygen toxicity.

Review of all the available evidence indicates that HBO has a definite place in the management of CO poisoning. COHb levels cannot be used as a guide for treatment as they do not correlate with the clinical severity of CO poisoning. The following approach is recommended for HBO treatment for CO poisoning:

- Patients with severe poisoning must receive HBO regardless of their COHb levels.
- Pregnant patients must be treated with HBO regardless of signs and symptoms.
- Administration of more than one course of HBO treatment to those who remain in coma remains controversial.

There is some controversy regarding the pressure of HBO. Use of pressures between 2.5 and 3 ATA seems appropriate for CO poisoning. Mg^{2+}, a physiological calcium antagonist, helps in the prevention of late sequelae of CO poisoning by blocking cellular calcium influx.

Cyanide Poisoning

Cyanide is one of the most rapidly acting and lethal poisons known. Cyanide exists as either a gas or as the liquid hydrogen cyanide (HCN), also known as prussic acid. It is one of the smallest organic molecules that can be detected: inhalation of as little as 100 mg of gas can cause instantaneous death. An oral dose of the sodium or potassium salt (lethal dose 300 mg) acts more slowly; symptoms may not appear for several minutes and death may not occur for 1 h. Cyanide poisoning is mostly suicidal, but exposure can occur in the electroplating industry, in laboratory procedures, and through smoke inhalation in fires. Propionitrile, a substituted aliphatic nitrile commonly used in manufacturing industry, is capable of generating cyanide. Cyanogenic glycosides are found in several plant species, including apricot kernels and bitter almonds. The iatrogenic source is sodium nitroprusside, which is used as a vasodilator and as a hypotensive agent. Cyanide is a metabolite of nitroprusside, and toxicity results from rapid infusion, prolonged use, or renal failure.

Pathophysiology

Cyanide combines with cytochrome-a3-oxidase and exhibits a great affinity for oxidized iron (Fe^{3+}). This complex inhibits the final step of oxidative phosphorylation and halts aerobic metabolism. The patient essentially suffocates from an inability to use oxygen.

Clinical Features of Cyanide Poisoning

Signs and symptoms of acute cyanide poisoning reflect cellular hypoxia and are often nonspecific. The central nervous system is the most sensitive target organ with initial stimulation followed by depression.

Laboratory Diagnosis

Blood cyanide levels are useful in confirming toxicity, but treatment has to be initiated before the results of this test are available. Changes in ECG and EEG are nonspecific.

Treatment

The basic treatment of cyanide poisoning is chemical (Cyanide Antidote Kit, Eli Lilly & Co). The object is to bind the cyanide in its harmless form as a stable cyanmethemo-globin by giving sodium nitrite. Cyanide is later liberated by dissociation of cyanmethemoglobin. To convert this to thiocyanate, a harmless substance, intravenous sodium thiosulfate is given. Theoretically, hydroxocobalamin is promising as antidote for cyanide poisoning because cobalt compounds have the ability to bind and detoxify cyanide. Limited data on human poisonings with cyanide salts suggest that hydroxocobalamin is an effective antidote; data from smoke inhalation are less clear-cut (Thompson and Marrs 2012). The rate of absorption may be greater with inhaled hydrogen cyanide and the recommended slow intravenous administration of hydroxocobalamin may severely limit its clinical effectiveness in these circumstances. Limitations of chemical treatment indicate the need for a supplemental approach and use of HBO has been explored for this indication. Acute cyanide poisoning in rats, combined administration of hydroxocobalamin and HBO has a beneficial and persistent effect on the disturbed cerebral metabolism due to cyanide intoxication (Hansen et al. 2013).

Rationale for Use of HBO in Cyanide Poisoning

Theoretically it appears unlikely that HBO would exert its effect in cyanide poisoning by competing with cyanide at a receptor site in cytochrome-a3-oxidase. Possible mechanisms for the positive effect of HBO are as follows:

- The equation "cytochrome oxidase + cyanide = cytochrome oxidase cyanide" is pushed to the left by high pO_2 levels.
- Increased detoxification of cyanide by elevated oxygen pressures.
- Sufficient cellular respiration may continue via cyanide insensitive pathways under hyperbaric conditions to counteract effects of hypoxia.

Animal experimental studies have shown HBO to be effective in cyanide poisoning. There are several anecdotal reports of patients with cyanide poisoning in whom HBO was useful for treatment.

Hydrogen Sulfide Poisoning

Hydrogen sulfide (H_2S) is a highly toxic, inflammable, colorless gas, readily recognized by its characteristic odor of "rotten eggs." The mechanism of toxicity is similar to that of cyanide and CO poisoning. Hydrogen sulfide is a mitochondrial toxin and inhibits cellular aerobic metabolism. Therapies for toxic exposures include removal from the contaminated environment, ventilation with 100 % oxygen, and nitrite therapy if administered immediately after exposure. The rationale for the use of HBO in H_2S poisoning is that nitrates aid the conversion of hemoglobin to methemoglobin. The latter, by binding free sulfide ions, spares intracellular cytochrome oxidase.

In rats poisoned with LD75 hydrogen sulfide, pure oxygen at 1 ATA was effective in preventing death, but oxygen at 3 ATA was more effective (Bitterman et al. 1986). The best therapy was the combination of oxygen at 3 ATA with sodium nitrite. The clinical usefulness of HBO in H2S poisoning is based on the relief of cerebral edema and protection of the vital organs from hypoxia. Several case reports have shown that HBO treatment is successful in treating H_2S poisoning. Five patients with severe H_2S poisoning were treated successfully with HBO in combination with the use of nitrates (Hsu et al. 1987). Delayed neurologic toxicity from H_2S was treated successfully in a patient by using HBO 3 ATA for 90 min during the initial treatment with significant improvement (Pontani et al. 1998). Daily treatments at 2.4 ATA were continued and neurological deficits resolved completely in 3 days. HBO therapy was used successfully in the management of H_2S toxicity in patients who had not responded to NBO (Belley et al. 2005).

Carbon Tetrachloride Poisoning

Carbon tetrachloride (CCl_4) poisoning is not an uncommon occurrence in clinical practice. In moderate cases, the clinical course is benign. When severe hepatorenal injury occurs, the prognosis is grave because of hepatic insufficiency.

Although ischemic anoxia can damage the sinusoidal capillaries, the popular theory of CCl_4-induced hepatic injury is based on free radicals. CCl_4 exerts its toxicity through its metabolites, including the free radicals CCl_3 and CCl_3OO. Oxygen strongly inhibits the hepatic cytochrome P-450-mediated formation of CCl_3 from CCl_4 and promotes the conversion of CCl_3 to CCl_3OO. Both of these free radicals can injure the hepatocyte by lipoperoxidation and by binding covalently to the cell structures. Under conditions of hypoxia most of the free radicals are CCl_3, whereas under hyperoxia most are CCl_3OO. A reduced glutathione (GSH)-dependent mechanism can protect against CCl_3OO but not against CCl_3, so there is an advantage in using HBO in CCl_4 poisoning. HBO at 2 ATA given 6 h after administration of CCl_4 to rats has been shown to improve the survival rate and inhibit the in vivo conversion of CCl_4 to its volatile metabolites $CHCl_3$ and CO_2. The predominant effect is on CO_2, which is quantitatively the more significant metabolite. Most of the animal experimental studies show that the mortality of the HBO-treated animals is lowered and there is less impairment of the liver function tests. Conclusions of controlled studies of the effects of HBO on rats poisoned with CCl_4 are as follows:

- HBO improves survival from CCl_4 poisoning.
- The response rate is time related. There is a better survival rate in animals treated within 1 h of poisoning compared with those treated after 4 h.
- The improved survival with HBO is the result of decreased hepatotoxicity.

Although the mechanism of the protective effect of HBO on the liver is not well understood, it has been used successfully in patients with CCl_4 poisoning. CCl_4 poisoning is rare these days as this toxic solvent is no longer used in the industry. However, when a case occurs there is no satisfactory conventional treatment. HBO has been shown to be useful, and free radical scavengers such as vitamin E seem to be effective only if given before or with HBO.

Methemoglobinemias

The reversible oxygenation and deoxygenation of Hb at physiological partial pressures of oxygen require that the heme iron of deoxyhemoglobin remain in the Fe^{2+} form. In methemoglobinemias iron is already oxidized to the Fe^{3+} form, rendering the molecule incapable of binding oxygen. When Hb is oxygenated during the process of respiration, an electron is transferred from the Fe^+ atom to the bound oxygen molecule. Thus, in oxyhemoglobin, the iron possesses some of the characteristics of the Fe^{3+} state, whereas the oxygen takes on the characteristic of the superoxide (O_2^-) anion, which is a free radical.

Methemoglobinemia results from exposure to oxidizing substances such as nitrates or nitrites. Many drugs and chemicals have toxic effects on the Hb molecule and produce methemoglobinemia, e.g., nitrobenzene and nitrites. The methemoglobinemia is usually asymptomatic. As methemoglobin levels increase, patients show evidence of cellular hypoxia in all tissues. Death usually occurs when methemoglobin fractions approach 70 % of total hemoglobin. The diagnosis depends upon the demonstration of methemoglobin and the causative agent.

Treatment

Methylene blue remains an effective treatment for methemoglobinemia, but HBO can be a useful adjunct. Comparison of antagonism to the lethal effects of sodium nitrite displayed by various combinations of methylene blue, oxygen, and HBO shows that HBO is the most effective agent, with or without methylene blue. Patients with drug-induced methemoglobinemia (methemoglobin levels 50–70 %), who are admitted in a comatose state, recover following treatment with HBO at 2.2 ATA as methemoglobin decreases at a rate of 5–8 % per hour of exposure to HBO. A patient, who was accidentally intoxicated with isobutyl nitrite by a threefold lethal dose, a blood exchange transfusion was performed under HBO and the patient recovered (Jansen et al. 2003). In a young male suffering from severe methemoglobinemia of 68 % after consumption of nitrites ('poppers') in association with considerable ethanol consumption, toluidine blue was administered as first-line antidotal therapy immediately followed by HBO therapy (Lindenmann et al. 2015). The result was enhanced reduction of methemoglobin, and rapid tissue reoxygenation by the oxygen dissolved in plasma, independent of the degree of methemoglobinemia.

Miscellaneous Poisons

Organophosphorus Compounds

Organophosphorus compounds have been used as pesticides and as chemical warfare nerve agents such as soman and sarin. The mechanism of toxicity of organophosphorus compounds is the inhibition of acetylcholinesterase, resulting in accumulation of acetylcholine and the continued stimulation of acetylcholine receptors. The management of poisoning with organophosphorous compounds consists of atropine sulfate and blood alkalinization with sodium bicarbonate and also magnesium sulfate as an adjunctive treatment. Neurotoxicity is a serious concern. Experiments on rabbits have shown that accumulated poisoning with paraoxon leads to development of hypoxia with a rapid fall in oxygen tension in the muscles and the venous blood, and a shift of the acid–base balance toward the uncompensated metabolic acidosis. HBO at 3 ATA for 2–4 h considerably prolongs the survival of the poisoned animals. Role of HBO in potential management of organophosphorus poisoning with neurotoxicity requires further investigation.

Conclusions: Poisoning Other Than with CO

There are only anecdotal reports of the use of HBO in cases of cyanide, hydrogen sulfide, and CCl$_4$ poisoning and methemoglobinemias; in situations like this one cannot have controlled studies. In a critical case HBO should be considered as a supplement to conventional methods. The liver is the target organ for injury caused by toxins that are activated by drug-metabolizing enzymes to reactive molecular intermediates. These intermediates cause cell injury by forming chemical bonds with cell proteins, nucleic acid, and lipids, and by altering the biological function of these molecules. The hepatocyte, in particular, is affected by toxic drug injury because it is the main site in the body where these toxins are activated. HBO has a marked effect on toxic liver damage by blocking the injury caused by toxins activated by oxidative biotransformation. HBO has no effect on damage caused by toxins that do not require biotransformation to induce liver damage. HBO may increase the hepatic necrosis induced by compounds which undergo oxidative biotransformation (e.g., thioacetamide, aflatoxin, dimethylnitrosamine), but this can be overcome and inhibited by prolonged hyperoxia.

References

Abramovich A, Shupak A, Ramon Y, Shoshani O, Bentur Y, Bar-Josef G, et al. Hyperbaric oxygen for carbon monoxide poisoning. Harefuah. 1997;132:21–4, 71.

Adamiec L, Kaminski B, Kwiatkowski H, et al. Hyperbaric oxygen in treatment of acute carbon monoxide poisoning. Anaesth Resusc Intensive Ther. 1975;3:305–13.

Annane D, Chadda K, Gajdos P, Jars-Guincestre MC, Chevret S, Raphael JC. Hyperbaric oxygen therapy for acute domestic carbon monoxide poisoning: two randomized controlled trials. Intensive Care Med. 2011;37:486–92.

Beard RR, Wertheim GA. Behavioral impairment associated with small doses of carbon monoxide. Am J Public Health. 1967;57:2012–22.

Belley R, Bernard N, Côté M, Paquet F, Poitras J. Hyperbaric oxygen therapy in the management of two cases of hydrogen sulfide toxicity from liquid manure. CJEM. 2005;7:257–61.

Bernard C. Lecons sur les effets des substances toxiques et medicamenteuses. Paris: Bailliere; 1857.

Bitterman N, Talmi Y, Lerman A, Melamed Y, Taitelman U. The effect of hyperbaric oxygen on acute experimental sulfide poisoning in the rat. Toxicol Appl Pharmacol. 1986;84:325–8.

Bonfiglioli R, Carnevali L, Di Lello M, Violante FS. Bilateral hearing loss after dichloromethane poisoning: a case report. Am J Ind Med. 2014;57:254–7.

Bothuyne-Queste E, Joriot S, Mathieu D, Mathieu-Nolf M, Favory R, Houfflin-Debarge V, et al. Ten practical issues concerning acute poisoning with carbon monoxide in pregnant women. J Gynecol Obstet Biol Reprod (Paris). 2014;43:281–7.

Chance B, Erecinska M, Wagner M. Mitochondrial responses to carbon monoxide toxicity. Ann NY Acad Sci. 1970;174:193–204.

Chen YG, Lin TY, Dai MS, Lin CL, Hung Y, Huang WS, et al. Risk of peripheral artery disease in patients with carbon monoxide poisoning: a population-based retrospective cohort study. Medicine (Baltimore). 2015;94:e1608.

Chen SY, Lin CC, Lin YT, Lo CP, Wang CH, Fan YM. Reversible changes of brain perfusion SPECT for carbon monoxide poisoning-induced severe akinetic mutism. Clin Nucl Med. 2016;41(5):e221–7.

Cho S-H, Lee DH, Yeun DR. Incidence of carbon monoxide intoxication. J Korean Med Assoc. 1986;29:1233–40.

Choi IS. Delayed neurologic sequelae in carbon monoxide intoxication. Arch Neurol. 1983;40:433–5.

Coburn RF. Endogenous carbon monoxide production. N Engl J Med. 1970;282:207–9.

Colignon M, Lamy M. Carbon monoxide poisoning and hyperbaric oxygen therapy. In: Schmutz J, editor. Proceedings of the 1st Swiss symposium on hyperbaric medicine. Basel: Foundation for Hyperbaric Medicine; 1986. p. 51–68.

Ducassé JL, Celsis P, Marc-Vergnes JP. Non-comatose patients with acute carbon monoxide poisoning: hyperbaric or normobaric oxygenation? Undersea Hyperb Med. 1995;22:9–15.

End E, Long CW. HBO in carbon monoxide poisoning. I. Effect on dogs and guinea pigs. J Ind Hyg Toxicol. 1942;24:302–6.

Friedman P, Guo XM, Stiller RJ, Laifer SA. Carbon monoxide exposure during pregnancy. Obstet Gynecol Surv. 2015;70:705–12.

Garrabou G, Inoriza JM, Morén C, Oliu G, Miró Ò, Martí MJ, et al. Mitochondrial injury in human acute carbon monoxide poisoning: the effect of oxygen treatment. J Environ Sci Health C Environ Carcinog Ecotoxicol Rev. 2011;29:32–51.

Gliner JA, Horvath SM, Mihevic PM. Carbon monoxide and human performance in a single and dual task methodology. Aviat Space Environ Med. 1983;54:714–7.

Gorman DF, Clayton D, Gilligan JE, Webb RK. A longitudinal study of 100 cases consecutive admissions for carbon monoxide poisoning to the Royal Adelaide Hospital. Anesth Intensive Care. 1992;20:311–6.

Goulon M, Barois A, Bapin M, Nouailhat F, Grosbuis S, Labrousse J. Intoxication oxycarbonée et anoxie aigue par inhalation de gaz de charbon et d'thydrocarbures. Ann Med Intern (Paris). 1969;120:335–49.

Grinker RR. Parkinsonism following carbon monoxide poisoning. J Neuro Ment Dis. 1926;6:18–28.

Haldane JS. The action of carbonic oxide on man. J Physiol. 1895;18:430.

Hampson NB. Treatment of mechanically ventilated patients poisoned with carbon monoxide: is "hyperbaric oxygenation" achieved. Undersea Hyperbaric Med 1998;25:17 (abstract).

Hampson NB, Dunford RG, Kramer CC, Norkool DM. Selection criteria utilized for hyperbaric oxygen treatment of carbon monoxide poisoning. J Emerg Med. 1995;13:227–31.

Hampson NB, Simonson SG, Kramer CC, Piantadosi CA. Central nervous system oxygen toxicity during hyperbaric treatment of patients with carbon monoxide poisoning. Undersea Hyperb Med. 1996;23:215–9.

Hansen MB, Olsen NV, Hyldegaard O. Combined administration of hyperbaric oxygen and hydroxocobalamin improves cerebral metabolism after acute cyanide poisoning in rats. J Appl Physiol (1985) 2013;115:1254–61.

Heyndrickx A, Scheiris C, Vercruysse A, Okkerse E. Gas chromatographic determination of carbon monoxide in blood and the hyperbaric oxygen treatment in carbon monoxide poisoning cases. J Pharm Belg. 1970;25(3):247–58.

Hsu P, Li HW, Lin YT. Acute hydrogen sulfide poisoning treated with hyperbaric oxygen. J Hyperbaric Med. 1987;2:215–21.

Icme F, Kozaci N, Ay MO, Avci A, Gumusay U, Yilmaz M, et al. The relationship between blood lactate, carboxy-hemoglobin and clinical status in CO poisoning. Eur Rev Med Pharmacol Sci. 2014;18:393–7.

Jain KK. Carbon monoxide poisoning. Green: St. Louis; 1990.

Jain KK. Carbon monoxide poisoning: neurologic aspects. In: Greenamyre JT, editor. Medlink neurology. San Diego: MedLink Corporation; 2016.

Jansen T, Barnung S, Mortensen CR, Jansen EC. Isobutyl-nitrite-induced methemoglobinemia; treatment with an exchange blood transfusion during hyperbaric oxygenation. Acta Anaesthesiol Scand. 2003;47:1300–1.

Jiang J, Tyssebotn I. Normobaric and hyperbaric oxygen treatment of acute carbon monoxide poisoning in rats. Undersea Hyperb Med. 1997;24:107–16.

Kienlen J, Alardo JP, Dimeglio G, et al. Traitement de l'intoxication oxycarbonée par l'oxygène hyperbare—propos de 370 observations. J Med Montpellier. 1974;9:237–43.

Klebs D. Ueber die Wirkung des Kohlenoxyds auf den tierischen Organismus. Arch Path Anat Physiol Klin Med. 1865;32:450–517.

Koren G, Sharav T, Pastuszak A, Garrettson LK, Hill K, Samson I, et al. A multicenter, prospective study of fetal outcome following accidental carbon monoxide poisoning in pregnancy. Reprod Toxicol. 1991;5:397–403.

Koyama K. Acute experimental carbon monoxide poisoning and hyperbaric oxygenation (HBO). Tokyo Jikeikai Med J. 1976;91:195–215.

Lilienthal JL, Fugitt CH. The effect of low concentrations of carboxyhemoglobin on the "altitude tolerance" of man. Am J Physiol. 1946;145:359–64.

Lindenmann J, Fink-Neuboeck N, Schilcher G, Smolle-Juettner FM. Severe methaemoglobinaemia treated with adjunctive hyperbaric oxygenation. Diving Hyperb Med. 2015;45:132–4.

Mathieu D, Nolf M, Durocher A, Saulnier F, Frimat P, Furon D, et al. Acute carbon monoxide poisoning risk of late sequelae and treatment by hyperbaric oxygen. Clin Toxicol. 1985;23:315–24.

Messier LD, Myers RA. A neuropsychological screening battery for emergency assessment of carbon-monoxide-poisoned patients. J Clin Psychol. 1991;47:675–84.

Mikulka P, O'Donnell R, Heinig P, Theodore J. The effect of carbon monoxide on human performance. Ann NY Acad Sci. 1973;174:409–20.

Mutluoglu M, Metin S, Arziman I, Uzun G, Yildiz S. The use of hyperbaric oxygen therapy for carbon monoxide poisoning in Europe. Undersea Hyperb Med. 2016;43:49–56.

Norkool DM, Kirkpatrick JN. Treatment of acute carbon monoxide poisoning with hyperbaric oxygen: a review of 115 cases. Ann Emerg Med. 1985;14:1168–71.

Ogawa M, Katsurada K, Sugimoto T, Sone S. Pulmonary edema in acute carbon monoxide poisoning. Int Arch Arbeitsmed. 1974;33:131–8.

Pace N, Strajman E, Walker EL. Acceleration of carbon monoxide elimination in man by high pressure oxygen. Science. 1950;111:652–4.

Pineas H. Klinischer und anatomischer Befund eines Falles von CO-Vergiftung. Z Neurol. 1924;93:36–8.

Pontani BA, Warriner RA, Newman RK, et al. Delayed neurologic sequelae after hydrogen sulfide poisoning treated with hyperbaric oxygen therapy. Undersea Hyperb Med 1998;25:10 (abstract).

Putnam TJ, McKenna JB, Morrison LR. Studies in multiple sclerosis. I. The histogenesis of experimental sclerotic plaques and their relation to multiple sclerosis. JAMA. 1931;97:1591–6.

Raphael JC, Elkharrat D, Jars-Guincestre MC, Chastang C, Chasles V, Vercken JB, et al. Trial of normobaric and hyperbaric oxygen for acute carbon monoxide intoxication. Lancet 1989;ii:414–9.

Roderique JD, Josef CS, Newcomb AH, Reynolds PS, Somera LG, Spiess BD. Preclinical evaluation of injectable reduced hydroxocobalamin as an antidote to acute carbon monoxide poisoning. J Trauma Acute Care Surg. 2015;79(4 Suppl 2):S116–20.

Sasaki T. One-half clearance time of carbon monoxide hemoglobin in blood during hyperbaric oxygen therapy (OHP). Bull Tokyo Dent Univ. 1975;22:63–77.

Schaad G, Kleinhanss G, Piekarski C. Zum Einfluss von Kohlenmonoxid in der Atemluft auf die psychophysische Leistungsfähigkeit. Wehrmed Mschr. 1983;27:423–30.

Scheinkestel CD, Bailey M, Myles PS, Jones K, Cooper DJ, Millar IL, et al. Hyperbaric or normobaric oxygen for acute carbon monoxide poisoning: a randomised controlled clinical trial. Med J Aust. 1999;170:203–10.

Schrot J, Thomas JR, Robertson RF. Temporal changes in repeated acquisition behavior after carbon monoxide exposure. Neurobehav Toxicol Teratol. 1984;6:23–8.

Schulte JH. Effects of mild carbon monoxide intoxication. Arch Environ Health. 1963;7:524–30.

Sloan EP, Murphy DG, Hart R, Cooper MA, Turnbull T, Barreca RS, et al. Complications and protocol considerations in carbon monoxide poisoned patients who require hyperbaric oxygen therapy. Ann Emerg Med. 1989;18:629–34.

Sluitjer ME. The treatment of carbon monoxide poisoning by the administration of oxygen at high pressure. Springfield: Thomas; 1963.

Smith G, Sharp GR. Treatment of carbon-monoxide poisoning with oxygen under pressure. Lancet. 1960;276:905–6.

Smith G, Ledingham IM, Sharp GR, Norman JN, Bates EH. Treatment of coal-gas poisoning with oxygen at 2 atmospheres pressure. Lancet 1962;i:816–8.

Thom SR. Dehydrogenase conversion to oxidase and lipid peroxidation in the brain after CO poisoning. J Appl Physiol. 1992;73:1584–9.

Thom SR, Taber RL, Mendiguren II, Clark JM, Hardy KR, Fisher AB. Delayed neuropsychologic sequelae after carbon monoxide poisoning: prevention by treatment with hyperbaric oxygen [see comments]. Ann Emerg Med. 1995;25:474–40.

Thompson JP, Marrs TC. Hydroxocobalamin in cyanide poisoning. Clin Toxicol (Phila). 2012;50:875–85.

Tirpitz D, Bakyara T. Hyperbare Oxygen bei CO-Intoxikationen. Der Inform Arzt. 1988;8:51–4.

Trouton D, Eysenck HJ. The effects of drugs on behavior. In: Eysenck HJ, editor. Handbook of abnormal psychology. New York: Basic Books; 1961. p. 634–96.

van Hoesen KB, Camporesi EM, Moon RE. Should hyperbaric oxygen be used to treat the pregnant patient for acute carbon monoxide poisoning? JAMA. 1989;261:1039–43.

Wattel F, Mathieu D, Neviere R, Mathieu-Nolf M, Lefèbvre-Lebleu N. L'intoxication au monoxyde de carbone. Presse Med. 1996;25:1425–9.

Wattel F, Mathieu D, Mathieu-Nolf M. A 25-year study (1983-2008) of children's health outcomes after hyperbaric oxygen therapy for carbon monoxide poisoning in utero. Bull Acad Natl Med. 2013;197:677–94; discussion 695–7.

Weaver LK, Hopkins RO, Chan KJ, et al. Hyperbaric oxygen for acute carbon monoxide poisoning. N Engl J Med. 2002;347:1057–67.

Weaver LK. Hyperbaric oxygen therapy for carbon monoxide poisoning. Undersea Hyperb Med. 2014;41:339–54.

Yastrebov VE, Kustov VV, Razinkin SM. Effect of a short-term exposure to carbon monoxide high concentrations on man's psychophysiological functions. Kosm Biol Aviakosm Med. 1987;21:47–50.

Youn BA, Kozikowski RJ, Myers RA. The development of treatment algorithm in methylene chloride poisoning based on a multicase experience. Undersea Biomed Res 1989;12(Suppl):20 Abstract #16.

Yun DR, Cho SH. Hyperbaric oxygen treatment in acute CO poisoning. Korean J Prev Med. 1983;16:153–6.

K.K. Jain

Abstract

HBO has been shown to be a valuable adjunct to the medical and surgical treatment of various infections. Host defense mechanisms against infection are impaired by hypoxia and oxygen has an adjunct effect with antibiotics particularly in anaerobic infections such as gas gangrene. HBO plays an important role in the treatment of other soft tissue infections and osteomyelitis.

Keywords

Hyperbaric oxygen (HBO) • Necrotizing fasciitis • Antibiotic • Osteomyelitis • Oxygen • Gas gangrene • Fungal infections • AIDS • Malignant otitis externa • Leprosy

Introduction

Host Defense Mechanisms Against Infection

Phagocytic leukocytes present the first and the most important line of defense against microorganisms introduced into the body. The capacity of the leukocytes to kill depends largely on the amount of oxygen available to them. Bacterial killing usually consists of two phases. The first phase involves degranulation, in which ingested bacteria are exposed to various antimicrobial substances derived from the leukocyte granules. The second phase is the oxidative phase (Fig. 14.1), which depends on the molecular oxygen captured by the leukocytes and converted to high energy radicals such as superoxide, hydroxyl radicals, peroxides, aldehyde hypochlorite, and hypochlorites. The rate of production of free radicals, which determines the oxidative bacterial killing, depends on the local oxygen tension. The killing sequence can be replicated to some extent in vitro by incubating bacteria in the presence of halide ions, hydrogen peroxide, and myeloperoxidases, a mixture that generates hypohalite-free radicals.

Impairment by Anoxia

The oxidative killing mechanism is related to the nonoxidative pathway. The energy for this pathway is provided by the hexose-mono-phosphate shunt. Absence of the enzyme primary oxidase (NADPH) means absence of the substrate on which it acts—oxygen—and is equal to anoxia. Therefore, lack of oxygen leads to loss of killing power of the leukocytes. The major loss of killing capacity occurs when tissue pO_2 levels fall below 30 mmHg.

Oxygen as an Antibiotic

The characteristics of oxygen as an antibiotic are shown in Table 14.1. The effect of hyperbaric oxygenation (HBO) in anaerobic infections is well recognized. The high levels of oxygen in the tissues are detrimental to organisms that thrive in the absence of oxygen. The aerobic bacteria, however, show a biphasic response on exposure to HBO. At pressures of 0.6–1.3 ATA the growth is enhanced, but above 1.3 ATA it

K.K. Jain, MD, FRACS, FFPM (✉)
Blaesiring 7, Basel 4057, Switzerland
e-mail: jain@pharmabiotech.ch

Fig. 14.1 Schema of oxidative killing mechanism and its relation to nonoxidative pathway. *HOCl* hypochlorite, *HOI* hypoiodite, *HMPS* hexose-monophosphate shunt. Reproduced with permission from Rabkin and Hunt. Infection and Oxygen. In: Davis JC, Hunt TK (Eds.): Problem Wounds—Role of Oxygen. New York: Elsevier; 1988

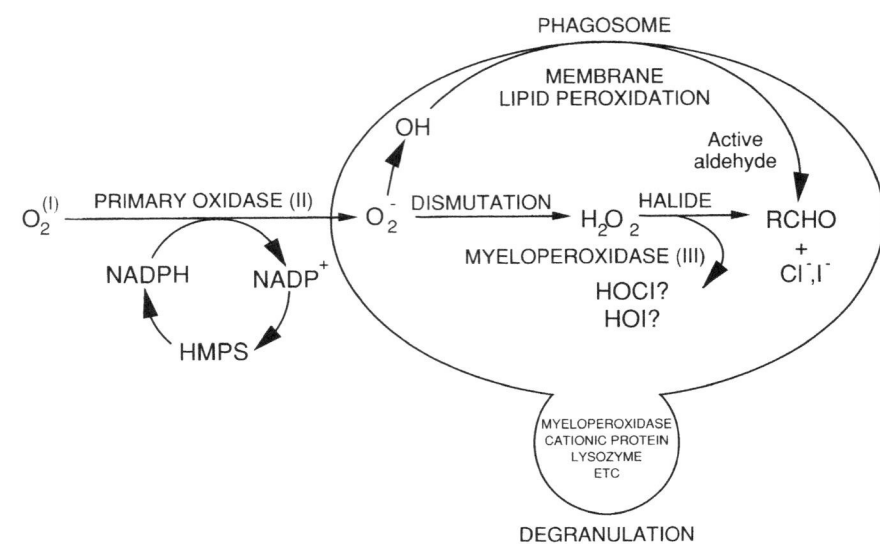

Table 14.1 Oxygen as an antibiotic and rationale for HBO therapy in infections

1. Oxygen acts as an antibiotic by impairing the bacterial metabolism. The effect of HBO is not selective but covers a broad spectrum of Gram positive as well as Gram negative organisms. It is most effective in anaerobic infections
2. HBO improves the phagocytosis, which is impaired by hypoxia
3. Hypoxia impairs the immune mechanism of the body, whereas HBO improves it
4. HBO produces free radicals which are toxic to the microorganisms
5. HBO has a synergistic effect when combined with sulfonamides and increases the effect five- to tenfold
6. HBO is effective in drug-resistant infections
7. Adequate tissue oxygen tension is required for achieving an optimal effect of the antibiotics. The effect of aminoglycosides is reduced in anoxic conditions as oxygen is needed for transporting the drug into bacteria
8. Oxygen has a direct bactericidal or bacteriostatic effect equal to that of some antibiotics
9. HBO inhibits the exotoxin production, e.g., alpha-toxin of *C. perfringens* or detoxifies the oxygen-labile exotoxins, e.g., theta-toxin of *C. perfringens*

is inhibited. The toxicity of oxygen to the microbes is time dependent. The aim is to have an exploitable difference in specificity to the drug between the host and the parasite. The greater the specificity of the drug for the parasite, the safer the drug is for clinical use. As a drug, oxygen acts indiscriminately, however; the quantities of oxygen required to raise tissue pO_2 to a level that would adversely affect the growth or metabolism (including toxin production) of the microorganisms is in the same range that produces symptoms of pulmonary and central nervous system toxicity. There are, therefore, two goals:

1. To expose the microorganisms to a given pO_2 for a time long enough to affect the microbial physiology adversely and give the host defense mechanisms an opportunity to prevail. The exposure should not be so long as to produce tissue toxicity.
2. To raise tissue pO_2 sufficiently to bolster the body's defense mechanisms without altering the physiology of the microbe simultaneously.

Bacteria in culture are exposed to intermittent HBO to simulate clinical situations and to determine the time-dose relationships. The growth of *Mycobacterium tuberculosis* is greatly retarded after twice-daily 3-h exposures to oxygen at 2.87 ATA for 5 days, while twice-daily 2-h exposures to 1.87 ATA are less effective. There are species differences in response to increased pO_2.

Oxygen may enhance the effects of other antimicrobial agents, particularly para-aminobenzoic acid (PABA) antagonists such as sulfonamides. HBO at 2.87 ATA increases the effectiveness of sulfisoxazole five- to tenfold. There is no oxygen enhancement of PABA analogs on *Corynebacterium diphtheriae*. The only drug-resistant organism that is susceptible to oxygen-induced synergy is *M. tuberculosis*.

Improving tissue oxygen by administration of normobaric oxygen decreases infectious necrosis as effectively as prophylactic antibiotics, and has an additive effect. In several animal models of peritonitis due to pathogenic organisms, HBO reduces mortality and has a synergistic effect with antibiotics which further reduce the mortality.

In a murine model of group A streptococcal myositis, HBO treatment alone does not decrease mortality significantly in vivo whereas penicillin therapy alone improves outcome significantly but the combined treatment of penicillin and HBO exerts synergistic effects in both decreasing bacterial counts in vivo and increasing survival in this model.

HBO as an Adjuvant to Antibiotics

Efficacy of several bactericidal antibiotics such as ciprofloxacin is enhanced by stimulation of the aerobic respiration of pathogens, and that lack of O_2 increases their tolerance. Chronic *Pseudomonas aeruginosa* lung infection is the most severe complication in cystic fibrosis patients. It is characterized by antibiotic-tolerant biofilms in the endobronchial mucus with zones of O_2 depletion mainly due to polymorphonuclear leucocyte activity. Re-oxygenation of O_2-depleted biofilms improves susceptibility to ciprofloxacin possibly by restoring aerobic respiration. As an example, re-oxygenation of O_2-depleted *P. aeruginosa* strain PAO1 agarose-embedded biofilms by HBO treatment using 100 % O_2 at 2.8 ATA, enhances the diffusive supply for aerobic respiration during ciprofloxacin treatment (Kolpen et al. 2016). Thus combining ciprofloxacin treatment with HBO therapy has the potential to improve treatment of *P. aeruginosa* biofilm infections.

In a controlled experimental study on rats combination of HBO with antibiotics vancomycin and tigecycline had a significant effect on mediastinitis resulting from methicillin-resistant *Staphylococcus aureus* (Kurt et al. 2015). Thus, methicillin-resistant *S. aureus* mediastinitis can be treated without requiring a multidrug combination, thereby reducing the medication dose and decreasing the side effects.

The expert panel on diabetic foot infection (DFI) of the International Working Group on the Diabetic Foot conducted a systematic review of all published reports, particularly randomized clinical trials, relating to any type of treatment for infection of the foot in persons with diabetes (Peters et al. 2016). Results of comparisons of different antibiotic regimens generally demonstrated that newly introduced antibiotic regimens appeared to be as effective as conventional therapy (and also more cost-effective in one study), but one study failed to demonstrate non-inferiority of a new antibiotic compared with that of a standard agent. This review revealed little evidence upon which to make recommendations for the treatment of DFIs and pointed the need for further well-designed trials that will provide robust data upon which to make decisions about the most appropriate treatment of both skin and soft tissue infection and osteomyelitis in diabetic patients.

HBO in the Treatment of Infections

For oxygen to be effective as a bactericidal agent, it has to be delivered to the infected areas. Normobaric oxygen may not reach the affected area, but HBO is more effective. The presence of normal blood flow and normal oxygen content of the blood does not exclude the possibility of hypoxia of the infected tissues, such as ulcers in the lower extremities. For most infections 100 % oxygen is used at 2.5 ATA for 1 h sessions, which can be given once a day or preferably twice a day. The treatment is continued until the infection subsides. There are two reasons for choosing 2.5 ATA:

1. It is a safe pressure well below the upper limit of 3 ATA. This is an important consideration because of the debilitated state of some patients and the lengthy treatment required.
2. The immune system is stimulated by oxygen pressures up to 2.5 ATA (see Chap. 26), whereas higher pressures have an immunosuppressive effect.

HBO exposures should be intermittent, as continual exposure of experimental animals to high oxygen pressures has been found to be detrimental to phagocytosis. Finally, it must be pointed out that HBO therapy is used as an adjunct to other well-recognized methods of treatment of infection, and it should not replace the antibiotics used in accordance with the results of the culture and sensitivity studies on the organisms.

Not all doses of HBO have an antibacterial effect. The use of HBO at pressures lower than 1.3 ATA promotes the growth of aerobic bacteria in vivo by enhancing oxygen delivery to bacteria in the injured tissues. Pressures have to be increased to sufficient levels for oxygen to be bacteriostatic or bactericidal.

Microbes with adequate antioxidant defenses are resistant to the toxic effect of oxygen-free radicals. Some bacteria even use free radical production to injure host cells. Two virulent strains of Listeria monocytogenes exhibit maximal production of H_2O_2 and O_2^-. Virulence can be correlated with survival of *L. monocytogenes* in macrophage monolayers. A virulent strain of *L. monocytogenes* and an isolate of *Staphylococcus aureus* do not release O_2 in significant amounts. Addition of exogenous H_2O_2 results in a significant loss of macrophage viability.

Bacterial antioxidant enzymes are important in resisting x-dependent microbicidal activity in human polymorphonuclear neutrophils (PMN). Surface-associated SOD and high levels of catalase act together to protect strains of Nocardia asteroides from the bactericidal effect of PMN. Interaction between oxygen-derived free radicals and antioxidant defense mechanisms may be a crucial factor in the establishment of bacterial infections. The outcome of in vitro or in vivo HBO treatment of aerobic bacteria depends on the particular organism and the experimental conditions.

HBO has been shown to be beneficial in septicemia. Although hyperoxia may lead to increased lipid peroxidation and free radical damage, it is also possible that lesser degrees of hyperoxygenation such as 2–3 ATA may antagonize lipid peroxidation, which has been implicated in tissue damage in septicemia.

Infections for which HBO has been studied and is recommended by the Undersea and Hyperbaric Medicine Society include necrotizing fasciitis, gas gangrene, chronic refractory osteomyelitis (including malignant otitis externa), mucormycosis, intracranial abscesses, and diabetic foot ulcers that have concomitant infections (Kaide and Khandelwal 2008). In all of these processes, HBO is used adjunctively along with antimicrobial agents and aggressive surgical debridement.

HBO in the Treatment of Soft Tissue Infections

These infections are usually necrotizing and occur in traumatic or surgical wounds, around foreign bodies; they affect patients who are compromised by either diabetes mellitus, vascular insufficiency, or both. Anaerobic soft tissue infections are still life threatening infections. Although their frequency is actually moderate; they remain severe because physicians are often insufficiently aware of them. Their origin is often traumatic or surgical but may also be secondary to an ulcer or a small wound in a high-risk patient with arteriosclerosis or diabetes mellitus. Hypoxia, traumatic muscle crush, heavy bacterial contamination as well as incorrect antibiotic prophylaxis are the major reasons for their occurrence. Management consists of antibiotics adapted to both anaerobic and associated aerobic bacteria, large and early surgical debridement, but with conservative excision, and intensive HBO therapy. Strict prevention measures must be applied to avoid their occurrence. Various factors influence outcome in a large group of patients presenting with necrotizing soft tissue infections and analyses of risk factors for mortality have been performed, producing conflicting conclusions regarding optimal care. In particular, there is some debate regarding the impact of concurrent physiologic derangements, type and extent of infection, and the role of HBO in treatment.

Logistic regression analysis based on retrospective chart review of 198 consecutive patients with documented necrotizing soft tissue infections, treated at a single institution in the USA during an 8-year period, tested the impact of characteristics of each patient and his/her clinical course on outcome (Elliott et al. 1996). The mortality rate among these patients was 25.3 %. The most common sites of origin of infection were the perineum (Fournier's disease; 36 % of cases) and the foot (in diabetics; 15.2 %). By logistic regression analysis, risk factors for death included age, female gender, extent of infection, delay in first debridement, elevated serum creatinine level, elevated blood lactate level, and degree of organ system dysfunction at admission. Diabetes mellitus did not predispose patients to death, except in conjunction with renal dysfunction or peripheral vascular disease. Myonecrosis, noted in 41.4 % of the patients who underwent surgery, did not influence mortality. The authors concluded that necrotizing soft tissue infections represent a group of highly lethal infections best treated by early and repeated extensive debridement and broad-spectrum antibiotics.

Various studies indicate that HBO appears to offer the advantage of early wound closure in necrotizing soft tissue infections. Certain biomarkers help in identifying individuals at increased risk for multiple-organ failure and death, thereby assisting in decisions to allocate intensive care resources. Common necrotizing soft tissue infections are described here.

Crepitant Anaerobic Cellulitis

This includes clostridial as well as nonclostridial cellulitis. It manifests itself as a necrotic soft tissue infection with abundant soft tissue gas. This condition usually occurs with local trauma and vascular insufficiency in the lower extremities. Multiple organisms isolated from these infections include bacteroides species, peptostreptococcus species, clostridium species, and enterobacteriaceae.

Progressive Bacterial Gangrene

This is a subacute to chronic ulcer formation on the abdominal or the thoracic wall with a zone of gangrene surrounding it. The major symptom is pain. Microorganisms found in the gangrenous margin are microaerophilic or anaerobic streptococci, and the central part of the lesion contains *Staphylococcus aureus* and enterobacteriaceae. This synergistic bacterial combination is necessary to produce gangrenous lesions.

Necrotizing Fasciitis

Necrotizing fasciitis (NF) is a rare infection of soft tissues considered to be due to streptococcal infection and first described as a generalized condition (Meleney 1924). Fournier's gangrene (described in this chapter) is considered to be a localized variant of it. Several hundred cases have been reported in the literature. Patients usually complain of pain which is disproportionate to minor skin changes in early phases. Deeper changes are more widespread than the skin changes. Shock with multiorgan failure can occur later in the course of the disease. Microscopic examination of tissue aspirates shows the infective organisms and imaging techniques show the infection spreading along tissue planes.

Primary, aggressive but tissue-saving debridement, and concomitant antibiotics are the cornerstones of therapy of NF. HBO therapy can oxygenate infected hypoxic tissues to help marginally viable tissues survive, reduce the inflammatory response, improve leukocyte bacterial oxidative killing capacity, and achieve infection control and healing (Flam et al. 2009).

A single-center, retrospective, case-controlled study of patients attending a hospital in Australia has assessed the effect of HBO therapy in reducing mortality or morbidity in 342 patients with necrotizing fasciitis (NF) over a 13-year period from 2002 to 2014 (Devaney et al. 2015). The most commonly involved sites were the perineum (33.7%), lower limb (29.9%), and trunk (18.2%). The commonest predisposing factor was diabetes mellitus (34.8%). Polymicrobial NF (Type I NF) occurred in 50.7% and Group A streptococcal fasciitis (Type II NF) occurred in 25.8% of patients. Overall, mortality was 14.4%; 12% in those treated with HBO, and 24.3% in those not treated with HBO. Mortality was linked to severity of illness at presentation. However when adjusted for severity score and need for intensive care management, HBO was associated with significant reduction in mortality.

Nonclostridial Myonecrosis

This is also a synergistic necrotizing cellulitis and is similar to clostridial myonecrosis because of extensive muscle and fascia involvement. It occurs most commonly in the perineal area and Fournier's gangrene is a variant of it. Multiple organisms that have been isolated include peptostreptococcus species, bacteroides species, and enterobacteriaceae.

Differential diagnosis and treatment of these infections is listed in Table 14.2. The treatment of these infections is a combination of aggressive surgery, debridement, appropriate antibiotics, good nutritional support, and optimal oxygenation of the infected tissues. HBO treatment has been used successfully as adjunctive therapy in mixed soft tissue infections. An objective evaluation of the use of HBO in these infections is difficult because of the multitude of variable factors in patients and other treatment methods used.

Fournier's Gangrene

Many controversial issues exist surrounding the disease pathogenesis and optimal management of Fournier's gangrene. In Fournier's original descriptions in 1883, the disease arose in healthy subjects without an obvious cause. Most contemporary studies, however, are able to identify definite urologic or colorectal etiologies in a majority of cases. Concurrent diseases include diabetes mellitus, ethanol abuse, and use of systemic immunosuppressants. Management involves prompt surgical debridement with initiation of broad-spectrum antibiotics. Multiple debridements, orchiectomy, urinary diversion, and fecal diversion are performed as clinically indicated. HBO is used as adjuvant therapy, with considerable reduction in overall mortality. Although a grim prognosis usually accompanies the diagnosis, significant improvement is reported by combining traditional surgical and antibiotic regimens with HBO therapy. Successful use of HBO in Fournier's gangrene has been

Table 14.2 Differentiation and treatment of the common necrotizing bacterial soft tissue infections[a]

	Crepitant anaerobic cellulitis	Progressive bacterial synergistic gangrene	Necrotizing fasciitis	Nonclostridial myonecrosis
Incubation	More than 3 days	2 weeks	1–4 days	Variable, 3–14 days
Onset	Gradual	Gradual	Acute	Acute
Toxemia	None or slight	Minimal	Moderate to marked	Marked
Pain	Absent	Moderate	Moderate to severe	Severe
Exudate	None or slight	None or slight	Serosanguinous	Profuse dishwater pus
Odor to exudate	+Foul	+Foul	Foul	+Foul
Gas	Abundant	May be present	Usually not present	Not pronounced
Muscle	No change	No change	Viable	Marked change
Skin	Little change	Shaggy ulcer, gangrenous margin	Pale red cellulitis	Minimal change
Mortality	5–10%	10–25%	30%	75%
Treatment				
Antibiotics	Yes	Yes	Yes	Yes
Surgery	I & D	I & D	I & D	Muscle removal
Adjunctive HBO	No	Yes (severe cases)	Yes (compromised host)	Yes

I & D incision and drainage

reported in several studies. In some cases, the infection was progressive in spite of surgery and antibiotics and was arrested only with the use of HBO treatment. It is concluded that HBO is very effective in the treatment of Fournier's gangrene.

Gas Gangrene

Gas gangrene is an acute painful necrotic condition of the soft tissues usually associated with trauma of surgery, but it may occur spontaneously. It is due to infection with various species of gas-forming anaerobic organisms and is also referred to as clostridial myonecrosis, and as Gasödem or Gasbrand in German. Although one-third of all wounds of violence are contaminated with such organisms, only 3% develop the clinical disease. The annual incidence in the USA is about 1000 cases.

Bacteriology and Pathogenesis

Clostridia are putrefactive, Gram-positive, anaerobic, spore-forming, and encapsulated bacilli comprising more than 150 species. They are mostly soil contaminants but have also been isolated from the human gastrointestinal tract and the skin. *Clostridium welchii* was first recognized as a cause of gas gangrene by Welch in 1892. Subsequently renamed *C. perfringens*, this organism is implicated in 50–100% of all cases of gas gangrene. Clostridia thrive in tissues that have low oxygen tensions as a result of trauma or ischemia. They release exotoxins that set a vicious circle in motion: there is tissue edema around the area of necrosis, which further diminishes the blood supply and oxygen tension and diminishes the numbers of leukocytes, leading to rapid spread of the necrotizing process. The patient may become moribund within 12 h and die.

Alpha-toxin, a C-lecithinase, is the major lethal toxin of *C. perfringens*; it precedes hemolysis and necrosis. It is stable under oxygen pressures of 2–3 ATA although there is experimental evidence that further production of toxin is halted. Other toxins assist in destroying, liquefying, and dissecting the adjacent tissues with resulting rapid spread of the process. Some toxins affect vascular permeability and cause edema. The proteolytic and saccharolytic enzymes are responsible for the production of hydrogen sulfide. The toxins produce dysfunction of the brain, heart, and kidneys. The local condition of the wound is far more important than the presence of clostridia and can be considered a deciding factor in the evolution of the infection and its clinical sequelae. Gas gangrene has been recorded after:

1. Soft tissue trauma
2. Foreign bodies, hemorrhage, or necrotic tissue in the wound

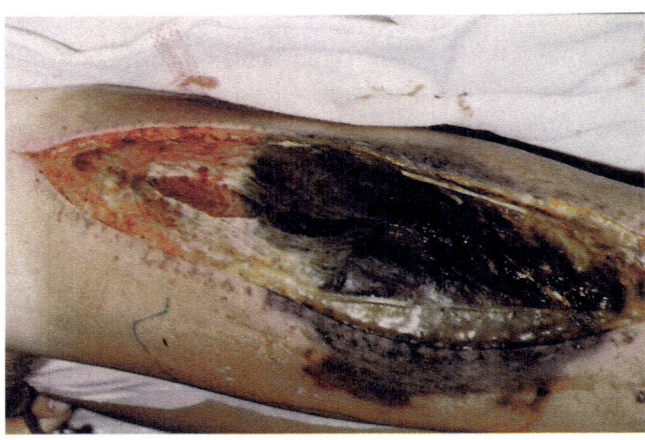

Fig. 14.2 Photograph showing the appearance of gas gangrene. Courtesy of Prof. D. Bakker, Amsterdam

3. High velocity missile wounds
4. Compound fractures
5. Deep contamination of wounds
6. Prolonged delay in surgery
7. Traumatic or surgical interruption of blood supply
8. Careless abortion procedure
9. Too-tight plaster casts or dressings
10. Any kind of surgery
11. Other (often minor) injuries in the immune-compromised host

Diagnosis

The clinical picture of gas gangrene is quite typical. There is a swollen wound with bronze, gray, or purple discoloration, bullae, and watery discharge (Fig. 14.2). Pain is an early symptom. Crepitation is a late sign. Signs of systemic toxicity may be fever, tachycardia, and mental impairment. A Gram stain of the wound is the most rapid method of diagnosis. Presence of Gram-positive bacteria with the typical symptoms and signs should be considered a case of gas gangrene unless proven otherwise. Treatment should be initiated before confirmation by culture can be obtained, as this requires 48–72 h. A rapid method of diagnosis involves measurement of sialidase activity in the serum or the muscle tissue of the patient.

X-rays will not reveal gas consistently, and when present, gas is not pathognomonic of gas gangrene. Gas distribution in a feathery pattern indicating spread along muscle fasciculi, however, is pathognomonic (Fig. 14.3). Large gas bubbles are usually associated with open wounds or necrotizing fasciitis. The classification of clostridial infections is presented in Table 14.3. This classification is used as a guide for initiating treatment: categories I and II require surgical treatment, whereas categories III and IV may be managed medically. Category III may progress to category II or I if not

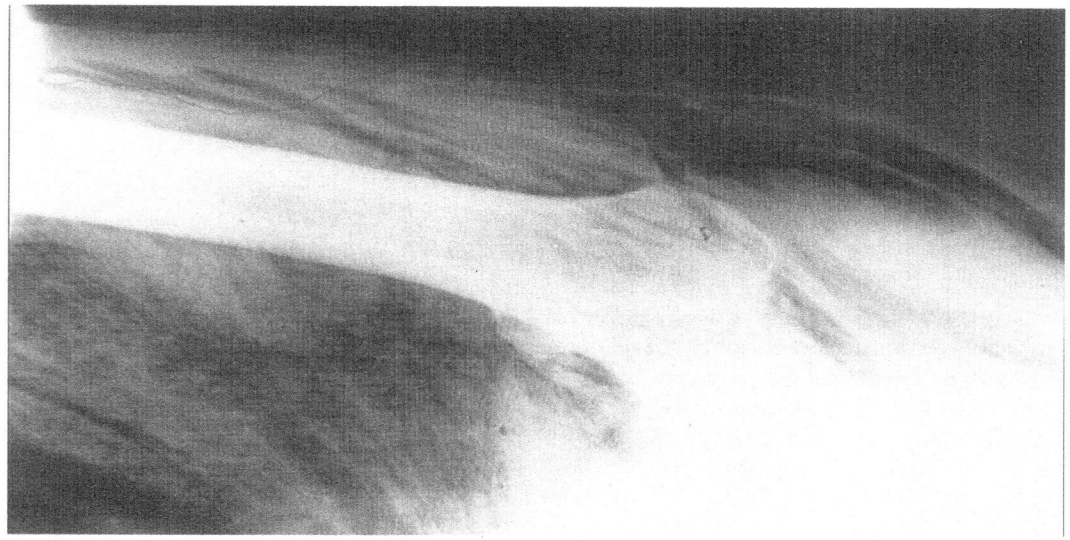

Fig. 14.3 X-ray of the affected limb in gas gangrene showing the typical pattern of distribution of gas in the tissues

Table 14.3 Classification of clostridial infections

Category	Type	Subtype		Examples
I	Clostridial myonecrosis (gas gangrene)	(a)	Spreading	Crepitant: edematous
		(b)	Diffuse	Noncrepitant
II	Primary organ involvement			Uterus, gallbladder
III	Clostridial cellulitis	(a)	Anaerobic toxemia	
		(b)	Localized	
IV	Clostridial contamination			

Table 14.4 Differential diagnosis of soft tissue gas

Bacterial		Nonbacterial
I	Aerobic aerogenic infections	Mechanical effect of trauma
	(a) Hemolytic staphylococcal fascitis	Air hose injury, injection
	(b) Hemolytic streptococcal gangrene	Hydrogen peroxide irrigation
	(c) Coliform	Injection of benzine
II	Anaerobic streptococcal infections	Barotrauma; dysbarism
III	*Bacteroides* infections	Postoperative
IV	Clostridia	Aberrant sexual activity
V	Mixed aerobic and anaerobic infections	

managed properly. The combination of gas in tissues and necrotizing myositis does not always mean gas gangrene. Differential diagnosis of soft tissue gas is given in Table 14.4. The history and the findings on physical examination assist in diagnosis. Extensive gas in the tissues in the absence of systemic toxicity suggests gas-forming fasciitis.

Treatment of Gas Gangrene

The essentials of treatment of gas gangrene are:

- General supportive measures for seriously ill patients. The patients usually require intensive care. Tissue perfusion, oxygenation, and fluid as well as electrolyte balance have to be maintained. Blood transfusions may be necessary because of hemolysis caused by clostridia. HBO may be used at this stage for a patient who is too ill to undergo surgery. A few treatment sessions may stabilize the condition of the patient so surgery may be carried out.
- High doses of antibiotics. Penicillin is preferred but other antibiotics may be combined depending on the nature of the superimposed infections.
- Surgery. This has an important place in the management of gas gangrene. The main object is the removal of necrotic tissue and blood because the erythrocytes containing catalase counteract the effect of HBO treatment.
- HBO is a useful adjunct to surgery and antibiotics.

HBO in the Treatment of Gas Gangrene: Clinical Results

The action of HBO in clostridial and other anaerobic infections is based on the formation of free radicals and the lack of free radical degrading enzymes such as superoxide dismutase, catalase, and peroxidases.

The first successful use of HBO at 3 ATA in the management of gas gangrene was reported more than half a century ago (Brummelkamp et al. 1961). The major benefit of HBO treatment in gas gangrene is the inhibition of toxin production, which stops at tissue oxygen tensions of 60 mmHg and above. HBO counteracts the hypoxic environments in which the clostridia thrive. Peroxidase develops within the organisms to inactivate or kill them, but the presence of catalase in muscle or blood inactivates the peroxidase. Hence, the removal of necrotic tissue by surgery is essential for the proper effect of HBO. Tissue pO_2 levels of 250 mmHg are required for inhibition of clostridia.

It is doubtful whether the toxins already formed by the bacteria can be eliminated any faster with the help of HBO. The use of HBO can be a guide to the demarcation of the necrotic and the viable tissue after initial debridement. A more definite excision can be performed after HBO treatments. HBO has no effect on the necrotic tissue itself. Neither oxygen nor antibiotics can penetrate such tissue, which should be surgically removed. HBO treatment results in a marked increase in tissue oxygenation in both healthy tissue and in the vicinity of infected tissue. The hyperoxygenated tissue zone surrounding the infected area may be of significance in preventing the extension of invading microorganisms.

For the initial management of gas gangrene the "Amsterdam therapeutic regimen." (Bakker 1988) is as follows. Before a patient suspected of gas gangrene is transferred to the hyperbaric unit, doctors from the referring hospital are advised to refrain from surgical intervention and to treat the patient with 1–2 million units of penicillin-G intravenously. Thereafter, the following protocol is carried out:

1. Wound inspection to evaluate the clinical picture, discoloration of skin, muscle necrosis, swelling of the infected area, discharge and smell from the wound, in order to ascertain whether gas gangrene is involved.
2. Removal of sutures and opening of the wound is performed in sutured postoperative or posttraumatic wounds. In cases of gas gangrene after injections or minor injuries, wounds are not surgically handled (i.e., no incision or excision).
3. Bacteriology, including a direct smear for Gram stain, aerobic and anaerobic blood and wound cultures, and tissue specimens for histology. A Gram stain with Gram-positive clostridial rods supports the clinical diagnosis of gas gangrene, and HBO treatment is indicated. However, before the results of cultures are known, treatment is

started because the alpha-toxin production has to be stopped as quickly as possible.
4. Demarcation of the boundaries of discoloration and crepitance.
5. Blood sampling for laboratory investigation, including hemoglobin, hematocrit, leukocytes, electrolytes, kidney and liver function tests, arterial blood gases, etc.
6. Infusion therapy and treatment for shock as soon as the patient arrives in the hospital.
7. X-rays for signs of clostridial myositis.
8. Antibiotics (6 × 1 million units penicillin-G/day).
9. Chloral hydrate as a sedative (1 g rectally) has proved useful. Interaction of other sedatives, and their use under hyperbaric conditions has been outlined in Chap. 9.
10. Myringotomy performed in patients (small children, very old, and seriously ill patients) who are not capable of "clearing the ears," to equalize the pressure on both sides of the eardrum during treatment. Myringotomy is easily and quickly performed under local anesthesia and is virtually without complications. The opening in the eardrum remains competent during the 3 days of treatment. If, for other reasons, HBO treatment has to be continued, tympanostomy tubes are inserted.

The HBO pressures recommended for gas gangrene vary from 2.5 ATA to 3 ATA while breathing oxygen and the treatment sessions should last about 90 min. This usually leads to an oxygen partial pressure of 200 mmHg in the infected tissues. Frequency of the treatments should vary from 3 to 4 per 24 h during the first 48 h and then two treatment sessions daily until the infection is controlled. More than 7 sessions in 3 days are seldom required.

The reported number of cases of gas gangrene where HBO treatment was used exceeds 2500. The true number is greater as HBO is an accepted mode of treatment for gas gangrene and many surgeons do not report such cases. With few exceptions, the reported results of HBO were favorable; details for some of the larger reported series are given in Table 14.5. Although there are no randomized trials of HBO in these infections, in vitro data and meta-analysis of clinical cases strongly support the use of HBO. It would be difficult to conduct randomized controlled clinical trials in a condition such as gas gangrene. A Cochrane database systematic review of randomized controlled trials failed to establish efficacy of HBO in gas gangrene because only 2 trials were available with total of 90 patients (Yang et al. 2015).

The emphasis should be on prophylaxis and prevention of gas gangrene by proper wound management. The use of gas gangrene antitoxins is obsolete. Patients with trauma and overwhelming infection should be transferred to a major trauma center with hyperbaric facilities. HBO should be used early, but it is worth a try even at a later stage before any ablative surgery of the limbs is undertaken.

Table 14.5 Results in some large series of cases of gas gangrene where HBO was used as an adjunctive therapy

Authors and year	Cases	Survival	Remarks
Hart et al. (1983)	139	70	Limb salvage rate 80 %
Tirpitz (1986)	480		Survival rate increased to 90 % with use of IgG therapy
Bakker (1988)	409	79.5	Amputation rate only 8.7 % after
Hirn and Niinikoski (1988)	32	72.9	All patients who died had been transferred from other hospitals in moribund condition
Desola (1990)	85	80	Multicenter study. Outcome was satisfactory in 67.1 % of survivors
Korhonen et al. (1999)	53	77.4 %	Conclusion was that patient survival can be improved if the disease is recognized early and appropriate therapy applied promptly

Fungal Infection

Actinomycosis

Actinomycosis is an anaerobic infection with four clinical forms: cervicofacial, thoracic, abdominal-pelvic, and disseminated. The cervicofacial form responds well to antibiotic treatment; the other forms often require surgical procedures. Due to low tissue oxygen levels, the prognosis for cure is low. An increase in the oxygen tension with subsequent oxygen radical formation is lethal for the actinomycosis organisms. HBO is recommended as an adjunct to surgical care and antimicrobial therapy.

Mucormycosis

Mucormycosis is a devastating fungal disease that occurs most commonly in immune-suppressed patients who have burns, who are on long-term corticosteroid therapy, or who present with diabetic acidosis. The major location of the infection is the rhinocerebral area, lungs, and intestine. The mortality rate prior to the advent of amphotericin B (AMB) was 70 %, but this decreased to 40 % with the use of AMB. Mucormycosis has been reported in patients who undergo multiple bone marrow transplant for thalassemia and are in advanced phase of disease with severe acquired hemochromatosis. HBO is used in fulminating mucormycosis on the following theoretical basis:

- To provide oxygen to the tissues distal to the occluded vessels in order to achieve local tissue survival
- To reduce acidosis
- To exercise a fungicidal effect

Rhinocerebral Mucormycosis

The disease is fatal when cerebral extension occurs. The mainstay of the treatment is surgery, AMB, and eradication of

the underlying cause. Several cases of rhinocerebral mucormycosis occur in immunocompromised states and patients with diabetes mellitus as a predisposing cause. Progressive loss of vision may occur in rhino-orbital-cerebral mucormycosis and CT-imaging reveals bony defects in sinus borders to orbits or endocranium. Immediate diagnosis and therapy are essential. Radical procedures like orbital exenteration must be considered in all cases. Therapeutic success can be achieved due to advances in antimicrobial therapy, HBO, and treatment of the underlying disease (Arndt et al. 2009).

HBO treatment has been used for patients with brain abscesses, secondary to mucormycosis where the disease progresses despite aggressive debridement, surgery, and AMB therapy.

Candida albicans

Effect of HBO treatment and antifungal agents on *Candida albicans* has been examined in vitro. There was no response to increased atmospheric pressure alone, but addition of 100 % oxygen under pressure led to growth inhibition of pO_2 of 900 mmHg and killing of organisms at a pO_2 value of 1800 mmHg. Clinical use of HBO for this infection and a study of the interaction of HBO with antifungal agents has been suggested by but not tested clinically.

Nocardia Asteroides

This opportunistic infection occurs in patients receiving chemotherapy. Patients with Nocardia asteroides abscesses respond dramatically to HBO therapy.

Phycomycotic Fungal Infections

Necrotizing fasciitis can occur in the extremities due to invasive phycomycotic fungal infection. A standard HBO gas gangrene protocol can be used to stop the progression of the fungal infection.

HBO in the Management of AIDS

Currently, this viral infection is receiving much attention and no cure for it has been found although combination chemotherapy can keep the infection under control for long periods. In 1987, I suggested the use of HBO as a supplement to chemotherapy for the following reasons:

- Free radicals generated by HBO and accelerated by mild hyperthermia (38.5 °C) can penetrate the lipid covering of the virus, particularly before its entry into the monocytes (free form) and after its entry into the brain after crossing the blood–brain barrier, whence it may be released from the monocytes and attack the neurons. The toxic effects of free radicals on the normal cells of the body can be blocked by the use of Mg^{2+}, a cell membrane protector (see Chap. 6).
- HBO increases the production of reactive oxygen intermediates (ROIs), responsible for producing cellular oxidative stress and their enhancement or diminution of viral replication. ROIs are veridical against enveloped viruses such as HIV.
- HBO treatment has been shown to be effective against opportunistic infections found in AIDS.
- HBO pressures up to 2.5 ATA have an immune-stimulating effect and bring about an increase in the number of lymphocytes.

The limitation of this therapy is that very little of the virus is found in a free form in the body, where it would be susceptible to the effect of free radicals. It is difficult to eradicate the virus entrenched in tissue cells without killing the cells. However, it is conceivable that HBO treatment in conjunction with drug therapy may reduce AIDS encephalopathy.

Some authors have reported on results of ex vivo and in vivo quantitative assays on HIV-infected plasma and peripheral blood mononuclear cells (PBMCs) at baseline and after treatment. Uninfected PBMCs have also been treated with HBO and then exposed to HIV at ambient pressure. HIV viral load was decreased in the infected cells, and few viruses entered uninfected PBMCs exposed to HBO. The results of such studies were used to support the theory that HBO has an antiviral effect, but these observations have not been reproduced on other experimental studies. However, several hundred AIDS patients have been treated with HBO.

Concluding Remarks

There is no doubt that HBO helps the secondary infections in AIDS patients and thus improves their condition and reduces the mortality. However, the direct effect in eradicating AIDS remains to be proven. At present, very many potent and effective chemotherapeutic agents are available for treating these patients and molecular diagnostics can enable viral loads to be estimated. HBO claims of efficacy have to be tested against other drug regimens as controls. The problem may be denying effective drugs to AIDS patients. HBO has a definite place as an adjunct to antimicrobial drugs for the treatment of secondary infections in AIDS patients but claims of a direct anti-HIV effect will have to be verified by properly designed studies in this field.

Miscellaneous Infections

Leprosy (Hansen's Disease)

Leprosy is a chronic infectious disease caused by *Mycobacterium leprae*. It principally affects the peripheral nerves and skin. The spinal cord and brain are not involved.

Leprosy is prevalent in tropical countries and the total number of leprosy patients in the world is estimated to be 12 million. Effective chemotherapy was introduced only in the 1950s and the number of patients currently under treatment remains less than 33 %. Endemic foci of the disease are found in the USA, where the number of leprosy sufferers is estimated to be about 5000; they are mainly refugees from the Far East and South America.

Effective chemotherapy is available in the form of dapsone, rifampicin, and clofazamine. Leprosy can be definitely controlled by the judicious use of these drugs, individually or in combination to overcome drug resistance. Duration of therapy ranges from 6 months to 2 years or until negative skin smears are obtained. Cell-mediated immunity to *M. leprae* is impaired in patients with leprosy, but there is no generalized immune deficiency. The procedures for immune therapy with significant long-term effects are still under development. A vaccine may prevent new cases; however, eradication of leprosy and rehabilitation of the patients is still a tremendous problem.

Role of HBO in Leprosy

The use of HBO therapy in conjunction with methylene blue in the treatment of leprosy was first reported in Brazil in 1938 (Ozorio de Almeida and Costa 1938). They treated nine patients using a variety of oxygen regimens for total treatment duration of 10 h (in several sessions), using pressures from 3 ATA to 3.5 ATA. Posttreatment changes consisted of a marked decrease of skin infiltration, disappearance of tubercles, and generalized improvement in the condition of the patients. In six of the nine cases, the bacilli disappeared completely from the lesions. This report is of interest for several reasons:

- Hyperbaric air had been used previously for the treatment of tuberculosis, but this is the first recorded use of HBO for an infectious disease.
- No effective chemotherapy for leprosy was available in 1938. The rationale for using methylene blue was that,

since this substance stains the tissues, it must fix the organisms for exposure to oxygen.

- The object of the treatment was to expose the organisms to oxygen. This was in line with the thinking of the time when tuberculosis patients were exposed to fresh air and oxygen inhalation.

Gottlieb in the USA, unaware of the work in Brazil, also suggested the use of HBO in leprosy 25 years later (Gottlieb 1963). In another study later on 50 patients suffering from leprosy were treated, each with 4 sessions of HBO at 3 ATA for 30 min (Wilkinson et al. 1970). The interval between the first and the second treatment was 24 h; that between the second and third was 30 days. All the 45 patients available for evaluation improved; definite improvement was observed in 51.11 %, moderate improvement in 40 %, and slight improvement in 8.88 %. A member of the same group later on reported the results of 200 cases of leprosy treated with HBO at 3 ATA for 60 min twice daily for 3 consecutive days (Rosasco 1974). Chemotherapy was stopped during this period and not resumed. Ten patients were available for follow-up examination 5 years later and showed no sign of recurrence of the disease. This is a very small percentage of the original number of patients and therefore has no statistical significance. It is difficult to explain why there was no further work on this subject for 30 years, following the original observation of the effectiveness of HBO treatment in leprosy in 1938. A controlled study of the effect of HBO in drug-resistant intractable leprosy was conducted in India in 1979, but the results were not published. Twenty leprosy patients were divided into two groups of ten each. Drug therapy was stopped and one group was treated with HBO at 2.5 ATA (1 h twice daily) for 3 days while the other group served as a control. These patients were followed for 1 year by periodic biopsy and smear examinations. The biopsy specimens of the patients treated with HBO became negative after 8 months, whereas there were no changes in the lesions of the patients not exposed to HBO.

A protocol for investigation of the effect of HBO on leprosy has been devised that included the following (Youngblood 1984):

- Pretreatment biopsy of the lesion and inoculation into the mouse footpad model.
- Repetition of (1) after 5 days of HBO treatment at 3 ATA (1-h session twice daily).
- Microscopic examination of the pre- and post-HBO inoculated footpads and comparison of the viability, morphology, and the relative number of bacteria in the treated group with those in the untreated controls. Only one patient was reported to have been treated according to this protocol and was shown to have improved clinically; no further information was published on this project.

In conclusion, it can be stated that no definitive study of the effect of HBO on leprosy has been carried out. There is need for such a study. The adjunctive role of HBO in the drug treatment of leprosy should be considered in the following situations:

- Patients who are severely anemic and have to wait until their blood hemoglobin levels improve before chemotherapy is started.
- In drug-resistant cases with drug toxicity.
- In patients with ulcers and those who require surgery.
- There is good evidence that HBO helps in wound-healing and shortens the recovery period after plastic surgery (see Chaps. 15 and 28).

It is doubtful whether enough HBO facilities can be provided on a scale large enough to deal with this problem for millions of patients in underdeveloped countries.

Nosocomial Infections

These are infections acquired in hospital. About 80 % of nosocomial infections are caused by aerobic bacteria. *Pseudomonas aeruginosa*, a Gram-negative bacterium pertaining to the Pseudomonas family, is responsible for 6–22 % of all hospital infections. In rats infected with *P. aeruginosa*, HBO at 2 ATA for 35 min/day for 8 days induces a significant reduction in mortality and morbidity with eradication of bacteria in blood cultures, bronchial aspirate, and skin biopsies. These effects are enhanced by the concomitant intraperitoneal use of amikacine—an antibiotic used for the treatment of Gram-negative bacteria. HBO is worth a clinical trial for nosocomial infections in humans.

Tuberculosis

It has been shown experimentally that HBO inhibits the growth of *Mycobacterium tuberculosis* and has a synergistic action with the antitubercular drugs isoniazid, P-aminosalicylic acid, and streptomycin. There is not much interest in clinical uses of HBO in tuberculosis, perhaps because the current drug therapy is adequate. HBO may, however, be considered for drug-resistant organisms.

Osteomyelitis

Osteomyelitis is an inflammatory process with bacterial infection involving the bone. Additionally, ischemia and hypoxia are present in the infected bone tissue. The condition may be acute, subacute, or chronic. Chronic osteomyelitis is defined as bone infection that persists beyond 6 months with exposed bone and drainage, histological or radiological evidence of infection, or a positive bone culture. The term "refractory osteomyelitis" refers to those cases that fail to heal in spite of surgical and antibiotic therapy.

Incidence of chronic osteomyelitis is increasing because of the prevalence of predisposing conditions such as diabetes mellitus and peripheral vascular disease. Plain X-rays are useful for initial diagnosis and potential complications. Improvements in imaging such as MRI and bone scintigraphy have improved diagnostic accuracy of osteomyelitis. Direct sampling of the wound for culture and antimicrobial sensitivity is essential for targeted treatment.

Management of Osteomyelitis

The basic principles of management of osteomyelitis are as follows:

1. Surgery:
   (a) Drainage of abscess
   (b) Removal of foreign bodies
   (c) Debridement of sequestrum
   (d) Removal of barrier to normal vascularization
   (e) Obliteration of dead spaces as a result of debridement
2. Antibiotics: appropriate antibiotics at optimal dosage to be administered for an adequate length of time.

The increased incidence of methicillin-resistant microorganisms in osteomyelitis such as *Staphylococcus aureus* complicates selection of antibiotics. Surgical debridement is usually necessary in chronic cases. The recurrence rate remains high despite surgical intervention and long-term antibiotic therapy. The optimal surgical objectives are not always achievable, and this is one of the common causes of refractory osteomyelitis. Surgical treatment is effective in 70–80 % of chronic osteomyelitis cases. (This does not include cases that are denied surgery because of poor prognosis.) One does not know how many of the remaining 20–30 % would benefit from HBO therapy. The role of HBO in the management of refractory osteomyelitis is shown in Fig. 14.4.

Fig. 14.4 Although antibiotics will help kill microorganisms in the nonossified tissues around the focus of infection and surgery will remove the macroscopic portions of dead, infected bone, HBO improves host responsiveness by making the environments more favorable to WBC oxidative killing, neovascularization, and resorption of dead, infected bone. Reproduced with permission from Strauss MB. Refractory osteomyelitis. J Hyperbaric Med 1987;2: 147–159

REFRACTORY OSTEOMYELITIS

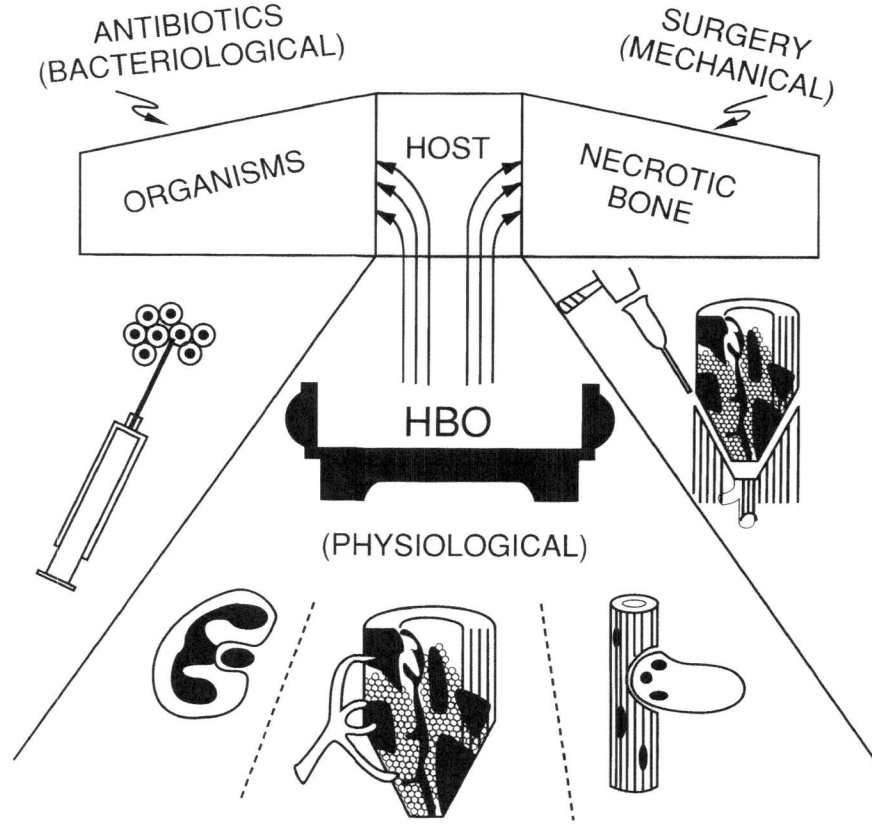

HBO Treatment of Osteomyelitis

Osteomyelitis is a hypoxic condition as shown by intramedullary pO_2 measurements, which usually give values below 30 mmHg. There are three possible causes of the hypoxia:

- Oxygen consumption by the microorganisms
- Oxygen consumption by inflammatory cells
- Interference with local perfusion due to tissue edema

The possible mechanisms of action of HBO in osteomyelitis are:

1. HBO can raise the tissue oxygen tension in partially ischemic, hypoxic tissues.
2. HBO, by providing adequate oxygen, enhances the leukocyte killing mechanisms that are oxygen dependent through hydrogen peroxide and superoxide production. HBO, by itself, has been shown to be as effective as cephalosporins in controlling staphylococcal osteomyelitis in the animal model.
3. Optimal wound pO_2 can enhance osteogenesis or neovascularization to fill the dead space with vascular or structurally sound bony tissue. Improved vascularity facilitates entry of leukocytes, antibodies, and antibiotics to the infective focus.
4. HBO enhances osteoclastic activity to remove bony debris.
5. The effectiveness of HBO in osteomyelitis may be due to the enhancement of host factors rather than to a direct effect on microorganisms causing the disease. Oxygen tensions in the infected tissues cannot always be raised to levels considered high enough to be directly toxic to the microorganisms.

The direct effect of HBO on bacteria is not important in osteomyelitis. The optimal pO_2 for these effects should be maintained at 100 mmHg. The effect of intermittent HBO on experimental staphylococcal osteomyelitis in rats was demonstrated nearly half a century ago (Hamblin 1968). Osteomyelitis was established with discharging sinuses or abscesses and confirmed radiologically. This was a controlled study and no animal received antibiotics or surgery. The treatment was given for 3 weeks and the treated animals were divided into groups according to the pressures of oxygen used. The best results were obtained in the group treated with HBO at 2 ATA for 2 h 3 times a day. Since HBO given prophylactically did not prevent the development of infections, it was concluded that the effectiveness of HBO on established osteomyelitis is due to the enhancement of host defenses and not to a direct effect on the organisms.

The effect on the intramedullary tension of 100 % oxygen exposure at 1, 2, 3, and 4 ATA pressure in rabbits with chronic right tibial osteomyelitis has been studied (Esterhai et al. 1986). The oxygen tensions were measured polarographically through implanted electrodes. The tension in the left tibia (normal, control) was low (below 30 mmHg), and the infected side still lower. It rose in response to HBO on both sides but returned to baseline in 15 min after cessation of therapy.

The effect of the following three modalities of treatment was compared in a rat tibia model of staphylococcal osteomyelitis (Mendel et al. 1999):

1. HBO alone
2. Antibiotic cefazolin
3. HBO and cefazolin

The infection rate in this model was 96 % and mortality was 0 %. HBO was found to be effective in that the number

Table 14.6 Clinical results of treatment of chronic osteomyelitis with HBO

Authors and year	Cases	Pressure	Results and comments
Slack et al. (1966)	5	2 ATA	Successful. Organisms included *Staphylococcus pyogenes* and *Proteus vulgaris*
Davis (1977)	98	2 ATA	Disease process arrested in 50 % and remained so at 5-year follow-up
Eltorai et al. (1984)	40[a]	2 ATA[b]	30 patients (68 %) were cured
Sheftel et al. (1985)	5		Methicillin-resistant staphylococcal osteomyelitis. Five of seven episodes were arrested in these patients by a combination of surgery, antibiotics, and HBO
Davis et al. (1986)	38	2 ATA[c]	34 (89.5 %) of these patients became free from clinical signs of osteomyelitis for 34 months. HBO plus wound debridement plus antibiotics

[a]Spine, ischia, hips sacrum and calcaneus
[b]Average 50 sessions
[c]48 daily HBO sessions

of colony-forming bacteria (CFB) per gram decreased from 106 to 105. Animals receiving cefazolin had a mean CFB count of 104. The best results were obtained in animals treated by a combination of HBO and cefazolin but bone sterilization was never recorded.

Clinical Results of HBO Treatment in Osteomyelitis

Clinical results of the treatment of chronic osteomyelitis are shown in Table 14.6.

There are many other reports of improvement of chronic osteomyelitis with HBO therapy, but there are no controlled studies. All the studies emphasize the important role of good surgical and antibiotic management and point out that HBO is not a substitute but a supplement to these treatments. The overall success rate in various studies ranges from 60 to 85 %. These are good results if one considers the severe nature of the cases treated with HBO. In some cases, the alternative to HBO was amputation of the involved extremity.

HBO therapy plays an important role in treatment of post-traumatic osteomyelitis following bone fractures. A combination of instrumentation removal, aggressive surgical irrigation and bone debridement, intravenous antibiotic treatment, and early HBO therapy are recommended for a compromised host who develops recurrent osteomyelitis (Delasotta et al. 2013).

HBO plays a vital role in treatment of osteomyelitis of the skull and the spine. In the latter, the involved bone cannot be removed entirely (see Chap. 21). There is only one reported study with negative effects of HBO in osteomyelitis (Esterhai et al. 1988).

Osteomyelitis of the Jaw

Osteomyelitis of the mandible is usually due to untreated odontogenic infections, post-extraction complications, and untreated or poorly managed mandibular fractures. Because the mandible receives less blood than the maxilla, it is more susceptible to infections. Nevertheless, the prognosis for osteomyelitis of the jaw is better than for osteomyelitis of the long bones. The reasons for this are the jaw's easy accessibility for debridement and its proximity to a richly vascular area with collateral circulatory pathways. The usual organisms found are:

• *Actinomyces israelii*, an obligatory anaerobe
• Eikenella corrodens
• *Bacteroides fragilis*
• *Staphylococcus aureus*

Treatment of osteomyelitis of the jaw should include the following measures:

1. Removal of the source of infection; tooth extraction or root canal therapy
2. Debridement of necrotic tissue
3. Staining and culture of the infected tissue
4. Insertion of drains and irrigation with Dakin's solution
5. Immobilization; use of fixation pins if necessary
6. Antibiotic therapy

Most cases of osteomyelitis of the jaw respond to appropriate debridement and antibiotic therapy, but some are refractory to all the measures outlined above. HBO treatment is indicated in these cases. There are few published reports of large series of patients of this type treated by HBO. Although successful treatment of patients with suppurative osteomyelitis of the jaw by surgery and antibiotics without HBO has been reported, it is difficult to eradicate diffuse sclerosing osteomyelitis, which is characterized by recurrent episodes of swelling, pain, and trismus, without abscess formation or discharge. Clinical trial of conventional therapy and of additional HBO treatments have shown that patients for whom additional HBO was used were fully relieved of symptoms, whereas those treated without HBO continued to have further minor recurrences. Adjuvant HBO is successful in the treatment of patients with chronic recurrent osteomyelitis of the mandible and is a treatment option that can avoid ablative surgery in some cases (Handschel et al. 2007).

Osteomyelitis of the Sternum

HBO has been used with good results in the treatment of chronic sternal osteomyelitis. Infectious sternal dehiscence is a serious complication after open heart surgery. Patients with infected sternal wounds can be successfully treated by a combination of surgical debridement, antiseptic irrigation, antibiotics, and HBO (2.8 ATA) with resolution of all cases of infected sternal dehiscence.

A retrospective analysis of osteomyelitis after sternotomy and cardiothoracic surgery compared 6 patients who received HBO to 6 who did not (Yu et al. 2011). The authors reported no treatment-related complications and the intensive care unit length of stay in patients who received HBO was ~40 days shorter. In addition, duration of invasive and noninvasive positive pressure ventilation was also decreased. Furthermore, they also noted that hospital mortality was lower in HBO patients.

Malignant Otitis Externa

This syndrome was first described as an antibiotic-resistant *Pseudomonas aeruginosa* infection of the external auditory meatus with osteomyelitis of the temporal bone (Chandler

1968). It usually affects patients with long-standing diabetes mellitus and a weakened immune system. Over 150 cases have been described in the literature since the original report in 1968. The overall mortality is 35%. Spread of infection beyond the external auditory meatus can produce lethal invasive osteomyelitis. Such patients should be investigated by using radiological procedures such as tomography of the temporal bone and intensive management with antibiotics, surgery, and HBO is recommended. The multimodal treatment approach of malignant otitis externa by surgical debridement, combinations of antibiotics, specific immunoglobulins, and adjunctive HBO has proved to be highly effective in improving the survival and quality of life of the patients, which justifies the high costs that this therapy may involve (Tisch and Maier 2006).

References

Arndt S, Aschendorff A, Echternach M, et al. Rhino-orbital-cerebral mucormycosis and aspergillosis: differential diagnosis and treatment. Eur Arch Otorhinolaryngol. 2009;266:71–6.

Bakker DJ. Clostridial myonecrosis. In: Davis JC, Hunt TK, editors. Problem wounds—role of oxygen. New York: Elsevier; 1988. p. 153–72.

Brummelkamp WD, Hogendijk J, Boerema I. Treatment of anaerobic infections (clostridial myositis) by drenching the tissues with oxygen under high pressure. Surgery. 1961;49:299.

Chandler JR. Malignant external otitis. Laryngoscope. 1968;78:1257.

Davis JC. Refractory osteomyelitis of the extremities and the axial skeleton. In: Davis JC, Hunt TK, editors. Hyperbaric oxygen therapy. Bethesda: Undersea Medical Society; 1977. p. 217–77.

Davis JC, Heckman JD, DeLee JC, et al. Chronic nonhematogenous osteomyelitis treated with adjuvant hyperbaric oxygen. J Bone Joint Surg. 1986;68A:1210–7.

Desola J, Escola E, Moreno E, et al. Combined treatment of gas gangrene with hyperbaric oxygen, surgery and antibiotics. National multicenter collaborative study. Med Clin (Barcelona). 1990;94:641–50.

Delasotta LA, Hanflik A, Bicking G, Mannella WJ. Hyperbaric oxygen for osteomyelitis in a compromised host. Open Orthop J. 2013;7:114–7.

Devaney B, Frawley G, Frawley L, Pilcher DV. Necrotising soft tissue infections: the effect of hyperbaric oxygen on mortality. Anaesth Intensive Care. 2015;43:685–92.

Elliott DC, Kufera JA, Myers RA. Necrotizing soft tissue infections. Risk factors for mortality and strategies for management. Ann Surg. 1996;224:672–83.

Eltorai IM, Hart GB, Strauss MB. Osteomyelitis in the spinal cord injured: a review and a preliminary report on the use of hyperbaric oxygen. Paraplegia. 1984;22:17–24.

Esterhai Jr JL, Clark JM, Morton HE, Smith DW, Steinbach A, Richter SD. Effect of hyperbaric oxygen exposure on oxygen tension within the medullary canal in the rabbit tibial osteomyelitis model. J Orthop Res. 1986;4:330–6.

Esterhai Jr JL, Pisarello J, Brighton CT, Heppenstall RB, Gelman H, Goldstein G. Treatment of chronic refractory osteomyelitis with adjunctive hyperbaric oxygen therapy. Orthop Rev. 1988;17:809–15.

Flam F, Boijsen M, Lind F. Necrotizing fasciitis following transobturator tape treated by extensive surgery and hyperbaric oxygen. Int Urogynecol J Pelvic Floor Dysfunct. 2009;20:113–5.

Gottlieb SF. The possible role of hyperbaric oxygen in the treatment of leprosy and tuberculosis. Dis Chest. 1963;44:215–7.

Hamblin DL. Hyperbaric oxygen: its effect on experimental staphylococcal osteomyelitis in rats. J Bone Joint Surg Am. 1968;50:1129–41.

Handschel J, Brüssermann S, Depprich R, Ommerborn M, Naujoks C, Kübler NR, et al. Evaluation of hyperbaric oxygen therapy in treatment of patients with osteomyelitis of the mandible. Mund Kiefer Gesichtschir. 2007;11:285–90.

Hart GB, Lamb RC, Strauss MB. Gas gangrene—a collective review. J Trauma. 1983;23:991–1000.

Hirn M, Niinikoski J. Hyperbaric oxygen in the treatment of clostridial gas gangrene. Ann Chir Gynaecol. 1988;77:37–40.

Kaide CG, Khandelwal S. Hyperbaric oxygen: applications in infectious disease. Emerg Med Clin North Am. 2008;26:571–95.

Kolpen M, Mousavi N, Sams T, Bjarnsholt T, Ciofu O, Moser C, et al. Reinforcement of the bactericidal effect of ciprofloxacin on Pseudomonas aeruginosa biofilm by hyperbaric oxygen treatment. Int J Antimicrob Agents. 2016;47:163–7.

Korhonen K, Klossner J, Hirn M, Niinikoski J. Management of clostridial gas gangrene and the role of hyperbaric oxygen. Ann Chir Gynaecol. 1999;88:139–42.

Kurt T, Vural A, Temiz A, Ozbudak E, Yener AU, Sacar S, et al. Adjunctive hyperbaric oxygen therapy or alone antibiotherapy? Methicillin resistant Staphylococcus aureus mediastinitis in a rat model. Rev Bras Cir Cardiovasc. 2015;30:538–43.

Meleney FL. Hemolytic streptococcus gangrene. Arch Surg. 1924;9:31.

Mendel V, Reichert B, Simanowski HJ, Scholz HC. Therapy with hyperbaric oxygen and cefazolin for experimental osteonyelitis due to staphylococcus auerus in rats. Undersea Hyperb Med. 1999;26:169–74.

Ozorio de Almeida A, Costa HM. Treatment of leprosy by oxygen at high pressure associated with methylene blue. Rev Bras Leprol. 1938;6:237–65.

Peters EJ, Lipsky BA, Aragón-Sánchez J, Boyko EJ, Diggle M, Embil JM, et al. Interventions in the management of infection in the foot in diabetes: a systematic review. Diabetes Metab Res Rev. 2016;32 Suppl 1:145–53.

Rosasco SA. Hyperbaric oxygen treatment of patients during resistant leprosy. In: Trapp WG, Banister EW, Davison AJ, editors. Proceedings of the 5th International Congress on Hyperbaric Medicine. Burnaby: Simon Fraser University; 1974.

Sheftel TG, Mader JT, Pennick JJ, Cierny G. Methicillin-resistant staphylococcus aureus osteomyelitis. Clin Orthop Relat Res. 1985;198:231–9.

Slack WK, Thomas DA, Dejode LRJ. Hyperbaric oxygen in treatment of trauma, ischemic disease of limbs and varicose ulcerations. In: Brown IW, Cox B, editors. Proceedings of the 3rd international congress on hyperbaric medicine. Washington, DC: National Academy of Sciences–National Research Council; 1966. p. 621–4.

Tirpitz D. The value of hyperbaric oxygenation in treatment of gas gangrene. In: Schmutz J, editor. Proceedings of the 1st Swiss symposium on hyperbaric medicine. Basel: Foundation for Hyperbaric Medicine; 1986. p. 169–93.

Tisch M, Maier H. Malignant external otitis. Laryngorhinootologie. 2006;85:763–9.

Wilkinson FF, Rosasco SA, Calori BA, et al. Conclusiones preliminares sobre el uso del oxigeno hiperbaro en lepra lepromatosa. Rev Leprol. 1970;7:459–79.

Yang Z, Hu J, Qu Y, Sun F, Leng X, Li H, et al. Interventions for treating gas gangrene. Cochrane Database Syst Rev 2015;12: CD010577.

Youngblood DA. Hyperbaric oxygen in the treatment of Hansen's disease. Hyperbaric Oxygen Rev. 1984;5:244–50.

Yu WK, Chen YW, Shie HG, Lien TC, Kao HK, Wang JH. Hyperbaric oxygen therapy as an adjunctive treatment for sternal infection and osteomyelitis after sternotomy and cardiothoracic surgery. J Cardiothorac Surg. 2011;6:141–6.

Hyperbaric Oxygen Therapy and Chronic Lyme Disease: The Controversy and the Evidence

15

Caroline E. Fife and Kristen A. Eckert

Abstract

Lyme disease, a bacterial infection caused by *Borrelia burgdorferi* and transmitted to humans by the bite of infected blacklegged ticks, is the most common vector-borne disease in the United States. The hallmark manifestation of Lyme disease, an erythema migrans around the tick bite, is found on most infected persons. Less than optimal laboratory testing is an unreliable diagnostic option for up to 20 % who present without objective symptoms. Antibiotics administered early on in the disease cure up to 90 % of infected persons. Persistent symptoms and reinfection may occur after antibiotic therapy. Patient groups advocate for chronic Lyme disease (CLD), a condition of persistent symptoms in patients which may or may not be related to *B. burgdorferi* infection, a diagnosis that is not promoted by the general medical and scientific community. The protean nature of Lyme disease in its presentation and response to conventional therapy has challenged research and driven patients, especially those with CLD, to seek alternative therapies, including hyperbaric oxygen therapy (HBOT). Neither Lyme disease nor CLD is an approved indication for HBOT, and evidence is scarce to support the use of HBOT on this confusing disease, although some dramatic cases of improvement have been reported. An HBOT registry for Lyme disease and CLD would be an important tool to better understand the number of patients treated and whether or not HBOT has a beneficial effect on this puzzling and controversial condition. This registry could serve as the vehicle to perform the prospective trials that are needed to generate potential evidence to support the use of HBOT on Lyme disease.

Keywords

Lyme disease • Chronic Lyme disease • Hyperbaric oxygen therapy • Off-label • Registry

This chapter is dedicated to the memory of William P. Fife, PhD

C.E. Fife, MD (✉)
CHI St. Luke's Wound Clinic, Lufkin, TX 75904, USA

Baylor College of Medicine, Houston, TX 77030, USA

Intellicure, Inc., 2700 Research Forest Dr., The Woodlands, TX 77381, USA
e-mail: cfife@intellicure.com

K.A. Eckert, MPhil
Strategic Solutions, Inc., 1143 Salsbury Ave., Cody, WY 82414, USA

Introduction to Lyme Disease vs. Chronic Lyme Disease: A Brief Overview

Lyme disease, a bacterial infection caused by *Borrelia burgdorferi* and transmitted to humans by the bite of infected blacklegged ticks, is the most common vector-borne disease in the United States (US) (http://www.cdc.gov/lyme/stats/index.html). The U.S. Centers for Disease Control and Prevention (CDC) reported up to a potential 36,307 cases of Lyme disease in 2013, 27,203 of which were confirmed diagnoses. The additional 9104 probable cases reported refer to patients diagnosed by a physician with serologic evidence of exposure but without any objective signs (Aucott et al. 2012;

© Springer International Publishing AG 2017
K.K. Jain, *Textbook of Hyperbaric Medicine*, DOI 10.1007/978-3-319-47140-2_15

Borgermans et al. 2014). Fourteen states of the Northeast and Midwest shared 95 % of the disease burden. Pennsylvania had the most number of confirmed cases, with 4981, while Maine had the highest incidence of Lyme in 84.8 people per 100,000 population (http://www.cdc.gov/lyme/stats/index.html).

Three to 30 days after an infected tick bites a person, an erythema migrans develops in the form of a bull's eye rash around the bite, with a circumference of up to 30 cm, in 70–80 % of infected persons (http://www.cdc.gov/lyme/signs_symptoms/index.html). Immediate symptoms include fever, chills, headache, fatigue, muscle and joint aches, and swollen lymph nodes. Months after an infection is left untreated, additional rashes may appear elsewhere on the body and the patient may have more serious symptoms, such as arthritis with severe joint pain and swelling, facial or Bell's palsy, and heart palpitations, among others.

The CDC recommends two-tier serologic testing for the diagnosis of Lyme disease. The initial testing is an immunoglobulin (Ig)M and IgG quantitative enzyme-linked immunosorbent assay, which—if positive—is then confirmed by IgG and IgM Western blots (Nelson et al. 2014; DeBiasi 2014). Since 2005, the CDC and the U.S. Food and Drug Administration (FDA) have warned against the use of other laboratory-developed tests given their potential for misdiagnosis, based on demonstrated false-positive results from laboratory contamination (Nelson et al. 2014). Unfortunately, this serologic testing has low sensitivity to early infection, in particular the IgM Western blot, and less than 50 % of patients with erythema migrans are positive (Molins et al. 2015; Marques 2015). Serologic testing sensitivity increases with the infection duration. To further complicate the matter, the two-tier serologic testing may not be effective for Lyme disease contracted outside of the US, as there are more diverse *Borrelia* species in Europe (Puri et al. 2014).

Antibiotics administered early on in the disease in 14- to 30-day courses cure 80–90 % of infected patients (Marques 2008; Smith et al. 2002), but more evidence is needed to better understand the efficacy of antibiotic therapy on Lyme disease due to the variable outcomes in the other 10–20 % of the patient population (Sapi et al. 2011; Dinser et al. 2005; Dersch et al. 2015). Persistent symptoms may still occur after primary therapy with antibiotics in some patients. Different antibiotics may be more appropriate to different *Borrelia* species, but doxycycline and ceftriaxone are more beneficial for adults and amoxicillin for children.

In the medical and scientific community, the chronic state of Lyme disease refers to ongoing infection, while posttreatment Lyme disease (PTLD) or post-Lyme disease syndrome (PLDS) is the term often used to describe patients with a clinical diagnosis of Lyme disease who have symptoms lasting for more than 6 months after stopping antibiotic therapy (Borgermans et al. 2014; Halperin 2015; Johnson et al. 2014; Aucott et al. 2013). Fatigue, myalgia, arthralgias, sleep dis-

turbances, cognitive disorders, and depression are just some of the long-term symptoms endured by this group of patients (Marques 2008). When chronic infection is left untreated, symptoms can persist in the long term and involve the nervous system in 10–15 % of patients (Halperin 2015). However, there is no evidence that nonspecific symptoms in these patients, such as fatigue and headache, reflect damage to the nervous system or are specific to and/or diagnostic of Lyme disease. In vitro studies have shown that different morphological forms of *B. burgdorferi* respond differently to antibiotics and persister *B. burgdorferi* cells when antibiotics were used have been confirmed (Sapi et al. 2011; Feng et al. 2015; Sharma et al. 2015). Round body forms and biofilm-like colonies may be resistant to antibiotics in vitro. However, there is no evidence that viable *B. burgdorferi* infection persists in humans following antimicrobial therapy, but rather, reinfection with different strains of the bacteria has been confirmed (Shapiro 2015; Oliveira and Shapiro 2015; Baker 2010). Regardless of the lack of clinical evidence of persistent infection in patients with PTLD/PLDS, there is a popular belief that extended and repeated antibiotic therapy is effective on this group of patients with persistent symptoms (Baker 2010), even though current treatment guidelines for PTLD/PLDS strongly recommend against retreatment with antibiotics (Delong et al. 2012; Fallon et al. 2012). These recommendations are based on the findings from four randomized controlled trials (RCTs) sponsored by the U.S. National Institutes of Health that demonstrated that antibiotics were not effective on persistent symptoms and that the intravenous method used caused serious adverse effects (Oliveira and Shapiro 2015; Delong et al. 2012; Fallon et al. 2012; Klempner et al. 2013) and are further supported by a more recent randomized, prospective, cross-over study (Sjöwall et al. 2012). Some argue that the original RCTs had serious enough design flaws with unrealistic primary outcomes, underpowering, and poor statistical methods (Delong et al. 2012), while others argue that repeated antibiotic therapy is effective, but not safe (Fallon et al. 2012); however, there is no credible evidence to support these claims (Klempner et al. 2013). The medical community overall feels that there is no justification of extended antibiotic therapy in the absence of infection, and there is more than sufficient evidence to disprove the use of antibiotics on patients with persistent symptoms (Halperin 2015; Baker 2010; Sjöwall et al. 2012).

Other than antibiotics, there is no other confirmed treatment option for Lyme disease. The development of a vaccine to prevent Lyme disease has not been without controversy. Two vaccines were taken off the market for a variety of reasons in the 1990s, but mainly due to low public demand and sales and safety issues (Aronowitz 2012; Plotkin 2011; Poland 2011). Recent evidence has supported the effective and safe use of an outer surface protein A (OspA) vaccine to prevent Lyme disease and reinfection and protect against most Borrelia species in humans, including one RCT that showed good results in 300 healthy adults (Comstedt et al. 2014; Wressnigg et al. 2013, 2014). However, larger confirmatory formulation studies still need to be done with infected individuals (Wressnigg et al. 2013).

Chronic Lyme Disease

The concept of chronic Lyme disease (CLD) has evolved over recent years by CLD advocates to mean a condition of persistent symptoms in patients, which may or may not be related to *B. burgdorferi* infection (Borgermans et al. 2014; Ali et al. 2014; Palmieri et al. 2013; Lymedisease.org/wp-content/uploads/2015/04/lymedisease.org-patient-survey-20151.pdf). CLD is not prolonged, untreated infection, nor is it a treated infection with persistent symptoms.

CLD is indirectly supported by the unreliability of serological testing. The confirmation of the eradication of *B. burgdorferi* is among the most challenging aspects of the management of Lyme disease (Fife and Fife 2009). The Western blot positive bands can disappear and reappear as the disease progresses. Positive bands may persist for more than a year after the disease appears to be clinically resolved (Fife and Fife 2009). Conversely, Lyme antibodies have been found present in a patient who was seronegative, because they did not appear in Western blot bands due to their sequestration in immune complexes (Schutzer et al. 1990). Clinical symptomology, therefore, might be a more accurate diagnostic endpoint then laboratory testing.

An individual who previously had acute Lyme disease that was successfully resolved with conventional therapy can develop the psychological and physical symptoms of CLD years later in the absence of (re-)infection (Garakani and Mitton 2015). In such cases, it is important to first consider the presence of other infections, recurrent infection, and pre-existing psychiatric conditions prior to diagnosing CLD.

CLD is generally promoted by patient advocacy groups, and not by the medical community (Baker 2010). Anyone can google "chronic Lyme disease" to better understand this science vs. nature debate. An example of patient advocacy is the group, LymeDisease.org. In 2015, this group provided 6104 responses from patients with Lyme disease to a patient perspective survey on Lyme disease (Lymedisease.org/wp-content/uploads/2015/04/lymedisease.org-patient-survey-20151.pdf). Ninety-seven percent of patients were diagnosed by a physician; 81 % had their diagnosis confirmed by laboratory testing. Delayed diagnosis of 6 months to longer than 2 years was reported by 78 % of patients. Common prior misdiagnoses included mood disorders (59 %), chronic fatigue (55 %), fibromyalgia (49 %), and rheumatoid arthritis—all conditions with nonspecific symptoms similar to those reported with Lyme disease. Nearly all patients (97 %) reported persisting symptoms, including fatigue (59 %), sleep impairment (50 %), muscle pain (47 %), joint pain, (46 %), depression (41 %), memory loss, cognitive impairment, and/or nerve pain (38 %), and headaches (32 %). Ninety percent reported that short-term therapy failed. Half of patients reported being ill for longer than 10 years. The survey methodology is not described (Lymedisease.org/wp-content/uploads/2015/04/lymedisease.org-patient-survey-20151.pdf), so it is difficult to interpret these results, such as why 90 % failed conventional treatment when antibiotics have been proven effective in 80–90 % of patients. Furthermore, reinfection is not discussed. However, this survey provides a better glimpse into the rationale advocacy groups have in supporting CLD as a disease, as well as the degree of patient frustration and long-term suffering. With more than 9000 probable cases of Lyme disease reported by the CDC in 2013 (http://www.cdc.gov/lyme/stats/index.html), the number of survey responses and experiences shared by these patients are not that unlikely, particularly if we assume that these individuals did not present with the erythema migrans, a factor that could have contributed to their delayed diagnosis.

Most patients of the LymeDisease.org survey respondents suffered from chronic fatigue, and more than half reported that they were misdiagnosed with chronic fatigue syndrome (CFS) (Lymedisease.org/wp-content/uploads/2015/04/lymedisease.org-patient-survey-20151.pdf). In British Columbia, where Lyme disease incidence is low, not a single patient suspected of having CLD tested positive for Lyme using serological testing, but rather, these patients had a similar phenotype to patients diagnosed with CFS (Patrick et al. 2015). Given that the sensitivity issues with serological testing resolve with a longer duration of the disease and are therefore more accurate with prolonged infection (Molins et al. 2015; Marques 2015), it is understandable that the medical community is as skeptical about CLD as is presented in the literature.

With up to 30 % of patients not presenting with the hallmark bull's eye rash and 25 % of the potential case load reported by the CDC being probable diagnoses (http://www.cdc.gov/lyme/stats/index.html; http://www.cdc.gov/lyme/signs_symptoms/index.html), Lyme disease is at the center of a polarized medical debate over its sub-optimal diagnostic methodologies, treatment limitations, and the controversy of whether or not a chronic form of the disease exists. The elephant in the CLD room is: how does one even treat a disease that may or may not exist? The protean nature of Lyme disease in its presentation and response to antibiotics has challenged research and driven patients, especially those with unconfirmed diagnoses and CLD, to seek alternative therapies. Lantos et al. recently identified more than 30 alternative, nonantimicrobial treatments for Lyme disease, which included hyperbaric oxygen therapy

(HBOT), as well as energy and radiation-based therapies, nutritional therapy, chelation and heavy metal therapy, and stem cell transplantation, among others (Lantos et al. 2015). They did not find that any of these treatments were supported by evidence in the medical literature. The use of HBOT on patients with CLD has been reported, albeit scarcely, in the literature since the 1990s (Fife and Fife 2009; Huang et al. 2014).

HBOT for Lyme Disease and CLD

Neither Lyme disease nor CLD is listed among the 14 HBOT indications approved by the Undersea & Hyperbaric Medical Society (UHMS) or FDA, which regulates the promotion of devices like hyperbaric chambers (http://uhms.org/resources/hbo-indications/html). Despite the fact that the promotion of hyperbaric oxygen therapy for Lyme Disease is considered False Advertising under the Food, Drug and Cosmetic Act, numerous facilities promote the use of HBOT for Lyme disease on the Internet. Beginning with a search on Google, we searched through online lists and databases of HBOT clinics in the US to identify clinics that promote the use of HBOT for Lyme disease and/or treated patients with Lyme disease. We identified three online lists/databases of HBOT clinics (http://hyperbariclink.com/treatment-centers/treatment-centers.aspx#.Vc9vizZRG3i; http://www.chroniclymedisease.com/hyperbaric_oxygen_chamber_treatment_location; http://www.healing-arts.org/children/hyperbaricoxygen therapy_hbot.htm). Using these links, we found 106 clinics in 29 states treating patients with Lyme disease and/or promoting the off-label use of HBOT for Lyme disease. Although our results are by no means complete, given the difficulty of tracking independent HBOT providers, these results provide a sense of the consumer healthcare market for HBOT for Lyme disease. Table 15.1 compares the CDC 2013 Lyme disease data with the results of our internet search. Interesting observations can be made. Maine, which has the highest incidence of Lyme disease, has no clinics treating Lyme disease with HBOT. Among the top five states with the most number of potential Lyme disease cases reported (Pennsylvania, Massachusetts, New York, New Jersey, and Connecticut), there are only one to six clinics listed per state. Meanwhile, California and Florida, with very low incidences reported or 0.2 per 100,000 population and 0.4 per 100,000 population, respectively, have the most number of HBOT clinics for Lyme disease combined (42 clinics, or 39.6 % of all clinics identified in Table 15.1). Thus, the results of our internet search imply that most providers promoting the use of HBOT for Lyme disease are in less endemic areas. With Lyme disease predominant in the Northeast, but not so in the West or Southeast, we cannot estimate how many from less endemic areas travel to more endemic areas. It is possible that the reason that there are fewer alternative therapies promoted for Lyme disease in the Northeast is because, given the higher risk of the population becoming infected, there are adequate Lyme disease diagnosis and management programs available. Healthcare providers in less endemic areas may not have the experience or sufficient knowledge to identify and treat Lyme disease well in the acute phase. This is further supported by the LymeDisease.org survey results, with 47 % of responders explaining that their diagnostic testing was delayed because they did not live in endemic areas (Lymedisease.org/wp-content/uploads/2015/04/lymedisease.org-patient-survey-20151.pdf). Perhaps, therefore, people in Florida and California, two states that reported 250 potential cases in 2013, are more likely to not be diagnosed and treated in a timely manner with Lyme disease and have persistent symptoms. Without any published evidence to support these patient trends towards HBOT, we can only speculate as to the reasons for the apparent regional disparity between the prevalence of disease and the popularity of HBOT.

There is no doubt that independent clinics in the US are promoting the use of HBOT for Lyme disease, as confirmed by most of their websites listed online (http://hyperbariclink.com/treatment-centers/treatment-centers.aspx#.Vc9vizZRG3i; http://www.chroniclymedisease.com/hyperbaric_oxygen_chamber_treatment_location; http://www.healing-arts.org/children/hyperbaricoxygen therapy_hbot.htm). The promotion of HBOT for Lyme disease has ethical implications for these independent providers. (See Chap. 49 for a further discussion of the ethical considerations of off-label use of HBOT.) The FDA prohibits the advertising of off-label use of marketed drugs, biologics, and medical devices (http://www.fda.gov/RegulatoryInformation/Guidances/ucm126486.htm). However, recent federal lawsuits have determined that the promotion of off-label use is protected as a form of "free speech," so long as the information regarding off-label use is provided in a "truthful and non-misleading" manner (Boumil 2013; http://insidehealthpolicy.com/login-redirect-no-cookie?n=84883&destination=node/84883). As a result of these recent legal cases, updated guidelines on off-label use are pending from the FDA.

Rationale for Using HBOT

HBOT Mechanism of Action

The effects of oxygen on a bacterial infection are well-studied. When a pathogen invades, the body's early response to infection involves the oxidative burst phenomenon, when reactive oxygen species are rapidly produced (Allen et al. 1997). The resulting lower levels of oxygen in the tissue inhibit the function of neutrophils, the phagocytes essential for the killing of foreign debris and bacteria. In the presence of osteomyelitis, neutrophil function was enhanced by increasing the tissue oxygen levels (Mader et al. 1978).

Table 15.1 United States Lyme disease statistics for 2013 and number of hyperbaric oxygen therapy (HBOT) clinics treating for Lyme disease

State	Confirmed cases (http://www.cdc.gov/lyme/stats/index.html.)	Incidence (cases per 100,000 population) (http://www.cdc.gov/lyme/stats/index.html)	Probable cases (http://www.cdc.gov/lyme/stats/index.html)	Total potential cases	Number of Lyme-treating HBOT clinics (http://hyperbariclink.com/treatment-centers/treatment-centers.aspx#.Vc9vizZRG3i; http://www.chroniclymedisease.com/hyperbaric_oxygen_chamber_treatment_location; http://www.healing-arts.org/children/hyperbaricoxygen therapy_hbot.htm)[a]
Alabama	11	0.2	13	24	2
Alaska	14	1.9	0	14	0
Arizona	22	0.3	10	32	1
Arkansas	0	0	0	0	0
California	90	0.2	22	112	28
Colorado	0	0	0	0	0
Connecticut	2111	58.7	814	2925	2
Delaware	400	43.2	109	509	0
District of Columbia	33	5.1	2	35	0
Florida	87	0.4	51	138	14
Georgia	8	0.1	0	8	3
Hawaii	0	0	0	0	0
Idaho	14	0.9	5	19	1
Illinois	337	2.6	0	337	4
Indiana	101	1.5	9	110	0
Iowa	153	5	94	247	0
Kansas	18	0.6	16	34	0
Kentucky	17	0.4	23	40	0
Louisiana	0	0	0	0	2
Maine	1127	84.8	246	1373	0
Maryland	801	13.5	396	1197	2
Massachusetts	3816	57	1474	5290	1
Michigan	114	1.2	54	168	4
Minnesota	1431	26.4	909	2340	0
Mississippi	0	0	0	0	0
Missouri	1	0	2	3	2
Montana	16	1.6	2	18	0
Nebraska	7	0.4	3	10	0
Nevada	11	0.4	5	16	3
New Hampshire	1324	100	363	1687	0

(continued)

Table 15.1 (continued)

State	Confirmed cases (http://www.cdc.gov/lyme/stats/index.html.)	Incidence (cases per 100,000 population) (http://www.cdc.gov/lyme/stats/index.html)	Probable cases (http://www.cdc.gov/lyme/stats/index.html)	Total potential cases	Number of Lyme-treating HBOT clinics (http://hyperbariclink.com/treatment-centers/treatment-centers.aspx#.Vc9vizZRG3i; http://www.chroniclymedisease.com/hyperbaric_oxygen_chamber_treatment_location; http://www.healing-arts.org/children/hyperbaricoxygen therapy_hbot.htm)[a]
New Jersey	2785	31.3	981	3766	2
New Mexico	0	0	6	6	1
New York	3512	17.9	1103	4615	6
North Carolina	39	0.4	141	180	3
North Dakota	12	1.7	17	29	0
Ohio	74	0.6	19	93	2
Oklahoma	1	0	2	3	3
Oregon	12	0.3	31	43	2
Pennsylvania	4981	39	777	5758	3
Rhode Island	444	42.2	280	724	0
South Carolina	33	0.7	9	42	2
South Dakota	3	0.4	1	4	0
Tennessee	11	0.2	14	25	1
Texas	48	0.2	34	82	3
Utah	10	0.3	5	15	1
Vermont	674	107.6	219	893	0
Virginia	925	11.2	382	1307	4
Washington	11	0.2	7	18	1
West Virginia	116	6.3	27	143	0
Wisconsin	1447	25.2	425	1872	3
Wyoming	1	0.2	2	3	0
Total	27,203	8.6	9104	36,307	106

[a]Twelve additional HBOT clinics treating Lyme disease were found when using Google to search for the websites of clinics listed in references (http://hyperbariclink.com/treatment-centers/treatment-centers.aspx#.Vc9vizZRG3i; http://www.chroniclymedisease.com/hyperbaric_oxygen_chamber_treatment_location; http://www.healing-arts.org/children/hyperbaricoxygen therapy_hbot.htm), which did not have websites listed

When *B. Burgdorferi* is confirmed in patients with Lyme disease, mitochondrial dysfunction in the immune cells results from oxidative stress and interrupted intracellular communication, observed as significantly low levels of cytosolic ionized calcium ($p < 0.0001$) compared to non-infected patients (Peacock et al. 2015). In vitro *B. Burgdorferi* cultures showed a decrease in infectivity when exposed to a partial pressure of oxygen and carbon dioxide equivalent to sea level atmospheric conditions ($PO_2 = 160$ mmHg, $PCO_2 = 0.3$ mmHg) (Austin 1993). Infectivity was viable when *B. Burgdorferi* was cultured in 4% O_2/5% CO_2 ($PO_2 = 30$ mmHg). The partial pressure of oxygen at the tissue level is approximately 30 mmHg under normal conditions; thus, it is unlikely that the bacteria could be suppressed by the host breathing normal air. However, the increase in tissue PO_2 that occurs during HBOT may have a suppressive effect on the bacteria (Austin 1993).

When breathing pure oxygen at 2.36 ATA, the inspired PO2 is 1794 mmHg. Tissue PO_2 has been variously reported, depending on whether it is measured transcutaneously or invasively, where on the body it is measured and with what instrument. However, it is reasonable to assume that tissue oxygen levels approach 300 mmHg respiring oxygen at 2.36 ATA. The elevated PO_2 may inhibit the function of *B. burgdorferi*, and the enhanced effectiveness of leukocyte function in response to elevated oxygen levels could further explain the reported beneficial effect of HBOT on patients with Lyme disease.

Treating Lyme Disease and CLD with HBOT: The Evidence

Providers who promote the use of HBOT for Lyme disease often cite the results of a 6-year Texas A&M University pilot program from the 1990s (Fife and Fife 2009). This case series involved patients with a serological diagnosis of Lyme disease, in accordance with CDC criteria, who were treated with intravenous antibiotics and deteriorated during and after treatment. We do not know for certain from the published materials if persisting or recurring infection was confirmed once patients finished their antibiotic rounds, but based on the current definitions and information we have, it appears these patients had PTLD or PSLD. Subjects underwent up to 40 1-h HBOT sessions at a pressure of 2.36 ATA. Within approximately 3 days of initiating HBOT, all subjects developed a Jarisch-Herxheimer reaction (suggesting that a competent immunological assault against the pathogen did occur), manifested by myalgias, chills, and a low-grade fever, which lasted for 2–3 weeks in most subjects. Improvement or resolution of symptoms was observed in 37 of 38 subjects within 3 weeks posttreatment and was sustained in approximately 70% of subjects for up to 6 years posttreatment. The delayed benefit may have been because of the time required to reduce chronic inflammation and cytokine hyperactivity to normal levels. Improved cognitive abilities and concentration and abated

depression were also reported in patients who had previous symptoms (Fife and Fife 2009).

We previously detailed three case examples from the pilot program at Texas A&M. These case reports are summarized in Table 15.2. They were all female patients who never presented with an erythema migrans, but who were diagnosed with Lyme disease by serological testing. All three women had many symptoms that recurred and/or persisted for 3 years to up to possible 14 years that greatly interfered with their physical and emotional well-being, with Case No. 3 having to be taken out of school as a result of her illness. Cases No. 1 and 3 both resided in areas known to be endemic for Lyme disease, and the patient history of Case No. 1 might suggest that this was a case of recurring infection. All reported that they were improved 5 months after stopping HBOT, with improvements already noticeable during the treatment period in Cases No. 2 and 3.

HBOT was also reported to benefit a 31-year-old patient with recurring Lyme disease and persistent symptoms in Taiwan (Huang et al. 2014). All symptoms of the nervous system, including irritability, mood swings, poor concentration, loss of short-term memory, sleep disturbance, facial tingling, blurred vision, and photophobia, and migrating arthralgias of the musculoskeletal system, were resolved following 30 HBOT sessions.

Fibromyalgia syndrome (FMS) is a persisting, nonspecific, and painful condition that is aggravated by Lyme disease (Efrati et al. 2015; Schmidt-Wilcke and Clauw 2011; Sarzi-Puttini et al. 2011). In a prospective, active control crossover trial of 60 female patients with FMS, HBOT administered in forty 90-min sessions, 5 days/week, using 100% oxygen at 2 ATA led to significant improvement in both treated and crossover groups (Efrati et al. 2015). Based on SPECT imaging analysis, it was found that HBOT induces neuroplasticity and can significantly rectify abnormal brain activity in areas affected by FMS-related pain. However, during the first 10–20 sessions, some subjects (29%) experienced intensified pain which later ameliorated and is not yet understood. The potential use of HBOT to treat patients with CLD who have FMS requires further research.

There have been intriguing reports of Lyme disease presenting as sudden hearing loss and responding to HBOT (Piper et al. 2011; Peltomaa et al. 2000; Espiney Amaro et al. 2015). Idiopathic sudden sensorineural hearing loss (ISSHL) is the most recently approved HBOT indication by the UHMS (Piper et al. 2011). It is defined as a hearing loss of at least 30 dB that occurs within 3 days over at least three contiguous frequencies. With a known annual US incidence of 5–20 cases per 100,000 population, the majority of ISSHL cases (65%) resolve spontaneously. In a subpopulation of patients with sudden hearing loss, it was discovered after serological testing that the prevalence of *B. burgdorferi* infection was six times more than the general patient population

Table 15.2 Case examples ($n = 3$) from the pilot hyperbaric oxygen therapy (HBOT) and Lyme disease program at Texas A&M University (Fife and Fife 2009)

#	Sex	Age (y)	Patient history	Age at diagnosis (y)	Method of diagnosis	Antibiotic treatment	Symptoms	Adverse reaction to HBOT	Status of HBOT benefit	Patient status, 5 months post-HBOT
1	F	40	• Past diagnosis of non-convulsive epilepsy and migraines • No history of tick bite or erythema migrans • Lived in Lyme disease-endemic area	35	(Positive) serological testing	• First clarithromycin[a] • Second cefixime[a] • Third intravenous ceftriaxone[a] • Fourth amoxicillin[a] and probenicid[a] • Fifth sodium divalproex,[a] clonazepam,[a] cefotaxime,[a] and imipenem-cilastatin	• Chronic fatigue • Limited walking distance • Constant joint pain • Serious cognitive difficulties • Suicidal ideation	• Severe JH reaction during 3-weeks of 32 HBOT sessions	• Improved walking distance and cognitive function at 2-months post-HBOT; antibiotics stopped	Many ADLs resumed at normal levels
2	F	39	• No history of tick bite or erythema migrans	33	(Positive) serological testing	• Regimen(s) not specified, but antibiotics caused a JH reaction	• Partial loss of vision in left eye • Paresthesia on left side • Generalized fatigue • Reduced mental alertness • Joint stiffness • Muscle pain • Left leg weakness	• Extreme fatigue after third HBOT session (possible JH reaction) • Tingling in left foot after 4–5 sessions	• More energy, decreased pain in left foot, and leg weakness resolved after sixth HBOT session • Stopped antibiotics 4 months post-HBOT	Improved with only episodic "down days"
3	F	16	• +10 years of recurring symptoms • No history of tick bite or erythema migrans • Lived in Lyme disease-endemic area	13	(Positive) serological testing	• Aggressive long-term treatment [regimen(s) not specified] that alleviated temporarily symptoms was but ended due to severe JH reaction	• Fatigue • Joint and muscle pain • Mood swings • Weight gain and loss • Insomnia • Encephalo-pathy • Short-term memory loss • Headaches[b]	• Fever and headache (possible JH reaction) after third HBOT session	• After 4–5 treatments, concentration increased from 30 min to 3 h	Continued to improve, allowing patient to excel in college

y years, *F* female, *JH* Jarisch Herxheimer, *ADL* activities of daily living

[a]Antibiotics were terminated prior to study due to lack of benefit

[b]All symptoms aggravated by stress; patient was removed from high school

(Peltomaa et al. 2000). There has been a case report of a patient with Lyme disease whose only presenting symptom was sudden hearing loss (initially without cause), which abated with HBOT and systemic corticosteroid therapy. Later serological testing confirmed Lyme disease, and systemic antibiotic therapy fully restored the patients' hearing and resolved the infection (Espiney Amaro et al. 2015).

The optimal HBOT regimen for CLD is unknown—whether treatments should be given once or twice daily, every day until all sessions are completed, or with days off in between session (Fife and Fife 2009).

The Need for a HBOT Medical Registry

Given the number of centers promoting the use of HBOT in CDL and the potential number of patients treated (based on current Lyme disease incidence data), the lack of information regarding the outcome of HBOT treated patients is troubling. Despite the paucity of evidence on the safety and efficacy of HBOT on Lyme disease and the questionable existence of CLD, patient advocacy groups and independent providers adamantly promote HBOT for Lyme disease to the public. HBOT is clearly a treatment option that is valued by a sub-set of the patient population with nonspecific symptoms and unconfirmed infection. However, if the scientific and medical community does not perform more research on HBOT and Lyme disease, then this alternative treatment will never be accepted for routine use in clinical practice and will never be covered by insurance. The challenges of performing research on Lyme disease are many—from unreliable diagnostic and laboratory methods that cannot with certainty identify the *B. burgdorferi* nor confirm its eradication in a treated patient, to the CLD controversy that divides the public and medical communities. So far, the evidence for HBOT in Lyme disease has been limited to small case series. RCTs are the gold standard to prove the efficacy of a treatment, but in Lyme disease, these are mainly undertaken by pharmaceutical companies investigating antibiotic therapies and that would have little financial incentive to investigate efficacy of HBOT on Lyme disease (Fife and Fife 2009). It has been suggested that the use of medical registries to assess the potential benefit of HBOT on understudied diseases would generate more data and better analysis of the effect of HBOT on Lyme (Fife and Fife 2009; Chan and Brody 2001).

An HBOT registry would immediately fill a long-term gap in knowledge on the number of patients with Lyme disease and CLD who are treated with HBOT. We can estimate from an internet search the number of providers that treat Lyme disease with HBOT (see Table 15.1), but we cannot know from this information how many patients are treated. A study in Tennessee demonstrated just how difficult it is to get accurate data on the number of patients with Lyme disease (Jones et al. 2013). Confirmed cases of Lyme disease were compared using data reported from the Tennessee Department of Health and a private managed care organization for 2000–2009. The private sector incidence of Lyme disease was 7.7 times higher than that reported by the public sector, which suggests underreporting of nearly 200 annual cases (Jones et al. 2013). National medical registries would enable the collection of more accurate data from both the public and private sector and help the medical community understand better the number of probable vs. confirmed cases and the issues concerning misdiagnoses. For example, the fact that there are more independent clinics promoting HBOT for Lyme disease in less endemic states (e.g., Florida and California) might be supported by medical registry data if it were found that more patients in those states are going undiagnosed, are misdiagnosed, or treated with inadequate treatment regimens.

Prior to developing a registry, there must be an established, defined treatment protocol that is approved by a sponsoring Institutional Review Board (IRB) (Fife and Fife 2009; Chan and Brody 2001). Participating facilities must have this protocol approved by their respective IRBs or an independent IRB. Participating patients also must sign a consent protocol. All participating patients with Lyme disease/CLD would receive HBOT as an adjunct to conventional therapy. A central repository would host patient outcome data for analysis. Registry data can be used to define treatment protocols, as well as to define a subset of patients who are unlikely to benefit from HBOT and/or should be excluded from clinical trials (Fife and Fife 2009; Chan and Brody 2001). These data could provide more evidence on the efficacy of HBOT for Lyme disease. They could also generate more analysis of patients diagnosed with CLD and help the medical community better understand and respond to this apparently increasing group of patients with frustrating physical and psychological symptoms.

Conclusion

Clearly, HBOT is valued by patients who have persistent symptoms after stopping conventional therapy for Lyme disease, and by patients who suspect they have Lyme disease or CLD. At the same time, Lyme disease remains an unproven indication for HBOT and CLD remains an unconfirmed condition in the medical community. It is necessary to generate more research on the efficacy of HBOT. It appears that HBOT at least ameliorates persistent symptoms in patients who have already undergone antibiotic therapy for Lyme disease. Whether or not this beneficial effect is a placebo, we cannot say. Until better data are available, HBOT will continue to be considered investigational for Lyme disease in all its presentations.

It is possible for HBOT to be provided in an ethical manner for off-label indications, including CLD. For the symptom of ISSHL, which can occur in patients with Lyme disease, HBOT would seem to be indicated. Lyme disease might be a rare (and undiagnosed) cause of ISSHL. Given the many nonspecific and persistent symptoms that can occur with Lyme disease and CLD, and that only Lyme *recurrence* has been scientifically confirmed (as opposed to a "chronic" infection), further research is needed. It is necessary for us to investigate the use of HBOT on nonspecific symptoms attributed to CDL, but which are also found in the general patient population. An HBOT registry for patients with Lyme disease and CLD would be an important tool to better understand the number of patients treated, especially those with CLD. Such a registry could facilitate the design of the prospective trials that will be needed to determine whether HBOT is effective in this difficult, frustrating, and confusing disease.

References

Ali A, Vitulano L, Lee R, Weiss TR, Colson ER. Experiences of patients identifying with chronic Lyme disease in the healthcare system: a qualitative study. BMC Fam Pract. 2014;15:79.

Allen DB, Maguire JJ, Mahdavian M, Wicke C, Marcocci L, Scheuenstuhl H, et al. Wound hypoxia and acidosis limit neutrophil bacterial killing mechanisms. Arch Surg. 1997;132:991–6.

Aronowitz RA. The rise and fall of the Lyme disease vaccines: a cautionary tale for risk interventions in American medicine and public health. Milbank Q. 2012;90:250–77.

Aucott JN, Seifter A, Rebman AW. Probable late Lyme disease: a variant manifestation of untreated Borrelia burgdorferi infection. BMC Infect Dis. 2012;12:173.

Aucott JN, Crowder LA, Kortte KB. Development of a foundation for a case definition of post-treatment Lyme disease syndrome. Int J Infect Dis. 2013;17:e443–9.

Austin FE. Maintenance of infective Borrelia burgdorferi Sh-2-82 in 4% oxygen–%% carbon dioxide in vitro. Can J Microbiol. 1993;29:1103–10.

Baker PJ. Chronic Lyme disease: in defense of the scientific enterprise. FASEB J. 2010;24:4175–7.

Borgermans L, Goderis G, Vandevoorde J, Devroey D. Relevance of chronic Lyme disease to family medicine as a complex multidimensional chronic disease construct: a systematic review. Int J Family Med. 2014;2014:138016.

Boumil MM. Off-label marketing and the First Amendment. N Engl J Med. 2013;368:103–5.

Chan EC, Brody B. Ethical dilemmas in hyperbaric medicine. Undersea Hyperb Med. 2001;28:123–30.

Chroniclymedisease.com. Location of hyperbaric oxygen treatment centers. http://www.chroniclymedisease.com/hyperbaric_oxygen_chamber_treatment_location. Accessed 15 Aug 2015.

Comstedt P, Hanner M, Schüler W, Meinke A, Lundberg U. Design and development of a novel vaccine for protection against Lyme borreliosis. PLoS One. 2014;9, e113294.

DeBiasi RL. A concise critical analysis of serologic testing for the diagnosis of Lyme disease. Curr Infect Dis Rep. 2014;16:450.

Delong AK, Blossom B, Maloney EL, Phillips SE. Antibiotic retreatment of Lyme disease in patients with persistent symptoms: a biostatistical review of randomized, placebo-controlled, clinical trials. Contemp Clin Trials. 2012;33:1132–42.

Dersch R, Freitag MH, Schmidt S, Sommer H, Rauer S, Meerpohl JJ. Efficacy and safety of pharmacological treatments for acute Lyme neuroborreliosis—a systematic review. Eur J Neurol. 2015. doi:10.1111/ene.12744. [Epub ahead of print].

Dinser R, Jendro MC, Schnarr S, Zeidler H. In vitro susceptibility testing of Borrelia burgdorferi sensu lato isolates cultured from patients with erythema migrans before and after antimicrobial chemotherapy. Antimicrob Agents Chemother. 2005;49:1294–301.

Efrati S, Golan H, Bechor Y, Faran Y, Daphna-Tekoah S, Sekler G, et al. Hyperbaric oxygen therapy can diminish fibromyalgia syndrome—prospective clinical trial. PLoS One. 2015;10, e0127012.

Espiney Amaro C, Montalvão P, Huins C, Saraiva J. Lyme disease: sudden hearing loss as the sole presentation. J Laryngol Otol. 2015;129:183–6.

Fallon BA, Petkova E, Keilp JG, Britton CB. A reappraisal of the U.S. clinical trials of Post-Treatment Lyme Disease Syndrome. Open Neurol J. 2012;6:79–87.

Feng J, Auwaerter PG, Zhang Y. Drug combinations against Borrelia burgdorferi persisters in vitro: eradication achieved by using daptomycin, cefoperazone and doxycycline. PLoS One. 2015;10, e0117207.

Fife WP, Fife CE. Textbook of hyperbaric medicine. In: Jain KK, editor. Hyperbaric oxygen therapy in chronic Lyme disease. 5th ed. Germany: Hogrefe & Huber; 2009. p. 149–55.

Garakani A, Mitton AG. New-onset panic, depression with suicidal thoughts, and somatic symptoms in a patient with a history of Lyme disease. Case Rep Psychiatry. 2015;2015:457947.

Halperin JJ. Chronic Lyme disease: misconceptions and challenges for patient management. Infect Drug Resist. 2015;8:119–28.

Healing-arts.org. Hyperbaric oxygen therapy providers and treatment centers in the United States treating autism, cerebral palsy and other neurological disorders. 2008. http://www.healing-arts.org/children/hyperbaricoxygen therapy_hbot.htm. Accessed 15 Aug 2015.

Huang CY, Chen YW, Kao TH, Kao HK, Lee YC, Cheng JC, et al. Hyperbaric oxygen therapy as an effective adjunctive treatment for chronic Lyme disease. J Chin Med Assoc. 2014;77:269–71.

Hyperbariclink. Hyperbaric oxygen treatment centers directory. Hyperbariclink, LLC. 2015. http://hyperbariclink.com/treatment-centers/treatment-centers.aspx#.Vc9vizZRG3i. Accessed 15 Aug 2015.

Inside Health Policy. Federal Judge Lets Amarin Promote Vascepa Off-Label, Say FDA Policies Violate 1st Amendment. 7 Aug 2015. http://insidehealthpolicy.com/login-redirect-no-cookie?n=84883&destination=node/84883. Accessed 10 Aug 2015.

Johnson L, Wilcox S, Mankoff J, Stricker RB. Severity of chronic Lyme disease compared to other chronic conditions: a quality of life survey. PeerJ. 2014;2, e322.

Jones SG, Coulter S, Conner W. Using administrative medical claims data to supplement state disease registry systems for reporting zoonotic infections. J Am Med Inform Assoc. 2013;20:193–8.

Klempner MS, Baker PJ, Shapiro ED, Marques A, Dattwyler RJ, Halperin JJ, et al. Treatment trials for post-Lyme disease symptoms revisited. Am J Med. 2013;126:665–9.

Lantos PM, Shapiro ED, Auwaerter PG, Baker PJ, Halperin JJ, McSweegan E, et al. Unorthodox alternative therapies marketed to treat Lyme disease. Clin Infect Dis. 2015;60:1776–82.

LymeDisease.org. Outcomes important to Lyme patients. Results of a LymeDisease.org patient survey conducted in 2015. Lymedisease.org/wp-content/uploads/2015/04/lymedisease.org-patient-survey-20151.pdf. Accessed 19 Aug 2015.

Mader JT, Adams KR, Couch LA, Sutton TE. Therapy of hyperbaric oxygen in experimental osteomyelitis due to Staphylococcus aureus in rabbits. J Infect Dis. 1978;138:312–28.

Marques AM. Chronic Lyme disease: a review. Infect Dis Clin North Am. 2008;22:341–60.

Marques AR. Laboratory diagnosis of Lyme disease: advances and challenges. Infect Dis Clin North Am. 2015;29:295–307.

Molins CR, Ashton LV, Wormser GP, Hess AM, Delorey MJ, Mahapatra S, et al. Development of a metabolic biosignature for detection of early Lyme disease. Clin Infect Dis. 2015;60:1767–75.

Nelson C, Hojvat S, Johnson B, Petersen J, Schriefer M, Beard CB, et al. Concerns regarding a new culture method for Borrelia burgdorferi not approved for the diagnosis of Lyme disease. MMWR Morb Mortal Wkly Rep. 2014;63:333.

Oliveira CR, Shapiro ED. Update on persistent symptoms associated with Lyme disease. Curr Opin Pediatr. 2015;27:100–4.

Palmieri JR, King S, Case M, Santo A. Lyme disease: case report of persistent Lyme disease from Pulaski County, Virginia. Int Med Case Rep J. 2013;6:99–105.

Patrick DM, Miller RR, Gardy JL, Parker SM, Morshed MG, Steiner TS, et al. Lyme disease diagnosed by alternative methods: a phenotype similar to that of chronic fatigue syndrome. Clin Infect Dis. 2015;61:1084–91. pii: civ470.

Peacock BN, Gherezghiher TB, Hilario JD, Kellermann GH. New insights into Lyme disease. Redox Biol. 2015;5:66–70.

Peltomaa M, Pyykkö I, Sappälä I, Viitanen L, Viljanen M. Lyme borreliosis, an etiological factor in sensorineural hearing loss? Eur Arch Otorhinolaryngol. 2000;257:317–22.

Piper SM, LeGros TL, Murphy-Lavoie H. Idiopathic sudden sensorineural hearing loss (New! approved on October 8, 2011 by the UHMS Board of Directors). Undersea & Hyperbaric Medical Society. https://www.uhms.org/14-idiopathic-sudden-sensorineural-hearing-loss-new-approved-on-october-8-2011-by-the-uhms-board-of-directors.html. Accessed 15 July 2015.

Plotkin SA. Correcting a public health fiasco: the need for a new vaccine against Lyme disease. Clin Infect Dis. 2011;52 Suppl 3:s271–5.

Poland GA. Vaccines against Lyme disease: what happened and what lessons can we learn? Clin Infect Dis. 2011;52 Suppl 3:s253–8.

Puri BK, Segal DR, Monro JA. Diagnostic use of the lymphocyte transformation test-memory lymphocyte immunostimulation assay in confirming active Lyme borreliosis in clinically and serologically ambiguous cases. Int J Clin Exp Med. 2014;7:5890–2.

Sapi E, Kaur N, Anyanwu S, Luecke DF, Datar A, Patel S, et al. Evaluation of in-vitro antibiotic susceptibility of different morphological forms of Borrelia burgdorferi. Infect Drug Resist. 2011;4:97–113.

Sarzi-Puttini P, Atzeni F, Mease PJ. Chronic widespread pain: from peripheral to central evolution. Best Pract Res Clin Rheumatol. 2011;25:133–9.

Schmidt-Wilcke T, Clauw DJ. Fibromyalgia: from pathophysiology to therapy. Nat Rev Rheumatol. 2011;7:518–27.

Schutzer SE, Coyle PK, Belman AL, Golightly MG, Drulle J. Sequestration of antibody to Borrelia burgdorferi in immune complexes in seronegative Lyme disease. Lancet. 1990;335:312–5.

Shapiro ED. Repeat or persistent Lyme disease: persistence, recrudescence or reinfection with Borrelia Burgdorferi? F1000Prime Rep. 2015;7:11.

Sharma B, Brown AV, Matluck NE, Hu LT, Lewis K. Borrelia burgdorferi, the causative agent of Lyme disease, forms drug-tolerant persister cells. Antimicrob Agents Chemother. 2015;59:4616–24. pii: AAC.00864-15.

Sjöwall J, Ledel A, Ernerudh J, Ekerfelt C, Forsberg P. Doxycycline-mediated effects on persistent symptoms and systemic cytokine responses post-neuroborreliosis: a randomized, prospective, crossover study. BMC Infect Dis. 2012;12:186.

Smith RP, Schoen RT, Rahn DW, Sikand VK, Nowakowski J, Parenti DL, et al. Clinical characteristics and treatment outcome of early Lyme disease in patients with microbiologically confirmed erythema migrans. Ann Intern Med. 2002;136:421–8.

U.S. Food and Drug Administration. "Off-label" and investigational use of marketed drugs, biologics, and medical devices—information sheet. Updated 25 June 2014. http://www.fda.gov/RegulatoryInformation/Guidances/ucm126486.htm. Accessed 10 Aug 2015.

Undersea & Hyperbaric Medical Society. Indications for hyperbaric oxygen therapy. http://uhms.org/resources/hbo-indications/.html. Accessed 7 Sept 2015.

United States Centers for Disease Control and Prevention. Lyme disease. data and statistics. http://www.cdc.gov/lyme/stats/index.html. Accessed 15 Aug 2015.

United States Centers for Disease Control and Prevention. Signs and symptoms of untreated Lyme disease. http://www.cdc.gov/lyme/signs_symptoms/index.html. Accessed 28 Aug 2015.

Wressnigg N, Pöllabauer EM, Aichinger G, Portsmouth D, Löw-Baselli A, Fritsch S, et al. Safety and immunogenicity of a novel multivalent OspA vaccine against Lyme borreliosis in healthy adults: a double-blind, randomised, dose-escalation phase 1/2 trial. Lancet Infect Dis. 2013;13:680–9.

Wressnigg N, Barrett PN, Pöllabauer EM, O'Rourke M, Portsmouth D, Schwendinger MG, et al. A novel multivalent OspA vaccine against Lyme borreliosis is safe and immunogenic in an adult population previously infected with Borrelia burgdorferi sensulato. Clin Vaccine Immunol. 2014;21:1490–9.

K.K. Jain

Abstract

This chapter describes the basics of how oxygen enhances wound healing. Hyperbaric oxygen (HBO) promotes wound healing by counteracting tissue hypoxia and is a valuable adjunct in the management of ischemic, infected, and nonhealing wounds. Important applications include ulcers in diabetic foot. In plastic surgery, HBO improves the survival of skin flaps. It reduces the mortality and morbidity in burns. Applications of HBO in management of skin disorders, frostbite, and spider bites are also discussed.

Keywords

Arterial insufficiency ulcers • Diabetic ulcer • Frostbite • Hyperbaric oxygen (HBO) • Nonhealing wounds • Plastic surgery • Skin diseases • Spider bite • Thermal burns • Venous ulcers • Wound healing

Introduction

These three topics are lumped together in this chapter because nonhealing wounds frequently come under the care of plastic surgeons and disorders of the skin form a common bond between plastic surgery and dermatology.

A wound is a disturbance in the continuity of intact tissue structures, mostly associated with loss of substance. The damage may be the result of mechanical, thermal, physical, surgical, or chemical influences. An ulcer is a local defect, or excavation of the surface of an organ or tissue, which is produced by sloughing of inflammatory necrotic tissue. The cutaneous wound is described as an ulcer if there is focal loss of dermis and epidermis.

The rapidly aging population and patients with multiple concomitant pathologies present an increasing population of patients with nonhealing and problem wounds causing an unwelcome challenge for all healthcare providers. Nonhealing wounds are a growing public health concern,

and >$25 billion per year in the USA are spent caring for patients with chronic wounds. Methods that may be used to heal soft tissue wounds are shown in Table 16.1.

Traditional surgical procedures have not solved the problem of nonhealing wounds. Many of the patients are not surgical candidates, and there are problems with healing of donor sites of the skin graft. Wound closure alone does not suffice as there is a high rate of wound dehiscence. Several nonsurgical methods are in development. A revolution in wound care has been the introduction of Apligraf® to cover the skin ulcer. It will be described further in the management of venous ulcers for which it has been approved and is in clinical trials for the management of diabetic and pressure ulcers. Keratinocyte growth factor (repifermin) is in phase II studies. It stimulates the growth of epithelial cells and might attract fibroblasts to the site of the wound, thereby stimulating the production of new connective tissue.

Hyperbaric medicine is only an adjunctive and rather slow method of promoting wound healing. Undue emphasis has been placed on this approach with some hyperbaric centers specializing only in wound healing. Application of HBO to wound healing has been recommended by the Undersea and Hyperbaric Medical Society and approved by the healthcare providers on the basis of economic studies carried out prior to

K.K. Jain, MD, FRACS, FFPM (✉)
1 Blaesiring 7, Basel 4057, Switzerland
e-mail: jain@pharmabiotech.ch

Table 16.1 Methods of treatment of ulcers

Surgical
- Surgical debridement and closure
- Conventional skin grafting

Nonsurgical
- Wound dressings with application of various chemicals
- Exogenous application of growth factors: keratinocyte growth factor, platelet-derived growth factor
- Application of bioengineered skin implant, e.g., Apligraf®
- Electrical stimulation
- Hyperbaric oxygen
- Vacuum-assisted closure system

Correction of underlying cause
- Stripping of varicose veins for venous ulcers
- Management of chronic venous insufficiency by drugs, e.g., Venoruton®
- Control of diabetes in case of diabetic ulcers
- Treatment of infections
- Eradication of underlying osteomyelitis
- Correction of malnutrition
- Counteracting vasoconstriction: idiopathic or drug induced
- Reduction of steroid use

the introduction of new methods. HBO will remain an important adjunct to wound healing but its role needs to be redefined. Because the focus of this textbook is on HBO, wound healing and the role of oxygen in this process will be described as a prelude to the discussion of the use of HBO in wound care.

Wound Healing

Wound healing is a complex process involving multiple interacting cell types and biochemical mediators. Following tissue injury, platelets and fibrin are attracted to the wound site. Macrophages, fibroblasts, smooth muscle cells, and endothelial cells follow. These cells become organized, interact, and produce cytokines that stimulate cell growth. Angiogenesis and collagen production follow. Macrophages phagocytize dead tissue and contaminants, and the wound becomes filled with granulation tissue. Finally the wound site is populated by cells normally present at that location, and the wound is considered to have healed.

Role of Oxygen in Wound Healing

Oxygen is a critical nutrient of the wound and plays an important role in wound repair. Fluctuations of oxygen tension within the physiological range control the proliferation of fibroblasts by altering the activity of a stable intermediate substance that regulates the cellular response to growth factors. Oxygen is required for hydroxylation of proline and lysine, a step that is necessary for the release of collagen from the fibroblasts and its incorporation into the healing wound matrix.

Some local hypoxia is an inevitable result of tissue injury and may act as a stimulus to repair. Wound perfusion also depends on angiogenesis. An angiogenic factor is produced by macrophages under hypoxic conditions or exposure to high lactate levels. This process is not inhibited by oxygen administration as tissue levels are maintained constantly at high oxygen tension to inhibit this process.

Pathophysiology of Nonhealing Wounds

A chronic (nonhealing) wound or the so-called problem wound is defined as any wound which fails to heal within a reasonable period by the use of conventional medical and surgical methods. Conditions associated with nonhealing of wounds include arterial insufficiency, diabetes, cancer, infections, stress, and use of corticosteroids. Nonhealing in a wound is mostly related to hypoxia and ischemia. The metabolic requirements of the dividing fibroblasts are increased. Since the energy needs for repair are the greatest at the time the local circulation is impaired, there is an energy crisis in the wound. Hypoxia thus impairs collagen synthesis, and the collagen fibers that are formed have low tensile strength. When the environmental oxygen tension is less than 10 mmHg, fibroblasts do not migrate properly. Anoxia leads to accumulation of metabolites such as ammonia that cause swelling of cells and impair healing. Hypoxia can activate enzymes that synthesize collagen. This paradox is partially explained by the observation that synthesis of collagen is doubled by elevation of lactate (5–15 mmol) induced by hypoxia. If the tissue pO_2 is raised to 40 mmHg, collagen production rises sevenfold. Wounds in ischemic areas are highly susceptible to infection which is known to interfere with wound healing.

Regardless of etiology, a common denominator of nonhealing wounds is tissue hypoxia. This has been confirmed by tissue oxygen studies. The extent of the "problem" is a clinical definition that is partially proportional to the degree of hypoxia. Ischemia is a common cause of nonhealing wounds, but ischemia and hypoxia are not the same. Ischemic wounds are usually hypoxic, but not all hypoxic wounds are ischemic. A wound with adequate perfusion may be relatively hypoxic as infection in the wound can raise the oxygen requirements.

Some common causes of cutaneous ulceration with examples are listed in Table 16.2.

Table 16.2 Some common causes of cutaneous ulcers

1.	Vascular: arterial or venous insufficiency
2.	Metabolic: diabetes
3.	Physical trauma: decubitus ulcers, burns, radiation, frostbite
4.	Infections: bacterial, fungal, etc.
5.	Neuropathic: tabes dorsalis and syringomyelia
6.	Neoplastic: squamous cell carcinoma
7.	Toxic: drug induced

Wound Healing Enhancement by Oxygen

Rationale of the Use of Oxygen

The rationale of using oxygen in wound healing can be summarized as follows:

1. Hypoxia in the wounds can be corrected by oxygen therapy, which varies from inhalation of 40 % oxygen at ambient pressure to 100 % oxygen at 2.5 ATA. High pressures are needed to oxygenate the hypoxic center of chronic nonhealing wounds.
2. Hypoxia can arise in a normally perfused tissue when it is the site of an inflammatory reaction, and HBO at 2 ATA has been shown to improve the tissue oxygenation in this situation.
3. Intermittent correction of wound hypoxia by oxygen therapy increases fibroblast replication and collagen production.
4. Improvement of oxygen supply raises the RNA/DNA ratio in the tissues, indicating increased formation of rough endoplasmic reticulum by the cells of the wounded area, and a higher degree of cellular differentiation.
5. Raising the wound oxygen tension increases the capability of the leukocytes to kill pathogenic bacteria (see Chap. 14).
6. The increased oxygen supply meets the increased oxygen needs of the healing wound.
7. Oxygen administered at 1–2 ATA promotes the rate of epithelialization in ischemic wounds.
8. HBO promotes neoangiogenesis in wounds.

The benefit of HBO in hypoxic wounds is depicted schematically in Fig. 16.1.

New tissues striving to fill the dead space of a wound need to be supplied by a new vasculature, which follows the formation of collagen. Capillaries grow into the hypoxic area, and collagen synthesis is carried further into the wound in this manner. Obliteration of the dead space proceeds in cyclical fashion. Increasing the capillary pO_2 tension by HBO increases the amount of oxygen reaching the advancing cells. These cells are able to migrate further and retain the ability to synthesize. This enables the vascular supply to advance more quickly, which ensures faster closure of the wound.

Experimental Studies

Wounds exposed to oxygen at 2.5 ATA show linear strength increase in the first week. Prolonged hyperoxygenation beyond the optimal needs can retard healing. HBO has been shown to reduce the severity of damage in cryobiologic wounds in rats and to stimulate faster and better tissue repair. The complex cell interaction involved in wound healing and the effect of HBO on this are not fully understood. The healing effect of O_2 in chronic wounds is not explained by increased phagocytosis or increased adhesions of macrophages. Results of a study in a rat model of ischemic wound indicate that HBO improves wound healing by downregulation of HIF-1a and subsequent target gene expression with attenuation of cell apoptosis and reduction of inflammation (Zhang et al. 2008).

Role of Nitric Oxide in HBO-induced Wound Healing

In controlled experiments, HBO (2.5 ATA for 2 h) used three times has been shown to increase the bursting strength and stimulate angiogenesis in the early stages of healing of incisions in

Fig. 16.1 Benefits of HBO to ischemic and hypoxic wounds. Note that HBO acts at the same points where hypoxia interferes with wound healing

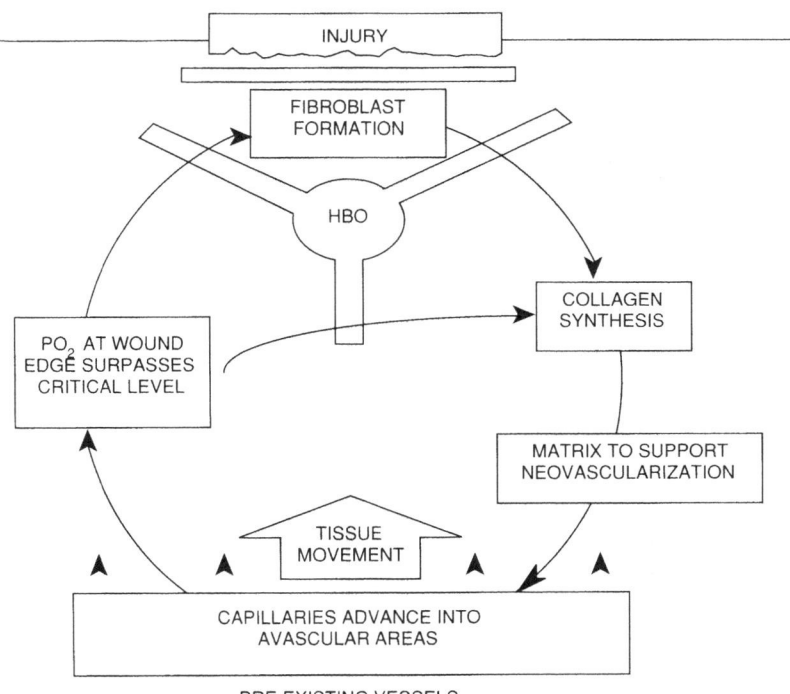

rats. HBO-induced Ang2 expression may occur through transcriptional stimulation and requires the nitric oxide (NO) signaling pathway, which may play an important role in HBO-induced angiogenesis. A study was conducted to document general somatic and wound NO levels during and after HBO treatment (Boykin and Baylis 2007). The study evaluated chronic wound patients that responded favorably to HBO treatment (20 treatments; 2 ATA×90 min). Successful HBO was associated with increased wound granulation tissue formation and significantly improved wound closure. Wound fluid and fasting plasma samples were obtained for measurement of nitrate and nitrite (NOx), the stable oxidation products of NO; plasma L-arginine (L-Arg); and asymmetric dimethylarginine (ADMA) . NOx measurements were obtained before treatment (baseline), after 10 and 20 treatments, and at 1 and 4 weeks after therapy. Wound fluid NOx levels tended to increase during treatments, were significantly elevated at 1 and 4 weeks after therapy, and correlated with reductions in wound area. Plasma L-Arg and ADMA were unchanged during and after HBO. This preliminary study documents a significant increase in local wound NO levels (by NOx measurements) after successful HBO and suggests that this mechanism may be an important factor in promoting enhanced wound healing and wound closure associated with this therapy. It is important to note that NO synthesis is transient, because although NO is required for wound healing to occur, too much hinders healing (Fosen and Thom 2014).

HBO for Impairment of Wound Healing by Stress

Psychological stress has been shown to dysregulate healing in both humans and animals. Stress launches a sequence of events that constrict blood vessels and deprive the tissues of oxygen, which is an important mediator of wound healing. Decreased oxygen supply combined with increased oxygen demand in the wounds of the stressed animals can impair healing rate by as much as 45 %. In the mouse model of impaired healing due to stress induced by confinement, HBO therapy during early wound healing significantly ameliorated the effects of stress, bringing healing to near-control levels. There is no significant effect of HBO on the wounds of control animals. Nitric oxide (NO) is critically involved in wound healing, by increasing blood flow and the delivery of oxygen. Gene expression of inducible nitric oxide synthase (iNOS) in the wound, modulated by psychological stress and oxygen balance, has been studied by real-time PCR. Expression of iNOS increases in stressed mice, and HBO treatment of the stressed animals decreases iNOS expression. Thus, methods aimed at increasing tissue oxygenation, such as HBO , have a high therapeutic potential.

HBO Therapy Guided by Tissue Oxygen Tension Measurement

The rational approach to treatment of nonhealing wounds by HBO should include monitoring of tissue oxygen tension. Tissue oxygen tensions during normobaric as well as HBO breathing are shown in Fig. 16.2 and Table 16.3.

Transcutaneous oxygen pressure ($tcpO_2$) is a noninvasive method, and its measurements have been shown to correlate with wound healing. These measurements are taken on the area surrounding the wound and not directly on the wound surface. It is generally considered that $tcpO_2$ greater than 20 mmHg in room air predicts a positive response to HBO. The value should double on 100 % oxygen and increase

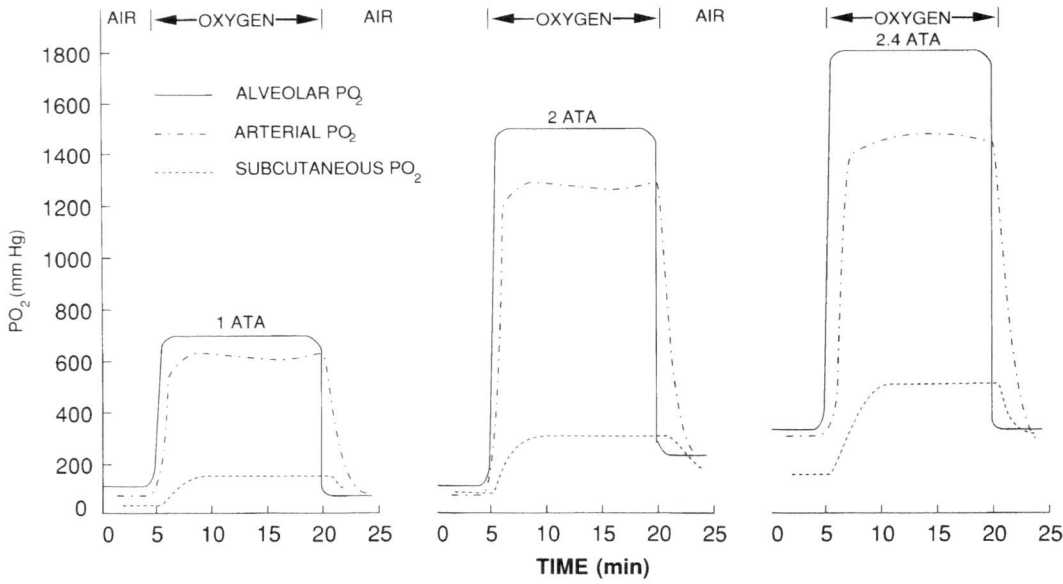

Fig. 16.2 Tissue oxygen tension during normobaric and hyperbaric oxygen breathing. Reproduced with permission from Sheffield & Heimbach: Respiratory Physiology. In: Dehart RL (ed). Fundamentals of Aerospace Medicine. Philadelphia: Lea & Febiger; 1985: 87

Table 16.3 Range of tissue oxygen tensions (mmHg) with HBO therapy

	1 ATA (air)	1 ATA (O$_2$)	2 ATA (O$_2$)	2.5 ATA (O$_2$)
Arterial pO$_2$	100	600	1400	1800
Transcutaneous pO$_2$	70–75	450–550	1200–1300	1400–1500
Muscle pO$_2$	30–35	60–75	220–300	No data available
Subcutaneous pO$_2$	30–50	90–150	200–300	300–500
Wound pO$_2$	5–20	200–400	600–800	800–1100

to 100 mmHg at 2 ATA. TcpO$_2$ has been measured in edematous wounds before and after a regimen of HBO therapy, in patients breathing normobaric air (AIR), 100 % normobaric oxygen (NBO), and 100 % O$_2$ at 2.36 ATA. Only during AIR is pre tcpO$_2$ of markedly edematous wounds significantly lower than that of moderately edematous and nonedematous wounds. After HBO therapy, wound severity score and periwound edema rating decrease significantly, and periwound edema ratings can no longer be distinguished by tcpO$_2$. Although pre-periwound tcpO$_2$ measured during both O$_2$ and HBO evaluations is significantly greater than that measured during AIR and is positively correlated with subsequent change in wound severity, regression analyses have failed to yield a significant prediction equation. The conclusions of such studies are:

- Dramatically marked increases in tcpO$_2$ of normally hypoxic edematous wounds during O$_2$ and HBO challenges demonstrate that periwound edema is an O$_2$ diffusion barrier during normal conditions.
- HBO therapy significantly reduces periwound edema in markedly edematous wounds.
- Despite significant correlations between pre-therapy periwound tcpO$_2$ measured during O$_2$ and HBO challenges and changes in wound severity, single tcpO$_2$ measurements are not predictive of changes in periwound edema or overall wound severity.

A retrospective analysis of 1144 patients with diabetic lower extremity ulcers treated by HBO shows that the reliability of in-chamber tcpO$_2$ as an isolated measure was 74 % with a positive predictive value of 58 % (Fife et al. 2002). Better results may be obtained by combining information about sea-level air and in-chamber oxygen. A sea-level air tcpO$_2$ < 15 mmHg combined with an in-chamber tcpO$_2$ < 400 mmHg predicts failure of HBO therapy with a reliability of 75.8 % and a positive predictive value of 73.3 %.

The oxidative phosphorylation process in the mitochondria requires a minimum oxygen tension of 0.5–3 mmHg in the mitochondria. Cytochrome c activity is reduced progressively as tissue pO$_2$ falls and is markedly reduced below 30 mmHg. These changes are reversible when the oxygen tension is elevated again. These basic metabolic functions are required for the tissues to heal.

Clinical Applications

The use of supplemental oxygen is recommended for all patients considered to be at high risk of infection who are either undergoing or recovering from surgery. Results of various controlled trials suggest that HBO is helpful for some wounds. The main criticism is that there are inadequate or no controls in most studies. Given the clinical nature of the problem, it is not possible to design optimal controlled studies. It is now established that HBO treatments in selected patients can facilitate healing by increasing tissue oxygen tension, thus providing the wound with a more favorable environment for repair. Therefore, HBO has become an important component of any comprehensive wound care program.

The optimal dose of oxygen for a nonhealing wound is not yet determined. The optimal pO$_2$ for the wound is about 50–100 mmHg. Oxygen is only an adjuvant treatment; the primary care of the wound by debridement and meticulous dressing is necessary. The primary cause of the ulcer should be eliminated where possible. Three methods of oxygen administration are usually available:

1. Normobaric oxygen (100 %) inhalation
2. Topical HBO
3. HBO by inhalation in a chamber

Normobaric Oxygen
Normobaric oxygen (100 %) inhalation is the most commonly used method and is usually adequate in acute wounds where the wound pO$_2$ is over 30 mmHg. Methods of oxygen inhalation have been described by Jain (1989).

Topical Hyperbaric Oxygen
Topical application by a small hyperbaric chamber (TOPOX) which encloses the affected limb has been described in Chap. 7. This technique has been used for treatment of leg ulcers. Four methods of topical application of oxygen are (Dissemond et al. 2015):

1. Delivery of pure oxygen under pressure
2. Delivery of pure oxygen under ambient condition
3. Chemical release of oxygen via an enzymatic reaction
4. Increase of oxygen by facilitated diffusion using oxygen-binding and oxygen-releasing molecules

Treatment with topical oxygen is associated with an induction of vascular endothelial growth factor (VEGF) expression in wound edge tissue and an improvement in wound size (Gordillo et al. 2008). Healing of leg ulcers under topically applied HBO was first described in 1969, and later on the same author described other patients with leg ulcers due to different causes (Fischer 1969; Fischer 1975). HBO was administered by a topical chamber applied to the affected extremity. Pressure of 1.03 ATA was not exceeded to avoid obstruction of capillary blood flow. The oxygen delivery was maintained at 4 L/min, and treatment was performed twice daily, each session lasting 2–3 h. Wound debridement was done as necessary. The patients served as their own controls, as they had been treated by other methods before with no success. Most of the ulcers healed well, but HBO failed to heal those associated with severe ischemia. There was absorption of oxygen through the ulcer as evidenced by the rise of capillary pO_2 in the area of the ulcer, without an increase of systemic capillary pO_2. In some cases the stimulation of the granulation tissue was so effective that it rose above the skin surface. These findings show that HBO is a simple, safe, and inexpensive treatment to reduce the time required for healing of ulcers and in some cases served as a good preparation for surgical intervention. A simple disposable polyethylene bag device for application of local HBO to leg ulcers is available.

A novel wound bandage based on microfluidic diffusion delivery of oxygen has been devised (Lo et al. 2013). In addition to modulating oxygen from 0 to 100 % in 60 s rise time, the microfluidic oxygen bandage provides a conformal seal around the wound. When 100 % oxygen is delivered, it penetrates wound tissues as measured in agar phantom and in vivo wounds. Treatment of murine diabetic wounds with this microfluidic oxygen bandage improved healing outcomes in the form of higher collagen maturity. These findings suggest that the microfluidic oxygen bandage may be a useful technique for studying poorly healing wounds.

Published data on the oxygen diffusion properties of skin indicate that the upper skin layers to a depth of 0.25–0.40 mm are almost exclusively supplied by external oxygen, whereas the oxygen transport of the blood has only a minor influence. This is almost 10 times deeper than previous estimates. This zone includes the entire outermost layer of living cells—the epidermis—and some of the dermis below, which contains sweat glands and hair roots. As a consequence, a malfunction in capillary oxygen transport cannot be the initiator of the development of superficial skin defects such as those observed in chronic venous incompetence and peripheral arterial occlusive disease. Peripheral vascular disease contributes to ulceration by poor blood supply, which starves tissues of nutrients. These concepts indicate that ulcer management should not involve bandaging but atmospheric exposure. Although environmental oxygen may suffice in superficial ulcers, nonhealing deep ulcers with hypoxic wounds would require supplemental exposure to oxygen, which may be more effective by topical application than systemic exposure to HBO. The advantages of topical application of HBO are:

1. The ischemic areas are separated from the oxygen by a thin layer of tissue only a few microns thick, whereas systemic oxygen must traverse a much larger distance to reach the ischemic tissue at the base of the ulcer.
2. This method avoids the toxicity of HBO.
3. No special equipment is required. Only a disposable polyethylene bag is used.
4. Low cost.

The limitations of this method are:

1. It is effective in open wounds. Encrustation of ulcers prevents the oxygen from diffusing to the base of the ulcer.
2. Pressure applied to the limb may impair the circulation of the limb.
3. Ulcers penetrating into deep tissues do not respond well to this method.

Electrical stimulation has been combined with HBO for promotion of wound healing. In an open study, no significant differences in healing were observed between patients receiving topical HBO alone and those receiving topical HBO/electrical stimulation (Edsberg et al. 2002). Preliminary data indicate that topical hyperbaric oxygen facilitates wound healing and full closure for pressure ulcers in patients with and without diabetes mellitus. Multicenter, prospective, randomized, double-blind controlled studies have also been carried out.

In 2011, the FDA reclassified the topical oxygen chamber for extremities from class III to class II (Food and Drug Administration 2011). This device is intended to surround a patient's limb and apply humidified oxygen topically at a pressure slightly greater than atmospheric pressure to aid healing of chronic skin ulcers, such as bedsores. This will enable the use of such devices under exemption and avoid the procedure of premarket authorization for class III devices.

Adjuncts to HBO for Wound Healing

Alpha-lipoic acid (LA) has been shown to accelerate wound repair in patients with chronic wounds who undergo HBO therapy. In a study, patients undergoing HBO therapy were randomized into two groups in a double-blind manner: the LA group and the placebo group (Alleva et al. 2008). Gene expression profiles for matrix metalloproteinases (MMPs) and for angiogenesis mediators were evaluated in biopsies collected at the first HBO session, at the seventh HBO session, and after 14 days of HBO treatment. ELISA tests were used to validate microarray expression of selected genes. LA supplementation in combination with HBO therapy downregulated the inflammatory cytokines and the growth factors which, in turn, affect expression of MMPs. LA regulates MMP expression in cells that are involved in wound repair The disruption of the positive autocrine feedback loops that maintain the chronic wound state promotes progression of the healing process.

Concluding Remarks on the Role of HBO in Management of Acute Wound Healing

HBO can augment healing in complicated acute wounds in combination with standard wound management principles. However, HBO is not routinely indicated in normal wound management, because when used by itself or if used only in the postoperative period, it is unlikely to have any benefit. Further investigations are needed before it can be recommended as a routine mainstay in adjuvant wound therapy (Dauwe et al. 2014).

Role of HBO in Nonhealing Wounds and Ulcers

If the wound pO_2 cannot be raised to above 30 mmHg by normobaric 100 % oxygen inhalation, HBO should be tried at pressures of 2–2.5 ATA. The treatments should last for 1–2 h and should be repeated every 24 h. Such a schedule correlates with the cell cycle of human fibroblasts, which lasts about 24 h, and the duration of mitosis, which takes about 1 h. Lack of rise of wound pO_2 in response to HBO therapy is usually an indicator that further treatments may be ineffective. HBO therapy is used in the following types of wounds and ulcers:

1. Ulcers due to arterial insufficiency
2. Diabetic foot ulcers
3. Venous stasis ulcers
4. Decubitus ulcers
5. Infected wounds
6. Frostbite
7. Intractable wounds associated with spider bite
8. Refractory perineal Crohn's disease

Ulcers Due to Arterial Insufficiency

Many of the peripheral vascular diseases reviewed in Chap. 25 are accompanied by ulceration of skin on the legs or even gangrene. Local rather than regional blood flow insufficiency is the cause of skin lesions in peripheral vascular disease. Satisfactory results are obtained with HBO at 2 ATA in ulcers typical of thromboangiitis obliterans. In arteriosclero-

sis the response is less satisfactory unless prolonged courses of treatment are instituted.

In a study of 22 patients with leg ulcers and pain due to chronic vascular insufficiency treated by means of HBO at 2–2.5 ATA for up to 70 sessions, 15 obtained relief of rest pain and 12 had healing of ulcers (Kidokoro et al. 1969). HBO at 2 ATA was used to treat 16 patients with arteriosclerotic ulcers that were refractory to conventional treatments, and in 75 % of cases, the ulcers healed completely (Hart and Strauss 1979).

Another study on 50 patients with arteriosclerotic ulcers treated with HBO alone (1.5–3.0 ATA) showed that healing was achieved in 52 % and improvement in 20 % (Perrins and Barr 1986). These were all geriatric patients, and amputation was avoided in 65 % of them. The same authors treated 8 further patients with split skin grafts and HBO; 7 of them healed, and no effect was observed on the 1 remaining patient. The conclusions reached by these authors were:

- Many patients with ulcers associated with peripheral vascular disease that have resisted treatment by other means can be healed by prolonged courses of HBO.
- The response is dose dependent. Some ulcers respond to 1.5 ATA, while others require up to 3 ATA. Some fail to respond to treatment for a total of 2 h per day; others heal with less than 1 h a day.
- The period required for healing can be reduced considerably if the ulcer base is prepared with a course of HBO before split skin grafting.
- Of all the different types of ulcers, those due to rheumatoid vasculitis showed the best results. Of the 15 patients, 73 % healed with HBO alone, and all of the three that had split skin grafts healed.

A study reported complete healing of arterial insufficiency ulcers in all patients where the distal transcutaneous pO_2 could be raised above 100 mmHg by HBO treatments at 2.5 ATA (100 % oxygen) with daily sessions of 90 min each (Wattel et al. 1991). An average of 46 sessions per patient were required. HBO was ineffective in those patients where the distal transcutaneous pO_2 could not be raised above 100 mmHg. A retrospective chart review of patients who received HBO for arterial insufficiency ulcers that failed to heal despite standard treatment showed that overall rate of healing was 43.9 % (Heyboer et al. 2014). The overall major amputation rate was 17.1 %; the amputation rate among those who healed was 0 % compared to 42.4 % among those not healed. These findings suggest that HBO is useful for management of arterial insufficiency ulcers that have failed standard treatment and point out the need for a prospective controlled study.

Diabetic Ulcers

Introduction and Epidemiology

Diabetic ulcers usually involve the foot and hence the term "diabetic foot." The US incidence of diabetic ulcers is about 80,000 per year of which 25–30 % are not healed by standard therapy. Approximately 20 % of all diabetics who enter hospital are admitted because of foot problems with ulcers. Even when hyperglycemia is controlled by insulin, the vascular pathology of diabetes continues to progress. It may result in large vessel occlusive disease or pathology of the microvasculature. An additional pathology is diabetic neuropathy, and the secondary infections in the wound lead to the term "diabetic foot syndrome." The whole lower extremity may become gangrenous and require amputation which carries a high mortality in the elderly diabetic patients. A diabetic has 15–20 higher chance of having an amputation of the lower extremity as a nondiabetic individual. According to the American Diabetes Association, 42 out of 10,000 diabetics in the USA have an amputation yearly because of diabetic foot syndrome. HBO has been shown to reduce the leg amputation rate in diabetic gangrene.

General Management

Standard care for diabetic ulcers includes good wound care, control of diabetes, and treatment of infections. Recent advances in the treatment of diabetic ulcers include the introduction of skin substitutes such as Apligraf (Organogenesis Inc.) to close the skin ulcer. A platelet-derived growth factor, Regranex (Janssen Pharmaceutica), has also been approved for the treatment of diabetic ulcers of the lower extremities in the USA. The growth factor stimulates the migration of cells to the ulcer site, encouraging the patient's body to grow new tissue to heal the ulcers. If gangrene sets in, the lower extremity is amputated below the knee.

Role of HBO in the Management of Diabetic Foot

HBO reduces insulin requirements in diabetics (see Chap. 28), but no effect on diabetic neuropathy has been demonstrated. HBO may have an important role in preventing gangrene by counteracting the vascular insufficiency, and this issue needs to be examined further. The rationale of HBO in diabetic wound is based on the known effect of HBO in counteracting hypoxia, edema, and infection. Before considering HBO treatment, one has to consider whether tissue oxygen in the ulcer can be augmented by HBO.

Whether or not the oxygen tension can be raised in the diabetic wound by HBO depends upon the patency of the vasculature around the ulcer. The decision regarding the use of HBO is made after vascular evaluation of the extremity involved and the transcutaneous pO_2 determination. A decision tree based on this is shown in Fig. 16.3. Oxygen tensions were measured transcutaneously in 10 diabetic patients

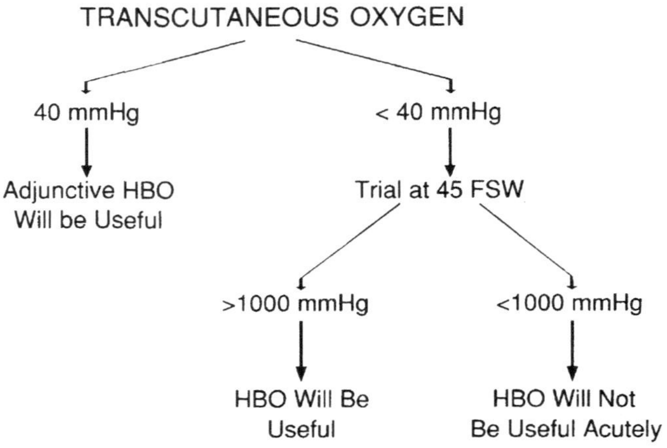

Fig. 16.3 Algorithm for decision-making in offering HBO as an adjunct to the diabetic patients. Reproduced with permission from Emhoff and Myers: Transcutaneous oxygen measurements in wound healing in the diabetic patient. In: Kindwall EP (ed). Proceedings of the Eighth International Congress on Hyperbaric Medicine. San Pedro, CA: Best Publishing Company; 1987

to assess the adequacy of microcirculation in the affected areas (Emhoff and Myers 1987). The normal range of pO_2 measured transcutaneously over the leg is 45–95 mmHg. Only two of these patients had pO_2 above this value, eight had a lower value. The authors believe that in diabetics, the pO_2 value has to be raised much higher for optimal healing. If pO_2 cannot be raised to 1000 mmHg when the patient breathes 100 % oxygen at 2.36 ATA, it can be stated that the patient's microcirculation is defective and would not allow adequate supply and flow of oxygen to the wound, and HBO may not be useful.

Adjuncts to HBO in the Management of Diabetic Ulcers

Endothelial progenitor cells (EPCs) are the key cellular effectors of neovascularization and play a central role in wound healing, but their circulating and wound-level numbers are decreased in diabetes, implicating an abnormality in EPC mobilization and homing mechanisms. The deficiency in EPC mobilization is presumably due to impairment of endothelial NOS-NO cascade in the bone marrow. Hyperoxia, induced by a clinically relevant HBO protocol, can significantly enhance the mobilization of EPCs from the bone marrow into peripheral blood. However, increased circulating EPCs failed to reach the wound tissues, partly as a result of downregulated production of SDF-1a in local wound lesions with diabetes. Administration of exogenous SDF-1a into wounds reverses the EPC homing impairment and, with HBO, synergistically enhances EPC mobilization, homing, neovascularization, and wound healing (Liu and Velazquez 2008).

Although HBO mobilizes stem cells in humans, animal experimental studies indicate that the specific target which initiates this process is NOS-3 in the stromal cell compartment of the bone marrow with subsequent liberation of stem cell factor. Contrary to many of the traditional agents which mobilize stem cells, HBO does not concomitantly elevate the circulating leukocyte count, which may be thrombogenic (Ma et al. 2011). Newly mobilized stem cells appear to have greater content of HIF-1, HIF-2, and thioredoxin, which in the murine model exhibit improved neovascularization (Thom et al. 2011). Subsequent to HBO treatments of diabetic patients, most wound margin HIFs and thioredoxin appear to be derived from localized stem cell suggesting that they may play an important role in supplying critical factors during wound healing in diabetic patients.

Clinical Use of HBO in Diabetic Foot

Various studies of the use of HBO in treating diabetic foot are summarized in Table 16.4. Most of the studies used HBO at 2–3 ATA and the number of sessions varied from 4 to 79. A standard problem wound protocol is 100 % oxygen at 2 ATA/2 h daily/5 days a week.

One study can be criticized for a low proportion of the patients who completed the study (Stone et al. 1995). A good example is the study that was done on 70 diabetic subjects who were consecutively admitted to a diabetology unit for foot ulcers (Faglia et al. 1996). Only two subjects, one in the arm of the treated group and one in the arm of nontreated group, did not complete the protocol and were therefore excluded from the analysis of the results. Finally, 35 subjects received HBO and another 33 did not. Of the treated group (mean session=38.8±8), three subjects (8.6 %) underwent major amputation: two below the knee and one above the knee. In the nontreated group, 11 subjects (33.3 %) underwent major amputation: 7 below the knee and 4 above the knee. The difference is statistically significant. The relative risk for the treated group was 0.26. The transcutaneous oxygen tension measured on the dorsum of the foot significantly increased in subjects treated with HBO therapy: 14.0±11.8 mmHg in the treated group and 5.0±5.4 mmHg in the nontreated group. Multivariate analysis of major amputation on all the considered variables confirmed the protective role of HBO therapy and indicated low ankle–brachial index values and high Wagner grade as negative prognostic determinants. It was concluded that HBO, in conjunction with an aggressive multidisciplinary therapeutic protocol, is effective in decreasing major amputations in diabetic patients with severe prevalently ischemic foot ulcers. The decision on using HBO is correlated with following classification of the diabetic foot:

Table 16.4 Studies of the use of HBO for diabetic foot

Authors and year	No. of patients	Success rate (%)	Comments
Hart and Strauss (1979)	11	18	All of the patients improved but ulcer healed completely only in 2
Perrins and Barr (1986)	24	67	Amputation was avoided in 18 % of the cases
Baroni et al. (1987)	26	83	
Davis et al. (1987)	168	70	
Wattel et al. (1991)	20	75	Mixed pathology: 9 patients with arterial insufficiency and 11 with diabetic ulcers
Doctor et al. (1992)	30	?	Prospective study. Thirty patients were randomized to a study group (HBO plus conventional treatment) and a control group (conventional treatment only). The treatment group showed better results in that the number of positive bacterial cultures decreased from 19 to 3 (in the control group from 16 to 12). Only 2 patients in the treatment group required amputations as compared to 7 patients in the control group
Oriani et al. (1992)	80	96	Prospective study. Sixteen of the patients in this study either refused HBO or had contraindications for the use of HBO and were identified as controls. Of the 62 who received HBO, 59 (96 %) recovered versus 12 (67 %) in the control group. Only 3 patients in the HBO group required amputation as compared to six in the control group
Stone et al. (1995)	87	72	Of the 501 patients in the study, 382 received conservative treatment. The end point was salvage of both lower extremities. Of the 119 treated patients, only 87 were available for follow-up
Faglia et al. (1996)	68	92.4	The end point was amputation. The amputation rate was 8.6 % in the HBO-treated patients and 33.3 % in the control group
Zamboni et al. (1992)	5	100[a]	Prospective with five controls for duration of 7 weeks
Landau and Schattner (2001)	100	81	Open study of topical hyperbaric oxygen and low energy laser radiation of the ulcer
Kalani et al. (2002)	38	76	Success rate in patients treated conventionally was 48 %. Seven patients (33 %) in this group compared to 2 patients (12 %) in HBO-treated group went to amputation
Ong (2008)	45	71	77 % of successful cases were at risk of amputation prior to treatment

[a]Reduction of wound size and no complete healing

- Grade I: Superficial lesions. No need for hyperbaric treatment.
- Grade II: Deep ulceration reaching tendons and bone. HBO is indicated as cost-effective treatment.
- Grade III: Involvement of deep tissues with infection. HBO is indicated as an adjunct to debridement.
- Grade IV: Gangrene of a portion of the foot. HBO treatments may reduce the size of the gangrenous portion which needs to be excised.
- Grade V: Gangrene of the whole foot. Usually amputation is required.

Guideline for the Use of HBO in the Treatment of Diabetic Foot Ulcers

Many of these patients are referred to specialized wound centers, where HBO therapy has become a mainstay in healing wounds, especially diabetic foot ulcers (DFUs). Response of DFU to HBO therapy is unaffected by glycemic control prior to treatment, and HBO treatment should not be delayed for suboptimal blood glucose control (Bakhtiani et al. 2015).

The Undersea and Hyperbaric Medical Society (UHMS), following the approach of the Grading of Recommendations Assessment, Development, and Evaluation (GRADE) working group, undertook a systematic review of the HBO literature in order to rate the quality of evidence and generate practice recommendations for the treatment of DFUs (Huang et al. 2015). Results of this analysis showed that HBO is beneficial in preventing amputation and promoting complete healing in patients with Wagner Grade 3 or greater DFUs who have just undergone surgical debridement of the foot as well as in patients with Wagner Grade 3 or greater DFUs that have shown no significant improvement after 30 or more days of treatment. In patients with Wagner Grade 2 or lower DFUs, there was inadequate evidence to justify the use of HBO as an adjunctive treatment. This provides a moderate level of evidence supporting the use of HBO for DFUs. Future research should be directed at improving methods for patient selection, testing various treatment protocols, and improving the existing estimates.

Critical Evaluation of HBO for Treatment of Diabetic Foot Ulcers

The Cochrane Database of controlled trials concluded that HBO therapy significantly improved healing of DFUs in the short term but not the long term and pointed out various flaws in design and/or reporting of trials that led to lack of confidence in the results. Further trials were suggested to properly evaluate HBO in persons with chronic wounds; these trials must be adequately powered and designed to minimize all kinds of bias (Kranke et al. 2012). A systematic review of randomized clinical trials to assess the additional

value of HBO in promoting the healing of DFUs and preventing amputations showed some evidence of the effectiveness of HBO in improving the healing of DFUs in patients with concomitant ischemia (Stoekenbroek et al. 2014). The authors suggested larger trials of higher quality before implementation of HBO in routine clinical practice for patients with DFUs can be justified.

As many as 30–40% of DFU patients with Wagner' Grades 3 and 4 ulcers treated with HBO fail to heal by 24 weeks. Unfortunately, the patient will have already received lengthy therapy (3–60 daily treatments over 6–10-week time period) before having the wound deemed nonresponsive. Currently, practitioners employ a combination of clinical markers, diagnostic testing, and a 4-week preliminary healing response, but this approach is inaccurate and delays definitive identification of HBO responder and nonresponder phenotypes (Johnston et al. 2016). These authors have questioned the underlying mechanisms of effectiveness of HBO in wound healing and suggested more advanced analyses of gene expression may help to improve understanding of wound healing.

Economic Analysis

Long-term HBO therapy is costly, with a typical course running into the tens of thousands of dollars. Estimation of the cost of hospitalization and rehabilitation associated with amputation has shown that the use of HBO as an adjunct in cases of problem wounds of the limbs has resulted in a high rate of salvage of the limbs, which would be expected to lower the cost of medical care. Experience with the use of HBO in nonhealing wounds both diabetic and those due to arterial insufficiency has been rather disappointing (Ciaravino et al. 1996). From 1989 to 1994, fifty-four patients with nonhealing lower extremity wounds resulting from underlying peripheral vascular disease and/or diabetes mellitus were treated with HBO at Orlando Regional Medical Center, Florida. Wounds were grouped into the following five categories: (1) diabetic ulcers, (2) arterial insufficiency, (3) gangrenous lesions, (4) nonhealing amputation stumps, and (5) nonhealing operative wounds.

Each patient received an average of 30 treatments. Outcomes for all 54 patients treated with HBO in this study were dismal. None of the patients experienced complete healing, six (11%) showed some improvement, 43 (80%) showed no improvement, and in five cases (9%) results were inconclusive because these patients underwent concomitant revascularization or amputation. Thirty-eight of the 43 patients who showed no improvement (88%) ultimately required at least one surgical procedure to treat their wounds. Thirty-four patients (63%) developed complications, most commonly barotrauma to the ears, which occurred in 23 patients (43%). The average cost of 30 HBO treatments was $14,000 excluding daily inpatient charges.

The authors found that it is difficult to justify such an expensive, ineffective, and complication-prone treatment modality for problem extremity wounds.

Concluding Remarks

No definitive studies on the usefulness of HBO in limb salvage have been carried out as yet. The Orlando study quoted above may also have been done poorly as the technique of HBO treatment may not have been proper as indicated by the high barotrauma rate. Hospitalization is not required for HBO treatment, and inpatient charges should not be included in any economic analysis as part of HBO therapy costs. Nevertheless, this study indicates a controversy surrounding the use of HBO for diabetic foot. Because most published studies suffer from methodological problems, there is an urgent need for a collaborative, international, randomized prospective clinical trial for the application of HBO in diabetic foot lesions, as part of a multidisciplinary treatment approach, before HBO can be recommended as standard therapy in patients with foot ulcers.

The problem of management of a diabetic foot should be divided into two parts: healing of ulcer and the limb salvage. For treatment of ulcer, the definitive primary treatment should be application of a skin substitute. One product, Apligraf® (Organogenesis, Inc.), which is a living skin equivalent engineered from human skin cells, is already approved for the treatment of venous ulcers and is commercially available. It is in clinical trials for diabetic and pressure ulcers. It is a one-time application as an outpatient at a wound center or similar facility. Another similar product which is in clinical trials is Dermagraft (Advanced Tissue Sciences). More promising than skin substitutes are the cell and gene therapies in development for wound healing (Jain 2016). If the foot is threatened with gangrene, the role of HBO should be investigated in controlled and well-designed studies. Current economic analyses favor HBO as it is less expensive than amputation in some countries. If prolonged HBO expenses exceed the one-time expense of amputation, the quality of life may be the only justification for the use of HBO which may help limb salvage.

Venous Ulcers

Pathophysiology

A review of various studies suggests that 1% of the general population will suffer from chronic venous ulcers at some point during life. A venous ulcer (also referred to as stasis ulcers) is one of the manifestations of chronic venous insufficiency (CVI), which is defined as hypertension involving either the superficial or both the superficial and the deep venous systems. The term CVI is also used to describe the stigmata of this disease: pigmentation, atrophie blanche, induration, varicose eczema, and ulceration. CVI is a common condition if one includes a related condition, varicose veins, which arise from the same underlying cause, i.e., incompetence of valves in the perforator veins.

Chronic venous hypertension and repeated pressure peaks, provoked by calf muscle contractions, which are transmitted to the skin microvasculature, lead to microangiopathy which is characterized by enlarged blood capillaries, reduced capillary numbers, microvascular thrombosis, and increased permeability of microlymphatics. These changes have been documented by using fluorescent videomicroscopy and microlymphography. Transcutaneous oxygen measurements and laser Doppler flowmetry have shown that transcutaneous oxygen tension is decreased, whereas Doppler reflux is enhanced. These findings indicate hypoperfusion of the superficial skin layers with paradoxical hyperperfusion of the deeper layers. Transcutaneous (tc) measurements show a decrease of $tcpO_2$ and this correlates with the degree of alterations of skin capillaries. Trophic changes leading to venous ulcerations are caused by microvascular ischemia, and edema is due to increased capillary permeability and deficient lymphatic drainage. Edema further hinders tissue nutrition and transdermal diffusion of oxygen. This mechanism is supported by the demonstration of decreased transcutaneous pO_2 (measured as postischemic response) in patients with severe venous disease. Pericapillary deposition of fibrin in response to venous hypertension acts as a diffusion barrier to oxygen and thus impairs the nutrition of the skin. However, it is not certain that venous ulceration is attributable to failure of diffusion of oxygen and other small nutritional molecules to the tissues of the skin. It is likely that neutrophils attach themselves to the cutaneous microcirculation, become activated, and produce endothelial injury by release of cytokines, oxygen free radicals, proteolytic enzymes, and platelet-activating factors. Repeated over many months or years, this process leads to chronic inflammation. The microvascular changes in the skin are characterized by activated endothelium and perivascular inflammatory cells. In conclusion, the exact pathomechanisms of venous ulcers remain to be resolved.

Treatment of Venous Ulcers

It appears that ulcers associated with CVI have a different pathomechanism, and the management of the ulcer should be based on treatment of the CVI. The venous ulcers need to be differentiated from several other types including those due to arterial insufficiency because the management strategies are different. General measures for all leg ulcer patients should include the following:

- Elevation of the leg at night. This diminishes the exudate from the ulcer and reduces edema.
- Compression: by special stockings or intermittent pneumatic compression. The compliance rate of compression stockings or bandage is quite poor.
- Ulcer dressing and topical treatment.

- Surgical treatment is directed at debridement of the ulcer and correction of the underlying cause. This may involve procedures to correct venous hypertension or stripping of varicose veins.
- Pharmacotherapy. Oxerutins (Venoruton, Novartis) is an established treatment for chronic venous insufficiency.
- Growth factors. Several growth factors are being evaluated for this purpose. One of these in clinical trials is keratinocyte growth factor.
- Apligraf® (Organogenesis Inc.) is approved for treatment of venous ulcers. Like human skin, Apligraf is composed of two layers. The outer epidermal layer is made of living keratinocytes and the dermal layer consists of fibroblasts, both derived from human donor tissue that is thoroughly screened to exclude pathogens. It is applied by a physician in an outpatient facility or a wound care center. Apligraf heals more ulcers faster than compression therapy alone and is expected to become the treatment of choice for this condition.

HBO for Treatment of Venous Ulcers

Rationale of HBO for venous ulcers is based on the hypoxia theory which has not been proven to be the sole pathomechanism. HBO promotes healing of venous ulcers but is not necessary for the healing. Oxygen tension measurements show low pO_2 values with microcirculatory disturbance of the ulcer tissue. After a compression bandage had been applied to the legs, the tissue oxygen tension of the ulcers increases markedly, probably as the result of diminished venous stasis. These ulcers heal without any special HBO treatment.

An example of a venous stasis ulcer treated by HBO and the results are shown in Fig. 16.4. HBO at 2.5 ATA once a day in a monoplace chamber was used for treatment of 17 patients with varicose ulcers of the legs until maximum benefit was achieved (Slack et al. 1966). Five patients healed completely, six showed marked improvement, and another four had slight improvement. In a series of 16 cases of ulcers due to venous stasis treated with HBO via topical application, improvement was noted within 8 h of starting treatment in all cases (Fischer 1969). Complete relief was obtained in 17 of 19 cases of venous stasis ulcers by the use of HBO at 2 ATA after conventional treatment had failed (Bass 1970).

Combination of HBO with skin grafting is more effective than HBO alone. Skin grafting is carried out for large ulcers, and HBO is also used as an adjunct to promote healing of skin grafts. In 12 patients treated with HBO (1.5–3 ATA), there was healing in 6 only; 6 patients required split skin grafts followed by treatment with HBO resulting in 100% healing (Perrins and Barr 1986). Saphenectomy wounds may not heal properly and HBO therapy is useful in the management of these.

Recommendations for management of nonhealing venous ulcers are as follows:

- Primary treatment by application of Apligraf® which is a substitute for skin graft.
- Supplementary treatment with HBO until the ulcer has healed.
- Prophylactic treatment of CVI with Venoruton to prevent recurrence of venous ulcer.
- The only one of these established by clinical trials is Apligraf®. Further clinical studies need to be carried out to support the supplementary use of HBO and Venoruton.

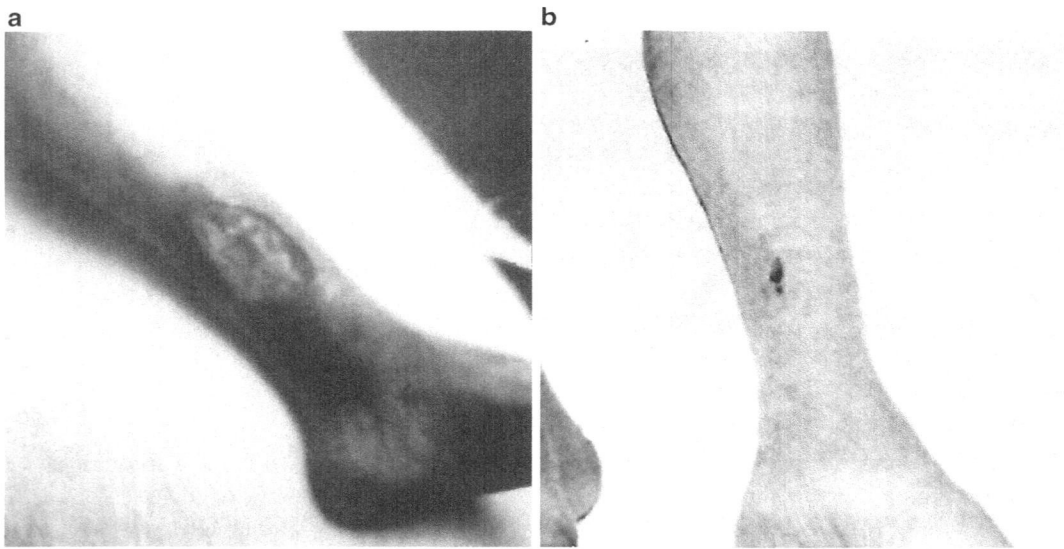

Fig. 16.4 Example of an arterial insufficiency ulcer of the leg treated by HBO (**a**) before treatment and (**b**) after treatment

Decubitus Ulcers

Pathophysiology

The cause of decubitus ulcers is pressure on the skin, which interferes with circulation at the point of contact. Prolonged rest or immobilization in one position, as with hemiplegics and paraplegics, may lead to this within a few hours. Poor skin hygiene, malnutrition, and debility are contributing factors. These ulcers are usually located over bony prominences such as the sacrum and the heel. The ulcer results from breakdown of the ischemic skin and subsequent bacterial invasion and inflammatory reaction. Persistence of the latter leads to microvascular thrombosis, which further aggravates ischemia. From the management point of view, they are considered as chronic wounds.

Role of HBO

Measurement of the oxygen tension of the tissues under pressure transcutaneously shows that pressure of 15 kPa on a point leads to anoxia and a pressure sore in 2 h. Treatment of 26 patients with pressure sores on the hips and the sacral areas using topical HBO at 1.03 ATA (practically NBO) led to improvement in almost all cases with 6 h of treatment (Fischer 1969). A pinkish color developed and the inflammatory reaction subsided. This was followed by granulation and epithelialization. Lesions less than 6 cm in diameter eventually healed, but in three patients where the lesions were larger than this, HBO suppressed bacterial growth and stimulated granulation tissue before plastic surgical repair. The National Institute for Health and Care Excellence (NICE) guidelines for the care of pressure sores in the UK exclude the use of HBO (Stansby et al. 2014).

Some cases of pressure sores treated conservatively because of anaerobic infections, osteomyelitis, and septic arthritis, which contraindicated surgical intervention, may heal completely. Patients with ulcers covered by inadequately vascularized flaps have ~75 % chance of healing completely if HBO is given shortly after surgery. HBO should be considered when a skin flap is in danger of ischemia during surgery for pressure sores.

Future Status of HBO for Pressure Ulcers

Introduction of skin substitutes such as Apligraf® may obviate the need for HBO treatments alone or as an adjunct to surgery for pressure ulcers. However, HBO may be useful for preparation of patients with infected pressure ulcers before a skin substitute is applied. In some cases it may be used as an adjunct to accelerate healing after application of the skin substitute. In any case, the role of HBO in the treatment of pressure ulcers needs to be redefined. Prevention of such ulcers will remain the most important part of medical management.

Infected Wounds

The role of HBO in the treatment of infections is described in Chap. 14. The use of HBO should be considered if an infected space cannot be sufficiently vascularized with debridement and flap construction. Infected ischemic ulcers usually heal in response to HBO therapy.

Frostbite

Pathogenesis

Frostbite usually results from exposure to temperatures below –2 °C. The extent of injury is determined by the duration of exposure, humidity, high altitude (decrease of oxygen tension), and the rapidity of cooling. Predisposing factors such as peripheral vascular disease may influence the extent of tissue damage in frostbite.

Damage to the tissues is caused by freezing or by ischemic changes that occur during rewarming. Intracellular ice formation leads to indirect damage from dehydration. The vascular complications are vasoconstriction, thrombosis, and ischemic swelling of soft tissues such as muscles, which can cause a compartment syndrome. The ischemic lesions may take several weeks to evolve.

Study of pathophysiology of frostbite has revealed marked similarities in inflammatory processes to those seen in thermal burns and ischemia–reperfusion injury. Evidence of the role of thromboxanes and prostaglandins has resulted in more active approaches to the medical treatment of frostbite wounds.

Clinical Features

Most of the clinical experience has been in the two world wars and the Korean conflict, representing >1 million cases. Clinically, frostbite can be classified into three stages:

1. Erythema, only superficial redness
2. Blistering of the skin
3. Necrosis of the skin and soft tissues

Laboratory Studies

The following laboratory studies have been found to be helpful in the assessment of such cases:

- Noninvasive vascular studies; Doppler and digital plethysmography.
- X-rays. Tissue edema is seen in early cases. Osteoporosis is noted in 50 % of the cases, 4–10 weeks following the injury. Damage to the epiphyseal plates can occur in children.
- EMG and nerve conduction studies may be useful in assessing the lesions of the peripheral nerves.

Management

This consists of the following measures:

1. Emergency management; rewarming
2. Chemical sympathectomy (reversible blocking by intra-arterial injection)
3. Vasodilators
4. Heparin and infusion of low molecular weight dextran to reduce the sludging in microcirculation
5. Wound care
6. Delayed debridement 1–3 months after demarcation
7. Hyperbaric oxygenation

HBO has been found to be useful in limiting tissue loss and enhancing healing after frostbite. The successful use of HBO has been reported in several cases. HBO is capable of improving nutritive skin blood flow in frostbitten areas more than 2 weeks after the injury. There are cases where HBO was started a few days after frostbite and amputation of the affected fingers had been considered, complete recovery occurred following HBO treatments. A case is reported of frostbite of all fingers of a mountain climber, who was treated by HBO, resulting in healing of all fingers to full function, except some cosmetic deformity of the tip of the most severely affected finger (Folio et al. 2007). There are no controlled clinical studies and the results of controlled animal studies are conflicting.

HBO counteracts tissue hypoxia and reduces tissue edema. It promotes wound healing and prevents infection. Eventually it helps to demarcate the necrotic area from the viable area so that a greater part of the involved tissue can be salvaged and restored to function. HBO is indicated when there is evidence of ischemia that is refractory to other measures, and where surgery is considered to cover soft tissue defects.

Spider Bite

Introduction

A significant number of persons are bitten by the brown recluse spider (*Loxosceles reclusa*) each year. It is widely distributed in the Central and Southern United States. The bite is accompanied by pain, pruritus, and erythema at the site of skin puncture. Most bites result in nothing more than a local reaction which is self-limiting and resolves spontaneously. A great majority of the remaining bites are followed by a vesicle formation a few hours later that ruptures, leading to the formation of an ulcer of with systemic sequelae. The bite may go unnoticed, which delays treatment until tissue necrosis occurs. The underlying tissue, including the muscle, is involved with enlargement of the ulcer. The cause of tissue necrosis may be hypoxia or vasospastic and thrombotic action of the venom. The necrotizing component of the brown spider

venom is considered to be the enzyme lipase sphingomyelinase D, which contains sulfhydryl groups that are susceptible to HBO. Systemic symptoms that may be present in 25 % of patients usually occur within 24–72 h. These include fever, chills, malaise, nausea, vomiting, myalgia, rash, jaundice, hemolytic anemia, renal failure, shock, and disseminated intravascular coagulation. Death has been reported in children. Antivenom for recluse spider bite reduces the size of the necrotic area and is useful if given during the first 4 h. Therapeutic options for wounds resulting from spider bites are controversial and include local care, corticosteroids, dapsone, and HBO therapy

Animal Experimental Studies

Brown recluse spider venom has been injected intradermally in albino rabbits, and the effect of HBO has been studied on the resulting ulcers. Although there is no difference in healing of lesions as assessed by measuring the lesion area, animals receiving HBO have complete reepithelialization, while those not receiving any HBO develop necrotic cavities extending into the dermis with myonecrosis. A prospective controlled study was performed on New Zealand rabbits to delineate the effects of HBO therapy on spider bites (Maynor et al. 1997). The animals were divided into five groups: (1) venom and no HBO, (2) venom and one immediate HBO treatment (100 % O_2), (3) venom and immediate HBO with ten treatments (100 % O_2), (4) venom and then delayed (48 h) HBO therapy with ten treatments (100 % O_2), and (5) venom and immediate hyperbaric treatment with normal inspired PO_2 for ten treatments (8.4 % O_2). Three animals in group 2 also received a control sodium citrate buffer injection. HBO treatments were at 2.5 ATA for 90 min twice daily. Daily measurements were made of the lesion diameter and skin blood flow using a laser Doppler probe. There was no significant effect of HBO on blood flow at the wound center or 1–2 cm from the wound center. Standard HBO significantly decreased wound diameter at 10 days, whereas hyperbaric treatment with normoxic gas had no effect. Histologic preparations from two animals in each group revealed that there were more polymorphonuclear leukocytes in the dermis of all the HBO-treated animals when compared with the venom-alone and sodium citrate controls. It was concluded that HBO treatment within 48 h of a simulated bite from *L. reclusa* reduces skin necrosis and results in a significantly smaller wound in this model. The mechanism appears unrelated to augmented local blood flow between treatments.

Treatment with HBO in Humans

Six cases of brown recluse spider bite have been described where HBO treatment (2 ATA, 90 min, twice daily for 1–3 days) was started 2–6 days postbite (Svendsen 1986). All the patients recovered without any surgery or hospitalization. A soldier who was bitten on the glans penis by a brown recluse spider and received HBO treatment within 24 h of the bite followed by twice daily for 5 days, recovered in a week without any sequelae (Broughton 1997). A patient with brown recluse spider bite to the left lower eyelid was treated by HBO in addition to canthotomy as well as administration of dapsone, antibiotics, and steroids (Jarvis et al. 2000). Complete recovery occurred with cicatrization at the site of the bite. Another case of brown recluse spider bit with necrotic wound and hemolysis was managed successfully with dapsone and HBO (Wilson et al. 2005). Results of HBO treatment in the reported cases shows that it is possible to avoid surgery and other sequelae of this spider bite.

HBO for Inflammatory Bowel Disease

Inflammatory bowel disease (IBD) is the term used for chronic inflammation of all or part of the digestive tract. IBD primarily includes ulcerative colitis (UC) and Crohn's disease (CD). Both usually involve severe diarrhea, pain, fatigue, and weight loss. IBD can be debilitating and sometimes leads to life-threatening complications. Anti-inflammatory and immune suppressor drugs are used initially. Infliximab, a TNF-α inhibitor, and similar drugs are used more recently. Patients who do not respond to or cannot tolerate medical therapy may be considered for HBO therapy, which is a relatively safe and potentially efficacious treatment option for IBD patients. A systematic review of various studies showed that the overall response rate was 86 % (Dulai et al. 2014). Of the 40 UC patients with endoscopic follow-up reported, the overall response rate to HBO was 100 %. However, to understand the true benefit of HBO in IBD, well-controlled, blinded, randomized trials are required.

Refractory Perineal Crohn's Disease

Perineal Crohn's disease (CD) is an extremely difficult condition to treat medically or surgically. Current surgical methods include procedures such as incision and drainage, debridement, fistulotomy, muscle flaps, colostomy, etc. Medical treatments involve the use of sulfasalazine, metronidazole, broad-spectrum antibiotics, and immunosuppressive agents. There are anecdotal case reports of patients who respond dramatically to HBO treatment after failure of multiple medical and surgical treatments. HBO, when integrated in a comprehensive management program including debridement and metronidazole therapy, results in a complete and sustained closure of the fistula.

Seven patients with perineal CD were subjected to daily sessions of HBO in a multiplace hyperbaric chamber with good clinical effects (Weisz et al. 1997). Each patient received a total of 20 sessions during a time period of 1 month. IL-1, IL-6, and TNF-α measurements were done several times during the initial sessions and after completing therapy. Pretreatment cyto-

kine levels were elevated in patients compared to age-matched normal controls. During the first 7 days of treatment, IL-1, IL-6, and TNF-α levels in supernatants of LPS-stimulated monocytes derived from patients' peripheral blood were decreased compared to pretreatment levels. Parallel measurements of serum IL-1 levels revealed an initial elevation and thereafter decreased levels, which remained low throughout the first week of HBO treatment. After completion of therapy, cytokine levels increased to pretreatment values. The authors concluded that alterations in secretion of IL-1, IL-6, and TNF-α may be related to the good clinical effect of HBO treatment in CD patients with perianal disease.

A systematic review showed that overall response rate for perineal CD to HBO therapy was 88 %; 18 of 40 patients had complete healing and 17 had partial healing (Dulai et al. 2014). The role of HBO in larger groups or less severely affected patients with perineal CD has not yet been studied, nor has the minimum number of treatments required for initial or complete healing of perineal disease in this population been described.

HBO as an Aid to the Survival of Skin Flaps and Free Skin Grafts

Basic Considerations

Skin coverage for open wounds is obtained by transposition of skin as a flap or a pedicle graft or by application of grafts of split or full-thickness skin. Naturally, there is some risk, as ischemia is an unavoidable consequence of these procedures. The tissue damage incurred may result in failure of 21 % of replants and 11 % of free flaps. The raising and transfer of a pedicle flap takes 2–3 months, and if even one stage fails, this period may be doubled.

The problem of closing large open wounds was partially solved by the introduction of split skin grafting. After excision, the vessels of the graft collapse, and the fibrinogen free fluid they contain bathes the graft to meet its metabolic requirements for some days. During this period, there is low oxygen tension in the wound area. Remarkably, this healing skin can survive with a flow of only 1–2 mL of blood per 100 g tissue per min, contrasting markedly with the flow to normal skin of 90 mL per 100 g per min.

Ischemic injury to the skin flaps plays a role in the evolution of skin necrosis. Free radicals contribute to ischemic damage; superoxide dismutase, given immediately after the injury, exerts a protective effect in the viable zones in the microvasculature, where free radicals are generated by neutrophils contained in the gaps between the endothelium and the vessel wall.

The chemical changes that occur in the skin, fat, and blood vessels of the skin flap, as well as the muscles in the myocutaneous flap, include a breakdown of the Na/K pump and inflammation of the perivascular tissue, with a concomitant increase in the number of free radicals. The edema resulting from these changes may cause constriction of the lumen, particularly in the microvasculature. Tissue levels of energy in the form of ATP and oxygen are usually depleted, leading to sequential necrosis of myocytes, smooth muscle cells, fat cells, and endothelial cells lining the vasculature. Endothelial damage may result in the exposure of subendothelial collagen, leading to platelet aggregation and thrombus formation after revascularization. Plasma levels of creatine kinase in the first 24 h postischemia are significantly higher in the ischemic flaps that fail, compared with those that survive. This parameter has been proposed as a means of predicting potential failure of the flap after an ischemic insult and an indication to take appropriate measures to remedy the situation.

Tissue hypoxia is the common denominator in the pathogenesis of ischemia and infection that can lead to skin flap necrosis. The effectiveness of HBO is based on relief of tissue hypoxia.

Animal Experimental Studies

HBO has been shown to be of definite value in preventing necrosis in the pedicle flaps and also limits the extent of necrosis in the free composite grafts. In various studies, all experimental flaps in rabbits exposed to HBO at 2 ATA for 2 h twice daily were reported to survive, whereas none of the flaps in the controls treated with hyperbaric air survived. Tissue oxygen tension of pedicle flaps, skin grafts, and third-degree burns in experimental rats are significantly lower at 24 h than in normal skin. There was no significant increase in tissue oxygen tension after exposure to 100% oxygen at ambient pressure. The response of these tissues to HBO at 2 ATA, however, is rapid and large in most cases. The high oxygen tensions returned to preexposure levels after discontinuation of HBO.

Studies in pigs with shallow wounds showed that treatment with HBO at 2 ATA for 16 h of a 48-h period resulted in 80% epidermal coverage, as against 49% in controls (Winter and Perrins 1970). Immediate postoperative HBO increases the flap survival area to twice that in nontreated control animals. Better results are obtained with HBO at 2 ATA than at 3 ATA. If the start of HBO is delayed by >24 h after surgery, the beneficial effect is diminished considerably. These findings are relevant to the healing of sites of skin graft removal in human patients, which epithelialize faster under HBO.

In a controlled study, HBO at 2 ATA for 2 h twice daily for 30 days had no effect on the healing of full-thickness wounds in rats if the circulation was intact (Kivisaari and Niinikoski 1975). When the circulation was interrupted locally, the control group had impaired healing, whereas healing in the HBO-treated group approached normal parameters. The results of their experiments indicate that HBO is not effective in improving the flap survival unless ischemia is a factor for nonhealing. The effect of HBO and air under pressure on skin survival in acute 8×8 cm neurovascular island flaps has been studied in rats (Tan et al. 1984). Skin flaps treated with 8% oxygen at 2.5 ATA (equivalent to room air at standard pressure) exhibited no improvement in skin survival. Skin flaps treated with hyperbaric air (21% oxygen) and hyperbaric 100% oxygen exhibited significant increase in survival.

The controversy in the literature between survival of flaps in rats and nonsurvival in pigs with HBO can be explained. The flap in a pig is a true random flap, while the one in a rat is a myocutaneous flap incorporating the panniculus cavernosum and has a different blood supply than the flap in the pig. Preoperative or postoperative HBO treatment has been shown to improve the survival rate of free flaps in rats to 66% as compared to 20% without the use of HBO (Kaelin et al. 1990). This beneficial effect was explained by the increase of superoxide dismutase activity induced by intermittent exposure to HBO and is an important factor in protection from reperfusion injury.

The number and size of blood vessels in the microvasculature are significantly greater in animals' skin flaps treated with HBO as compared with controls, and HBO enhances flap survival by this mechanism. HBO treatment of ischemic rat skin flaps in the acute phase improves distal microvascular skin perfusion as measured by laser Doppler flowmetry, and this correlates with improvement of skin flap survival (Zamboni et al. 1992).

The effect of HBO on pedicled skin flap in the cat based on the caudal superficial artery which was ligated was tested (Kerwin et al. 1992). There was no significant difference in the total flap survival between treated and nontreated control animals. The limitation of this study was that HBO at 2 ATA was used for 90 min once a day instead of the usual twice daily treatments. However, HBO did improve the color and decrease the exudate produced by the skin flap in the early postoperative period, factors that may be important in skin flap survival in less controlled conditions. The authors suggested the use of larger samples and a more sensitive model for future studies.

Intensive and tapering HBO therapy has been shown to demonstrate 35% less necrosis as compared with controls in random skin flaps in swine (Pellitteri et al. 1992).

Survival of free flaps of rats stored under HBO conditions increased from 10% (in room air) to 60% after 18 h of preservation. Inhibition of xanthine oxidase system was postulated to be one of the mechanisms of improved success of skin flap transplantation with HBO (Tai et al. 1992). HBO treatment significantly increases flap survival in rat axial skin flap model and reduces deleterious effects of ischemia–reperfusion injury (Agir et al. 2003).

Comparison and Combination of HBO with Other Methods for Enhancing Flap Survival

Some drugs and biological preparations when administrated alone have shown a favorable effect on flap survival. Combinations of HBO with these agents have also been investigated to look for synergistic effects.

Corticosteroids

In the rat dorsal skin flap model, perioperative corticosteroids improve the skin viability. This therapy alone was as efficacious as HBO or HBO combined with corticosteroids.

N-acetylcysteine

N-acetylcysteine (NAC) is a prodrug that supplies bioavailable cysteine for replenishment of glutathione, a powerful active radical scavenger that is depleted in ischemia-reperfusion injury. A study has investigated the role of HBO alone, NAC alone, and combination of both on the necrosis area of random rat's skin flaps. Results showed that HBO alone is associated with reduced area of necrosis of skin flap. NAC alone was associated with poor results, and combination with HBO did not produce better results than the use of HBO alone. These findings suggest that the diffusion of oxygen through the interstitial space was the determining factor of more favorable results of HBO or combination with NAC (da Rocha et al. 2012).

Nicotinamide

Nicotinamide, which is considered to be angiogenic, can provide benefit equal to that of HBO in improving survival rate of skin flaps in rats. No additive effect between nicotinamide and HBO has been observed.

Vascular Endothelial Growth Factor

Combination of vascular endothelial growth factor (VEGF)-loaded microspheres and HBO improved random skin flap survival in rats compared with the effect of VEGF or HBO alone, suggesting these two agents exhibited a synergistic effect (Xie et al. 2015).

Clinical Applications

With the use of HBO as an adjunct to flaps in a plastic surgery unit, the usual failure rate for such operations was 10 and was reduced significantly to 4.5 % (Perrins and Barr 1986). The authors recommended starting HBO treatment as soon as there is any doubt about the viability of the flap, rather than as a last resort. The pressure should be raised until the flap is pink and held at that level for 60–90 min. During this time the edema usually resolves, although it reappears between treatments, and additional treatments are required. These authors had also carried out a controlled study that revealed contrasting effects on patients undergoing split skin grafting. After surgery, these patients were treated either conventionally or by exposure to 100 % oxygen at 2 ATA for 2 h twice daily for 3 days. The better results were obtained in the HBO-treated group of 24 patients, where 92 % of the surface area of the graft survived compared with 63 % in the controls. A complete and successful graft occurred in 65 % of the treated patients but only 17 % of the controls. In certain situations pedicle skin grafts can be replaced by full-thickness grafts with intensive HBO. Complete survival of full-thickness grafts has been achieved in patients in whom free skin transfer would not normally have been contemplated.

With interruption of blood supply, the mechanism by which free skin grafts are revascularized is not fully understood. They either connect to the existing vessels of the host or atrophy and are replaced by vessels invading the graft. In any case the graft is hypoxic in the initial stages and may not survive. HBO applied in this situation can penetrate the skin to a depth of up to 70 μm by direct diffusion. Oxygen permeability of the skin is a function of the richness and pressure of the oxygen: 100 % oxygen at ambient pressure applied topically does not elevate the tissue oxygen tension of the dermis, while HBO can elevate the tissue oxygen tension of the superficial layers of the dermis only. Skin color changes under HBO can be noted even in dead animals, indicating transdermal diffusion of the oxygen.

Under HBO treatment, the donor site from which the grafts are taken heals remarkably quickly. Although HBO improves the success rate of skin grafting, routine use of HBO is not recommend, but it is valuable in treating cases of severe burns in children by making it possible to obtain further grafts from donor sites sooner than is normally practicable.

It is generally accepted that composite grafts of full-thickness skin and cartilage are unreliable for tissues farther than 0.75 cm from a viable source of blood. However, successful reattachment by microvascular anastomosis of an avulsed ear using HBO as an adjunct therapy has been reported. HBO has been found to be a useful adjunct to microvascular transfer of free osteocutaneous flaps, pedicled on deep circumflex iliac vessels, for mandibular reconstruction.

A retrospective review was conducted of patients who received HBO therapy for a failing or threatened post-reconstructive flap from 2008 to 2012 to identify treatment variables associated with positive clinical outcomes (Larson et al. 2013). Patients who were treated successfully demonstrated an average improvement in flap area of 68.3%. Variables significantly associated with a favorable treatment outcome included a high percentage of treatment completion and high pretreatment transcutaneous oxygen measurements.

Tissue expansion has been widely used to provide additional soft tissue for clinical reconstruction. Rapid expansion requires a much shorter clinical period than conventional expansion; however, less natural skin growth occurs resulting in a larger stretch-back ratio and insufficient extra soft tissue for clinical use. An experimental study in rabbits has shown that the use of HBO in the inflation phase of rapid expansion can effectively promote blood flow in the expanded skin, increase its natural skin growth, and reduce the instant stretch-back ratio and tension of expanded skin (Ju et al. 2012).

Conclusion

There is considerable disparity in the results of animal experiments carried out to evaluate the effect of HBO on the survival of graft flaps. Apart from the controversy regarding the rat versus the pig experimental model, there are other variations in the experiment designs that make comparison of various studies impossible. Various studies indicate that when ischemia threatens the viability of a graft, HBO improves the chances of survival mainly by one or more of the following mechanisms:

- Relief of hypoxia/ischemia of the tissues
- Diminished metabolic disturbances in the ischemic/hypoxic tissues
- Improvement of the microcirculation and reduction of platelet aggregation
- Increase in the number and size of blood vessels within the microvasculature
- By counteracting free radical-mediated reperfusion injury
- By accelerating the formation of healthy granulation tissue over the bone

HBO is not recommended for routine use as an adjunct to flaps and grafts. Indications for its use are:

1. Significant local ischemia/hypoxia
2. Graft in an irradiated field
3. Previous graft failure

HBO appears to be most effective when given within the first 24 h following surgery. Usually pressures of 2–2.4 ATA are used for 90 min twice a day, and the treatment duration varies from 3 to 10 days depending on the flap type and its condition of viability. It would be difficult to carry out double-blind, prospective studies under the circumstances in which HBO is used in these highly variable wounds.

HBO as an Adjunct in the Treatment of Thermal Burns

Basic Considerations

Thermal injury results in coagulation necrosis of the cellular elements of the epidermis and dermis; the depth of injury is determined by the intensity and duration of heat exposure. With tissue injury, vessels are disrupted or thrombosed and cells destroyed; interstitial fluid, cellular elements, and connective tissues interact. Adjacent intact vessels soon dilate and platelets and leukocytes begin to adhere to the vascular endothelium as an early event in the inflammatory response. Increased capillary permeability is then observed as plasma leaks from the microvasculature into the area of damage. Wound edema is followed by influx of numerous polymorphonuclear neutrophilic leukocytes and monocytes that accumulate at the site of injury. Following these initial inflammatory events, new capillaries, immature fibroblasts, and newly formed collagen fibrils appear within the wound. The neovasculature and other components of wound repair support the rapidly regenerating epithelium that covers a partial-thickness injury. With full-thickness burns, these elements form a luxurious bed of granulation tissue that readily accepts a split-thickness skin graft. Normal repair processes do not proceed smoothly in third-degree burns. Ischemic process in the tissues can increase threefold during the 48 h following injury. Burns are at risk for infection for the following reasons:

- There is loss of integrity of the skin, which is a barrier against invading microorganisms.
- There is impairment of the immune system.
- The presence of necrotic tissue predisposes to infection.

Due to increased vascular permeability, there is extravasation of plasma in burns. This response is not limited to the burned area, as there may be systemically released vasoactive mediators (prostaglandins). It has been suggested that oxygen-induced vasoconstriction may limit the perfusion of the tissues having increased vascular permeability. There is animal experimental evidence that plasma extravasation decreases after HBO exposure.

Most of the recent research on burn wound pathophysiology has been directed toward the third-degree component of the burn wound. The accepted clinical approach is excision of the third-degree burn and coverage of the debrided area.

In partial-thickness (second-degree) burns, not covered by stratum corneum, there is massive fluid loss. The resulting dehydration deepens the wound and may convert it into a full-thickness loss. Efforts have been directed at salvaging the viable tissue. Desiccation can be prevented by keeping the wound covered. Epithelialization of a burn wound depends upon (a) the total cell population surviving the injury, (b) migration, and (c) mitosis. HBO appears to affect the burn wound by allowing earlier reversal of capillary stasis. There is lessening of desiccation and increased oxygen supply to the hypoxic, thermally damaged cells, which might not survive otherwise. There is, therefore, a larger surviving mass of epithelial cells to resurface the wound. The major effect of HBO is facilitation of normal healing, whether by stimulation of mitosis or by migration remains to be seen.

Experimental Studies

Healing takes 30 % less time in burned rabbits treated with HBO than in controls. HBO also accelerates revascularization of full-thickness burn wounds in rats. There is faster epithelialization of blister-removed second-degree burn wounds in guinea pigs treated by HBO (2 ATA) with early return of capillary patency. Investigations of the effect of HBO on burns of different depths in guinea pigs show spontaneous healing, as well as good integration of the graft, regardless of the depth of the burn (second or third degree). Immediate and consistent application of HBO to burn wounds in guinea pigs infected with *Pseudomonas aeruginosa* resulted in better healing than in those animals not treated by HBO.

The following effects of HBO have been demonstrated in a rat scald burn model:

* Reduction of tissue edema
* Repletion of depleted ADP and PCr stores
* Decrease of elevated lactate levels
* Prevention of reduction of phosphorylase activity, a sensitive marker for muscle cell damage

In standardized third-degree burns in guinea pigs, untreated animals show a considerable increase in the wound area as compared to the initial lesions, whereas the wound area is reduced in animals treated with HBO. In several studies, HBO has been shown to have a beneficial effect on superficial dermal lesions caused by ultraviolet radiation in human volunteers. Edema, exudation, and hyperemia decreases but rate of epithelialization is not accelerated.

Clinical Applications

Clinical application of HBO in burns is based on first observation that burned coal miners with CO poisoning who were treated with HBO appeared to do better than those treated conventionally (Wada et al. 1965). Their wounds dried earlier, had fewer infections, and healed faster.

A randomized double-blind study of 191 burn patients concluded that application of HBO within the first 24 h

decreases the healing time, morbidity, and mortality significantly (Hart 1974). The healing time is related directly to the percentage of burns. The monoplace chamber is recommended as a safe, economical, and convenient means of HBO treatment for burn patients. HBO therapy in burns is an adjunctive measure: it does not replace resuscitative, topical, or surgical care and is not a panacea. Based on HBO treatment of burns in 800 patients during 6 years at Sherman Oaks Community Hospital in California, treatment recommended schedule was as follows (Grossman 1978):

* Treatment was given within 4 h of admission of the patient to the burn unit.
* Treatment was given in a monoplace chamber at 2–2.5 ATA (100 % oxygen) for varying periods of time.
* Tissue pO_2 was monitored. In second-degree burns, the tissue pO_2 achieved at 2 ATA was 1200 mmHg compared with 25 mmHg at 1 ATA. This value dropped to 40 mmHg 2 h after treatment. In third-degree burns, the tension achieved at 2 ATA was 1500 mmHg, dropping to 400 mmHg 2 h after treatment.

The results were reductions in (1) patients' fluid requirements; (2) second-degree burn healing time; (3) eschar separation time; (4) donor graft harvesting time; (5) length of hospital stay; (6) complications such as Curling's ulcer, infections, pulmonary emboli, etc.; and (7) mortality (by 10 % compared with the non-HBO-treated patients). These good results continued at the Sherman Oaks Community Hospital as reported later in the accumulated experience with 1130 burn patients (Grossman and Grossman 1982). In a comparative study, human patients with burns are treated by adjunctive HBO therapy at 2.5 ATA, for a 90- to 120-min session, which was repeated two to three times daily in the first 24 h and then 1–2 times per day (Niu et al. 1987). The overall mortality in the HBO-treated and non-HBO-treated patients was not different, but in a high-risk group of patients, the mortality was reduced considerably. There was less fluid loss and earlier reepithelialization in the HBO-treated patients.

Conclusions from a historically controlled study of HBO in burns patients were (Cianci et al. 1989):

* In patients with burns involving 18–39 % of total body surface, there was a 37 % reduction in the length of hospital stay.
* In patients with partial- to full-thickness burns involving 40–80 % of total body surface, there was a reduction of the number of surgical procedures for debridement and grafting.
* HBO-treated patients showed a reduction of fluid requirements. The authors recommended HBO in a carefully controlled setting and in combination with a recognized burn care program.

The following protocol for the treatment of burn patients has been used in several studies by the authors (Hart and Grossman 1988):

- General supportive care: care of the airway, intravenous buffered Ringer's lactate solution for rehydration, and avoidance of morphine and narcotics prior to HBO session.
- Silver sulfadiazine is applied to the burn wound every 8 h. Mafenide (Sulfamylon) cream should be carefully removed before placing the patient in the hyperbaric chamber (see Chap. 9).
- HBO is applied in a monoplace chamber at 2 ATA for 90-min sessions that are repeated every 8 h during the first 24 h postburn and then twice a day until all the wounds are epithelialized.
- Debridement and grafting procedures are performed when eschars start to separate. This occurs characteristically from the 10th to the 14th day. HBO is applied again after recovery from the anesthetic.

Conclusion

There are adequate experimental studies to support the beneficial effect of HBO in thermal burns. The rationale for HBO therapy in thermal burns is summarized in Table 16.5. The Undersea and Hyperbaric Medical Society approves the treatment of patients with burns by HBO provided the treatment is carried out in an approved facility for care of burns according to a strict protocol which involves the use of HBO at 2 ATA for 90 min twice daily. HBO as an adjunct to comprehensive management of patients with burns has resulted in a statistically significant 25 % reduction in the length of hospital stay ($p < 0.012$), and 19 % reduction in overall cost of care (Cianci et al. 1989, 1990).

Applications of HBO in Dermatology

The role of HBO in leprosy is described in Chap. 14 (Infections). Some of the other skin conditions where HBO is useful are briefly described here.

Necrobiosis Lipoidica Diabeticorum

This is chronic cutaneous complication of diabetes mellitus but similar lesions may appear in nondiabetics as well. The characteristic typical plaques with indurated periphery and central atrophy are prone to ulceration which may be refractory to medical and surgical treatment. Corticosteroids have been used but this therapy may not be tolerated by some diabetic patients.

Diabetic microangiopathy is an important factor in the pathophysiology of this disease, and there is significant hypoxia in the wound. HBO was used in a diabetic patient with necrobiosis lipoidica of 7 year's duration that had remained refractory to medical treatment (Weisz et al. 1993). The lesions healed after 98 daily sessions of HBO at 2.5 ATA for 90 min. The reported case of a 28-year-old insulin-dependent diabetic woman with disease duration of 23 years who spontaneously developed ulcerated necrobiosis lipoidica on pretibial skin was treated with HBO (Bouhanick et al. 1998). The disease progressively improved during 113 sessions of HBO therapy and local corticosteroids.

Pyoderma Gangrenosum

This disease is characterized by the appearance of one or more bluish-black, boggy, undermined ulcers, which appear most frequently on the legs. Vasculitis, wound ischemia, and infections are common in this disease. The pathogenesis of pyoderma gangrenosum is obscure. Frequently misdiagnosed

Table 16.5 Summary of rationale for HBO therapy in thermal burns

During the first 24 h	After the first 24 h
1. HBO counteracts vasodilatation and exudation of plasma by its vasoconstricting effect and prevents burn shock	1. It relieves paralytic ileus
2. It inhibits wound infection	2. It has a beneficial effect on stress ulceration of the stomach (Curling's ulcers)
3. It promotes epithelialization of the wound	3. It reduces hypertrophic scarring and ulcerations
4. It is a useful adjunct to survival of skin grafts and flaps	4. It counteracts burn encephalopathy/cerebral edema
5. It is effective against other serious problems accompanying serious burns, such as smoke inhalation injury and CO poisoning	5. It reduces the length of hospitalization
6. It reduces fluid requirements	6. It reduces the need for surgical procedures
7. It counteracts ischemia of the tissues	
8. It helps to maintain the integrity of the wound by minimizing RBC aggregation and platelet thrombi and their propagation from the zone of heat coagulation	

as a necrotizing infection, the elusive nature of its etiology and pathogenesis has hindered the establishment of a standardized management algorithm, leaving therapies as the mainstay of treatment. Conventional management of this disease consists of local treatment of the wound, immunosuppressants, and treatment of any underlying disease.

The rationale for the use of HBO in pyoderma gangrenosum is based on the effectiveness of HBO in skin wound healing and as an adjunct to antibiotics. Several successful cases have been reported in the literature. Skin grafting can fail in this condition because of the rejection of the autograft. HBO was used in four patients with pyoderma gangrenosum to prepare the wound for skin grafting, which was successful in all the cases (Davis et al. 1987).

A 61-year-old woman who presented with temporally discrete bilateral dorsal hand pyoderma gangrenosum lesions was successfully managed with a multimodality therapy including HBO. The initial treatment was a combination of HBO therapy and skin grafting with a negative-pressure dressing, both individually demonstrated to be effective for prompt wound stabilization and coverage (Mowlds et al. 2013). Stabilization and eventual resolution was achieved using intravenous and topical steroids followed by HBO therapy.

Purpura Fulminans

Purpura fulminans is an acute and often fatal disease of children characterized by the sudden occurrence of ecchymotic lesions on the lower extremities that rapidly progress to necrotic gangrene. Disseminated intravascular coagulation is a major component of the disease. Cases treated successfully with HBO, along with other standard treatments, have been reported (Waddell et al. 1965; Kuzemko and Loder 1970; Dudgeon 1971). In a case of a pneumococcal sepsis complicated by disseminated intravascular coagulation and purpura fulminans, adjunctive HBO therapy resulted in reduction of ischemic tissue and sparing of much of the at-risk tissue from gangrene (Cooper et al. 2014).

Toxic Epidermal Necrolysis

HBO (2 ATA, 1–2 h sessions once a day) was used in 3 patients with drug-induced epidermal necrolysis (Ruocco et al. 1986). Reepithelialization occurred in all the patients with ~10 treatments. The reasons stated for the beneficial effect of HBO in this condition are:

- Activation of dermal metabolism
- Antibacterial action
- Possibly an immunosuppressive effect

Psoriasis

Psoriasis is a chronic inflammatory skin disease resulting from immune dysregulation. Several cases of psoriasis have been reported to be successfully treated by HBO. HBO has been used as an adjunct to phototherapy in the treatment of 45 patients (Shakhtmeister and Savrasov 1987). The treatment was well tolerated, and the course of the disease was shortened as compared with the results of conventional treatment. The average duration of remission of the disease was 1.5 years. In another report, 5 patients were treated with psoriasis using HBO (Maulana and Djonhar 1987). Good results were obtained in two patients with lessening of desquamation and erythema after 2 weeks, and disappearance of the lesions after 4 weeks. Treatment failed in one patient and two patients were lost to follow-up. No conclusions can be drawn from this report. Two patients with long histories of psoriasis showed marked improvement with the use of multiple sessions of HBO at 2.8 ATA for 60 min (Butler et al. 2009). The authors described the pathogenesis of psoriasis as chronic inflammation related to its effects on secretion of IL-1, IL-6, and TNF-α. The selective anti-inflammatory effects of HBO on prostaglandin, nitric oxide, and cytokines involved in wound pathophysiology as well as the immunosuppressive effects of HBO contribute to the beneficial effect of HBO. Validation of this beneficial effect requires controlled clinical studies on a larger number of patients.

Because of the involvement of the immune system, regulatory T cells (Tregs) are important in the prevention of psoriasis. Treg function was closely associated with tissue ROS level, which is raised by HBO. An experimental study has investigated Treg function in imiquimod-induced psoriatic dermatitis in association with both in elevated and lowered levels of ROS by using knockout mice, such as glutathione peroxidase-1(−/−) as well as by using HBO or chemicals such as N-acetylcysteine (Kim et al. 2014). Results showed that appropriately elevated levels of ROS might prevent psoriasis through enhancing Treg function.

Scleroderma

Diffuse and progressive scleroderma is one of the connective tissue disorders. A frequent complication is ulcers on the digits of the limbs. Ninety percent of these patients suffer from Raynaud's phenomenon. Five patients with scleroderma were treated using HBO (Zhou 1986). In all cases there was improvement in the symptoms of peripheral vascular disturbances. Further investigations of the long-term effect are required.

Study of electron microscopic changes in patients with scleroderma treated by HBO showed that some of the abnormalities of mitochondria improved and a larger number of "energy" mitochondria appeared after the HBO treatments (Delektorsky et al. 1987). Local ischemia was identified using transcutaneous oximetry in 2 patients with scleroderma and intractable bilateral extremity ulcers (Markus et al. 2006). Each patient then underwent 30 treatments of HBO using 2.4 ATA with resulting wound healing.

References

Agir H, Mersa B, Aktas S, Olgac V. Histologic effects of hyperbaric oxygen therapy administered immediately after or two hours after ischemia-reperfusion injury: a rat abdominal skin flap model. Kulak Burun Bogaz Ihtis Derg V. 2003;10:18–124.

Alleva R, Tomasetti M, Sartini D, Emanuelli M, Nasole E, Di Donato F, et al. alpha-Lipoic acid modulates extracellular matrix and angiogenesis gene expression in non-healing wounds treated with hyperbaric oxygen therapy. Mol Med. 2008;14:175–83.

Bakhtiani P, Mansuri O, Yadav A, Osuoha C, Knight P, Baynosa R, et al. Impact of hyperbaric oxygen on diabetic ulcers is unaffected by glycemic control. Undersea Hyperb Med. 2015;42:183–90.

Bass BH. The treatment of varicose leg ulcers by hyperbaric oxygen. Postgrad Med J. 1970;46:407.

Bouhanick B, Verret JL, Gouello JP, Berrut G, Marre M. Necrobiosis lipoidica: treatment by hyperbaric oxygen and local corticosteroids. Diabetes Metab. 1998;24:156–9.

Boykin Jr JV, Baylis C. Hyperbaric oxygen therapy mediates increased nitric oxide production associated with wound healing: a preliminary study. Adv Skin Wound Care. 2007;20:382–8.

Broughton G. Management of brown recluse spider bite to the glans penis. Military Medicine. 1997;161:627–9.

Butler G, Michaels JC, Al-Waili N, Finkelstein M, Allen M, Petrillo R, et al. Therapeutic effect of hyperbaric oxygen in psoriasis vulgaris: two case reports and a review of the literature. J Med Case Rep. 2009;3:7023.

Cianci P, Lueders H, Lee K, et al. Current status of adjunctive hyperbaric oxygen in the treatment of thermal burns. In: Schmutz J, Bakker D, editors. Proceedings of the 2nd Swiss symposium on hyperbaric medicine. Basel: Foundation for Hyperbaric Medicine; 1989.

Cianci P, Williams C, Lueders H, Lee H, Shapiro R, Sexton J, et al. Adjunctive hyperbaric oxygen in the treatment of thermal burns: an economic analysis. J Burn Care Rehabil. 1990;11:140–3.

Ciaravino ME, Friedell ML, Kammerlocher TC. Is hyperbaric oxygen a useful adjunct in the management of problem lower extremity wounds? Ann Vasc Surg. 1996;10:558–62.

Cooper JS, Allinson P, Keim L, Sisson J, Schuller D, Sippel J, et al. Hyperbaric oxygen: a useful adjunct for purpura fulminans: case report and review of the literature. Undersea Hyperb Med. 2014;41:51–7.

da Rocha FP, Fagundes DJ, Pires JA, da Rocha FS. Effects of hyperbaric oxygen and N-acetylcysteine in survival of random pattern skin flaps in rats. Indian J Plast Surg. 2012;45:453–8.

Dauwe PB, Pulikkottil BJ, Lavery L, Stuzin JM, Rohrich RJ. Does hyperbaric oxygen therapy work in facilitating acute wound healing: a systematic review. Plast Reconstr Surg. 2014;133:208e-15e.

Davis JC, Landeen JM, Levine RA. Pyoderma gangrenosum: skin grafting after preparation with hyperbaric oxygen. Plast Reconstr Surg. 1987;79:200–7.

Delektorsky VV, Antonyev AA, Nomoeva TN. Ultrastructural changes in the mitochondria in scleroderma patients in the course of hyperbaric oxygenation. Vestn Dermatol Venerol. 1987;11:20–7.

Dissemond J, Kröger K, Storck M, Risse A, Engels P. Topical oxygen wound therapies for chronic wounds: a review. J Wound Care. 2015;24:53–4, 56–60, 62–3.

Doctor N, Pandya S, Supe A. Hyperbaric oxygen therapy in diabetic foot. J Postgrad Med. 1992;38:112–4.

Dudgeon DL, Kellogg Dr, Gilchrist GS, Woolley MM Purpura fulminans Arch Surg. 1971;103:351–8.

Dulai PS, Gleeson MW, Taylor D, Holubar SD, Buckey JC, Siegel CA. Systematic review: The safety and efficacy of hyperbaric oxygen therapy for inflammatory bowel disease. Aliment Pharmacol Ther. 2014;39:1266–75.

Edsberg LE, Brogan MS, Jaynes CD, Fries K. Topical hyperbaric oxygen and electrical stimulation: exploring potential synergy. Ostomy Wound Manage. 2002;48:42–50.

Emhoff TA, Myers RA. Transcutaneous oxygen measurements and wound healing in diabetic patients. In: Kindwall EP, editor. Proceedings of the 8th International Congress on Hyperbaric Medicine. San Pedro: Best; 1987. p. 309–13.

Faglia E, Favales F, Aldeghi A, Calia P, Quarantiello A, Oriani G, et al. Adjunctive systemic hyperbaric oxygen in treatment of severe prevalently ischemic diabetic foot ulcer – A randomized study. Diabetes Care. 1996;19:1338–43.

Fife CE, Buyukcakir C, Otto GH, Sheffield PJ, Warriner RA, Love TL, et al. The predictive value of transcutaneous oxygen tension measurement in diabetic lower extremity ulcers treated with hyperbaric oxygen therapy: a retrospective analysis of 1,144 patients. Wound Repair Regen. 2002;10:198–207.

Fischer BH. Topical hyperbaric oxygen treatment of pressure sore and skin ulcers. Lancet. 1969;2(7617):405–9.

Fischer BH. Treatment of ulcers on the legs with hyperbaric oxygen. J Dermatol Surg. 1975;1:55–8.

Folio LR, Arkin K, Butler WP. Frostbite in a mountain climber treated with hyperbaric oxygen: case report. Mil Med. 2007;172:560–3.

Food and Drug Administration. Medical devices; reclassification of the topical oxygen chamber for extremities. Final rule. Fed Regist. 2011;76:22805–7.

Fosen KM, Thom SR. Hyperbaric oxygen, vasculogenic stem cells, and wound healing. Antioxid Redox Signal. 2014;21:1634–47.

Gordillo GM, Roy S, Khanna S, Schlanger R, Khandelwal S, Phillips G, et al. Topical oxygen therapy induces vascular endothelial growth factor expression and improves closure of clinically presented chronic wounds. Clin Exp Pharmacol Physiol. 2008;35:957–64.

Grossman AR. Hyperbaric oxygen in the treatment of burns. Ann Plast Surg. 1978;1:163–71.

Grossman AR, Grossman AJ. Update on hyperbaric oxygen and treatment of burns. Hyperbaric Oxygen Rev. 1982;3:51–9.

Hart GB. Exceptional blood loss anemia. Treatment with hyperbaric oxygen. JAMA. 1974;288:1028–9.

Hart GB, Grossman AR. Thermal burns. In: Kindwall EP, Goldman RW, editors. Hyperbaric medicine powers. Milwaukee: St. Luke's Medical Center; 1988. p. 98–109.

Hart GB, Strauss MB. Responses of ischemic ulcerative conditions to OHP. In: Smith G, editor. Hyperbaric medicine. Aberdeen: Aberdeen University Press; 1979. p. 312–4.

Heyboer 3rd M, Grant WD, Byrne J, Pons P, Morgan M, Iqbal B, et al. Hyperbaric oxygen for the treatment of nonhealing arterial insufficiency ulcers. Wound Repair Regen. 2014;22:351–5.

Huang ET, Mansouri J, Murad MH, Joseph WS, Strauss MB, Tettelbach W, Oversight Committee UHMSCPG, et al. A clinical practice guideline for the use of hyperbaric oxygen therapy in the treatment of diabetic foot ulcers. Undersea Hyperb Med. 2015;42:205–47.

Jain KK. Oxygen in Physiology and Medicine. Charles C. Thomas: Springfield, IL; 1989.

Jain KK. Cell therapy. Basel: Jain Pharma Biotech; 2016. p. 1112.

Jarvis RM, Neufeld MV, Westfall CT. Brown recluse spider bite to the eyelid. Ophthalmology. 2000;107:1492–6.

Johnston BR, Ha AY, Brea B, Liu PY. The mechanism of hyperbaric oxygen therapy in the treatment of chronic wounds and diabetic foot ulcers. R I Med J. 2016;99:24–7.

Ju Z, Wei J, Guan H, Zhang J, Liu Y, Feng X. Effects of hyperbaric oxygen therapy on rapid tissue expansion in rabbits. J Plast Reconstr Aesthet Surg. 2012;65:1252–8.

Kaelin CM, Im MJ, Myers RAM, Manson PN, Hoopes JE. The effects of hyperbaric oxygen on free flaps in rats. Arch Surg. 1990;125:607–9.

Kalani M, Jorneskog G, Naderi N, Lind F, Brismar K. Hyperbaric oxygen (HBO) therapy in treatment of diabetic foot ulcers. Long-term follow-up. J Diabetes Complications. 2002;16:153–8.

Kerwin SC, Hosgood G, Strain GM, Vice CC, White CE, Hill RK. The effect of hyperbaric oxygen treatment on a compromised axial pattern flap in the cat. Vet Surg. 1992;22:31–6.

Kidokoro M, Sakakibara K, Rakako T, et al. Experimental and clinical studies upon hyperbaric oxygen therapy for peripheral vascular disorders. In: Wada J, Iwa T, editors. Hyperbaric Medicine. Baltimore: Williams & Wilkins; 1969. p. 462–8.

Kim HR, Lee A, Choi EJ, Hong MP, Kie JH, Lim W, et al. Reactive oxygen species prevent imiquimod-induced psoriatic dermatitis through enhancing regulatory T cell function. PLoS One. 2014;9, e91146.

Kivisaari J, Niinikoski J. Effects of hyperbaric oxygenation and prolonged hypoxia on the healing of open wounds. Acta Chir Scand. 1975;141:14–9.

Kranke P, Bennett MH, Martyn-St James M, Schnabel A, Debus SE. Hyperbaric oxygen therapy for chronic wounds. Cochrane Database Syst Rev. 2012;4, CD004123.

Kuzemko JA, Loder RE. Purpura fulminans treated with hyperbaric oxygen. Br Med J. 1970;4:157.

Landau Z, Schattner A. Topical hyperbaric oxygen and low energy laser therapy for chronic diabetic foot ulcers resistant to conventional treatment. Yale J Biol Med. 2001;74:95–100.

Larson JV, Steensma EA, Flikkema RM, Norman EM. The application of hyperbaric oxygen therapy in the management of compromised flaps. Undersea Hyperb Med. 2013;40:499–504.

Liu ZJ, Velazquez OC. Hyperoxia, endothelial progenitor cell mobilization, and diabetic wound healing. Antioxid Redox Signal. 2008;10:1869–82.

Lo JF, Brennan M, Merchant Z, Chen L, Guo S, Eddington DT, et al. Microfluidic wound bandage: localized oxygen modulation of collagen maturation. Wound Repair Regen. 2013;21:226–34.

Ma YH, Lei YH, Zhou M, Li X, Zhao HY. Effects of hyperbaric oxygen therapy in the management of chronic wounds and its correlation with CD34(+) endothelial progenitor cells. Zhonghua Yi Xue Za Zhi. 2011;91:3214–8.

Markus YM, Bell MJ, Evans AW. Ischemic scleroderma wounds successfully treated with hyperbaric oxygen therapy. J Rheumatol. 2006;33:1694–6.

Maulana O, Djonhar D. Some experience in hyperbaric oxygenation therapy for dermatological cases in Naval Hospital Jakarta. In: Presented at the 9th International Congress on Hyperbaric Medicine. Sydney, Australia, 1–4 March 1987.

Maynor ML, Moon RE, Klitzman B, Fracica PJ, Canada A. Brown recluse spider envenomation: A prospective trial of hyperbaric oxygen therapy. Acad Emerg Med. 1997;4:184–92.

Mowlds DS, Kim JJ, Murphy P, Wirth GA. Pyoderma gangrenosum: A case report of bilateral dorsal hand lesions and literature review of management. Can J Plast Surg. 2013;21:239–42.

Niu AKC, Yang C, Lee HC, et al. Burns treated with adjunctive hyperbaric oxygen therapy: a comparative study in humans. J Hyperbaric Med. 1987;2:75–85.

Ong M. Hyperbaric oxygen therapy in the management of diabetic lower limb wounds. Singapore Med J. 2008;49:105–9.

Oriani G, Michael M, Meazza D, et al. Diabetic foot and hyperbaric oxygen therapy: a ten year experience. J Hyperbaric Med. 1992;7:213–22.

Pellitteri PK, Kennedy TL, Youn BA. The influence of intensive hyperbaric oxygen therapy on skin survival in a swine model. Arch Otolaryngol Head Neck Surg. 1992;118:1050–4.

Perrins JD, Barr PO. Hyperbaric oxygenation and wound healing. In: Schmutz J, editor. Proceedings of the 1st Swiss symposium on HBO. Basel: Foundation for Hyperbaric Medicine; 1986. p. 119–32.

Ruocco V, Bimonte D, Luongo C, Florio M. Hyperbaric oxygen treatment of toxic epidermal necrolysis. Cutis. 1986;38:267–71.

Shakhtmeister IA, Savrasov VP. Experience with the photochemotherapy of psoriasis combined with hyperbaric oxygenation. Vestn Dermatol Venerol. 1987;7:35–6.

Slack WK, Thomas DA, Dejode LRJ. Hyperbaric oxygen in treatment of trauma, ischemic disease of limbs and varicose ulcerations. In: Brown IW, Cox B, editors. Proceedings of the 3rd International Congress on Hyperbaric Medicine. Washington, D.C.: National Academy of Sciences – National Research Council; 1966. p. 621–4.

Stansby G, Avital L, Jones K. Marsden G. Guideline Development Group Prevention and management of pressure ulcers in primary and secondary care: summary of NICE guidance BMJ. 2014;348:g2592.

Stoekenbroek RM, Santema TB, Legemate DA, Ubbink DT, van den Brink A, Koelemay MJ. Hyperbaric oxygen for the treatment of diabetic foot ulcers: a systematic review. Eur J Vasc Endovasc Surg. 2014;47:647–55.

Stone JA, Scott R, Brill RL, et al. The role of hyperbaric oxygen in the treatment of diabetic foot wounds. Diabetes. 1995;44 suppl 1:71A.

Svendsen FJ. Treatment of clinically diagnosed brown recluse spider bites with hyperbaric oxygen: a clinical observation. J Arkansas Med Soc. 1986;83:199–204.

Tai YJ, Birely BC, Im MJ, Hoopes JE, Manson PN. The use of hyperbaric oxygen for preservation of skin flaps. Ann Plast Surg. 1992;28:284–7.

Tan CM, Im MJ, Myers RAM, Hoopes JE. Hyperbaric oxygen therapy and hyperbaric air on the survival of island skin flaps. Plast Reconstr Surg. 1984;73:27–30.

Thom SR, Milovanova TN, Yang M, Bhopale VM, Sorokina EM, Uzun G, et al. Vasculogenic stem cell mobilization and wound recruitment in diabetic patients: increased cell number and intracellular regulatory protein content associated with hyperbaric oxygen therapy. Wound Repair Regen. 2011;19:149–61.

Wada J, Ikeda T, Kamada K, et al. Oxygen hyperbaric treatment for severe CO poisoning and severe burns in coal mines (Hokutan-Yubari) gas explosion. Igaku Jpn. 1965;54:68.

Waddell W, Saltzman HA, Fuson RL, Harris J. Purpura gangrenosa treated with hyperbaric oxygenation. JAMA. 1965;191:971–4.

Wattel FE, Mathieu MD, Fossati P, Rettenmaier G. Hyperbaric oxygen in the treatment of diabetic foot lesions search for healing predictive factors. J Hyperbaric Med. 1991;6:263–8.

Weisz G, Ramon Y, Waisman D, Melamed Y. Treatment of necrobiosis lipoidica diabeticorum by hyperbaric oxygen. Acta Derm Venereol (Stockh). 1993;73:447–8.

Weisz G, Lavy A, Adir Y. Modification of in vivo and in vitro TNF-alpha, IL-1, and IL-6 secretion by circulating monocytes during hyperbaric oxygen treatment in patients with perianal Crohn's disease. J Clin Immunol. 1997;17:154–9.

Wilson JR, Hagood Jr CO, Prather ID. Brown recluse spider bites: a complex problem wound. A brief review and case study. Ostomy Wound Manage. 2005;51:59–66.

Winter GD, Perrins DJD. Effects of hyperbaric oxygen treatment on epidermal regeneration. In: Wada J, Iwa T, editors. Proceedings of the 4th International Congress on Hyperbaric Medicine. London: Baillere; 1970. p. 363–8.

Xie XG, Zhang M, Dai YK, Ding MS, Meng SD. Combination of vascular endothelial growth factor-loaded microspheres and hyperbaric oxygen on random skin flap survival in rats. Exp Ther Med. 2015;10:954–8.

Zamboni WA, Roth AC, Russel RC, Smoot EC. The effect of hyperbaric oxygen on reperfusion of ischemic axial skin flaps: a laser doppler analysis. Ann Plast Surg. 1992;28:339–41.

Zhang Q, Chang Q, Cox RA, Gong X, Gould LJ. Hyperbaric oxygen attenuates apoptosis and decreases inflammation in an ischemic wound model. J Invest Dermatol. 2008;128:2102–12.

Zhou LS. Hyperbaric oxygen in treatment of diffusing scleroderma: report of 5 cases. Presented at the 5th Chinese Conference on Hyperbaric Medicine, Fuzhow, China, 26–29 Sept 1986.

K.K. Jain

Abstract

Hyperbaric oxygen (HBO) therapy has been used with good results in the management of radionecrosis—the term used for radiation-induced tissue necrosis. This chapter reports on the applications after discussing important background topics such as physics, biology, and pathology. HBO therapy for radionecrosis is considered according to involvement of various types of tissues such as soft tissues and bones (osteoradionecrosis). Special consideration is given management of radionecrosis of the central nervous system (CNS). Because radiation therapy is used for treatment of cancer, the effect of HBO on cancer recurrence is also discussed.

Keywords

HBO effect on cancer • Hyperbaric oxygen (HBO) • Osteoradionecrosis • Radiation encephalopathy • Radiation therapy • Radionecrosis

Intoduction

Radiation therapy has proven to be effective in the treatment of malignancies. The goal is to irradiate tumors with minimal adverse effects on the surrounding normal tissue. This is difficult to achieve, and in practice there is usually some degree of residual damage to the tissues after radiotherapy. Theoretically it is possible to destroy all malignancies if the dosage of radiation is raised to high levels. With the limitations of the human body's tissue tolerance to radiation, optimal dosage schedules are followed that provide an acceptable benefit/damage ratio for the patient. Radiation-induced tissue necrosis is a complication even when accepted dosage schedules are followed. The late effects of radiation therapy following the treatment of cancer are a well-known consequence. A basic knowledge of radiation physics and radiation biology is essential for understanding the pathology of radionecrosis.

K.K. Jain, MD, FRACS, FFPM (✉)
1 Blaesiring 7, Basel 4057, Switzerland
e-mail: jain@pharmabiotech.ch

Radiation Physics

There are two types of ionizing radiations with significant biological effects:

1. Electromagnetic radiation: a combination of electric and magnetic fields, consisting of bundles of energy called photons. This form of radiation is termed gamma rays if it originates from the atomic nucleus and X-rays if it originates from the shell around the nucleus.
2. Particulate radiation. Examples of this are the heavy radiation particles such as protons and neutrons.

Unit of Radiation

A rad is the amount of radiation of any type that results in deposition of 100 ergs of energy/g of tissue. Directly ionizing radiation transfers energy to the tissue by direct disruption of the atomic structure of the tissue. Indirectly ionizing radiations such as neutrons transfer energy by being absorbed by the tissue atom nuclei, which, in turn, give off directly ionizing charged particles as well as gamma rays and X-rays.

© Springer International Publishing AG 2017
K.K. Jain, *Textbook of Hyperbaric Medicine*, DOI 10.1007/978-3-319-47140-2_17

X-rays scatter in tissues, whereas heavy radiation particles like proton beams can be focused on targets at depths with peak effect. The tissues in the path of the beam receive minimal radiation.

Radiation Biology

In the initial stages of radiation tissue interaction, there are several metastable states and energy transfer processes that precede chemical changes in the tissues. The indirect effects of radiation are due to reactive species (free radicals derived from water molecules). The chemical changes resulting from radiation are:

- Damage to the protein structure
- Lipid peroxidation
- DNA damage

The cell DNA is a critical target. There is breakage of hydrogen bonds between the strands of DNA and formation of cross links with other DNA molecules and chromosomal proteins. There is some correlation between DNA molecules and chromosomal proteins and between DNA damage and cellular radiosensitivity. The radiosensitivity of a cell depends upon the stage of the cell cycle at the time of radiation and is greatest just prior to mitosis. The radiosensitivity of the cells is directly proportional to their mitotic activity and inversely proportional to their level of specialization.

The effect of ionizing radiation on the tissues is the sum of the damage to cells in the tissues: damage to the critical cell components of a certain tissue can cause death of the whole tissue or even the whole organ. Connective tissue (including vascular epithelium) has a radiosensitivity that is intermediate between differentiating intermitotic cells and reverting postmitotic cells. Damage to vascular epithelium with obliteration of the vessels may be responsible for the delayed necrosis following radiation.

Radiation Pathology

Clinicopathological Correlations

The clinicopathological correlation of the sequence of events following radiation is divided into four periods:

1. Acute period. First 6 months. During this period there is accumulation of acute organ damage, which may be clinically silent.
2. Subacute period. Second 6 months. This is the end of the recovery from the acute period. Persistence and progression of permanent tissue damage are evident during this period.
3. Chronic period. Second to fifth year. There is further progression of chronic progressive residual damage. There is deterioration of microvasculature with resulting hypoperfusion, parenchymal damage, and reduced resistance to infections.
4. Late clinical period. After the fifth postirradiation year. Further progression of changes in the chronic period with additional effects of aging (premature) and radiation carcinogenesis may manifest during this period.

Whole body irradiation may cause acute radiation sickness, but the localized radiation-induced damage that manifests during the subacute and the chronic periods is relevant to our discussion in this chapter. Radiation damage progresses slowly and continues long after the radiotherapy has been discontinued. Damaged cells do not reproduce and otherwise normal cells may fail to reproduce because of loss of vascularity. There is loss of collagen and increased fibrosis in the radiated tissues due to low oxygen gradient. Oxygen tension at the center of an uncomplicated radiated area is 5–10 mmHg.

Effect of Radiation on Blood Vessels

Radiation has been shown to produce swelling, degeneration, and necrosis of the endothelium with resulting thickening of the vessel wall. These vascular changes progress slowly after radiation and have been referred to as proliferative endarteritis and necrotizing vasculitis. The arterioles and the capillaries suffer the most damage, whereas the larger vessels are spared.

Effect on Soft Tissues

The skin is the tissue that has been most extensively studied for the effects of radiation in the acute, subacute, and chronic periods. Skin atrophy occurs in the chronic stages and the skin is prone to ulceration with minor trauma. Skin incisions made through previously irradiated areas heal poorly. The underlying soft tissues undergo necrosis due to microvascular occlusion. Radiation may directly affect the mucosal cells of the gastrointestinal and genitourinary tracts producing gastroenteritis and cystitis, respectively. A case of laryngeal radionecrosis was treated successfully with HBO (Hsu et al. 2005).

Radiation Effects on the Nervous System

The effects of radiation on the nervous system vary considerably. The normal neurons are fairly resistant to the usual doses of radiation. Radiation necrosis is thought to result from complex dynamic interactions between parenchymal and vascular endothelial cells within the CNS.

Radiation Effects on the Bone

The bone is 1.8 times as dense as soft tissues and absorbs a larger portion of the incident radiation than do soft tissues. Radiation affects both the vascular and the cellular components of the bone. High doses of radiation damage the blood vessels passing between the periosteum and the surface of the bone, leading to bone death. Radiation upsets the balance between the constantly occurring osteoclastic destruction and osteoblastic construction of the adult bone. This leads to osteoporosis and finally osteonecrosis, which usually takes place 4 months to several years following radiation. The usual sites of necrosis are:

- The mandible, generally following radiotherapy of soft tissue tumors of the head and the neck. The mandible absorbs more radiation than the maxilla because of its greater density and shows more necrosis due to its lesser vascularity.
- The ribs, the clavicle, and the sternum, usually following radiotherapy of breast cancer.
- The skull, usually following radiotherapy of brain tumors and soft tissue tumors of the scalp.
- Vertebral column, usually following radiation of spinal cord tumors.
- The pelvis and femoral head following radiation of pelvic tumors.

HBO Therapy for Radionecrosis

Effect of HBO on Radiation Damage to Skin and Mucous Membranes

A study has evaluated the effect of HBO on vascular function and tissue oxygenation in irradiated facial skin and gingival mucosa (Svalestad et al. 2014). Patients with history of radiotherapy (50–70 Gy) to the orofacial region 2–20 years previously were randomly allocated to a treatment or control group. Vascular perfusion was measured with laser Doppler flowmetry (LDF), and tissue oxygenation was recorded by transcutaneous oximetry ($TcPO_2$). Measurements were made prior to HBO exposure as well as 3 and 6 months after an average of 28 HBO sessions with partial pressure of oxygen of 240 kPa for 90 min. Blood flow in the mucosa and the skin after heat provocation increased significantly following HBO. $TcPO_2$ increased significantly in the irradiated cheek, but not at reference points outside the field of radiation. There were no differences between the 3- and 6-month follow-ups. The study concluded that oxygenation and vascular capacity in irradiated facial skin as well as gingival mucosa are enhanced by HBO and these effects persist for at least 6 months.

Rationale for Clinical Application

There is no satisfactory treatment of radiation necrosis using the available conventional methods. It is difficult to provide adequate nutrients and oxygen to the devascularized tissues. Radiation ulcers are painful and the use of narcotic analgesics can lead to addiction. Reconstructive surgery in the radiated areas has a high failure rate due to healing problems. Frustration with the use of conventional methods has led to the trial use of HBO in the management of radiation necrosis.

However, only approximately one-third of patients in the USA receive HBO for delayed radiation injury. More than 600,000 patients receive radiation for malignancy in the USA annually, and about one-half will be long-term survivors. Serious radiation complications occur in 5–10 % of survivors. A large population of patients is therefore at risk for radiation injury. HBO has been applied to treat patients with radiation injury since the mid-1970s. Published results are consistently positive, but the level of evidence for individual publications is usually not high level because it consists mostly of case series or case reports and randomized controlled trials are rare. Radiation injury is one of the UHMS-"approved" indications, and third-party payers usually reimburse for this application (Feldmeier 2012).

HBO raises the tissue pO_2 to within the normal range and stimulates collagen formation at wound edges. This, in turn, enhances the formation of new microvasculature. This provides reepithelialization of small ulcers and provides a better nutritive bed to support grafts and pedicle flaps. Tissue oxygen studies have shown that angiogenesis becomes measurable after eight treatments with HBO, reaches a plateau at 80–85 % of non-radiated tissue vascularization after 20 treatments, and remains at this level whether or not HBO is continued (Marx et al. 1985).

The rationale of the use of HBO for nonhealing wounds also applies to radiation necrosis. Osseous implants are sometimes required for reconstruction of bone in radionecrosis. In rabbit tibias exposed to tumoricidal doses of radiation, adjuvant HBO therapy was shown to improve the amount of histologic integration of the implants in this compromised situation as compared with contralateral control implants (Larsen et al. 1993).

HBO is not used in the early postradiation period as it may potentiate the effects of radiation. HBO may have no effect as a prophylactic for radionecrosis because a certain amount of vascular damage should be evident before HBO effect can be observed. In some situations, HBO, by resolution of the swelling of the involved tissues, permits a better definition of the tumor tissue, which can be resected surgically. The presence of residual tumor in an ulcer bed, on the other hand, would lead to failure of a skin graft, even if HBO is used.

The benefit of treating radiation injuries in patients by the use of HBO was first reported in 1973 (Mainous et al. 1973; Greenwood and Gilchrist 1973). In a later study of treatment of 378 patients with this diagnosis, 336 patients completed the treatment course of HBO after exclusion of deaths and drop-outs for various reasons (Hart and Strauss 1986). The reasons for discontinuance of the therapy (contraindications) were recurrence of the tumor, viral infections, and smoking by patients. HBO was considered as an adjunct to surgery and other appropriate medical regimens. Each patient was treated at 2 ATA for 2 h daily in the case of outpatients or 1.5 h twice daily in the case of inpatients for a total of 120 h or less. If healing was not adequate, the treatment was repeated after a rest period of 3–6 months. As HBO immediately following radiation may have deleterious effects, the authors did not start HBO therapy until 2 months after the last radiotherapy treatment. They concluded that HBO combined with other appropriate treatments reduces the morbidity of radiation injury.

It is concluded that the clear physiological basis, supported by experimental data of usefulness of HBO in radiation necrosis and confirmed by almost identical beneficial results in multiple centers, makes the use of adjunctive HBO in soft tissues radionecrosis as well as osteoradionecrosis compelling indications. Review of a cumulative 14-year experience with 124 patients has shown that HBO therapy led to significant improvement in 94% of the cases (Slade and Cianci Med 1998). The average number of treatments for these patients was 33.1 and the average HBO treatment costs were $15,800. The patient material covered a wide range of soft tissues affected by radiation necrosis, and the treatment protocol was HBO at 2 ATA for 90–120 min daily and occasionally twice daily. The authors feel that a minimum of 30 treatments are necessary, and there is need to develop more definite outcome predictors and treatment protocols for soft tissue radiation damage indicators.

The role of HBO in radiation necrosis in the adults is well established now. In order to evaluate this approach in the pediatric population, a study reviewed experience at the University of Pennsylvania, Philadelphia (Ashamalla et al. 1996). Between 1989 and 1994, 10 patients who underwent radiation therapy for cancer as children were referred for HBO therapy. Six patients underwent HBO therapy as a prophylactic measure prior to maxillofacial procedures, dental extractions and/or root canals (4 patients), bilateral coronoidectomies for mandibular ankylosis (1 patient), and wound dehiscence (1 patient). Therapeutic HBO was administered to 4 other patients, 1 patient for vasculitis resulting in acute seventh cranial nerve palsy, and the other 3 after sequestrectomy for osteoradionecrosis (mastoid bone, temporal bone, and sacrum, respectively). Osteoradionecrosis was diagnosed both radiologically and histologically after exclusion of tumor recurrence. The number of treatments

ranged between 9 and 40 (median, 30). Treatments were given once daily at 2 ATA for 2 h each. Adjunctive therapy in the form of debridement, antibiotics, and placement of tympanotomy tubes was administered to 2 patients. Ages at HBO treatment ranged from 3.5 to 26 years (median, 14 years). The most commonly irradiated site was the head and neck region. The interval between the end of radiation therapy and HBO treatment ranged between 2 months and 11 years (median, 15 years). The median follow-up interval after HBO therapy was 2.5 years (range, 2 months to 4 years). Except for 2 patients who had initial anxiety, nausea, and vomiting, HBO treatments were well tolerated. In all but 1 patient, the outcome was excellent. All of the 6 patients who received HBO continued to demonstrate complete healing of their orthodontal scars at the last follow-up. In the 4 patients who received HBO as a therapeutic modality, all 4 had documented disappearance of signs and symptoms of radionecrosis, and 2 patients demonstrated new bone growth on follow-up CT scan. One patient with vasculitis and seventh cranial nerve palsy had transient improvement of hearing; however, subsequent audiograms returned to baseline. It was concluded that the use of HBO for children with radiation-induced bone and soft tissue complications is safe and results in few significant adverse effects. It is a potentially valuable tool both in the prevention and treatment of radiation-related complications.

Management of Osteoradionecrosis

Basic Studies

Several studies have been carried out to demonstrate the protective effect of HBO on osteoradionecrosis. Animal experiments were conducted to test for a protective effect of HBO and basic fibroblast growth factor (bFGF) on bone growth (Wang et al. 1998). Control C3H mice received hind leg irradiation at 0, 10, 20, or 30 Gy. HBO-treated groups received radiation 1, 5, or 9 weeks before beginning HBO. The remaining groups began bFGF±HBO 1 or 5 weeks after 30 Gy. HBO treatments were given 5 days/per week for 4 weeks at 2 ATA for 3 h/day. At 18 weeks control tibia length discrepancy was 0.0, 4.2, 8.2, and 10.7% after 0, 10, 20, and 30 Gy, respectively. HBO beginning in weeks 1, 5, and 9 following 10 Gy decreased these discrepancies to 2.0%, 1.8%, and 2.4%, respectively. After 20 Gy, HBO decreased these discrepancies to 7.0%, 4.9%, and 3.6%, respectively. At 30 Gy, HBO alone had no effect on bone shortening. bFGF improved tibia length discrepancy with or without HBO. At 18 weeks length discrepancies were 6.5% and 7.3 and after bFGF alone were 6.8% and 7.3% for treatment beginning in week 1 or 5, respectively. Tibial growths at 18 and 33 weeks following radiation were similar. This study showed that bone growth impairment by radiation can be significantly reduced by HBO after 10 or 20 Gy, but not after 30 Gy. At 30 Gy bFGF still significantly reduced the degree of bone shortening, but HBO provided no added benefit to bFGF therapy.

HBO therapy was found to be effective in the treatment of complications of irradiation for cancer in head and neck area (Narozny et al. 2005). Impact of perioperative HBO therapy on the quality of life of maxillofacial patients who undergo surgery in irradiated fields has been assessed in 66 patients (Harding et al. 2008). The head and neck sub-modules identified significant improvements in teeth, dry mouth, and social contact. It was recommended that adjunctive HBO should be considered for the treatment and prevention of some of the long-term complications of radiotherapy.

Osteoradionecrosis of the Mandible

Mandibular osteoradionecrosis is a late complication of radiotherapy for cancers of the head and neck, particularly of the oral cavity. Mandibular osteoradionecrosis is also the most frequently reported radiation injury—235 of 378 patients (62.2 %) in one series (Hart and Strauss 1986). This high frequency is because of the singularity of the blood supply running through the matrix of the bone and the proximity of the tumor to the mandible. Radiation decreases the number of osteoclasts and osteoblasts in the irradiated mandible, and if the mandible is fractured, the healing is delayed. In a normal mandible, after fracture, the alveolar processes remodel, and tooth sockets will heal in 9–12 months.

X-rays of the mandible in osteonecrosis show a variety of lesions including osteolysis and pathological fracture. In some cases, X-rays do not show any abnormalities, and when present, the abnormalities do not necessarily correlate with the clinical severity of the disease. In the past, infection was considered to play a role in the pathogenesis of osteoradionecrosis, although it is now considered essentially a nonbacterial process. The following conventional treatments have been used in the past on the assumption that osteoradionecrosis is an infection:

- Irrigation of the wound with a variety of solutions ranging from saline to hydrogen peroxide and other disinfectants
- Antibiotic therapy
- Superficial sequestrectomy

The abovementioned treatments are obsolete now, and HBO has an important role in the management of osteoradionecrosis of the mandible (Fattore and Strauss 1987; Patel et al. 1989). Of the 206 patients of Hart and Strauss (1986) who underwent treatment with HBO as an adjunct, 72 % had an excellent result, 10 % a good result, and 15 % a fair

response. The remaining 3 % were failures. There are some variations in the technique of combination of HBO with surgery. The Marx/University of Miami protocol consists of three stages (Marx and Johnson 1988):

Stage I
This includes all patients having osteoradionecrosis of the jaw with three exceptions: cutaneous fistulae, pathological fractures, and radiological evidence of bone absorption at the inferior border of the mandible. Patients with these exceptions are allocated to stage III. Treatment of stage I includes daily HBO treatments at 2.4 ATA (90 min), wound care by saline rinses, no bone removal, and discontinuance of antibiotics. If improvement continues, ten further sessions of HBO are given. If there is no improvement, the patient is considered a nonresponder in stage I and moved to stage II.

Stage II
A local wound debridement is attempted to identify patients with only cortical bone involvement who do not require jaw resection. A transoral alveolar sequestrectomy is performed. If healing continues satisfactorily, ten further HBO treatments are given. If the wound dehisces, the patient is considered to be a nonresponder in stage II and is moved to stage III.

Stage III
The patient is given 30 HBO treatments followed by transoral partial jaw resection and a stabilization procedure (extraskeletal or mandibulomaxillary fixation). A further ten HBO treatments are given and the patient is advanced to stage III-R (reconstruction).

Stage III-R
The emphasis in this stage is on early reconstruction and rehabilitation. Ten HBO sessions are given in the postoperative period and jaw fixation is maintained for 8 weeks.

This protocol was used for the treatment of 268 patients over a period of 8 years (Marx et al. 1985). Resolution of the lesions was achieved in 38 patients in stage I (14 %), 48 patients in stage II (18 %), and 182 patients in stage III (68 %). The authors carried out a randomized clinical trial of HBO vs. penicillin for prevention of radiation-induced osteoradionecrosis after tooth extraction in a high-risk population. One group received only penicillin before and after extraction; the other group received no antibiotics, but did receive HBO at 2.4 ATA for 20 daily sessions of 90 min each. One-half of the sessions were given before the extractions and the other half afterwards. The incidence of osteoradionecrosis was 29.9 % in the antibiotic group and only 5.4 % in the HBO group. The conclusion was that HBO should be considered as a prophylactic measure when post-radiation dental care (e.g., tooth extraction) involving trauma to the tissues is necessary.

A retrospective analysis of 41 patients with osteoradione-crosis of the mandible treated at the Hyperbaric Chamber Unit of the Toronto Hospital showed that 83 % of these patients had a significant improvement (Mounsey et al. 1993). These authors concluded that HBO is of benefit in the management of these cases and that mild cases will heal with HBO alone, but in severe cases surgery is necessary to remove the dead tissue. The authors recommended that such patients should receive dental evaluation, local wound care, and a strict oral hygiene. Diseased teeth should be removed prior to radiotherapy, and any teeth that develop abscesses subsequently should be extracted in conjunction with pro-phylactic HBO.

A study was carried out to assess the long-term progress of 26 patients who experienced postradiation osteonecrosis of the jaw between 1975 and 1989 (Epstein et al. 1997). Of 26 patients who had been previously managed with HBO ther-apy as a part of their treatment for postradiation osteonecrosis of the jaw, 20 were evaluated to determine their current status of the condition: resolved, chronic persisting (unresolved), or active progressive (symptomatic). Two of 20 patients experi-enced recurrences of the condition. In one of these patients, surgical treatment was identified as the stimulus of postradia-tion osteonecrosis. In the other patient, the recurrence appeared to be related to periodontal disease activity. In 60 % (12 of 20) of the patients, the condition remained resolved, improvement in clinical staging occurred in 10 % (2 of 20) (from symptomatic to unresolved or resolved), and 20 % (5 of 20) of the patients continued to demonstrate chronic persist-ing postradiation osteonecrosis at the end of the long-term follow-up period. This study supports the contention that postradiation osteonecrosis can occur at any time after radia-tion therapy and that patients remain at risk up to 231 months after treatment of the cancer and probably indefinitely after radiation therapy. These findings also suggest that risk of sec-ond episodes of the condition after management of an initial episode is low. In addition, the follow-up study revealed that chronic nonprogressive postradiation osteonecrosis can remain stable without extensive intervention including com-bined HBO therapy and surgery.

Results of a retrospective study of 33 patients with man-dibular osteoradionecrosis who were treated by the use of HBO during periods 2009–2011 in a medical center in India have been reported (Gupta et al. 2013). Treatments were car-ried out in a multiplace hyperbaric chamber at 2.4 ATA, for 90 min once a day for up to 30 sessions, and 85 % of patients showed improvement.

Osteonecrosis of the Temporal Bone

Temporal bone is susceptible to the development of osteora-dionecrosis because it is covered by a thin layer of skin, has a limited blood supply, and is composed mainly of compact bone. The latent period for the development of clinically manifest osteoradionecrosis of the temporal bone is 8 months to 23 years with an average of 8 years (Ramsden et al. 1975). Surgical treatment involves removal of all necrotic bone. A patient with osteoradionecrosis of the temporal bone was treated using HBO as an adjunct, and the result was complete resolution (Rudge 1993).

Osteoradionecrosis of the Chest Wall

One series of osteonecrosis of the chest wall included 20 cases, which developed following radiation therapy for can-cer of the breast, lung, or mediastinum and involved the ster-num and/or ribs (Hart and Strauss 1986). All the patients recovered. Three cases of postradiation osteomyelitis of the chest wall were treated successfully by a combination of HBO and surgery (Kaufman et al. 1979).

Osteoradionecrosis of the Vertebrae

Four cases of necrosis of the vertebrae in the series of Hart and Strauss were treated by HBO and minor debridements (Hart and Strauss 1986). All 4 patients recovered, and 3 had spontaneous fusions.

Management of Radionecrosis of CNS

Radiation Myelitis

Radiation myelitis of the cervical spinal cord was first reported more than 60 years ago following radiation therapy for pharyngeal cancer (Ahlbom 1941). The pathology of radi-ation injury usually involves interstitial tissue damage and microvascular endothelial injury causing thrombosis with secondary regional ischemia. Provision of HBO during the period of ischemia should, theoretically, minimize the effect of radiation injury. However, HBO has also been shown to potentiate the effects of radiation. One of the practical prob-lems is that adverse neurological effects of radiation may not manifest clinically for several months following exposure.

The use of HBO was investigated in rats with radiation-induced myelitis (Poulton and Witcofski 1985). The animals were randomized into HBO treatment and control groups. Eight weeks following radiation therapy, the animals in the treatment group were given HBO at 2.5 ATA for 30 min 5 times a week for 4 weeks. Serial neurological examinations did not show any benefit or harm as a result of HBO therapy.

An animal experimental study, in which all animals received identical amounts of radiation, was carried out to investigate HBO as a treatment or prophylaxis for radiation myelitis (Feldmeier et al. 1993). Group I received no HBO, group II began HBO at onset of myelitis, group III received HBO as prophylactic beginning 6 weeks after radiation, and group IV received HBO and radiation on the same day but following it after no less than 4 h. HBO consisted of 90 min sessions at 2.4 ATA for 20 daily treatments. All animals progressed to myelitis but it was least severe in group III and most severe in group IV.

Efficiency of HBO for established radiation myelitis has also been investigated (Glassburn et al. 1977). They reported 9 patients in whom radiation myelitis had appeared 5–21 months after receiving 400–6300 rads for a variety of tumors in or overlying the spinal cord. Patients were treated 2–5 times weekly for 2–30 min at 2.5–3.0 ATA. The total number of treatments ranged from 21 to 61. They concluded that 6 of the 9 patients improved as a result of therapy. Cerebral hemodynamic changes under HBO were studied in 23 patients with brain vascular pathology in the late period of radiation-induced disease (Torubarov et al. 1983). Clinical improvement was observed in all patients.

Results have been reported in 10 patients (8 males and 2 females, average age 46 ± 8 years) who had radiation myelitis and were given HBO at 2 ATA for 90 min twice daily for 2 weeks. Three patients with established neurological deficit did not show any response (Hart and Strauss 1986). Three patients who were treated within 1 year of onset showed cessation of progression of disease and slight improvement. Four patients who had symptoms for less than 6 months showed marked improvement in function. The authors concluded that HBO is useful in radiation myelopathy; however, patients should not be given treatment immediately following the radiation, but at least 2 months after the last radiation treatment.

In a retrospective analysis of 9 patients with radiation myelopathy treated with HBO, 6 (66 %) were stabilized or improved by HBO (Angibaud et al. 1995). There are few case reports of the use of HBO for radiation myelitis in recent years. One report describes a case of radiation myelitis with a progressive improvement in the clinico-radiologic picture following HBO that was documented by MRI (Calabro and Jinkins 2000). Controlled studies are required to prove the value of HBO in this disease.

Radiation Encephalopathy

Radiation encephalopathy has been reported following radiation therapy for brain tumors and is sometimes difficult to differentiate from the recurrence or extension of the brain tumor. It can occur in up to 10 % of brain radiotherapy cases, and the incidence depends on radiation dose and exposed area of the brain. Available treatments for radiation encephalopathy include steroids, vitamin E, vasodilators, and HBO. An investigational treatment is intravenous bevacizumab, a monoclonal antibody for VEGF, which is a known mediator of cerebral edema in radiation encephalopathy.

Two patients with radiation-induced encephalopathy who were treated with a combination of vasodilators and HBO showed marked improvement in cerebral function (Hart and Strauss 1986). Radiation-induced necrosis (RIN) of the brain is a complication associated with the use of aggressive focal treatments such as radioactive implants and stereotactic radiosurgery. Ten patients who presented with new or increasing neurologic deficits associated with imaging changes after radiotherapy received HBO treatments (Chuba et al. 1997). Necrosis was proven by biopsy in 8 of these cases. HBO was comprised of 20–30 sessions at 2–2.4 ATA, for 90–120 min. Initial improvement or stabilization of symptoms and/or imaging findings was documented in all 10 patients studied, and no severe HBO toxicity was observed. Four patients died, with the cause of death attributed to tumor progression. Five of six surviving patients were considered to be improved by clinical and imaging criteria; 1 patient was alive with tumor present at the last follow-up. The authors concluded that HBO is an important adjunct to surgery and steroid therapy for RIN of the brain.

Two patients with arteriovenous malformations, who developed radiation encephalopathy following treatment with Gamma Knife, were treated by HBO at 2.5 ATA in sessions of 60 min per day (Leber et al. 1998). This treatment was repeated 40 times in cycles of ten sessions. Both patients responded well to HBO, one lesion disappeared and the other was reduced significantly in size. No adjuvant steroids were given. Although these results provide evidence for the potential value of HBO in treating radiation encephalopathy, further experience will be needed to confirm its definite benefit.

The use of HBO therapy has been described to manage radiation necrosis of the brain, which developed after two treatments with stereotactic radiosurgery to the same lesion (Kohshi et al. 2003). Treatment was continued with steroids alone for 2 months, but the patient started to deteriorate clinically and radiographically. Improvement started again following the resumption of HBO therapy. A retrospective review of 10 patients who underwent HBO therapy for post-radiation injury to the CNS concluded that there was improvement in subjective, clinical, and radiologic outcomes (Valadão et al. 2014). However, the results were not consistent across all patients as HBO did not lead to any improvement in those with nonspecific delayed radiation injury.

Radiation-Induced Optic Neuropathy

Radiation-induced optic neuropathy (RION) is a devastating complication of radiotherapy to the head and neck. Cumulative doses of radiation that exceed 50 Gy or single doses to the anterior visual pathway or greater than 10 Gy are usually required for RION to develop. RION has been reported years after external beam radiation therapy. Patients commonly present with unexplained, painless visual loss in one or both eyes, visual field defects, pupillary abnormalities, and defective color vision. Various theories of pathomechanism implicate vascular occlusion, demyelination, free radical injury, direct damage to cellular DNA, and damage to the blood–brain barrier. MRI with or without contrast is an important diagnostic tool. Visual outcome is poor and there is no established treatment. Corticosteroids and free radical scavengers show some efficiency in treatment, especially in acute phases.

HBO treatment of RION has been suggested. A series of 13 patients with RION were treated using a combination of corticosteroids and HBO (Roden et al. 1990). Recurrence of tumor and other causes of loss of vision were ruled out by appropriate studies. There was no improvement of vision in any of these patients. However, other cases have been reported of RION where visual recovery occurred after HBO therapy (Borruat et al. 1993; Liu 1992). Partial visual recovery from RION after HBO has been reported in a patient with Cushing disease treated with stereotactic radiosurgery of the pituitary gland (Boschetti et al. 2006).

The 27th reported case of RION was a 78-year-old female with RION who received HBO, and she was the first one treated without concomitant steroids (Li et al. 2014). She had improvement of visual acuity throughout her first course of 30 treatments, including regaining the ability to ambulate independently, but subsequently deteriorated following completion. A second course of 40 additional HBO treatments was prescribed resulting in subjective improvement in patient's visual symptoms once more followed with subsequent decline after treatment. Posttreatment MRI, as compared to pretreatment MRI, showed resolution of previously visible optic nerve contrast enhancement.

Management of Radionecrosis of Soft Tissues

Delayed Radiation Injuries of the Extremities

Radiation injuries of the extremities usually present as nonhealing wounds within the radiation fields of previously treated skin cancer. The experience with management of 17 such patients has been reported (Feldmeier et al. 1998). They were treated in a multiplace chamber at 2.4 ATA daily and wound care was maintained. Eleven of these patients had complete resolution of the wounds, and 1 had improvement but not complete healing, while 4 failed to heal and went on to have amputations. The success rate of HBO in this setting was 65 % and nonresponders to HBO had 80 % rate of going on to amputations. It is thus important that these patients should have an adequate trial with HBO as the first-line treatment.

Soft Tissue Necrosis of the Head and Neck

Radiotherapy, which is often used for cancer in the head and neck, leads to damage of tissue cells and vasculature. Surgery in such tissues has an increased complication rate, because wound healing requires angiogenesis and fibroplasia as well as white blood cell activity, all of which are jeopardized. HBO raises oxygen levels in hypoxic tissue, stimulates angiogenesis and fibroplasia, and has antibacterial effects. All of the 48 patients with soft tissue necrosis of the head and neck in one series presented after operative procedures with breakdown (Hart and Strauss 1986). With the exception of one lethal aspiration, all the patients improved.

In a consecutive retrospective study, 15 patients with soft tissue wounds without signs of healing after surgery in fulldose (64 Gy) irradiated head and neck regions were treated with HBO and adjuvant therapy (Neovius et al. 1997). The patients in this study were also compared with patients examined in an earlier study, with corresponding wounds treated without HBO. The healing processes seemed to be initiated and accelerated by HBO. In the HBO group, 12 of 15 patients healed completely, 2 patients healed partially, and only 1 patient did not heal at all. There were no life-threatening complications. In the reference group, only 7 of 15 patients with corresponding wounds without signs of healing eventually healed without surgical intervention, and 2 patients had severe postoperative hemorrhage, which in one case was fatal. Evaluation of results supports the hypothesis that HBO therapy has a clinically significant effect on initiation and acceleration of healing processes in irradiated soft tissues.

Radionecrosis of the Larynx

Radiation therapy is the treatment of choice for early stages of laryngeal cancer, and the larynx is often included in the field of radiation of head and neck cancer. Postradiation edema of the larynx usually resolves spontaneously but occasionally persists as long as 6 months. Laryngeal radionecrosis is an uncommon complication of radiotherapy for carcinoma of the head and neck. The interval between conclusion of radiation therapy and development of radionecrosis ranges from 3 to 12 months. Neither computed tomography nor magnetic resonance imaging differentiates between necrotic tissue and recurrent tumor. Tissue ischemia and hypoxia play an important role in its pathogenesis. This is a debilitating disease with pain, dysphagia, and respiratory obstruction. Biopsy is required to differentiate it from recurrent cancer. The pathological changes are fibrosis, endarteritis, and chondroradionecrosis. Tracheostomy and laryngectomy are required in some cases.

Chandler's grading system is a useful guide to the evaluation of the therapy of laryngeal necrosis. It is summarized as follows (Feldmeier et al. 1993b):

- Grade 1: Slight hoarseness. Laryngeal edema and telangiectasia.
- Grade II: Moderate hoarseness. Slight impairment of vocal cord mobility and moderate edema.
- Grade III: Severe hoarseness with dyspnea and dysphagia. Severe impairment of cord mobility.

- Grade IV: Respiratory distress. Fistula, fixation of the skin to the larynx, laryngeal obstruction.

Humidification, broad spectrum antibiotics, steroids, and hyperbaric oxygen, with or without surgery, are successful in many cases. Of the 8 patients with advanced radionecrosis of the larynx who were treated with adjuvant HBO therapy, 4 were Chandler's grade IV laryngeal necrosis (Ferguson et al. 1987). Signs and symptoms of radionecrosis were markedly ameliorated in 7 of the 8 patients. Only one patient required laryngectomy. As compared with a previous series of cases where HBO was not used, there was a definite improvement of the outcome in these cases treated by HBO therapy as an adjunct. In another series of 9 patients with laryngeal necrosis that were treated by using HBO, 8 were Chandler's grade IV, and the ninth was grade III (Feldmeier et al. 1993a). All the 9 patients were able to maintain their voice until death or the last follow-up. All patients with tracheostomies could be decannulated and the fistulae were closed. The authors recommended HBO as a therapeutic option whenever laryngeal necrosis occurs, and there is a chance to save the larynx.

A case of laryngeal radionecrosis was reported to be successfully treated by the use of HBO therapy, and laryngectomy was avoided (Abe et al. 2012). This was an elderly male who received radical chemoradiotherapy (CRT) for mesopharyngeal cancer and developed dyspnea with throat pain 9 months after completion of CRT. Laryngoscopy revealed vocal cord impairment because of severe laryngeal edema. He initially received conservative therapy combined with antibiotics, steroids, and prostaglandins. Because his dyspnea was persistent despite this treatment, HBO therapy was administered and 20 sessions resulted in complete remission of the dyspnea. HBO therapy, therefore, is regarded as an effective conservative therapeutic option for laryngeal radionecrosis.

Delayed Radiation Injuries of the Abdomen and Pelvis

Radiation therapy is less commonly applied for malignancies of the abdomen but is still used for some cancers of the pancreas, biliary tree, stomach, and colon. Radiation doses are limited due to poor tolerance of normal organs located in the abdomen. Whole abdomen radiation for ovarian cancer with local spread can have about 20 % risk of complications. The most serious complications usually occur after a period of 6 months or longer and result from vascular compromise and hypoxia secondary to reactive fibrosis in the irradiated tissue. Some of these complications require surgical interventions. In a review of 44 patients with radiation injury involving the abdomen and pelvis, 41 of them were available for follow-up examination (Feldmeier et al. 1996). Twenty-six of these patients healed, 6 failed to heal, and 9 patients had inadequate HBO therapy (<20 treatments). Overall, the

success rate in patients receiving at least 20 treatments was 81 %.

Clinical improvement of malabsorption due to radiation enteritis has been reported following HBO therapy (Neurath and Branbrink 1996). A patient who developed severe diarrhea with blood and pain in the rectum following postoperative radiation therapy for uterine cancer was advised to have a colostomy but declined (Hamour and Denning 1996). After 98 h of HBO treatments (2.5 ATA) over a period of 4 weeks, she improved and the rectal ulceration decreased in size until it healed completely 2 months later. The patient did not have any recurrence of these symptoms.

Radiation-Induced Hemorrhagic Cystitis

This is an adverse effect of therapeutic radiation administered for a variety of pelvic malignancies. Clinical features are:

- Recurrent hemorrhage (hematuria)
- Urinary urgency
- Pain

Bladder biopsy in these cases shows the following:

- Mucosal edema
- Vascular telangiectasis
- Submucosal hemorrhages
- Obliterative endarteritis
- Smooth muscle fibrosis

It is a progressive disease and does not resolve spontaneously. Conventional treatment of this complication has included the following modes of treatment:

- Intravascular instillation of formalin, alum, and silver nitrate
- Systemic use of steroids and aminocaproic acid (inhibitor of fibrinolysis)
- Antibiotics
- Cauterization of bleeding vessels
- Bilateral ligation of the hypogastric arteries

Most of these approaches treat symptoms, but none of these promote healing and may even have undesirable side effects. Because these complications are partially due to endothelial damage as well as to decreased vascularity and oxygenation to pelvic tissues, HBO may be able to improve oxygenation and induce angiogenesis in damaged organs, resulting in recovery from radiation injury. Ten patients with radiation-induced cystitis were treated with HBO at 3 ATA (90-min sessions/day, 5 days/week) for an average of 20 sessions (Rijkmans et al. 1989). In 6 patients, hematuria stopped after 12 sessions of HBO. In another 4 patients where there was only partial resolution of hematuria, residual tumor was found in the bladder mucosa and was better defined after resolution of the edema of the surrounding tissue. The tumor was resected in these patients.

Series of Hart and Strauss included 15 patients with radiation cystitis, 11 of whom were relieved of symptoms of tenesmus and hematuria by a combination of HBO and surgery (Hart and Strauss 1986). In another series, each of the 8 patients suffering from radiation-induced cystitis was treated with a series of 60 HBO sessions (2 h at 2 ATA daily), and improvement in 7 of these patients was document by cystoscopy (Weiss and Neville 1989). The hypervascularity of the bladder wall was diminished. The authors stated that the symptomatic relief was accompanied by a significant reversal of tissue injury. Clinical remissions were an average of 24 months (range 6–43 months). Only 1 patient failed to respond. The authors recommended HBO as the primary treatment for patients with symptomatic radiation-induced hemorrhagic cystitis.

Other cases of radiation-induced cystitis treated successfully by the use of HBO have been reported by other authors (Velu and Myers 1992, Kindwall 1993, Nakada et al. 1992, Shameem et al. 1992, Morita et al. 1994). In the largest series, 14 patients were treated with radiation-induced cystitis using HBO at 2.4 ATA for 90 min daily sessions for an average of 28 treatments per patient (Norkool et al. 1993). There was complete resolution or marked improvement in 10 of these (74 %). Of the 4 patients with poor outcome, 3 had recurrence of malignancy that was not present before HBO treatment. The cost of HBO therapy compared favorably with that of conservative treatment.

A retrospective analysis of clinical records of 176 patients with refractory radiation-induced hemorrhagic cystitis treated at the Portuguese Navy Center for Underwater and Hyperbaric Medicine, during a 15-year period, shows that this condition can be successfully as well as safely treated with HBO (Ribeiro de Oliveira et al. 2015). Treatment effectiveness seems to be correlated to the number of sessions performed as well as with reduction in need for transfusion therapy.

In conclusion, HBO has been shown to have a favorable effect on the course of radiation-induced cystitis as observed in numerous published cases and several other cases which have not been reported. There is a difference in pressure used. It appears that the use of 2.4 ATA instead of 2 ATA reduces the number of treatments from about 60 to about 30. Open clinical studies have shown beneficial effect of HBO on radiation cystitis. There is a lack of randomized trials to definitively demonstrate the effectiveness of HBO for cystitis. Concern still exists regarding the durability of the beneficial effects.

Radiation Proctitis

Chronic proctitis is a well-known complication of therapeutic irradiation. Most patients had previously been treated with radiotherapy for prostate carcinoma. Radiation-induced proctitis is a difficult clinical problem to treat and will probably become more significant with the rising incidence of diagnosis of prostate cancer. Patients with proctitis mainly suffer from bleeding, diarrhea, incontinence, and pain. A male patient suffering from severe radiation-induced hemorrhagic proctitis was reported to have healed after HBO therapy (Charneau et al. 1991). In a prospective observational study on 14 patients with radiation-induced soft tissue necrosis following treatment of pelvic malignancy, wounds had failed to heal after 3 months of conservative therapy (Williams et al. 1992). All of the patients received 15 courses of HBO. All those with radiation necrosis of the vagina or rectovaginal fistula healed. There was only one treatment failure.

In a series of 14 patients with chronic radiation-induced proctitis, 9 were treated with HBO in a monoplace chamber at 2 ATA, and 5 patients were treated at 2.36 ATA (Warren et al. 1997). Eight patients experienced complete resolution of symptoms, and 1 patient had substantial improvement for a total response rate of 64 %. Follow-up ranged from 5 to 35 months. Five patients (36 %) were classified as nonresponders. Three experienced significant improvement during treatment but relapsed soon after therapy was discontinued, whereas two had no symptomatic improvement. Responders who had sigmoidoscopy after therapy showed documented improvement, whereas no nonresponders showed improvement. The authors concluded that HBO therapy should be considered in patients with chronic radiation proctitis.

In more than half of the patients with radiation proctitis, symptoms partially or completely resolve after HBO treatment (Woo et al. 1997). HBO should be considered in the treatment of radiation-induced proctitis. Further prospective trials with strict protocol guidelines are warranted to definitively demonstrate the effectiveness of HBO for proctitis.

Both hemorrhagic cystitis and proctitis with hematochezia may occur secondary to pelvic- and prostate-only radiotherapy. A series of 19 patients received 100 % oxygen at 2 ATA pressure for 90–120 min per treatment in a monoplace chamber (Oliai et al. 2012). Complete resolution of hematuria was seen in 81 % ($n=9$) and partial response in 18 % ($n=2$). Recurrence of hematuria occurred in 36 % ($n=4$) after a median of 10 months. Complete resolution of hematochezia was seen in 50 % ($n=2$), partial response in 25 % ($n=1$), and refractory bleeding in 25 % ($n=1$). The conclusion was that HBO is appropriate for radiation-induced cystitis and proctitis once less time-consuming therapies have failed to resolve the bleeding.

Effect of HBO on Cancer Recurrence

Because there may be residual cancer in some of the patients treated for radiation necrosis, there is some concern that

HBO may promote cancer growth or recurrence. A historical review of the effects of HBO on malignancy reported 3 cases of occult carcinoma that manifested clinically after HBO was started and presumably led to the proliferation of the tumor in all 3 cases (Eltorai et al. 1987). The authors considered HBO therapy to be contraindicated in malignancy. There is no evidence to substantiate this view.

Squamous cell carcinoma, transplanted in mice, neither progresses nor regresses when the animals are exposed to HBO (Sklizovic et al. 1993). Other studies suggest that HBO may even have an inhibitory effect on cancer growth (Ehler et al. 1991, Headley et al. 1991, Mestrovic et al. 1996). The effect of HBO on dimethylbenzathracene-induced oral carcinogenesis has been studied in an animal model (McMillan et al. 1989). The group that received simultaneous HBO had fewer tumors, but these were larger than those in the non-HBO group. They concluded that HBO has a tumor-suppressive effect during the induction phase of oral carcinoma and appears to have a stimulatory effect during the proliferative phase. In a survey of this topic, majority of the hyperbaric practitioners who responded did not consider HBO to have cancer-promoting or cancer-accelerating properties (Feldmeier et al. 1993b).

A review of the pertinent literature to answer the question "Does HBO have a cancer-causing or -promoting effect?" reveals conflicting results (Feldmeier et al. 1994). Several of the studies showed a positive effect of HBO in suppressing tumor growth, whereas other studies failed to demonstrate this effect. One explanation of this difference is that generation of free radicals by HBO may diminish superoxide dismutase and affect the susceptibility of tumor cells to HBO (Mestrovic 1996).

Conclusion

Radiation wounds are difficult to treat and in the past there have been few nonsurgical options. Now, there is considerable evidence of the beneficial effect of HBO on radiation necrosis, and it has become a useful adjunct to surgery. Among the bony structures, the effect on osteoradionecrosis of the mandible is most striking. Among the soft tissues, the effect on laryngeal necrosis is impressive. The effect on the radionecrosis of the neural tissues other than the brain is not striking.

There are no controlled studies to prove the efficacy of HBO in radionecrosis. Apart from the variations in clinical presentation, there is difficulty in controlling other methods of treatment.

A review of 74 publications reported results of applying HBO in the treatment or prevention of radiation injuries and appraised these in an evidence-based fashion (Feldmeier and Hampson 2002). All but seven of these publications report a positive result when HBO is delivered as treatment for or prevention of delayed radiation injury. These results are particularly impressive in the context of alternative interventions. Without HBO, treatment often requires radical surgical intervention, which is likely to result in complications. Other alternatives including drug therapies are rarely reported and for the most part have not been the subject of randomized controlled trials.

However, evidence increasingly supports the use of HBO as an adjunctive treatment in a variety of radiation injuries. The positive outcomes in 94 % of 411 patients collected prospectively over 8 years at a single center strongly supports the efficacy of HBO treatment for chronic radiation tissue injury (Hampson et al. 2012). The conditions evaluated in this study included osteoradionecrosis of the jaw, cutaneous radionecrosis with open wounds, laryngeal radionecrosis, radiation cystitis, and gastrointestinal radionecrosis. A new registry of radiation injuries has been established to evaluate the outcomes and treatment parameters of HBO treatment. A total of 2538 patient entries with 10 types of radiation injuries were analyzed (Niezgoda et al. 2016). The five most common injuries were osteoradionecrosis (33.4 %), dermal soft tissue radionecrosis (27.5 %), radiation cystitis (18.6 %), radiation proctitis (9.2 %), and laryngeal radionecrosis (4.8 %). HBO therapy resulted in improvement or resolution of symptoms in 76.7–92.6 % of cases, depending on type of injury. These outcomes from a large patient registry of radiation-induced injuries support the continued therapeutic use of HBO therapy for radiation injuries. HBO is recommended for delayed radiation injuries for soft tissue and bony injuries of most sites. A systematic review of randomized controlled trials found only small trials indicating that HBO is associated with improved in patients with late radiation tissue injury affecting tissues of the head, neck, anus, and rectum (Bennett et al. 2016). HBO also appears to reduce the chance of osteoradionecrosis following tooth extraction in an irradiated field.

Future research should continue on the effect of HBO on radiation injuries. Growth factors show promise in the management of chronic irradiated tissues, and it would be worthwhile to investigate the effect of combination of HBO with growth factors.

References

Abe M, Shioyama Y, Terashima K, Matsuo M, Hara I, Uehara S. Successful hyperbaric oxygen therapy for laryngeal radionecrosis after chemoradiotherapy for mesopharyngeal cancer: case report and literature review. Jpn J Radiol. 2012;30:340–4.

Ahlbom HE. Results of radiotherapy of hypopharyngeal cancer at Radium-hemmet, Stockholm. Acta Radiol. 1941;22:155–71.

Angibaud G, Ducasse JL, Baille G, Clanet M. Potential value of hyperbaric oxygenation in the treatment of post-radiation myelopathies. Rev Neurol (Paris). 1995;151:661–6.

Ashamalla HL, Thom SR, Goldwein JW. Hyperbaric oxygen therapy for the treatment of radiation-induced sequelae in children. The University of Pennsylvania experience. Cancer. 1996;77:2407–12.

Bennett MH, Feldmeier J, Hampson NB, Smee R, Milross C. Hyperbaric oxygen therapy for late radiation tissue injury. Cochrane Database Syst Rev. 2016;4, CD005005.

Borruat FX, Schatz NJ, Glass JS, Feun LG, Matos L. Visual recovery from radiation-induced optic neuropathy: role of hyperbaric oxygenation. J Clin Neuroophthalmology. 1993;13:98–101.

Boschetti M, De Lucchi M, Giusti M, Spena C, Corallo G, Goglia U, et al. Partial visual recovery from radiation-induced optic neuropathy after hyperbaric oxygen therapy in a patient with Cushing disease. Eur J Endocrinol. 2006;154:813–8.

Calabro F, Jinkins JR. MRI of radiation myelitis: a report of a case treated with hyperbaric oxygen. Eur Radiol. 2000;10:1079–84.

Charneau J, Bouachour G, Person B, Burtin P, Ronceray J, Boyer J. Severe hemorrhagic radiation proctitis advancing to gradual cessation with hyperbaric oxygen. Dig Dis Sci. 1991;36:373–5.

Chuba PJ, Aronin P, Bhambhani K, Eichenhorn M, Zamarano L, Cianci P, et al. Hyperbaric oxygen therapy for radiation-induced brain injury in children. Cancer. 1997;80:2005–12.

Ehler WJ, Marx RE, Kiel J, et al. Induced regression of oral carcinoma by oxygen radical generating systems. J Hyperbaric Med. 1991;6:111–8.

Eltorai IM, Hart GB, Strauss MB, et al. Does hyperbaric oxygen provoke occult carcinoma in man? In: Kindwall EP, editor. Proceedings of the 8th International congress on hyperbaric medicine. San Pedro: Best Publishing; 1987. p. 18–29.

Epstein J, van der Meij E, McKenzie M, Lepawsky M, Stevenson-Moore P. Postradiation osteonecrosis of the mandible: a long-term follow-up study. Oral Surg Oral Med Oral Pathol Oral Radiol Endod. 1997;83:657–62.

Fattore L, Strauss RA. Hyperbaric oxygen in the treatment of osteoradionecrosis: a review of its use and efficacy. Oral Surg Oral Med Oral Pathol. 1987;63:280–6.

Feldmeier JJ. Hyperbaric oxygen therapy and delayed radiation injuries (soft tissue and bony necrosis): 2012 update. Undersea Hyperb Med. 2012;39:1121–39.

Feldmeier JJ, Hampson NB. A systematic review of the literature reporting the application of hyperbaric oxygen prevention and treatment of delayed radiation injuries: an evidence based approach. Undersea Hyperb Med. 2002;29:4–30.

Feldmeier JJ, Lange JD, Cox SD, et al. Hyperbaric oxygen as a prophylactic or treatment for radiation myelitis. Undersea Hyperbaric Med. 1993;20:249–55.

Feldmeier JJ, Heimbach RD, Davolt DA, Brakora MJ. Hyperbaric oxygen as an adjunctive treatment for severe laryngeal necrosis: a report of nine consecutive cases. Undersea Hyperbaric Med. 1993a;20:329–35.

Feldmeier JJ, Heimbach RD, Davolt DA, Brakora MJ. Hyperbaric oxygen and the cancer patient: a survey of practice patterns. Undersea Hyperbaric Med. 1993b;20:337–45.

Feldmeier JJ, Heimbach RD, Davolt DA, Brakora MJ, Sheffield PJ, Porter AT. Does hyperbaric oxygen have a cancer-causing or -promoting effect? A review of the pertinent literature. Undersea Hyperbaric Med. 1994;21:467–75.

Feldmeier JJ, Heimbach RD, Davolt DA, Court WS, Stegmann BJ, Sheffield PJ. Hyperbaric oxygen as an adjunctive treatment for delayed radiation injuries of the abdomen and pelvis. Undersea Hyperbaric Med. 1996;23:205–13.

Feldmeier JJ, Heimbach RD, Davolt DA, et al. Hyperbaric oxygen as an adjunct in the treatment of delayed radiation injuries of the extremities. Undersea Hyperbaric Med. 1998;25:9 (abstract).

Ferguson BJ, Hudson WR, Farmer JC. Hyperbaric oxygen therapy for laryngeal radionecrosis. Ann Otol Rhinol Larnygol. 1987;96:1–6.

Glassburn JR, Brady LW, Plenk HP. Hyperbaric oxygen in radiation therapy. Ann Cancer. 1977;39:751–65.

Greenwood TW, Gilchrist AG. Hyperbaric oxygen and wound healing in postirradiation head and neck surgery. Br J Surg. 1973;50:394.

Gupta P, Sahni T, Jadhav GK, Manocha S, Aggarwal S, Verma S. A retrospective study of outcomes in subjects of head and neck cancer treated with hyperbaric oxygen therapy for radiation induced osteoradionecrosis of mandible at a tertiary care centre: an Indian experience. Indian J Otolaryngol Head Neck Surg. 2013;65 Suppl 1:140–3.

Hamour A, Denning DW. Hyperbaric oxygen therapy in a women who declined colostomy. Lancet. 1996;348:197.

Hampson NB, Holm JR, Wreford-Brown CE, Feldmeier J. Prospective assessment of outcomes in 411 patients treated with hyperbaric oxygen for chronic radiation tissue injury. Cancer. 2012;118: 3860–8.

Harding SA, Hodder SC, Courtney DJ, Bryson PJ. Impact of perioperative hyperbaric oxygen therapy on the quality of life of maxillofacial patients who undergo surgery in irradiated fields. Int J Oral Maxillofac Surg. 2008;37:617–24.

Hart GB, Strauss MB. Hyperbaric oxygen in the management of radiation injury. In: Schmutz J, editor. Proceedings 1st Swiss symposium on hyperbaric medicine. Basel: Stiftung für Hyperbare Medizin; 1986. p. 31–51.

Headley DB, Gapany M, Dawson DE, Kruse GD, Robinson RA, McCabe BF. The effect of hyperbaric oxygen on growth of human squamous cell carcinoma xenografts. Arch Otolarngol Head Neck Surg. 1991;117:1269–72.

Hsu YC, Lee KW, Ho KY, Tsai KB, Kuo WR, Wang LF, et al. Treatment of laryngeal radionecrosis with hyperbaric oxygen therapy: a case report. Kaohsiung J Med Sci. 2005;21:88–92.

Kaufman T, Hirshowitz B, Monies-Chass I. Hyperbaric oxygen for postirradiation osteomyelitis of the chest wall. Harefuah. 1979;97:220–2. 271.

Kindwall EP. Hyperbaric oxygen treatment of radiation cystitis. Clin Plast Surg. 1993;20:589–92.

Kohshi K, Imada H, Nomoto S, Yamaguchi R, Abe H, Yamamoto H. Successful treatment of radiation-induced brain necrosis by hyperbaric oxygen therapy. J Neurol Sci. 2003;209:115–7.

Larsen PE, Stronczek MJ, Beck FM, et al. Osteointegration of implants in radiated bones with and without adjunctive hyperbaric oxygen. J Oral Maxillofac Surg. 1993;51:280–7.

Leber KA, Eder HG, Kovac H, Anegg U, Pendl G. Treatment of cerebral radionecrosis by hyperbaric oxygen therapy. Stereotact Funct Neurosurg. 1998;70 Suppl 1:229–36.

Li CQ, Gerson S, Snyder B. Case report: hyperbaric oxygen and MRI findings in radiation-induced optic neuropathy. Undersea Hyperb Med. 2014;41:59–63.

Liu JL. Clinical analysis of radiation optic neuropathy. Chung Hua Yen Ko Tsa Chih. 1992;28:86–8.

McMillan T, Calhoun KH, Mader JT, et al. The effect of hyperbaric oxygen on oral mucosal carcinoma. Laryngoscope. 1989;99: 241–4.

Mainous EG, Boyne PJ, Hart GB. Hyperbaric oxygen treatment of mandibular osteomyelitis: report of three cases. J Am Dent Assoc. 1973;87:1426–30.

Marx RE, Johnson RP. Problem wounds in oral and maxillofacial surgery: the role of hyperbaric oxygen. In: Davis JC, Hunt TK, editors. Problem wounds, the role of oxygen. New York: Elsevier; 1988. p. 65–123.

Marx RE, Johnson RP, Kline SN. Prevention of osteoradionecrosis: a randomized prospective clinical trial of hyperbaric oxygen versus penicillin. J Am Dent Assoc. 1985;111:49–54.

Mestrovic J. Does hyperbaric oxygen have a cancer-causing or promoting effect? Undersea Hyperbaric Med 1996;23: 55–56 (letter).

Mestrovic J, Kosuta D, Gosovic S, Denoble P, Radojković M, Angjelinović S, et al. Suppression of rat tumour colonies in the lung by oxygen at high pressure is a local effect. Clin Exp Metastasis. 1996;8:113–9.

Morita T, Takahashi K, Kitani Y, et al. Treatment of radiation cystitis with hyperbaric oxygen. In: Proceedings of the XI International Congress on Hyperbaric Medicine. San Pedro, Best Publishing; 1994.

Mounsey RA, Brown DH, O'Dwyer TP, Gullane PJ, Koch GH. Role of oxygen therapy in the management of mandibular osteoradionecrosis. Laryngoscope. 1993;103:605–8.

Nakada T, Yamaguchi T, Sasagawa I, Kubota Y, Suzuki H, Izumiya K. Successful hyperbaric oxygenation for radiation cystitis due to excessive irradiation to uterus cancer. Eur Urol. 1992;22:294–8.

Neovius EB, Lind MG, Lind FG. Hyperbaric oxygen therapy for wound complications after surgery in the irradiated head, and neck: a review of the literature and a report of 15 consecutive patients. Head Neck. 1997;19:315–22.

Narozny W, Sicko Z, Kot J, Stankiewicz C, Przewozny T, Kuczkowski J. Hyperbaric oxygen therapy in the treatment of complications of irradiation in head and neck area. Undersea Hyperb Med. 2005;32:103–10.

Neurath MF, Branbrink A, Meyer zum Büschenfelde KH, Lohse AW. A new treatment for severe malabsorption due to radiation enteritis. Lancet 1996;347: 1302.

Niezgoda JA, Serena TE, Carter MJ. Outcomes of radiation injuries using hyperbaric oxygen therapy: an observational cohort study. Adv Skin Wound Care. 2016;29:12–9.

Norkool DM, Hampson NB, Gibbons RP, Weissman RM. Hyperbaric oxygen therapy for radiation-induced hemorrhagic cystitis. J Urology. 1993;150:332–4.

Oliai C, Fisher B, Jani A, Wong M, Poli J, Brady LW, et al. Hyperbaric oxygen therapy for radiation-induced cystitis and proctitis. Int J Radiat Oncol Biol Phys. 2012;84:733–40.

Patel P, Raybould T, Maryama Y. Osteoradionecrosis of the jaw bones at the University of Kentucky Medical Center. J Kentucky Med Assoc. 1989;87:327–31.

Poulton TJ, Witcofski RL. Hyperbaric oxygen therapy for radiation myelitis. Undersea Biomed Res. 1985;12:453–8.

Ramsden RT, Bulman CH, Lorigan BP. Osteoradionecrosis of the temporal bone. Otolaryngol Head Neck Surg. 1975;89:941–55.

Ribeiro de Oliveira TM, Carmelo Romão AJ, Gamito Guerreiro FM, Matos Lopes TM. Hyperbaric oxygen therapy for refractory radiation-induced hemorrhagic cystitis. Int J Urol. 2015;22:962–6.

Rijkmans BG, Bakker DJ, Dabhoiwala NF, Kurth KH. Successful treatment of radiation cystitis with hypealianic oxygenation. Eur Urol. 1989;16:354–6.

Roden D, Bostley TM, Fowble B, Clark J, Savino PJ, Sergott RC, et al. Delayed radiation injury to the retrobulbar optic nerves and chiasm. Ophthalmology. 1990;97:346–51.

Rudge FW. Osteoradionecrosis of the temporal bone: treatment with hyperbaric oxygen therapy. Military Med. 1993;158:196–8.

Shameem IA, Shimabukuro T, Shirataki S, Yamamoto N, Maekawa T, Naito K. Hyperbaric oxygen therapy for the control of intractable cyclophosphamide-induced hemorrhagic cystitis. Eur Urol. 1992;22:263–4.

Sklizovic D, Sanger J, Kindwall EP, Fink JG, Grunert BK, Campbell BH. Hyperbaric oxygen therapy and squamous cell carcinoma cell line growth. Head Neck. 1993;5:236–40.

Slade B, Cianci P. Outcomes in 124 patients after monoplace hyperbaric oxygen therapy for radiation tissue damage—a 14 year experience. Undersea Hyperbaric Med 1998;25: 9 (abstract).

Svalestad J, Thorsen E, Vaagbø G, Hellem S. Effect of hyperbaric oxygen treatment on oxygen tension and vascular capacity in irradiated skin and mucosa. Int J Oral Maxillofac Surg. 2014;43:107–12.

Torubarov FS, Pakhomov VI, Krylova IV, Agapova EV. Changes in cerebral hemodynamics in patients with vascular pathology in the late stages of radiation sickness treated with hyperbaric oxygenation. Zh Nevropatol Psikhiatr Im S S Korsakova. 1983;83(1): 28–33.

Valadão J, Pearl J, Verma S, Helms A, Whelan H. Hyperbaric oxygen treatment for post-radiation central nervous system injury: a retrospective case series. Undersea Hyperb Med. 2014;41:87–96.

Velu SS, Myers RAM. Hyperbaric oxygen treatment of radiation induced hemorrhagic cystitis (abstract). Undersea Biomed Res. 1992;19(suppl):85.

Wang X, Ding I, Xie H, Wu T, Wersto N, Huang K, et al. Hyperbaric oxygen and basic fibroblast growth factor promote growth of irradiated bone. Int J Radiat Oncol Biol Phys. 1998;40:189–96.

Warren DC, Feehan P, Slade JB, Cianci PE. Chronic radiation proctitis treated with hyperbaric oxygen. Undersea Hyperbaric Med. 1997;24:181–4.

Weiss JP, Neville EC. Hyperbaric oxygen: primary treatment of radiation-induced hemorrhagic cystitis. J Urol. 1989;142:43–5.

Williams Jr JA, Clarke D, Dennis WA, Dennis 3rd EJ, Smith ST. The treatment of pelvic soft tissue radiation necrosis with hyperbaric oxygen. Am J Obstet Gynecol. 1992;167:412–5; discussion 415–6.

Woo TC, Joseph D, Oxer H. Hyperbaric oxygen treatment for radiation proctitis. Int J Radiat Oncol Biol Phys. 1997;38:619–20.

K.K. Jain

Abstract

Hyperbaric oxygen (HBO) has several effects that are useful for treating neurological disorders. This chapter reviews evidence concerning the effect of HBO on cerebral metabolism, cerebral blood flow, blood–brain barrier, and oxygen tension in the cerebrospinal fluid. Rationale for the use of HBO in neurological disorders is based on this evidence.

Indications for the use of HBO are listed. Clinical examination as well as the diagnostic procedures used for assessing the effect of HBO are described, particularly brain imaging. HBO has been used in thousands of cases of neurological disorders. Although controlled clinical trials are limited, the rational basis of HBO as well as good clinical results are strong arguments for use of HBO for treating neurological disorders.

Keywords

Blood–brain barrier • Brain imaging • Cerebral edema • Cerebral hypoxia • Cerebral ischemia • Cerebral metabolism • HBO effect on brain function • HBO effect on CNS • HBO in neurology • Hyperbaric oxygen (HBO)

Introduction

Since hypoxia and ischemia are involved in the pathophysiology of many disorders of the nervous system, hyperbaric oxygen (HBO) therapy has an important role in their management. To understand the role of HBO in neurological disorders, a basic knowledge of cerebral metabolism, cerebral blood flow, and the neurophysiology of the brain is essential.

Effect of HBO on Cerebral Metabolism

The effect of HBO on cerebral metabolism in the healthy state has been described in Chap. 2. The response of the injured brain to HBO is quite different. There is evidence for a Pasteur effect (inhibition of glycolysis by oxygen) with

hyperoxia in the case of carbohydrate metabolism in cerebrovascular disease. Inhalation of 100 % oxygen significantly decreased cerebral metabolic rate (CMR) for lactate and pyruvate. Since cerebral blood flow (CBF) decreased and cerebral pO_2 increased slightly, total glycolysis was decreased. Cerebral pO_2 plotted against CMR lactate showed evidence of the Pasteur effect.

Holbach et al. (1977) studied the effect of HBO on cerebral metabolism in cases of brain injury. They noted that normally there is aerobic glycolysis with phosphofructokinase as the regulating enzyme. The activity of this enzyme and the glycolysis are inhibited when, through the oxidation of glucose, citrate concentration and adenosine triphosphate rises (the Pasteur effect). Conversely, glycolysis is stimulated when ATP and citrate levels fall from high energy use, as in hypoxia (reverse Pasteur effect). Since 1 mL of oxygen oxidizes 1.34 mg of glucose, the glucose oxidation quotient (GOQ) is

$$\text{AVD of glucose} - \text{AVD of lactate} = 1.34\,\text{AVD of oxygen,}$$

where AVD is the arteriovenous difference.

K.K. Jain, MD, FRACS, FFPM (✉)
1 Blaesiring 7, Basel 4057, Switzerland
e-mail: jain@pharmabiotech.ch

© Springer International Publishing AG 2017
K.K. Jain, *Textbook of Hyperbaric Medicine*, DOI 10.1007/978-3-319-47140-2_18

The normal GOQ is 1.34 because the brain consumes oxygen almost exclusively from the oxidative metabolism of glucose. GOQ increases in anaerobic glycolysis as there is too high an amount of glucose still available for oxidation, even after subtracting the considerably increased AVD lactate. In patients treated with 100 % oxygen at 1.5 ATA (measurements made 10–15 min after the exposure), there was a moderate increase in AVD glucose and AVD lactate. The AVD oxygen remained constant. This resulted in a balancing of the cerebral glucose metabolism as reflected in the normal or near normal GOQ values. In trials of HBO at 2 ATA in similar situations, there was an increase of AVD glucose and a decrease of AVD oxygen compared with the values measured prior to the treatment (Holbach et al. 1977). The GOQ increased. The authors concluded that in the injured brain, HBO at 1.5 ATA has beneficial effects, whereas raising the pressure to 2 ATA has deleterious effects.

Contreras et al. (1988) measured cerebral glucose utilization using the autoradiographic 2-deoxyglucose technique in rats injured by focal cortical freeze lesions. They treated these animals with HBO at 2 ATA (90-min sessions) for 4 consecutive days. There was an overall increase of cerebral glucose utilization measured 5 days after injury when compared with the lesioned control animals exposed only to air (Fig. 18.1). The data indicate that the changes in cerebral glucose metabolism persist beyond the period of exposure to HBO. This observation is important as it explains the persistence of clinical improvement in patients after exposure to HBO.

Preclinical and clinical investigations indicate that the positive effect of HBO for severe traumatic brain injury (TBI) occurs after rather than during treatment. The brain appears better able to use baseline O_2 levels following HBO treatments. In a phase II clinical trial, in comparison with standard care (control treatment), combined HBO/normobaric hyperoxia (NBH) treatments significantly improved biomarkers of oxidative metabolism in relatively uninjured brain as well as pericontusional tissue, reduced intracranial hypertension, and showed improvement in biomarkers of cerebral toxicity (Rockswold et al. 2013). There was significant reduction in mortality and improved favorable outcome by combination of HBO and NBH therapy as compared with the two treatments in isolation.

HBO and intravenous hydroxocobalamin (OHCob) have synergistic effect as both abolish cyanide (CN)-induced surges in interstitial brain lactate and glucose concentrations. Whereas HBO delays an increase in whole-blood CN concentrations, OHCob acts as an intravascular CN scavenger. An experimental study in rats has shown that combined administration of OHCob and HBO has a beneficial and persistent effect on the cerebral metabolism during CN poisoning (Hansen et al. 2013).

Effect of HBO on Cerebral Blood Flow

Various studies of the effect of HBO on CBF are shown in Table 18.1. It is generally recognized that oxygen has a vasoconstrictive action and reduces CBF, though the

Fig. 18.1 Color-coded transformation of autoradiographs of brain sections at the level of the auditory cortex into a quantitative map of glucose utilization. Three of these areas that demonstrate a statistically significant interaction between the lesion and the HBO therapy are the auditory cortex (AC), the medial geniculate body (MGB), and the mammillary body (MB). The lesion was performed on the right side of the brain and is shown on the right side of these photographs. From Contreras FL, Kadekaro M, Eisenberg HM. The effect of hyperbaric oxygen on glucose utilization in a freeze-traumatized rat brain. J Neurosurg 1988;68: 137. With permission from JNS Publishing Group

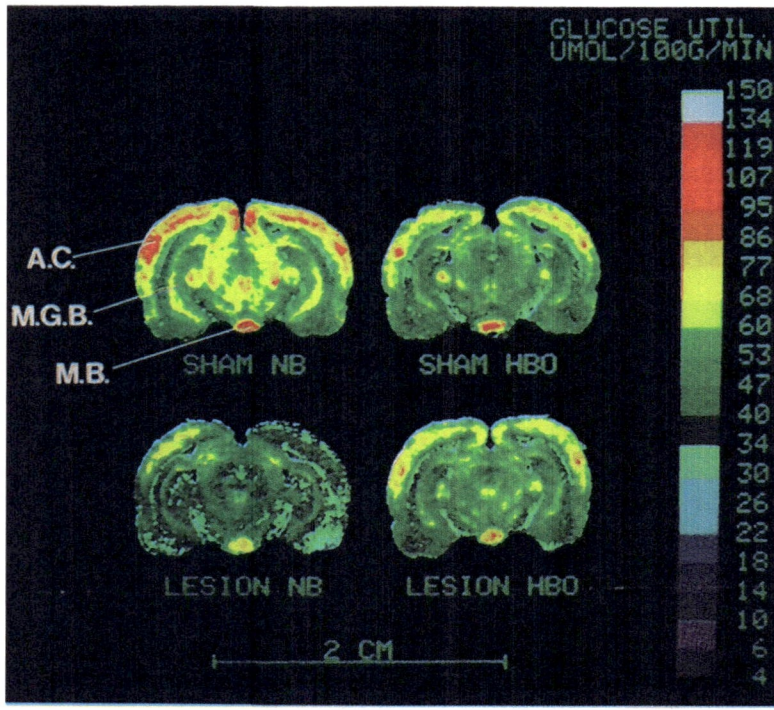

Table 18.1 Summary of cerebral blood flow under HBO as reported by various authors

Authors and year	Method	Material	Inhalant	Pressure	Change
Kety and Schmidt (1948)	Nitrous oxide	Man	O_2 85–100 %	1 ATA	Decrease 13 %
Lambertson et al. (1973)	Nitrous oxide	Man	O_2 100 %	3.5 ATA	Decrease 25 %
Jacobson and Lawson (1963)	Krypton-85 clearance	Dog	O_2 100 %	1 ATA 2 ATA	Decrease 12 % Decrease 21 %
Tindall et al. (1965)	Electromagnetic flowmeter	Baboon, internal carotid (5 min)	O_2 90 %	1 ATA 3 ATA 3 ATA	Decrease 9 % Decrease 13 % Decrease 18 % (10 min)
Harper et al. (1965)	Krypton-85 clearance	Dogs made hypotensive by bleeding	O_2 100 %	2 ATA	No change
Di Pretoro et al. (1968)	Rheography	Man	O_2 100 % Air	2 ATA 2 ATA	Reduced No change
Wuellenweber et al. (1969)	Thermal probes	Patients with brain injuries	O_2 100 %	2.5 ATA	Increase
Miler et al. (1970)	rCBF	Dogs, cryogenic probe lesions	O_2 100 %	2 ATA	
Hayakawa (1974)	Ultrasonic rheography	Man, internal carotid	O_2 100 %	1 ATA 2 ATA	Decrease 1 % Decrease 8 %
Artru et al. (1976)	^{133}Xe clearance	Patients with brain injury	O_2 100 %	2.5 ATA	Increase (in patients with cerebral edema)
Ohta et al. (1987)	^{133}Xe	Healthy volunteers	O_2 100 %	1 ATA 1.5 ATA 2 ATA 3 ATA	Decrease 9 % Decrease 23 % Decrease 29 % Decrease 14 %
Omae et al. (1998)	Transcranial Doppler	Human volunteers	O_2 100 %	HBO 2 ATA, control with hyperbaric air	Velocity of blood flow in the middle cerebral artery decreased with HBO as compared to hyperbaric air
Demchenko et al. (1998)	Hydrogen (H_2) clearance method	Rats	O_2 100 %	HBO 3 ATA	Decrease 26–39 %
Di Piero et al. (2002)	SPECT	Divers Healthy non-diver controls	O_2 100 %	HBO 2.8 ATA	Normobaric O_2 (NBO) No difference in CBF distribution between controls and divers in both NBO and HBO
Demchenko et al. (2005)	Platinum electrodes in globus pallidus	Rats	Air 100 % O_2	2–6 ATA	Doubling of CBF with HBO led to 13–64-fold increase in pallidum in a linear manner
Meirovithz et al. (2007)	Fiber-optic probe	Awake restrained rats	100 % O_2	1.75–6 ATA	The maximal level of microcirculatory HBO at 2.5 ATA is double the normoxic level

mechanism is unknown. Extracellular superoxide dismutase plays a critical role in the physiological response to oxygen in the brain by regulating nitric oxide (NO) availability. CBF responses in genetically altered mice to changes in PO_2 demonstrate that SOD3 regulates equilibrium between superoxide (O_2^-) and "NO", thereby controlling vascular tone and reactivity in the brain. That SOD3 opposes inactivation of NO is shown by the absence of vasoconstriction in response to PO_2 in the hyperbaric range in SOD3+/+mice, whereas NO-dependent relaxation is attenuated in SOD3−/− mutants (Demchenko et al. 2002). Thus, extracellular SOD promotes NO vasodilation by scavenging O_2^-, while hyperoxia opposes NO and promotes constriction by enhancing endogenous O_2^- generation and decreasing basal vasodilator effects of NO. The explanation of increase of CBF in some reports is as follows:

- If the probe was measuring flow in the area of the damaged brain, the increase in flow could be an "inverse steal phenomenon" due to vasoconstriction elsewhere.

- The area of brain under the probe might have lost its power of autoregulation, and the increase of blood flow could be due to an increase of perfusion pressure owing to a decrease of intracranial pressure (ICP) consequent upon vasoconstriction elsewhere in the brain.

The conflict among the reports in the literature on this subject arises from the variable effect of HBO on the normal versus the injured brain. If CBF is impaired by cerebral edema or raised ICP, it can be improved by HBO. Leninger-Follert and Hossmann (1977) made observations on the microcirculation and cortical oxygen pressure, during and after prolonged cerebral ischemia, that are relevant to the effect of HBO. According to these authors, complete cerebral ischemia of 1 h in cats followed by reactive hyperemia and recirculation as well as reoxygenation of the brain can occur. However, there is a critical phase of a few hours after the recommencement of circulation as soon as reactive hyperemia ceases. If brain swelling occurs during this period, cerebral hypoxia may develop. If brain swelling can be prevented, however, the distribution of oxygen pressure in the cortex can be restored to normal. HBO has a beneficial effect on cerebral edema.

Bean et al. (1971) suggested that HBO had a dual influence on the central vasculature initial vasoconstriction followed by vasodilatation and that prolonged exposure to HBO results in the loss of oxygen vascular constrictive controls. Based on the evidence available, it may be concluded that HBO generally causes vasoconstriction and results in a reduction of CBF. The detailed response of cerebral vessels to HBO, however, varies according to the degree of compression, exposure time, region of the brain, and pathological process in the brain and blood vessels. Ohta et al. (1987) believe that too much oxygen disturbs the regulatory oxygen response of CBF and may explain the pathogenesis of oxygen toxicity. These investigators state that reduced CBF under HBO is a protective response against oxygen toxicity.

Bergö et al. (1993) measured the changes in CBF distribution during HBO (5 ATA for 5 and 35 min) exposure in rats with unilateral frontal decortication lesions. CBF was reduced in most cerebral regions on the lesioned side. Brainstem showed reduction of CBF below the increased oxygen content after 35 min of HBO. The hypoxia as well as the disturbed balance between glutaminergic and GABAergic neurotransmitter systems was considered to have contributed to the increased frequency of convulsions in these animals. CBF decreases during HBO treatment at a constant $PaCO_2$. Hypercapnia prevents this decline, and elevated $PaCO_2$ augmented oxygen delivery to the brain, but increases the susceptibility to oxygen toxicity (Bergö and Tyssebotn 1999).

Omae et al. (1998) conducted a study to clarify the relationship between HBO and CBF in humans. Middle cerebral arterial blood flow velocity (MCV) was measured using tran-

scranial Doppler (TCD) technique in a multiplace hyperbaric chamber. The Doppler probe was fixed on the temporal region by a head belt, and the transcutaneous gas measurement apparatus ($tcPO_2$ and $tcPCO_2$) was fixed on the chest wall. MCV and transcutaneous gas were measured continuously in eight healthy volunteers under four various conditions: 1 ATA air, 1 ATA O_2, 2 ATA air, and 2 ATA O_2. Next, the effect of environmental pressure was studied in another eight healthy volunteers, in whom the $tcPO_2$ was kept at almost the same level under conditions of both 1 ATA and 4 ATA by inhaling oxygen at 1 ATA. MCV of 1 ATA O_2, 2 ATA air, and 2 ATA O_2 decreased, and $tcPO_2$ increased significantly in comparison with that of 1 ATA air. A significant difference in MCV was observed between the O_2 group and the air group under the same pressure circumstance. On the other hand, there were no differences in MCV or $tcPO_2$ between 4 ATA air and 1 ATA plus O_2, and the influence for the MCV of the environmental pressure was not observed. The authors concluded that hyperoxemia caused by HBO reduces the CBF, but the high atmospheric pressure per se does not influence the CBF in humans.

A decrease in nitric oxide (NO) availability in the brain tissue due to the inhibition of nitric oxide synthase (NOS) activity during the early phases of HBO exposure is involved in hyperoxic vasoconstriction leading to reduced rCBF. Increased levels of asymmetric dimethylarginine, an endogenous inhibitor of NOS, have been demonstrated in rat brains exposed to HBO (Akgül et al. 2007).

Effect of HBO on the Blood–Brain Barrier

Some earlier animal experimental studies indicated that HBO increases the permeability of the cerebral vessel walls in normal animals. These findings were not substantiated in later studies. Blood–brain barrier (BBB) is disturbed in certain disorders such as cerebrovascular ischemia, and HBO may serve to decrease the permeability of BBB. Intra-ischemic HBO therapy reduces early and delayed postischemic BBB damage and edema after focal ischemia in rats and mice (Veltkamp et al. 2005).

Effect of HBO on Oxygen Tension in the Cerebrospinal fluid

Oxygen tension of cerebrospinal fluid (CSF) usually reflects the arterial pO_2 tension. However, in severe brain injury, intracranial arteriovenous shunts or capillary blocks may prevent the rise of CSF oxygen tension with a rise of respiratory oxygen, and this difference may be an index of the degree of injury to the brain. This may also mean that in a brain with multiple injuries, oxygen may not reach the damaged part resulting in hypoxia.

Rationale for the Use of HBO in Neurological Disorders

The following are the main mechanisms of the effectiveness of HBO in neurological disorders:

- Relief of hypoxia
- Improvement of microcirculation
- Relief of cerebral edema by vasoconstrictive effect
- Preservation of partially damaged tissue and prevention of further progression of secondary effects of cerebral lesions
- Improvement of cerebral metabolism

Relief of hypoxia is the most significant effect of HBO. Hypoxia has been described in Chap. 5. Hypoxemia can be corrected by normobaric 100 % oxygen inhalation, but hypoxia of some lesions of the CNS requires HBO for correction. The beneficial effect of HBO on cerebral hypoxia has been shown by biochemical studies. It is well known that there is an increase of lactate in brain and CSF in cerebral injury and anoxia. There is a decrease in the CSF lactate/pyruvate ratio during HBO exposure leading to reduction of anaerobic in favor of aerobic metabolism.

The rational basis of the use of HBO in some neurological disorders is understandable in view of the pathogenesis of multiple sclerosis. According to one concept, the following phenomena may occur in multiple sclerosis (James 1987, 2007):

- Failure of pulmonary filtration of fat microemboli
- Blood–brain barrier dysfunction that allows access of fat emboli to the brain parenchyma
- Focal areas of perivenous edema preceding demyelination

Vascular disturbances in the pathogenesis of multiple sclerosis may provide the rational basis for HBO therapy in this disease.

Cerebral Hypoxia

Oxygen is vital for the brain, and oxygen deficiency, regardless of the cause, starts a vicious circle of pathological changes in brain tissue:

Primary brain damage → hypoxia edema → aggravation of hypoxia → secondary brain damage

The object of HBO therapy in brain injuries is to supply the brain tissue with adequate oxygen and to interrupt this process.

Cerebral Edema

Brain edema is divided into three types:

- Vasogenic. There is cerebral vasomotor paresis with transudation of plasma proteins into the extracellular space of the brain, e.g., brain injury, abscess, tumor, or infarction.
- Cytotoxic. Swelling in the intracellular space, e.g., CO poisoning and hyposmolarity.
- Interstitial. Fluid escapes from the ventricle to enter the extracellular space of the periventricular white matter. This is unique to hydrocephalus.

Cerebral edema is a frequent finding in many disorders of the CNS. Its pathogenesis is depicted in Fig. 18.2.

Generalized edema is a life-threatening process due to the rise of intracranial pressure (ICP) associated with it. The role of localized edema in aggravating the neurological deficits resulting from focal vascular and demyelinating lesions is generally not well recognized. With modern neuroimaging techniques, it has become possible to demonstrate focal brain edema in vivo.

The ICP represents the sum of three components: the volume of the brain substance, the CSF, and the blood present in the cranial cavity at any time. Reduction of any of these components can lower ICP. The conventional treatments for brain edema and raised ICP include corticosteroids, osmotic diuretics, hyperventilation, barbiturate coma, and ventricular drainage.

Experimental Studies

Most of the research regarding the effect of HBO on cerebral edema and raised ICP has been done on experimental animals. These studies are shown in Table 18.2. Since these studies were published, further experimental work continues in this area.

Effect of HBO preconditioning (HBO-PC) on peri-hemorrhagic focal edema and aquaporin-4 (AQP-4) expression has been studied in an experimental rat model of intracerebral hemorrhage (ICH). The results show that HBO-PC may downregulate AQP-4 expression to reduce the intracerebral edema, thus strengthening tolerance to ICH and protecting the neurons (Fang et al. 2015). Peri-hemorrhagic edema exacerbates the mass effect of hematoma and contributes to early neurological deterioration after intracerebral hemorrhage (ICH). Because oxygen therapy has a protective effect on the BBB, a study examined the effects of oxygen therapy on edema formation and BBB permeability after ICH in a mouse model (Zhou et al. 2015). NBO and HBO (3 ATA for 1 h) initiated within 30 min of ICH induction attenuated edema formation and BBB disruption, whereas delayed oxygen therapy had no effect. Early oxygen therapies prevented occludin degradation, MMP-9 activation, and reduced HIF-1α

Fig. 18.2 Pathophysiology of
cerebral edema

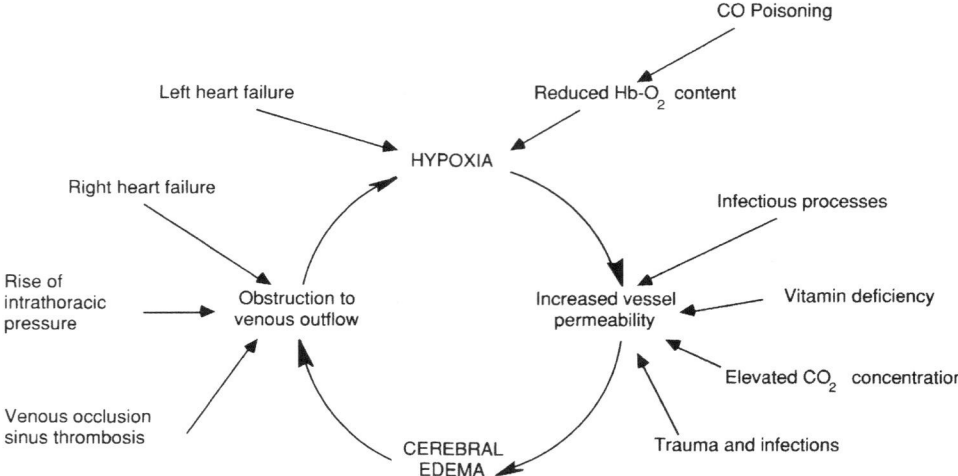

expression. Although early oxygen therapy can attenuate edema formation and BBB disruption after ICH, the brief therapeutic time window limits the translational potential.

Clinical Studies

Clinical studies of the effect of HBO on cerebral edema are shown in Table 18.3. A classical concept of the role of HBO in cerebral edema, which is still valid, is as follows (Pierce and Jacobson 1977):

> "This therapy directly decreases vasogenic brain edema and due to improvement of O_2 delivery to anoxic tissue acts on cytotoxic brain edema as well. The mechanism underlying the potentially beneficial action of HBO appears clear and is well supported by animal and clinical studies. HBO should be considered an adjunct for patients who are not sufficiently responsive to standard methods. Treatment levels should not exceed 2 ATA and an effort should be made to prevent the rebound phenomenon by titrating pO_2 downwards, preferably by varying O_2 concentrations while maintaining hyperbaric pressure levels."

The favorable results of HBO on cerebral edema in experimental animals have been confirmed by the clinical use of HBO for the relief of traumatic cerebral edema. HBO (1.5 ATA) treatment of patients with severe brain injury reduces raised intracranial pressure and improves aerobic metabolism (Rockswold et al. 2001; Sukoff 2001).

Application of HBO during the early phase of severe fluid percussion brain injury in rats significantly diminishes ICP elevation rate and decreased mortality level (Rogatsky et al. 2005). In conclusion, it can be stated that HBO relieves cerebral edema by the following mechanisms as shown in Fig. 18.3:

- Reduction of CBF but maintenance of cerebral oxygenation.
- HBO counteracts the effects of ischemia and hypoxia associated with cerebral edema and interrupts the cycle of hypoxia/edema.

HBO lowers raised ICP in traumatic cerebral edema as long as the cerebral arteries are reactive to CO_2. It is ineffective in the presence of vasomotor paralysis and is contraindicated in terminal patients with this condition. The effects of HBO can persist after the conclusion of a session, and there is no rebound phenomenon, as is the case with the use of osmotic diuretics. If the ICP is elevated due to obstruction in the CSF pathways, as is the case in intraventricular hemorrhage, HBO and dehydrating agents have only a temporary effect in lowering ICP. Ventricular drainage is important in these patients, not only to lower the ICP but also to improve the CBF that decreases as an effect of raised ICP. Persistence of raised ICP can cause further cerebral damage. Studies of the effect of HBO on raised ICP in patients with brain tumors and cerebrovascular disease indicate that reduced ICP is initially due to direct vasoconstriction caused by hyperoxia but tends to rise again. However, the secondary rise can be prevented by induced hypocapnia.

The injured brain is susceptible to oxygen toxicity if high pressures are used. This is usually not a problem as the pressures seldom exceed 2.5 ATA; 1.5 ATA is used for most neurological indications.

Role of HBO in Neuroprotection

The concept of neuroprotection is now important in many neurological disorders that were once only treated symptomatically and in which a disease-modifying approach is desirable. Neuroprotective agents have an important role in the management of neurodegenerative disorders as well as acute insults such as CNS trauma, cerebral ischemia, and iatrogenic hypoxia/ischemia during surgical procedures. Neuroprotective strategies are also required to protect the brain against toxic effects of chemicals and drugs. There are numerous

Table 18.2 Experimental studies of the effect of HBO on cerebral edema

Authors and year	Experimental animals and methods	Results and comments
Jamieson and Van Den Brenk (1963)	Rats. Oxygen tension measured in the brain under HBO (2 ATA)	Decrease of edema. Increase of brain oxygen tension in spite of vasoconstriction
Coe and Hayes (1966)	Rats. Two groups with brain injury by liquid nitrogen One group treated by HBO at 3 ATA	Treated group survived longer and had less cerebral edema and less neuronal damage than the untreated group
Dunn and Connolly (1966)	Dogs. One group treated by HBO, the other by normobaric 100%. Single 2 h treatment	Reduction in mortality in both groups equal. Authors concluded that any additional benefits from HBO was not manifest because of vasoconstriction
Jinnai et al. (1967)	Cats and rabbits	Extradural balloons and intracarotid injections. Group tested by HBO at 3 ATA for 1 h
Sukoff et al. (1967)	Dogs. Psyllium seed injections in the brain	HBO at 3 ATA given at every 8 h starting 25 h after injury Decreased mortality and morbidity in treated animals as compared with untreated ones
Moody et al. (1970)	Dogs. Injuries simulating extradural hematoma. Assisted respiration with 100% oxygen (1 ATA) in one group and 100% oxygen at 1 ATA or 2 ATA in other groups with spontaneous respiration	Best reduction in mortality was in animals breathing spontaneously with 100% oxygen at 2 ATA for 4 h
Hayakawa et al. (1971)	Dogs with and without brain injury at HBO 3 ATA CSF pressure measurements	In dogs without brain damage, CSF pressure decreased initially but rose later due to CBF disturbances. There was more consistent decrease in brain-injured animals
Dunn (1974)	Freeze lesions to produce cerebral edema. Four groups 1. Control 2. Ventilated for 2–3 h with air 3. 3 h of 97% oxygen + 3% CO_2 hyperventilation 4. 3 h of HBO at 3 ATA (97% oxygen + 3% CO) + hyperventilation	The lowest mortality (29%) was in group 4 (mean survival 5.3 days). The highest mortality was in group 3 (mean survival 2 days). HBO with hyperventilation was shown to reduce ICP definitely
Nagao et al. (1975)	25 dogs. Anesthetized and ventilated	ICP raised by extradural balloons. HBO reduced ICP only when cerebral circulation was responsive to CO_2 In animals treated by HBO, CO_2 reactivity was maintained until high levels of ICP
Miller (1979)	Dogs. Cerebral edema by liquid nitrogen. Effect of HBO on CBF and ICP	HBO caused a 30% reduction of ICP and 19% reduction of CBF so long as the cerebral vessels remained responsive to CO_2
Gu (1985)	Rabbits. Experimental edema. Treated by various mixtures of nitrogen and oxygen as well as 100% O_2 at 1 and 4 ATA	No effect of mixtures of oxygen and nitrogen 100% caused a drop of ICP at both 1 and 4 ATA
Isakov and Romasenko (1985)	30 rabbits. Head injury, 15 treated by HBO. The rest were controls	Ten sessions of HBO led to significant reduction of tissue water in the brain of animals treated by HBO
Nida et al. (1995)	Fluid percussion (FP) injury or cortical injury (CI) in rats. Treated with HBO (1.5 ATA for 60 min), starting 4 h after head trauma	HBO reduced edema produced by FP but not by CI although both were equally severe

neuroprotective agents from several pharmacological as well as nonpharmaceutical categories (Jain 2011). HBO is an important neuroprotective agent.

A study on cultured cortical neurons has shown that HBO-PC has a directly beneficial effects on cortical neurons subjected to oxygen–glucose deprivation by the activation of peroxisome proliferator-activated receptor gamma (PPAR-γ) subsequent to the production of 15-deoxy-Δ(12,14)-prostaglandin J(2) (an endogenous ligand with a high affinity for PPAR-γ), which in turn increases the downstream antioxidant enzymatic activities (Zeng et al. 2012).

Role of HBO in neuroprotection against spinal cord injury (SCI) has been investigated in a rat model. Nitric oxide and induced NO synthase (iNOS) are involved in this mechanism. The study concluded that HBO therapy can promote

Table 18.3 Clinical studies of the effect of HBO on cerebral edema

Authors and year	Diagnosis and no. of patients	Results and comments
Jinnai et al. (1967)	Head injuries, 7; postoperative neurosurgery, 8	Neurological and EEC improvement but not long lasting
Hayakawa et al. (1971)	Brain trauma or neurosurgery, 15 continuous monitoring of ICP and CBF before, during, and after HBO at 2 ATA	Three types of responses: I CSF pressure decreased initially and then rose ($n=9$) II ICP was lowered and remained so ($n=2$) III Little or no response of ICP to HBO ($n=4$)
Miller (1973)	Head injury patients, 30% reduction of ICP at 2 ATA (PAO$_2$ 1227 mmHg)	No further education when pressure raised to 3 ATA
Sukoff and Ragatz (1982)	Head injury patients, 50	Considerable reduction of cerebral edema as shown by CT scan and clinical evaluation

Fig. 18.3 Mechanism of effectiveness of HBO in cerebral edema

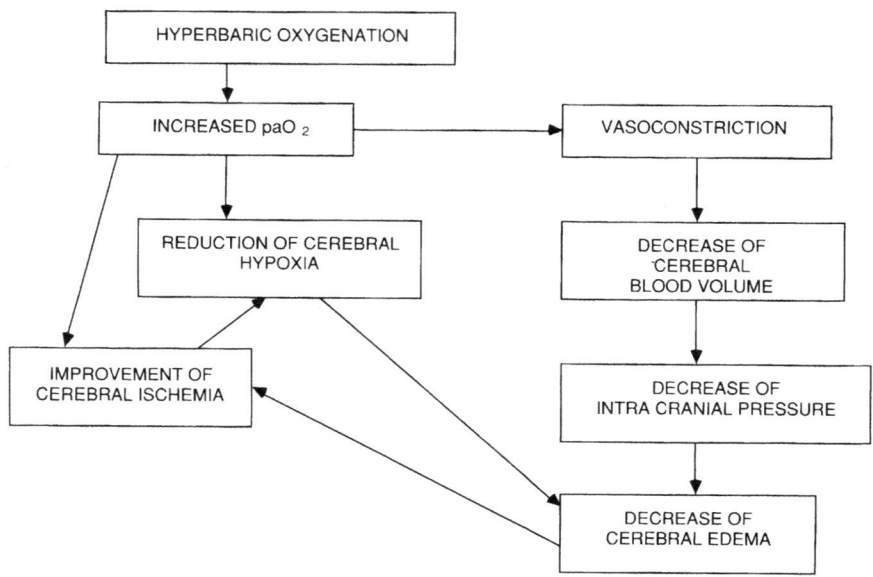

neuroprotection following SCI, which may be related to the effect of HBO on the iNOS mRNA–iNOS–NO signaling pathway (Huang et al. 2013).

Interleukin-10 (IL-10) plays a role of in the neuroprotection of HBO against TBI in a mouse model (Chen et al. 2014). HBO (100 %) given for 1 h at 2 ATA enhanced IL-10 levels in the serum and brain tissues. Sirtuin 1 (Sirt1) is a class III histone deacetylase involved in neuroprotection induced by HBO-PC in animal models of cerebral ischemia. HBO-PC was shown to increase the expression of Sirt1 and reduced infarct volume ratio and neurobehavioral deficit in a rat model of middle cerebral artery occlusion (Xue et al. 2016). HBO-PC also increased expression of nuclear factor erythroid 2-related factor 2 (Nrf2), heme oxygenase 1 (HO-1), and superoxide dismutase 1 (SOD1) concomitant with decrease in the level of malondialdehyde (a biomarker of oxidative stress). Furthermore, either Sirt1 or Nrf2 knockdown by short interfering RNA inhibited the expression of Nrf2, HO-1, and SOD1 and eliminated the neuroprotective effects of HBO-PC. These results suggest

that the Nrf2/antioxidant defense pathway is involved in the long-lasting neuroprotective effects of Sirt1 induced by HBO-PC against transient focal cerebral ischemia.

Indications for the Use of HBO in Neurological Disorders

Various neurological conditions where HBO has been reported to be useful are listed in Table 18.4. Most of these are based on a review of the literature. There are few controlled clinical studies. The Undersea and Hyperbaric Medical Society (UHMS) USA does not list any of these conditions (with the exception of cerebral air embolism) as approved for payment by third-party insurance carriers. The role of HBO in cerebrovascular disease is described in Chap. 19. HBO for the management of anoxic encephalopathies is dealt with in Chap. 20, neurosurgical disorders in Chap. 21, HBO as an adjunct to the management of multiple sclerosis is discussed in Chap. 22, cerebral palsy in

Table 18.4 Neurological indications for the use of HBO therapy

1. Cerebrovascular disease
Acute cerebrovascular occlusive disease
Chronic poststroke stage
Treatment of spasticity
Aid to rehabilitation
Adjunct to cerebrovascular surgery
Selection of patients for intracranial/extracranial bypass operation
Postoperative complications of intracranial aneurysm surgery: cerebral edema and ischemia
Carotid endarterectomy under HBO as a cerebral protective measure
2. Cerebral air embolism
3. Head injuries: cerebral edema and raised intracranial pressure
4. Spinal cord lesions
Acute traumatic paraplegia within 4 h of injury
Spinal cord decompression sickness (spinal cord "hit")
Ischemic disease of the spinal cord
Aid to the rehabilitation of paraplegia and quadriplegia
Residual neurological deficits after surgery of compressive spinal lesion
5. Cranial nerve lesions
Optic nerve ischemia: occlusion of the central artery of the retina
Facial palsy
Sudden deafness
Vestibular disorders
6. Peripheral neuropathies
7. Multiple sclerosis
8. Cerebral insufficiency (decline of mental function): multi-infarct dementia
9. Infections of the CNS and its coverings: brain abscess, meningitis
10. Radiation-induced necrosis of the CNS: radiation myelopathy and encephalopathy
11. CO poisoning
12. Migraine headaches
13. Cerebral palsy

Chap. 23, and miscellaneous disorders in Chap. 24. The rationale for the use of HBO is discussed, along with the indications.

Clinical Neurological Assessment of Response to HBO

Neurological examination in the hyperbaric chamber is important in determining the effect of hyperbaric oxygen. Some of the effects are transient and may not be seen after removal of the patient from the chamber. It is not necessary to have a specialist provide a simple brief neurological examination, because any physician should be able to carry out such an investigation. Due to constraints of space and time, the examination should be limited to less than 5 min and repeated as often as possible, but at least three times during a hyperbaric session—once during the compression phase, once during the oxygenation phase, and once during decompression. A simple procedure such as measurement of the handgrip by a hand dynamometer can be done more often. The following are some examples as guide-

lines. Each hyperbaric center should develop its own protocol for the minimum neurological testing acceptable to the attending neurologist.

Comatose Patients

For comatose patients, the following should be included in the testing:

1. Reaction to painful stimuli by movement of limbs.
2. The presence or absence of decerebrate rigidity.
3. Pupil size and reaction to light.
4. Fundoscopic examination—look for any vasoconstriction.
5. Glasgow coma scale in the case of patients with head injury.

Paraplegics

1. Mark the level below which the sensory loss begins and chart the sensory loss, if partial.

2. Grading of the major muscle group power if incomplete lesion.
3. In subacute or chronic cases with spasticity, clinical grading of spasticity by passive range of motion.

Hemiplegics (Stroke Patients)

1. Fundoscopic examination, visual acuity, and visual fields by confrontation
2. Motor power testing, proximal muscles of the arm and the leg; test the time it takes for the stretched-out (in sitting position) and the raised leg (in supine position) to drift; measurement of the handgrip by a hand-held dynamometer
3. Testing for spasticity, clinical grading of spasticity (see Chap. 19), measurement of spasticity of fingers by a handy muscle tonometer

A patient's response to a single HBO treatment is sometimes used for determining the response to HBO therapy and to make a decision regarding continuation of the therapy, but this may not be adequate. In some patients, the improvement resulting from HBO therapy is noticeable only after several treatments.

Diagnostic Procedures Used for Assessing the Effect of HBO

Routine neurological procedures are not necessarily useful in assessing the effects of HBO therapy, but the following are worthy of consideration.

Electrophysiological Studies

The EEG has been found to be useful in assessing the response of patients to HBO treatment. A technique of interval amplitude EEG analysis (power spectrum) of patients during HBO therapy sessions has been described (Wassmann 1980). Two examples of the use of EEG in evaluating the response to HBO are shown in Figs. 18.4 and 18.5. Slow waves tended to decrease and alpha activity tends to increase on the side of the lesion in patients undergoing HBO at 2 ATA. Topographic EEG mapping is an acceptable objective parameter of the effect of HBO on the brain. In normal subjects somatosensory evoked potentials (SSEP) are reproducible under hyperbaric conditions and can be used to assess the response of spinal cord injury patients to HBO therapy. EEG is used little now for the evaluation of HBO treatment effects. The emphasis is now on brain imaging methods.

Recording biological signals inside a hyperbaric chamber poses technical challenges (the steel walls enclosing it greatly attenuate or completely block the signals), practical (lengthy cables creating eddy currents), and safety (sparks hazard from power supply to the electronic apparatus inside the chamber), which can be overcome with new wireless technologies. A Bluetooth system has been developed for EEG recording inside a hyperbaric chamber and enables EEG signal transmission outside the chamber (Pastena et al. 2015a). In contrast to older systems, this technology allows the online recording of amplified signals, without interference from eddy currents. This technology has been applied to measure EEG activity in professional divers under experimental conditions in a hyperbaric chamber to determine how oxygen, at a constant pressure of 2.8 ATA, affects the electrical activity

Fig. 18.4 HBO therapy of a patient with severe cerebral edema and raised intracranial pressure (ICP). Continuous recording. Courtesy of Wassman and Holbach, 1988

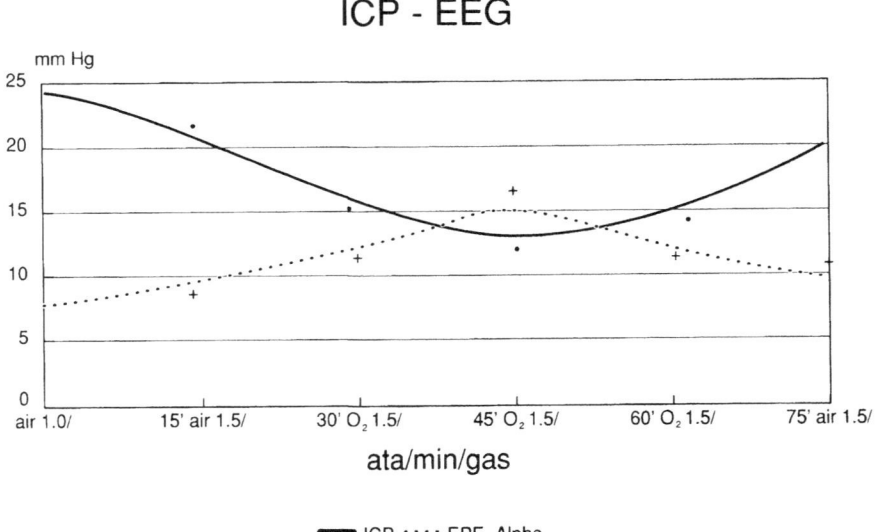

Fig. 18.5 Illustration of EEG power spectrum during HBO treatment of a patient suffering from cerebral hypoxia. A definite increase of alpha activity is seen during the rise of oxygen partial pressure. Courtesy of Wassmann and Holbach, 1988

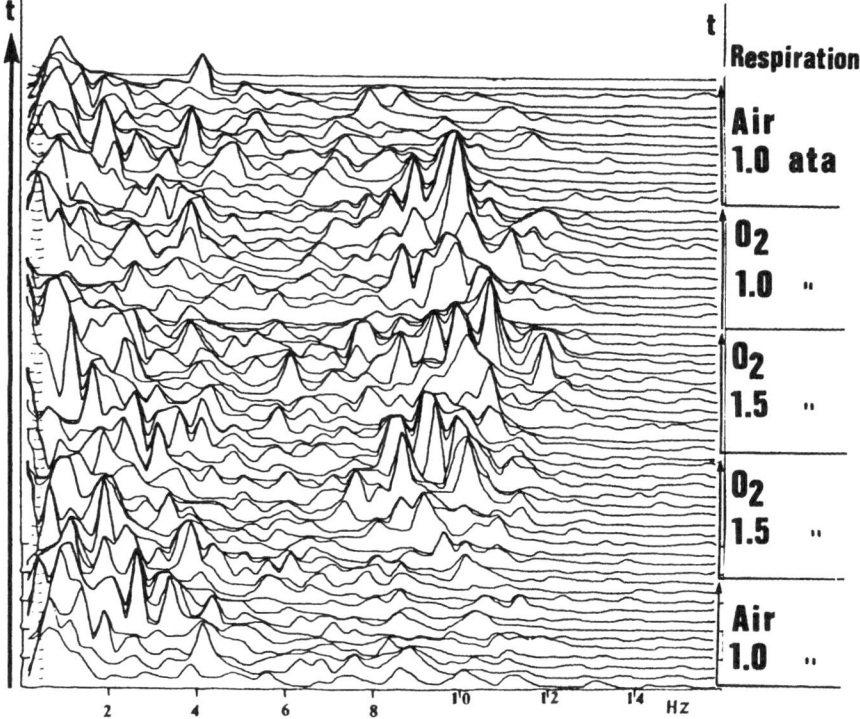

of the brain. A 32-channel EEG recording with Bluetooth showed that during oxygen breathing, brain activity showed an early fast delta decrease in the posterior regions, with a synchronous and significant increase in alpha in the same regions. After decompression, the delta relative power decrease was uniformly distributed over the cerebral cortex until minute 8, and the alpha relative power was maximal in the posterior regions during the first 2 min (Pastena et al. 2015b). This system has the potential to detect early signs of possible oxygen toxicity during HBO treatment.

Cerebral Blood Flow

This is most relevant to stroke and its management using HBO. Brain dysfunction after stroke closely relates to the site and extension of lesions and thus correlates with the degree of reduction of CBF and metabolism. The most commonly used method in the past few years has been the [133]xenon (Xe) inhalation method. The technique is based on gamma scintillation counting on NaI crystals after inhalation of [133]xenon. This gives the values for regional CBF (rCBF), More recently positron emission tomography (PET) has been used for measuring rCBF. Relations between rCBF, glucose metabolism, oxygen consumption, and the structural lesions have been studied in the acute stroke to assess the

impact of various treatments on the evolution of stroke during the first few hours after the onset. rCBF is also useful in the subacute and chronic phases of stroke. The severity of hemiparesis correlates with degree of asymmetry of CBF. Bilateral reductions of CBF are more likely to be associated with cognitive impairment. Quantitative CBF in acute ischemic stroke can be determined by XeCT, and these measurements correlate with early CT findings. This system is commercially available, and the advantages of this method are that CBF can be determined by the CT staff along with routine CT without waiting for the CBF staff. Results are available within 20 min.

A study in healthy volunteers has shown that CBF distribution increases during HBO in sensory motor and visual cortices with a higher perfusion tracer distribution in areas involved in dorsal attention system and in default mode network (Micarelli et al. 2013). These findings indicate both the externally directed cognition performance improvement related to the HBO and the internally directed cognition states during resting-state conditions, suggesting possible beneficial effects in TBI and stroke patients.

A study aimed to characterize changes in rCBF in patients with CO poisoning who subsequently developed severe delayed neuropsychiatric sequelae (DNS) with akinetic mutism as well as improvement with HBO (Chen et al. 2016). All recovered to nearly normal daily function after initial treatments. However, after a "lucid interval" DNS progressed to akinetic mutism. The SPECT images acquired at the onset of akinetic mutism demonstrated variable hypoperfusion in frontal–temporal–parietal regions, with the greatest severity in the left temporal–parietal regions. Functional neuropsychiatric tests were performed in parallel. After HBO treatment, the brain SPECT showed significantly fewer hypoperfusion regions, and neuropsychiatric tests showed dramatically improved function. Improvement in rCBF correlated well with functional recovery after treatment.

Computerized Tomography

Principles

Computerized tomography (CT) permits the examination of tissue by the same principle as conventional X-ray imaging, except that the radiation passes successively through tissue from multiple different directions, detectors measure the degree of attenuation of the exiting radiation relative to the incident radiation, and computers integrate the information and construct the image in cross section. Administration of a contrast agent increases X-ray attenuation owing to the high atomic number and electron density of the iodinated compounds used. Use of intravenous contrast agent enables the assessment of the integrity of the BBB. CT angiography (CTA) can also be performed after intravenous infusion of a nonionic contrast agent. Contrast CT can detect cytotoxic edema.

Advantages and Disadvantages

Advantages of CT are the widespread availability, short study time, and sensitivity for detection of calcification and acute hemorrhage. It can be used in situations where MRI cannot be used in persons with intracranial metallic clips, pacemakers, and other metal prostheses. It is preferred in rapidly evolving neurologic disorders where direct observation of the patient and life support systems is essential during scanning procedure. CT usually costs about half as much the MRI scan. Main disadvantages of CT scan are that it involves radiation and is less sensitive than MRI. Most of the hospitals in the USA with 200 or more beds have this equipment. The distribution of this diagnostic facility is much lower in Europe, and rare is confined mostly to large medical centers in developing countries.

Uses. This is the most widely used diagnostic procedure in neurological disorders. CT scan is the method of choice for assessment of ischemic injury to the brain. It is done without contrast to determine whether the stroke is hemorrhagic or ischemic. It is absolutely essential because all subsequent therapeutic decisions depend on the results of this examination. It can detect almost all of intracranial hematomas more than 1 cm in diameter and more than 95% of subarachnoid hemorrhages. Definite changes of infarction are usually not seen for 24–48 h after onset, but subtle signs of ischemia may appear before 3 h.

CT scan is used for detecting traumatic hematomas, brain tumors, abscesses, and other infectious granulomas such as tuberculomas. Edema surrounding intracranial lesions such as those due to brain tumor and injury can be detected. Changes from cerebral edema include a local mass effect with distortion of the ventricular system.

Magnetic Resonance Imaging

Principle

A tissue, when placed in a strong magnetic field, causes certain naturally occurring isotopes (atoms) within the tissue to line up within the field, orienting the net tissue magnetization in the longitudinal direction. Current magnetic resonance imaging (MRI) uses signals derived from 1H, the most plentiful endogenous isotope. Within a magnetic field, these atoms do not orient precisely with the axis of the field, but wobble a few degrees off center. Application of a radio-frequency pulse perpendicular to the applied magnetic field reorients the net tissue magnetization from the longitudinal to the transverse plane. When the radio-frequency pulse is turned off, the net tissue magnetization returns to its previous orientation, resulting in a magnetic resonance signal that can be detected by receiver coils. Application of different-gradient magnetic fields to the tissue under study permits reconstruction of the signal from individual volume units in space. The result is a clear image of the tissue in space.

Sequences such as T1 and T2, proton density, and spin-echo-weighted images enhance the utility of the MRI. Use of intravascular contrast material gadolinium-diethyleneamine pentaacetic acid with MRI enhances the magnetic susceptibility of the adjacent tissue, thereby providing information about the integrity of the BBB. Diffusion-weighted imaging can detect cytotoxic edema and is sensitive to early ischemic changes in the brain. Magnetic resonance angiography (MRA) enables noninvasive visualization of the cerebral and extracerebral vessels. Magnetic resonance spectroscopy provides a noninvasive method of studying brain metabolites, brain pH, and some neurotransmitter without the use of ionizing radiation. Functional MRI is a method of imaging the oxygen status of hemoglobin in order to visualize local changes in CBF that reflect changes in neuronal activity in response to a specific sensory stimulus or motor task.

Advantages and Disadvantages

The advantages of MRI are the absence of ionizing radiation, sensitivity to blood flow, high soft tissue contrast resolution, and capacity to produce images in any plane. MRI is superior to CT for detecting most CNS lesions including cerebral infarction but is not as effective as CT for detecting subarachnoid hemorrhage. MRI may show evidence of ischemic stroke sooner than CT. Drawbacks of MRI include the lack of general availability and difficulty in monitoring seriously ill patients during the examination and the time needed to perform it which is longer than that for unenhanced CT scan. SAH can be missed by MRI scan.

Uses

A study measured T1 from MRI under normobaric oxygen and HBO conditions as a biomarker of tissue pO_2 since dissolved molecular oxygen acts as an endogenous contrast agent (Muir et al. 2016). Brain tissue T1 decreased corresponding to increased pO_2 with increasing inhaled oxygen concentrations. MRI-derived tissue pO_2 was markedly lower than the arterial pO_2 but was slightly higher than venous pO_2. This approach may prove useful in evaluating tissue oxygenation in disease states such as stroke.

With newer MRI techniques such as diffusion-weighted and perfusion-weighted imaging, immediate identification of ischemic injury is possible, and reversible ischemia can be estimated. MRI is superior to CT in detecting cerebral edema and for detecting small lacunar lesions, particularly those located deep within the cerebral hemispheres and in the brain stem.

MRI is also used for evaluating the progression or regression of lesions of multiple sclerosis.

MRI and diffusion-weighted imaging have been used to evaluate the efficacy HBO in experimental TBI in rabbits (Wei et al. 2014). Results show that HBO can improve the impaired BBB and cytotoxic edema after TBI and promote the recovery of neural function.

A retrospective analysis of patients suffering from chronic neurocognitive impairment from TBI treated with HBO was done pre- and post-HBO by using objective computerized cognitive tests and brain perfusion MRI (Tal et al. 2015). Post-HBO whole-brain perfusion analysis showed significantly increased CBF and cerebral blood volume. Clinically, HBO induced significant improvement in the global cognitive scores with most prominent improvements in information processing speed, visual spatial processing, and motor skills indices. The improvement was attributed to HBO-induced cerebral angiogenesis, which improves perfusion to the chronic damage brain tissue even months to years after the injury.

Positron Emission Tomography

This is a method of radionuclide scanning which requires the intravenous radioligand with a positron-emitting isotope, accumulation of the ligand in the brain, and subsequent emission of the positrons from the ligand into the adjacent tissue during radioactive decay. Positrons are the antimatter equivalent of electrons. The collision of an electron and a positron annihilates both particles, converting their masses to energy in

the form of two photons (gamma rays) that leave the brain at an angle of 180° to each other and can be decayed. The radioligands that are most frequently used are 18F-fluorodeoxyglucose and ^{15}O-water for determining cerebral blood flow. The use of PET is limited by a high cost, the need for a nearby cyclotron to produce radioisotopes with short half-lives, and its restricted spatial and temporal resolution. Routine use for neurodiagnostics is not currently practical. PET is referred to as functional imaging because, by using appropriate tracers, one can determine CBF and regional cerebral metabolic rate for oxygen (CMR O_2) and CMR for glucose (CMR glu). These techniques are extremely sensitive in the early detection of a cerebrovascular disturbance and can delineate the natural course of an episode that can lead to cerebral infarction. Evidence of ischemia is clearly demonstrated by substantial reduction in CBF and elevated CMR O_2 and CMR glu. The effect of a therapeutic intervention can be assessed by demonstrating the complete or partial reversal of these physiological and biochemical parameters.

Permanently and irreversibly damaged cortex in acute stroke can be detected by flumazenil PET. Evidence of tissue damage might be of relevance in selection of individualized therapeutic strategies. PET can be utilized in pilot trials for selection of patients who might benefit from particular therapeutic strategies and can be used to evaluate therapeutic effects in an experimental setting which then might form the basis for large clinical trials.

PET with radioactive ^{15}O (^{15}O-PET) has been used to compare CBF and regional cerebral oxygen consumption in patients with CO poisoning and patients with acute cerebral ischemia treated by HBO. The findings are useful as a guide to the prognosis of HBO as well as to HBO treatment. The results suggested that HBO confers protection against ischemic brain damage. PET is expensive, not easily available, and its use is limited.

Single Photon Emission Computed Tomography

This is a useful tool for assessing the effect of HBO in neurological disorders. SPECT (single photon emission computed tomography) is very similar to PET in its use of radioactive tracer and detection of γ-rays. However, unlike PET the radioisotopes used for SPECT emit only a single γ-ray during decay that is measured directly. Moreover, SPECT scans are significantly less expensive than PET scans partly due to that the nuclides used in SPECT have a longer half-life and are relatively easily obtained than PET. Conventional SPECT uses highly polar radiopharmaceuticals such as ^{99}mTc-pertechnetate. These tracers do not penetrate the normal brain but can cross a damaged BBB and appear as focal areas of increased activity in the region of the brain pathology. The long half-life of these tracers is a disadvantage. A radiolabeled lipid-soluble amine, iofetamine (^{123}I-IMP), is an indirectly agonistic amphetamine derivative that readily crosses the BBB and is taken up by the functioning neurons, and its distribution in the brain mirrors that of the CBF. Brain activity is observed within a minute after injection and can be detected for up to 4–5 h. The areas of the brain affected by stroke show a reduced uptake of the tracer material and can be used to document the pathophysiology in stroke patients. This test has been used in many of the studies to monitor the natural recovery and effect of therapy on stroke patients. The ^{123}I SPECT scan is ideal for evaluating the effect of HBO on stroke patients for the following reasons:

1. It is more widely available and less costly than PET scan. Any nuclear medicine facility with a gamma camera has the capability for this procedure.
2. There is a short waiting period for uptake of the isotope.
3. The procedure can be integrated with HBO sessions and a post-HBO scan can be done with the same injection as for the pre-HBO scan.
4. This scan documents the area of cerebral infarction as diminished uptake, and any improvement is easy to document by noting the increased uptake of the tracer.
5. Improvement in the scan can be correlated with clinical improvement, which is not always the case when CT scan is used.
6. Two areas, the central area representing the infarct core and the peripheral area or the peri-infarct zone, may be differentiated during the subacute period of the stroke. The pathophysiology and outcome are different in these two areas, and studies of subacute infarction should refer to the area involved. The central area is the site of wide variations of rCBF and IMP uptake during the development of necrosis. The peripheral area, with its slight decrease in rCBF and IMP uptake without morphological changes, appears stable because it is present early after stroke and may persist for years. Knowledge of the spontaneous changes in rCBF and IMP uptake in these two areas during the subacute period will facilitate the evaluation of new treatment for cerebral infarction.
7. SPECT performed within 24 h may be helpful in predicting outcome in clinical practice and in appropriately categorizing patients into subgroups for clinical trials.

IMP is no longer available commercially, and its use has been replaced by ^{99}mTc in hexamethylpropyleneamine oxime (HM-PAO). In HM-PAO scans half of the dose of the tracer is given initially and the brain is imaged. The patient is then exposed to HBO for 60–90 min, and the other half of the dose is given followed by brain imaging. Alternatively, the second scan using full-dose HM-PAO can be done at a later time, 24–48 h after the initial scan (also using full dose) followed by the HBO session. The difference between the two

scans helps to determine whether there is potentially recoverable brain tissue present. Hypometabolic but potentially viable areas in the brain can be identified using HM-PAO SPECT in conjunction with HBO. Idling neurons are capable of reactivation when given sufficient oxygen (Neubauer et al. 1992). Changes in tracer distribution after HBO may be a good prognostic indicator of viable neurons. Recoverable brain tissue can be identified and improved with cerebral oxygenation using HBO, and the results can be documented with SPECT (Neubauer and James 1998).

One study has used archival data to compare 25 older and 25 younger subjects who were investigated with SPECT scans for evaluation of HBO for chronic neurological disorders: pretherapy, midtherapy, and posttherapy (Golden et al. 2002). ANOVAs using the SPECT scans as a within-subjects variable and age as a between-subjects variable confirmed the hypothesis that the cerebral measures all changed but that the cerebellar and pons measures did not. Post hoc t-tests confirmed that there was improvement in blood flow from the beginning to the end of the study. An age effect was found on only two of the five measures; however, there were no interactions. Analysis by post hoc t-tests showed that the younger group had higher blood flows, but not more improvement than the older group. The results provided the first statistical research data to show the effectiveness of HBO in improving blood flow in chronic neurological disorders.

SPECT imaging with ^{99}mTc-ECD brain perfusion has been used for the assessment of brain perfusion treated with HBO (Asl et al. 2015). It showed decreased cerebral perfusion in different types of cerebral palsy patients. The study also showed that HBO improved cerebral perfusion in a few cerebral palsy patients. This is useful information in view of controversy about the effectiveness of HBO in cerebral palsy.

References

Akgül EO, Cakir E, Ozcan O, Yaman H, Kurt YG, Oter S, et al. Pressure-related increase of asymmetric dimethylarginine caused by hyperbaric oxygen in the rat brain: a possible neuroprotective mechanism. Neurochem Res. 2007;32:1586–91.

Artru F, Philippon B, Gauf BM, Deleuze R. Cerebral blood flow, cerebral metabolism and cerebrospinal fluid biochemistry in brain-injured patients after exposure to hyperbaric oxygen. Eur Neurol. 1976;14:351–64.

Asl MT, Yousefi F, Nemati R, Assadi M. 99mTc-ECD brain perfusion SPECT imaging for the assessment of brain perfusion in cerebral palsy (CP) patients with evaluation of the effect of hyperbaric oxygen therapy. Int J Clin Exp Med. 2015;8:1101–7.

Bean JE, Lingnell J, Coulson J. Regional cerebral blood flow oxygen tension and EEG in exposure to oxygen at high pressure. J Appl Physiol. 1971;31:235.

Bergö GW, Engelsen B, Tyssebotn I. Unilateral frontal decortication changes in cerebral blood flow distribution during hyperbaric oxygen exposure in rats. Aviat Space Environ Med. 1993;64:1023–31.

Bergö GW, Tyssebotn I. Cardiovascular effects of hyperbaric oxygen with and without addition of carbon dioxide. Eur J Appl Physiol Occup Physiol. 1999;80:264–75.

Chen SY, Lin CC, Lin YT, Lo CP, Wang CH, Fan YM. Reversible changes of brain perfusion SPECT for carbon monoxide poisoning-induced severe akinetic mutism. Clin Nucl Med. 2016;41:e221–7.

Chen X, Duan XS, Xu LJ, Zhao JJ, She ZF, Chen WW, et al. Interleukin-10 mediates the neuroprotection of hyperbaric oxygen therapy against traumatic brain injury in mice. Neuroscience. 2014;266:235–43.

Coe JE, Hayes TM. Treatment of experimental brain injury by hyperbaric oxygenation. A preliminary report. Am Surg. 1966;32:493–5.

Contreras FL, Kadekaro M, Eisenberg HM. The effect of hyperbaric oxygen on glucose utilization in a freeze-traumatized rat brain. J Neurosurg. 1988;68:137.

Demchenko IT, Boso AE, Natoli MJ, et al. Measurement of cerebral blood flow in rats and mice by hydrogen clearance during hyperbaric oxygen exposure. Undersea Hyperbaric Med. 1998;25:147–52.

Demchenko IT, Luchakov YI, Moskvin AN, et al. Cerebral blood flow and brain oxygenation in rats breathing oxygen under pressure. J Cereb Blood Flow Metab. 2005;25:1288–300.

Demchenko IT, Oury TD, Crapo JD, Piantadosi CA. Regulation of the brain's vascular responses to oxygen. Circ Res. 2002;91:1031–7.

Di Piero V, Cappagli M, Pastena L, et al. Cerebral effects of hyperbaric oxygen breathing: a CBF SPECT study on professional divers. Eur J Neurol. 2002;9:419–21.

Di Pretoro L, Forti G, Adami V. Effet dell'iperbarismo e dell'ossigneazione iperbarica sul circolo cerebrale. Acta Anaesthesiol (Padova). 1968;19 Suppl 9:73–84.

Dunn JE. An evaluation of HBO, hypocapnic hyperventilation and methyl prednisolone therapy in cold induced cerebral swelling. In: Paper presented at the 5th International congress on hyperbaric medicine, Simon Fraser University, Burnaby, Canada, 1974.

Dunn JE, Connolly JM. Effects of hypobaric and hyperbaric oxygen on experimental brain injury. In: Brown IW, Cox BG, editors. Hyperbaric medicine. Washington, DC: National Research Council; 1966. p. 447–54.

Fang J, Li H, Li G, Wang L. Effect of hyperbaric oxygen preconditioning on peri-hemorrhagic focal edema and aquaporin-4 expression. Exp Ther Med. 2015;10:699–704.

Golden ZL, Neubauer R, Golden CJ, Greene L, Marsh J, Mleko A. Improvement in cerebral metabolism in chronic brain injury after hyperbaric oxygen therapy. Int J Neurosci. 2002;112:119–31.

Gu ZZ. Effect of oxygen at various pressures on intracranial pressure. Chung Hua Shen Ching Ching Shen Ko Tsa Chih. 1985;18:17–20.

Hansen MB, Olsen NV, Hyldegaard O. Combined administration of hyperbaric oxygen and hydroxocobalamin improves cerebral metabolism after acute cyanide poisoning in rats. J Appl Physiol (1985). 2013;115:1254–61.

Harper AM, Ledingham IM, McDowall DG. The influence of hyperbaric oxygen on the blood flow and oxygen uptake of the cerebral cortex in hypovolemic shock. In: Ledingham IM, editor. Proceedings of the 2nd International congress on clinical applications of hyperbaric medicine. Edinburgh: Livingstone; 1965. p. 342–6.

Hayakawa T. Hyperbaric oxygen treatment in neurology and neurosurgery. J Life Sci. 1974;4:1–25.

Hayakawa T, Kanai N, Kuroda R, et al. Response of cerebrospinal fluid pressure to hyperbaric oxygenation. Neurol Neurosurg Psychiatry. 1971;34:580–6.

Holbach KH, Caroli A, Wassmann ZH. Cerebral energy metabolism in patients with brain lesions at normo and hyperbaric oxygen pressure. J Neurol. 1977;217:17–30.

Huang H, Xue L, Zhang X, Weng Q, Chen H, Gu J, et al. Hyperbaric oxygen therapy provides neuroprotection following spinal cord injury in a rat model. Int J Clin Exp Pathol. 2013;6:1337–42.

Isakov IV, Romasenko MV. Effect of hyperbaric oxygenation on the water content of brain tissue in experimental toxic cerebral edema. Zh Nevropatol Psikhiatr. 1985;85:1786–9.

Jacobson I, Lawson DD. The effect of hyperbaric oxygen on experimental cerebral infarction in the dog. J Neursurg. 1963;20:849.

Jain KK. A handbook of neuroprotection. New York: Humana/Springer; 2011.

James PB. Hyperbaric oxygenation in fluid microembolism. Neurol Res. 2007;29:156–61.

James PB. The scientific basis for hyperbaric oxygen therapy in focal oedema. In: Rose FC, Jones R, editors. Multiple sclerosis. London: Libbey; 1987. p. 223–8.

Jamieson D, van den Brenk HA. Measurement of tension in cerebral tissues of rats exposed to high pressures of oxygen. J Appl Physiol. 1963;18:869–76.

Jinnai D, Mogami H, Ioko M, et al. Effect of hyperbaric oxygenation on cerebral edema. Neurol Med Clin. 1967;9:260–1.

Kety SS, Schmidt CF. The effects of altered arterial tensions of carbon dioxide and oxygen on cerebral blood flow and cerebral oxygen consumption of normal young men. J Clin Invest. 1948;27:484–92.

Lambertsen CJ, Gelfand R, Lever MJ, et al. Respiration and gas exchange during a 14-day continuous exposure to 5.2 per cent O_2 in N_2 at pressure equivalent to 100 FSW (4 ATA). Aerosp Med. 1973;44:844–9.

Leninger-Follert E, Hossmann KA. Microflow and cortical oxygen pressure during and after prolonged cerebral ischemia. Brain Res. 1977;124:158–61.

Meirovithz E, Sonn J, Mayevsky A. Effect of hyperbaric oxygenation on brain hemodynamics, hemoglobin oxygenation and mitochondrial NADH. Brain Res Rev. 2007;54:294–304.

Micarelli A, Jacobsson H, Larsson SA, Jonsson C, Pagani M. Neurobiological insight into hyperbaric hyperoxia. Acta Physiol (Oxf). 2013;209:69–76.

Miller JD. The effects of hyperbaric oxygen at 2 and 3 atmospheres: absolute and intravenous mannitol on experimentally increased intracranial pressure. Eur Neurol. 1973;10:1–10.

Miller JD. The management of cerebral oedema. Br J Hosp Med. 1979;21:152–66.

Moody RA, Mead CO, Ruamsuke S, Mullan S. Therapeutic value of oxygen at normal and hyperbaric pressure in experimental head injury. J Neurosurg. 1970;32:51–4.

Muir ER, Cardenas DP, Duong TQ. MRI of brain tissue oxygen tension under hyperbaric conditions. Neuroimage. 2016;133:498–503.

Nagao S, Okmura S, Nishimoto A. Effect of hyperbaric oxygenation on vasomotor tone in acute intracranial hypertension: an experimental study. Resuscitation. 1975;4:51–9.

Neubauer RA, Gottlieb SF, Miale A. Identification of hypometabolic areas in the brain using brain imaging and hyperbaric oxygen. Clin Nucl Med. 1992;17:477–81.

Neubauer RA, James P. Cerebral oxygenation and the recoverable brain. Neurol Res. 1998;20 Suppl 1:S33–6.

Nida TY, Biros MH, Pheley AM, et al. Effect of hypoxia or hyperbaric oxygen on cerebral edema following moderate fluid percussion or cortical impact injury in rats. J Neurotrauma. 1995;12:77–85.

Ohta H, Nemoto M, Kawamura S, et al. The effects of hyperoxemia on cerebral blood flow in subarachnoid hemorrhage patients. No To Shinkei. 1987;39:649–56.

Omae T, Ibayashi S, Kusuda K, Nakamura H, Yagi H, Fujishima M. Effects of high atmospheric pressure and oxygen on middle cerebral blood flow velocity in humans measured by transcranial Doppler. Stroke. 1998;29:94–7.

Pastena L, Formaggio E, Faralli F, Melucci M, Rossi M, Gagliardi R, et al. Bluetooth communication interface for EEG signal recording in hyperbaric chambers. IEEE Trans Neural Syst Rehabil Eng. 2015a;23:538–47.

Pastena L, Formaggio E, Storti SF, Faralli F, Melucci M, Gagliardi R, et al. Tracking EEG changes during the exposure to hyperbaric oxygen. Clin Neurophysiol. 2015b;126:339–47.

Pierce EC, Jacobson JH. Cerebral edema. In: Davis JC, Hunt TK, editors. Hyperbaric oxygen therapy. Bethesda: Undersea Medical Society; 1977. p. 287–302.

Rockswold SB, Rockswold GL, Vargo JM, Erickson CA, Sutton RL, Bergman TA, et al. Effects of hyperbaric oxygenation therapy on cerebral metabolism and intracranial pressure in severely brain injured patients. J Neurosurg. 2001;95:544–6.

Rockswold SB, Rockswold GL, Zaun DA, Liu J. A prospective, randomized Phase II clinical trial to evaluate the effect of combined hyperbaric and normobaric hyperoxia on cerebral metabolism, intracranial pressure, oxygen toxicity, and clinical outcome in severe traumatic brain injury. J Neurosurg. 2013;118:1317–28.

Rogatsky GG, Kamenir Y, Mayevsky A. Effect of hyperbaric oxygenation on intracranial pressure elevation rate in rats during the early phase of severe traumatic brain injury. Brain Res. 2005;1047:131–6.

Sukoff MH, Hollin SA, Jacobson JH. The protective effect of hyperbaric oxygen in experimentally produced cerebral edema and compression. Surgery. 1967;62:40–6.

Sukoff MH, Ragatz RE. Hyperbaric oxygenation for the treatment of acute cerebral edema. Neurosurgery. 1982;10:29–38.

Sukoff MH. Effects of hyperbaric oxygenation. J Neurosurg. 2001;95:544–6.

Tal S, Hadanny A, Berkovitz N, Sasson E, Ben-Jacob E, Efrati S. Hyperbaric oxygen may induce angiogenesis in patients suffering from prolonged post-concussion syndrome due to traumatic brain injury. Restor Neurol Neurosci. 2015;33:943–51.

Tindall GT, Wilkins RH, Odom GL. Effect of hyperbaric oxygenation on cerebral blood flow. Surg Forum. 1965;16:414–6.

Veltkamp R, Siebing DA, Sun L, Heiland S, Bieber K, Marti HH, et al. Hyperbaric oxygen reduces blood-brain barrier damage and edema after transient focal cerebral ischemia. Stroke. 2005;36:1679–83.

Wassmann W. Quantitative Indikatoren des hirnelektrischen Wirkungsverlaufs bei hyperbarer Oxygenierung. EEG EMG. 1980;11:97–101.

Wassmann H, Holbach KH. Zerebrale Insuffizienz durch ischsche Hypoxie unter hyperbarer Sauerstoff-Behandlung. Geriatr Rehabil. 1988;1:143–50.

Wei XE, Li YH, Zhao H, Li MH, Fu M, Li WB. Quantitative evaluation of hyperbaric oxygen efficacy in experimental traumatic brain injury: an MRI study. Neurol Sci. 2014;35:295–302.

Xue F, Huang JW, Ding PY, Zang HG, Kou ZJ, Li T, et al. Nrf2/antioxidant defense pathway is involved in the neuroprotective effects of Sirt1 against focal cerebral ischemia in rats after hyperbaric oxygen preconditioning. Behav Brain Res. 2016;309:1–8.

Zeng Y, Xie K, Dong H, Zhang H, Wang F, Li Y, Xiong L. Hyperbaric oxygen preconditioning protects cortical neurons against oxygen-glucose deprivation injury: role of peroxisome proliferator-activated receptor-gamma. Brain Res. 2012;1452:140–50.

Zhou W, Marinescu M, Veltkamp R. Only very early oxygen therapy attenuates posthemorrhagic edema formation and blood-brain barrier disruption in murine intracerebral hemorrhage. Neurocrit Care. 2015;22:121–32.

K.K. Jain

Abstract

HBO, by counteracting the hypoxia of ischemic brain tissue, aids the recovery of stroke patients. As a background, epidemiology, pathophysiology, and conventional management of stroke patients are described. The role of HBO in the management of acute as well as chronic poststroke stages is discussed. Various preclinical and clinical studies are reviewed. Controversies about the use of HBO in stroke are also mentioned. Finally, the value of HBO as a supplement to physical therapy and for the relief of spasticity in rehabilitation of patients in the chronic poststroke stage is emphasized based on the study done by the author at Fachklinik Klausenbach in Germany.

Keywords

Cerebral hypoxia • Cerebral infarction • Cerebral ischemia • Chronic poststroke stage • Hyperbaric oxygen (HBO) • Neuroprotection • Oxygen carriers • Penumbra zone • Spasticity in stroke • Stroke • Stroke rehabilitation • Vascular dementia

Introduction

"Stroke" is the term commonly used to describe the sudden onset of a neurological deficit such as weakness or paralysis due to disturbance of the blood flow to the brain. The term is applied loosely to cover ischemic and hemorrhagic episodes. The preferred terms are "ischemic stroke" or "cerebral infarction." A completed (established) stroke is an acute, nonconvulsive episode of neurological dysfunction that lasts longer than 24 h. A transient ischemic attack is a focal, nonconvulsive episode of neurological dysfunction that lasts less than 24 h and often lasts less than 30 min. An ischemic stroke occurs when a thrombus or an embolus blocks an artery to the brain, blocking or reducing the blood flow to the brain and consequently the transport of oxygen

and glucose which are critical elements for brain function. Ischemic strokes may also occur due to spasm of the cerebral arteries without any obstruction of the lumen such as in patients with migraine. Cerebral infarction can also occur as a result of obstruction to the venous outflow from the brain. Two distinct types of hemorrhage are intracerebral hemorrhage due to hypertension and subarachnoid hemorrhage due to rupture of an aneurysm (ballooning of the intracranial artery).

The World Health Organization (WHO) defines stroke as "rapidly developing clinical signs of focal (or global) disturbance of cerebral function with symptoms lasting 24 h or longer or leading to death, with no apparent cause other than of vascular origin." This definition includes subarachnoid hemorrhage but excludes transient ischemic attacks and brain hemorrhages or infarctions due to nonvascular causes. Fundamentals of epidemiology, pathophysiology, diagnosis, and current management of stroke are described briefly in this chapter as a background to discuss the role of HBO. The role of HBO as an adjunct to surgery for cerebrovascular disease is described in Chap. 21.

K.K. Jain, MD, FRACS, FFPM (✉)
1 Blaesiring 7, Basel 4057, Switzerland
e-mail: jain@pharmabiotech.ch

Epidemiology of Stroke

According to the World Health Organization, 15 million people suffer stroke worldwide each year. Of these, five million die and another five million are permanently disabled. Stroke is the third leading cause of death and an important cause of hospital admissions in most industrialized countries. Stroke accounts for 10 % of deaths in all industrialized countries. It is the most common cause of disability worldwide. There are over two million stroke survivors in the USA, and about 500,000 patients are discharged annually from acute care hospitals. It has been estimated that only 10 % of the stroke survivors return to work without disability, 40 % have mild disability, 40 % are severely disabled, and 10 % require institutionalization (Fig. 19.1). The incidence of stroke in the USA is ~800,000 cases per year. More than four million Americans are living with the consequences of stroke currently. The incidence of stroke in Western Europe is 600,000 cases per year. In the year 2016, over two million new stroke patients are expected in the USA, Europe, and Japan. About half of these will be in the USA. Stroke is less common in developing countries. In spite of the improvement in the care of stroke, the incidence is rising by 2 % per year. The incidence rate in India is 119–145/100,000 based on the recent population-based studies. In China, with a population of 1.4 billion, there are 2.5 million new stroke cases each year and 7.5 million stroke survivors.

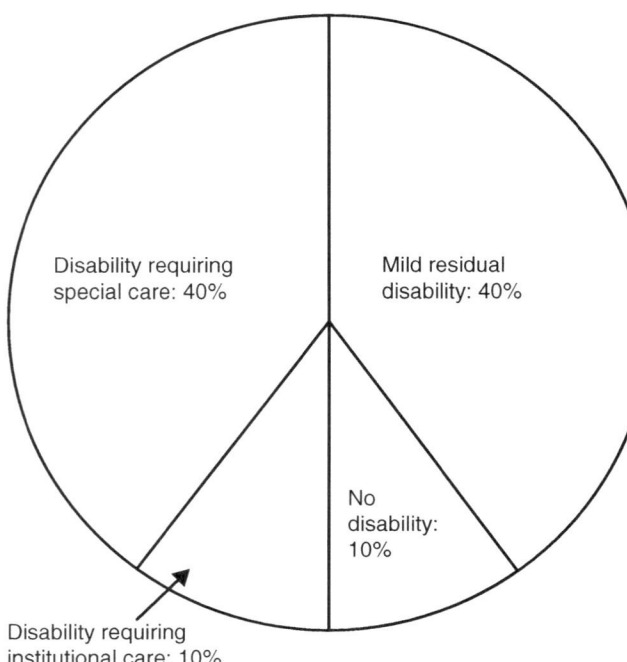

Fig. 19.1 Functional results for stroke survivors

Risk Factors for Stroke

Various risk factors for stroke are:

- Aging
- Alcohol
- Atherosclerosis involving major vessels
  - Atherosclerosis of aortic arch
  - Carotid stenosis
- Cardiovascular
  - Heart disease
  - Atrial fibrillation
  - Endocarditis
  - Left ventricular hypertrophy
  - Mitral valve prolapse
  - Myocardial infarction
  - Patent foramen ovale
- Coagulation disorders
- Cold
- Endocrine disorders
  - Diabetes mellitus
  - Hypothyroidism
- Female sex
- Genetic
  - Angiotensin-converting enzyme gene deletion polymorphism
  - Genetically determined cardiovascular, hematological, and metabolic disorders causing stroke
- Hemorheological disturbances
  - Increased blood viscosity
  - Elevated hematocrit
  - Red blood cell disorders
  - Leukocytosis
- Heredity: parental history of stroke associated with increased stroke risk in the offspring
- Hyperlipidemia
- Hypertension
- Hypotension
- Lack of physical activity
- Metabolic disorders
  - Hyperuricemia
  - Hyperhomocysteinemia
- Migraine
- Nutritional disorders
  - High salt intake
  - Malnutrition
  - Vitamin deficiency
- Obesity
- Psychosocial factors: anger, aggression, stress
- Pregnancy
- Race: strokes more common in black Americans than whites

- Raised serum fibrinogen levels
- Sex: strokes more common in men than in women
- Sleep-related disorders: snoring and sleep apnea
- Smoking
- Transient ischemic attacks

Pathophysiology of Stroke

The term "cerebrovascular disease" is used to mean any abnormality of the brain resulting from pathological processes of the blood vessels. The "pathological processes" are defined as lesions of the vessel wall, occlusion of the vessel lumen by an embolus or a thrombus, rupture of the vessel, altered permeability of the vessel wall, and increased viscosity or other changes in the quality of blood.

Causes of Stroke

The causes and risk factors for ischemic stroke overlap. Causal relationship is more definite than a risk factor which implies an increase in the chance of stroke in the presence of that factor. The interaction between risk factors and causes of stroke is shown in Fig. 19.2. Various causes of stroke are:

- Atherosclerosis of arterial wall
  - Atherosclerotic occlusion of cerebral arteries
  - Carotid stenosis
- Arterial occlusion secondary to infections
  - Bacterial meningitis: *H. influenzae* and tuberculosis
  - Meningovascular syphilis
  - Cysticercosis
  - Cerebral malaria
  - Herpes zoster
  - Viral infections: AIDS
- Arterial occlusion secondary to head and neck trauma
  - Closed head injury
  - Blunt trauma to neck
- Fractures and dislocations of the cervical spine
  - Chiropractic manipulations of the neck
  - Beauty parlor stroke syndrome
- Cervical spondylosis with compression of vertebral arteries
- Congenital abnormalities of the cerebral vessels: hypoplasia of arteries
- Coagulation disorders
- Drug-induced stroke
  - Therapeutic drugs
  - Drug abuse
- Embolism
  - Cardiogenic embolism: atrial fibrillation

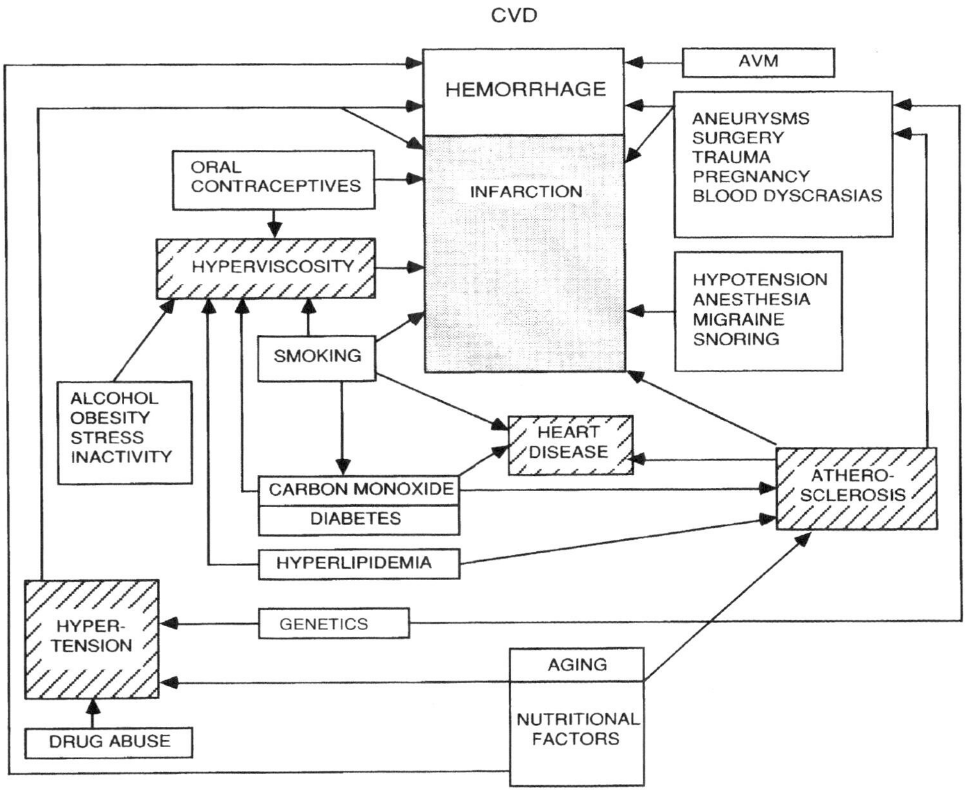

Fig. 19.2 Interaction of risk factors for stroke

- – Embolism from peripheral arteries
- – Tumor emboli
- Hematological disorders, e.g., sickle cell anemia
- Genetic
- Iatrogenic as complications of:
  - – Anesthesia
  - – Cerebral angiography
  - – Cardiovascular surgery
  - – Neurosurgical procedures
- Infections AIDS
  - – Bacterial meningitis
  - – Chickenpox
  - – Cysticercosis
  - – Subacute bacterial endocarditis
  - – Syphilis
- Inflammatory diseases
  - – Systemic, e.g., rheumatoid arthritis and systemic lupus erythematosus of the cranial arteries:
  - – Temporal arteritis
  - – Aortic branch arteritis (Takayasu's disease)
  - – Granulomatous intracranial arteritis
- Myocardial infarction
- Nonatherosclerotic vasculopathies
  - – Moyamoya disease
  - – Thromboangiitis obliterans (Buerger's disease)
  - – Radiation vasculopathy
  - – Spontaneous cervical artery dissection
  - – Fibromuscular dysplasia
  - – Cerebral amyloid angiopathy

Among the different causes of stroke, 70 % are due to an ischemic infarct, of which 9 % are due to large artery occlusion, 5 % are due to tandem arterial pathology, 26 % are lacunar, 19 % are from a cardiac source, and 40 % are of uncertain cause. The three disease processes responsible for most ischemic strokes are:

1. Large vessel atherothrombotic disease, which accounts for about 14 % of the cases
2. Small vessel atherothrombotic disease (lacunar stroke), accounting for about 27 % of the cases
3. Embolic disease, accounting for about 59 % of the cases

Changes in the Brain During Ischemic Stroke

Changes that occur in the brain during a stroke are both histological and biochemical (metabolic). The brain requires 500–600 mL oxygen/min (25 % of the total body consumption). One liter of blood circulates to the brain each minute. If this flow is interrupted completely, neuron metabolism is disturbed after 6 s, brain activity ceases after 2 min, and brain damage begins in 5 min. Brain tissue deprived of its oxygen supply undergoes necrosis or infarction (also called "zone of softening" or encephalomalacia). The infarct may be pale if devoid of blood, or hemorrhagic if blood extravasates from small vessels in the area of infarction. Depending on the degree of ischemia, the changes are reversible up to a few hours, and some recovery of function can take place after days, weeks, months, or even years. The first 3 h after acute stroke are usually considered to be the therapeutic window during which therapeutic interventions can stop the progression of stroke and reverse the biochemical disturbances to some extent.

Two major types of strokes are ischemic and hemorrhagic. Most ischemic lesions (infarcts) are due to occlusion of cerebral vessels, although they may occur in the absence of demonstrable occlusion of the vessels. The pathophysiology of cerebral ischemia is shown in Fig. 19.3, and various factors influencing the size of a cerebral infarct are shown in Table 19.1.

Clinicopathological Correlations

Various stages in the evolution of stroke are shown in Table 19.2.

The symptoms of a stroke vary according to the arterial system or the branch involved. Most stroke syndromes are designated by the name of the artery supplying the area of the brain that is infarcted. Neurological deficits due to stroke depend upon the type and location of the disease process. A common presentation is hemiplegia due to occlusion of the carotid artery or the middle cerebral artery, with aphasia if the dominant hemisphere is involved. In vertebral–basilar territory strokes, the neurological picture is more varied with involvement of cranial nerves and the sensory pathways. In the most severe form, the patient becomes comatose.

There are variations in the arterial supply and collateral circulation, and sometimes an artery may be occluded without any infarction, or infarction may not be clinically manifest. The major cause of cerebrovascular disease is atherosclerosis, a noninflammatory degenerative disease that can affect segments of almost any artery in the body. Atherosclerosis is the commonest vascular disorder, although other diseases also affect the cerebral circulation. Some of these are embolic occlusion of the cerebral arteries by detached thrombi from the heart or major vessels, intracranial vascular malformations, and microvascular disorders.

Structure of a Cerebral Infarct

There are three phases of evolution of morphological changes with infarction: coagulation necrosis, liquification necrosis, and cavitation. The three zones of histological alterations within an infarct are:

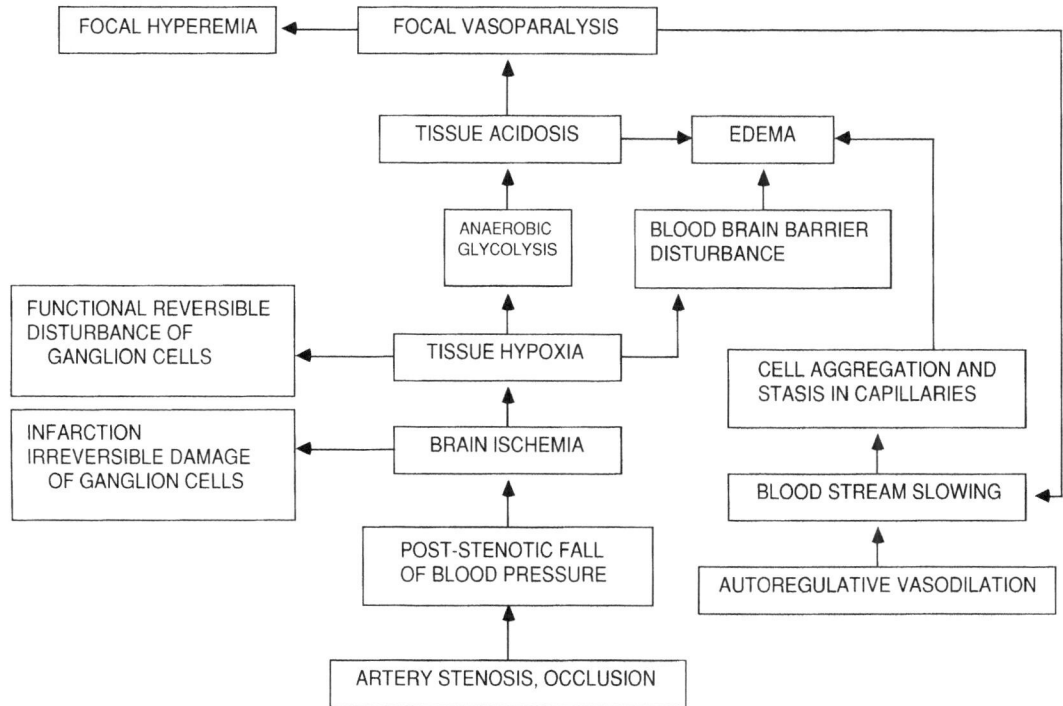

Fig. 19.3 Pathophysiology of cerebral ischemia

Table 19.1 Factors that influence the extent of infarction

Factors that increase infarction	Factors that decrease infarction
Hypotension; reduction of cardiac output	Increase of pressure
Lack of collaterals	Adequate collaterals
Hypoxia	Oxygenation
Sudden occlusion of the vessel	Gradual occlusion of the vessel
Increased viscosity of blood	Decreased viscosity of blood
Increased metabolism; hyperthermia	Decreased metabolism; hypothermia; sedation
Cerebral edema	Absence of cerebral edema

Table 19.2 Stages in the evolution of a cerebral ischemic episode

I. Transient ischemic attacks (TIA)	Minutes to 24 h
II. Reversible ischemic neurological deficit (RIND)	Hours
III. Prolonged reversible ischemic neurological deficit (PRIND) (stroke in evolution)	Days
IV. Brain infarction with fixed neurological deficit (completed stroke)	Hours to months
V. Chronic poststroke stage	More than 1 year after onset

1. A central zone with variable neuronal necrosis ranging from pale ghost cells to shrunken neurons with pyknotic nuclei.
2. A reactive zone at the periphery of the central zone within which there is neuronal necrosis and leukocytic infiltration and neovascularization.
3. A marginal zone peripheral to the reactive zone within which there are shrunken neurons and swollen astrocytes in various stages of hyperplasia and hypertrophy.

The traditional concept of infarction that the brain tissue dies from a shortage of blood and oxygen lasting more than a few minutes is no longer valid. The interruption of blood flow is seldom total, and a drop of CBF to as low as 50 % can maintain function. The neuronal structure can be preserved with CBF as little as 15–20 % of the normal (Fig. 19.4). Between the zones of infarction and normal brain is a third zone referred to as the "penumbra" (Fig. 19.5) containing the so-called dormant or idling neurons (Symon 1976). These neurons are nonfunc-

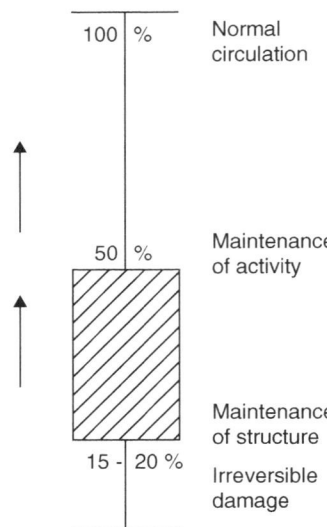

Fig. 19.4 Critical levels of cerebral blood flow required for maintenance of structure and function

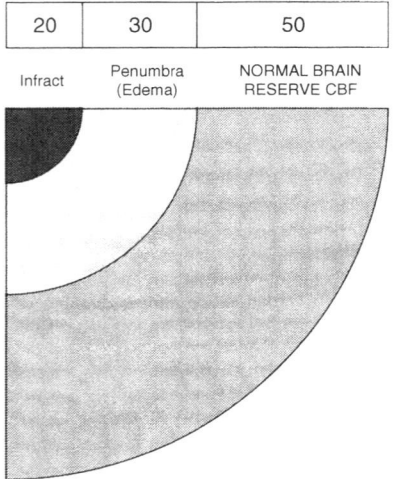

Fig. 19.5 Penumbra zone in cerebral infarction. Numbers indicate the percentage of cerebral blood flow in this model to correlate with that in Fig. 19.4

tional but anatomically intact and can be revived. The presence of viable brain tissue in the penumbra explains why the acute clinical presentation of a stroke is a rather poor predictor of the outcome (Astrup et al. 1981). A trickle of blood flow is maintained to the penumbra zone, which is hypoxic. It can be presumed that the critical parameter for cellular function is oxygen availability rather than blood flow.

Cerebral Metabolism in Ischemia

The cascade of biochemical events following cerebral ischemia is shown in Fig. 19.6. The outcome of cerebral ischemia depends on cerebral metabolic reactions to the failing circulation.

Although ischemia is a circulatory disorder, its impact on the brain is determined by neurochemical events at the subcellular level. Several investigative therapies for stroke are based on an attempt to prevent detrimental biochemical events. The correlation between the metabolic changes and hemodynamic changes in an ischemic focus is shown in Table 19.3.

Glutamate as a Biomarker of Stroke

Excitotoxic injury, triggered by inappropriately high levels of extracellular glutamate and possibly other excitatory amino acids, has been identified as the dominant mechanism underlying calcium-mediated injury of gray matter in a number of experimental models. Glutamate levels are elevated in the CSF of patients with progressive cerebral infarcts. Glutamate levels in patients with cortical infarcts have been found to be higher than in patients with deep infarcts. The explanation of this may be that underlying molecular mechanisms of anoxic/ischemic injury are different in the white and the gray matter. These results also suggest that there may be different molecular signatures of different types of stroke.

Role of Oxygen Free Radicals in Cerebral Ischemia

Free radicals are formed during normal respiration and oxidation. Oxidation is a chemical reaction in which a molecule transfers one or more electrons to another. Stable molecules usually have matched pairs of protons and electrons, whereas free radicals have unpaired electrons and tend to be highly reactive, oxidizing agents. Damage to cells caused by free radicals includes protein oxidation, DNA strand destruction, increase of intracellular calcium, activation of damaging proteases and nucleases, and peroxidation of cellular membrane lipids. Furthermore, such intracellular damage can lead to the formation of prostaglandins, interferons, TNF-α, and other tissue-damaging mediators, each of which can lead to disease if overproduced in response to the oxidative stress. Free radicals can be measured in vivo and some of the antioxidant mechanisms have been studied in transgenic mice. Free radicals have been linked to numerous human diseases including ischemia/reperfusion injury resulting from stroke. Reoxygenation provides oxygen to sustain neuronal viability and also provides oxygen as a substrate for numerous enzymatic oxidation reactions that produce reactive oxidants. In addition reflow following oxidation also increases oxygen to a level that cannot be utilized by mitochondria under normal physiological conditions.

Damaging effect of free radicals is controlled to some extent by the antioxidant defense systems and cellular repair mechanisms of the body but at times it is overwhelmed. Enzymes such as superoxide dismutase, catalase, and glutathione peroxidase and vitamins such as tocopherol, ascorbate, and beta-carotene act to quench radical chain reactions. Many of these agents have been investigated as potential therapeutic agents. Unfortunately, most studies testing naturally

Fig. 19.6 Sequence of
biochemical events following
cerebral ischemia. *CBF*
cerebral blood flow, *FFA* free
fatty acids, *Ke* extracellular
potassium ion, *Cai* intracellular
calcium ion, *Nai* intracellular
sodium io, *GABA* gamma-
aminobutyric acid (Welch and
Barkley 1986)

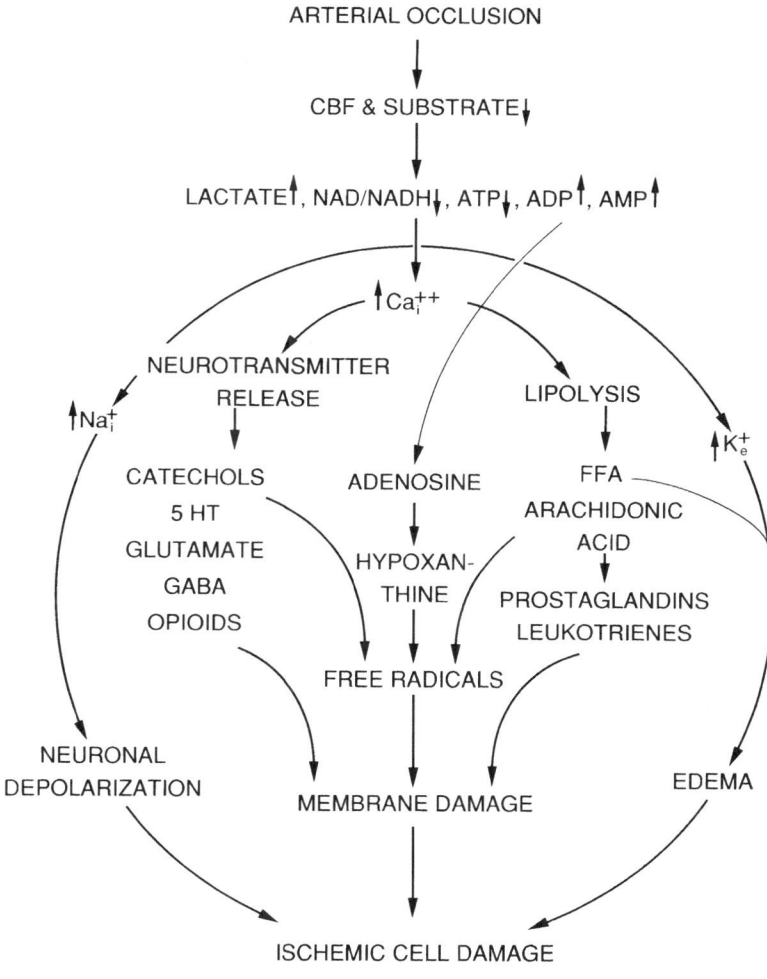

Table 19.3 Hemodynamic and metabolic changes in an ischemic focus

Area	Cerebral blood flow	Characteristics
Central zone	<0.10 mL/g/min	Rise of extracellular K; fall of ATP; increase of lactate and intracellular acidosis
Boundary	0.10–0.15 mL/g/min	Extinction of neuronal electrical activity; limited rise of extracellular K
Collateral	>0.15 mL/g/min	Undisturbed metabolism, hyperemia

occurring antioxidants have resulted in disappointing
results. Generally, natural antioxidants must be produced on
site within the cell to be effective in disease prevention. Free
radicals are normally scavenged by superoxide dismutases
(SODs) and glutathione peroxidases. Vitamin E and ascorbic
acid are also likely to be involved in the detoxification of
free radicals but these mechanisms may be overwhelmed
during reperfusion and damage may occur to the brain
parenchyma.

Free radicals have been a topic of discussion in relation to
HBO therapy because oxygen administration is considered
to increase oxidative stress. This issue remains unresolved.

There is no convincing evidence that HBO induces any oxidative stress that is harmful to the patient with stroke.

Reperfusion Injury

Reperfusion implies resumption of the blood flow either
spontaneously or as a result of thrombolysis or surgical procedures, there is resumption of the principal functions of
tissue perfusion: oxygen delivery, provision of substrates
for metabolism, and clearance of metabolic wastes. This has
beneficial effects as well as a dark side-reperfusion injury.
Interactions between blood and the damaged tissues can
lead to further tissue injury. Major mechanisms postulated

to participate in this injury are loss of calcium homeostasis, free radical generation, leukocyte-mediated injury, and acute hypercholesterolemia.

Molecular Mechanism in the Pathogenesis of Stroke

Various molecular mechanisms are involved in the pathophysiology of ischemic stroke and form the basis of experimental interventions. It is beyond the scope of this textbook to describe these in detail but some important ones are as follows.

Gene Expression in Response to Cerebral Ischemia

During the early postischemic stages, protein synthesis in the brain is generally suppressed, but specific genes are expressed, and their corresponding proteins may be synthesized. There is expression of a range of genes in cerebral ischemia which may have either a beneficial or a detrimental effect on the evolution of neuronal injury. The first set of genes to be activated following neuronal injury in focal cerebral ischemia are the c-fos/c-jun complex which are involved in the induction of target genes that regulate cell growth and differentiation. According to the excitotoxic hypothesis, ischemic neuronal death is induced by the release of excitatory amino acid glutamate. Activation of the NMDA receptor-operated and voltage-sensitive calcium channels causes calcium influx which activates degrading enzymes leading to disintegration of nuclear and cell membranes and generation of oxygen free radicals. Calcium influx also induces expression of c-fos. The induction of neurotrophin genes by c-fos/c-jun has been demonstrated although the role of these induced proteins in the overall adaptive response is not certain. Gene regulation, including immediate early genes is required for programmed neural death after trophic factor deprivation and is predicted to be involved in apoptosis triggered by cerebral ischemia. Novel therapies following cerebral ischemia may be directed at genes mediating either recovery or apoptosis.

Induction of Heat Shock Proteins

Heat shock protein (HSP) concentrations increase in the brain after experimentally induced strokes. Induction of HSP 70 does not occur until reperfusion for 24 h following cerebral ischemia and occurs only in areas with earlier induction of c-fos/c-jun, suggesting that induction of HSP occurs in neurons that survive to that point. HSP does not participate in early response for neuronal survival after global cerebral ischemia. Although the proteins are known to protect cells against damage caused by various stresses, it was not known that they were doing anything

useful. It is now realized that HSPs may be factors in ischemia tolerance and neuroprotection against ischemia. Insertion of gene for HSP 72 into the brain of rats, using a viral vector, has been shown to protect against ischemia, and this forms the basis of a potential gene therapy approach.

Role of Cytokines and Adhesion Molecules in Stroke

Inflammatory–immunologic reactions are involved in the pathogenesis of cerebral ischemia. In addition to this, cells such as astrocytes, microglia, or endothelial cells have been found to be activated by cerebral injuries including stroke. These cells then become immunologically reactive and interact with each other by producing substances including cytokines and adhesion molecules. Three major cytokines, tumor necrosis factor (TNF)-α, interleukin (IL)-1, and IL6, are produced by cultured brain cells after various stimuli. Increased expression of adhesion molecules such as ICAM-1 and VCAM are observed in cultured microglial cells after treatment with TNF-α. ELAM and P-selectin were also found to be expressed. The induction of these adhesion molecules in the ischemic brain is time-locked and appears to be controlled in a highly regulated manner during the process of ischemic cascade. An understanding of the cytokine-adhesion molecule cascades in the ischemic brain may allow us to develop new strategies for the treatment of stroke. Further work is required to define the role of these cytokines and other signaling molecules in cerebral ischemic infarcts. This may open the way for gene therapy of cerebral infarction: antisense methods and the use of genetically engineered overexpressors.

DNA Damage and Repair in Cerebral Ischemia

There is evidence of DNA damage in experimental stroke, and this is an important factor in the pathophysiology of stroke. DNA repair may be an important mechanism for the maintenance of normal physiological function. Research in the science of DNA injury and repair will likely provide new and important information on mechanisms of cell damage and provide opportunities for the development of novel and effective therapies to reduce CNS injury in stroke. Techniques for measuring DNA damage are available that are applicable to in vitro and in vivo models of cerebral ischemia.

Role of Neurotrophic Factors

Neurotrophic factors (NTFs) are polypeptides which regulate the proliferation, survival, migration, and differentiation of cells in the nervous system. By definition, a neurotrophic factor is synthesized by and released from target cells of the neurons, bound to specific receptors, internalized and retrogradely transported by the axon to the cell soma where multiple survival-promoting effects are initiated. The major hypotheses for the functional effects of cerebral insult-induced neurotrophin changes are protection against neuronal damage and stimulation of neuronal sprouting as well as synaptic reorganization. Basic fibroblast growth factor (bFGF) is one of the NTFs that has been studied extensively in relation to stroke and is in clinical trials.

Role of poly(ADP-ribose) polymerase (PARP) gene. DNA damage can lead to activation of the nuclear enzyme PARP, which catalyzes the attachment of ADP ribose units from NAD to nuclear proteins following DNA damage. Excessive activation PARP can deplete NAD and ATP, which is consumed in regeneration of NAD, leading to cell death by energy depletion. Genetic disruption of PARP provides profound protection against glutamate-NO-mediated ischemic insults in vitro and major decreases in infarct volume after reversible middle cerebral artery occlusion. This provides evidence for a primary involvement of PARP activation in neuronal damage following focal cerebral ischemia and suggests that therapies designed toward inhibiting PARP may provide benefit in the treatment of cerebrovascular disease.

Classification of Ischemic Cerebrovascular Disease

A practical comprehensive classification of stroke is needed for evaluation of new therapies. With many variations in the initial presentations, pathology, brain imaging, and the clinical course, it is essential that a patient with stroke be labeled with these variables. This status would change in the natural course of the disease as well as by modifications with treatment. A proposed classification of ischemic cerebrovascular disease is shown in Table 19.4.

The case summary of a patient should include information on these essential points which can be coded under the letters and numerals for sorting out categories from a large series.

The patient presented with right hemiplegia (I1), showed an infarct on CT (II2), severe atherosclerotic narrowing of left internal carotid artery (III–A1, B1, C3), recovered partially over a period of 3 weeks, and was found to have hypertension (V1).

Recovery from Stroke

It is well recognized that spontaneous, often dramatic, improvement occurs in patients with acute ischemic stroke. Recovery from stroke depends upon several factors, listed in Table 19.5. Recovery varies according to:

Table 19.4 A practical classification of ischemic cerebrovascular disease for evaluating therapy

I	Initial clinical features	
	1. Asymptomatic	
	2. TIA	
	3. Neurological deficits: hemiplegia, aphasia	
II	Brain imaging studies	
	1. Normal	
	2. Infarction	
	3. None carried out	
III	Vascular pathology	
	A. Location	
	1. Cerebral arteries (including neck arteries)	
	2. Heart and the great vessels	
	3. Blood elements (coagulation disorders)	
	B. Type	
	1. Atherosclerotic occlusive disease	
	2. Thromboembolic	
	3. Other	
	C. Severity	
	1. Minimal	
	2. Moderate	
	3. Severe	
IV	Clinical course (state time period)	
	1. Single event. No recurrence	
	2. Partial recovery	
	3. Complete recovery	
	4. Fixed neurological deficits	
V	Major risk factors	
	1. Hypertension	
	2. Heart disease	
	3. Atherosclerosis	
	4. Old age	
	5. Diabetes	
	6. Smoking	
	7. Other risk factors	
	8. None identified	

Table 19.5 Factors that influence the recovery from stroke

1. Neurological status of the patient:
   (a) Prior to stroke
   (b) Immediately following stroke
2. Age
3. Type of stroke
4. Location of lesion in the cerebral arteries
5. Risk factors of stroke
6. Treatment of stroke

- Presence of collateral blood supply. The degree of motor improvement has been shown to correlate significantly (positively) with CBF values in the undamaged motor cortex of the opposite cerebral hemisphere.
- Regression of cerebral edema.

- Volume of penumbra that escapes infarction offers opportunities for secondary perifocal neuronal reorganization. Mapping of the extent of penumbra enables prediction for potential of recovery and select the most appropriate candidates for therapeutic trials.
- There is considerable scope for functional plasticity in the adult human cerebral cortex. Cortical reorganization is associated with functional recovery in stroke. Retraining after stroke can extend cortical representation of the infarcted area and improve skilled motor performance.

Recovery of cerebral energy metabolism is a prerequisite for the recovery of brain function and depends, to some extent, on the restoration of blood flow following ischemia. Postischemic resynthesis of ATP is limited. The recovery process is far more complex than the simple process of reversal of ischemia by revascularization.

The size of the penumbra zone is an important factor in the recovery of brain function. In the patient with an acute stroke, it is difficult to distinguish between the deficits due to areas of infarction and those due to the penumbra zone with potential for recovery. The duration of survival of neurons in the penumbra zone is not known but can extend to years, as evidenced by the recovery following HBO.

The time course of clinical recovery from stroke is variable and controversial. Most of the motor recovery usually occurs in the first 3 months, and functional recovery can continue for 6 months to 1 year after stroke. The following are important neurophysiological mechanisms underlying recovery from stroke.

About one-fourth of patients with acute ischemic stroke show some degree of spontaneous improvement by 1 h, and nearly half of the patients show some improvement by 6 h. Few of these patients, however, show complete motor recovery. Ninety percent of these patients remain improved on long-term follow-up indicating that improvement during the first 48 h after acute ischemic stroke is a predictor of favorable long-term outcome. This is correlated with absence of early hypodensity seen on CT. This improvement should be taken into consideration in design of any clinical trial of acute treatment of stroke. Mechanisms of recovery following acute ischemic stroke are:

- Unmasking or release from inhibition of previously ineffective pathways
- Synaptic sprouting and formation of new dendritic connections for pathways for transmission of neural messages

These mechanisms are the basis of the concept of neuroplasticity, which is the term used for the ability of the central nervous system (CNS) to modify its own structural organization and function.

Complications of Stroke

Various complications of stroke have been reported in the literature. These can be divided into neurological and medical or systemic complications. They have an adverse effect on the outcome of stroke and many are preventable. Deterioration of the neurological status, including a decrease in consciousness or progression of neurological deficits, occurs during the first week in 26–43 % of the patients with acute stroke. In some the causes are extension or hemorrhagic transformation of the infarct. Other causes are metabolic disturbances such as hypoglycemia and hyponatremia and adverse effects of drugs. Early deterioration is associated with a poor prognosis. Determinants of neurological worsening may include causative aspects rather than just the evolution of the ischemic or hemorrhagic process itself. Acute neurological complications of ischemic stroke are:

- Progressive neurological deficits
- Cerebral edema with transtentorial herniations
- Extension of infarction or appearance of a new infarct
- Hemorrhagic transformation of infarct
- Seizures

Stroke may be aggravated by treatment. Examples of this are complications of surgery on the cerebral blood vessels. Adverse effects of several drugs used in stroke patients may aggravate the condition. One example of this is cerebral hemorrhage resulting from anticoagulant or thrombolytic therapy in patients with ischemic infarction.

Sequelae of Stroke

The chronic poststroke stage may manifest some neuropsychological sequelae, as shown in Table 19.6. These are an extension of the neurological deficits seen in the acute phase

Table 19.6 Neuropsychological sequelae of stroke

- Persistence of neurological deficits
- Epilepsy
- Spasticity
- Central pain syndrome
- Neuropsychological disturbances
  Memory disturbances
  Intellectual and cognitive impairment
  Dementia
  Depression
  Pseudodepressive manifestations
  Anxiety
  Apathy
  Pathological laughing and crying
  Mania

of stroke. These are important but not always detected or emphasized. Two of them—spasticity and dementia—are important and will be considered here as they are amenable to treatment with hyperbaric oxygen.

Spasticity. This is the most troublesome complication of stroke and interferes with the physical rehabilitation of the patients. Spasticity is defined as a velocity-dependent response of a muscle to passive stretching, increased resistance to passive manipulation of the paretic limb, and is most marked in the antigravity muscles. Spasticity does not bear any definite relation to the degree of paralysis or the time of onset of the stroke; usually it becomes noticeable a few weeks after the onset of stroke. The underlying mechanism is controversial. The final common pathway for the expression of muscle tone is the anterior horn cells and myoneural junction. Spasticity may be viewed as alpha overactivity. A slight amount of spasticity of the paretic leg may be helpful in ambulation, but spasticity in the hand interferes with fine movements. Persistent spasticity can lead to contractures of muscles, tendons, and joint capsules.

Vascular Dementia

Dementia is defined as deterioration in intellectual function which is sufficient to interfere with customary affairs of life, which is not isolated to a single category of intellectual performance and is independent of level of consciousness. Vascular dementia may be the leading cause of cognitive impairment in the world, but there is no general agreement as to its definition. The term "vascular" may be obsolete and "dementia" implies that a patient has reached a state from which recovery is unlikely. The alternative term of vascular cognitive impairment has been used. Another term used in the literature is multi-infarct dementia but vascular dementia has a broader connotation and is the most widely used to describe cognitive impairment after stroke. Poststroke dementia is another term used to describe this condition. The only catch to this is that a patient with vascular disease may develop dementia without any manifest stroke.

Stroke patients are at risk for dementia. The prevalence of dementia 3 months after an ischemic stroke in patients over the age of 60 years is over 25 % and about ten times that in controls. Poststroke dementia is the second most common cause of dementia after Alzheimer's disease in Europe and the USA. In Asia and many other countries, it is more common than the dementia of Alzheimer's disease. Vascular risk factors are dominant in this form of dementia although there may be some genetic factors and some overlap with Alzheimer's disease. Treatable vascular risk factors occur more frequently in patients with vascular cognitive impairment than in patients with Alzheimer's disease. The importance of this distinction is that the vascular risk factors are

more amenable to treatment. A single explanation for poststroke dementia is not adequate; rather, multiple factors including stroke features (dysphasia, major dominant stroke syndrome), host characteristics (level of education), and prior cerebrovascular disease each independently contribute to the risk. Dementia is relatively frequent after a clinical first stroke in persons younger than 80 years, and aphasia is very often associated with poststroke dementia.

Two main causes of infarction in vascular dementia are hypoperfusion and vessel obstruction resulting in different types of lesions. Hypoperfusion is due to blood pressure fall in combination with vascular stenosis. Most of these infarcts are of an incomplete nature, i.e., an attenuation of the tissue leaving some axons with axon sheaths or intact neurons with scarring. Vascular obstruction may involve both the large extracerebral arteries as well as the small intracerebral vessels. Small vessel disease is usually due to hypertensive angiopathy, amyloid angiopathy, or microembolism.

Diagnosis of Stroke

The diagnosis of stroke is basically clinical, but confirmation requires laboratory procedures. In the case of acute stroke, the primary diagnosis at site of occurrence is important as it affects the treatment decisions. With the availability of treatment for acute stroke, the reliability of prehospital diagnosis has been examined. In a study in Ohio, emergency medical dispatchers correctly identified 52 % and paramedics 72 % of patients with stroke (Kothari et al. 1995). At the physician's level, neurologists obviously make a more accurate diagnosis than primary care physicians. False-positive rate without supplementary laboratory investigations varies from 1 to 5 %. This increases if the patient is unable to give a history because of impairment of consciousness or loss of speech. Diagnostic errors are most likely to arise in patients with atypical presentations and those with other diseases associated with cerebrovascular complications. Diagnosis of stroke depends on the clinical stage. Clinical diagnosis is important for classification of stroke which is an important part of clinical research for testing new therapies.

The diagnosis of stroke should be confirmed by laboratory investigations. Various laboratory diagnostic procedures used for stroke patients are:

- General laboratory examination
  - Hematology: full blood count, thrombophilia screen, erythrocyte sedimentation rate, etc.
  - Biochemistry: blood glucose, electrolytes, etc.
- Lumbar puncture and CSF examination
- Biomarkers of stroke in blood and CSF
- Doppler ultrasound
- Radioisotope imaging of atherosclerotic plaques

- Electroencephalography (EEG)
- Magnetoencephalography
- Neuro-ophthalmic examination: fundoscopy and ophthalmodynamometry
- Cerebral blood flow
- Cerebral angiography
- Brain imaging studies
  - Computerized tomography (CT)
  - Magnetic resonance imaging (MRI)
  - Positron emission tomography (PET)
  - Single-photon emission computerized tomography (SPECT)
- Cardiac investigations
  - Electrocardiography (ECG)
  - Transthoracic echocardiography
  - Transesophageal echocardiography

The most important of the imaging methods in relation to acute ischemic stroke are the brain imaging methods. These are discussed in Chap. 10. Currently CT scans and MRI are done routinely, and SPECT is still limited to certain centers. The last is the most relevant for evaluation of the effects of HBO on acute ischemic stroke.

Stroke Scales

The most commonly used functional scales in stroke patients, which measure only basic activities of daily living, are the Barthel Index and the Rankin Scale. Two global scales frequently used in clinical trials are the Unified Neurological Stroke Scale (UNSS) and the National Institutes of Health (NIH) Stroke Scale. These will be described in the following pages.

Barthel Index

The Barthel Index scores the patient's performance in ten basic activities of daily life, chosen and weighted as to reflect the amount of help required. For example, 15 points are given for walking and transfers; 10 points for feeding, bowel, bladder, toileting, and dressing; and 5 points for bathing and grooming. The maximum score is 100, which corresponds to full independence, and the lowest score is 0, which corresponds to bedridden state with full dependence. Most of the patients being discharged home have a score of 60 or above at that time. At a score of 85, most patients can dress themselves and transfer from bed to chair without help. The scores are not arbitrary but represent a definite average level of autonomy. The advantage of the thresholds of the Barthel Index is that they can be used in different types of statistical analyses. The reliability of the Barthel Index is high as reflected by an

interobserver agreement of more than 85 %. It is a more reliable and less subjective scale for assessing disability, from which a Rankin Handicap score can then be derived to enable those managing the stroke patients to assess aspects of handicap as well as disability.

Rankin Scale

This scale has the following scoring system:

0: No symptoms at all
1: No significant disability despite symptoms, able to carry out all usual duties and activities
2: Slight disability, unable to carry out all previous activities but able to look after own affairs without assistance
3: Moderate disability, requiring some help, but able to walk without assistance and attend to own body needs without assistance
4: Moderately severe disability, unable to walk without assistance, and unable to attend to body needs without assistance
5: Severe disability, bedridden, incontinent, and requiring constant nursing care and attention
6: Dead

National Institutes of Health Stroke Scale

National Institutes of Health (NIH) Stroke Scale is a standardized measure of neurological function to assess outcome after investigative therapy for acute stroke. It has 15 items which cover level of consciousness, pupillary response, best motor, limb ataxia, sensory, visual, neglect, and dysarthria items. This scale was used for the earlier tPA studies.

Unified Neurological Stroke Scale

The Unified Neurological Stroke Scale (UNSS) is composed of the Neurological Scale for Middle Cerebral Artery Infarction (MCANS) and Scandinavian Neurological Stroke Scale (SNSS). This scale is constructed specifically to assess patients with hemiparesis due to MCA infarction. Most of the items deal with testing the motor function. Consciousness and verbal communication are rated, but it excludes sensory and cognitive dysfunction items which are known to be less reliable and difficult to assess in evaluation of stroke in general. Disability evaluation items are omitted as they are included in scales for functional evaluation. The Unified Neurological Stroke Scale demonstrates good reliability and high construct and predictive validity, and its use is supported in ischemic and hemorrhagic stroke. Structural equation modeling is an appropriate technique for use with scales of this type.

Canadian Neurological Scale

The Canadian Neurological Scale (CNS) is a highly reliable and validated stroke scoring system. Long-term outcome can be predicted soon after acute stroke with a simple mathematical model based on the patient's age and initial CNS score. In contrast to other scales, which include assessment of neglect, coordination, sensation, and gait, the CNS focuses on level of consciousness, speech, and strength. Because impairment of these modalities is basic to the evaluation of any stroke patients, the data required for retrospective application of the CNS is more likely to be available in hospital records. Retrospective scoring of initial stroke severity using an algorithm based on the CNS is valid and can be reliably performed using hospital discharge summaries.

Evaluation of Various Scales

Stroke scales were originally devised to quantify disturbances in neurological function explained by stroke-induced brain lesions. In the course of evolution of these scales disagreements have arisen as to the weighting of certain elements in these scales. For example, coma is considered more serious than sensory disturbances of a limb. Considerable controversy still exists regarding the utility of these scales. The main finding of these analyses supports that the scales in popular use share many items but emphasize different features of the standard clinical examination. The scales most closely approximate one another for assessment of sensorimotor function. They vary widely when it comes to assessment of higher cerebral function.

Stroke scales only partially explain functional health and the impact of impairment on functional outcome seems to be underestimated by stroke scale weights. In an appraisal of reliability and validity of 9 stroke scales, the following were found to be the most reliable, based on interobserver agreement: NIH Scale, CNS Scale, and the European Stroke Scale. The Barthel Index is considered to be the most reliable disability scale. In the NIH tissue plasminogen activator (tPA) stroke trial, no measure of disability was found to describe all dimensions of recovery for stroke patients at 90 days. To compare treatments, the NINDS tPA Stroke Trial Coordinating Center proposed the use of a global statistical test, which allowed an overall assessment of treatment efficacy for a combination of correlated outcomes (Tilley et al. 1997).

An Overview of the Conventional Management of Stroke

The management of stroke will be discussed according to whether it is the acute phase or chronic poststroke stage. Treatment of acute ischemic stroke is more critical because there is a chance to prevent or limit irreversible damage to the brain. This is a challenge because of the limitations of feasible methods and of the short time window, which is considered to be no more than 3 h. The management of poststroke stage is more rehabilitation oriented and is aimed at recovery of the lost function.

Acute Ischemic Stroke

Until the approval of thrombolytic therapy by tissue plasminogen activator (tPA) in 1996, there was no definite treatment of acute stroke. The availability of thrombolytic therapy has opened the door for improved and more definitive care for acute stroke patients. It is now considered important to bring the acute stroke patients to a medical center within the first few hours following stroke. The ideal place for a patient is a stroke center, and if this is not available, a major general hospital with neurological service would be adequate. Objectives of acute stroke therapy are:

- To reduce the mortality rate in those who survive stroke to below 20 %
- Restoration of normal cerebral blood flow
  - Thrombolysis of blood clot obstructing cerebral arteries
  - Surgical procedures such as carotid endarterectomy
- Cerebral protection against the effects of cerebral ischemia
  - Hyperbaric oxygen
  - Neuroprotectives
- Supportive medical care
  - Maintenance of airway and oxygenation
  - Management of concomitant diseases such as heart disease and hypertension
  - Maintenance of fluid and electrolyte balance
  - Prevention of complications such as aspiration pneumonia
- Preservation of life and management of systemic effects of stroke
- Neurologic intensive care
  - Monitoring for increased intracranial pressure
  - Management of neurological complications, e.g., cerebral edema and seizures
- Prevention of disease extension and recurrence
- Anticoagulation/antiplatelet therapy
  - Risk factor management
- Rehabilitation: to enable 70 % of the stroke survivors to live independently 3 months after stroke

These goals are ideal but extremely difficult to attain. To achieve these objectives, all patients with acute ischemic stroke should be treated on an emergency basis within 1 h of occurrence. The current management of acute stroke is summarized in Table 19.7.

The acute stroke is a medical emergency and most of these patients are transported by ambulance to a hospital. Trained and experienced ambulance attendants are able to recognize stroke in

Table 19.7 Current management of acute stroke

• Medical therapies
Thrombolytic therapy
Anticoagulant therapy
Antiplatelet agents
Hemorheological agents: trental
Drugs for reduction of cerebral edema
Management of hypotension
Complementary medical therapies: herbs and acupuncture
Hyperbaric oxygen
• Management of concomitant disorders
Antihypertensive medications
Drugs for cardiac disorders
• Surgical therapies
Evacuation of intracerebral hematomas
Decompressive craniotomy
Carotid endarterectomy
Embolectomy
Transluminal angioplasty
Surgical procedures for revascularization
• Start of rehabilitation

fair percentage of patients. In some countries a physician accompanies the ambulance. Care during transport varies according to the type of medical attendants in the ambulance. Most of the patients receive basic medical care according to the condition. Unconscious patients are observed and airway is maintained if necessary with intubation. Supplementary oxygen is usually given and an intravenous line is established. Monitoring of cardiovascular function varies in different countries. Blood pressure is checked regularly and ECG monitoring is done in some countries. The emergency medical facility is notified to have necessary personnel and equipment ready on arrival, including the readiness of emergency CT scan and alerting the emergency physician for the possibility of the patient as a candidate for tPA therapy. On arrival in the emergency department, the level of care varies according to the facility, e.g., a stroke center or a small general hospital. Airway and circulation are checked. Supplemental oxygen and intravenous saline or lactate Ringer solution is started. An eyewitness history of the onset is obtained as the patient's account may not be reliable. Establishing the time and mode of onset is important. A careful clinical neurovascular examination is done. Neurological dysfunction is recorded and examination repeated to see if it is recovering, stable, or increasing. Most of the acute care in the USA is done by emergency room physicians who also administer tPA.

Major questions that remain unanswered and are under investigation for treatment of acute stroke are:

- Redefinition of indications and modifications of thrombolytic therapy
- Value of early intravenous heparin following acute ischemic stroke
- Value of antiplatelet therapy given during the first 6 h after stroke onset

- Neuroprotective therapy for acute stroke
- Value of hyperbaric oxygenation in acute ischemic stroke
- Value of hypothermia in acute ischemic stroke
- Combination of various therapies

Over 200 compounds are in various stages of development for acute stroke by the pharmaceutical industry. These fall into the following categories and are discussed in detail elsewhere (Jain 2016).

- Thrombolytics
- Anticoagulants
- Defibrogenating agents
- Agents to improve hemorheology
- Neuroprotectives
  - Adenosine analogs
  - Anti-inflammatory agents
  - Apoptosis inhibitors
    Calpain inhibitors
    Cycloheximide
- Ion channel modulators
  - Ca+ channel blockers
  - Na+ channel blockers
- NMDA antagonists
  - NMDA receptor antagonists—competitive and noncompetitive
  - AMPA antagonists
  - Glycine-site antagonists
- Non-NMDA excitatory amino acid antagonists 5-HT agonist
  - GABA agonists
  - Opioid receptor antagonists
- Nitric oxide scavengers
- Free radical scavengers
- Drugs counteracting lactate neurotoxicity
- Agents for regeneration and repair
  - Neurotrophic factors
  - Nootropic agents
  - Phosphotidylcholine synthesis
- Hormonal modulators of cerebral ischemia
- Anti-edema agents
- Antihypoxic agents
- Miscellaneous agents
- Oxygen carriers
- Cell therapy
- Gene therapy

Neuroprotectives

A neuroprotective agent is one that aims to prevent neuronal death by inhibiting one or more of the pathophysiological steps in the processes that follow occlusion (or rupture) of a cerebral artery (Jain 2011). Neuroprotection is an important part of acute therapy of stroke to protect the neural tissues from the ischemic cascade that increases the damage. Even if the ischemia is reversed by thrombolytic therapy, reperfusion injury may be responsible for further tissue damage.

The time window during which initiation of treatment with neuroprotective agents may rescue brain tissue is limited. The ideal time window for thrombolytic therapy is considered to be <3 h, and most of the neuroprotectives in clinical trials are used in a time window of >3 h. Ideally a neuroprotective should be given as soon as possible after the ischemic insult, i.e., within the first 3 h. It should precede the use of thrombolytic therapy and at least overlap it.

Oxygen Carriers

Two main categories of pharmaceutical agents have been used for delivery of oxygen to the tissues: perfluorocarbons (PFCs) and hemoglobin-based oxygen carriers. Both are primarily blood substitutes. Here we are interested in the use of these substances as oxygen carriers to the ischemic brain in stroke. Theoretically, cell-free carriers should transfer oxygen to the tissues more efficiently than red cells but so far, this has not been readily demonstrable. A third category is liposome-encapsulated Hb where Hb is entrapped in a bilayer of phospholipid. A modifier of heme function is also enclosed to adjust the oxygen-carrying capacity of HB. The half-life of this product can be increased by coating the liposome surface with sugar. Some of the oxygen carriers are:

Hemoglobin-based Oxygen Carriers (HBOCs). Preparation of HBOCs involves the removal of the cellular capsule of Hb and modifying the structure of Hb to prevent it from degradation, to enable it to function in simple electrolyte solutions and avoid toxic effects in the body.

Diaspirin cross-linked hemoglobin. Purified diaspirin cross-linked hemoglobin (DCLHb) is a cell-free hemoglobin that is intramolecularly cross-linked between the two alpha subunits, resulting in enhanced oxygen offloading to tissues and increased half-life. It is prepared from outdated human red cells. Because Hb molecules are minute compared with red cells, free Hb may perfuse into capillaries that have been shut down and thus prevent secondary damage.

Perfluorocarbons (PFCs). PFCs are inert organic substances produced by substituting fluorine for hydrogen in specific positions within highly stable carbon chains. They are not metabolized by the body and are excreted via the lungs, urine, and feces although a small amount may be stored in the reticuloendothelial system. The two major mechanisms underlying the efficacy of PFCs for oxygen transport and delivery are (1) a high solubility coefficient for oxygen and CO_2 and (2) PFCs release O_2 to the tissues more effectively because their O_2 binding constant is negligible. They have been investigated intensively over the past 30 years. PFC-based oxygen carriers, while more recent than HBOCs, have some advantages over HBOCs. They are synthetic, chemically inert, and inexpensive. PFCs have a high affinity for oxygen and carbon dioxide. PFCs can substitute for red blood cells transport oxygen as a dissolved gas rather than as chemi-

cally bound as in the case of HBOCs. This makes a difference to the way the oxygen is presented to the tissues. It is not yet certain if PFCs can provide more oxygen to the tissues than simple oxygen inhalation. Other drawbacks are adverse characteristics such as instability, short intravascular half-life, and uncertainty concerning toxic effects.

Cell Therapy

Cell therapy is the prevention or treatment of human disease by the administration of cells that have been selected, multiplied, and pharmacologically treated or altered outside the body (ex vivo). Cells may repair the damage or release therapeutic molecules. The scope of cell therapy can be broadened to include methods, pharmacological as well as non-pharmacological, to modify the function of intrinsic cells of the body for therapeutic purposes. Various types of cells have been used for this purpose, but most of the current interest in cell therapy centers on stem cells. Cell therapy can be combined with HBO. HBO can promote the mobilization and multiplication of stem cells. Examples of some of the strategies are (Jain 2013):

- Implantation of genetically programmed embryonic stem cells
- Intravenous infusion of marrow stromal cells
- Intravenous infusion of umbilical cord blood stem cells
- Intracerebral administration of multipotent adult progenitor cells
- Neural stem cell therapy for stroke

Gene Therapy

Gene therapy can be broadly defined as the transfer of defined genetic material to specific target cells of a patient for the ultimate purpose of preventing or altering a particular disease state. Carriers or delivery vehicles for therapeutic genetic material are called vectors which are usually viral but several non-viral techniques are being used as well. The broad scope of gene therapy covers implantation of genetically engineered cells, repair of defective gene in situ, excision or replacement of the defective gene by a normal gene, and inhibition of gene expression by antisense oligodeoxynucleotides. Examples of some of the strategies that are under investigation to reduce cerebral infarction are (Jain 2013):

- Transfer of glucose transporter gene to neurons/HSV vector.
- Adenovirus vector coding for bFGF1–154 may be used to induce angiogenesis in vivo.
- Intracerebroventricular injection of antisense c-fos oligonucleotides.
- Intracerebroventricular injection of oligonucleotide antisense to NMDA-Ra receptor.
- Intracerebroventricular injection of adenovirus vector carrying a human IL-2 receptor antagonist protein.
- Intraparenchymal injection of HSV-packaged amplicon vector expressing bcl-2.

Combination of approaches to management of stroke. In view of the multiple choices available for experimental therapies of stroke, some thought has been given to combination therapies. This has been done within the same category and also between compounds from different categories. Some examples of potential combinations are:

- Thrombolytics and neuroprotectives. The two therapies address different problems. Can be used simultaneously. Neuroprotectives may counteract reperfusion injury as a sequelae of thrombolysis.
- Thrombolytics and HBO. HBO may protect the brain against ischemia/hypoxia during the first hour until the patient can be transported and investigated to have thrombolytic therapy. Should improve the results in survivors. Also counteracts edema associated with stroke.

Management of the Chronic Poststroke Stage

In contrast to the tremendous efforts being made for the management of acute stroke, little is done for the patients in the chronic poststroke stage. Most of the patients have been discharged to home at this stage and very few receive regular physical therapy. Physicians are seldom interested in these patients who are considered to have fixed neurological deficits due to irreversible brain damage. They come to the attention of physicians only because of neurological and systemic complications which sometimes require hospitalization and surgery. However, conventional and sometimes innovative efforts have been made in patients in the chronic poststroke stage for the management of spasticity, for improvement of motor deficits, and for the treatment of dementia.

Management of Spasticity

Current methods for the management of spasticity are shown in Table 19.8. None of these methods is satisfactory in the long term: all the drugs have toxic effects. Physical therapy helps, but the effects are of short duration.

Strategies to facilitate motor recovery in the chronic poststroke stage. The following measures have been used in an attempt to improve motor deficits:

- Drugs that may improve motor function
  - ACH chlorohydrate
  - Amphetamine
  - Apomorphine
  - Caffeine
  - Carbaminol choline
  - Fluoxetine
  - GM1 gangliosides
  - Levodopa
  - Neostigmine
  - Norepinephrine
  - Phenylpropanolamine
  - Piracetam
  - Selective serotonin reuptake inhibitors
  - Yohimbine
- Promotion of neural regeneration and enhancement of synaptic plasticity
- Surgical procedures
  - Cerebral revascularization
  - Neural transplantation

It is generally believed that there is a significant interaction between acetylcholine (ACh) and norepinephrine (NE) in the CNS. NE modulates the direct release of ACh from the cerebral cortex by way of alpha-1 receptors. This release is also mediated by gamma-aminobutyric acid (GABA). There are anatomical connections between the locus coeruleus (LC) located in the floor of the fourth ventricle and the cholinergic cells in the septum, hippocampus, and cerebral cortex. The current hypothesis is that release of NE from LC is the integral factor in recovery of motor function after stroke.

Currently the use of these pharmacologic agents for motor recovery in stroke is not supported by class I evidence (Keser and Francisco 2015). Of all the drugs studied in animal models, amphetamine was most consistently reported to accelerate recovery of function. Amphetamine has a variety of effects primarily on the brain neurons releasing NE. Intraventricular infusions of NE mimic the effect of amphetamine, whereas similar infusions of dopamine have no effect. In a rat model of cerebral infarction, amphetamine appears to promote alternate circuit activation—a pharmacological property that may be advantageous for recovery after stroke. There is experimental evidence for fibroblast growth factor-2 as a mediator of amphetamine-enhanced motor improvement following stroke (Wolf et al. 2014). Evidence that amphetamine combined with physical therapy promotes recovery of motor function was provided by a double-blind pilot study (Crisomoto et al. 1987). A review of eight clinical trials performed since then shows that the results are unimpressive, conflicting, and far from successful results demonstrated in animal experiments (Walker-Batson 2013). Although amphetamine has been

Table 19.8 Currently used methods for the management of spasticity

1. Physical medicine:
Physical modalities: heat, cold, vibration, electrical stimulation
Physical therapy: use of proper splints, proper positioning of patient, spasm inhibiting exercises, slow and prolonged stretch
2. Drugs: dantrolene, baclofen, diazepam, phenytoin plus chlorpromazine
3. Surgery:
Orthopedic: lengthening, sectioning, release and transposition of tendons
Neurosurgical: intramuscular neurolysis and rhizotomy, spinal cord stimulation, intrathecal baclofen, tizanidine

reported to promote recovery of motor function in some stroke patients, the objections to this approach are:

- Amphetamine aggravates rather than improves spasticity.
- Amphetamine is contraindicated in several conditions including hypertension, which is frequent in stroke patients.
- Amphetamine is habit-forming and has other undesirable side effects.

For further investigation of clinical potential of neuropharmacological agents for motor recovery in stroke, better-designed clinical trials are needed. Patients who are likely to benefit from this approach need to be identified as well as integration of drugs into multidisciplinary stroke rehabilitation. The role of surgical procedures in the chronic poststroke stage is described in Chap. 20.

Treatment of Vascular Dementia

It is important to determine the type of dementia before starting the treatment. Vascular dementia is potentially preventable and more responsive to treatment than degenerative dementias such as Alzheimer's disease. Effective and early treatment of risk factors for stroke is likely to prevent recurrent cerebral infarctions and progression of dementia. The main form of therapy is prevention, but several pharmacotherapeutic approaches are:

- Antiplatelet therapy
- Agents for improving hemorheology
- Cerebral blood flow enhancers
- Nootropics (cerebral metabolic enhancers)
- Neuroprotectives
- Ergot derivatives

There is no hard evidence that any of these drugs can improve dementia significantly.

Treatment of Poststroke Depression

Poststroke depression occurs in one-third of patients after the acute stage and persists in the chronic poststroke stage. HBO has been reported to improve depression during recovery after acute stroke. A clinical trial has evaluated the effectiveness of hyperbaric oxygen (Yan et al. 2015). Patients were randomized into three groups: fluoxetine group, HBO therapy group, and HBO combined with fluoxetine group. Combined HBO with fluoxetine was more effective than the other treatment methods.

Role of HBO in the Management of Acute Stroke

Scientific Basis

The role of HBO in relieving ischemia and hypoxia has already been described in Chap. 18. These are the most important reasons for using HBO in cerebral ischemia. HBO also has an important role in improving the microcirculatory disturbances. Logistic problems in the use of HBO in the management of stroke have been reviewed (Jain and Toole 1998).

The resistance to blood flow is greater in vessels in which the diameter is less than 1.5 mm, e.g., the capillaries. The viscous effect is less, because the red blood cells (RBC) are aligned in a column as they pass through the lumen (Fahraeus–Lindqvist effect) instead of moving randomly. In microcirculatory disturbances, such as occur with clumping of RBC and slowing of circulation, the viscosity of the blood increases tremendously. RBC can get stuck where the endothelial cells protrude into the lumen of the capillary. The blood flow can become totally blocked for a fraction of a second or a longer period. Some plasma may, however, seep across the obstruction. HBO has a beneficial effect in cerebral ischemia through the following mechanisms:

1. Oxygen dissolved in plasma under pressure raises pAO_2 and can nourish the tissues even in the absence of RBC (Boerema et al. 1959).
2. Oxygen can diffuse extravascularly. Diffusion is facilitated by the gradient between the high oxygen tension in the patent capillaries and the low tension in the occluded ones. The effectiveness of this mechanism depends upon the abundance of capillaries in the tissues. Because the brain is a very vascular tissue, this mechanism can provide for the oxygenation of the tissues after vascular occlusion.
3. The supply of oxygen to the tissues can be facilitated by decreasing the viscosity of the blood and reducing platelet aggregation and increasing RBC deformability.
4. HBO relieves brain edema. By its vasoconstricting action, HBO counteracts the vasodilatation of the capillaries in the hypoxic tissues and reduces the extravasation of fluid.
5. Blood–brain barrier (BBB) is disturbed in cerebrovascular ischemia, and HBO may serve to decrease the permeability of BBB. Intra-ischemic HBO therapy reduces early and delayed postischemic BBB damage and edema after focal ischemia in rats and mice (Veltkamp et al. 2005).
6. HBO also reduces the swelling of the neurons by improving their metabolism.
7. HBO, by improving oxygenation of the penumbra that surrounds the area of total ischemia, prevents glycolysis and subsequent intracellular lactic acidosis and maintains cerebral metabolism in an otherwise compromised area.
8. In a rat model of ischemic stroke, HBO treatments mobilize bone marrow stem cells to an ischemic area, stimulate expression of trophic factors, and improve neurogenesis and gliosis (Lee et al. 2013). These effects may help in neuronal repair after ischemic stroke.

HBO in Relation to Cerebral Ischemia and Free Radicals

Free radical generation and possible relation to hyperbaric oxygen have been discussed in Chap. 2. The role of free radicals in mediating oxygen toxicity has been discussed in Chap. 6. Free radical generation is increased during reperfusion following ischemia. This may result in damage to the myelin although neurons and axons are preserved by hyperoxic perfusion. Various free radical scavengers may be useful adjuncts to HBO therapy in acute stroke. In experimental studies, administration of HBO to rabbits after global ischemia showed no evidence of aggravation of the brain injury even though free radical production was increased.

Animal Experiments

Animal Models of Stroke

Investigation of pathophysiology and therapy of cerebral ischemia requires animal experimental models where effects of ischemia can be produced under controlled conditions. This goal is not easy to achieve because of the diversity of the scientific issues related to brain ischemia research that are relevant to therapy. Although larger animals (cats, dogs, and subhuman primates) have been used to study brain ischemia, rats are the most popular and desirable animals for this purpose. The important features are low cost, resemblance to the human brain vasculature, small brain size that is suited to whole brain fixation procedures, and their greater acceptability (e.g., in comparison with subhuman primates). The last is an important point with the current trends in animal rights movement. Transgenic models of stroke are also available. One example is of nitric oxide synthase knockout mice that are more resistant to ischemic stroke. These models may be helpful for understanding the pathophysiology of ischemic stroke but are not relevant to HBO. Models of focal ischemia are most relevant to human stroke and involve the occlusion of a selected artery. The methods used for occlusion vary. Middle cerebral artery occlusion (MCAO) in the rat is a standard model of experimental focal vascular ischemia and has gained increasing acceptance because of its predictive validity. It is used for studying the pathophysiology of stroke as well as for efficacy of neuroprotective agents. A convenient method to evaluate the therapeutic effect is the measurement of infarct volume by brain sectioning. MRI has also been used in animal stroke models for in vivo evaluation of neuroprotective effects of various compounds in cerebral ischemia. Traditional T2-weighted MRI has a very limited use in identifying ischemic issue destined for infarction because accurate measurements can only be made at time points of >4 h. Diffusion-weighted MRI has enabled accurate assessment of early ischemic changes occurring within 30–40 min of temporary or permanent MCA occlusion in animals.

No animal model can exactly represent human stroke, and there are fallacies of testing neuroprotective compounds in animal models. Some of these results are difficult to translate into human clinical trials. One advantage, however, of these models is that a standard model can be used to compare various therapies. Stroke models may be quite appropriate for evaluating the effects of HBO in acute cerebral infarction.

Animal Experimental Evidence for Effectiveness of HBO in Cerebral Ischemia

Animal experimental evidence for the effect of HBO in ischemia/hypoxia is summarized in Table 19.9. These are mostly studies of focal cerebral ischemia. Experimental studies of global ischemia/hypoxia are described in Chap. 23. In one of the earlier studies showing the protective effect of HBO against cerebral ischemia, HBO at 2 ATA facilitated recovery of dogs made hypoxic by CO_2 inhalation (Smith et al. 1961). In another series of animals, the same authors observed the diameter of cortical vessels through burr holes. They noted no changes in arterial diameter whether the animals breathed room air or oxygen at 2 ATA, as long as the arterial pCO_2 was kept at 40 mmHg. Of the eight studies, only one failed to find any beneficial effect of HBO. Another seven studies, done on different animals and different time periods (1961–1987), have shown the beneficial effect of HBO in cerebral ischemia.

Breathing 100 % oxygen at ambient pressures does not appear to have the same effect. In one study it has been shown to lead to a threefold increase in mortality in gerbils when administered 3–6 h after 15 min of ischemia induced by vascular occlusion (Mickel et al. 1987). The explanation given was that oxygen free radical toxicity aggravates the lipid peroxidation following ischemia. Apparently this aggravation does not occur with oxygen at 1.5 ATA. Oxygen toxicity may, however, occur at higher pressures and after prolonged application. Survival rates were 30 % in control group versus 70 % in the group treated with HBO. Neurological recovery with slight disability was in 1 of 10 control animals versus 6 out of 9 animals in the HBO-treated group.

In one study of the use of HBO in rat MCAO model, the percentage of infarcted area increased significantly in animals treated 12 and 23 h following arterial occlusion as compared to the beneficial effect of HBO within 6 h after the occlusion (Badr et al. 2001a, b). The results of this study suggest that applying HBO within 6 h of ischemia-reperfusion injury could benefit the patient but that applying HBO 12 h or more after injury could harm the patient.

Hyperglycemia is known to aggravate cerebral infarction and hemorrhagic transformation after ischemic stroke in which oxidative stress and matrix metalloproteinases play an important role. Preconditioning rats with HBO prior to inducing a stroke by occlusion of the middle cerebral artery attenuated hemorrhagic transformation of infarct (Soejima et al. 2013). HBO for the chronic phase of stroke

Table 19.9 Animal experimental studies regarding the effect of HBO in cerebral ischemia/anoxia

Authors and year	Animal model	Technique of ischemia/anoxia	Treatment protocol	Measurements and results
Smith et al. (1961)	Dogs	CO inhalation	HBO 2 ATA, 100% oxygen controls, no treatment	Neurological recovery facilitated; cortical vessel diameter, no change if CO2 is 40 mmHg
Jacobson and Lawson (1963)	Dogs anesthetized	Middle cerebral artery clipping, transcranial	1. HBO 2 ATA	Decreased CBF; less protection than hypothermia
			2. Controls, no clipping	Decreased CBF with vasoconstriction
			3. Hypothermia + air	Protective effect
			4. Hypothermia + HBO	Protective effect same as in 3 (breathing air)
Moore et al. (1966)	Dogs	Total circulatory arrest with hypothermia	HBO 3 ATA, 100% oxygen; controls room air	Extension of safe period of occlusion from 1 to 2 min under normothermia to 2–3 min with hypothermia
Whalen et al. (1966)	Dogs	Induced cardiac fibrillation	HBO 3 ATA, 100% oxygen controls, no treatment	Prolonged the period from fibrillation to cessation of EEG activity; cerebral protection
Corkill et al. (1985)	Gerbils	Carotid ligation	HBO 1.5–2 ATA with 100% oxygen; controls air	Calorimetric videodensimetric estimation of cerebral ischemia through intact cranium; best results obtained in HBO groups
Shiokawa et al. (1986)	Rats— spontaneous hypersensitive	Bilateral carotid ligation	HBO 2 ATA, 100% oxygen; controls, room air	HBO prevented increase in cerebral lactate and prolonged survival time if started 3 h after ligation but no effect if started 1 h post ligation
Weinstein et al. (1986)	Cats (awake)	Temporary occlusion of middle cerebral artery for 6 or 24 h (from previously implanted vessel occluder via transorbital approach)	HBO 1.5 ATA 100% oxygen for 40 min during or after 6 h occlusion and before, during, or after 24 h occlusion; controls room air	Neurological assessment, grade 0–10. Brain examined after cats killed on day 10
				1. HBO during first 3 h of 6 h occlusion results in a 4 grade improvement which persisted during rest of the occlusion period
				2. Average grade of neurological deficit 94% less with HBO than in controls
				3. Infarct size in HBO group was 58% less than in controls in 6 h group and 40% less in 24 h group
Burt et al. (1987)	Gerbils	Right carotid ligation	HBO 1.5 ATA, 100% oxygen	Neurologic; brain staining with tetrazolium
			1. 36 h with 5 min air breaks/h treatment	1. Infarcts in 26% but all animals died within 24–36 h from oxygen toxicity
			2. 36 h with 1 h air break/h treatment	2. 44% Had cerebral infarcts
			3. 18 h with 5 min air breaks/h treatment	3. 11% Had infarcts during the first 18 h; no infarcts during the next 18 h
			4. Controls; room air unligated controls	4. 72% Had cerebral infarcts; no mortality when subjected to protocol 1
Kawamura et al. (1990)	Rats	Middle cerebral artery occlusion for 4 h	HBO at 2 ATA 100% oxygen for 30 min. Treatment given between 2.5 and 3.5 h following ischemic insult	HBO reduced ischemic neuronal injury and brain edema
Reitan et al. (1990)	Gerbils	Unilateral carotid artery interruption	HBO at 2.5 ATA 100% oxygen for 2–4 h after occlusion. Controls: pentobarbital and superoxide dismutase	Increased survival in HBO-treated group

(continued)

Table 19.9 (continued)

Authors and year	Animal model	Technique of ischemia/anoxia	Treatment protocol	Measurements and results
Yatsuzuka (1991)	Dogs	Complete cerebral ischemia for 18 min	HBO at 2 ATA for 170 min	CBF, EEG, and indicators of oxidative stress
				HBO reduced brain damage without increasing oxidative stress
Takahashi et al. (1992)	Cats	Global ischemia induced by occlusion of the ascending aorta and caval veins for 15 min	HBO at 3 ATA 100 % oxygen for 1 h at 3, 24, and 29 h after ischemia	Survival rates were 30 % in control group versus 70 % in group treated with HBO. Neurological recovery with slight disability was in 1 of 10 control animals versus 6 out of 9 animals in the HBO-treated group
			Controls: room air	
Wada et al. (1996)	Gerbils	Occlusion of both common carotid arteries under anesthesia	1 h to male Mongolian gerbils either for a single session or every other day for five sessions. Two days after HBO pretreatment, the gerbils were subjected to 5 min of forebrain ischemia	Seven days after recirculation, neuronal density per 1 mm length of the CA1 sector in the hippocampus was significantly better preserved in the five-session HBO pretreatment group. Tolerance against ischemic neuronal damage was induced by repeated HBO pretreatment, which is thought to occur through the induction of HSP-72 synthesis
Krakovsky et al. (1998) (0 %). Even among the animals that did not survive the 14 day period, those exposed to HBO	Rats	Acute global ischemia by four-vessel occlusion	Two groups: (1) control animals that breathed air at atmospheric pressure and (2) rats exposed to oxygen at 3 ATA	Survival rate was significantly higher (45 %) in the HBO group than in the control group survived longer than the control animals
Roos et al. (1998)	Rats	Middle cerebral artery occlusion	Group I received a single 30-min HBO treatment at 2 ATA	Daily neurologic examinations and computerized quantal bioassay were used to determine the ET50—the occlusion time required to cause a neurologic abnormality in half of the animals
			Group II received 30-min HBO treatments at 2 ATA daily for 4 consecutive days	HBO therapy showed no apparent benefit in a rat model as a treatment modality for acute cerebral ischemia with reperfusion
Atochin et al. (2000)	Rats	Reversible occlusion of the middle cerebral artery	HBO (2.8 ATA 100 % oxygen for 45 m)	HBO reduced functional neurological deficits and cerebral infarct volume by inhibiting neutrophil accumulation
Chang et al. (2000)	Rats	Occlusion of the middle cerebral artery	HBO (3 ATA) 2 × 90 min at a 24-h intervals	Also hyperbaric air at similar schedule
Prass et al. (2000)	SV129 or C57BL/6 mice	Focal cerebral ischemia induced 1 day after the fifth HBO session	HBO (3 ATA, 1 h daily/5 days), 100 % oxygen	HBO can induce tolerance to focal cerebral ischemia, but this effect is strain dependent
Sunami et al. (2000)	Rats	Ligation of the right middle cerebral and right common carotid arteries	HBO (3 ATA) 2 h initiated 10 min after onset of ischemia	Reduced infarct volume by increasing oxygen supply to the ischemic periphery without aggravating lipid peroxidation
Veltkamp et al. (2000)	Rats	Reversible occlusion of middle cerebral artery	HBO 1.5 or 2.5 ATA	Controls with 100 % normobaric oxygen
Badr et al. (2001a)	Freely moving rats	Middle cerebral artery occlusion	HBO (3 ATA, 1 h), 100 % oxygen	Neuroprotective effect as HBO normalized brain energy metabolites and excitatory amino acids disturbances that occur during cerebral ischemia
		After 2 h of occlusion, the suture was removed and reperfusion was allowed		

(continued)

Table 19.9 (continued)

Authors and year	Animal model	Technique of ischemia/anoxia	Treatment protocol	Measurements and results
Yang et al. (2002)	Rats	Focal cerebral ischemia was by occlusion of the middle cerebral artery	HBO (2.8 ATA 100% oxygen) during ischemia. Room air for control animals	HBO offered significant neuroprotection. The mechanism seems to partly imply reduced level of dopamine
Hjelde et al. (2002)	Wistar rats	Right middle cerebral occluded for 4 h	HBO (2 ATA, 100% oxygen for 230 min)	HBO did not reduce tissue damage
Yin et al. (2002)	Rats	Transient middle cerebral artery occlusion with focal ischemia	HBO (3 ATA, 100% oxygen for 1 h) given 6 h after reperfusion	HBO within 6 h reduced infarction. There was inhibition of COX-2 over-expression in cerebral cortex accompanying the neuroprotective effect
Qin et al. (2007)	Rat	Middle cerebral artery occlusion	3 ATA for 1 h 30 min after	Reduction of hemorrhagic transformation
Hou et al. (2007)	Rat	Middle cerebral artery occlusion with ischemia/reperfusion	NBO control	The infarct size after HBO was smaller than for NBO
			HBO at 2 ATA	
Eschenfelder et al. (2008)	Rat	Middle cerebral artery occlusion with ischemia/reperfusion	HBO at 1.5, 2, 2.5, or 3 ATA for 1 h	Reduction in infarct volume with HBO 2.5 and 3.0 ATA over 1 week
Sun et al. (2008)	Rat	Filament-induced middle cerebral artery occlusion for 2 h	HBO at 3 ATA for 95 min	HBO improves penumbral oxygenation in focal ischemia by modification of the hypoxia-inducible factor-1α

has been studied in rat models that survive for 1 week after 2 h occlusion of the middle cerebral artery, and treatment is continued for 6 weeks (Hu et al. 2014). In this model, HBO enhances endogenous neurogenesis and improves neurofunctional recovery in the possibly mediated by reactive oxygen species/HIF-1 α/β-catenin pathway. A single treatment of HBO immediately after MCAO in mice followed by 24 h of reperfusion was shown to significantly reduce cerebral edema and improve perfusion (Pushkov et al. 2016). Toll-like receptor 4 knockout also protects mice from ischemic damage, but to a lesser extent than HBO treatment, as shown in this study.

HBO therapy and memantine, a noncompetitive NMDA antagonist, are both promising treatment strategies for improving stroke prognosis. However, HBO's narrow therapeutic time window, <6 h poststroke, and the adverse effect of high-dose memantine administration limit the use of these therapeutic interventions. Combination of memantine treatment 15 min after the onset of ischemic event in MCAO rats and HBO therapy 12 h post-reperfusion significantly restored neurologic scores as well as decreased infarct volume and increased antioxidant activity (Wang et al. 2015). These results imply that the combination of memantine and HBO therapy not only prolongs the therapeutic window of HBO treatment but also lowers the dosage requirement of memantine. The mechanism underlying the neuroprotective effects of the combined treatment may lie in alleviated BBB permeability, inhibited inflammatory response, and upregulated antioxidant enzyme activity.

In a systematic review of experimental studies of the effect of HBO on stroke, 51 that met the inclusion criteria were identified among the 1198 studies examined (Xu et al.

2016). When compared with control group data, HBO therapy resulted in infarct size reduction or improved neurological function (32% decrease in infarct size). Mortality was 18.4% in the HBO group and 26.7% in the control group. Subgroup analysis showed that a maximal neuroprotective effect was reached when HBO was administered immediately after MCAO with an ATA of 2 and >6 h of HBO treatment.

Neuroprotective Effect of HBO Preconditioning

HBO-induced neuroprotective effect possibly depends on the time when treatment starts. The application of HBO before or in the early phase of an ischemic injury can increase ischemic tolerance, inducing at first a hypoxic/ischemic like effect stimulating endogenous mechanisms for cell survival and to prevent further damage (synthesis of HIF-1α, etc.) resulting in increased hypoxic tolerance (Gu et al. 2008; Li et al. 2008). This is referred to as HBO preconditioning (HBO-PC).

In an experimental study to verify the possible pathways involved in neuroprotection in HBO-PC, hyperglycemic MCAO rats received 1 h daily HBO sessions for 5 consecutive days, and occlusion was induced 24 h after the last HBO treatment (Guo et al. 2016). HBO-PC decreased infarction volume and improved neurobehavioral function. In addition, it provided additional protective effects in hemorrhagic transformation of infarct, which was independent of infarction volume. These beneficial effects were reversed after blocking the ROS/thioredoxin-interacting protein/Nod-like receptor protein 3 pathway.

Neuroprotection in cerebral ischemia involves sirtuin 1 (Sirt1), a class III histone deacetylase, which is induced by HBO-PC. In rats with middle cerebral artery occlusion (MCAO) as an ischemic stroke model, HBO-PC increased the expression of Sirt1, nuclear factor erythroid 2-related factor 2 (Nrf2), heme oxygenase 1 (HO-1), and superoxide dismutase 1 (SOD1) after 1 week (Xue et al. 2016). There was decrease of infarct volume ratio, neurobehavioral deficit, and malondialdehyde content (a measure of oxidative stress). Furthermore, either Sirt1 or Nrf2 knockdown by short interfering RNA (siRNA) inhibited the expression of Nrf2, HO-1, and SOD1 and eliminated the neuroprotective effects of HBO-PC. These results suggest the involvement of Nrf2/antioxidant defense pathway in the long-lasting neuroprotective effects of Sirt1 induced by HBO-PC in transient focal cerebral ischemia.

Intracerebral hemorrhage (ICH) results in secondary brain injury due to neuroinflammation. Results of a study in rat model of ICH indicate that motor dysfunction and brain water content are alleviated by HBO-PP along with reduction in degeneration of neurons (Yang et al. 2015). The growth of Iba-1-positive microglia and TNF-α were reduced in the HBO-PC group compared with the untreated ICH group. CD11b-Iba-1 double staining demonstrated that the ratio of CD11b and Iba-1 was significantly decreased in the HBOP group. Overall, the data demonstrated that HBO-PC can significantly alleviate the ICH-induced neuroinflammation by regulating microglial changes and represent a novel target for ICH treatment.

Review of Clinical Studies

Most of the studies of HBO in acute stroke are uncontrolled. Only a few controlled studies have been done in recent years and further studies are planned. Considerable background information can be extracted from the uncontrolled studies reported in the literature.

Uncontrolled Clinical Studies

Various studies on the clinical applications of HBO in cerebrovascular disease, as reported in the literature, are summarized in Table 19.10. The total number of cases reported in the literature is >1000. The reported rate of improvement is 40–100% and is much higher than the natural rate of recovery, particularly because many of the reported cases were in a chronic poststroke stage with stable neurological deficits. A major criticism of these studies is that none of them was a randomized controlled study. The report of Lebedev (1983) was labeled a controlled study but it did not meet the usual criteria of such studies; therefore, it is included among the uncontrolled studies.

Illingworth et al. (1961) were the first to suggest that HBO could be beneficial in cerebrovascular disease. Ingvar and Lassen (1965) were the first to use HBO for treatment of patients with cerebral ischemia and proposed the following rationale:

- An acute ischemic lesion implies a rapid fall to zero of the oxygen tension within the central part of the lesion.
- There is little chance of reaching this anoxic part by any form of currently available therapy.
- With HBO at 2–2.5 ATA, diffusion of oxygen into the nonvascularized part of the brain is enhanced.

The authors treated four patients, and three improved. The fourth, who died with extensive thrombotic lesions of the brain stem, showed dramatic initial improvement with recovery from coma. Although the authors obtained good results, the argument about the extravascular diffusion of oxygen is questionable. The maximum distance that oxygen may have to diffuse in the extravascular tissue from the capillary to the neuron is 0.1 mm. Even at 3 ATA of oxygen, this diffusion distance extends to only 0.075 mm.

Neubauer and End (1980) used HBO in 122 patients with strokes due to thrombosis in both the acute and the chronic stages. The patients were investigated thoroughly with EEG, CT scan, and CSF examination, as indicated. Generally, the patients with completed stroke had previously been given the conventional medical and physical therapy. HBO was given at 1.5–2 ATA, and the duration and frequency of treatments were adjusted according to current signs after improvement with initial HBO sessions. The duration of the sessions was as long as 1 h, and the sessions were as frequent as every 12 h. Of 79 patients who received treatment, 5 months to 9 years after onset of stroke, 65% reported improvement in the quality of life. It was also shown that patients treated with HBO spent fewer days in the hospital (standard treatment 287 days, versus HBO 177 days). The authors noted that using HBO in this way as a supplement to other methods of treatment makes appraisal of the role of HBO difficult. They could not identify the type of patient that would benefit most from HBO, but stated that a significant number of patients would benefit to some extent. They suggested randomized controlled studies. Neubauer continued to treat stroke patients with HBO since his 1980 report and documented the effects using rCBF measurements (Neubauer 1983) and MRI, as well as SPECT (Neubauer 1988). HBO is used for stroke in clinical practice at the discretion of the treating physician. Prompt use of HBO in some situations can save considerable disability. An example is a case reported from Saudi Arabia, in which HBO was used to treat a young woman who developed hemiplegia and seizures after accidental catheterization of the right common carotid artery and infusion of parenteral nutrition by Bohlega and McLean (1997). Carotid angiography and MRI showed

Table 19.10 Uncontrolled studies of the application of HBO in cerebrovascular disease

Authors and year	Diagnosis	No. of patients	HBO protocol	Method of evaluation and results
Ingvar and Lassen (1965)	Focal cerebral ischemia	4 single treatment	2 2.5 ATA 1.5–2.5 h	Improvement in 3 patients; clinical and EEG
Saltzman et al. (1966)	Acute cerebrovascular insufficiency	25	2–3 ATA, 1 h; single session	8 improved dramatically; 5 improved during but regressed later; 12 did not improve
Hart and Thompson (1971)	Occlusion of right middle cerebral A	1	2.5 ATA, 2 h/day; 15 treatments	Patient improved during 15 treatments but regressed during the following month; improvement recurred following resumption of HBO treatments
Sarno et al. (1972)	Cerebrovascular disease, most of patients were aphasics; at least 3 months poststroke	32	2 ATA, 90 min; single session	Patients served as their own controls while breathing 10.5 % oxygen (instead of 100 % in the treated group); no improvement in aphasia
Charcornac et al. (1975)	Cerebrovascular insufficiency	26	2.5 ATA, 1 h; single session	Clinical assessment and EEG; improvement in 20 patients
Larcan et al. (1977)	Acute cerebral artery occlusion; both acute and chronic cases	36	2 ATA + urokinase	17 recovered and 18 died (52 % compared with 77 % deaths in those treated by intensive care alone)
Holbach and Wassman (1979)	Internal carotid and MCA occlusion; both acute and chronic cases	131	1. 5 ATA, 1 h/day	Clinical, neurological, and EEG power spectrum; improvement in 80 % of acute and 43 % of chronic cases
Kapp (1981)	Cerebral infarction	22	1.5 ATA, 40 min/day; 14 days	Clinical assessment, 10 patients improved during HBO, 9 had surgical revascularization, 6 of these maintained improvement; neurological deficits recurred in 3 patients with unsuccessful operations
Neubauer and End (1980)	Stroke; acute and chronic cases	122	1.5–2 ATA, 1 h/day 10 sessions acute, 20 sessions chronic	Total hospitalization stay of treated patients was 177 days (287 days in untreated patients); 65 % of chronic patients (5 months to 9 years) improved
Newman and Manning (1980)	Vertebrobasilar occlusion (?air embolism); locked in syndrome	1	6 ATA for 1 h within 1 h of onset of stroke	Full recovery
Gismondi et al. (1981)	Acute stroke	4	2 ATA	All patients improved
Isakov et al. (1981)	Ischemic stroke	140	1.6–2 ATA, 1 h/day; 6–15 sessions	Clinical, neurological, and cardiovascular assessment; rheoencephalography; 80 % improved; in 52 % improvement coincided with HBO treatment
Nagakawa et al. (1982)	Occlusive CVD	22	2 ATA, 1 h/day; 12 treatments	Excellent recovery in 6, moderate in 7, slight in 6, and 3 patients were unchanged
Shalkevich (1981)	Vertebrobasilar insufficiency	54	2–3 ATA, 1 h/day; 10–15 sessions	Clinical, EEG, and vestibular testing; 47 patients improved
Lebedov et al. (1983)	Acute occlusive CVD	124	2 ATA; duration?	Improved level of consciousness and alpha activity in HBO-treated patients as compared with controls
Akimov et al. (1985)	Cerebrovascular disease	104	2 ATA 6–15 sessions	Clinical, electrophysiological, psychological, and biochemical assessment; 74 patients showed good results, 22 satisfactory, and in 8 the results were doubtful; 3–5 year follow-up

(continued)

Table 19.10 (continued)

Authors and year	Diagnosis	No. of patients	HBO protocol	Method of evaluation and results
Ohta et al. (1985)	CVD including infarction and hemorrhage	134	2 ATA	Overall improvement in 72 % of patients; CBF decreased with decrease in intracranial pressure; EEG and SSEP improved
Jia et al. (1986)	Cerebral thrombosis 1 month to 3 years after onset	104	2.5 ATA, two 40 min sessions per day, with 10 min air breaks per day; 30–50 treatments	Recovery in 33 patients (31.7 %), marked improvement in 32 cases (30.8 %), improvement in 35 cases (33.7 %), and ineffective in 4 cases (3.8 %); recovery coincided with HBO treatment
Kazantseva (1986)	Acute ischemic stroke	60	1.6–2 ATA; variable schedule	Clinico-polygraphic study: EEG, ECG, rheoencephalography, sphygmography of the temporal arteries, phlebography
Hao and Yu (1987)	Cerebral thrombosis (782) Cerebral embolism (16) TIA (31) Cerebral arteriosclerosis (149)	978	Pressure and duration? 20–30 sessions	Improvement in 82.3 % of cases
Sugiyama and Kamiyama (1987)	Cerebral infarction 1–3 months after onset	142	2 ATA for 75 min; 20 daily sessions	Very good results in 15 %, moderate improvement in 33 %, and 20 % showed no effect
Jain and Fischer (1988)	Hemiplegia; chronic poststroke	21	1.5 ATA, 45 min/day; 6 weeks	Neurological assessment during HBO treatments; measurement of handgrip with dynamometer; improvement of handgrip and spasticity in all patients during HBO and maintained by use of physical therapy and repeated treatments
Gusev et al. (1990)	Acute stroke	220	1.2–1.3 ATA	Normalization of EEG, acid–base balance, and decrease of raised free radicals by activation of lipid peroxidation

evidence of arterial occlusion and ischemic infarction. HBO treatment at 2.5 ATA was instituted 6 h after this episode, and the patient showed improvement considerably within a few hours of the treatment. This was followed by daily HBO treatments for 1 week and she recovered with minimal residual neurological deficit. MRI showed considerable regression of the infarct.

Controlled clinical trials. Such trials are considered necessary because the value of HBO therapy in acute stroke remains controversial. Controlled trials will be required for proving the efficacy of HBO in acute stroke because it is difficult to prove that the recovery is due to treatment and not natural recovery. The other issue is demonstrating the safety of HBO in acute stroke patients. For a number of logistical problems, it has not been easy to carry out clinical trials of HBO in acute stroke. There have been only three controlled trials reported at the time of writing (Table 19.11), and others are in progress.

Anderson et al. (1991) administered HBO in a double-blind prospective protocol to 39 patients with acute ischemic cerebral infarction. They aborted the study when no dramatic improvement was noted in the HBO-treated patients. Rather, there was a trend favoring the control patients (treated with air only) who have less severe neurological deficits and smaller infarcts. This trend was considered to be an artifact of randomization process. The treatment protocol was broken in 19 of the 39 patients, and 8 patients refused to continue treatment. The results of this trial neither prove or disprove the usefulness of HBO in acute stroke and can be disregarded. They merely point out the difficulties in carrying out such trials.

Nighogossian et al. (1995) reported the results of a randomized trial on 34 patients. These were enrolled over a period of 3 years. Half of these received HBO, whereas the other half were treated in hyperbaric air. There was no significant difference at inclusion between the two groups regarding age, time from stroke onset to randomization, and Orgogozo scale. The mean score of the HBO group was better at 1 year, but no statistically significant improvement was observed in the HBO group on the Rankin score. The authors concluded that HBO was safe in these patients and there was an outcome trend favoring HBO therapy. They recommended large-scale controlled trials. In a later review, these authors suggested a large double-blind trial of HBO, possibly in combination with thrombolytic therapy (Nighogossian and Trouillas 1997).

Table 19.11 Controlled clinical trials of the application of HBO in acute ischemic cerebral infarction

Authors and year	No. of patients	Study design	HBO protocol	Results
Anderson et al. (1991)	39	Double-blind prospective study	Patients treated within 2 w of onset	Same schedule of hyperbaric air in sham group. Study aborted as no dramatic improvement was noted in the HBO-treated patients
			HBO 1 h at 1.5 ATA repeated every 8 h for total of 15 treatments	
Nighogossian et al. (1995)	34	Randomized: half of the patients received HBO; the other half were treated in hyperbaric air. Patients treated within 24 h of onset	HBO 40 m at 1.5 ATA, daily for 10 treatments	Control group received hyperbaric air
				HBO was safe in these patients and there was an outcome trend favoring HBO therapy
Rusyniak et al. (2003)	33	Randomized, prospective, double-blind, sham-controlled study	HBO 1 h at 2.5 ATA (100% O2) or 1.14 ATA in the sham group	No differences between the groups at 24 h. At 3 months sham patients had a better outcome as defined by their stroke scores
Vila et al. (2005)	26	Randomized but not blinded	Daily 45 min exposures of HBO for 10 d or hyperbaric air in controls	Improvement of function in HBO-treated patients
Imai et al. (2006)	38	Randomized, prospective	HBO combined with intravenous edaravone (free radical scavenger)	6/19 patients in the HBO group, but 1/19 in the control group, had favorable outcomes

Rusyniak et al. (2003) conducted a randomized, prospective, double-blind, sham-controlled pilot study of 33 patients presenting with acute ischemic stroke who did not receive thrombolytics over a 24 month period. Patients were randomized to treatment for 60 min in a monoplace hyperbaric chamber pressurized with 100% O_2 to 2.5 ATA in the HBO group or 1.14 ATA in the sham group. Primary outcomes measured included percentage of patients with improvement at 24 h using NIHSS scale and 90 days (NIHSS, Barthel Index, modified Rankin Scale, Glasgow Outcome Scale). Secondary measurements included complications of treatment and mortality at 90 days. Results revealed no differences between the groups at 24 h. At 3 months, however, a larger percentage of the sham patients had a good outcome defined by their stroke scores compared with the HBO group (NIHSS, 80% versus 31.3%; $P=0.04$; Barthel Index, 81.8% versus 50%; $P=0.12$; modified Rankin Scale, 81.8% versus 31.3%; $P=0.02$; Glasgow Outcome Scale, 90.9% versus 37.5%; $P=0.01$) with loss of statistical significance in a intent-to-treat analysis. It was concluded that HBO does not appear to be beneficial and in fact may be harmful in patients with acute ischemic stroke. The design of this study, however, invalidates any conclusions because HBO at 1.5 ATA has been established to be a safe pressure to treat patients with acute stroke. The control group was closer to this parameter. This study should have included a group treated with HBO at 1.5 ATA (Jain 2003).

HBO dose is adjusted either by changing the pressure or the duration of exposure and number of treatments. In a ret-rospective analysis of the published data of clinical studies performed in different hyperbaric centers (a total of 265 patients), the total dose of HBO therapy (D_{HBOT}) was calculated as follows (Rogatsky et al. 2003):

$$D_{HBOT} = pO_2 \times T_s \times N_t,$$

where pO_2 is measured as ATA, T_s is the duration of a single treatment, and N_t is the number of treatments.

This method was used to analyze the HBO dose-effect relationship in patients with acute ischemic stroke. D_{HBOT} can be easily understood and analyzed when measured within a limit of 50 units defined as unit medical dose (UMD) of HBO therapy. Efficacy of HBO (EfHBOT) represents the percentage of the total number of patients who showed significant clinical improvement of their neurological status in the course of the treatment. The level of EfHBOT in each study was compared with a corresponding value of D_{HBOT}. A comparison of the data shows a pronounced tendency for higher values of EfHBOT as the level of the average values of the total D_{HBOT} increases. The coefficient of correlation between these parameters appears to be fairly high ($r=0.92$). The maximum possible value of EfHBOT is 100%, which corresponded to the average values of D_{HBOT} at a level of no less than 30 agreed units. The examined data suggest that applying optimal total D_{HBOT} may provide a maximum possible EfHBOT in treating patients with acute ischemic stroke.

Controlled Clinical Studies

In a prospective, randomized, controlled trial on 74 patients who suffered a stroke 6–36 months prior to inclusion, HBO therapy led to significant neurological improvements, implying that neuroplasticity can still be activated in the chronic poststroke stage (Efrati et al. 2013).

The conclusion of the latest publication from The Cochrane Database of Systematic Reviews of HBO for stroke is that "evidence from the 11 randomized clinical trials is insufficient to provide clear guidelines for practice, the possibility of clinical benefit has not been excluded. Further research is required to better define the role of hyperbaric oxygen in this condition" (Bennett et al. 2014).

As of May 2016, two clinical trials of HBO for stroke are ongoing in Canada. One of these, HOPES Study at the University of British Columbia, is a double-blind, randomized trial (HBO with 100 % oxygen versus sham HBO) in post established stroke (referred to as poststroke stage in this book) to test the effectiveness of HBO (daily 2 h treatments, 5 days a week) in improving neurological function in patients who are 6–36 months postischemic stroke (ClinicalTrials.gov identifier: NCT02582502). In the second trial pilot, randomized controlled trial at Toronto University Health Network, investigators are comparing the combination of HBO therapy and the focused rehabilitation exercise program versus exercise program alone on recovery of arm function in patients with chronic stroke (ClinicalTrials.gov identifier: NCT02666469).

Reasons for difficulty of translating results of animal experimental studies to clinical application as well as the lack of proven evidence for effectiveness HBO therapy in stroke are summarized as follows along with suggestions to improve the methods (Fischer et al. 2010):

- In contrast to experimental animal studies in standardized models, the human clinical trials include patients with diverse range of localization of the ischemic injury and its causative pathology. Therefore, it seems to be essential before including a patient in a trial, to evaluate not only his clinical symptoms but to verify the exact localization of artery occlusion and extension of brain infarction with widely available modern neuroimaging techniques to get comparable study groups (Lee et al. 2008).
- HBO is sometimes used with varying parameters such as starting point of therapy, ATA pressure, and the frequency of HBO treatments to suit individual requirements, but to have comparable study groups, it is essential to use lesser variations in therapeutic interventions.
- Blinding of the therapy is very difficult in conscious patients, but it can be solved by performing multiple, low-level pressure changes that are difficult to perceive by the patients.
- It is important to evaluate the data in pilot studies before starting extensive and expensive advanced phase clinical trials.

HBO as a Supplement to Rehabilitation of Stroke Patients

The objective neurological improvement in chronic poststroke patients undergoing HBO therapy was first documented by Jain in 1987 (Jain and Fischer 1988), and a long-term follow-up was presented (Jain 1989). This was also the first documentation of relief of spasticity due to stroke by HBO. Wassmann (1980) has reported the power spectrum of the EEG recording during an HBO session and the improvement of this parameter in responders. The neurological assessment of his patients was not done until after the HBO session. The transient neurological improvement of these patients, which might have occurred in the chamber and reversed afterward, may have been overlooked. Under these circumstances, the allocation of a patient to the "nonresponder" group may not be justified.

The Klausenbach Study

The study conducted by Jain at the Fachklinik Klausenbach in Germany was aimed at assessing the effect of HBO on motor deficits in strokes objectively, using a simple repeatable method that could be applied in the hyperbaric chamber. The protocol was such that it did not interfere with the application of two other methods—mental training and physical exercise—used in the hyperbaric chambers, which have been found to be useful adjuncts in previous studies.

Fifty patients with occlusive cerebrovascular and residual hemiparesis or hemiplegia were investigated during the period December 1987–May 1989. There was no selection of patients as the HBO therapy has become a standard procedure in the rehabilitation of stroke patients in the Fachklinik Klausenbach. Only those patients were included in this study who were available to the author for examination prior to HBO treatment, during the sessions in the chamber, and subsequently. Data on other patients treated during the author's absence were available but not included in this study. Neurological and functional assessment was done on admission and at discharge, but the most constantly measured parameter was the handgrip, using a handheld dynamometer, which recorded pressures up to 1 kg or more. Motor power and spasticity of the hand were graded clinically according to the scales shown in Tables 19.12 and 19.13. The duration of stay of the patients was limited to 6 weeks by hospital rules. During the first week following admission, the patient underwent investigative procedures and assessment and received the standard medical treatment and physical therapy. The visit to the hyperbaric chamber was limited to familiarization and a session of breathing 100 % normobaric oxygen. Dynamometer readings during this week and during a visit to the hyperbaric chamber were used as baseline values. Repeated measurements made with a handheld dynamometer on the paralyzed side are considered to be reliable.

Daily HBO sessions were started during the second week. Each session lasted 45 min (10 min compression plus 30 min at 1.5 ATA plus 5 min decompression). Handgrip and spasticity were measured every 5 min during the stay in the chamber. In the first 8 patients, physical therapy was initially given immediately following the HBO session. When it was observed that a trial session of physical therapy in the chamber prolonged the relief from spasticity, physical therapy was routinely given in the chamber during the HBO session.

Most of the patients were transferred to the Fachklinik Klausenbach from acute care facilities for stroke, including university hospitals. Those where surgery was indicated had been operated on. The shortest period of time from the stroke episode to the admission was 3 weeks and the longest 5 years. Most of the patients were in a chronic poststroke stable condition with no day-to-day neurological changes during the first week of admission to the hospital.

Results of the Study

The overall results of this study are summarized in Table 19.14, and the effect on spasticity is shown in Table 19.15. The course of 1 patient at various phases before, during, and after HBO treatments is shown with regard to motor power and spasticity (Fig. 19.7). An example of the effect of HBO on spasticity of the hand is shown in Fig. 19.8. The near normal posture of the hand after HBO demonstrates the effectiveness of HBO in spasticity. The overall improvement of mobility and gait was shown by videotapes before and after HBO.

At 1-year follow-up, patients continued to maintain the improvement noted at the time of discharge without any further HBO treatments. There were no complications resulting from this treatment. Other patients treated by a similar protocol by other clinic staff members during this period showed a response to HBO by an increase of handgrip power in all cases. Those with aphasia and cognitive deficits also improved during this period.

Discussion of Klausenbach Study

All of the 50 patients in this series showed response to HBO by improvement of neurological status. The degree of improvement varied according to the extent of neurological deficit at onset and the interval between the onset of stroke and the institution of HBO therapy. The most marked improvement was in those patients where the treatment was started earlier, the neurological deficits were less severe, and the spasticity was minimal. Twenty-one of the patients had significant spasticity between grades 2–5 (on a scale of 1–5). In all these, the spasticity was reduced during HBO sessions by 1–2 grades. This improvement was transient initially and started to regress during 1–8 h following HBO treatment. However, the beneficial effect of HBO on spasticity was prolonged by conducting physical therapy exercises against spasticity in the chamber during HBO.

The treatment has a cumulative effect, as shown in Fig. 19.9. However, as the "ceiling" of improvement is reached, the peaks of improvement with each session become smaller. After a patient has reached the peak, further HBO treatments are superfluous.

Table 19.14 Long-term results of treatment of stroke patients with combined HBO and physical therapy

Neurological dysfunction	No. with dysfunction	No. improved
Impairment of mental function	35	30 (86%)
Impairment of gait	24	10 (41%)
Motor power impairment	50	50 (100%) (paralysis)
Spasticity	21	21 (100%)
Speech impairment	8	2 (25%)
Total number of patients	50	Some had more than one deficit

Table 19.12 Grading of motor power of the hemiplegic hand

Grade 0: no movement
1. Flicker of finger movement
2. Measurable handgrip: 1–5 kg
3. Measurable handgrip: 5–15 kg
4. Handgrip 15 kg but less than that of the healthy hand
5. Full strength with normal movements

Table 19.13 Grading of spasticity in the hemiplegic hand

Grade 0: normal tone and movements
1: Stiffness of fingers, slow finger tapping
2: Partially closed fist, minimal force required to open it
3: Partially closed fist, moderate force required to open it
4: Fully closed fist, can be partially opened with moderate force
5: Clenched fist, can be partially opened with extreme force

Table 19.15 Effect of HBO on grades of hand spasticity in stroke in 21 patients

Pre-HBO	No.	During HBO	After 6 weeks of HBO	At 6 months to 1 year
5	1	4	4	4
	1	2	3	3
4	4	2	3	3
	2	3	3	3
3	6	1	1	1
	3	2	2	2
2	4	1	1	1

Fig. 19.7 Course of
spasticity and motor power of
the paralyzed left hand of a
patient with right middle
cerebral artery occlusion.
Initial spasticity was grade 5
and motor power 0. At 6 m
follow-up, the spasticity was
reduced to grade 3, and the
motor power rose to grade 3.
Broken lines indicate
measurements made in the
hyperbaric chamber. *PT*
physical therapy, *HBA*
hyperbaric air at 1.5 ATA for
45 min, *NBO* 100 %
normobaric oxygen by face
mask for 45 min, *HBO*
hyperbaric oxygen (100 %) at
1.5 ATA for 45 min

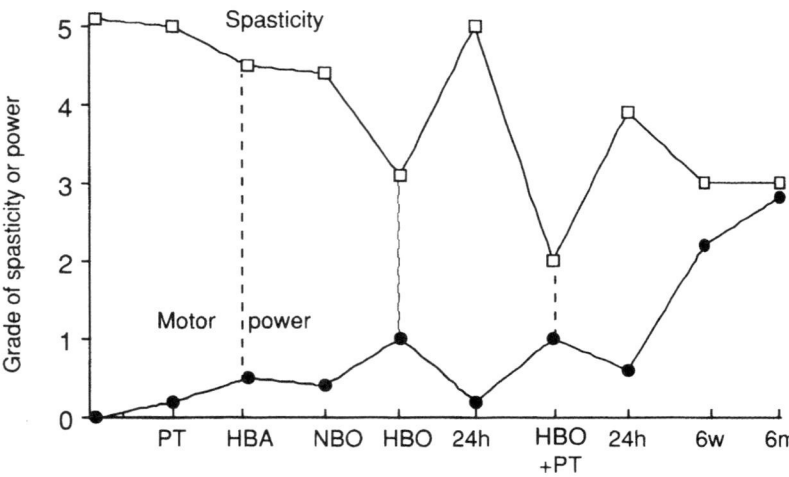

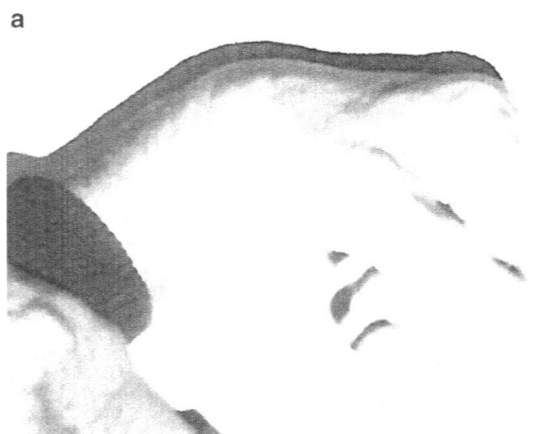

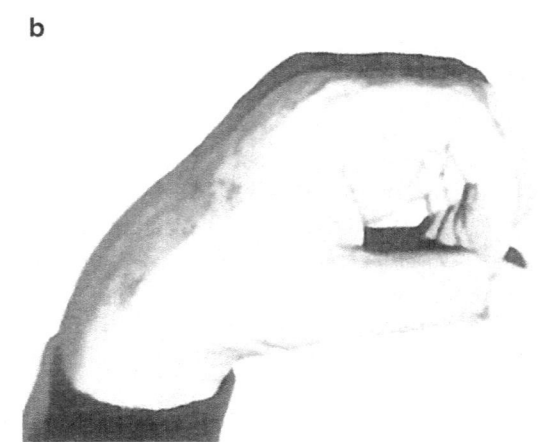

Fig. 19.8 (**a**) Posture of the left hand before HBO (grade 5). (**b**) Posture of the hand after HBO therapy alone (grade 3)

Concluding Remarks on Klausenbach Study

1. All patients with neurological deficits due to occlusive cerebrovascular disease showed a response to HBO at 1.5 ATA by measurable increases of power of handgrip on the paralyzed side.
2. The response to HBO was initially transient but reproducible with sessions repeated daily. After 6 weeks, the improvement was maintained in most of the patients.
3. The peaks of response to HBO got smaller as the plateau of maximum improvement was reached. When there was no further measurable response to HBO, the treatments were terminated.
4. The benefit from HBO was limited by the size of the penumbra and the total neuronal damage done during the insult.
5. The spasticity was reduced during the HBO session and improvement maintained for longer periods if physical therapy was carried out simultaneously.

6. Some of the improvement in motor power was due to relief of spasticity, but considerable improvement was also noted in patients without spasticity.
7. Patients who respond to HBO therapy and are considered candidates for the EC/IC bypass operation may improve with long-term HBO therapy and may not require surgery. HBO, by improving oxygenation, may be more effective than an EC/IC bypass operation.
8. HBO therapy should be instituted early in the management of stroke. In our series, those treated within 3 months of the initial episode did not develop spasticity. Since the number of these patients is small, a larger number of patients should be treated with HBO in the first week following stroke, to test the hypothesis that early HBO therapy may prevent the development of spasticity.
9. Hyperbaric oxygen therapy at 1.5 ATA is safe and well tolerated by stroke patients. So far we have no evidence that higher pressures would extend the improve-

Fig. 19.9 Pattern of recovery of stroke patients treated by combination of HBO therapy and physical therapy

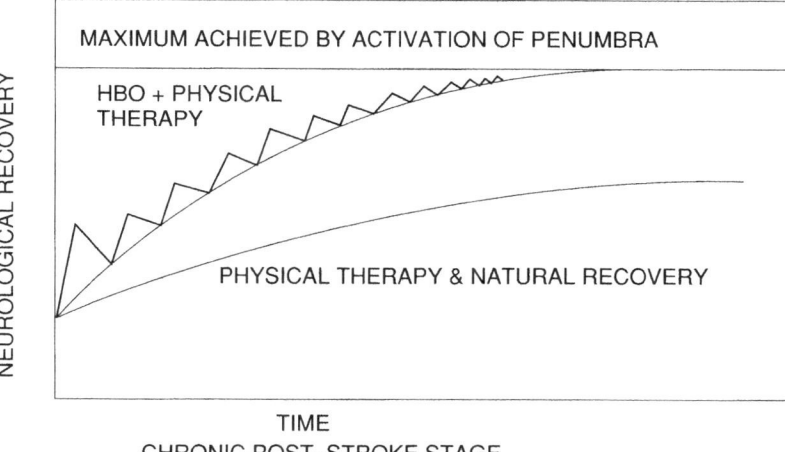

ment in patients who have reached a "ceiling" effect with 1.5 ATA.

10. In view of the 100 % response rate and the limitation of length of stay of our patients, we cannot justify a randomized controlled study where one-half of the patients would not receive HBO. Longitudinal studies, however, are in progress, to compare simultaneous HBO and physical therapy with the two treatments given separately.

11. Response to HBO is not necessarily seen during the first session. A few treatments may be required for the initial improvement to be demonstrated.

12. Fixed neurological deficits persisting for years after stroke are no contraindication of HBO therapy. Neubauer and End (1980) and Holbach et al. (1977) have shown response to HBO in these cases. One patient showed response 5 years after stroke and fixed neurological deficits.

13. If a patient is seen at a stage where there are no potentially viable neurons or if the maximum possible recovery has taken place through other methods of treatment, no response to HBO would be expected. Since the start of the present study, we have not yet encountered such a patient.

14. Effort was made to control the risk factors for stroke in these patients, such as obesity, smoking, and hyperlipidemia. Those with high hematocrit had venesection for lowering the hematocrit. All these measures were already in effect at the time of admission or were instituted during the first week. These measures may contribute to the overall improvement of the patients and the lack of any recurrence of stroke during the period of observation. The role of HBO only in the prevention of stroke recurrence remains to be determined by properly designed studies and longer follow-up.

15. Although natural recovery may still occur in the chronic poststroke stage, in no case treated by any other method did the recovery of motor function take place so dramatically as it did during HBO therapy.

16. HBO is superior to the currently used methods for the control of spasticity, the duration of the effect is longer, and no side effects have been encountered.

17. A hyperbaric chamber with 100 % oxygen at 1.5 ATA is the ideal place to combine physical therapy with mental training and should be included in the routine management of stroke patients. Under HBO conditions, physical exercise improves cerebral blood perfusion and oxygenation. This leads to improved mental performance.

Conclusions of the Effects of HBO in Stroke Patients

Modern concepts of the pathophysiology of stroke provide a rational basis for using HBO in stroke management. Conventional methods of stroke management are not satisfactory, and the role of many surgical procedures for stroke remains controversial. Animal experimental studies and uncontrolled human trials have shown the effectiveness and safety of HBO therapy after stroke. At the Fachklinik Klausenbach (FRG), simultaneous HBO and physical therapies were used in the rehabilitation of stroke patients. Objective evaluation of patients during the HBO session showed a 100 % response rate (improvement of spasticity or motor power or both). The improvement was initially transient but could be maintained, following a course of daily treatments (1.5 ATA for 45 min) for 6 weeks, in most of the cases. The most significant finding was the striking reduction of spasticity under HBO conditions and the prolongation of this benefit if physical therapy was combined with HBO therapy and repeated daily. The mechanism of relief of spasticity has not been demonstrated conclusively. At present the most likely explanation is that it is related to improvement of function of the neurons in the affected areas of the brain. The rise of tissue pO_2 in the spastic, inactive, and hypoxic muscles affected by spasticity seems to play a secondary role.

The response to HBO has been considered a criterion for selecting patients for the EC/IC bypass operation (see Chap. 20). There are some patients in the chronic poststroke stage who can be managed by the long-term combination of physical therapy and HBO without the need for an operation. HBO does not change the vascular pathology, but improves the cerebral function by activation of the partially affected neurons in the penumbra zone that survive the insult due to a trickle of blood supply by collaterals. The hypothesis that long-term alterations of ischemia/hypoxia with hyperoxia may promote collateral circulation remains to be proven.

Objective measurement of spasticity and motor power as well as the SPECT scan has provided the evidence for the improvement following HBO therapy in poststroke patients with fixed neurological deficits. With the evidence available, it may not be necessary to carry out randomized double-blind studies in such patients to evaluate the effect of HBO therapy.

However, the role of HBO in acute stroke is not well defined. Because recovery spontaneously takes place in this stage, controlled studies should be done to assess the effect of HBO. The three controlled clinical trials completed to date have not been encouraging, and the methodology needs to be improved. Two important issues are the time window and pressure at which the treatments should be conducted. As HBO is used for neuroprotective effect in acute stroke, it should be ideally used within the 3 h window and not over 6 h following the initial insult. The use of HBO as an aid to rehabilitation in the subacute and chronic phase is safe because some of the initial biochemical disturbances following initial insult are stabilized by that time. There is animal experimental evidence that the use of HBO in the acute stage after the 6 h time window may be harmful.

HBO at or below a pressure of 2 ATA was used in the majority of >2000 stroke patients that have been treated in published studies. Pressure of 1.5 ATA is optimal for recovery of the cerebral ischemic injury. Higher pressures used in animal studies cannot be transposed into humans. Rehabilitation of stroke patients should also be planned during the first few months following stroke. Long-term follow-up studies are required to determine whether such measures would reduce the chronic disability from stroke and reduce the incidence of severe spasticity in stroke patients. The use of HBO may also reduce the need for some surgical procedures.

There has been ongoing study of HBO for cerebral ischemia, and a review of the current publications supports further investigation of this therapy for stroke (Al-Waili et al. 2005). The failure of some clinical trials of HBO in stroke is probably attributable to factors such as delayed time to therapy, inadequate sample size, and the use of excessive chamber pressures (Singhal 2007).

Future Prospects

Basic and clinical data suggest that HBO could be a safe and effective treatment option in the management of acute stroke, but further studies are needed to clarify its clinical utility when applied within the treatment window of 3–5 h (Sanchez 2013). The FDA has approved the use of HBO therapy for central retinal artery occlusion, and treatments for this indication are reimbursed by healthcare insurance and Medicare. It is hoped that HBO use for stroke, which is currently off-label in the USA, will be approved in the near future.

Previous trials did not assess long-term benefit in patients with tissue reperfusion. In this modern era of stroke thrombolysis and advanced neuroimaging, HBO may have renewed significance. If applied within the first few hours after stroke onset or in patients with imaging evidence of salvageable brain tissue, HBO could be used to lengthen the window for the administration of thrombolytic or neuroprotective drugs.

References

Al-Waili NS, Butler GJ, Beale J, Abdullah MS, Hamilton RW, Lee BY, et al. Hyperbaric oxygen in the treatment of patients with cerebral stroke, brain trauma, and neurologic disease. Adv Ther. 2005;22:659–78.

Akimov GA, Lobzin VS, Sapov IA, et al. Assessment of the efficiency of hyperbaric oxygen therapy in early forms of cerebrovascular disorders. Neurosci Behav Physiol. 1985;15:13.

Anderson DC, Bottini AG, Jagiella WM, Westphal B, Ford S, Rockswold GL, et al. A pilot study of hyperbaric oxygen in the treatment of human stroke. Stroke. 1991;22:1137–42.

Astrup J, Siesjö BK, Symon L. Thresholds in cerebral ischemia; the ischemic penumbra. Stroke. 1981;12:723–5.

Atochin DN, Fisher D, Demchenko IT, Thom SR. Neutrophil sequestration and the effect of hyperbaric oxygen in a rat model of temporary middle cerebral artery occlusion. Undersea Hyperb Med. 2000;27:185–90.

Badr AE, Yin W, Mychaskiw G, Zhang JH. Effect of hyperbaric oxygen on striatal metabolites: a microdialysis study in awake freely moving rats after MCA occlusion. Brain Res. 2001a;916:85–90.

Badr AE, Yin W, Mychaskiw G, Zhang JH. Dual effect of HBO on cerebral infarction in MCAO rats. Am J Physiol Regul Integr Comp Physiol. 2001b;280:R766–70.

Bennett MH, Weibel S, Wasiak J, Schnabel A, French C, Kranke P. Hyperbaric oxygen therapy for acute ischaemic stroke. Cochrane Database Syst Rev. 2014;(11):CD004954.

Boerema I, Meyne NG, Brummelkamp WH, Bouma S, Mensch MH, Kamermans F, et al. Life without blood. Arch Chir Neer. 1959;11:70–83.

Bohlega S, McLean DR. Hemiplegia caused by inadvertent intracarotid infusion of total parenteral nutrition. Clin Neurol Neurosurg. 1997;99:217–9.

Burt JT, Kapp JP, Smith RR. Hyperbaric oxygen and cerebral infarction in the gerbil. Surg Neurol. 1987;28:265.

Chacornac R, Martin YN, Fournier-Jenoudet MT, Deleuze R. Hyperbaric oxygen therapy in cerebral circulatory insufficiency. Ann Anesthesiol Fr. 1975;16:485–500.

Chang CF, Niu KC, Hoffer BJ, Wang Y, Borlongan CV. Hyperbaric oxygen therapy for treatment of postischemic stroke in adult rats. Exp Neurol. 2000;166:298–306.

Corkill G, Van Housen K, Hein L, Reitan J. Videodensimetric estimation of the protective effect of hyperbaric oxygen in the ischemic gerbil brain. Surg Neurol. 1985;24:406.

Crisomoto E, Duncan PE, Propst M, Dawson DV, Davis JN. Evidence that amphetamine with physical therapy promotes recovery of motor function in stroke patients. Ann Neurol. 1987;23:94.

Efrati S, Fishlev G, Bechor Y, Volkov O, Bergan J, Kliakhandler K, et al. Hyperbaric oxygen induces late neuroplasticity in post stroke patients—randomized, prospective trial. PLoS One. 2013;8, e53716.

Eschenfelder CC, Krug R, Yusofi AF, et al. Neuroprotection by oxygen in acute transient focal cerebral ischemia is dose dependent and shows superiority of hyperbaric oxygenation. Cerebrovasc Dis. 2008;25:193–201.

Fischer BR, Palkovic S, Holling M, Wölfer J, Wassmann H. Rationale of hyperbaric oxygenation in cerebral vascular insult. Curr Vasc Pharmacol. 2010;8:35–43.

Gismondi A, Micalella F, Metrangolo C, et al. Treatment of cerebral ischemia with hyperbaric oxygen therapy. Minerva Med. 1981;72:1417.

Gu GJ, Li YP, Peng ZY, Xu JJ, Kang ZM, Xu WG, et al. Mechanism of ischemic tolerance induced by hyperbaric oxygen preconditioning involves upregulation of hypoxia-inducible factor-1alpha and erythropoietin in rats. J Appl Physiol. 2008;104:1185–91.

Guo ZN, Xu L, Hu Q, Matei N, Yang P, Tong LS, et al. Hyperbaric oxygen preconditioning attenuates hemorrhagic transformation through reactive oxygen species/thioredoxin-interacting protein/nod-like receptor protein 3 pathway in hyperglycemic middle cerebral artery occlusion rats. Crit Care Med. 2016;44:e403–11.

Gusev EI, Kazantseva NV, Nifontova LA, et al. Mechanisms of the therapeutic effects of hyperbaric oxygenation in minor differential pressures in stroke. Zh Nevropatol Psikhiatr. 1990;90:34–40.

Hao M, Yu CK. An outline of hyperbaric oxygen therapy in treatment of ischemic cerebrovascular disease in China. J Chin Med Univ. 1987;16:56–8.

Hart GB, Thompson RE. The treatment of cerebral ischemia with hyperbaric oxygen therapy. Stroke. 1971;2:247.

Hjelde A, Hjelstuen M, Haraldseth O, Martin D, Thom R, Brubakk O. Hyperbaric oxygen and neutrophil accumulation/tissue damage during permanent focal cerebral ischaemia in rats. Eur J Appl Physiol. 2002;86:401–5.

Holbach KH, Wassmann H, Hohelochter KL, Jain KK. Differentiation between reversible and irreversible poststroke changes in brain tissue. Surg Neurol. 1977;7:325.

Holbach KH, Wassmann H. Neurochirurgische Therapie der zerebralen Mangeldurchblutung. Neurol Psychiat (Bucur). 1979;5:347.

Hou H, Grinberg O, Williams B, et al. The effect of oxygen therapy on brain damage and cerebral pO(2) in transient focal cerebral ischemia in the rat. Physiol Meas. 2007;28:963–76.

Hu Q, Liang X, Chen D, Chen Y, Doycheva D, Tang J, et al. Delayed hyperbaric oxygen therapy promotes neurogenesis through reactive oxygen species/hypoxia-inducible factor-1α/β-catenin pathway in middle cerebral artery occlusion rats. Stroke. 2014;45:1807–14.

Illingworth CFW, Smith G, Lawson DD, Ledingham IMCA, Sharp GR, Griffith JC. Surgical and physiological observations in an experimental pressure chamber. Br J Surg. 1961;49:22.

Imai K, Mori T, Izumoto H, et al. Hyperbaric oxygen combined with intravenous edaravone for treatment of acute embolic stroke: a pilot clinical trial. Neurol Med Chir (Tokyo). 2006;46:373–8.

Ingvar D, Lassen NA. Treatment of focal cerebral ischemia with hyperbaric oxygen. Acta Neurol Scand. 1965;41:92.

Isakov YV, Pravdenkova GV, Ananiev IS, et al. Hyperbaric oxygenation in acute period of cerebral stroke and craniocerebral injury. In: Abstracts of the 7th International congress of hyperbaric medicine, Moscow, 2–6 September 1981. p. 295–6.

Jacobson I, Lawson DD. The effect of hyperbaric oxygen on experimental cerebral infarction in the dog. J Neurosurg. 1963;20:849.

Jia SJ, Zhang JD, Qu ZK. Experience on the clinical use of HBO treatment in cerebral thrombosis: a report of 104 cases. In: Presented at the 5th Chinese conference on hyperbaric medicine, Fuzhou, China, 26–29 Sept 1986.

Jain KK. Effect of hyperbaric oxygenation on spasticity in stroke patients. J Hyperb Med. 1989;4:55–61.

Jain KK. Hyperbaric oxygen in acute ischemic stroke (letter). Stroke. 2003;34(9), e153.

Jain KK. Handbook of neuroprotection. New York: Springer; 2011.

Jain KK. Applications of biotechnology in neurology. New York: Springer; 2013.

Jain KK. Neuroprotection. Basel: Jain PharmaBiotech; 2016.

Jain KK, Fischer B. New aspects of the use of hyperbaric oxygenation for rehabilitation of stroke patients. Geriatr Rehabil. 1988;1:45.

Jain KK, Toole JF. Hyperacute hyperbaric oxygen therapy for cerebral ischemia (Edited Proceedings of a Conference, Winston-Salem, NC, November 1997). Bethesda: Undersea Hyperbaric Medical Society; 1998.

Kapp JP. Neurological response to hyperbaric oxygen—a criterion for cerebral revascularization. Surg Neurol. 1981;15:43–6.

Kawamura S, Yasui N, Shirasawa M, Fukasawa H. Therapeutic effects of hyperbaric oxygenation on acute focal cerebral ischemia in rats. Surg Neurol. 1990;34:101–6.

Kazantsev NV. Mechanism of action of hyperbaric oxygenation in ischemic stroke. Zh Nevropatol Psikhiatr. 1986;86:1315–20.

Keser Z, Francisco GE. Neuropharmacology of poststroke motor and speech recovery. Phys Med Rehabil Clin N Am. 2015;26:671–89.

Kothari R, Barsan W, Brott T, Broderick J, Ashbrock S. Frequency and accuracy of prehospital diagnosis of acute stroke. Stroke. 1995;26:937–41.

Krakovsky M, Rogatsky G, Zarchin N, Mayevsky A. Effect of hyperbaric oxygen therapy on survival after global cerebral ischemia in rats. Surg Neurol. 1998;49:412–6.

Larcan A, Laprevote-Heully MC, Lambert H, et al. Indications des thrombolytiques au cours des accidents vasculaires cérébraux thrombosants traités par ailleurs. Therapie. 1977;32:259.

Lebedov VV, Isakov IV, Pravdenkova SV. Effect of hyperbaric oxygenation on the clinical course and complications of the acute period of ischemic strokes. Zh Vopr Neirokhir Im N N Burdenko. 1983;3:37.

Lee JI, Wittsack HJ, Christaras A, Miese FR, Siebler M. Normalization of brain tissue lactate after hyperbaric oxygen therapy in a progressive stroke patient. Cerebrovasc Dis. 2008;26:447–8.

Lee YS, Chio CC, Chang CP, Wang LC, Chiang PM, Niu KC, et al. Long course hyperbaric oxygen stimulates neurogenesis and attenuates inflammation after ischemic stroke. Mediators Inflamm. 2013;2013:512978.

Li J, Liu W, Ding S, Xu W, Guan Y, Zhang JH, et al. Hyperbaric oxygen preconditioning induces tolerance against brain ischemia-reperfusion injury by upregulation of antioxidant enzymes in rat. Brain Res. 2008;1210:223–9.

Mickel HS, Yashesh N, Vaishnav N, von Lubitz D, Weiss JF, Feuerstein G. Breathing 100% oxygen after global brain ischemia in Mongolian gerbils results in increased lipid peroxidation and increased mortality. Stroke. 1987;18:426–30.

Moore GF, Fuson RL, Margolis G, Brown Jr IW, Smith WW. An evaluation of the protective effect of hyperbaric oxygenation on the central nervous system during circulatory arrest. J Thorac Cardiovasc Surg. 1966;52:618.

Nagakawa Y, Kinomoto H, Mabuchi S, et al. Significance of oxygenation at high pressure (OHP) as a therapeutic method for occlusive cerebrovascular disease. No Shinkei Geka. 1982;10:1067–74.

Neubauer RA. Certain neurological indications for hyperbaric oxygen. Presented at the meeting of the International Society of Hyperbaric Medicine, Oxford, UK, 1–3 Sept 1988.

Neubauer RA. Regional cerebral blood flow studies of the effect of hyperbaric oxygen in acute stroke and chronic neurologic deficits of stroke. Paper presented at the first European conference on hyperbaric medicine, Amsterdam; 7–9 Sept 1983.

Neubauer RA, End E. Hyperbaric oxygenation as an adjunct therapy in strokes due to thrombosis. Stroke. 1980;11:297.

Newman RP, Manning EJ. Hyperbaric chamber treatment for "locked-in" syndrome. Arch Neurol. 1980;37:529.

Nighogossian N, Trouillas P. Hyperbaric oxygen in the treatment of acute ischemic stroke: an unsettled issue. J Neurol Sci. 1997; 150:27–31.

Nighogossian N, Trouillas P, Adeleine P, Salord F. Hyperbaric oxygen in the treatment of acute ischemic stroke. A double-blind pilot study. Stroke. 1995;26(8):1369–72.

Ohta H, Yasui N, Kawamura S, et al. Choice of EIAB operation candidates by topographic evaluation of EEG and SSEP with concomitant RCBF studies under hyperbaric oxygenation. In: Spetzler RF, Carter LP, Selman WR, Martin NA, editors. Cerebral revascularization for stroke. New York: Thieme Stratton; 1985. p. 208–16.

Prass K, Wiegand F, Schumann P, Ahrens M, Kapinya K, Harms C, et al. Hyperbaric oxygenation induced tolerance against focal cerebral ischemia in mice is strain dependent. Brain Res. 2000;871:146–50.

Pushkov D, Nicholson JD, Michowiz S, Novitzky I, Weiss S, Ben Hemou M, et al. Relative neuroprotective effects hyperbaric oxygen treatment and TLR4 knockout in a mouse model of temporary middle cerebral artery occlusion. Int J Neurosci. 2016;126(2):174–81.

Qin Z, Karabiyikoglu M, Hua Y, et al. Hyperbaric oxygen-induced attenuation of hemorrhagic transformation after experimental focal transient cerebral ischemia. Stroke. 2007;38:1362–7.

Reitan JA, Kien ND, Thorup S, Corkill G. Hyperbaric oxygen increases survival following carotid ligation in gerbils. Stroke. 1990;21:119–23.

Rogatsky GG, Shifrin EG, Mayevsky A. Optimal dosing as a necessary condition for the efficacy of hyperbaric oxygen therapy in acute ischemic stroke: a critical review. Neurol Res. 2003;25:95–8.

Roos JA, Jackson Friedman C, Lyden P. Effects of hyperbaric oxygen on neurologic outcome for cerebral ischemia in rats. Acad Emerg Med. 1998;5:18–24.

Rusyniak DE, Kirk MA, May JD, Kao LW, Brizendine EJ, Welch JL, et al. Hyperbaric oxygen therapy in acute ischemic stroke: results of the Hyperbaric Oxygen in Acute Ischemic Stroke Trial Pilot Study. Stroke. 2003;34:571–4.

Saltzman HA, Anderson B, Whalen RE, et al. Hyperbaric oxygen therapy of acute cerebral vascular insufficiency. In: Brown IW, Cox BG, editors. Hyperbaric medicine. Washington, DC: National Research Council; 1966.

Sanchez EC. Mechanisms of action of hyperbaric oxygenation in stroke: a review. Crit Care Nurs Q. 2013;36:290–8.

Sarno JE, Rusk HA, Diller L, et al. The effect of hyperbaric oxygen on the mental and verbal ability of stroke patients. Stroke. 1972;2:10.

Shalkevich VB. Use of hyperbaric oxygenation in the therapy of transient cerebral circulatory disturbances in the vertebro-basilar system. In: Yefuni SN, editor. Abstracts of the 7th International congress on HBO medicine. Moscow: USSR Academy of Sciences; 1981. p. 294–5.

Shiokawa D, Fujishima M, Yanai T, Ibayashi S, Ueda K, Yagi H. Hyperbaric oxygen therapy in experimentally induced acute cerebral ischemia. Undersea Biomed Res. 1986;13:337.

Singhal AB. A review of oxygen therapy in ischemic stroke. Neurol Res. 2007;29:173–83.

Smith G, Lawson DD, Renfrew S, Ledingham IM, Sharp GR. Preservation of cerebral cortical activity by breathing oxygen at 2 ATA pressure during cerebral ischemia. Surg Gynecol Obstet. 1961;113:13.

Soejima Y, Hu Q, Krafft PR, Fujii M, Tang J, Zhang JH. Hyperbaric oxygen preconditioning attenuates hyperglycemia-enhanced hemorrhagic transformation by inhibiting matrix metalloproteinases in focal cerebral ischemia in rats. Exp Neurol. 2013;247:737–43.

Sugiyama H, Kamiyama K. The effectiveness of hyperbaric oxygenation on cerebral ischemia. In: Presented at the 9th International congress on hyperbaric medicine, Sydney, Australia, 1–4 March 1987.

Sun L, Marti HH, Veltkamp R. Hyperbaric oxygen reduces tissue hypoxia and hypoxia-inducible factor-1 alpha expression in focal cerebral ischemia. Stroke. 2008;39:1000–6.

Sunami K, Takeda Y, Hashimoto M, Hirakawa M. Hyperbaric oxygen reduces infarct volume in rats by increasing oxygen supply to the ischemic periphery. Crit Care Med. 2000;28:2831–6.

Symon L. The concept of threshold of ischemia in relation to brain structure and function. J Clin Pathol. 1976;11(Suppl):149–54.

Takahashi M, Iwatsuki N, Ono K, Tajima T, Akama M, Koga Y. Hyperbaric oxygen therapy accelerates neurologic recovery after 15-minute complete global cerebral ischemia in dogs. Crit Care Med. 1992;20:1588–94.

Tilley BC, Lyden PD, Brott TG, Lu M, Levine SR, Welch KM. Total quality improvement method for reduction of delays between emergency department admission and treatment of acute ischemic stroke. Arch Neurol. 1997;54:1466–74.

Veltkamp R, Warner DS, Domoki F, Brinkhous AD, Toole JF, Busija DW. Hyperbaric oxygen decreases infarct size and behavioral deficit after transient focal cerebral ischemia in rats. Brain Res. 2000;853:68–73.

Veltkamp R, Siebing DA, Sun L, Heiland S, Bieber K, Marti HH, et al. Hyperbaric oxygen reduces blood-brain barrier damage and edema after transient focal cerebral ischemia. Stroke. 2005;36:1679–83.

Vila JF, Balcarce PE, Abiusi GR, et al. Improvement in motor and cognitive impairment after hyperbaric oxygen therapy in a selected group of patients with cerebrovascular disease: a prospective single-blind controlled trial. Undersea Hyperb Med. 2005;32:341–9.

Wada K, Ito M, Miyazawa T, Katoh H, Nawashiro H, Shima K, et al. Repeated hyperbaric oxygen induces ischemic tolerance in gerbil hippocampus. Brain Res. 1996;740:15–20.

Walker-Batson D. Amphetamine and post-stroke rehabilitation: indications and controversies. Eur J Phys Rehabil Med. 2013;49:251–60.

Wang F, Liang W, Lei C, Kinden R, Sang H, Xie Y, et al. Combination of HBO and memantine in focal cerebral ischemia: is there a synergistic effect? Mol Neurobiol. 2015;52:1458–66.

Wassmann W. Quantitative Indikatoren des hirnelektrischen Wirkungsverlaufs bei hyperbarer Oxygenierung. EEG EMG. 1980;11:97–101.

Weinstein PR, Hameroff SR, Johnson PC, Anderson GG. Effect of hyperbaric oxygen therapy or dimethyl sulfoxide on cerebral ischemia in unanesthetized gerbils. Neurosurgery. 1986;18:528.

Welch KMA, Barkley GL. Biochemistry and pharmacology of cerebral ischemia. In: Barnett HJM et al., editors. Stroke. New York: Churchill Livingston; 1986. p. 75–90.

Whalen R, Heyman A, Saltzman H. The protective effect of hyperbaric oxygen in cerebral ischemia. Arch Neurol. 1966;14:15.

Wolf WA, Martin JL, Kartje GL, Farrer RG. Evidence for fibroblast growth factor-2 as a mediator of amphetamine-enhanced motor improvement following stroke. PLoS One. 2014;9, e108031.

Xu Y, Ji R, Wei R, Yin B, He F, Luo B. The efficacy of hyperbaric oxygen therapy on middle cerebral artery occlusion in animal studies: a meta-analysis. PLoS One. 2016;11, e0148324.

Xue F, Huang JW, Ding PY, Zang HG, Kou ZJ, Li T, et al. Nrf2/antioxidant defense pathway is involved in the neuroprotective effects of Sirt1 against focal cerebral ischemia in rats after hyperbaric oxygen preconditioning. Behav Brain Res. 2016;309:1–8.

Yan D, Shan J, Ze Y, Xiao-Yan Z, Xiao-Hua H. The effects of combined hyperbaric oxygen therapy on patients with post-stroke depression. J Phys Ther Sci. 2015;27:1295–7.

Yang ZJ, Camporesi C, Yang X, Wang J, Bosco G, Lok J, et al. Hyperbaric oxygenation mitigates focal cerebral injury and reduces striatal dopamine release in a rat model of transient middle cerebral artery occlusion. Eur J Appl Physiol. 2002;87:101–7.

Yang L, Tang J, Chen Q, Jiang B, Zhang B, Tao Y, et al. Hyperbaric oxygen preconditioning attenuates neuroinflammation after intracerebral hemorrhage in rats by regulating microglia characteristics. Brain Res. 2015;1627:21–30.

Yatsuzuka H. Effects of hyperbaric oxygen therapy on ischemic brain injury in dogs. Masui. 1991;40:208–23.

Yin W, Badr AE, Mychaskiw G, Zhang JH. Down regulation of COX-2 is involved in hyperbaric oxygen treatment in a rat transient focal cerebral ischemia model. Brain Res. 2002;926:165–71.

Paul G. Harch

Abstract

Hyperbaric oxygen (HBO) therapy has been used in a number of conditions characterized by global ischemia (as opposed to focal ischemia of stroke), and anoxia, and leading to impairment of consciousness. Conditions such as coma due to brain injury and anoxia associated with drowning and hanging are discussed under the following headings: (1) pathophysiology, (2) rational basis of HBO therapy, (3) review of animal experimental studies, and (4) review of human clinical studies. Finally case studies are given.

Keywords

Brain injury • Cerebral anoxia • Cerebral hypoxia • Cerebral ischemia • Coma • Global ischemia/anoxia • Hyperbaric oxygen (HBO) • Impairment of consciousness

Introduction

For a discussion of the effectiveness of hyperbaric oxygen (HBO) therapy in global cerebral ischemia/anoxia and coma, we define HBO as a medical treatment that uses increased atmospheric pressure and increased oxygen as drugs by fully enclosing a person or animal in a pressure vessel and then adjusting the dose of the drugs to treat pathophysiologic processes of the diseases. Like all drugs, the dose of HBO is crucial and should be customized to each patient's response. It is dictated by the pathological target and is determined by the amount of increase in pressure and pressure of oxygen above ambient pressure and oxygen pressure (Harch 2013), duration of exposure, frequency, total number of treatments, and timing of the dose in the course of the disease. As diseases and their pathologies evolve, different doses of HBO are required at different times. In addition, patients have

individual susceptibilities to drugs and manifest side effects and toxicity. Unfortunately, due to the lack of dosing tools, the ideal dose of HBO for an individual patient in acute or chronic global ischemia/anoxia and coma is unknown. The studies reviewed later suggest higher pressures (2 ATA or higher) and lesser numbers of treatments very early in the disease process whereas lower pressures (2 ATA or lower) and a greater number of treatments have been used as the brain injury matures. While this general trend seems justified, the absolute or effective pressures delivered to the patients in these reports may be slightly less than what is stated since many studies do not specify the HBO delivery system that was employed. For example, an oxygen pressurized chamber has an effective HBO pressure equal to the plateau pressure administered during the treatment, whereas an air pressurized chamber in which oxygen is administered by aviators mask can achieve a far lower effective HBO pressure, depending on the fit of the mask and the amount of its air/oxygen leak. In the later cases, the dose of oxygen is less. This concept is particularly important when analyzing the studies in this chapter performed prior to the late 1980s when the aviator mask dominated delivery systems in multiplace chambers.

In reviewing the data in this chapter, it is surprising that HBO has not enjoyed widespread use for neurological diseases

P.G. Harch, MD (✉)
Department of Medicine, Section of Emergency and Hyperbaric Medicine, University Medical Center, Louisiana Children's Medical Center, 2000 Canal Boulevard, New Orleans, LA 70112, USA

Louisiana State University School of Medicine, New Orleans, LA, USA
e-mail: paulharchmd@gmail.com

© Springer International Publishing AG 2017
K.K. Jain, *Textbook of Hyperbaric Medicine*, DOI 10.1007/978-3-319-47140-2_20

in the United States. This has been partly due to institutional reservations and overt therapeutic nihilism for neurological injuries, both of which are presently waning. To assume that HBO could have efficacy and benefit when liberally applied to various "accepted" indications which are more appropriately defined as "typically reimbursed," yet have none in the great majority of neurological conditions, is perplexing. After all, the brain is enclosed within the same body in the same pressure vessel and is exposed to the same elevated oxygen and atmospheric pressure. To justify this distinction, one would have to postulate an entire set of pathophysiological HBO-insensitive brain processes that are distinctly different from those in the rest of the body's HBO-sensitive organ systems to which we routinely apply HBO. This is illogical and unlikely. Such reasoning is indefensible when one considers the "typically reimbursed" neurological indications include carbon monoxide poisoning, brain decompression sickness, cerebral air embolism, brain abscess, and cyanide poisoning. We conclude that HBO should benefit other hypoxic/ischemic conditions of the brain, provided the dose is correct, i.e., target specific.

Other reasons for nonrecognition of HBO in neurological conditions concern methodologies. The standard for proof in scientific medicine has been the randomized prospective controlled double-blinded clinical trial. While some of the studies in this chapter meet this rigor (except for double blinding), many do not. Some are randomized, prospective, and controlled and thus exceed the quality of studies used to sanction reimbursement for most HBO indications in the United States. Other studies are uncontrolled series, case-controlled, or individual cases. Case-controlled series with chronic neurological maladies make powerful statements of efficacy from the statistical (Glantz 1992) and logical perspectives where the counterargument of placebo effect is minimized (Kienle and Kiene 1996). Furthermore, reviews of treatment effects in randomized controlled trials vs. observational studies with control groups have shown no quantitative or qualitative difference (Benson and Hartz 2000; Concato et al. 2000). All of this clinical data, in conjunction with the animal data, makes a strong case for at least attempting HBO in what are otherwise untreatable conditions with debilitating, tragic, and expensive outcomes, especially when the visual medium is used to prove single-case causality (Kiene and von Schön-Angerer 1998; Harch et al. 1996a). If these considerations are kept in mind when analyzing this chapter, it appears that the bulk of data is solidly in favor of a beneficial effect of HBO in global ischemia/anoxia and coma.

Pathophysiology

The effect of global ischemia/hypoxia on the brain has been discussed in Chap. 5. Oxidation of glucose is the primary energy source for the brain. Deprivation of oxygen causes deep psychological unresponsiveness in patients while glu-

cose and energy stores take a few minutes to exhaust (Plum and Pulsinelli 1986). Global deprivation of oxygen delivery can be achieved by reduction in blood flow (ischemia), oxygen (hypoxia/anoxia), or both (hypoxic or anoxic ischemia). Hypoxia to even an extreme degree can be tolerated for some time (mountain climbers), but ischemia cannot (Schmidt-Kastner 2015). It appears that the combination of reduction in both oxygen and blood metabolic substrates is critically injurious. Since the insult, oxygen deprivation is similar whether by lowered blood flow or oxygen content the two are often considered as a single type of insult and this concept will be followed in this chapter.

Complete global brain ischemia/anoxia is a severe transient insult to the brain best exemplified by cardiac arrest. It causes a stereotypic pathophysiology characterized by reperfusion hyperemia followed by progressive ischemia which is often heterogeneous (Safar 1986; Dirnagl 1993). The extent and pattern of injury is governed by a complex interplay of systemic and local respiratory, electrical, biochemical, and circulatory factors and selective vulnerability of cells (Myers 1979). Selective vulnerability of the CA1 hippocampal cells is a primary finding in complete global ischemia and is felt to be due to both intrinsic neuronal factors and hippocampal vascular features (Schmidt-Kastner 2015).

Most animal models of global brain ischemia/anoxia are not complete. Five models of global ischemia are commonly used in experimental work: (1) four vessel occlusion in rats, (2) two vessel occlusion with severe hypotension in rats, (3) two vessel occlusion in the gerbil, (4) two vessel occlusion combined with other insults in mice, and (5) and cardiac arrest in mice or rats (Schmidt-Kastner 2015). Two additional models are included in this chapter, a model commonly used for cerebral palsy (Rice et al. 1981), unilateral common carotid artery occlusion followed by 8% systemic hypoxia, and a birth asphyxia model whereby a pregnant uterus is harvested from a rat (Bjelke et al. 1991). Only the first and seventh models are complete; the others result in about 5% residual blood flow to the forebrain. The brainstem is usually not affected. Because of the differences in the various models findings in each study are difficult to generalize to other models and clinical syndromes.

The different models of global ischemia, especially the five incomplete models, result in differing severities of ischemia/hypoxia for differing periods of time that are differentially distributed to various regions of the brain. The primary insult of severe reduction in blood flow causes the depletion of ATP, failure of membrane ion pumps, cell swelling, and finally necrosis (Borgens and Liu-Snyder 2012). This is typified by the core or umbra in the focal ischemia model of stroke. Secondary injury then ensures with an early electrical repolarization injury (Borgens and Snyder 2012) followed by the inflammatory process, a component of which is reperfusion injury (Pundik et al.

2012). Lesser degrees of ischemia/hypoxia and ATP depletion appear to primarily affect the mitochondria, especially during the reperfusion period, where mitochondrial membrane hyperpolarization causes a burst of reactive oxygen species that launches apoptotic cascades through intracellular signaling mechanisms (Sanderson et al. 2013). This is typified by the penumbra in an ischemic stroke (Sanderson et al. 2013). Still lesser degrees of ischemia/hypoxia stimulate gene responses that are neuroprotective (preconditioning) for subsequent more severe ischemic/hypoxic insults (Bai and Lyden 2015). Due to the heterogeneity and distribution of the ischemic/hypoxic insult all of these processes are involved simultaneously with evidence of crosstalk between the processes leading to cell death along a spectrum between necrosis and apoptosis (Sanderson et al. 2013). Idiosyndratic features of a given patient's brain insult (near drowning without arrest, with arrest, vs. no arrest and prolonged low hypotension and hypoxia vs., etc.) combine with idiosyncratic vascular anatomical features, genetic factors, and the above degrees of ischemia and hypoxia to manifest heterogeneous brain injuries.

Superimposed upon this complexity is inflammation (Kunz et al. 2010; Iadecola and Anrather 2011) and variable activation of the microcirculation, common components of reperfusion injury and the secondary injury process. During ischemia there is injury to the vascular endothelium and blood–brain barrier which exposes the subendothelial extracellular matrix (Bai and Lyden 2015). Platelets, leukocytes, complement, pericytes, astrocytes, and microglia are all activated leading to postischemic hypoperfusion (Bai and Lyden 2015). The inflammatory process changes over months to years with infiltration of different cell types that elaborate different bioactive proteins. These proteins mediate multiple degradatory and repair processes. Accordingly, therapies must be highly specific in time and space (Borgens and Snyder 2012), thus explaining the failure of nearly all clinical therapeutic trials. The only therapy with broad effects on the immune system (Rossignol 2007) and widespread genomic activation of anti-inflammatory genes and suppression of pro-inflammatory genes is hyperbaric oxygen therapy (Godman et al. 2009).

Coma, on the other hand, is a neurological state resulting from a wide variety of cerebral insults that is caused by diffuse disruption (functional or anatomical) of the bilateral cerebral cortices, proximal brainstem (reticular activating system), or both (Rossor 1993). Coma is characterized by an alteration in the level of awakeness, ranges from mild somnolence to deep coma, and is graded on a number of scales, the best known of which is the Glasgow Coma Scale (Teasdale and Jennett 1974). In the studies reviewed later, coma usually refers to the more severe end of the continuum: unresponsiveness, posturing, and neurovegetative signs, however, a number of studies are unclear about the exact level of coma.

Rational Basis of HBO Therapy

HBO in acute global ischemia/anoxia is complicated by a lack of knowledge of the exact pathological targets and their oxygen sensitivity. It has been postulated that postischemic hypoperfusion may be a neurogenic reflex (Dirnagl 1993) and/or characterized by a block in the transduction of physiologic stimuli and hence protein synthesis (Siesjö et al. 1995). Assuming short-lived (minutes) global ischemia/anoxia and cell death independent of the microcirculation (Dirnagl 1993), positive effects of HBO acutely are shown later in multiple studies to be due to reversal of hypoxia and effects on cellular energy metabolism, mitochondria, ion homeostasis, membrane integrity, gene induction, and a plethora of as yet unidentified targets. The dramatic effect of even one HBO exposure on recovery of brain function, as indicated in many of the studies later, implies a powerful on/off drug effect that simultaneously quenches a degradative process and energizes the cell. It is easy to envision HBO acting at some or multiple points of blockade in the above-mentioned reflex or at a physiologic impasse.

One of the primary sites of action of HBO appears to be pressure and oxygen-sensitive genes and gene products (Harch 2015). In the chronic state, a single HBO may be responsible for the awakening of idling neurons (Neubauer et al. 1990), and when delivered both singly and repetitively considered a signal transducer (Siddiqui et al. 1995). The signal transduction mechanism is inferred in multiple noncerebral HBO wound models where trophic tissue changes result from repetitive HBO (Hyperbaric Oxygen Therapy Indications 2014), measured molecularly in two studies (Wu and Mustoe 1995; Buras et al. 2000), suggested in a replicated chronic traumatic brain injury rat model (Harch and Kriedt 2007), reaffirmed in a controlled human trial of HBO in chronic traumatic brain injury directed by Harch in Texas (Barrett et al. 1998), and powerfully demonstrated over the past 70 years in innumerable studies on the biological effects of increased pressure (Macdonald and Fraser 1999). In the past 15 years HBO has demonstrated up- and down-regulation of individual and mass numbers of genes with separate and overlapping clusters of gene activation determined by the different degrees of increase in both pressure and oxygen (Harch 2015; Oh et al. 2008; Chen et al. 2009a). A single exposure to human endothelial cells at 2.4 ATA effects expression and suppression of 8,101 genes (Godman et al. 2009). In the rat model of HBOT and chronic traumatic brain injury repetitive 1.5 ATA/90 min HBOT induced increased blood vessel density and cognitive function in injured hippocampus. While not measured, this trophism strongly implies gene activation effects of HBOT. Moreover, these findings likely underpin much of the trophic effect of HBOT in chronic brain injury and represent the first ever improvement of chronic brain injury in animals. Future studies should be focused on elucidating the molecular effects of HBO in this model and in global cerebral ischemia/anoxia.

With prolongation of global ischemia/anoxia, and especially incomplete global ischemia, or the recovery phase of reperfusion pretherapeutic intervention the microcirculation is disturbed (Dirnagl 1993; Kunz et al. 2010) and the pathophysiology begins to resemble that in acute traumatic brain injury (Cormio et al. 1997; Kunz et al. 2010): lipid peroxidation, edema, arterial spasm, cellular reperfusion injury, and anaerobic metabolism in the setting of penumbral lesions (Cormio et al. 1997). HBO has been shown to have positive effects on all of these: ischemic penumbra (Neubauer et al. 1990; Neubauer and James 1998; Barrett et al. 1998), cerebral edema (Sukoff and Ragatz 1982), arterial spasm (Kohshi et al. 1993; Kawamura et al. 1988), anaerobic metabolism (Holbach et al. 1977a), and peroxidation/cellular reperfusion injury (Thom 1993a). This last HBO sensitive pathophysiological target is most exciting since it seems to be a generic ischemic model-, species-, and organ-independent HBO effect (Harch 2000; Buras and Reenstra 2007). In a carbon monoxide rat model Thom (1993b) showed a powerful inhibitory action of HBO on white blood cell mediated brain lipid peroxidation when delivered 24 h before the poisoning or 45 min after removal from carbon monoxide. Zamboni et al. (1993) demonstrated a similar finding in a four hour global ischemic rat gracilis muscle model, using intravital microscopy. Follow-up work by (Khiabani et al. 2008) identified a plasma mediator(s) of this phenomenon.

HBO inhibition of WBCs is also inferred in brain decompression sickness and cerebral air embolism (Harch 1996) when one combines the Dutka et al. (1989), Helps and Gorman (1991) and Martin and Thom (2002) data, which implicates WBCs in the pathogenesis of these disorders, with the Thalmann (1990) review, which shows a 90 % single treatment cure rate in decompression sickness when hyperbaric recompression is delivered within the first 1–2 h of injury. Similarly, the data of Bulkley and Hutchins (1977) and Engler et al. (1986a, b) that document a WBC-mediated pathogenesis in cardiac reperfusion injury, in conjunction with the Thomas et al. (1990) tissue plasminogen activator/HBO/acute myocardial infarction dog model and the congruent human study of Shandling et al. (1997) strongly suggest an HBO-directed action on cellular reperfusion injury, among other effects. Lastly, Rosenthal et al. (2003) demonstrated a positive effect on the microcirculation similar to the findings of Zamboni et al. (1993). The beneficial effect of HBOT in most, if not all, of these studies is thought to be due to HBOT effects on endothelial-neutrophil interactions (Buras and Reenstra 2007). All of the earlier actions of HBO on the pathophysiology in acute traumatic brain injury should sum to provide a beneficial effect. In fact, such is the case as a review of the studies in

Table 20.2 shows a convincing argument for the use of HBO in acute severe traumatic brain injury. Similarly, if global ischemia/anoxia is prolonged or incomplete, e.g., unsuccessful hanging, microcirculatory disturbances are incomplete. Under these circumstances, HBO-induced inhibition of cellular reperfusion injury may partly explain the very positive results of the studies listed in Tables 20.1 and 20.2.

For HBO to be effective in coma it must be directed at diffuse targets in the bilateral hemispheric gray and white matter, the brainstem, or both. Acutely, regardless of the nature of the targets, e.g., microcirculatory, nonvascular, cellular, or other, HBO can conceivably act equally effectively on the hemispheres, brainstem, or both, and likely does. As the pathology matures, a significant HBO effect on hemispheric coma is very unlikely because of the large tissue volumes and low ratios of umbra to penumbra. Smaller tissue volumes are favored such that brainstem coma would be expected to have better results. This is suggested by the positive HBO data in the large traumatic mid-brain report of Holbach et al. (1974), the brainstem contusion subgroup of Artru et al. (1976a), the GCS 4–6 group of Rockswold et al. (1992, 2013), and the coma patients of Heyman et al. (1966) and Neubauer (1985). In all of these clinical trials, a recovery of just a few millimeters of reticular activating system can translate intofar-reaching effects in the hemispheres, e.g., awakening. Additional work will be necessary to confirm this hypothesis.

In chronic global ischemia/anoxia and coma the pathological targets become more speculative. The ischemic penumbra (Astrup et al. 1981) argument of (Neubauer et al. 1990) and sympathetic hibernating myocardium concept of (Swift et al. 1992) remain, but given the numbers of treatments reported later the element of time enters the equation and implies a trophic effect. This effect, which could include stimulation of axon sprouting, or possibly an alteration or redirection of blood flow as suggested earlier (Harch et al. 2007), or both, may be indiscriminately effective on the final common pathway of a variety of brain injuries similar to HBOT's generic effect on reperfusion injury (Harch 2000). Given the diversity of reports (Neubauer 1985; Neubauer et al. 1990, 1992, Neubauer 1995, Neubauer et al. 1998, Neubauer et al. 2004, Neubauer and James 1998; Harch et al. 1994a, b; Harch 1996; Harch and Neubauer 1999, 2004) and the multitude of studies listed later this maybe so. Regardless of the nature of this generic effect, in the past 29 years (PGH) and 38 years (RAN) these authors have noted an upward sawtooth response (Chap. 19, Stroke, Figs. 19.7 and 19.9) during HBOT in subacute and chronic brain injury with a partial regression once each round of HBOT ends. This implies permanent and transient components to the treatment (see Chap. 44, Neuroimaging). While the net HBO result appears uniform, the biochemical, molecular, cellular, and anatomic complexities of the transient, permanent, and final effects will need to be developed in the future.

Table 20.1 Hyperbaric oxygen therapy in global ischemia, anoxia, and coma—animal studies

Authors and year	Model	Animal species	Length of ischemia/anoxia	Initiation of HBO	HBO protocol	Results and conclusions
Moody et al. (1970)	Temporary complete global ischemia/anoxia using bilateral extradural balloons	50 dogs (20 controls)	Flattening of EEG for 3 min plus spontaneously rising intracranial pressure to equal systolic blood pressure. Evaluation after 10 days	Immediately after balloon deflation	Group 1: Controls 1 ATA air, spontaneous respiration Group 2: 1 ATA O_2/4 h on a ventilator Group 3: 1 ATA O_2/4 h, spontaneous respiration, no ventilator Group 4: 2 ATA O_2/4 h, spontaneous respiration, no vent	Group 1: 95 % mortality within 30 h after ischemia Group 2: 30 % mortality Group 3: 70 % mortality within 72–96 h after ischemia Group 4: 50 % mortality within 72–96 h after ischemia Quality of survivors was poor in Group 2 and good in Groups 3 and 4
Kapp et al. (1982)	Temporary complete global ischemia/anoxia. Total circulatory arrest with occlusion of aorta, superior vena cava, and inferior vena cava	10 cats	5 min	3–5 min after ischemia release	Group 1: 5 controls, 1 ATA O_2/2.5 h Group 2: 5 HBO, 1.5 ATA O_2/2.5 h	Beneficial effect of HBOT with significant reduction in EEG recovery time
Ruiz et al. (1986)	Temporary complete global ischemia/anoxia. Ventricular fibrillation and no ventilation for 12 min then cardiac resuscitation. Evaluate survival times, cardiac function, and neurological scoring 7 days postarrest	16 dogs	12 min	Approximately 13 min after end of arrest (resuscitation within 6 min + 7 min of hemodilution)	Group 1: Controls No treatment Group 2: Normovolemic hemodilution with hetastarch/MgSO4 to hematocrit of 20–30 % Group 3: Group 2: plus 2 ATA O_2/1 h	No significant difference in survival, cardiac function, or neurological scoring between control and HBO. Decreased hematocrit due to hemodilution felt to possibly be detrimental
Shiokawa et al. (1986)	Permanent incomplete global ischemia/anoxia. Bilateral carotid artery ligation. Measure survival times and lactate/ATP	60 Spontaneously hypertensive rats	1.5 or 3.5 h for survival experiment, 2.5 or 4.5 h for metabolic studies	At 1 h or 3 h postligation	Group 1: (Survival) (a) 1 ATA air/1.5 h (b) 1 ATA air/3.5 h (c) 2 ATA O_2/30 min at 1 h postligation (d) 2 ATA O_2/30 min at 3 h postligation Group 2: (Metabolic) Same as for survival experiment but assays at 2.5 (a and c) and 4.5 h (b and d) of ligation	All HBOT animals survived at least 1.5 or 3.5 h. Control animals that died in less than these times were excluded from analysis Animals with HBOT at 3 h survived significantly longer than controls with significantly less lactate accumulation. Trend toward more ATP accumulation in HBO Group D

(continued)

Table 20.1 (continued)

Authors and year	Model	Animal species	Length of ischemia/anoxia	Initiation of HBO	HBO protocol	Results and conclusions
Weinstein et al. (1986)	Temporary incomplete global ischemia/anoxia. Permanent unilateral carotid occlusion Temporary opposite carotid artery occlusion for 2, 5, 10, 20, or 60 min. Autopsy studies. Separate DMSO experiment	30 gerbils	2, 5, 10, 20, or 60 min	After 20 min of temporary occlusion	Group 1: Controls at 2, 5, 10, 20, or 60 min with bilateral carotid artery occlusion Group 2: HBO 1.5 ATA/15 min after 20 min of occlusion Group 3: Intraperitoneal DMSO at 5 or 10 min of bilateral occlusion Group 4: Controls–surgery without carotid occlusion	Mortality: Group 1: 2 min 0%, 5 min 33%, 10 min 33%, 20 min 100%, 60 min 100% Group 2: HBO 16% (p <.001) Extent of damage much less in HBO survivors Group 3: DMSO 86% mortality each
Van Meter et al. (1988)	Temporary complete global ischemia/cardiac arrest. Measured return of cardiac function by EKG and thermodilution cardiac output	Guinea pig	15 min	Immediately after 15-min arrest period	Group 1: Control. 1, 2.8 or 6 ATA air/maximum 30 min Group 2: HBOT at 1, 2.8, or 6 ATA oxygen/30 min maximum	Maximum initial postresuscitation survival at 2.8 ATA O$_2$ >6 ATA air or 6 ATA O$_2$, maximum mean postresuscitation survival time with 6 ATA O$_2$ >2.8 ATA O$_2$ >1 ATAO$_2$ >6 ATA air
Mickel et al. (1990)	Temporary incomplete global ischemia. Bilateral carotid artery occlusion. Histological evaluation at death or up to 28-day limit	60 gerbils	15 min	None	Group 1: 1 ATA O$_2$/first 3 h of reperfusion Group 2: 1 ATA air for 3 h of reperfusion	In the oxygen group: (1) Increased myelin damage, but better preservation of axons (2) Better preservation of neurons in the deeper laminae of the cerebral cortex (3) Increased mortality
Yatsuzuka (1991)	Temporary complete global ischemia. Cross clamp of ascending aorta. Measure intracranial pressure, cerebral blood flow, EEG, and oxidative stress (metabolites) before, during, and after HBO 34 dogs	34 dogs	18 min	60 min postischemic release	Group 1: Ischemic controls Group 2: HBOT without global ischemia Group 3: HBO 2 ATA/170 min	Significant decrease in intracranial pressure and oxidative stress metabolites in HBOT
Grigor'eva et al. (1992)	Permanent incomplete global ischemia. Bilateral carotid artery occlusion. Survival and histology measurements of cortical neurons	Approximately 60 rats	24 h	2 h after occlusion	Group 1: HBOT 2 ATA/1 h Group 2: Air 2 ATA/1 h Group 3: HBOT 1.2 ATA/30 min Group 4: Controls, sham, operation, sacrifice at 2.5 h Group 5: Controls, operation, air treatment, sacrifice at 2.5 h	At 24 h: Group 1: 30% survival with 25–30% sparing of neurons Group 2: 50% spared neurons (did not mark mortality) Group 3: 50% survival with 50–60% sparing of neurons Group 4: Used for baseline histologic studies Group 5: 100% mortality, when allowed to proceed to 24 h Pronounced protective effect in HBO groups with preservation of transcription and increased survival; 1.2 ATA was superior to 2 ATA

Takahashi et al. (1992)	Temporary complete global ischemia/anoxia. Occlusion of the ascending aorta and caval veins. EEG and neurological recovery scores measured over a period of 14 days postischemia	19 dogs	15 min	3, 24, and 29 h after release of ischemia	Group 1: 3 ATA O_2/1 h at 3, 24, and 29 h. Group 2: Controls air 1 ATA	Survival: 30% in control group 78% in hyperbaric group with significantly greater EEG and neurological recovery scores
Iwatsuki et al. (1994)	Temporary complete global ischemia. Same model as Takahashi's study	19 dogs	15 min	3, 24, and 29 h after release of ischemia	Group 1: nicardipine bolus immediately at the end of ischemia then nicardipine drip × 3 days plus HBOT—3 ATA/1 h at 3, 24, and 29 h after ischemia. Group 2: no nicardipine or HBOT	Survival rate and time, neurological recovery, and EEG scores all significantly better in HBOT/nicardipine group
Mink and Dutka (1995a)	Temporary complete global ischemia. CSF infusions to increase intracranial pressure to mean arterial pressure. Measure cortical somatosensory-evoked potentials and oxyradical brain damage	18 rabbits	10 min	Immediately on reperfusion	Group 1: 1 ATA air for 75 min. Group 2: 2.8 ATA O_2/75 min with air breaks	HBOT significantly increased evoked potentials and free radical generation but lipid peroxidation was unchanged
Mink and Dutka (1995b)	Same model as above 10 min 30 min after the end of ischemia	22 rabbits	10 min	30 min after the end of ischemia. On room air during the 30 min	Group 1: 2.8 ATA O_2/125 min with air breaks then 1 ATA O_2/90 min. Group 2: Control 1 ATA O_2/215 min	HBO significantly reduced brain vascular permeability and blood flow while somatosensory-evoked potentials were unchanged
Yaxi et al. (1995)	Temporary incomplete global ischemia. Temporary clamping of bilateral common carotid arteries (CCA) plus (?) internal jugular veins. Histochemical analysis of LDH, isocitrate dehydrogenase: (ICD H), cytochrome a3, ATPase, and cAMP. Also pathological study of tissue	52 rabbits	20 min (?)	Immediately after release of clamp	Group 1: Control. Room air × 20, 40, or 120 min. Group 2: (HBA-hyperbaric air): 8.4% O_2 at 2.5 ATA/20, 40, or 120 min. Group 3: HBOT at 2.5 ATA (by "mask")/20, 40, or 120 min. Tissue analysis immediately posthyperbaric treatment	Improvement in LDH, ICDH, cytochrome a3, and ATPase levels in 40 and 120-min HBO groups with concomitant reduced tissue injury on pathological examination

(continued)

Table 20.1 (continued)

Authors and year	Model	Animal species	Length of ischemia/anoxia	Initiation of HBO	HBO protocol	Results and conclusions
Yiqun et al. (1995)	Temporary incomplete global cerebral ischemia. Bilateral common carotid artery (CCA) clamping. Measured Na, K-ATPase activity in groups 1, 2, 3, 4, and 5 and histologic and electron microscope analysis in groups 1, 2, and 4	98 gerbils	60 min (?)	Immediately after treatment	Group 1: Control. Skin incision only. Group 2: Control CCA clamping plus 80-min. room air exposure. Group 3: CCA clamping plus 1 ATAO$_2$/80 min. Group 4: CCA clamping plus 2.5 ATA O$_2$/80 min. Group 5: CCA clamping plus 2.5 ATA air/80 min. Group 6: CCA clamping plus immediate sacrifice	Significant decrease ATPase activity in all groups except group 4 HBO. Least pathological changes in same group
Konda et al. (1996)	Temporary incomplete global ischemia/anoxia. Bilateral common carotid artery ligation. Histological exam of hippocampal neurons 3 weeks post-op and histochemical examination of heat shock proteins 36 h post-op	47 gerbils	10 min	2, 6, or 24 h post-op.	Group 1: 6 h postischemia: 2 ATAO$_2$/60 min t.i.d. × 7 days, then q.d. × 14. Group 2: 24 h postischemia: 2 ATAO$_2$/60 min 1 × day/14 days. Group 3: surgery, no HBO. Group 4: 2 ATA O$_2$/60 min 1 × day for 14 days. No surgery. Group 5: No HBO, no surgery. Sacrifice at 36 h: Group 6: Surgery, single HBO 2 ATA/60 at 2 h post-op. Group 7: Surgery, single HBO at 2 ATA/60 min 24 h post-op. Group 8: Surgery, no HBO	Preservation of hippocampal neurons in HBO animals (6 h animals > than 24 h animals) with less heat shock protein induction in HBO animals than controls. Increase in lysosomes and myelinoid structures in hippocampal neurons in HBO group. HBO prevented delayed neuronal death without oxygen toxicity
Wada et al. (1996)	Temporary incomplete global ischemia/anoxia, bilateral common carotid artery occlusion. Evaluate neuronal density 7 days postischemia and heat shock protein production in the hippocampus	49 gerbils	5 min (2 days after last HBOT)	Preischemia	Group 1: 2 ATA O$_2$/1 h × 1 treatment. Group 2: 2 ATA O$_2$/1 h every other day × 5 treatments. Group 3: Sham operation, no HBO. Group 4: Surgery, no HBO. Group 5: Groups 1, 2, and 3 without ischemia; measurement of heat shock proteins	Significant preservation of neurons in the 5 HBO pretreatment group with significant increase in heat shock protein production. Repetitive HBOT protects against ischemia neuronal damage possibly through heat shock protein induction
Krakovsky et al. (1998)	Temporary complete global ischemia (cauterization of bilateral vertebral arteries then temporary occlusion of the bilateral common carotid arteries). Measure brain blood flow by direct laser/Doppler flowmetry and 14-day survival	18 rats	60 min	"Brief delay to transfer to HBO chamber"	Group 1: Control. Room air. Group 2: HBOT: 3 ATA/1 h	Significantly increased survival in HBO (45%) vs. controls (0%). In <14-day survival, significant increase in survival time with HBO (59.8 h) vs. controls (17.9 h)

Van Meter et al. (1999b)	Temporary complete global ischemia/cardiac arrest. Measure initial return of circulation with BP >90/50 and sustained circulation for 2 h	36 swine	25 min	Immediately after the 25-min arrest period	Group 1: Control. 1 ATA O$_2$/maximum 30 min Group 2: 2 ATA O$_2$/maximum 30 min Group 3: 4 ATA O$_2$/maximum 30 min	Initial return of circulation and sustained return of circulation at 2 h only present in group 3; 4 ATA HBOT groups at 80% and 67%, respectively. All animals in all other groups failed to be resuscitated
Hai et al. (2002)	Temporary incomplete global ischemia/hypoxia (?) Right common carotid artery, internal carotid artery, and external carotid artery ligation (?) then 5.5% oxygen environment (same model as Calvert et al. 2002 study). Measure brain fibroblastic growth factor (bFGF) and bFGF mRNA after ten-day treatment period	44 rats (<7 days old)	2 h	7 days	Group 1: Control Room air for 10 days Group 2: HBOT 2.5 ATA/90 min q.d. × 10 Group 3: HBA (hyperbaric air) 2.5 ATA/90 min q.d. × 10 ("concentrations oxygen controlled under 25%") Group 4: "Untreated". "Free growing × 10 days" Group 5: Sham operation	Increased bFGF levels in HBA and HBO groups, especially in precortex and hippocampus. Increased bFGF mRNA only in HBO group
Van Meter et al. (2001a)	Temporary complete global ischemia/cardiac arrest. Measure initial return of circulation with BP >90/50 and sustained circulation for 2 h. Measure malondialdehyde	36 swine	25 min	Immediately after the 25-min arrest period	Group 1: Control. 1 ATA O$_2$/maximum 30 min Group 2: 2 ATA O$_2$/maximum 30 min Group 3: 4 ATA O$_2$/maximum 30 min	Significant reduction in brain lipid peroxidation in 4 ATA HBOT group only
Van Meter et al. (2001b)	Temporary complete global ischemia/cardiac arrest. Measure initial return of circulation with BP >90/50 and sustained circulation for 2 h. Measure myeloperoxidase content	36 swine	25 min	Immediately after the 25-min arrest period	Group 1: Control. 1 ATA O$_2$/maximum 30 min Group 2: 2 ATA O$_2$/maximum 30 min Group 3: 4 ATA O$_2$/maximum 30 min	No effect of any treatment group on myeloperoxidase content. Implies the target of ischemia reperfusion injury reduction with HBOT in this model is not leukocytes
Calvert et al. (2002)	Temporary incomplete global ischemia. Right common carotid artery ligation then 8% oxygen exposure. Measure brain weights and examine with light microscopy and electron microscopy at 24, 48, and 72 h., and 1, 2, and 6 weeks, and perform sensory motor functional test 5 weeks posthypoxia	229 rats (7 days old)	2½ h of hypoxia post-2 h carotid ligation	1 h after hypoxia	Group 1: Control Group 2: Ischemia/hypoxia plus room air recovery Group 3: HBOT 3 ATA/60 min	Significant preservation of brain weight in the right hemisphere of HBO rats at 2 and 6 weeks with less atrophy and apoptosis on light and electron microscopy. Sensory motor function also significantly improved at 5 weeks in HBO group

(continued)

Table 20.1 (continued)

Authors and year	Model	Animal species	Length of ischemia/anoxia	Initiation of HBO	HBO protocol	Results and conclusions
Rosenthal et al. (2003)	Temporary complete global ischemia (cardiac arrest/resuscitation). Measure neurological deficit score 23 h after resuscitation, sacrifice at 24 h and measure apoptosis in hippocampus and cerebral neocortex, arterial and sagittal sinus oxygenation and cerebral blood flow (CBF), cerebral oxygen extraction ratio (ERc), oxygen delivery (DO_2c), and metabolic rate for oxygen ($CMRO_2$) at baseline, 2, 30, 60, 120, 180, 240, 300, and 360 min after restoration of spontaneous circulation	20 dogs	1 h	1 h	Group 1: Control Room air resuscitation Group 2: HBO 2.7 ATA/60 min	Improvement in neurological deficit score in HBO group with significantly fewer dying neurons. Magnitude of neuronal injury correlated with the neurodeficit score. HBO decreased the oxygen extraction ratio without a change in oxygen delivery or $CMRO_2$
Zhou et al. (2003)	Temporary complete global ischemia. Bilateral carotid occlusion. Measure Nogo-A, Ng-R, and RhoA proteins at 6, 12, 24, 48, 96 h, and 7 days	78 rats	10 min	1 h after ischemia	3 ATA/2 h. Thirteen groups: 1 sham, 6 global ischemia, 6 global ischemia + HBO	HBO significantly reduced neurological injury (neuronal loss) and the levels of Nogo-A, Ng-R, and RhoA in injured cortex
Mrsic-Pelcic et al. (2004a)	Temporary complete global ischemia (vertebral cautery + transient bilateral carotid occlusion). Measure hippocampal SOD or Na, K ATPase	84 rats	20 min	2, 24, 48, or 168 h after ischemia (for SOD), or .5, 1, 2, 6, 24, 48, 72, or 168 h after ischemia (for ATPase)	2 ATA/1 h daily for 7 days	HBO significantly increased hippocampal SOD only when delayed 168 h and prevented ATPase decline only if begun during 1st 24 h of reperfusion
Mrsic-Pelcic et al. (2004b)	Temporary complete global ischemia (vertebral cautery + transient bilateral carotid occlusion). Measure optic nerve SOD or Na, K ATPase	84 rats	20 min	2, 24, 48, or 168 h after ischemia (for SOD), or .5, 1, 2, 6, 24, 48, 72, or 168 h after ischemia (for ATPase)	2 ATA/1 h daily for 7 days	HBO prevented ATPase decline in the optic nerve only if begun during 1st 6 h of reperfusion and no effect on SOD regardless of time of initiation
Gunther et al. (2004)	Complete global ischemia (brain slices postdecapitation). Measure purine nucleotide content and morphological changes	Rat(s)	5 or 30 min	After 5 or 30 min of anoxia	2.5 ATA/1 h, 1 ATA/1 h, 2.5 ATA air/1 h, or 1 ATA air/1 h	HBO and NBO equally effective at 5 min. Less so after 30 min hypoxia while only HBO lessened morphological cell injury

Reference	Model and measurements	Subjects	Duration	Timing	HBO protocol	Results
Li et al. (2005)	Temporary incomplete global ischemia (bilateral common carotid occlusion + hypotension to 30–35 mmHg). Measure HIF-1 alpha, p53, caspase-9, 3, and 8, bcl-2 and cell death at 6, 12, 24, 48, 96 h, and 7 days	78 rats	10 min	1 h after ischemia	3 ATA/2 h Thirteen groups: 1 sham, 6 global ischemia, 6 global ischemia + HBO	HBO reduced HIF-1 alpha, p53, caspase 9 and 3, and apoptosis, yet increased proapoptotic caspase 8 and decreased antiapoptotic bcl-2
Calvert and Zhang (2005)	Temporary incomplete global ischemia (unilateral carotid ligation + 8% oxygen exposure). Measure ATP, creatine, phosphocreatine, glucose at 4 and 24 h. Brain weight at 2 weeks	7-day-old rat pups	2 h	1 h after ischemia	3 ATA/2 h or 1 ATA/2 h	Significant reduction of brain injury and increase in ATP, cr, Pcr over controls with HBO and NBO
Yu et al. (2006)	Temporary incomplete global ischemia (unilateral carotid ligation + 8% oxygen exposure). Measure neural stem cells and myelin in hippocampus at 3 weeks	7-day-old rat pups	2 h	1 h after ischemia	2 ATA/? Oxygen or air daily × 7 days	HBO increased hippocampal stem cells and nestin expression. Both HBO and hyperbaric air mitigated myelin damage
Liu et al. (2006b)	"Hypoxic/ischemic brain damage." Article in Chinese. Model not described in English abstract. Measure hippocampal and cortical cell density at 48 h and neurobehavioral testing at 5 and 6 weeks	7-day-old rat pups ($n = 84$)	1 h	1, 3, 6, 12, or 24 h after ischemia	2.5 ATA/1.5 h at 1, 3, 6, 12, or 24 h	Neuronal density, sensorimotor, grip test, and treadmill were significantly increased over controls when HBO was delivered up to 6 h after ischemia
Liu et al. (2006a)	Temporary incomplete global ischemia (unilateral common carotid ligation + hypoxia). Measure spatial learning/memory 37 and 41 days and morphology 42 days after ischemia	7-day-old rat pups ($n = 52$)	2 h	.5–1 h after ischemia, daily × 2 days	2 ATA/?	HBO significantly improved spatial learning/memory and alleviated morphological and histological damage
Calvert et al. (2006)	Temporary incomplete global ischemia (unilateral carotid ligation + 8% oxygen exposure). Measure HIF-1 alpha, glucose transporter, LDH, aldolase, and p53	7-day-old rat pups	2 h	1 h after ischemia	2.5 ATA or 1 ATA oxygen	HBOT >NBOT significantly reduced elevated HIF-1 alpha, promoted a transient increase in glucose transporter, LDH, Ald, and decreased HIF-1 alpha-p53 interaction and expression of p53

(continued)

Table 20.1 (continued)

Authors and year	Model	Animal species	Length of ischemia/anoxia	Initiation of HBO	HBO protocol	Results and conclusions
Yang et al. (2008)	Temporary incomplete global ischemia (unilateral carotid ligation + 8 % oxygen exposure). Measure hippocampal stem cells at 7 and 14 days and nestin 6 h–14 days, myelin basic protein and pathological changes at 28 days	7-day-old rat pups	2 h	Within 3 after ischemia	2 ATA/? daily × 7 days	HBOT caused proliferation of stem cells which peaked at 7 days and migrated to the cerebral cortex at 14 days. New neurons, oligodendrocytes, and myelin basic protein was seen in the HBO group at 28 days
Wang et al. (2007a)	Temporary incomplete global ischemia: ligation left common carotid plus 8 % O_2 exposure for 2 h. Measure Wnt-3 protein expression and endogenous neural stem cell proliferation @ 6 and 24 h, 3, 7 and 14 days in subventricular zone	7-day-old rats	2 h	3 h posthypoxic insult	Group 1: Control Group 2: Hyp/Isch Group 3: Hyp/Isch + HBOT (2 ATA/?, once/day × 7 days (total of 7 HBOTs	Neural stem cells increased 3 h after HBOT, peaked at 7 days and remained higher at 14 days. Wnt-3 increased 3 h post-HBOT, peaked at 3 days, remained higher at 14 days. Neural stem cells and Wnt-3 significantly correlated and increased in both hemispheres Conclusions: HBO promotes proliferation of stem cells and is correlated with Wnt signaling
Wang et al. (2007b)	Temporary incomplete global ischemia as earlier. Measure T-maze, foot-fault test, and radial arm maze test 14 days and myelin basic protein (MBP) in the callositas and corpora striata 28 days after hypoxia/ischemia	7-day-old rats	2 h	3, 6, 12, 24, or 72 h after hypoxia/ischemia and 72 h after Hyp–Isch. 2.0 ATA/?, once/day × 7 days (total of 7 HBOTs)	Group 1: Hyp–Isch Experimental Groups: 3, 6, 12, 24, and 72 h after hypoxia/ischemia 2.0 ATA/?, once/day × 7 days (total of 7 HBOTs)	Significantly better performance on all 3 behavioral tests and elevated MBP for rats with HBOT up to 12 h after Hyp–Isch Conclusion: HBO w/I 12 h after Hyp–Isch can alleviate white matter damage
Liu et al. (2007)	Temporary incomplete global ischemia: left common carotid ligation, then 2 h 8 % O_2. Measure step-down inhibitory avoidance at 6 weeks; Morris Water Task and hippocampal cell density at 8 weeks	7-day-old rats (18)	2 h	1 h after hyp-ischemia	Group 1: Sham Group 2: Hyp-ischemia Group 3: HBO 2.5 ATA/1.5 h	In HBO group: significantly longer step-down and shorter latencies to reach plat form, less time spent in quadrant, diminished brain injury, and decreased cell loss of hippocampal CA1 region Conclusion: HBOT improves long-term learning-memory deficits and attenuates brain injury
Wang et al. (2008)	Temporary incomplete global ischemia. Left common carotid ligation then 2 h 8 % O_2. Measure stem cells 10 days, T-maze, foot-fault, and radial arm maze tests at 14, 22, 26 days, and morphology 28 days after hypoxia/ischemia	7-day-old rats	2 h	3, 6, 12, 24, or 72 h after hypoxia/ischemia after hyp-ischemia (2.0 ATA/60 min once/day × 7 days)	Group 1: Control Group 2: Hyp-Isch Groups 3–7: HBO 3, 6, 12, 24, and 72 h after hyp-ischemia 3–12 h groups	Significantly increased stem cells in 3–24 h groups, better performance, and less neuron loss in hippocampal CA1 in 3–12 h groups Conclusion: HBO therapeutic window in HIE can be delayed up to 12 h with decreased effect up to 24 h

Wang, et al. (2009)	Temporary incomplete global ischemia. Left common carotid ligation then 2 h 8% O$_2$. Measure apoptosis and neuronal cell population in cortex and CA1 of hippocampus 31 days after hypoxia/ischemia	7-day-old rats (88)	2 h	2, 48, 96 h after hyp-ischemia	Group 1: Control Group 2: Hyp-Isch Group 3: HBO, 2 h post-H-I Group 4: HBO, 48 h post-H-I Group 5: HBO, 96 h post-H-I HBO: 2 ATA/1 h, 1×/day × 7 days, 3 days res within each HBO group had 3 groups, receiving either 1 Conclusion: 1 course HBO receiving either 1 (7 HBOTs), 2 (14 HBOTs), or 3 courses (21 HBOTs)	Apoptosis inhibition and neuronal protection decreased with increasing delay to single course of HBO, but increased with increasing courses of HBO at 48 and 96 h after hypoxia/ischemia. The number of apoptotic cells and neurons was nearly equal in H–I and control after 1 course HBO Conclusion: 1 course HBO receiving either 1 w/l 2 h H–I can effectively inhibit apoptosis and protect neurons, but less so with delay to HBO. With delay to HBO protection can be increased with increasing number of HBOTs
Chen et al. (2009a)	Complete global isch: delayed Caesarean section model—harvest pregnant uterus from term rats, submerge in water bath for anoxia, deliver pups. Measure brainstem auditory-evoked potentials, pathological change, and number of neurons in hippocampus 4 weeks of age	Term rat pups (male) ? number	15 min	24 h after isch–hypox	Group 1: Isch–Hyp Group 2: H-I plus HBO @ 2 ATA/1 h, 1×/day × 14 days Group 3: Sham operated Group 4: Sham operated + HBO	HBO H-I group: shorter peak latency waves II and IV and interpeak latencies peaks I–IV, less pathological changes and more neurons in hippocampus. HBO control group more neurons than control group Conclusion: HBO improves synaptic transmission efficiency, electrophysiologic conduction velocity, and reduces neuronal death in neonatal rats with H-I injury
Chen et al. (2009b)	Temporary incomplete global ischemia: left common carotid ligation, then 2 h 8% O$_2$. Measure histopathological damage, Caspase-3, Nogo-A expression, Morris Water Maze in control, ephedrine, HBO, and combined HBO-ephedrine groups	7-day-old rats (80)	2 h	1 h after hyp–ischemia	Group 1: Sham operated Group 2: Hyp-Ischemia Group 3: Ephedrine Group 4: HBO Group 5: ephedrine + HBO HBO @ 2.5 ATA/2 h at depth	Caspase-3 and Nogo-A reduced in treatment groups, greater reduction in combined treatment group. Escape latency shorter and platform location crossings greater in combined group vs. single treatment groups Conclusion: combination treatment enhances neuroprotective effect partially by inhibiting Caspase-3 and Nogo-A pathways
Chen and Chen (2010)	Complete global isch: delayed Caesarean section model-harvest pregnant uterus from term rats, submerge in water bath for anoxia, deliver pups. Measure hippocampal ultrastructure P38 expression, and water maze test at 4 weeks of age	Term rat pups (male, 30)	15 min	24 h after isch–hypox	Group 1: Isch–Hyp Group2: H-I plus HBO @ 2 ATA/1 h, 1×/day × 14 days Group 3: Sham operated Group 4: Sham operated + HBO	Water maze test, hippocampal ultrastructure, and P38 significantly better than ischemic/hypoxic group for control and HBO groups with no difference between HBO and control Conclusion: HBO induces synaptic plasticity and reduces ultrastructural damage in perinatal hypoxia/ischemia

(continued)

Table 20.1 (continued)

Authors and year	Model	Animal species	Length of ischemia/anoxia	Initiation of HBO	HBO protocol	Results and conclusions
Liu, et al. (2013)	Temporary incomplete global ischemia: Unilateral carotid ligation, 8 % O_2 for 2 h. Measure apoptosis, caspase-3, apoptosis inducing factor 60 days post and cognitive and sensorimotor tests 28–60 days postinsult	7-day-old rats (108)	2 h	1 h post-hyp–ischemia	Group 1: Sham operated; Group 2: Hyp–ischemia; Group 3: HBO, 2.5 ATA/90 min once	Significant cognitive and sensorimotor improvements in HBO correlated with reduction size of hippocampal and cortex lesions. HBO decreased apoptosis, caspase-3, and AIF. Conclusion: HBO promoted long-term functional and histological improvement which is associated with suppression of apoptosis by inhibiting caspase-3 and AIF
Malek, et al. (2013)	Temporary Incomplete global ischemia. Bilateral temporary occlusion of both common carotid arteries. Measure hippocampal CA1 neuronal survival, brain temperature, nesting behavior in control, HBO, hyperbaric air, and normobaric oxygen groups	12–13 weeks gerbils	3 min	1,3, or 6 h after isch	Group 1: Sham; Group 2: Ischemia; Group 3: HBO-2.5 ATA/60 min, 1×/day × 3; Group 4: HBA, 2.5 ATA/60 min, 1×/day × 3; Group 5: 100 % O_2 1 ATA/60 min, 1×/day × 3	HBO and HBA significantly increased neuronal survival, behavioral performance, and abolished brain temperature increase when treated 1, 3, 6 h after ischemia. NBO only effective 1 h postischemia. Conclusion: HBO, HBA prevent neuronal damage primarily by pressure inhibition of brain temperature increase
Yin, et al. (2013)	Temporary incomplete global ischemia: Left common carotid ligation, 8 % O_2 for 2.5 h. Measure bone morphogenetic protein-4, nestin, and their mRNA expression, and apoptosis in hippocampus 7 days after HBO	7-day-old rats (30)	2.5 h	6 h post-hyp–ischemia	Group 1: Normal Control; Group 2: Hyp–ischemia; Group 3: HBO, 2.0 ATA/40 min, 1×/day × seven days	BMP-4, nestin, and their mRNA expression were highest in HBO group. Number of apoptotic cells significantly lower in HBO group vs. hypox–ischemia group and higher than control. Conclusion: HBO may promote neurorecovery in HIE due to increased protein and mRNA expression of BMP-4, nestin, and inhibition of apoptosis
Zhu, et al. (2015)	Temporary incomplete global ischemia: Unilateral carotid ligation, 8 % O_2 for 2 h. Measure cell density, apoptosis rate, Fas-L, caspase-8, caspase-3 + cells, nitric oxide, malondialdehyde, super-oxide dismutase in hippocampus 14 days post. Morris Water Maze 28 days post-hyp–ischemia	7-day-old rats (126)	2 h	6, 24, 48, 72 h, and 1 week post	Group 1: Sham operated; Group 3: 6 h HBO; Group 4: 24 h HBO; Group 5: 48 h HBO; Group 6: 72 h HBO; Group 7: 1 week HBO; All HBO: 2 ATA/60 min, 1×/day × 7 days	Significant improvements cell density, apoptosis, oxidative stress, Fas-L, caspases, and Water-Maze for HBO w/I 72 h, declining in time-dependent fashion. Conclusion: HBO inhibits oxidative stress and apoptosis in HIE; optimal therapeutic window is 72 h

Table 20.2 Hyperbaric oxygen therapy in global ischemia, anoxia, and coma—human studies

Authors and year	Diagnosis	No. of patients	Length of coma/neuroinsult prehyperbaric oxygen therapy (HBOT)	Timing of HBOT	HBOT protocol	Results and conclusions
Category I: Hyperacute Period (0–3 h postcerebral injury)						
Hutchison et al. (1963)	Global ischemia/anoxia. Asphyxiated neonates (apnea). No in chamber ventilator support available	65	3–38 min	3–38 min	2–4 ATA/30 × 1, 14 patients treated more than 1	79% resuscitation rate (25% died later of other causes). Overall, 55% discharged from hospital as well. Most deaths due to Hyaline membrane
Ingvar and Lassen (1965)	Coma: Progressive thrombotic CVA of the brainstem. Patient was preterminal	1	Not mentioned	At signs of failing circulation	2.0–2.5 ATA ... for 1.5–2.5 h	Rapid awakening in chamber with increase in blood pressure and decrease in heart rate. Death shortly after the end of 1 HBOT
Saltzman et al. (1966)	Various forms of cerebral ischemia. Some in coma but only 5 of 25 is level of consciousness specifically identified	25 (2 patients in coma in hyperacute or acute coma, 23 patients a few hours to 30 days after CVA)	1. 5 h 61-year-old patient with stupor and hemiplegia, suspected embolic clot. 2. 2.5 h 58-year-old with deep coma and hemoplegia, suspected air embolism	1. 5 h 2. 2.5 h	1. 2.02 ATA/>1 h, 1 treatment 2. 2.36 ATA/5 h, 1 treatment	First patient dramatic awakening 5 min into HBO with improvement of hemiplegia. Discharged from hospital with mild residual deficit. Second patient dramatic awakening 10 min into HBO with improvement of hemiplegia. Discharged from hospital with only partial paralysis of the right leg. Remainder of patients probably described in Heyman study: 3 patients dramatic temporary improvement, 8 patients less dramatic temporary improvement, 12 patients no change during HBOT. 24 of 25 patients with only 1 treatment. One patient with 3 treatments
Viart et al. (1970)	Hepatic coma infants (2 viral, 1 toxic); HBOT plus exchange transfusions	3	Not mentioned	Not mentioned	Not mentioned, but extreme profile implied	One died of pulmonary oxygen toxicity with 36 h of HBOT, two survived. All three with normalization of consciousness, EEG, and neurological examination, (One transient, two permanent) Cardiac conduction abnormalities during HBO in the two survivors? Difficult to assess the effect of HBO; authors feel high complication rate of HBOT makes exchange transfusion standard of care

(continued)

Table 20.2 (continued)

Authors and year	Diagnosis	No. of patients	Length of coma/ neuroinsult prehyperbaric oxygen therapy (HBOT)	Timing of HBOT	HBOT protocol	Results and conclusions
Hayakawa et al. (1971)	Acute coma: 9 TBI, 4 post-op brain tumor 7 patients ventilator dependent Measure CSF pressure pre, during, and post-one HBOT	13	Acute posttrauma and immediately post-op. Exact time not mentioned	Acute posttrauma and immediately post-op. Exact time not mentioned	2 ATA/1 h × 1	Three patterns of response: (1) 9 patients: CSF pressure decreased at beginning of HBOT and rose at end of HBOT (2) 2 patients: CSF pressure decreased with HBO and remained significantly lower at end of HBOT (3) 2 patients: no change in CSF pressure Conclusion: HBOT has two actions, decreases edema in injured brain and produces edema in normal brain. If HBOT produced significant change in CSF pressure, clinical improvement was remarkable and neurological deficit was mild. If no change CSF pressure with HBOT, severe brain damage and little clinical improvement
Voisin et al. (1973)	Global ischemia/anoxia/coma: Near hanging	35 (33 by suicide attempt)	14 controls with normobaric oxygen (NBO) prior to installation of HBO chamber in 1968	(2/3 of cases: <3 h from discovery to hospitalization	Exact timing not stated	(1) HBO 2 ATA/1 h × 1 or more Rxs. Total 51 Rxs in 35 patients (2) Control: NBO
Larcan et al. (1977)	Coma: Thrombotic CVA (HBOT + Urokinase)	77 (36 in varying degrees of coma, 10/36 in severe coma)	Only reported for urokinase/HBO group 16 patients <24 h 20 patients >24 h Only 1 patient treated in less than 3 h	Only reported for urokinase/HBO group 16 patients <24 h 20 patients >24 h	2.0 ATA/60–90 BID: 5 groups: (1) standard medical treatment (2) HBOT (3) HBOT + urokinase + heparin (4) HBOT + urokinase + plasma or heparin (5) HBOT + heparin	1 patient (<2 h) had excellent outcome. All 10 patients with profound coma (Grades III and IV) died. HBO treatment alone ineffective. Very complicated article—difficult to assess group assignment, time to initiation of treatment, etc. Incomplete data Conclusion: Urokinase plus HBO did the best, especially coma Grades I, II, and III, and the best results were in those patients treated in less than 6 h
Baiborodov (1981)	(1) Newborns with birth asphyxia (2) Syndrome of respiratory disturbance (3) Aspiratory syndrome	1555 2165 3110	>15 or >1030 min	1–5 min after artificial pulmonary ventilation (APV) or 1030 min after APV	HBOT 23 ATA/1.52 h for 10–15 min and 1.41.5 ATA/1.5–2.5 h	HBOT decreased cerebral circulatory disorders by 4 times and/or mortality by 8 times

Study	Condition	N	Time	Time	Treatment	Results
Mathieu et al. (1987)	Global ischemia/anoxia: Posthanging suicide attempt 88% in coma or brain dead	170 (136 HBO 34 NBO) HBO only for patients with impaired consciousness NBO patients with minor neurological problems	81% <3 h 19% >3 h	81% <3 h 19% >3 h	(1) 2.5 ATA/90 Q6H with NBO intervening until normal (2) Controls NBO	Worse coma requires more HBO. Recovery without neurological sequelae significantly better when HBO initiated <3 h posthanging (85 vs. 56%)
Kohshi et al. (1993)	Subarachnoid hemorrhage, status postaneurysm surgery Grade III and IV coma. Measure infarct incidence and Glasgow Outcome Scale on all, SPECT and EEG on some	43	Soon after onset of symptomatic vasospasm; exact time not mentioned	Soon after onset of symptomatic vasospasm; exact time not mentioned		(1) Control: mild hypertensive hypervolemia (2) HBOT 2.5 ATA/70 QD to BID. 2–21 treatments, avg. 10
Shn-Rong (1995)	Coma (95 cerebral ischemia/hypoxia: 23 near drownings, 44 near hangings, 2 electrocution, 14 narco-operation accidents, 1 Stokes–Adams, 4 barbital poisoning, 2 asphyxia, 5 Cover-Bedding syndrome; 56 of 95 with cardiac arrest). Moderate acute CO poisoning 156; serious acute CO 70 (up to 3 months coma); 12 hydrogen sulfide (2 h–20 days), 3 TBI (10, 20, and 30 days post)	336	Variable: Implied early treatment—first day	Variable: Implied early treatment—first day	(1) Ischemia/hypoxia: 2–2.5 ATA/120 × 2–3 days BID. Then 2 ATA/ variable time × up to 40 to 60 treatments (average 2–7) (2) Carbon monoxide: 2 ATA/120 BID × 1–2 days then 2 ATA/2 h QD (Avg 1–3 treatments moderate cases, 2–5 serious up to 40 total). One case, 3 months of coma treated 30, 60, and 60 treatments for a total of 150	Ischemia/hypoxia: 75% recovery of consciousness (62.5% of those with cardiac arrest, 92% without cardiac arrest) Carbon monoxide: 100% recovery in moderate poisoning, 93% in serious poisoning. Eleven of 12 recovery. TBI: 3 of 3 recovery
Sanchez et al. (1999)	Intestinal ischemia, necrotizing enterocolitis, or anoxic encephalopathy	7 neonates (3 with anoxic brain injury) over 34 weeks of age and 1200 g. All ventilator dependent	<6 h to >24 h	<6 h to >24 h	HBOT 2.0 ATA/45 min b.i.d.	All patients treated within 6 h of delivery resolved with only one treatment. Those treated after 24 h required more than one treatment, two of whom developed pulmonary oxygen toxicity which was easily treated. Sepsis, DIC, and cerebral edema resolved after one treatment. Three-month follow-up was performed

(continued)

Table 20.2 (continued)

Authors and year	Diagnosis	No. of patients	Length of coma/ neuroinsult prehyperbaric oxygen therapy (HBOT)	Timing of HBOT	HBOT protocol	Results and conclusions
Van Meter et al. (1999a)	Cardiac arrest with massive decompression illness and (?) near drowning	1	<22 min	22 min	US Navy Treatment Table 6A with 100% oxygen at 6 ATA. Converted to US Navy Treatment Table 7 air saturation decompression with intermittent 3 ATA oxygen-breathing periods	Returned to functional life. Twenty-year follow-up: patient married with children and works as a custom furniture carpenter
Mathieu et al. (2000)	Near hanging	305 (136 in Mathieu et al. 1987 study)	All patients irrespective of delay to treatment	All patients irrespective of delay	HBOT 2.5 ATA/90 min t.i.d. in the 1st 24 h then b.i.d. to total of 5 treatments	76% total recovery with 16% death rate, persistent neurological sequelae in 8%. Best results of HBO <3 h postrescue
Liu et al. (2006c)	Neonatal Hyp–Ischemic Encephalopathy; randomized and quasi-randomized controlled trials	Review–20 trials	- Birth–24 days	As soon as possible to 24 days of age	1.3–2.0 ATA/60–100 min (mostly 70 min), 1×/day, most commonly for 10 days, (exact protocol not stated or confused by use of term "courses")	Better outcomes than comparator in almost all trials. Odds ratio for mortality .26 and neurological sequelae .41 Conclusion: HBO possibly reduces mortality and neurological sequelae in neonatal HIE, however poor quality trials and reporting
Category II: Acute (>3–48 h postcerebral insult)						
Illingworth (1961)	Coma: Barbiturate overdose	1	13 h	13 h	2 ATA/95 min	Immediate benefit …later course uncomplicated
Koch and Vermeulen-Cranch (1962)	Global ischemia/anoxia after 3 min cardiac arrest	1	6 h	6 h	3 ATA/103 min (includes 60 min at 3 ATA)	Rapid recovery. Minimal visual field defect at discharge
Sharp and Ledingham (1962)	Pentobarbital overdose	1	>12 h. Patient brought to emergency room in coma; 12 h later, significant deterioration with low blood pressure, cyanosis, and assisted ventilation for 25 min. Resuscitative efforts failing	>12 h	2 ATA/65 min at depth	Rapid improvement within a few min in chamber. Discharged from hospital four days later well

Study	Condition	No. patients			HBO protocol	Results
Saltzman et al. (1966)	See earlier hyperacute period					
Heyman et al. (1966)	Coma: Various forms of cerebral ischemia	22 (2 in coma with quadriplegia, 2 stuporous or semicomatose)	(1) 4 h (2) 7 h (3) 7 days (4) 11 days	(1) 4 h (2) 7 h (3) 7 days (4) 11 days	(1) 2.36 ATA/79 × 1 (2) 2.36 ATA/45 × 1 (3) 2.0 2 ATA/26 min (4) 2.02 ATA/32 min	(1) Partial transient improvement during HBO (2) No significant change during HBO (3) No mention of immediate effect of HBOT; patient died 3 months later (4) No mention of immediate effect of HBOT; patient died 2 days later
Holbach and Caroli (1974)	Coma: Neurosurgical cases (43 traumatic brain injury (TBI), 47 CVA, 7 tumor, 3 infection, 2 ischemia); life-threatening TBI, acute CVA, severe post-op and post-TBI brain edema	102	Questionably in first 48 h	Questionably in first 48 h	(1) 52 patients: 2–3 ATA/not mentioned (2) 50 patients: 1.5 ATA/not mentioned. Overall average 2.6 HBOTs per patient	1.5 ATA group showed a significant 92 % increase in number of markedly improved patients over the 2–3 ATA group
Dordain et al. (1969)	Hepatic coma due to viral hepatitis	1	12 h	12 h	2.4 ATA/not mentioned × 3 in 24 h	Patient became normal
Mogami et al. (1969)	Coma: Severe acute cerebral damage. Measure EEG in 24 patients, CSF pressure, lactate, and pyruvate in 13	66 (51 severe acute trauma, 10 tumor, 2 CVA, 3 cerebral ischemia) Most in coma, 26 on vent	Acute cases, but length of coma not mentioned.	Acute cases, but time of initiation of HBOT not mentioned.	2 ATA/1 h QD or BID; 6 treatments at 3 ATA/30. Average 2 treatments per patient	Neurological improvement in 50 % of cases, EEG in 33 %, mostly during HBO with regression posttreatment. Best response in least injured; least response in coma patients. High variation in CSF fluid pressure, but mostly decreased during treatment with rebound posttreatment. Mixed carbon dioxide/oxygen inhalation treatment gas dangerous. Slight decrease in lactate: pyruvate in CSF
Viart et al. (1970)	See earlier hyperacute period					
Hayakawa et al. (1971)	See earlier hyperacute period. TBI patients most likely in acute period					
Voisin et al. (1973)	See earlier hyperacute period					
Holbach et al. (1974a)	Acute mid-brain syndrome with coma (traumatic brain injury)	99	Between 2nd and 10th day of intensive care	Between 2nd and 10th day of intensive care	(1) Controls-standard intensive care (2) HBOT: 1.5 ATA/45 × 1–7	Survival rate and time increased in HBO group, especially less than or equal to 30 years old. 21 % decrease in mortality and apallic state with HBO with 450 % increase in complete recovery

(continued)

Table 20.2 (continued)

Authors and year	Diagnosis	No. of patients	Length of coma/neuroinsult prehyperbaric oxygen therapy (HBOT)	Timing of HBOT	HBOT protocol	Results and conclusions
Sheffield and Davis (1976)	Prolonged cerebral hypoxia: Blind, disoriented, combative, severe thrashing disoriented with severe visual impairment at time of HBO	1	6–8 min	6.5 h	2.8 ATA (US Navy TT 6) ® US Navy TT 6A	Clearing of symptoms at 1.9 ATA, mild cognitive residual at end of 6 h treatment. Patient normal after 1.5 days
Holbach et al. (1977a)	Coma: 7 CVA, 23 TBI, all somnolent to stuporous	30	Few days	Few days postaccident		(1) Room air ® 1 ATA O₂ ® 1.5 ATA O₂ × 35–40 min ® 1 ATA O₂ room air. 10 min each stop (2) Room air ® 1 ATA O₂ ® 1.5 ATA O₂ ® 2.0 ATA O₂ ® 1.5 ATA O₂ ® 1.0 ATA O₂ ® room air
Holbach et al. (1977b)	Coma: TBI patients. High severity and acuity implied by ICP monitor and reference to comparable severe TBI patients in Holbach study earlier who were evaluated a few days postaccident. Measure CBF, blood pressure, temperature, EKG, arterial blood gases, pyruvate, and lactate. 5 % CO₂ test used to verify CO₂ reactivity of cerebral blood vessels	14	Exact time not mentioned	Exact time not mentioned	(1) 6 patients: room air ® 1 ATAO₂ ® 1.5 ATA O₂ ® 2 ATAO₂/30 min ® 1.5 ATA O₂ ® 1.0 ATA ® Room air. 15 min stops at each pressure except highest pressure (2) 8 patients: room air ® 1 ATAO₂ ® 1.5 ATA O₂ ® 2 ATAO₂ ® 2.5 ATA O₂/30 min ® 2.0 ATA O₂ ® 1.5 ATA O₂ ® 1.0 ATA O₂ ® Room air. 15 min stops at each pressure except highest pressure	Oxygen causes vasoconstriction up to 2 ATA. After about 15 min at 2 ATA and 2.5 ATA vasoconstriction is lost and 11 of 17 show marked increase in CBF with 4 of 11 having persistent increase after HBOT. This effect is nearly reversible on return to room air, but is a function of pressure and duration of oxygen exposure. CO₂ levels were stable. Simultaneously lactate decreased as proceeded to 2–2.5 ATA, but after 30 min at these pressures, no further change in lactate
Holbach (Companion to above article Holbach et al. (1977b, c)	Same as Holbach (1977b). Measure EEG	14	Same as Holbach (1977a)	Same as Holbach (1977a)	Same as Holbach (1977a)	Correlation between CBF and EEG up to 1.5 ATA with decrease in CBF and improvement in EEG. At 2.0 and 2.5 ATA there is a dissociation of vasoconstriction and EEG with severe alterations in EEG while CBF generally increases, due to oxygen toxicity. Upon return to room air, the changes are mostly reversible
Larcan et al. (1977)	See earlier hyperacute period					

Reference	N	Condition	Time	Time	Treatment	Comments
Isakov et al. (1982)	53	Coma: Acute ischemic stroke (some status postsurgery for subarachnoid hemorrhage). Includes 11 internal carotid artery and 10 vertebral-basilar artery strokes. Thirty patients in coma of varying degree. Authors measured a variety of pulmonary function parameters	<6 days poststroke or two days postsurgery	<6 days poststroke or 2 day postsurgery		Based on patients age, severity, and associated diseases. 1.6–2.0 ATA/55–90 min (exact total bottom time unclear by description) × 6–10 treatments Groups and data assignment unclear at times, but improved neurological condition in all groups and normalization of initial abnormal external respiration by eliminating pathological rhythms and decreasing hyperventilation. This effect occurred with a variable number of HBOT sessions. In the vertebral basilar artery group, significant decrease in respiratory volume and minute respiratory volume. (In 50 % stabilization of external respiration by the middle of the HBO course)
Sukoff and Ragatz (1982)	50	Coma: Acute severe traumatic cerebral edema	Approximately 6 h	Less than 6 h after admission		Group 1: 40 patients, 2 ATA/45 Q8 h × 48–96 h. Group 2: 10 patients, 2 ATA/45 Q8 h × 48 if ICP >15 after Osmitrol. Group 1: 22/40 improved. Better and more sustained results in lesser injured patients. Group 2: significant reduction in ICP
Smilkstein et al. (1985)	1	Hydrogen sulfide coma	10 h	10 h	2.5 ATA/45 initially then 2.0/75 × 1, then 2.0/90–120 TID initially to QD. Total 12 treatments	Asymptomatic at discharge, but bilateral Babinski and slight difficulty with complex tasks
Hsu et al. (1987)	1	Hydrogen sulfide coma	6 h	6 h	2.5 ATA/80 TID in first 24 h, then QD for a total of 15 treatments	Normal neurologically
Mathieu et al. (1987)		See earlier hyperacute period				
Belokurov et al. (1988)	23	Coma. Pediatrics (13 TBI, 2 subarachnoid hemorrhage, 7 hypoxia, 1 diabetic coma), measured coma score	4 h–17 days, when exclude 3 cases greater than 1 week old each, average =21.6 h	21.6 h	1.7–2.0 ATA/60 × 1/day 1–11 treatments	

(continued)

Table 20.2 (continued)

Authors and year	Diagnosis	No. of patients	Length of coma/ neuroinsult prehyperbaric oxygen therapy (HBOT)	Timing of HBOT	HBOT protocol	Results and conclusions
Rockswold et al. (1992)	Coma: Acute TBI (Glasgow Coma Scale 9 for 6 h)	168 (Randomized prospective controlled)	Average 26 h postinjury	Average 26 h postinjury	(1) 1.5 ATA/60 Q8 h × 2 weeks until brain dead or awake (avg. 21 treatments) (2) Control group: no HBO	Nearly 60 % reduction in mortality in HBO group, especially for those with ICP > 20 or GCS of 4–6
Thomson et al. (1992)	CO poisoning with persistent coma after 1st HBO treatment and normal carboxyhemoglobin	1	5.5 h	5.5 h	3 ATA × 1 2 ATA/90 BID × 3 days, QD × 10 days with 1 day break. Total 17 treatments	Normal at 5 weeks with maintenance of recovery measured by neuropsychometric testing
Dean et al. (1993)	Coma: Carbon monoxide poisoning	1	Day of poisoning	Day of poisoning	2.4 ATA/90 BID × 3 days, total 6 treatments	Awakening after 6 HBO. No evidence of significant neurological sequelae at 1 month
Kohshi et al. (1993)	See earlier hyperacute period					
Shn-Rong (1995)	See earlier hyperacute period					
Snyder et al. (1995)	Hydrogen sulfide poisoning coma, GCS = 3	1	11–12 h postexposure	11–12 h postexposure	3 ATA/60 then 2.5 ATA/90 BID × 1 day, 2.0 ATA/90 BID × 5, 2.0 ATA/90 QD × 10 23 total	Stepwise neurological improvement with HBOT. Significant cognitive residual
Yangsheng et al. (1995)	Respiratory and heart sudden stopping	27 (13 hanging, 7 electric shock, 2 cardiomyopathy, 1 overdose, 1 encephalitis-B, 1 severe CO, 1 acute anoxia, 1 severe crush injury. (Part of group of 324 patients which included CO/H2S/CN and severe TBI)	Cardiac and/or respiratory arrest, 211 min, 7 patients unknown. (?)		HBOT 2.5 ATA/60 min q.d. ×10 = 1 course. Repeat course as needed. Average 29 treatments (range, 4–50)	59 % cured, 37 % died, 4 % improved
Liu et al. (2006c)	Hypoxic/ischemic encephalopathy	Review of Chinese literature	Hours to 24 days	Hours to 24 days	1.2–2.0 ATA/60–100 min, daily, 5–50 treatments	Significant reduction in mortality and neurological sequelae
Liu et al.	See earlier Hyperacute Period					

Study	Condition / Measures	N			Treatment	Results / Conclusion
Zhou et al. (2008)	Hypoxic-Isch. Encephalopathy; Measure malondialdehyde (MDA), super-oxide dismutase (SOD), nitric oxide (NO), NO synthase, neonatal behavioral neuro assessment, (NBNA), and eye ground examination pre and post-HBO	60 neonates			Randomly administered 1.4, 1.5, or 1.6 ATA/ unstated period of time, 1×/day × 7 days	SOD higher and MDA, NO, and NOS lower in all 3 groups: all values for 1.6 group signif. better than 1.4 group while SOD and MDA signif. better 1.6 vs. 1.5 group. NBNA signif. incr. in all groups. None showed abnormal eye grounds. Conclusion: HBO with 1.4,1.5, 1.6 ATA safe and effective for neonatal HIE. Antioxidant capacity increases with increasing HBO pressure
Niu et al. (2009)	Heat Stroke/Coma. Measure GCS and laboratory values	1	Not stated		Several hours postconventional treatment in emergency department	GCS 5 on Day 1 progressed to GCS 8 on Day 4, extubated with normal core temperature and blood pressure. Discharged from hospital Day 12 with all laboratory normal
Rockswold et al. (2010)	Acute severe TBI, GCS ≤ 8, avg. 5.8 Cerebral Blood flow, Arterial-venous O_2 diff., cerebral metabolic rate of O_2, ICP, CSF lactate, F2-isoprostane, bronchial IL-6 and 8 measured pre, 1 h, and 6 h posttreatment	69	57 of 69 < 24 h, 12 < 48 h	57 of 69 < 24 h, 12 < 48 h	Group 1: Control standard care Group 2: Normobaric 100% O_2 for 3 h Group 3: HBO @ 1.5 ATA/60 min at depth NBO and HBO delivered 1×/24 h × 3 days (3 total)	HBO and NBO increase PO_2, HBO persists for at least 6 h posttreatment HBO increases CBF and $CRMO_2$ for 6 h HBO and NBO decrease CSF lactate, HBO for 5 h posttreatment. Lac/pyruv. decreased post-HBO and NBO. All parameters had most improvement when $PO_2 > 200$ (HBO). ICP lower after HBO and persists. Oxygen toxicity biomarkers no effect Conclusion: Dose–response oxygen benefit in acute severe TBI: HBO maximal No oxygen toxicity
Rockswold et al. (2013)	Acute severe TBI, GCS ≤ 8, avg. 5.7 Measure markers of cerebral metabolism, oxygen toxicity, ICP before, during, and up to 24 h posttreatment and clinical outcome after 6 months	42	37 of 42 < 24 h, 5 < 48 h	37 of 42 < 24 h, 5 < 48 h	Group 1: Control standard care Group 2: HBO @ 1.5 ATA/60 min at depth + 100% O_2 1 ATA/3 h, 1×/24 h × 3 days (3 total)	HBO/NBO: increased PO_2 normal and pericontusional brain during and posttreatment; decreased lac/pyruv. in normal brain; decreased ICP until next treatment; improved oxygen toxicity markers; improved mortality and favorable outcome Conclusion: combined HBO/NBO has better effect than either treatment alone

(continued)

Table 20.2 (continued)

Authors and year	Diagnosis	No. of patients	Length of coma/neuroinsult prehyperbaric oxygen therapy (HBOT)	Timing of HBOT	HBOT protocol	Results and conclusions
Category III: Subacute (49 h–1 month postcerebral insult)						
Heyman et al. (1966)	See earlier acute period and Saltzman study					
Holbach and Caroli (1974)	See earlier acute period					
Holbach et al. (1974)	See earlier acute period					
Artru et al. (1976a)	Coma (TBI). Measure cortical blood flow, cerebral metabolic rate for oxygen, cerebral metabolic rate glucose and lactate, glucose, lactate, and CSF parameters, (PO₂, glucose, lactate), pre and 2 1/3 h after HBO₂ 133Xenon technique	6 (3 post-op. plus 3 brainstem contusion) 12 normals plus controls with multiple sclerosis, and medical literature normal controls, all for cortical blood flow measurement	5–47 days postinjury	5–47 days postinjury	2.5 ATA/90 × 1; 1 patient 2.2 ATA 1 patient 3 studies, 1 patient 2 studies, 4 patients 1 study	Arterial PO₂ decrease in 8 of 9 patients, cortical blood flow variable due to differential effects on normal and injured brain
Artru et al. (1976b)	Coma (TBI)	60 (57 intubated or with tracheostomy) 9 subgroups	4.5 days	4.5 days	(1) 2.5 ATA/90 min QD × 10, 4 day break, repeat sequence until recovery of consciousness or die (2) No HBO	One subgroup (brainstem contusion) significantly higher rate of recovery of consciousness at 1 month with HBO and lower rate of persistent coma
Holbach et al. (1977b)	See earlier acute period					
Holbach et al. (1977c)	See earlier acute period					
Larcan et al. (1977)	See earlier hyperacute period					
Isakov et al. (1982)	See earlier acute period					
Belokurov et al. (1988)	See earlier acute period					
Kawamura et al. (1988)	Subarachnoid hemorrhage after operative intervention: 81% with vasospasm on angiography. Measure SSEPs pre, during, and after HBO. The during and postmeasurements were done on different HBOTs	26 patients (some in coma)	2–62 days after the last subarachnoid hemorrhage	2–62 days after last subarachnoid hemorrhage	HBOT 2 ATA/70 min? 1.3 ATA/10 min (loosely fitted mask during HBO treatment)	Significantly improved SSEPs during HBO in 57% of cases between 2 and 14 days posthemorrhage. Retention of effect highest in those treated within first 5 days of SAH and those with mild neurological deficits or mild brain swelling. Minimal effect in moderate to severe cases

Author	Condition	N	Timing	Timing	HBOT protocol	Results
Satoh et al. (1989)	Global ischemia/anoxia: posthanging patient in coma	1	5th hospital day	5th hospital day	Not mentioned in English abstract of Japanese author	Gradual progress
Shn-Rong (1995)	See earlier hyperacute period					
Neubauer et al. (1998)	Global ischemia/anoxia 1 Status epilepticus/hypoglycemia, 1 patient near drowning, SPECT brain imaging performed	2	Patient 1: over 1 week postinsult ambulatory, poor speech, agitated, combative Patient 2: 1.5 months post-near drowning	Patient 1: over 1 week postinsult ambulatory, poor speech, agitated, combative Patient 2: 1.5 months post-near drowning	(1) 1.5 ATA/60 total 88 (2) 154 treatments	Improved SPECT and neurological outcome in both patients
Rockswold et al. (2001)	Acute severe TBIs. GCS <8. Measure CBF, $AVDO_2$, $CMRO_2$, CSF lactate, ICP pre-, during, and post-HBOT	37	Average 23 h (9–49 h)	Delayed HBOT averaged 23 h (9–49 h)	HBO 1.5 ATA/60 min at depth q 24 h × 7 maximum, average 5/patient. 2nd Rx began >8 h after 1st treatment	Improved $CMRO_2$, and CSF lactate, especially in patients with decreased CBF or ischemia, recoupling of flow and metabolism, persistent effect lasting >6 h. reduction elevated ICP and CBF. Rec: shorter, more frequent sessions
Ren et al. (2001)	Acute severe TBI. Average GCS = 5.3 (controls), 5.1 (HBOT)	55 (20 control, 35 HBOT), randomized	"On the third day"	"On the third day"	2.5 ATA/40–60 min, ×10/4 days (1 course), × 3–4 courses	Significant improvement of: GCS and BEAM (with successive courses of HBOT), Glasgow Outcome Scale at 6 months, and morbidity and mortality
Liu et al. (2006c)	Hypoxic/ischemic encephalopathy	Review of Chinese literature	Hours to 24 days	Hours to 24 days	1.2–2.0 ATA/60–100 min, daily, 5–50 treatments	Significant reduction in mortality and neurological sequelae
Liu et al	See earlier Hyperacute Period					
Nakamura et al. (2008)	Severe TBI Initial GCS ≤ 8 Only 1 with GCS ≤ 8 at Time of HBOT Measure transcranial Doppler Mean flow velocity, and pulsatility index, arterio-jugular venous O_2 difference and jugular venous lactate	1 of 7	Subacute, after acute therapy in the ICU"	Subacute, after acute therapy in the ICU"	2.7 ATA/60 min. once/day × 5 days (total 5 treatments)	Sole patient still in coma at time of treatment. This patient and 2/6 had unfavorable outcomes. Data presented as group data so not possible to extract this patient's data. Significant group reduction in jugular venous lactate (JVL) and correlation of JVL with pulsatility index. No significant change mean flow velocity or AV O_2 difference
Zhang et al. (2009)	Coma from central pontine myelinosis postliver transplant. Moderate coma, GCS-Pittsburgh score of 20	1	9 days	9 days	? ATA/2 h, 1×/day × 14 days	Mild coma, GSC-Pittsburgh score 26 pupillary reaction, increased autonomic activities and muscle tone after HBO. At 6 months, mild coma

(continued)

Table 20.2 (continued)

Authors and year	Diagnosis	No. of patients	Length of coma/neuroinsult prehyperbaric oxygen therapy (HBOT)	Timing of HBOT	HBOT protocol	Results and conclusions
Category IV: Chronic (>1 month postcerebral injury)						
Neubauer (1985)	TBI. Prolonged coma, random selection	17	7.5 months	7.5 months	HBO 1.5 ATA/60 min, ×40–120 treatments	Average 88 % improvement on Glasgow Coma Scale. Twelve of 17 substantial improvement on GCS, five of 17 qualitatively improved
Kawamura et al. (1988)	See earlier subacute period					
Eltorai and Montroy (1991)	Coma: TBI plus anoxia	1	48 days	48 days	2 ATA/90 daily × 24	Recovery of consciousness; cognitive deficits. Extubated at day treatment center
Neubauer et al. (1989)	Global ischemia/anoxia/carbon monoxide and natural gas	1	2 years postinsult	2 years postinsult	1.5 ATA/60 × 21 treatments	Dramatic cognitive improvement and decrease in spasticity
Neubauer et al. (1992)	Global ischemia/anoxia: 12 years previously	1	12 years	12 years	1.5 ATA/60 QD, 61 treatments in 5 months	Marked neurological and cognitive improvement
Harch et al. (1994a)	Global ischemia/anoxia	4	Average age 3.25 years	Average age 3.25 years	1.5 ATA/90 QD × 80	All patients improved, some substantially. SPECT brain imaging improved
Neubauer (1995)	TBI: Coma, semiapallic	1	12 months	12 months	1.5 ATA/60 × 188	Improved from coma to ambulation and self-sufficiency
Shn-Rong (1995)	See earlier hyperacute period					
Neubauer et al. (1998)	Severe anoxic/ischemic encephalopathy: Abruptio placenta (1), near drowning (4), chokehold (1), natural gas + CO (1), and CO (1). Measured clinical outcomes and performed SPECT brain imaging before and after at least one hyperbaric treatment. SPECT and clinical outcomes measured	8	Unknown	3 months to 12 years postevent	HBOT 1.5 ATA, occasional 1.75 ATA/1 h q.d. to b.i.d. × 1, 27, 122, 181, 27, 200, 19, and >200 treatments	Clinical improvement in all patients and on SPECT
Neubauer and James (1998)	See earlier subacute period					
Montgomery et al. (1999)	Cerebral palsy. Measure gross motor functional measures (GMFM), Jebsen hand test, Ashworth spasticity scale, and video exams pre- and posttreatment	25	Unknown	Average age 5.6 years	Control each patient served as his own control	HBOT: 1.75 ATA 95 % oxygen/60 min at depth q.d., 5 days per week × 20 treatments or 1.75 ATA 95 % oxygen/60 min at depth b.i.d., 5 days per week × 20 treatments

Reference	Condition/measures	N	History	Age	Treatment	Results
Collet et al. (2001)	Cerebral palsy measure GMFM, psychometric test, and PEDI questionnaire pre, post, and 3 months after treatment	111	History of perinatal hypoxia	Average age = 7.2 years	Control 1.3 ATA air/60 min at depth q.d., 5 days per week × 40 HBOT 1.75 ATA 100 % oxygen/60 min at depth q.d., 5 days per week ×40	Improvement in GMFM in both groups which persisted at 3 months. Greatest changes in children with lowest scores which were independent of age. Improvement in language production, attention, memory, and PEDI in both groups. Caregiver scores for PEDI favored the air group. Improvement in oral facial structure and functional speech and language test in the air group
2nd International Symposium on Hyperbaric Oxygenation and the Brain Injured Child (authors: Neubauer, Harch, Chavdarov, Lobov, Zerbini 2002)	Chronic brain injury: Great majority of patients were cerebral palsy or global ischemia, anoxia and coma. Variety of tests performed including physical exam, laboratory testing, and functional brain imaging with SPECT	361	(?)	Vast majority <10 years of age	1.5–2 ATA oxygen/60–90 min q.d. to b.i.d., × 1 to >500 treatments (rare case)	Average 50 % of patients with noticeable improvements in different tests
Golden et al. (2002)	Chronic neurological disorders: CP 30 %, TBI 26 %, anoxic/ischemic encephalopathy 16 %, CVA 12 %, lyme disease 6 %, other 10 %. Measure SPECT pre, after at least 15 HBOTs, and after a course of at least 50 HBOTs	50 (25 under 18 years old and 25 over 18 years old)	Unknown	Average 5–1/3 years postinsult	HBOT 1.25–2.5 ATA/60 min b.i.d. (12 × per week)	Improvement in SPECT from first to last scan for both hemispheres and cortex with the 3rd SPECT showing more improvement than the 2nd SPECT, which was improved over the 1st. Main increase in blood flow didn't occur until after 2nd SPECT scan and a substantial number of treatments (>15). No change in blood flow to the pons and cerebellum
Hardy et al. (2002)	Cerebral palsy. Psychometric testing pre- and posttreatment	75	(?)	3–12 years of age. No average age given	Control 1.3 ATA air/60 min at depth q.d., 5 days per week × 40. HBOT 1.75 ATA oxygen/60 min at depth q.d., 5 days per week × 40	Better self-control and significant improvements in auditory attention, and visual working memory both groups. No difference between groups. Sham group significantly improved on 8 dimensions of parent rating scale vs. 1 dimension in HBO. No change in verbal span, visual attention, and processing speed in either group

(continued)

Table 20.2 (continued)

Authors and year	Diagnosis	No. of patients	Length of coma/neuroinsult prehyperbaric oxygen therapy (HBOT)	Timing of HBOT	HBOT protocol	Results and conclusions
Miura et al. (2002)	Overdose with loss of consciousness and cyanosis × unknown amount of time. Secondary deterioration fifteen days later with akinetic mutism. Measure EEG, MRI, MRS, and SPECT	1	(?)	50 days	HBO 2.0 ATA/90 min, 5 days a week × 71	Progressive improvement through 33 Rxs. Deterioration with strange behavior by 47th Rx. 52nd Rx disoriented, restless, and agitated with decreased memory. Excitability by 71st Rx requiring Valium, Tegretol, and Haldol. Behavior improved post-HBOT but disorientation and amnesia worsened. Nine months later patient better than pre-HBO. MRI, MRS, and EEG tracked patients course
Waalkes et al. (2002)	Cerebral anoxia: 8 with CP, 1 near drowning. Measured GMFM, spasticity, WEEFIM, video exams, parent questionnaire, and time spent in any 24-h. period by caregivers	9	(?)	6.4 years average age	1.7 ATA oxygen/60 min q.d., 5 days a week × 80	58 % average improvement in GMFM, minimal improvement WEEFIM. Significant reduction in time spent with caregiver in 24-h period. Patients still improving at end of study
Golden et al. (2006)	Chronic brain injury (Children: CP 29 %, TBI 26 %, HIE 17 %, Stroke 12 %, Lyme 7 %, other 9 %; adults: TBI 26 %, stroke 26 %, anoxia 21 %, hypoxia 7 %, other 20 %	21 children, 21 adults, each compared to 42 untreated brain injured and normal children or adults. Prospective, nonrandomized	Not stated	Static level of function for at least 1 year, but many patients were years postinsult. Adults were at least 2y postinsult	Not stated, but HBOT protocol well known at this clinic: 1.15–<2.0 ATA/60 q.d–b.i.d. Children: avg. 28 Rx's in 28 days. Adults: avg. 35 Rx's in 35 days	Children: significant improvement in measures of daily living, socialization, communication, and motor skills. Adults: significant improvements on all neuropsychological measures, including attention, motor, tactile, receptive and expressive language, word fluency, and immediate and delayed memory
Senechal et al. (2007)	Cerebral palsy	Review of literature	Not mentioned	Years postinsult	All published HBOT studies. Compared HBOT studies using the Gross Motor Functional Measures (GMFM) outcome to standard therapies using the GMFM	Significantly greater rate of GMFM improvement compared to all but one study which used dorsal rhizotomy. HBOT was the only therapy that also improved cognition

Study	Description	N	Age	Age	HBO protocol	Results
Harch et al. (1996a, b); Harch and Neubauer (1999; 2004)	Severe chronic TBI, near drowning, CP/autism disorder, CP, battered child. Measure clinical improvement by video. SPECT imaging, and cognitive tests in one	8	6 months–8 years	6 months–8 years	1.5 ATA/60 or 90 min total drive time 1–2×/day × 80 with 3–4 weeks break at approximately halfway point	Significant clinical gains in all patients with concomitant improvement in SPECT or cognitive tests. Reduction in seizures in one, normalization of seizure activity on EEG in another patient
Jiang et al. (2004)	Severe TBI, GCS 3–8. Measure Consciousness Recovery	175	1–12 months	1–12 months	Not stated. HBOT was 1×/day for 90 days	63% recovered consciousness: 73% w/1–3 months. Coma, 48% 4–6 months. Coma, 27% 6-12 months. Coma. 57% vs.78% with/vs. w/o brainstem injury; 46% vs. 75% with vs. w/o cerebral herniation. 53% w/ GCS 3–5, 75% w/GCS 6–8
Liu et al. (2009)	Persistent coma: trauma (9), CO (1), electrocution (1), ruptured AVM (1). All had 3 months of median nerve stimulation and were still in coma. Patients administered HBO and cervical spinal cord stimulation. Measure EEG, SPECT, GCS, and persistent vegetative state scores	12 patients 12 control	3–12 months	3–12 months	2.5 ATA/90, 1×/day, 5 days/week × 4 weeks, 1 week break, repeat (total 60 HBOTs). Spinal cord electr. stimulation 14 h/day, every day × year. Control: 3 months medial nerve stimulation before 1 year observation	6 patients in HBO emerged from coma, none in control. GCS, SPECT, PVS signif. increased in HBO grp. No tracheostomy or ventilator needed and only 1/12 with nasogastric feeding tube. No apparent improvement in control patients. Conclusion: Increase in GCS, cerebral blood perfusion in coma patients with spinal cord stimulation and HBO
Churchill et al. (2013)	Chronic anoxia, stroke, or TBI. Many with initial severe injury (54%) required inpatient rehabilitation. Measure feasibility, cognition, questionnaires, neuro exam, physical function some with speech evaluation and neuroimaging	63	1–29.3 years	1–29.3 years	1.5 ATA/60 min once/day × 60 (60 total HBOTs)	Feasibility was confirmed, although 44% required additional time to complete. Many reported symptom improvement, but generally not confirmed on standardized testing. Some significant cognitive and speech improvements, but not "clinically significant." Majority of imaged patients with significant improvement in functional imaging. 93% would participate again. No significant side effects

Review of Animal Experimental Studies

A review of the studies listed in Table 20.1 leads to the conclusion that HBO is unequivocally beneficial in acute global ischemia/anoxia regardless of treating pressure, frequency, duration, or number of treatments, but is sensitive to time to onset of HBO postinsult. Since the first publication of this chapter in the third edition of the Textbook in 1999, the data has been fortified with each successive edition of the text. Forty-five of forty-seven studies gave positive results, one study did not show any benefit, and one study used normobaric oxygen. In the complete ischemia models nearly all of the studies were performed at 2 ATA. Moody et al. (1970) showed a nearly 50 % reduction in mortality without the benefit of artificial ventilation using a prolonged 2 ATA exposure (4 h). Mrsic-Pelcic et al. (2004a) performed two metabolic studies assessing delay to HBOT as long as 168 h and found that HBOT at 2 ATA could prevent decline of ATPase and increase SOD in hippocampus if initiated as late as 24 h and 168 h, respectively. When they looked at the optic nerve (Mrsic-Pelcic et al. 2004b), however, HBO was effective with ATPase only if begun within 6 h of ischemia and had no effect on SOD regardless of time of initiation. Clinical parameters were not measured in either study, but it appears that optic nerve is more sensitive to complete global ischemia. Yatsuzuka (1991) generated a significant decrease in ICP and oxidative stress metabolites with a 2 ATA/170 min staged protocol. The sole lower pressure study by Kapp et al. (1982) measured EEG recovery time and CSF lactate change, demonstrating significant improvement at 1.5 ATA, for a prolonged 2.5 h. Ruiz et al. (1986) was the only insignificant result with a 2 ATA/1 h exposure, but this lack of efficacy may be partially explained by hemodilution with hetastarch prior to HBO.

The studies with possibly the greatest clinical implication for neonatal ischemic/hypoxic birth injury were the two studies by J. Chen et al. (2009), Chen and Chen 2010). Using the pregnant uterine harvest/global ischemia model of Bjelke et al. (1991), Chen demonstrated that HBOT at 2 ATA begun 24 h after ischemia and continued daily for 14 days improved synaptic transmission efficiency, electrophysiologic conduction velocity, reduced neuronal death and improved ultrastructure in the hippocampus, and improved cognition in rats 4 weeks after the hypoxic/ischemic insult. The HBO salvage effect was so extensive that no statistical difference could be measured between control rats and HBO-treated hypoxic/ischemic rats in cognition, hippocampal ultrastructure, and synaptic plasticity. These studies reaffirm the clinical studies in Table 20.2, especially the review of Chinese HBOT neonatal ischemic/hypoxic encephalopathy studies.

Using higher pressures, Takahashi et al. (1992), Iwatsuki et al. (1994), Krakovsky et al. (1998), and Zhou et al. (2003) at 3 ATA, Mink and Dutka (1995a, b) at 2.8 ATA, and Rosenthal et al. (2003) at 2.7 ATA obtained statistically sig-

nificant positive results on survival, neurological recovery, and various physiological or metabolic measures. In the Rosenthal experiment survival improved with increased oxygen extraction ratio but without a change in oxygen delivery or cerebral metabolic rate for oxygen, suggesting an improvement of the microcirculation similar to the Zamboni et al. (1993) HBO/peripheral global ischemia reperfusion model in rats. The Zhou experiment underscored the more permanent gene-signaling trophic effects of early HBO by showing a persistent elevation of Ng-R and RhoA, which are both associated with the inhibition of growth cone collapse, i.e., improvement of growth. Despite the tissue slice model of the (Gunther et al. 2004) experiment the results were interesting because they suggested equal sensitivity of pathological targets to both HBO and NBO very early after ischemia (5 min), but only HBO had a positive effect after 30 min of ischemia. In addition, only the HBO dosage had any effect on morphology regardless of early or later initiation. These results reinforce the points made in the introduction to this chapter about hyperbaric dosage differences with evolving pathology and the possible difference in efficacy of HBO depending on the route of delivery. The dose by aviator mask is lower than by oxygen hood or in a pure oxygen environment. Similarly, the dose of HBO in tissue slices is markedly different when 1 ATA and 3 ATA oxygen are used. Lastly, the study by Mink and Dutka (1995b) had conflicting results with a simultaneous decrease in brain vascular permeability and blood flow while somatosensory evoked potentials were unchanged. This implies concomitant beneficial and detrimental effects which are difficult to explain without more data.

The five Van Meter et al. (1988, 1999b, 2001a, b, 2008) studies are unique in that they showed resuscitation of animals using HBO, rather than delivering HBO after resuscitation as in the Rosenthal article. These combined experiments were dose–response evaluations of HBO at 1.0, 2.0, 2.8, 4.0, and 6.0 ATA. The swine study proved the ability of 4 ATA HBO to resuscitate animals after 25 min of cardiac arrest, simultaneously truncating white blood cell-independent brain lipid peroxidation. This is the longest successful arrest/resuscitation reported in the medical literature and has profound implications for application to human cardiac arrest (see Chaps. 42 and 43, HBO in Emergency Medicine). In 14 of the 20 studies the benefit of HBO was generated with one treatment, in two studies with three treatments, in two studies with seven treatments, and in the remaining two studies with 14 treatments. No consensus emerges for the ideal dose of HBO after complete global ischemia since only one study was done at less than 2.0 ATA, but the Van Meter dose–response study suggests that, at least in one model the maximal beneficial effect may be at doses nearly double the maximal clinical dose (6 ATA). More importantly, in the 20 studies, a beneficial effect on global ischemia, anoxia, and coma was demonstrated even when the ischemic insult was as long as 1 h (two studies) and the delay to treatment as long as 24 h after the ischemic insult (Zhou et al. 2003; J. Chen et al. 2009, Chen and Chen 2010).

The results are similarly impressive and uniformly positive in the group of incomplete global ischemia/anoxia experiments. As in the complete models no consensus emerges as to best HBO pressure, duration, frequency, or number of treatments, but time to intervention remains a dominant theme. With greater delay to treatment the beneficial effect of HBOT is less; however, this effect can be increased by increasing numbers of treatments out to 96 h postinsult (Wang et al. 2009). Shiokawa et al. (1986) demonstrated an improvement in survival with 2 ATA HBO for only 30 min, with best results at three hours postinsult as opposed to one hour. Weinstein et al. (1986) achieved an 84 % reduction in mortality with a 15 min 1.5 ATA treatment and Grigor'eva et al. (1992) demonstrated a superior effect of 1.2 ATA/30 min over 2 ATA/60 min on survival and preservation of neuronal transcription. Yaxi et al. (1995) and Yiqun et al. (1995) both showed improvements in brain enzymatic function from a single HBO treatment at 2.5 ATA with the Yaxi article suggesting a minimum 20–40 min duration of HBO exposure for efficacy. Konda et al. (1996), meanwhile, showed that repetitive HBO at 2 ATA/60 preserves hippocampal neurons and decreases heat shock proteins; there was a greater effect when the HBO was started at 6 h instead of 24 h. Essentially, HBO prevented delayed cell death (apoptosis) without oxygen toxicity. This antiapoptotic effect or preservation of neurons was also proven by Calvert et al. (2002, Calvert and Zhang 2005), Li et al. (2005)), indirectly by Liu XH (2006b), Liu M-N (2006a), Liu et al. (2007), Wang et al. (2008), Wang et al. (2009), S Chen et al. (2009), Liu et al. (2013), Malek et al. (2013), Yin et al. (2013), and Zhu et al. (2015). The Zhu study showed that this effect occurred in the absence of oxidative stress despite 7 HBOTs. The Wang et al. (2009) study extended the time window to 96 h postischemia, but showed a waning time-dependent effect that could be increased with repetitive course of HBOT. All of these studies were performed at 2–3 ATA. The Li and S Chen (2009) articles underscored the complexity of the microscopic brain injury milieu and the myriad of possible targets by its beneficial effect on apoptosis while increasing pro-apoptotic Caspase 8 and decreasing antiapoptotic bcl-2 (Li) and the Caspase-3 and Nogo-A pathways (S Chen). In Calvert's 2005 article the antiapoptotic effect occurred with both 3ATA and 1ATA.

All remaining incomplete global ischemia models used 1.2-3 ATA and varying numbers of treatments, indicating that the intermittency of dosing pioneered in HBO therapy maybe more important than the actual dose of oxygen. One study (Malek et al. 2013) suggested that the effect on neuronal survival was secondary to the prevention of brain temperature increase after ischemia which was primarily due to the increase in pressure, not oxygen. The data in these multiple studies suggests that early after incomplete or complete global ischemia pathological targets may be sensitive to a wide range of oxygen and pressure doses as long as they are short.

The clinical importance of all of these incomplete global ischemia studies is that, along with the Hai et al. (2002) study, they used similar animal models to simulate human neonatal ischemia/hypoxia, a research and clinical subject of intense interest that has been heightened by review of the important neonatal resuscitation paper by Hutchison et al. (1963) in the 1999 edition of this textbook. In the Hai study repetitive 2.5 ATA HBO delivered 7 days postinsult had a signal induction effect on brain fibroblastic growth factor (bFGF) while also increasing the amount of bFGF; bFGF increase also occurred in the hyperbaric air group. Most importantly, the studies that concurrently measured apoptosis, neuronal density, and functional (cognitive, motor, and behavior) outcomes showed that the histological improvements co-occurred with the functional improvements. Calvert et al. (2002), Liu XH (2006b), Liu M-N (2006a), Liu et al. (2007), S Chen et al. (2009), and Liu et al. (2013) all showed that the short-term effect on apoptosis, neuronal density, and improved morphology/histology with either one or two early HBO treatments translated to improved behavioral/neurological outcomes at 5–6 weeks. Wang et al. (2008) demonstrated the same effect with seven HBOTs up to 12 h after ischemia, Malek et al. (2013) with three treatments and a 6 h delay, and Zhu et al. (2015) with seven treatments and 72 h delay. Chen and Chen (2009) was able to demonstrate a similar histological effect paired with improved electrophysio-logical function using 14 treatments 24 h after ischemia, while Wang et al. (2007b) demonstrated white matter preservation and improved cognition/motor function 12 h after ischemia. These studies underscore the Hutchison clinical findings and strongly argue for additional human application of these animal findings. In particular, the white matter preservation in Wang et al. (2007b) has significant implication for the periventricular leukomalacia in cerebral palsy CP.

The remaining significant anatomic benefit of HBOT in the incomplete global ischemia models is the effect on stem cells. The studies by Yu et al. (2006), Wang et al. (2007a), Wang et al. (2008), Yang et al. (2008), and Yin et al. (2013) are important for the demonstration of increased stem cells with 7 HBO' treatments at 2 ATA up to 24 h after ischemia. In the Yang study these stem cells migrated to cerebral cortex by 14 days and new tissue growth was seen at 28 days. These findings underscore the known trophic effects of HBOT in noncentral nervous system models and suggest a similar process in the chronic brain injury study of HBO (Harch et al. 2007). The underlying mechanism in the acute phase of injury may be due to HBO effects on HIF-1α, which was demonstrated at both 2.5 and 1 ATA (Calvert et al. 2006), the Wnt-3 signaling pathway (Wang et al. 2007a), and the bone morphogenetic protein-4 and nestin pathways (Yin et al. 2013).

The only equivocal study (Mickel et al. 1990) showed that normobaric oxygen (NBO) gave mixed results: increased production of white matter lesions while sparing cortical neurons. Lastly, the Wada et al. (1996) study, the only model with preischemic HBO, proved an antiapoptotic effect of HBO. This is somewhat similar to the protective effect of precarbon monoxide exposure HBO in the Thom (1993a) model. Despite the inability to establish clear guidelines regarding HBO parameters in incomplete global ischemia/anoxia, the results of HBO treatment have been uniformly positive across the range of ischemic exposures (up to 3.5 h), with delays in starting HBO treatments up to 7 days, treatment pressures as low as 1.2 ATA and HBO durations as short as 15 min.

Most of the earlier studies initiated HBO within three hours of insult and showed positive results with a maximum of seven treatments and in most cases only one. The exceptions, however, represent 20 % of the studies and they demonstrate HBOT-induced improvements in anatomic, biochemical, histological, and genomic parameters with delay to treatment up to 96 h after ischemia and functional improvements up to 72 h after ischemia. Simultaneously, no overt oxygen toxicity has been demonstrated. The near uniform success of all of the earlier animal experiments suggests that preischemic HBO or single HBO soon after ischemia, possibly as late as 6 h, is highly beneficial and probably the most important factor in positive outcomes while the absolute HBO pressure is less important. With increasing delays to treatment greater numbers of treatment are required to obtain the same or near-same result. Even NBO appears to have a positive effect in some models, but the effect is generally much less than the HBO effect. The consistency of data reinforces the earlier discussion (vide supra) where global ischemia may activate the microcirculation and when this occurs, provides a convenient HBO target, white blood cells, however a great diversity of targets is suggested by the gene studies (Godman et al. 2009). The only exceptions to this conclusion are the Van Meter studies which strongly suggest that HBO pressures of at least 2.8 ATA and ideally 4–6 ATA are necessary for resuscitation from cardiac arrest. Interestingly, this model showed no effect on a derivative pathology of WBC involvement, myelopreoxidase.

Review of Human Clinical Studies

The human HBO experience in cerebral ischemia/anoxia and coma is extensive, complicated, incomplete at times, and spread across multiple medical conditions. Despite the heterogeneous group of studies, the data shows a beneficial effect of HBO, especially in the large series and particularly in traumatic brain injury (TBI).

Since the last edition of this chapter a number of important reviews have been published that support HBO across the time spectrum in pediatric neurologic injury. This data is consistent with previous reports and the above-mentioned animal studies. To facilitate review of the literature all reports have been categorized somewhat arbitrarily by amount of time delay to initiation of HBO. Some reports span multiple categories and are unclear about exact times of HBO intervention. In these a rough estimate was attempted based on the implications and inferences in the study, and references to companion articles. The four categories are hyperacute (less than or 3 h postinsult), acute (4–48 h post), subacute (49 h to 1 month post), and chronic (greater than 1 month after insult).

The studies of Mathieu et al. (1987, 2000), Voisin et al. (1973), Hutchison et al. (1963), Kohshi et al. (1993), Shn-Rong (1995), Larcan et al. (1977), Viart et al. (1970), Hayakawa et al. (1971), Saltzman et al. (1966), Ingvar and Lassen (1965), Baiborodov (1981), Sanchez et al. (1999), and Van Meter et al. (1999a) address the hyperacute period of global ischemia/anoxia and coma. The most clear-cut of these are the studies reported by Mathieu et al. (1987) and Hutchison et al. (1963). Mathieu used HBO in 170 cases of unsuccessful hanging, 34 of whom received NBO and 136 HBO, and found statistically significant greater recovery without sequelae if HBO was delivered <3 h posthanging (85 vs. 56 %). Worse coma required more treatment, but even the worst only averaged 3.9 HBOs. The 34 NBO patients were those with minor neurological problems; only patients with impaired consciousness received HBO. The pressure used in this study was 2.5 ATA/90 min. HBO for near hanging had become the standard of care at Mathieu's facility in northern France following installation of the HBO chamber in 1968 and the results of their historically controlled study of 1973 (Voisin). The study compared 14 patients with standard treatment (normobaric oxygen) pre-1968 to 35 patients with HBO after 1968. HBO reduced mortality by 39 % and neurological sequelae by 59 %. The authors stated that HBO provided "a recovery both quicker and of better quality." This series of 170 patients has been extended to 305 patients (Mathieu et al. 2000) with nearly identical results, again strongly arguing for HBO-responsive pathology within the first few hours of rescue from near hanging. These are similar to the initial results (79 %) reported by Hutchison et al. (1963) in resuscitation from neonatal asphyxia, but one-third of those patients regressed after the first treatment. Overall, 54 % were discharged from the hospital as "well." HBO was used at 2–4 ATA in this study and treatment was initiated 2–38 min after birth. These findings were replicated by Baiborodov (1981) at 2 to 3 ATA and 1.4–1.5 ATA in 555 infants. Although the HBO protocol is confusing and the details of the paper are limited due to publication of only the abstracts [the manuscripts were too numerous (300) and subsequently lost in a fire at one of the editors' homes] the eightfold reduction in mortality is compelling and consistent with Hutchison's data. More recently (Sanchez et al. 1999) has reported the same positive findings at 2 ATA in a small number of infants. Altogether these experiences with HBO in neonatal ischemia/hypoxia/"asphyxia" are remarkable and significantly supported by the animal data, particularly the Calvert et al. (2002) model.

Most of the other papers in this group imply hyperacute and acute treatment or do not state the time of HBO intervention. Kohshi et al. (1993) initiated HBO soon after onset of symptomatic vasospasm in subarachnoid hemorrhage postneurosurgical comatose patients using 2.5 ATA and an average 10 treatments which decreased subsequent progression to infarcts. Shn-Rong (1995) applied HBO in 336 cases of cardiac arrest, near drowning, unsuccessful hanging, electrocution, carbon monoxide, TBI, and other toxic and asphyxial coma patients, implying at least some treatment hyperacutely, with 75–100 % recovery rates at 2–2.5 ATA. Best results were with earlier treatment; delays to treatment required greater numbers of HBOs. Most remarkable was the 62.5 % resuscitation from cardiac arrest, a rate far exceeding the resuscitation rate from cardiac arrest in developed countries. In the Larcan et al. (1977) paper it appears that only one patient was treated in the hyperacute period with both urokinase and HBO. The result was excellent and the best in their study, but the effect cannot be necessarily attributed to HBO alone. The Viart et al. (1970) paper does not mention time to HBO in the three cases of infant hepatic coma, but the profile of HBO seemed extreme since 1 patient died of pulmonary oxygen toxicity with 36 h of HBO and the other two experienced cardiac conduction abnormalities during HBO, an extremely rare complication of HBO. Despite the apparent complications, all 3 patients had normalization of consciousness, EEG, and neurological exam with HBO, two permanently and one transiently. Hayakawa et al. (1971) performed a single 2ATA/1 h HBO immediately after surgery on four comatose brain tumor patients and 9 acute TBI patients. The time to initiation of HBO was not stated but was probably <3 h in the postoperative patients. The authors found 3 patterns of CSF pressure and clinical response that corresponded to differential effects on normal and injured brain; HBO decreases edema in injured brain and produces edema in normal brain. Most patients had an initial decrease of CSF pressure with HBO and then return to pre-HBO level at the end of HBO. The patients with a major decrease in CSF pressure during HBO had remarkable clinical improvement and a mild neurological deficit If there was no change in CSF pressure the reverse was true. The duration of the HBO neurological improvement was not mentioned.

The coma case reported by Ingvar and Lassen (1965) showed a transient rapid awakening of a patient with "failing circulation" but died at the conclusion of a 2–2.5 ATA/1.5–2.5 h HBO. This could be the natural history of the patient's disease and/or an oxygen toxicity effect. The other single case reports are of a "dramatic" near-complete cure of a suspected air embolism patient treated with a 2.36 ATA/5 h session of HBO (Saltzman et al. 1966) and the example of AGE, massive DCS, and cardiac arrest (Van Meter et al. 1999a). The Saltzman treatment was similar to the United States Navy Treatment Table VI for air embolism and serious decompression sickness and may explain the near-complete cure without oxygen toxicity after a higher pressure very prolonged oxygen exposure (5 h). The Van Meter case also used a very prolonged deep oxygen exposure, 6 ATA pure oxygen on a modified US Navy TT6A extended to a US Navy TT7 with oxygen breathing periods at 3 ATA. This case spawned the guinea pig and swine resuscitation experiments (Van Meter et al. 1988, 1999b, 2001a, b, 2008). The success of the Saltzman and Van Meter cases are likely due to the large proportion of the pathology caused by intravascular gas. Overall, the preponderance of data in these 14 HBO studies and 1,388 global ischemia/anoxia and coma patients is strongly positive with pressures greater than or equal to 2 ATA and a minimum of 1–7 treatments.

The publication of (Liu Z 2006c) deserves particular attention since it is a review of 20 randomized or "quasi-randomized" controlled Chinese studies. While there are many methodological criticisms of the studies, there is an overwhelming consistency of the results between the 20 studies and with the earlier 14 studies in this category, which show a reduction in mortality and neurological sequelae with HBO in term neonates (>36 weeks gestation) with hypoxic/ischemic encephalopathy. It appears likely that most of the patients treated were beyond the 3 h time limit of this category, falling into the acute category. The pressures used were 1.3–1.7 ATA, which is supportive more of the pressures used in the acute category, particularly for TBI. These lower pressures are similar to the pressure (<2 ATA) used by Baiborodov in his pediatric study.

Thirty-six studies fall into the second or acute category. Once again the preponderance of data is positive, either transiently or permanently, regardless of the etiology of coma. Kohshi et al. (1993), Mathieu et al. (1987), Voisin et al. (1973), Shn-Rong (1995), Viart et al. (1970), and Liu Z et al. (2006c) papers span this and the hyperacute period and were already reviewed. The Larcan et al. (1977) study had one patient in the hyperacute period mentioned earlier and 35 coma patients in the acute period. HBO appeared to have no effect and, in fact, was no different from the medical treatment group, but the data is incomplete, lacking a pure urokinase group and exact times to initiation of treatment. All ten severe coma patients died with lesser coma grades I–III showing the best response to combined urokinase plus HBO, and minimization of time to treatment the best predictor of success. The Saltzman et al. (1966) report also had one patient in both the hyperacute and acute periods. The acute patient had an embolic clot CVA and was treated 5 h post-CVA at 2.02 ATA/>1 h with near total permanent improvement. Lastly, nine TBI patients of (Hayakawa et al. 1971) 13 patients were most likely in the acute period, but the results have already been summed earlier.

Of the remaining 24 studies, 15 were at pressures greater than or equal to 2 ATA (Sharp and Ledingham 1962, Heyman et al. 1966; Mogami et al. 1969, Sukoff and Ragatz 1982, Thomson et al. 1992, Dean et al. 1993; Snyder et al. 1995, Yangsheng 1995, Dordain et al. 1969, Illingworth et al. 1961, Koch 1962, Hsu and Li 1987, Smilkstein et al. 1985, Sheffield and Davis 1976); 10 used 1.5 ATA (Holbach et al. 1974, Holbach and Caroli 1974, Holbach et al. 1977a, b, c; Rockswold et al. 1992; Rockswold et al. 2001; Niu et al. 2009; and Rockswold et al. 2010, 2013); 1 used 1.4, 1.5, or 1.6 ATA; and two used 1.6–2 ATA (Belokurov et al. 1988; Isakov et al. 1982); with near uniform transient or permanent positive results. Four of the ten 1.5 ATA reports (Holbach and Caroli 1974; 1977a, b, c) compared 1.5 ATA to either 2, 2.5, or 2–3 ATA and demonstrated better results at 1.5 ATA, using a variety of clinical, biochemical, and physiological outcome measures. Six of the ten studies (Holbach et al. 1974, 1977a, b, c; Rockswold et al. 1992, 2001) initiated treatment >24 h after injury. Three of these (Holbach and Caroli 1974; Holbach et al. 1977b, c) do not mention time to treatment, but imply treatment in the acute period since the patients are neurosurgical cases and they are reported incidentally in the study on cerebral glucose metabolism in acute brain-injured patients which is a preliminary version of patients who were a "few days" postinjury (Holbach et al. 1977a). The fourth and fifth 1.5 ATA papers of Holbach (Holbach et al. 1977b, c; Rockswold et al. 2010, 2013) span the acute and subacute periods and are similar patients to those in the other Holbach and Rockswold papers, respectively. In Holbach and Caroli (1974) 1.5 ATA had significantly better clinical results than 2–3 ATA. This is confirmed with CBF measurements (Holbach et al. 1977b), EEG (Holbach et al. 1977c), and cerebral glucose metabolism (Holbach et al. 1977a) where 15–30 min excursions to 2 and 2.5 ATA caused deterioration in the measured parameters. While the Holbach et al. (1977a) experiment did not explore pressures between1.5 and 2 ATA, the Belokurov study affirmed the efficacy of 1.7–2 ATA pressures in 23 comatose children with 100 % recovery of consciousness. Their results were maximal in TBI (13 of 23 patients) and if initiated <24 h postcoma. Similarly, Isakov et al. (1982) experienced good results between 1.6 and 2 ATA in patients with cerebrovascular accidents.

The final two studies in this category suggest HBOT benefit in a single case of heat stroke using 1.5 ATA for 6 treatments (Niu et al. 2009) and reaffirm HBO benefit in neonatal ischemic/hypoxic encephalopathy (Zhou, et al. 2008). Zhou, et al. (2008) compared 1.4, 1.5, and 1.6 ATA HBOT 1×/day for 7 days and showed improvement in neonatal behavioral neuro assessment in all groups and an improvement in antioxidant and decrease in lipid peroxidation indices. The great-

est effect on antioxidant defense and least lipid peroxidation was in the 1.6 ATA group. These results are consistent with the Liu Z et al. (2006c) review and suggest a beneficial clinical and biochemical effect of HBOT in neonatal ischemic/hypoxic encephalopathy.

The importance of the studies in the Acute Period is the dominant data on HBOT in acute severe TBI. The Rockswold and Holbach studies deserve special emphasis. Both represent a series of progressive studies by independent neurosurgical groups on the same clinical entity, acute severe traumatic brain injury. Holbach demonstrated the benefit of 1.5 ATA HBOT vs. higher doses of HBOT. Rockswold reaffirmed the benefit of 1.5 ATA and refined the dosing of HBOT. Rockswold et al. (2001) was an elegant follow-up study to Rockswold et al. (1992)) to evaluate the cerebral and biochemical physiological effects of 1.5 ATA HBO on acute severe TBI. The authors demonstrated that 30 min total dive time had achieved the maximum reduction of elevated ICP in chamber, one HBO recoupled flow/metabolism in injured brain and reduced lactate levels, and the HBO changes persisted at least six h after HBOT. The importance of the study is its duplication of the Holbach studies" elucidation of HBO effects on pathophysiology in acute severe TBI and the underpinning of all of the clinical studies, most notably the Rockswold et al. (1992) study with its HBO induced 47–59 % reduction in mortality. Rockswold et al. (2010) refined the dosing by investigating the combined effects of HBOT and normobaric oxygen vs. HBOT and normobaric oxygen alone. HBO/NBO had the greatest metabolic improvement without signs of oxygen toxicity. Rockswold et al. (2013) confirmed the clinical benefit of improved metabolic indices with a reduction in mortality and improvement in functional outcomes. The TBI studies of Holbach, Rockswold, and Ren et al. (2001) all demonstrated a 50–60 % reduction in mortality and improved clinical outcome with HBOT that emphatically argue for HBO in acute severe TBI. 629 of the 877 patients reviewed in this category (excluding Kohshi, Mathieu, Voisin, Shn-Rong, and Viart) had TBI; the data strongly argues for the routine use of HBO in TBI at 1.5 ATA. Overall, treatment courses tended to be longer in the acute category than the hyperacute, using higher HBO pressures earlier (less than or equal to 24 h) and lower pressures later, with overall positive effects regardless of coma etiology: chemical/toxic gas, trauma, CVA, surgery, etc.

In the third category, subacute (49 h–1 month) 16 studies are presented. The papers of Holbach et al. (Holbach and Caroli 1974; Holbach et al. 1974, Holbach et al. 1977b, c), Larcan et al. (1977), Shn-Rong (1995), Isakov et al. (1982), Belokurov et al. (1988), and Liu Z et al. (2006c) were discussed earlier, but to reiterate, many of the TBI cases of Holbach started HBO 2–10 days postinjury. Results were positive and favored treatment at 1.5 ATA for 1–7 times. Lareng et al. (1973) reported two additional late TBI coma cases and had excellent outcomes with prolonged treatment at 2.0 ATA. In the Shn-Rong series a number of carbon monoxide cases presented with > 6 days of coma. In general, they required more treatment, and one case of 90 day coma was cured finally with normal EEG after 150 treatments in three stages. Three patients with TBI coma of 10, 20, and 30 days regained consciousness after 7–20 treatments. Almost all except the initial few treatments were at 2 ATA. Two additional TBI studies by (Artru et al. 1976a, b) and a study by Nakamura et al. (2008) had mixed results. The first involved 60 TBI patients 4.5 days postinjury, HBO at 2.5 ATA, and an average 10 treatments with multiple breaks in protocol, and few receiving much treatment in the first week. Only one of nine subgroups (brainstem contusion) achieved significant improvement with HBO (see earlier discussion on penumbra/umbra size considerations in brainstem vs. cortical coma). The second study with 6 patients, 5–47 days postinsult, examined blood flow, metabolism, and CSF biochemistry before and after 2.5 ATA HBO. Results were inconclusive, but arterial partial pressure of oxygen declined in 8 of 9 patients, CSF oxygen remained elevated above baseline for 2 h after HBO, and the authors concluded that HBO has different effects on normal and injured brain circulation. Nakamura studied 7 TBI patients with initial GCS less than or equal to 8 with five 2.7 ATA HBOTs. The sole patient still in coma at time of treatment and 2/6 other patients had unfavorable outcomes, despite group improvement in some nonclinical indices All three of these studies featured high pressure, 2.5 or 2.7 ATA, later in the course of illness and are consistent with an oxygen toxicity effect as Holbach demonstrated in multiple reports earlier.

In contrast, the randomized, prospective-controlled Ren et al. (2001) study reported significant positive results in acute severe TBI using a high-pressure protocol and intensive dosing of HBOT. The treatment regimen was ten 2.5 ATA/60 min HBO treatments in 4 days, repeated in blocks up to a total of 40 HBO treatments. The patients experienced improvement in BEAM, GCS, and Glasgow Outcome Scale. The results are hard to reconcile with the Holbach and Artru data, and questions are raised about the uneven numbers of patients in the control (20) and HBO (35) groups for a randomized study. Despite this intensive high dose of HBO, there was no report of complications in the study.

The final five studies involve subacute global ischemia or coma cases. (Heyman et al. 1966), subarachnoid hemorrhage with postoperative vasospasm (Kawamura et al. 1988), posthanging (Satoh et al. 1989), status epilepticus/hypoglycemia (Neubauer and James 1998), and central pontine myelinosis coma status postliver transplant (Zhang, et al. 2009). Heyman did not mention immediate effects at 2.02 ATA, Kawamura noted sustained improvement in SSEPs at 2 ATA, Satoh noted "gradual progress" of his unsuccessful hanging patient, Neubauer found significant progress at 1.5 ATA, and Zhang

noted benefit but does not mention the dose of HBOT. In summary, with delay to treatment of 2–30 days generally positive results are achieved with HBO with a tendency to lower pressures and longer treatment courses.

The final category, chronic (>1 month), now has 22 studies, most of which address pediatric brain injury. Six of these are single cases and the remainder are prospective and retrospective case series, prospective controlled and uncontrolled trials, and a review article. All of the reports used 1.5– 2.0 ATA oxygen with most <1.75 ATA, except for Golden et al. (2002, 2006) and Miura et al. (2002), which used 1.25–2.5 ATA (2002) or <2.0 ATA (2006) and 2.0 ATA, respectively, Liu et al. (2009) which used 2.5 ATA, and Jiang et al. (2004), which did not mention pressure. Treatment times were mostly <60 min at depth and extended from 1 to over 500 treatments; most involved 40–80 treatments. The 2nd International Symposium studies were grouped together due to their heterogeneity of subjects, protocols, and hypotheses. For example, the Harch (2002) article addressed and identified oxygen toxicity and/or negative side effects of lower pressure HBO in chronic brain-injured patients with prolonged treatment courses at 1.5 ATA (average 119 treatments) and 1.75 ATA (91 treatments) or early in treatment at 1.75 ATA or greater. In addition, a withdrawal syndrome (4 patients) was described in brain-injured individuals habituated to 1.75 ATA HBO. In two of these four cases the author intervened and truncated the neurological deterioration with additional HBO at a lower pressure. These toxicity findings were reaffirmed by Miura et al. (2002) in a case of delayed neuropsychiatric sequelae from drug overdose complicated by hypoxia. The patient recovered acutely then deteriorated to akinetic mutism. The authors initiated HBO at 2.0 ATA/ 90 min and the patient improved then worsened during prolonged HBO, identical to cases in Harch (2002). The behavioral problems slowly abated upon cessation of HBO, but his cognitive decline continued. The case suggests overtreatment with HBO resulting in transient and permanent negative side effects against a background of permanent clinical improvement. MRI FLAIR, MRS, and EEG tracked the clinical course in a manner that was almost identically to the SPECT findings in the cases of Harch (2002). The Liu report is difficult to reconcile with this body of data in that the patients were treated at 2.5 ATA for 60 treatments. Nevertheless, Liu reported improvement in his patients.

The Churchill Study (2013) deserves special mention because it was a prospective study with numerous and detailed functional outcome measures that was designed to test feasibility and to replicate the functional imaging and clinical outcomes reported by Neubauer and Harch in multiple case series and case reports. The study utilized the same 1.5 ATA/60 min dose of HBOT used by Neubauer and Harch, but for only 60 HBOTs instead of the blocks of 40 (typically 80) used by Harch in the Perfusion/Metabolism Encephalopathy Study from 1994 to 1999 (Harch 2010). The majority of patients were survivors of severe anoxia, stroke, or TBI. The results generally duplicated the results reported by Neubauer and Harch with symptomatic improvement, some cognitive and speech improvement, and importantly, functional imaging improvements with the same pattern of normalization of blood flow seen in SPECT images in this text (Harch et al. 1996b; Harch and Neubauer 1999, 2004, Neubauer et al. 2004) and other publications (Harch, et al. 2012, all Neubauer studies earlier). The article concluded that clinically significant improvements were not achieved, but this may be more a reflection of the authors' definition of significant clinical improvement. Patients with chronic neurological residua from severe anoxic, ischemic, and traumatic injuries have lost significant amounts of brain tissue. Although HBOT has trophic stimulatory effects through gene modulation it is unreasonable to expect reinnervation of significantly denervated brains in 3 months, especially long white matter tract growth. It suggests that more treatment and a longer followup may generate further gains.

One of the most important additions to this category is the (Senechal report 2007). This study is described in detail in the chapter on cerebral palsy. In short, improvements in gross motor functional measures were the highest, fastest, and most durable in HBOT studies compared to studies using the GMFM for other types of therapies with the exception of two dorsal rhizotomy studies. The second important addition is the Golden et al. (2006) study, a controlled nonrandomized study of HBOT in a group of children and adults with chronic stable brain injury. Both groups showed significant improvements in nearly all measures after 28–35 HBO treatments at low pressure.

In conclusion, additional experience with HBO in chronic global ischemia, anoxia and coma that was supported by SPECT, standardized motor, and psychometric testing has accumulated in the past 5 years, strongly suggesting a positive trophic effect of HBO. These results are underpinned by the addition of the sole animal study in the literature that demonstrated a highly correlated improvement in vascular density and cognition using an HBO protocol originally designed for humans and used in many of the human studies earlier (Harch et al. 2007). This animal study strongly reinforces the human studies, especially in TBI, and argues for further application of HBO to other chronic forms of brain injury. The consistent findings in all of these studies in the late period were recovery of consciousness and that the longer to initiation of HBOT in patients with persistent coma, the less likely is recovery of consciousness.

Case Studies

To illustrate the effect of HBO in both acute and chronic global cerebral ischemia/anoxia and coma several cases treated by these authors are presented later. In each case the

visual medium of SPECT brain blood flow imaging on a high resolution scanner (7 mm; Picker Prism 3000) registers in a global fashion the neurocognitive clinical improvement experienced by the patients and witnessed by the authors. The SPECT brain scans presented later are CT technology with the patient's left brain on the reader's right and vice versa, with the 30 frame images registering transverse slices from the top of the brain in the left upper corner to the base of the brain in the lower right corner. Images are approximately 4 mm thick. Brain blood flow is color coded from white-yellow to yellow to orange to purple, blue and black from highest brain blood flow to lowest. Normal human brain shows predominantly yellows and oranges, but, more importantly, has a fairly smooth, homogeneous appearance. The companion image (B) to the 30 slice transverse set of images is a three-dimensional surface reconstruction of the transverse images. Abnormalities in perfusion are registered as defects and as coarseness of the brain's surface.

Patient 1: HBO Treatment for Coma Due to Traumatic Brain Injury

A 19-year-old male was inadvertently ejected from a motor vehicle at 65 mph with impact on the left frontal/parietal region of the skull. Within one-half hour Glasgow coma scale was 6–7 and the patient was ventilator dependent. CT of the brain revealed diffuse edema, midline shift, petechial hemorrhages, subarachnoid hemorrhage, small subdural hematoma, and basilar skull fracture. HBO was given 19 h postinjury at 1.75 ATA/90 b.i.d. On the first treatment the patient began to fight the ventilator. Initial SPECT brain imaging obtained 5 days postinjury on a single-head low-resolution scanner was "normal." Repeat SPECT imaging on a triple-head high-resolution scanner occurred 30 days postinjury (Fig. 20.1a, b) and now clearly demonstrated the significant injury to the left frontal area as well as the contra coup injury to the right parietal/occipital area characterized by luxury perfusion. Nine days later and two hours after a fifth additional HBO, SPECT was repeated (Fig. 20.2a, b) and showed a dramatic "filling in" of the injured areas thus giving functional neurophysiological support to the clinical decision to continue HBO. The patient, meanwhile, progressed rapidly on twice daily HBO for 4 weeks with often new neurological or cognitive findings occurring in the chamber and then continued on HBO 4 times a day for 7 weeks, at which time he was conversant and independently ambulatory with slight spasticity. At 11 weeks the patient was transferred to a re habilitation center and his HBO discontinued by the new medical team. SPECT imaging at this time (Fig. 20.3a–c) registers the patient's clinical progress with a persistent increase in flow to the left frontal region while some deterioration occurs to the area of previous

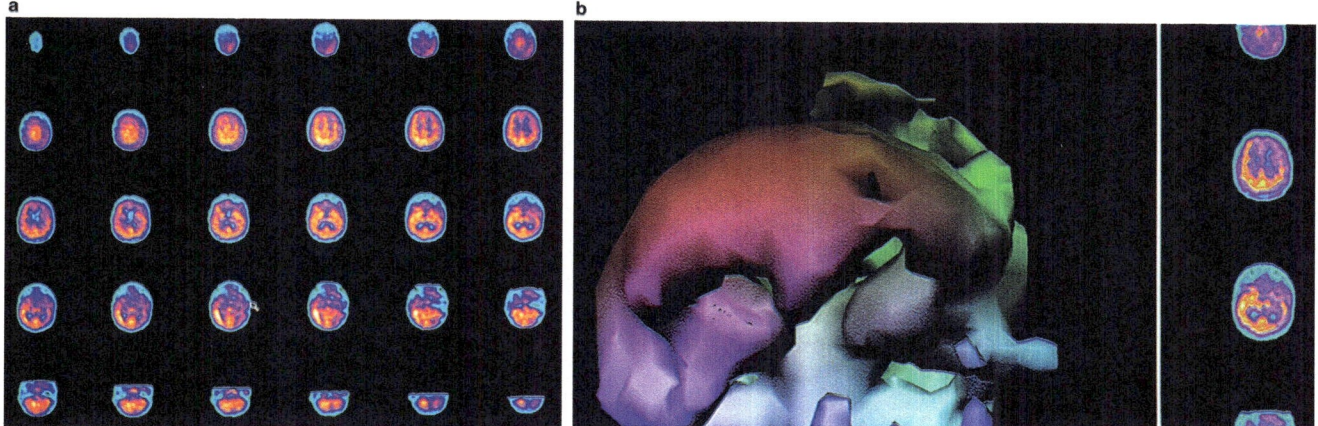

Fig. 20.1 (**a**) HMPAO SPECT brain imaging, transverse slices, 1 month postinjury. Note severe reduction in left frontal, parietal, and temporal brain blood flow with luxury perfusion in the right occipital parietal region. (**b**) Frontal projection three-dimensional surface reconstruction of Fig. 20.1a. Noncerebral uptake is shown in scalp and neck soft tissues

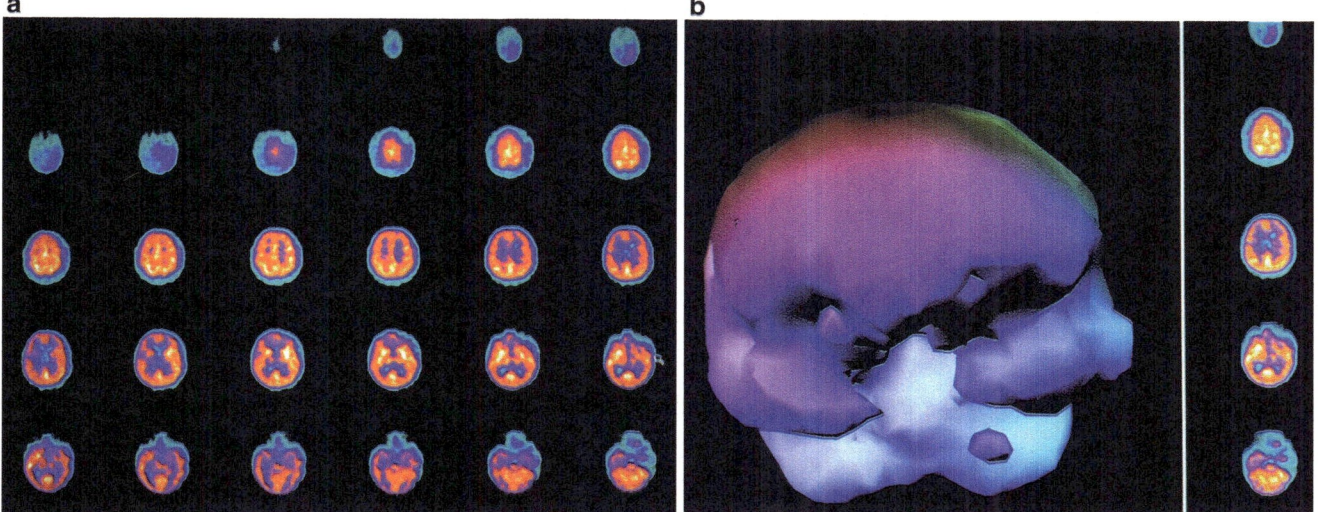

Fig. 20.2 (**a**) HMPAO SPECT brain imaging, transverse slices, 9 days after Fig. 20.1a, b and 2 h post 5th additional hyperbaric treatment. Note improvement in flow to the left frontal, parietal, and temporal regions while defects begin to appear in the right frontal and parietal area. Luxury perfusion is no longer evident. (**b**) Frontal projection three-dimensional surface reconstruction of Fig. 20.2a

luxury perfusion on the posterior right. The patient made transient limited initial progress at the rehabilitation center then quickly leveled off cognitively while his spasticity and balance worsened. Three months after discontinuance of HBO the patient's father requested further HBO and repeat SPECT brain scan (Fig. 20.4a, b), psychometric, and motor testing were obtained. SPECT now demonstrates a significant deterioration in the right frontal and posterior areas, while the left frontal normalization persists. The right posterior area has infarcted on simultaneous MRI. To assess recoverable brain tissue the patient underwent a single 1.75 ATA/90 min HBO followed by SPECT imaging (Fig. 20.5a, b); SPECT showed improvement in the right frontal and parietal/occipital lesions along the ischemic penumbral

margins. HBO was resumed for an additional 80 treatments, once/day at 1.75 ATA/90 min. The patient made a noticeable improvement in cognition (40 percentile gain in written computational mathematics), insight (the patient now verbalized for the first time the understanding that he had sustained a brain injury and could no longer aspire to be a surgeon), and balance (improvement in gait and progression from a 3-wheel tricycle to a 2-wheel bicycle). HBO (188 treatments total) was discontinued when the patient desired enrollment in remedial courses at a community college. SPECT imaging at this time (Fig. 20.6a, b) shows improvement in perfusion in the ischemic penumbral areas of the right-sided lesions. The left hemisphere remains intact. In summary, HBO, when reinstituted following SPECT and

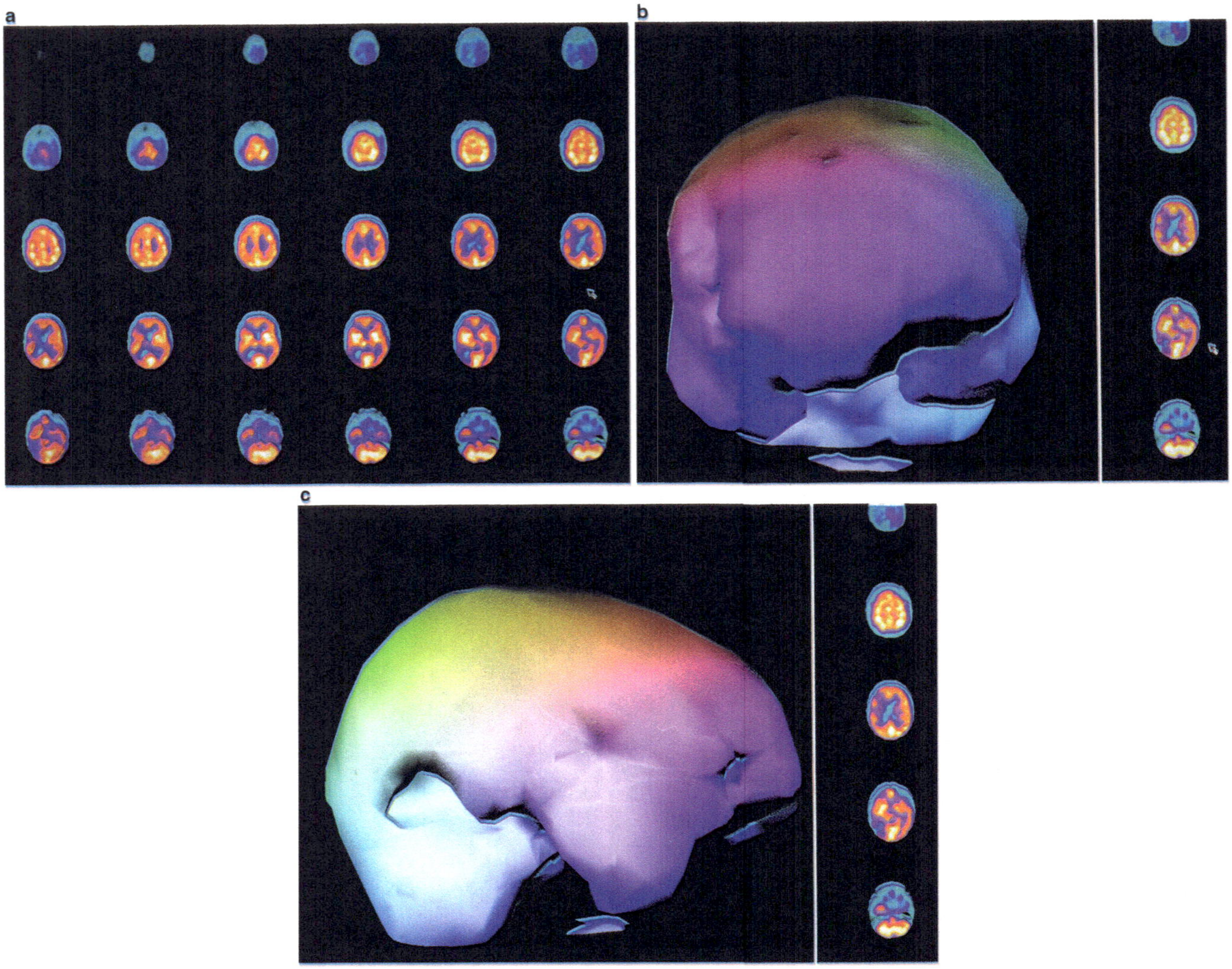

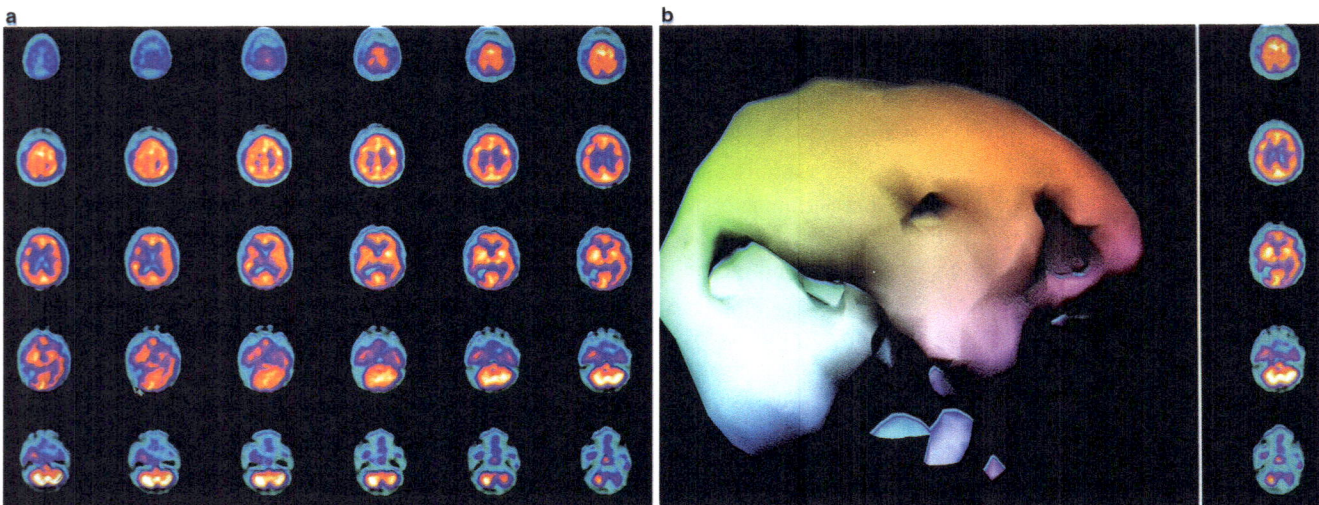

Fig. 20.3 (**a**) HMPAO SPECT brain imaging, transverse slices, 11 weeks and 108 hyperbaric treatments postinjury. Note maintenance of perfusion in the left frontal, parietal, and temporal regions with further progression of defects in the right frontal-parietal and posterior parietal-occipital areas. (**b**) Frontal projection three-dimensional surface reconstruction of Fig. 20.3a. (**c**) Right lateral projection three-dimensional surface reconstruction of Fig. 20.3a

Fig. 20.4 (**a**) HMPAO SPECT brain imaging, transverse slices, 3 months after Figs. 20.3a–c. Left frontal, parietal, and temporal perfusion is maintained with further deterioration of the right frontal and posterior defects. (**b**) Right lateral projection three-dimensional surface reconstruction of Fig. 20.4a

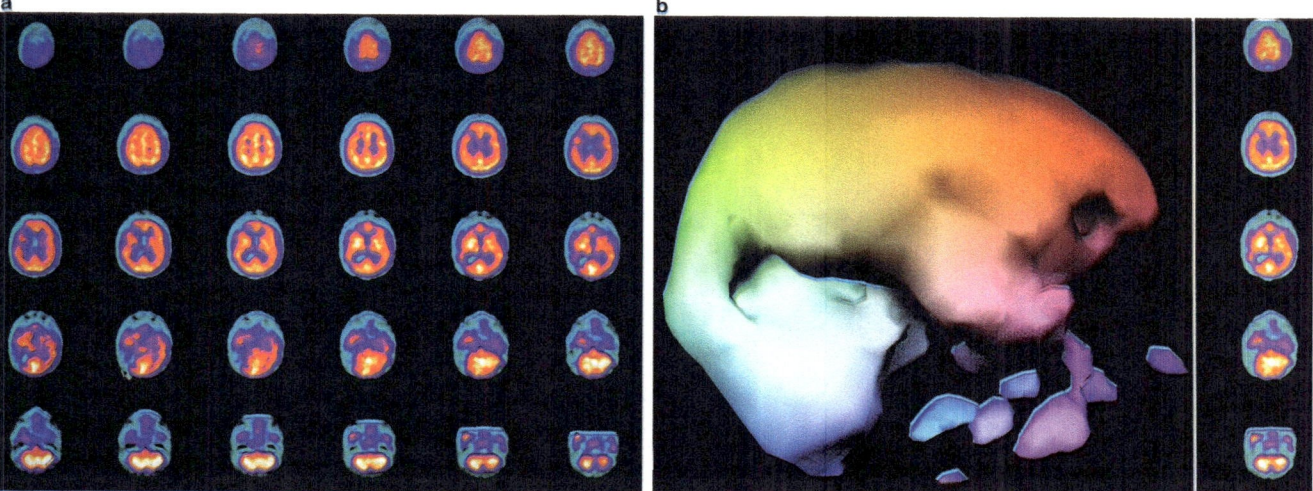

Fig. 20.5 (**a**) HMPAO SPECT brain imaging, transverse slices, 2 h following single HBO at 1.75 ATA/90 min. Note improvement in the right frontal and posterior defects. (**b**) Right lateral projection three-dimensional surface reconstruction of Fig. 20.5a

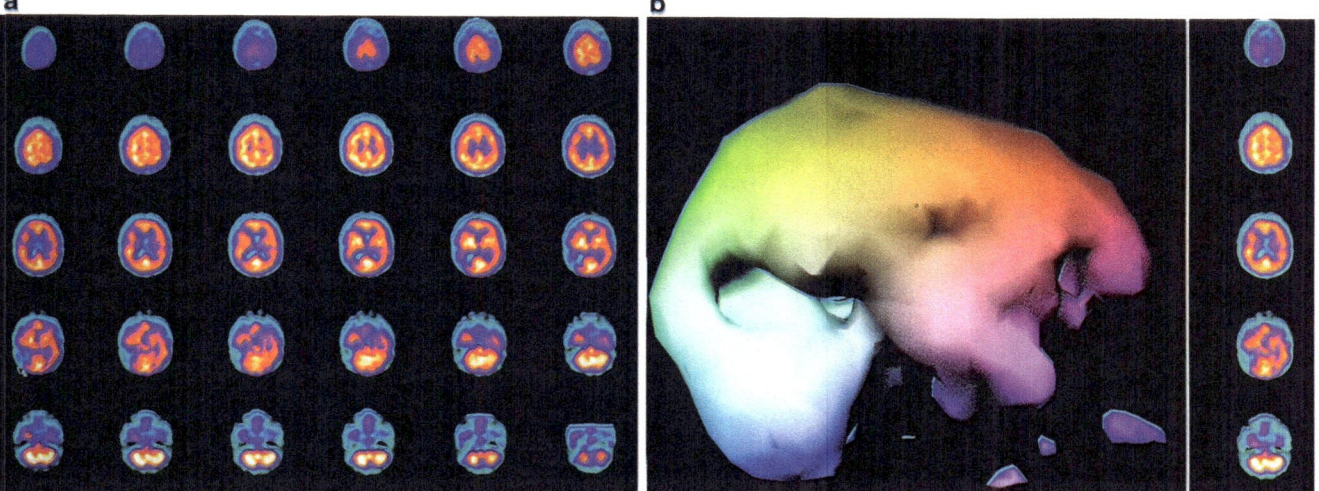

Fig. 20.6 (**a**) HMPAO SPECT brain imaging, transverse slices, 5 months and 80 HBO's after Fig. 20.4a. Note improvement in flow to the ischemic margins of the right frontal and posterior defects. (**b**) Right lateral projection three-dimensional surface reconstruction of Fig. 20.6a

relapse after discontinuation of HBO, prevented further deterioration and improved SPECT image as well as neuro-cognitive function in TBI, demonstrating the benefit of HBO in the chronic stage of TBI. To see a video of this case from the day of injury go to: https://www.youtube.com/watch?v=OM_omRuWYC4.

Patient 2: Near Drowning, Chronic Phase

The patient is a 4-year-old male who was found at the bottom of a swimming pool after an estimated 5 min of submersion. Resuscitation measures were instituted and a pulse was regained 45 min after removal from the pool. Two years after the injury, the patient was wheelchair bound with significant motor disabilities, inability to speak and communicate, and problems with drooling, attention span, and swallowing. SPECT brain imaging was performed on a high resolution scanner before (Fig. 20.7a, b) and 2 h after (Fig. 20.8a, b) a session of HBO at 1.5 ATA/60 min. The baseline scan in Fig. 20.7a shows a severe reduction in blood flow to the frontal lobes, while Fig. 20.8a shows a generalized improvement in brain blood flow, particularly to the frontal lobes, and denotes recoverable brain tissue after the single hyperbaric treatment. The patient embarked on a course of 80 hyperbaric treatments at 1.5 ATA/60 min one time/day, 5 days per week with a 3 week break at the 40 treatment point. At the end of 80 treatments, he returned for evaluation and was noted to have a generalized

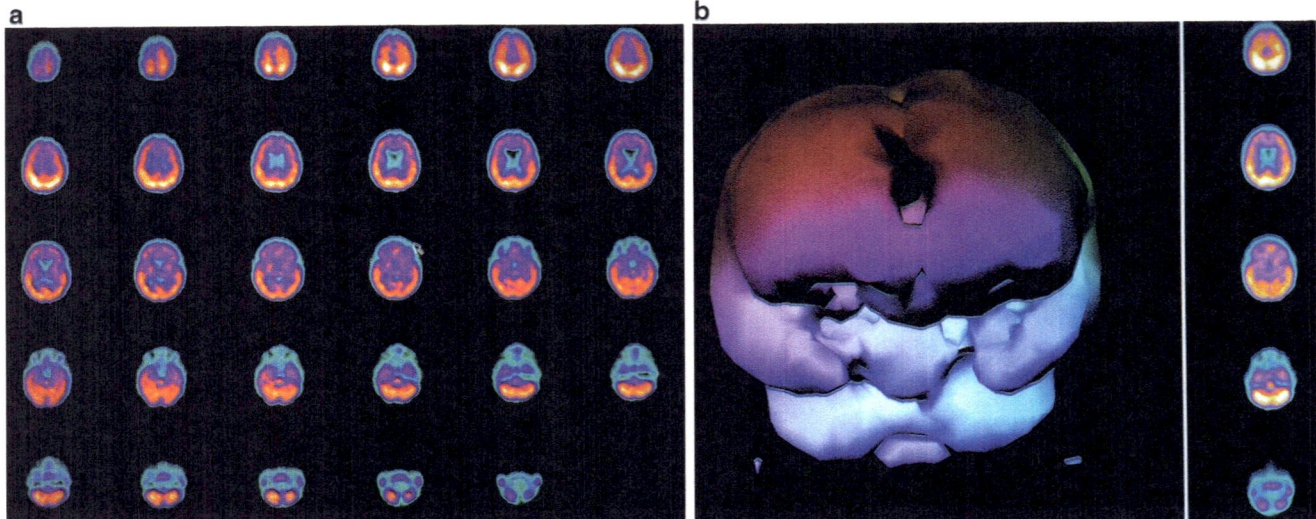

Fig. 20.7 (a) HMPAO SPECT brain imaging transverse slices, baseline study 2 years status post near drowning. Note considerable reduction in frontal blood flow. (b) Frontal projection three-dimensional surface reconstruction of Fig. 20.7a

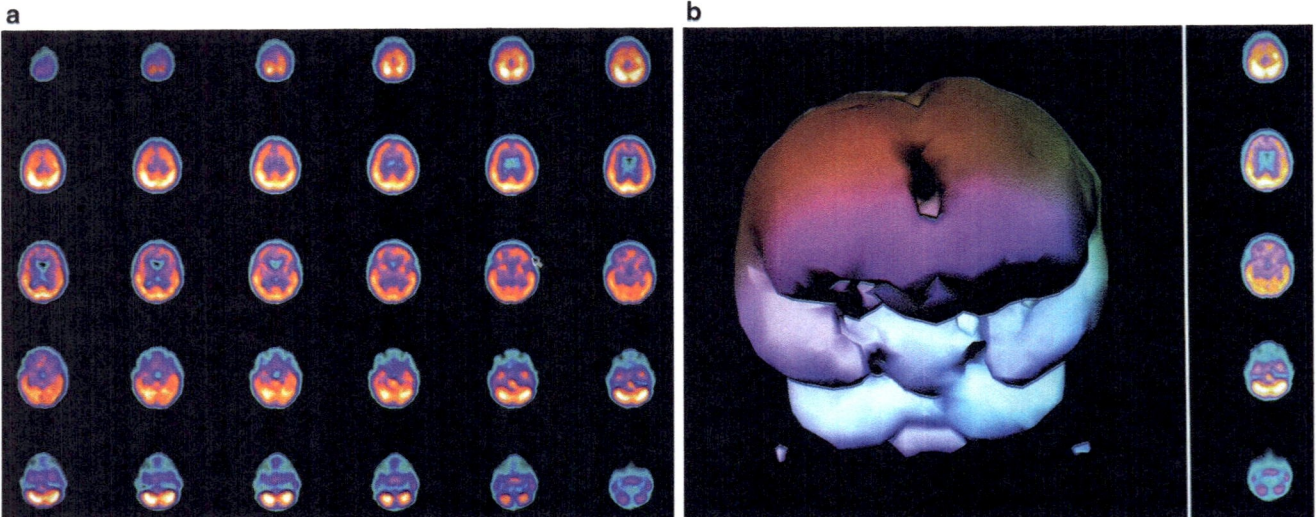

Fig. 20.8 (a) HMPAO SPECT brain imaging, transverse slices, 1 day after Fig. 20.8a and 2 h following single HBO at 1.5 ATA/60 min. Note diffuse increase in perfusion to the frontal lobes and improvement in overall brain blood flow. (b) Frontal projection three-dimensional surface reconstruction of Fig. 20.8a

improvement in spasticity, movement of all 4 extremities, increase in trunk and head control as well as improvements in swallowing, awareness, nonverbal communication, and attention span. There was a global increase in blood flow on SPECT brain imaging performed at that time (Fig. 20.9a, b).

Patient 3: Near Drowning, Chronic Phase

Case 3: The patient is a 4-year-old boy who is 2 years status post 30 min submersion in a pond. Resuscitation regained a pulse 45 min after removal from the water. Two years later, the child is severely disabled with almost no cognition, frequent postur-

ing, inconsistent tracking, extreme difficulty swallowing fluids, choking, and 10 petit mal seizures a day. Baseline SPECT brain imaging is shown in Fig. 20.10 with prominent abnormalities in the inferior frontal lobes. The patient underwent a single HBO at 1.5 ATA/60 min with repeat SPECT imaging 2 h after chamber exit (Fig. 20.11). A generalized improvement in flow is noted, particularly to the frontal lobes, identifying potentially recoverable brain tissue. The patient underwent a course of 80 hyperbaric oxygen treatments at 1.5 ATA/60 min QD, 5 days per week with approximately 1 month break after 40 treatments. On return evaluation, SPECT brain imaging was repeated (Fig. 20.12). Improvement in frontal lobe blood flow is noted over the baseline scan. The child exhibited greater awareness,

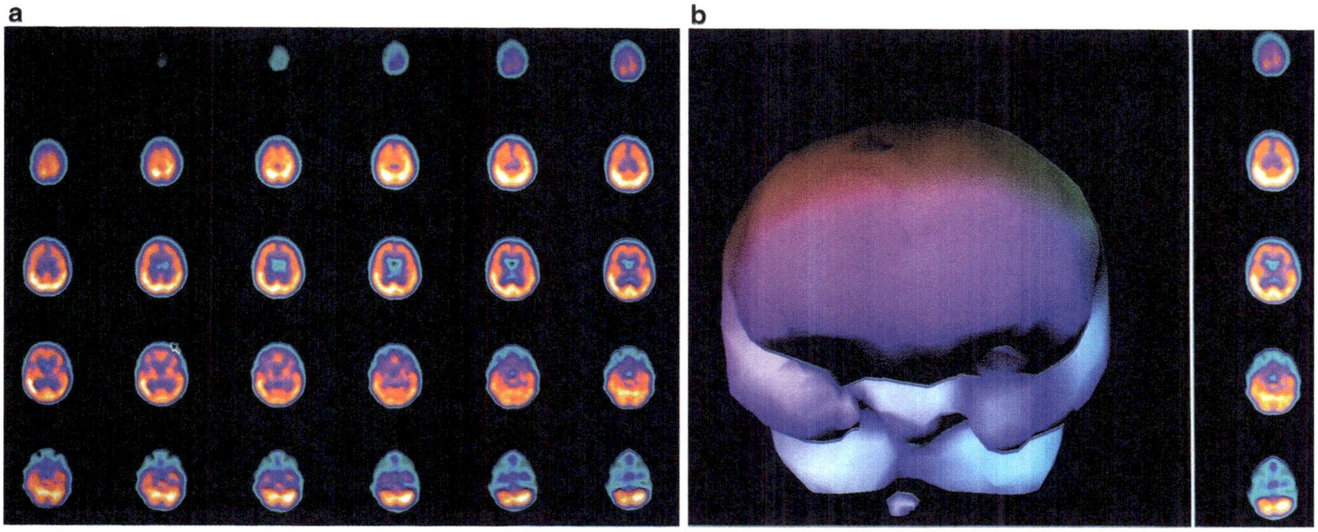

a

b

Fig. 20.9 (**a**) HMPAO SPEC' brain imaging, transverse slices, 4 months and 80 HBO's following Fig. 20.9a. Note persistent increase in perfusion to the frontal lobes. (**b**) Frontal projection three-dimensional surface reconstruction of Fig. 20.9a

Fig. 20.10 HMPAO SPECT brain imaging, transverse slices, baseline study 2 years post near drowning

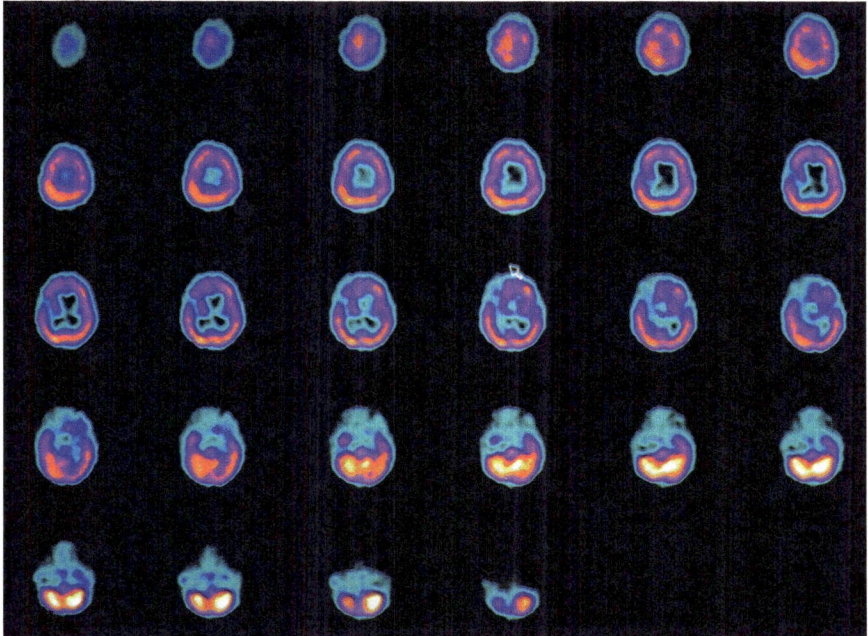

control of his head, eye tracking, alertness, nonverbal communication, performance of some simple commands, improvement in swallowing, and decrease in seizure frequency.

Patient 4: Battered Child Syndrome

Case 4: The patient is a 6-month-old girl who was slammed against the mattress of her crib by her father on multiple occasions over a 4-day period at 2 months of age. One of the first episodes was characterized by a short period of apnea; paramedics arrived at the house and found the child to be apparently normal. Three days later another episode of shaking ended with deliberate suffocation and cardiac arrest. Resuscitation was complicated by multiple recurrent arrests en route to and at the hospital. CT of the brain revealed bilateral subdural hematomas and subarachnoid hemorrhage and CT of the cord, L1 to L4 subdural hematoma. The child was ventilator dependent for 12 days. Seizures developed. Repeat CT 18 days after arrest showed severe diffuse encephalomalacia, bilateral infarcts, and bilateral hemorrhages with sparing of the basal ganglia,

Fig. 20.11 HMPAO SPECT brain imaging transverse slices 1 day after Fig. 20.10 and 2 h after a single HBO treatment at 1.5 ATA/60 min. Note generalized improvement to frontal lobe brain blood flow

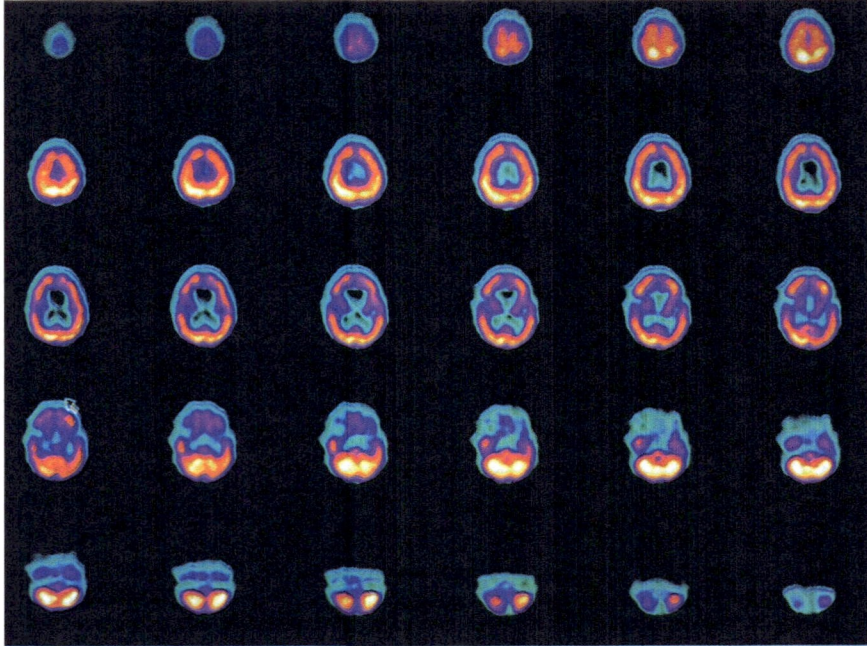

Fig. 20.12 HMPAO SPECT brain imaging transverse slices 4 months and 80 HBO treatments after Fig. 20.10. Note persistent improvement to blood flow to the frontal lobes over baseline scan of Fig. 20.10a

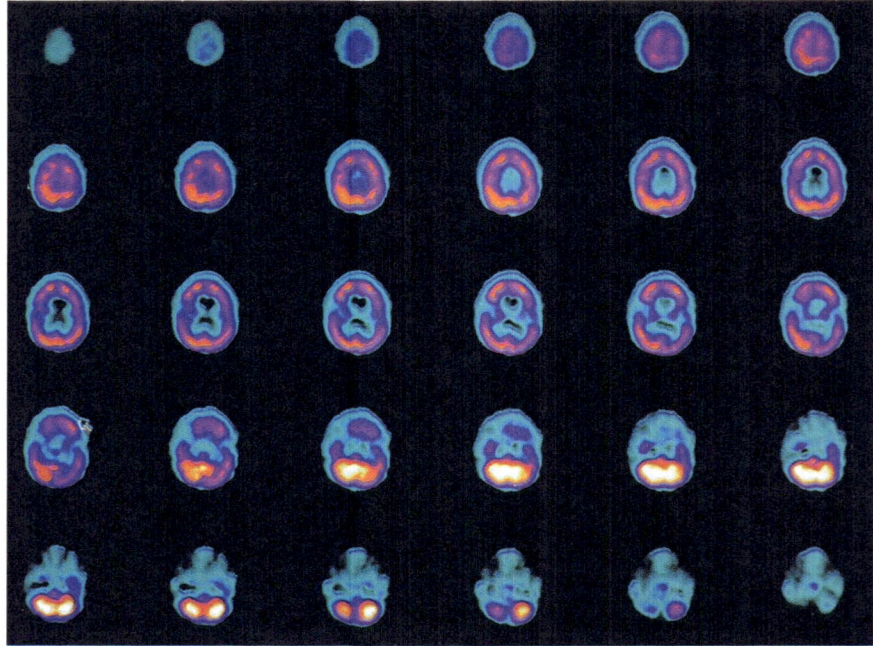

posterior fossa, and brainstem. EEG showed seizure activity on a background of minimal electrical activity. The mother unsuccessfully sought HBO therapy. Four months after the injury the child was stable enough to travel to New Orleans where she was found to be paraplegic with rectal prolapse secondary to loss of sphincter tone. She was unable to suck and was dependent on a feeding tube. She had 5–8 seizures/day and was unable to interact socially. The patient received 38 HBO sessions at 1.5

ATA/60 min TDT, 5 days/week with progressive neurological improvement. She was more awake and aware, starting to interact with her mother, had better head control, use of her arms, and no seizures. SPECT brain imaging reflects this improvement in Fig. 20.13; baseline scan is on the right and one after 38 HBOs is on the left. There is a remarkable diffuse increase in cortical blood flow after HBO with a relative absence of flow on the baseline scan, consistent with the EEG.

Fig. 20.13 ECD SPECT brain imaging transverse slices. Baseline study is on the right and after 38 HBO treatments on the left. Note the predominant thalamic, midbrain, brainstem, and posterior fossa flow and lack of cortical flow on the first study which is augmented by cortical flow on the after HBO study

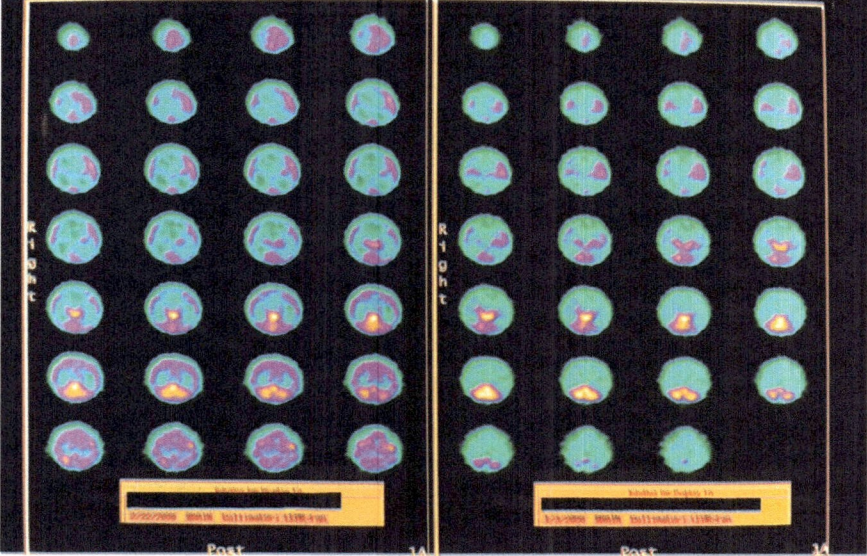

Fig. 20.14 ECD SPECT brain imaging transverse slices. Baseline study is on the right again and study after 80 HBO treatments is on the left. Note the improvement in cortical blood flow after HBO

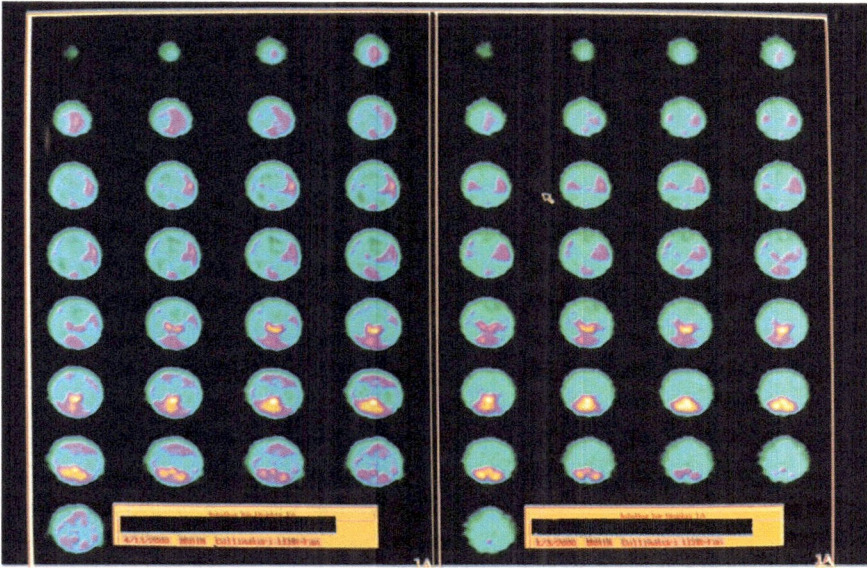

The day after her 38th HBO treatment the patient began a four-week phenobarbital taper. HBO was reinstituted at 1.5ATA/60 q.d., six treatments in 5 days/week for 42 more treatments (total of 80 HBO treatments) 2 weeks into the taper. By the 80th HBO treatment, the patient had begun a phenytoin taper, was eating baby food, had been weaned off Propulsid for her reflux disorder, was much more alert, had increased motor activity, truncal balance, improved social interaction/early smile, much less irritability, a return of rectal tone, and resolution of rectal prolapse, but was still paraplegic. Repeat SPECT brain imaging after 80 HBO treatments again captures this increased clinical activity with increased cortical blood flow in Fig. 20.14 (baseline scan is again on the right and after 80 HBO treatments on the left). Three-

dimensional surface reconstructions of the three scans are shown in chronological order in Figs. 20.15, 20.16, and 20.17. Repeat EEGs after 65 HBO treatments (patient off phenobarbital, now only on phenytoin) and 1 month after her 80th HBO treatment (off all anticonvulsants) showed no seizure activity. EEG also showed new background rhythm and bursts of frontal activity.

Conclusion

There are several causes of coma and global cerebral ischemia/anoxia. HBO has been used in a variety of animal models and in over 2800 patients with these conditions worldwide.

Fig. 20.15 Frontal projection three-dimensional surface reconstruction of baseline study in Fig. 20.13. Note the relative absence of cortical and striatal flow

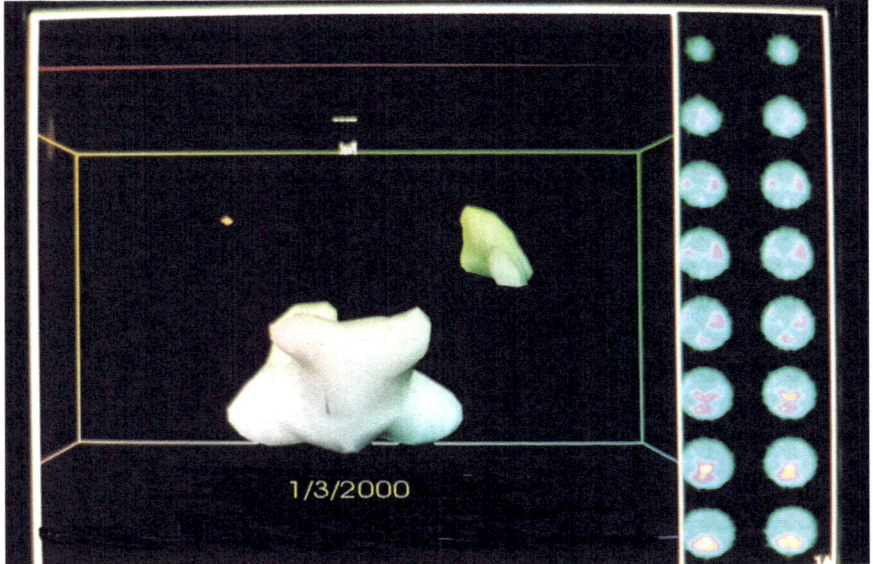

Fig. 20.16 Frontal projection three-dimensional surface reconstruction of second study (after 38 HBO treatments) in Fig. 20.13. The patient has developed some cortical blood flow

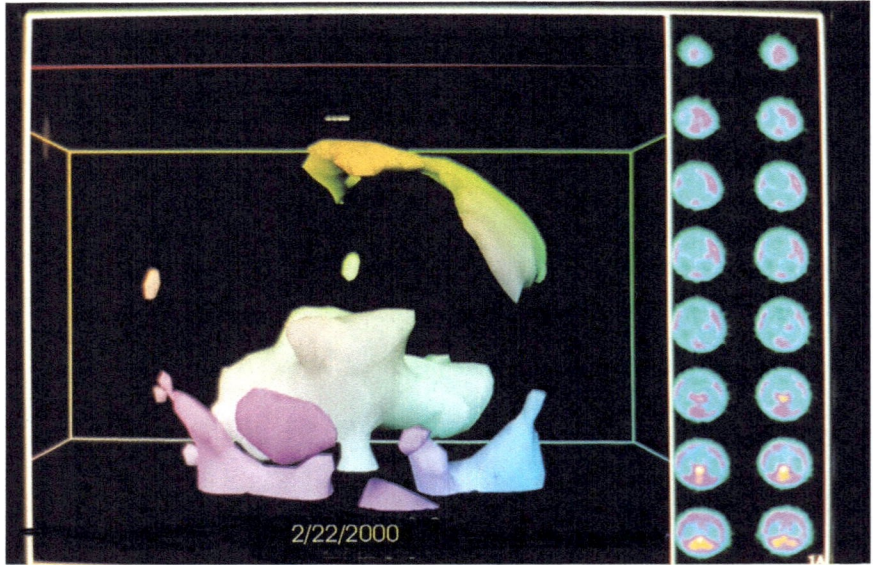

Although HBO protocols have varied, the results have been remarkably consistently positive with improvement in a variety of physiological and biochemical measures and outcomes, the most important of which was improvement in overall clinical condition and conscious ness. This consistent success rate suggests a generic effect of HBO on common brain pathophysiological processes at different stages in global ischemia/anoxia and coma. Importantly, this review excluded thousands of cases of acute carbon monoxide (CO) coma in the medical literature treated with HBO because of the confusion over HBO effects on the metabolic poison and COHb dissociation vs. hypoxia and other pathophysiology. No doubt hypoxia is a major contributing insult to the patient's overall condition in CO and reperfusion injury is a significant component of the pathophysiology, and both of these are treated definitively by HBO early after extrication, but many patients arrive for HBO hours after extrication (Thom et al. 1995; Goulon et al. 1969; Raphael et al. 1989), adequately oxygenated, with low or normal COHb levels, and outside the 45 min HBO window identified in Thom's rat model of CO reperfusion injury. Clearly, HBO is effective treatment for CO coma, irrespective of COHb and hypoxia, and it is acting on yet unidentified pathological targets (see Chap. 13). Cerebral arterial gas embolism (CAGE) of diving and nondiving etiology (thousands of cases) similarly was excluded because of the argument that bubbles are the primary pathophysiological target and not ischemia/hypoxia (for discussion see Chap. 12). It has been proposed that most bubbles in CAGE/cerebral decompression sickness have passed the cerebral circulation by the time of HBO and the primary pathological target of

Fig. 20.17 Frontal projection three-dimensional surface reconstruction of third study (after 80 HBO treatments) in Fig. 20.13. Note persistence of cortical blood flow

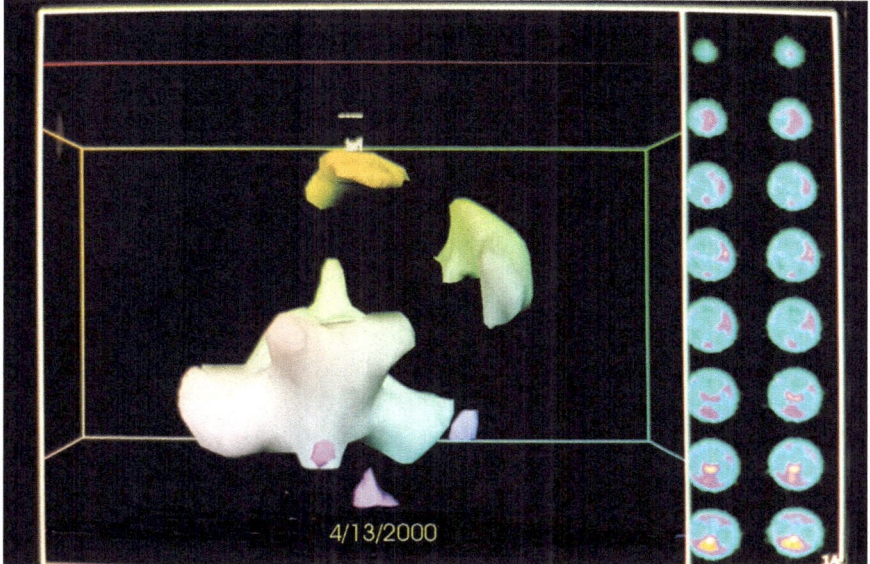

4/13/2000

treatment is reperfusion injury which is responsive to HBO (Harch 1996). In conclusion, the collective experience of HBO in many of the cases of coma due to CO (especially with delayed treatment 6 h or so) and CAGE is strongly positive and further bolsters the earlier conclusion on usefulness of HBO in coma and global ischemia/anoxia.

Another conclusion drawn from this review is that the earlier the HBO intervention the more impressive the results. In particular, if HBO is instituted within about 3 h of cerebral insult, over 75 % of patients will be noticeably improved or cured. This finding very strongly suggests targets that are both inhibited and stimulated by oxygen. A single hyper-acute HBO greater than or equal to 2 ATA is possibly quenching an on-going injurious cascade, reenergizing stunned neurons similar to the hibernating myocardium reactivation by HBO (Swift et al. 1992), and simultaneously reversing any hypoxia or anoxia. The best examples of this are the resuscitation experiments of (Van Meter et al. 1988, 1999b, 2001a, b) and (Calvert et al. 2002). The Van Meter experiments resuscitated arrested animals 25 min after arrest and truncated brain lipid peroxidation, but had no effect on any white blood cell mediated pathology. The Calvert experiment was a neonatal asphyxia model which inhibited apoptosis. When ischemia is incomplete, prolonged, or treatment is delayed >45 min HBOT likely inhibits reperfusion injury as demonstrated by the animal data of Thom, Zamboni, and other models (Harch 2000).

As treatment is delayed to 6 h, pressures above 2 ATA are still very effective, but they lose their effectiveness as delays approach 24 h. At this time lower pressures and more treatment are required and suggest treatment of different pathology. Most of the data in this time period derives from TBI studies performed at 1.5 ATA; the results show a dramatic reduction in mortality. With delays longer than 1 month, HBO assumes a

trophic role stimulating brain repair and possibly manipulating brain blood flow and metabolism as demonstrated in the Harch et al. (1996a) animal study, which was replicated in Harch et al. (2007). In both of these experiments (same model, larger numbers in the 2007 experiment) a human low pressure (1.5 ATA) protocol successfully employed from 1990 to 1994 was applied to rats with chronic traumatic brain injury. A series of 80 HBO treatment improved cognition and increased blood vessel density in the injured hippocampus. This study duplicates the known trophic effect of HBO in chronic shallow perfusion gradient radionecrosis head wounds (Marx et al. 1990) and likely underpins the mechanism of action of HBO in the multiple subacute and chronic neurological conditions reported in this chapter.

A more obscure point from this chapter that merits attention is the suggestion of an upper limit to HBO dosing in chronic brain injury (Harch 2002). Acute oxygen toxicity (overdose) is well known in HBO such that proper dosing requires a balance of therapeutic benefit with a minimum of negative side effects. Oxygen toxicity in chronic brain injury at pressures <2 ATA has been considered nonexistent in clinical HBO. The 35 examples in the Harch (2002) article and the case of Miura et al. (2002) suggest the opposite in a dose–response fashion. In general, this is consistent with the known oxygen toxicity inverse relationship of pressure and duration at pressure, but this finding requires further confirmation by other authors.

HBO in acute cerebral ischemia/anoxia and coma appears to satisfy the cardinal rule of medicine, primum non nocere. In the multitude of cases earlier and those not reviewed (CO and CAGE) the incidence of serious side effects of HBO is surprisingly small. In one review of nearly 1,000 CO poisoned patients (Hampson et al. 1996), the maximum seizure frequency was 3 % and only occurred at the highest pressures,

2.8–3 ATA, which is greater than the pressure in the great majority of the human studies in Table 20.2. The rate dropped tenfold to 0.3% with pressures of 2.4 ATA. These facts alone argue overwhelmingly for a reasonable attempt, without endangering patients in transport, to perform HBO in acute cerebral ischemia/anoxia and coma, especially where no other treatment modality exists or has shown clearcut superiority. In essence, HBO is a simple treatment with potentially profound impact after a single hyperacute administration on devastating incurable neurological conditions that generate monumental long-term tolls of material and human capital and suffering. An increasing number of animal and human experiments/articles are drawing attention to this potential.

HBO in acute cerebral ischemia/anoxia and coma satisfies the second cardinal rule of medicine—treat until the patient no longer benefits from treatment. In many of the hyperacute and acute studies HBO benefit was observed on the first or second treatment and was a prelude to further improvement with 1–2 weeks of treatment. The advance in care levels of such patients makes a powerful cost/effectiveness argument from human and financial perspectives. Unfortunately, the tradition in hyperbaric medicine has been to treat once or twice based on the US Navy's miraculous early results with hyperacute treatment of decompression sickness and air embolism, results not attained equally in the sport scuba diving arena. This stereotyped thinking has subsequently governed the approach to treatment of carbon monoxide poisoning, stroke, and other neurological maladies, ignoring the fact that HBO initiated at different times after a neurological insult is treating different neuropathology as has been discussed in this chapter. Such an approach may explain the limited positive results of (Saltzman et al. 1966; 11 of 25 patients with temporary improvement after single HBO), and (Rockswold et al. 1992; 47–59% reduction in mortality with 21 treatments, but no long term effect on functional outcome), among others. The greater consideration of the fixed HBO approach to neurologic injury and the finite, predetermined endpoint of the prospective controlled clinical trial is raised by asking the question of why stop HBO when the patient is continuing to benefit from treatment or showing neurological gains in the chamber at depth (see Patient 1). New neurological activity at depth strongly suggests ischemic neurological tissue, e.g., ischemic penumbra that would benefit from further HBO. This arbitrariness is most evident in DCI and CO poisoning where after 5–10 treatments a treating physician is asked how he knows that the patient would not continue to improve on his own. No one knows for sure with each individual case. However, we ask why this factor is not considered at the outset, or after the 2nd, 4th, 7th, 11th, or any other subsequent HBO treatment when the patient is making stepwise improvement with each or a few HBO treatments, it is known that it takes at least 1 year for a human tissue injury to mature (e.g., wound healing

tensile strength and time for neurological injury to be considered chronic), smoldering inflammatory cascades are the underlying pathology, and the analogy of a single HBO "jump starting a failed engine with a dead battery" is grossly inadequate. In fact, the deciding factor in determining the number of HBO treatments may be the point in the injury process at which HBO is initiated, not financial considerations, a factor increasingly dominating medical decision-making in the United States today.

In our accumulating extensive experience, repetitive HBO appears to be trophic, stimulatory to brain repair, and may not be complete in some cases until 200–300 treatments (see Patient 1). Perhaps the best and most expedient method to assess the HBO potential and endpoint of treatment at any time after injury for any brain pathology is SPECT brain imaging on a high resolution camera (see Figs. 20.1–20.6). SPECT before and after any single HBO at any point in the treatment process may help identify the injured brain's potential for any or further HBO. HBO can then be initiated or continued and combined with multiple other treatment modalities. This approach may help document cost-effectiveness of prolonged HBO by choosing endpoints. Currently, there are over 1200 hyperbaric centers in the United States but it is estimated that less than 5% of these routinely treat the neurological conditions addressed in this chapter with the exception of decompression sickness and CO poisoning. In the last edition of this chapter, we wrote that "As hyperbaric medicine continues to experience a resurgence in use and expansion of applications and research, the proliferation of chambers and increasing ease of access will facilitate use of HBO in acute cerebral ischemia/anoxia and coma and will be driven by ever greater lay public and physician knowledge of the earlier data through widespread computer-assisted dissemination." These words were prophetic as we are now seeing an Internet driven increase in HBO application to chronic neurological conditions. Efforts are currently underway to collect this massive amount of accruing data, publicize the results, leverage scientific proof of efficacy, and achieve reimbursement. The ultimate result will be a retrospective look and application of HBO to the highest impact targets, acute ischemic/hypoxic brain injury and resuscitation. The outcome will be a large scale dramatic improvement in mortality, morbidity, and quality of life. We predict that this will revolutionize the treatment of brain injury.

References

Artru F, Chacornac R, Deleuze R. Hyperbaric oxygenation for severe head injuries. Eur Neurol. 1976a;14:310–8.
Artru F, Philippon B, Gau F, Berger M, Deleuze R. Cerebral blood flow, cerebral metabolism and cerebrospinal fluid biochemistry in brain-injured patients after exposure to hyperbaric oxygen. Eur Neurol. 1976b;14:351–64.

Astrup J, Siesjo BK, Symon L. Thresholds in cerebral ischemia-the ischemic penumbra. Stroke. 1981;12(6):723–5.

Bai J, Lyden PD. Revisiting cerebral postischemic reperfusion injury: new insights in understanding reperfusion failure, hemorrhage, and edema. Int J Stroke. 2015;10(2):143–52.

Baiborodov BD. Some peculiarities in application of hyperbaric oxygenation during the treatment of acute respiratory insufficiency in newborn infants. In: Abstracts VII Int Cong HBO Medicine, Moscow September 2–6, 1981. p. 368.

Barrett K, Harch P, Masel B, Pattterson J, Corson K, Mader J. Cognitive and cerebral blood flow improvements in chronic stable traumatic brain injury induced by 1.5 ATA hyperbaric oxygen (abstract). Undersea and Hyperbaric Med. 1998;25:9.

Belokurov MI, Stepankov AA, Kirsanov BI. Hyperbaric oxygenation in the combined therapy of comatose states in children. Pediatriia. 1988;2:84–7.

Benson K, Hartz AJ. A comparison of observational studies and randomized, controlled trials. N Engl J Med. 2000;342:1878–86.

Bjelke B, Andersson K, Ogren SO, Bolme P. Asphyctic lesion: proliferation of tyrosine hydroxylase-immunoreactive nerve cell bodies in the rat substantia nigra and functional changes in dopamine neurotransmission. Brain Res. 1991;543:1–9.

Borgens RB, Liu-Snyder P. Understanding secondary injury. Q Rev Biol. 2012;87(2):89–127.

Bulkley BH, Hutchins GM. Myocardial consequences of coronary artery bypass graft surgery: The paradox of necrosis in areas of revascularization. Circulation. 1977;56(6):906–13.

Buras JA, Reenstra WR. Endothelial-neutrophil interactions during ischemia and reperfusion injury: basic mechanisms of hyperbaric oxygen. Neurol Res. 2007;29(2):127–31.

Buras JA, Stahl GL, Svodoba KKH, Reenstra WR. Hyperbaric oxygen downregulates ICAM-1 expression induced by hypoxia and hypoglycemia: the role of NOS. Am J Physiol Cell Physiol. 2000;278:C292–302.

Calvert JW, Zhang JH. Hyperbaric oxygenation restores energy status following hypoxia-ischemia in a neonatal rat model. FASEB Journal. 2005;4,S-1(4):A481.

Calvert JW, Yin W, Patel M, Bader A, Mychaskiw G, Parent AD, et al. Hyperbaric oxygenation prevented brain injury induced by hypoxia-ischemia in a neonatal rat model. Brain Res. 2002;951(1):1–8.

Calvert JW, Cahill J, Yamaguchi-Okada M, Zhang JH. Oxygen treatment after experimental hypoxia-ischemia in neonatal rats alters the expression of HIF-1alpha and its downstream target genes. J Appl Physiol. 2006;101(3):853–65.

Chen J, Chen YH. Effects of hyperbaric oxygen on intrauterine hypoxic-ischemic brain damage in neonatal rats. (article in Chinese). Zhongguo Dang Dai Er Ke Za Zhi. 2009;11(5):380–3.

Chen J, Chen YH. Effects of hyperbaric oxygen on synaptic ultrastructure and synaptophysin expression in hippocampus of neonatal rats with hypoxic-ischemic brain damage. Chin J Pediatr. 2010;48(3):199–204.

Chen Y, Nadi NS, Chavko M, Auker CR, McCarron RM. Microarray analysis of gene expression in rat cortical neurons exposed to hyperbaric air and oxygen. Neurochem Res. 2009a;34:1047–56.

Chen S, Xiao N, Zhang X. Effect of combined therapy with ephedrine and hyperbaric oxygen on neonatal hypoxic-ischemic brain injury. Neurosci Lett. 2009b;465:171–6.

Churchill S, Weaver LK, Deru K, Russo AA, Handrahan D, Orrison WW, et al. A prospective trial of hyperbaric oxygen for chronic sequelae after brain injury (HYBOBI). Undersea Hyperb Med. 2013;40(2):165–93.

Collet JP, Vanasse M, Marois P, Amar M, Goldberg J, Lambert J, et al. Hyperbaric oxygen for children with cerebral palsy: a randomized multicentre trial. Lancet. 2001;357:582–6.

Concato J, Shah N, Horwitz RI. Randomized, controlled trials, observational studies, and the hierarchy of research designs. N Engl J Med. 2000;342:1887–92.

Cormio M, Robertson CS, Narayan RK. Secondary insults to the injured brain. J Clin Neurosci. 1997;4(2):132–48.

Dean BS, Verdile VP, Krenzelok EP. Coma reversal with cerebral dysfunction recovery after repetitive hyperbaric oxygen therapy for severe carbon monoxide poisoning. Am J Emerg Med. 1993;11(6):616–8.

Dirnagl U. Cerebral ischemia: the microcirculation as trigger and target. In: Kogure K, Hossmann KA, Siesjö BK, editors. Progress in brain research, Neurobiology of ischemic brain damage, vol. 96. Amsterdam: Elsevier; 1993. p. 49–65.

Dordain M, Humbert G, Robert M, Leroy J, Delaunay P. Coma hepatique par hepatite virale traite avec success par l'oxygene hyperbare. Therapeutique. 1969;45(2):184–9.

Dutka AJ, Kochanek PM, Hallenbeck JM. Influence of granulocytopenia on canine cerebral ischemia induced by air embolism. Stroke. 1989;20:390–5.

Eltorai I, Montroy R. Hyperbaric oxygen therapy leading to recovery of a 6-week comatose patient afflicted by anoxic encephalopathy and posttraumatic edema. J Hyperbaric Med. 1991;6:189–98.

Engler RL, Dahlgren MD, Morris DD, Peterson MA, Schmid-Schonbein GW. Role of leukocytes in response to acute myocardial ischemia and reflow in dogs. Am J Physiol. 1986a;251(2 Pt 2):H314–23.

Engler RL, Dahlgren MD, Peterson MA, Dobbs A, Schmid-Schonbein GW. Accumulation of polymorphonuclear leukocytes during 3-h experimental myocardial ischemia. Am J Physiol. 1986b;251(1 Pt 2):H93–100.

Glantz SA. Experiments when each subject receives more than one treatment. In: Primer of bio-statistics. New York: McGraw-Hill; 1992. p. 278–319.

Godman CA, Chheda KP, Hightower LE, Perdrizet G, Shin DG, Giardina C. Hyperbaric oxygen induces a cytoprotective and angiogenic response in human microvascular endothelial cells. Cell Stress Chaperones. 2009. doi:10.1007/s12192-009-0159-0.

Golden ZL, Neubauer R, Golden CJ, Greene L, Marsh J, Mleko A. Improvement in cerebral metabolism in chronic brain injury after hyperbaric oxygen therapy. Int J Neurosci. 2002;112:119–31.

Golden Z, Golden CJ, Neubauer RA. Improving neuropsychological function after chronic brain injury with hyperbaric oxygen. Disabil Rehabil. 2006;28(22):1379–86.

Goulon M, Barois A, Rapin M, Nouailhat F, Grosbuis S, Labrousse J. Carbon monoxide poisoning and acute anoxia due to inhalation of coal gas and hydrocarbons: 302 cases, 273 treated by hyperbaric oxygen at 2 ata. Ann Med Interne (Paris). 1969;120(5):335–49.

Grigor'eva AV, Kazantzeva NV, Bul'chuk OV, Vikulova TA. Effects of different doses of hyperbaric oxygenation on morphology and transcription of cortical neurons of rats with experimental cerebral ischemia. Biull Eksp Biol Med. 1992;113(4):419–21.

Gunther A, Manaenko A, Franke H, Wagner A, Schneider D, Berrouschot J, et al. Hyperbaric and normobaric reoxygenation of hypoxic rat brain slices—impact on purine nucleotides and cell viability. Neurochem Int. 2004;45(8):1125–32.

Hai YU, Tian RL, Pan XW, Luan Z, Song LW. Effects of hyperbaric oxygen on brain bFGF and bFGF mRNA expression of neonatal grafts after hypoxia/ischemia injury. In: Joiner JT, editor. Proceedings of the 2nd international symposium on hyperbaric oxygenation for cerebral palsy and the brain injured child. Flagstaff: Best Publishing; 2002. p. 57–65.

Hampson NB, Simonson SG, Kramer CC, Piantadosi CA. Central nervous system oxygen toxicity during hyperbaric treatment of patients with carbon monoxide poisoning. Undersea Hyperb Med. 1996;23(4):215–9.

Harch PG. Late treatment of decompression illness and use of SPECT brain imaging. In: Moon RE, Sheffield PJ, editors. Treatment of Decompression Illness, 45th Workshop of the Undersea and Hyperbaric Medical Society. Kensington: UHMS; 1996. p. 203–42.

Harch PG. Generic inhibitory drug effect of hyperbaric oxygen therapy (HBOT) on reperfusion injury (RI) (abstract). Eur J Neurol. 2000;7 Suppl 3:150.

Harch PG. The dosage of hyperbaric oxygen in chronic brain injury. In: Joiner JT, editor. The Proceedings of the 2nd International Symposium on Hyperbaric Oxygenation for Cerebral palsy and the Brain-Injured Child. Flagstaff: Best Publishing; 2002. p. 31–56.

Harch PG. Hyperbaric oxygen therapy in the treatment of chronic traumatic brain injury: from Louisiana boxers to U.S. veterans, an American Chronology. Wound Care Hyperbaric Med. 2010;1(4):26–34.

Harch PG. Hyperbaric oxygen therapy for post-concussion syndrome: contradictory conclusions from a study mischaracterized as sham-controlled. J Neurotrauma. 2013;30:1995–9.

Harch PG. Hyperbaric oxygen in chronic traumatic brain injury: oxygen, pressure, and gene therapy. Med Gas Res. 2015;5:9. doi:10.1186/s13618-015-0030-6.

Harch PG, Neubauer RA. Hyperbaric oxygen therapy in global cerebral ischemia/anoxia and coma, Chapter 18. In: Jain KK, editor. Textbook of Hyperbaric Medicine. Gottingen: Hogrefe & Huber; 1999. p. 318–49.

Harch PG, Neubauer RA. Hyperbaric oxygen therapy in global cerebral ischemia/anoxia and coma, Chapter 18. In: Jain KK, editor. Textbook of hyperbaric medicine, 4th revised and expanded. Gottingen: Hogrefe & Huber; 2004. p. 223–61.

Harch PG, Gottlieb SF, Van Meter KW, Staab P. HMPAO SPECT brain imaging and low pressure HBOT in the diagnosis and treatment of chronic traumatic, ischemic, hypoxic and anoxic encephalopathies. Undersea Hyperb Med. 1994a;21(Suppl):30.

Harch PG, Van Meter KW, Gottlieb SF, Staab P. HMPAO SPECT brain imaging of acute CO poisoning and delayed neuropsychological sequelae (DNSS). Undersea Hyperb Med. 1994b;21(Suppl):15.

Harch PG, Kriedt CL, Weisend MP, Van Meter KW, Sutherland RJ. Low pressure hyperbaric oxygen therapy induces cerebrovascular changes and improves complex learning/memory in a rat open head bonk chronic brain contusion model. Undersea & Hyperbaric Med. 1996a;23(Suppl):48.

Harch PG, Van Meter KW, Neubauer RA, Gottlieb SF. Appendix 2, Use of HMPAO SPECT for assessment of response to HBO in ischemic/hypoxic encephalopathies. In: Jain KK, editor. Textbook of hyperbaric medicine, 2nd Revised edn. Gottingen: Hogrefe & Huber; 1996b. p. 480–91.

Harch PG, Kriedt C, Van Meter KW, Sutherland RJ. Hyperbaric oxygen therapy improves spatial learning and memory in a rat model of chronic traumatic brain injury. Brain Res. 2007;1174:120–9.

Harch PG, Andrews SR, Fogarty EF, Amen D, Pezzullo JC, Lucarini J, et al. A phase I study of low-pressure hyperbaric oxygen therapy for blast-induced post-concussion syndrome and post-traumatic stress disorder. J Neurotrauma. 2012;29(1):168–85.

Hardy P, Collet JP, Goldberg J, Ducruet T, Vanasse M, Lambert J, et al. Neuropsychological effects of hyperbaric oxygen therapy in cerebral palsy. Dev Med Child Neurol. 2002;44:436–46.

Hayakawa T, Kanai N, Kuroda R, Yamada R, Mogami H. Response of cerebrospinal fluid pressure to hyperbaric oxygenation. Nuerol Neurosurg Psychiatry. 1971;34:580–6.

Helps SC, Gorman DF. Air embolism of the brain in rabbits pretreated with mechlorethamine. Stroke. 1991;22:351–4.

Heyman A, Saltzman HA, Whalen RE. Use of HBO in treatment of cerebral ischemia and infarction. Circulation. 1966;33-34(Suppl II):II-20–7.

Holbach KH, Caroli A. Oxygen tolerance and the oxygenation state of the injured human brain. In: Trapp WG et al., editors. Procedures of the 5th international congress on hyperbaric medicine. Burnaby: Simon Fraser University; 1974. p. 350–61.

Holbach KH, Wassmann H, Kolberg T. Verbesserte reversibilitat des traumatischen mittelhirusyndromes bei anwendung der hyperbaren oxygenierung. Acta Neurochir. 1974;30:247–56.

Holbach KH, Caroli A, Wassmann H. Cerebral energy metabolism in patients with brain lesions at normo- and hyperbaric oxygen pressures. J Neurol. 1977a;217:17–30.

Holbach KH, Wassmann H, Caroli A. Continuous rCBF measurements during hyperbaric oxygenation. In: Procedures of the 6th International congress on hyperbaric medicine. Aberdeen: Aberdeen University Press; 1977b. p. 104–11.

Holbach KH, Wassmann H, Caroli A. Correlation between electroencephalographical and rCBF changes during hyperbaric oxygenation. In: Procedures of the 6th International congress on hyperbaric medicine. Aberdeen: Aberdeen University Press; 1977c. p. 112–7.

Hsu P, Li H-W, Lin Y-T. Acute hydrogen sulfide poisoning treated with hyperbaric oxygen. J Hyperbaric Med. 1987;2(4):215–21.

Hutchison JH, Ker MM, Williams KG, Hopkinson WI. Hyperbaric oxygen in the resuscitation of the newborn. Lancet. 1963;2:1019–22.

Hyperbaric Oxygen Therapy Indications, 13th Edition: The Hyperbaric Oxygen Therapy Committee Report. In: Weaver LK (ed.). Undersea and Hyperbaric Medical Society. North Palm Beach, FL: Best Publishing; 2014.

Iadecola C, Anrather J. The immunology of stroke: from mechanisms to translation. Nat Med. 2011;17:796–808.

Illingworth CFW, Smith G, Lawson DD, Ledingham IMcA, Sharp GR, Griffiths JC. Surgical and physiological observations in an experimental pressure chamber. Br J Surg. 1961;49:222–7

Ingvar DH, Lassen NA. Treatment of focal cerebral ischemia with hyperbaric oxygen. Acta Neurol Scand. 1965;41:92–5.

Isakov IV, Pravdenkova SV, Ioffe IS. Effect of hyperbaric oxygenation on respiration in acute cerebral circulatory disorders. Zh Vopr Neirokhir Im N N Burdenko. 1982;1:34–9.

Iwatsuki N, Takahashi M, Ono K, Tajima T. Hyperbaric oxygen combined with nicardipine administration accelerates neurologic recovery after cerebral ischemia in a canine model. Crit Care Med. 1994;22(5):858–63.

Jiang JY, Bo YH, Yin YH, Pan YH, Liang YM, Luo QZ. Effect of arousal methods for 175 cases of prolonged coma after severe traumatic brain injury and its related factors. Chin J Traumatol. 2004;7(6):341–3.

Kapp JP, Phillips M, Markov A, Smith RR. Hyperbaric oxygen after circulatory arrest: modification of postischemic encephalopathy. Neurosurgery. 1982;11(4):496–9.

Kawamura S, Ohta H, Yasui N, Nemoto M, Hinuma Y, Suzuki E. Effects of hyperbaric oxygenation in patients with subarachnoid hemorrhage. J Hyperbaric Medicine. 1988;3(4):243–55.

Khiabani KT, Bellister SA, Skaggs SS, Stephenson LL, Nataraj C, Wang WZ, et al. Reperfusion-induced neutrophil CD18 polarization: effect of hyperbaric oxygen. J Surg Res. 2008;150(1):11–6.

Kiene H, von Schön-Angerer T. Single-case causality assessment as a basis for clinical judgment. Alt Ther. 1998;4(1):41–7.

Kienle GS, Kiene H. Placebo effect and placebo concept: a critical methodological and conceptual analysis of reports on the magnitude of the placebo effect. Alt Ther. 1996;2(6):39–54.

Koch A, Vermeulen-Cranch DME. The use of hyperbaric oxygen following cardiac arrest. Br J Anaesth. 1962;34:738–40.

Kohshi K, Yokota A, Konda N, Munaka M, Yasukouchi H. Hyperbaric oxygen therapy adjunctive to mild hypertensive hypervolemia for symptomatic vasospasm. Meurol Med Chir (Tokyo). 1993;33:92–9.

Konda A, Baba S, Iwaki T, Harai H, Koga H, Kimura T, et al. Hyperbaric oxygenation prevents delayed neuronal death following transient ischaemia in the gerbil hippocampus. Neuropathol App Neurobiol. 1996;22(4):350–60.

Krakovsky M, Rogatsky G, Zarchin N, Mayevsky A. Effect of hyperbaric oxygen therapy on survival after global cerebral ischemia in rats. Surg Neurol. 1998;49:412–6.

Kunz A, Dirnagl U, Mergenthaler P. Acute pathophysiological processes after ischaemic and traumatic brain injury. Best Pract Res Clin Anaesthesiol. 2010;24:495–509.

Larcan A, Laprevote-Heully MC, Lambert H, Alexandre P, Picard L, Chrisment N. Indications des thrombolytiques au cours des accidents vasculaires cerebraux thrombosants traits par ailleurs par O.H.B (2 ATA). Therapie. 1977;32:259–70.

Lareng L, Brouchet A, Plat JJ. Experience of hyperbaric oxygen therapy in 2 cases of traumatic coma. Anesth Reanim. 1973;30:525–32.

Li Y, Zhou C, Calvert JW, Colohan AR, Zhang JH. Multiple effects of hyperbaric oxygen on the expression of HIF-1 alpha and apoptotic genes in a global ischemia-hypotension rat model. Exp Neurol. 2005;191(1):198–210.

Liu M-N, Zhuang S-Q, Zhang H-Y, Qin Z-Y, Li X-Y. Long-term effects of early hyperbaric oxygen therapy on neonatal rats with hypoxic-ischemic brain damage. Zhongguo Dang Dai Er Ke Za Zhi. 2006a;8(3):216–20.

Liu XH, Zhao YL, Ma QM, Zhou XH, Wang Y. Optimal therapeutic window of hyperbaric oxygenation in neonatal rat with hypoxic-ischemic brain damage. Zhonghua Er Ke Za Zhi. 2006b;44(3):177–81.

Liu Z, Xiong T, Meads C. Clinical effectiveness of treatment with hyperbaric oxygen for neonatal hypoxic-ischaemic encephalopathy: systematic review of Chinese literature. BMJ. 2006c;333(7564):374.

Liu XH, Zhao YL, Ma QM, Zhou XH, Wang Y. Hyperbaric oxygen improves long-term learning-memory deficits and brain injury in neonatal rat with hypoxia-ischemia brain damage. Sichuan Da Xue Xue Bao Yi Xue Ban. 2007;38(1):73–7.

Liu JT, Lee JK, Tyan YS, Liu CY, Chen YH, Lin TB. Neuromodulation on cervical spinal cord combined with hyperbaric oxygen in comatose patients—a preliminary report. Surg Neurol. 2009;72 Suppl 2:S28–34.

Liu XH, Yan H, Xu M, Zhao YL, Li LM, Zhou XH, et al. Hyperbaric oxygenation reduces long-term brain injury and ameliorates behavioral function by suppression of apoptosis in a rat model of neonatal hypoxia-ischemia. Neurochem Int. 2013;62:922–30.

Macdonald AG, Fraser PJ. The transduction of very small hydrostatic pressures. Comp Biochem Physiol A Mol Integr Physiol. 1999;122(1):13–36.

Malek M, Duszczyk M, Zyszkowski M, Ziembowicz A, Salinska E. Hyperbaric oxygen and hyperbaric air treatment result in comparable neuronal death reduction and improved behavioral outcome after transient forebrain ischemia in the gerbil. Exp Brain Res. 2013;224:1–14.

Martin JD, Thom SR. Vascular leukocyte sequestration in decompression sickness and prophylactic hyperbaric oxygen therapy in rats. Aviat Space Environ Med. 2002;73(6):565–9.

Marx RE, Ehler WJ, Tayapongsak P, Pierce LW. Relationship of oxygen dose to angiogenesis induction in irradiated tissue. Am J Surg. 1990;160:519–24.

Mathieu D, Wattel F, Gosselin B, Chopin C, Durocher A. Hyperbaric oxygen in the treatment of posthanging cerebral anoxia. J Hyper Med. 1987;2(2):63–7.

Mathieu D, Bocquillon N, Charre S. Wattel F Hyperbaric oxygenation in acute ischemic encephalopathy (near-hanging) (abstract). Eur J Neurol. 2000;7 Suppl 3:151.

Mickel HS, Kempski O, Feuerstein G, Parisi JE, Webster HD. Prominent white matter lesions develop in Mongolian gerbils treated with 100% normobaric oxygen after global brain ischemia. Acta Neuropathol. 1990;79(5):465–72.

Mink RB, Dutka AJ. Hyperbaric oxygen after global cerebral ischemia in rabbits does not promote brain lipid peroxidation. Crit Care Med. 1995a;23(8):1398–404.

Mink RB, Dutka AJ. Hyperbaric oxygen after global cerebral ischemia in rabbits reduces brain vascular permeability and blood flow. Stroke. 1995b;26:2307–12.

Miura S, Ohyagi Y, Ohno M, Inoue I, Ochi H, Murai H, et al. A patient with delayed posthypoxic demyelination: a case report of hyperbaric oxygen treatment. Clin Neurol Neurosurg. 2002;104:311–4.

Mogami H, Hayakawa T, Kanai N, Kuroda R, Yamada R, Ikeda T, et al. Clinical application of hyperbaric oxygenation in the treatment of acute cerebral damage. J Neurosurg. 1969;31:636–43.

Montgomery D, Goldberg J, Amar M, Lacroix V, Lecomte J, Lambert J, et al. Effects of hyperbaric oxygen therapy o children with spastic diplegic cerebral palsy: a pilot project. Undersea Hyperb Med. 1999;26(4):235–42.

Moody RA, Mead CO, Ruamsuke S, Mullan S. Therapeutic value of oxygen at normal and hyperbaric pressure in experimental head injury. J Neurosurg. 1970;32(1):51–4.

Mrsic-Pelcic J, Pelcic G, Peternel S, Pilipovic K, Simonic A, Zupan G. Effects of the hyperbaric oxygen treatment on the Na+, K+-ATPase and superoxide dismutase activities in the optic nerves of global cerebral ischemia-exposed rats. Prog Neuropsychopharmacol Biol Psychiatry. 2004a;28(4):667–76.

Mrsic-Pelcic J, Pelcic G, Vitezic D, Antoncic I, Filipovic T, Simonic A, et al. Hyperbaric oxygen treatment: the influence on the hippocampal superoxide dismutase and Na+, K+-ATPase activities in global cerebral ischemia-exposed rats. Neurochem Int. 2004b;44(8):585–94.

Multiple authors (Chavdarov, Harch, Lobov, Neubauer, Zerbini). In: Joiner JT (ed.). The Proceedings of the 2nd International Symposium on Hyperbaric Oxygenation for Cerebral palsy and the Brain-Injured Child. Flagstaff, AZ: Best Publishing; 2002.

Myers RE. A unitary theory of causation of anoxic and hypoxic brain pathology. Adv in Neurol. 1979;26:195–213.

Nakamura T, Kuroda Y, Yamashita S, Kawakita K, Kawai N, Tamiya T, et al. Hyperbaric oxygen therapy for consciousness disturbance following head injury in subacute phase. Acta Neurochir Suppl. 2008;102:21–4.

Neubauer RA. The effect of hyperbaric oxygen in prolonged coma. Possible identification of marginally functioning brain zones. Medicina Subacquea ed Iperbarica. 1985;5(3):75–9.

Neubauer RA. Interventional brain scanning in neurologic dysfunction. Lauderdale-by-the-Sea: Ocean Hyperbaric Center; 1995. p. 22.

Neubauer RA, James P. Cerebral oxygenation and the recoverable brain. Neurol Res. 1998;20 Suppl 1:S33–6.

Neubauer RA, Kagan RL, Gottlieb SF, James P. Delayed metabolism, reperfusion or redistribution in iofetamine brain imaging after exposure to hyperbaric oxygen, clinical correlations. In: Proceedings of the XV Annual Meeting of the European Undersea Biomedical Society, EUBS, Eilat, Israel. 1989. p. 237–43.

Neubauer RA, Gottlieb SF, Kagan RL. Enhancing "idling" neurons. Lancet. 1990;335:542.

Neubauer RA, Gottlieb SF, Miale A. Identification of hypometabolic areas in the brain using brain imaging and hyperbaric oxygen. Clin Nucl Med. 1992;17:477–81.

Neubauer RA, Gottlieb SF, Pevsner NH. Long-term anoxic ischemic encephalopathy: predictability of recovery. In: Oriani G, Wattel F, editors. Proceedings of the twelfth international congress on hyperbaric medicine. Flagstaff, AZ: Best Publishing; 1998. p. 417–29.

Neubauer V, Harch PG, Neubauer RA. Hyperbaric oxygen therapy in global cerebral ischemia/anoxia and coma, Chapter 21. In: Jain KK, editor. Textbook of hyperbaric medicine, 4th revised and expanded. Gottingen: Hogrefe & Huber; 2004. p. 287–96.

Niu KC, Chang CK, Lin MT, Huang KF. A hyperbaric oxygen therapy approach to heat stroke with multiple organ dysfunction. Chin J Physiol. 2009;52(3):169–72.

Oh S, Lee E, Lee J, Lim Y, Kim J, Woo S. Comparison of the effects of 40% oxygen and two atmospheric absolute air pressure conditions on stress-induced premature senescence of normal human diploid fibroblasts. Cell Stress Chaperones. 2008;13(4):447–58.

Plum F, Pulsinelli WA. Cerebral metabolism and hypoxic-ischemic brain injury, Chapter 90. In: Asbury AK, McKhann GM, McDonald WI, editors. Diseases of the nervous system, Clinical neurobiology, vol. 1. Philadelphia: WB Saunders; 1986. p. 1086–100.

Pundik S, Xu K, Sundararajan S. Reperfusion brain injury. Neurology. 2012;79 Suppl 1:S44–51.

Raphael JC, Elkharrat D, Jars-Guincestre MC, Chastang C, Chasles V, Vercken JB, et al. Trial of normobaric and hyperbaric oxygen for acute carbon monoxide intoxication. Lancet. 1989;2(8660):414–9.

Ren H, Wang W, Zhaoming CE. Glasgow Coma Scale, brain electric activity mapping and Glasgow Outcome Scale after hyperbaric oxygen treatment of severe brain injury (English Edition). Chin J Traumatol. 2001;4(4):239–41.

Rice JE, Vannucci RC, Brierley JF. The influence of immaturity on hypoxic-ischemic brain damage in the rat. Ann Neurol. 1981;9:131–41.

Rockswold GL, Ford SE, Anderson DC, Bergman TA, Sherman RE. Results of a prospective randomized trial for treatment of severely brain-injured patients with hyperbaric oxygen. J Neurosurg. 1992;76:929–34.

Rockswold SB, Rockswold GL, Vargo JM, Erickson CA, Sutton RL, Bergman TA, et al. Effects of hyperbaric oxygenation therapy on cerebral metabolism and intracranial pressure in severely brain injured patients. J Neurosurg. 2001;94:403–11.

Rockswold SB, Rockswold GL, Zaun DA, Zhang X, Cerra CE, Bergman TA, et al. A prospective, randomized clinical trial to compare the effect of hyperbaric to normobaric hyperoxia on cerebral metabolism, intracranial pressure, and oxygen toxicity in severe traumatic brain injury. J Neurosurg. 2010;112:1080–94.

Rockswold SB, Rockswold GL, Zaun DA, Liu J. A prospective, randomized Phase II clinical trial to evaluate the effect of combined hyperbaric and normobaric hyperoxia on cerebral metabolism, intracranial pressure, oxygen toxicity, and clinical outcome in severe traumatic brain injury. J Neurosurg. 2013;118:1317–28.

Rosenthal RE, Silbergleit R, Hof PR, Haywood Y, Fiskum G. Hyperbaric oxygen reduces neuronal death and improves neurological outcome after canine cardiac arrest. Stroke. 2003;34(5):1311–6. Epub 2003 Apr 3.

Rossignol DA. Hyperbaric oxygen therapy might improve certain pathophysiological findings in autism. Med Hypotheses. 2007;68:1208–27.

Rossor MN. Headache, stupor, and coma, Chapter 3.2. In: Walton J, editor. Brain's diseases of the nervous system. Oxford: Oxford University Press; 1993. p. 134–41.

Ruiz E, Brunette DD, Robinson EP, Tomlinson MJ, Lange J, Wieland MJ, et al. Cerebral resuscitation after cardiac arrest using hetastarch hemodilution, hyperbaric oxygenation and magnesium ion. Resuscitation. 1986;14:213–23.

Safar P. Cerebral resuscitation after cardiac arrest: a review. Circulation. 1986;74(Suppl IV):IV-138–53.

Saltzman HA, Anderson B, Whalen RE, Heyman A, Sieker HO. Hyperbaric oxygen therapy of acute cerebral vascular insufficiency. In: Brown IW, Cox BG, editors. Proceedings of the third international conference on hyperbaric medicine, publication 1404. Washington, DC: National Academy of Sciences National Research Council; 1966. p. 440–6.

Sanchez EC, Montes G, Oroz G, Garcia L. Management of intestinal ischaemia, necrotizing enterocolitis and anoxic encephalopathies of neonates with hyperbaric oxygen therapy. Undersea Hyperb Med. 1999;26(Suppl):22.

Sanderson TH, Reynolds CA, Kumar R, Przyklenk K, Huttemann M. Molecular mechanisms of ischemia-reperfusion injury in brain: pivotal role of the mitochondrial membrane potential in reactive oxygen species generation. Mol Neurobiol. 2013;47:9–23.

Satoh J, Murase H, Tukagoshi H. Hanging survivor showing alpha coma—a case report. Rinsho Shinkeigaku. 1989;29(5):612–6.

Schmidt-Kastner R. Genomic approach to selective vulnerability of the hippocampus in brain ischemia-hypoxia. Neuroscience. 2015;309:259–79.

Senechal C, Larivee S, Richard E, Marois P. Hyperbaric oxygenation therapy in the treatment of cerebral palsy: a review and comparison to currently accepted therapies. J Am Phys Surg. 2007;12(4):109–13.

Shandling AH, Ellestad MH, Hart GB, Crump R, Marlow D, Van Natta B, et al. Hyperbaric oxygen and thrombolysis in myocardial infarction: the "hot MI" pilot study. Am Heart J. 1997;134(3):544–50.

Sharp GR, Ledingham I. McA, Norman, JN. The application of oxygen at 2 atmospheres pressure in the treatment of acute anoxia. Anaesthesia. 1962;17(2):136–44.

Sheffield PJ, Davis JC. Application of hyperbaric oxygen therapy in a case of prolonged cerebral hypoxia following rapid decompression. Aviat Space Environ Med. 1976;47(7):759–62.

Shiokawa O, Fujishima M, Yanai T, Ibayashi S, Ueda K, Yagi H. Hyperbaric oxygen therapy in experimentally induced acute cerebral ischemia. Undersea Biomed Res. 1986;13(3):337–44.

Shn-Rong Z. Hyperbaric oxygen therapy for coma (a report of 336 cases). In: Proceedings of the international congress of hyperbaric medicine. 1995. p. 279–85.

Siddiqui A, Davidson JD, Mustoe TA. Ischemic tissue oxygen capacitance after hyperbaric oxygen therapy: a new physiologic concept. Plast Reconstr Surg. 1995;99:148–55.

Siesjö BK, Katsura K, Zhao Q, Folbergrova J, Pahlmark K, Siesjo P, et al. Mechanisms of secondary brain damage in global and focal ischemia: a speculative synthesis. J Neurotrauma. 1995;12(5):943–56.

Smilkstein MJ, Bronstein AC, Pickett HM, Rumack BH. Hyperbaric oxygen therapy for severe hydrogen sulfide poisoning. J Emerg Med. 1985;3:27–30.

Snyder JW, Safir EF, Summerville GP, Middleberg RA. Occupational fatality and persistent neurological sequelae after mass exposure to hydrogen sulfide. Am J Emerg Med. 1995;13(2):199–203.

Sukoff MH, Ragatz RE. Hyperbaric oxygenation for the treatment of acute cerebral eedema. Neurosurg. 1982;10(1):29–38.

Swift PC, Turner JH, Oxer HF, O'Shea JP, Lane GK, Woollard KV. Myocrdial hibernation identified by hyperbaric oxygen treatment and echocardiography in postinfarction patients: comparison with exercise thallium scintigraphy. Am Heart J. 1992;124:1151–8.

Takahashi M, Iwatsuki N, Ono K, Tajima T, Akama M, Koga Y. Hyperbaric oxygen therapy accelerates neurologic recovery after 15-minute complete global cerebral ischemia in dogs. Crit Care Med. 1992;20(11):1588–94.

Teasdale G, Jennett B. Assessment of coma and impaired consciousness. A practical scale. Lancet. 1974;2:81–4.

Thalmann ED. Principles of U.S. navy recompression treatments for decompression sickness. In: Diving accident management, 41st Undersea and Hyperbaric Medical Society Workshop. Undersea and Hyperbaric Medical Society publication 78 (DIVACC). 12/1/90. p. 194–221

Thom SR. Leukocytes in carbon monoxide-mediated brain oxidative injury. Toxicol Appl Pharmacol. 1993a;123(2):234–47.

Thom SR. Functional inhibition of leukocyte B 2 integrins by hyperbaric oxygen in carbon monoxide-mediated brain injury in rats. Toxicol Appl Pharmacol. 1993b;123:248–56.

Thom SR, Taber RL, Mendiguren II, Clark JM, Hardy KR, Fisher AB. Delayed neuropsychologic sequelae after carbon monoxide poisoning: prevention by treatment with hyperbaric oxygen. Ann Emerg Med. 1995;25(4):474–80.

Thomas MP, Brown LA, Sponseller DR, Williamson SE, Diaz JA, Guyton DP. Myocardial infarct size reduction by the synergistic effect of hyperbaric oxygen and recombinant tissue plasminogen activator. Am Heart J. 1990;120(4):791–800.

Thomson LF, Mardel SN, Jack A, Shields TG. Management of the moribund carbon monoxide victim. Arch Emerg Med. 1992;9(2):208–13.

Van Meter K, Gottlieb SF, Whidden SJ. Hyperbaric oxygen as an adjunct in ACLS on guinea pigs after 15 minutes of cardiopulmonary arrest. Undersea Biomed Res. 1988;15(Suppl):55.

Van Meter K, Weiss L, Harch PG. Hyperbaric oxygen in emergency medicine, Chapter 36. In: Jain KK, editor. Textbook of hyperbaric medicine. 3rd ed. Gottingen: Hogrefe & Huber; 1999a. p. 586–8.

Van Meter KW, Sheps SS, Swanson HT, Wilson JP, Barratt DM, Kodu U, Roycraft EL, Moises JP, Nolan TA, Harch PG. A controlled prospective randomized pilot open chest cardiopulmonary resuscitation

(CPR) comparing use of 100% oxygen in mechanical ventilation of swine at one, two, and four atmospheres ambient pressure after a 25 minute normothermic cardiopulmonary arrest at one atmosphere. Ann Emerg Med. 1999b;34(4 Pt. 2):S11.

Van Meter K, Moises J, Marcheselli V, Murphy-Lavoie H, Barton C, Harch P, Bazan N. Attenuation of lipid peroxidation in porcine cerebral cortex after a prolonged 25-minute cardiopulmonary arrest by high-dose hyperbaric oxygen (HBO). Undersea Hyperb Med. 2001a;28(Suppl):83–4.

Van Meter K, Xiao F, Moises J, Barratt D, Harch P, Murphy-Lavoie H, Bazan N. No difference in leukocyte adherence in the microvasculature in a porcine cerebral cortex by use of normobaric oxygen or low or high-dose hyperbaric oxygen in resuscitation after a prolonged 25 minute cardiopulmonary arrest. Ann Emerg Med. 2001b;38(4):S39.

Van Meter K, Sheps S, Kriedt F, Moises J, Barratt D, Murphy-Lavoie H, et al. Hyperbaric oxygen improves rate of return of spontaneous circulation after prolonged normothermic porcine cardiopulmonary arrest. Resuscitation. 2008;78(2):200–14.

Viart P, Blum D, Thys JP, Dubois J. Exsanguino-transfusions and hyperbaric oxygen in the treatment of hepatic coma in children. Arch Fr Pediatr. 1970;27(4):444–5.

Voisin C, Wattel F, Pruvost P, et al. Interet de l'oxygenotherapie hyperbare dans le traitement de la strangulation par pendaison. A propos de 35 observations. Maroc Med. 1973;53:302–5.

Waalkes P, Fitzpatrick DT, Stankus S, Topolski R. Adjunctive HBO treatment of children with cerebral anoxic injury. Army Med Dept J PB. 2002;8:13–21.

Wada K, Ito M, Miyazawa T, Katoh H, Nawashiro H, Shima K, et al. Repeated hyperbaric oxygen induces ischemic tolerance in gerbil hippocampus. Brain Res. 1996;740:15–20.

Wang XL, Yang YJ, Wang QH, Xie M, Yu XH, Liu CT, et al. Changes of Wnt-3 protein during the proliferation of endogenous neural stem cells in neonatal rats with hypoxic-ischemic brain damage after hyperbaric oxygen therapy. (article is Chinese). Zhongguo Dang Dai Er Ke Za Zhi. 2007a;9(3):241–6.

Wang XL, Yang YJ, Wang QH, Yu XH, Xie M, Liu CT, et al. Effect of hyperbaric oxygen therapy administered at different time on white matter damage following hypoxic-ischemic brain damage in neonatal rats. Zhongguo Dang Dai Er Ke Za Zhi. 2007b;9(4):308–12.

Wang XL, Zhao YS, Yang YJ, Xie M, Yu XH. Therapeutic window of hyperbaric oxygen therapy for hypoxic-ischemic brain damage in newborn rats. Brain Res. 2008;1222:87–94.

Wang QH, Yang YJ, Chen CF, Yao Y, Li M. Protective effects of delayed multiple course hyperbaric oxygen treatment against hypoxic-ischemic brain damage in neonatal rats. Chin J Contemp Pediatr. 2009;11(6):464–70.

Weinstein PR, Hameroff SR, Johnson PC, Anderson GG. Effect of hyperbaric oxygen therapy or dimethyl sulfoxide on cerebral ischemia in unanesthetized gerbils. Neurosurg. 1986;18(5):528–32.

Wu L, Mustoe TA. Effect of ischemia on growth factor enhancement of incisional wound healing. Surgery. 1995;117:570–6.

Yang YJ, Wang XL, Yu XH, Wang X, Xie M, Liu CT. Hyperbaric oxygen induces endogenous neural stem cells to proliferate and differentiate in hypoxic-ischemic brain damage in neonatal rats. Undersea Hyperb Med. 2008;35(2):113–29.

Yangsheng T. Hyperbaric oxygen treatment of acute ischemic and anoxic cerebral injury. In: Proceedings of the Eleventh International Congress on Hyperbaric Medicine, President Wen-ren Li, M.D., Secretariat Frederick S. Cramer, M.D. Flagstaff: Best Publishing; 1995. p. 21822.

Yatsuzuka H. Effects of hyperbaric oxygen therapy on ischemic brain injury in dogs. Japanese J Anesthesiol. 1991;40(2):208–23.

Yaxi Q, Anquan Y, Guangkai G, Yansheng T The study of the effect of hyperbaric oxygen on cerebral metabolic enzymes and cAMP during acute cerebral ischemia in rabbits. Proceedings of the Eleventh International Congress on Hyperbaric Medicine, President Wen-ren Li, M.D., Secretariat Frederick S. Cramer, M.D. Flagstaff: Best Publishing; 1995. p. 194–7.

Yin X, Meng F, Wang Y, Wei W, Li A, Chai Y, et al. Effect of hyperbaric oxygen on neurological recovery of neonatal rats following hypoxic-ischemic brain damage and its underlying mechanism. Int J Clin Exp Pathol. 2013;6(1):66–75.

Yiqun F, Jingchang L, Weiguang T, Haihong J, Peizhu X, Shilong L, Fenzhou S Effect of hyperbaric oxygen on brain Na, K-ATPase and ultrastructure of cerebral ischemia gerbils. Proceedings of the Eleventh International Congress on Hyperbaric Medicine, President Wen-ren Li, M.D., Secretariat Frederick S. Cramer, M.D. Flagstaff, AZ: Best Publishing; 1995. p. 269–78.

Yu XH, Yang YJ, Wang X, Wang QH, Xie M, Qi BX, et al. Effect of hyperbaric oxygenation on neural stem cells and myelin in neonatal rats with hypoxic-ischemic brain damage. Zhongguo Dang Dai Er Ke Za Zhi. 2006;8(1):33–7.

Zamboni WA, Roth AC, Russell RC, Graham B, Suchy H, Kucan JO. Morphologic analysis of the microcirculation during reperfusion of ischemic skeletal muscle and the effect of hyperbaric oxygen. Plast Reconstr Surg. 1993;91(6):1110–23.

Zhang ZW, Kang Y, Deng LJ, Luo CX, Zhou Y, Xue XS, et al. Therapy of central pontine myelinolysis following living donor liver transplantation: report of three cases. World J Gastroenterol. 2009;15(31):3960–3.

Zhou C, Li Y, Nanda A, Zhang JH. HBO suppresses Nogo-A, Ng-R, or RhoA expression in the cerebral cortex after global ischemia. Biochem Biophys Res Commun. 2003;309(2):368–76.

Zhou BY, Lu GJ, Huang YQ, Ye ZZ, Han YK. Efficacy of hyperbaric oxygen therapy under different pressures on neonatal hypoxic-ischemic encephalopathy. Zhongguo Dang Dai Er Ke Za Zhi. 2008;10(2):133–5.

Zhu M, Lu M, Li QJ, Zhang Z, Wu ZZ, Li J, et al. Hyperbaric oxygen suppresses hypoxic-ischemic rain damage in newborn rats. J Child Neurol. 2015;30(1):75–82.

K.K. Jain

Abstract

This chapter covers the applications of HBO in various conditions encountered in neurosurgical practice. These include traumatic brain injury (TBI) as well as its sequelae, and spinal cord injury (SCI). HBO has an important role in management of cerebral edema. HBO is a useful adjunct to management of ischemic and compressive lesions of the spinal cord as well as rehabilitation of the patient with SCI. HBO has important applications in cerebrovascular surgery based on its beneficial effect in cerebral ischemia including sequelae of ruptured intracranial aneurysms. In addition to its neuroprotective effect in procedures involving interruption of cerebral circulation, HBO has as an important application in selecting patients who are likely to benefit from cerebral revascularization procedures. Experimental studies as well as clinical applications are described. HBO is used either as a primary therapy or adjunct to other treatments such as radiotherapy of brain tumors and management of various complications of neurosurgery such as postoperative infections.

Keywords

Carotid endarterectomy • Cerebral edema • Cerebrovascular surgery • Extra-intracranial bypass • Hyperbaric oxygen • Neurosurgery • Postoperative complications • Spinal cord injury (SCI) • Stroke • Traumatic brain injury (TBI)

Introduction

Investigations of applications of hyperbaric oxygenation (HBO) in neurosurgery continue to evolve. A number of new publications have confirmed the efficacy of HBO in cerebral edema, which was initially reported over 40 years ago. Uncertainty among clinicians about using HBO in the therapy of cerebral pathology because definitive established mechanisms of action are still lacking has been addressed (Calvert et al. 2007).

The use of hyperbaric oxygenation (HBO) for diseases of the central nervous system is based on the ability of HBO to increase oxygenation and reduce cerebral blood flow. The pathophysiological sequelae of both head and spinal cord trauma include hypoxia and hyperemia. However, the complexity of central nervous system trauma involves events at multiple levels: cellular integrity and metabolism, blood flow, enzymatic disruption, and all their implications. Consequently, not only is multimodality therapy essential in central nervous system trauma, but also the specific effects must be carefully monitored inasmuch as the treatment of the brain and spinal cord with HBO is somewhat paradoxical, and carries with it the potential for therapeutic success as well as aggravation.

Role of HBO in the Management of Traumatic Brain Injury: TBI

Therapy for traumatic brain injury (TBI) must address the cascade of events that occurs subsequent to brain injury. The rationale for success must first be based on the potential of the

K.K. Jain, MD, FRACS, FFPM (✉)
Blaesiring 7, Basel 4057, Switzerland
e-mail: jain@pharmabiotech.ch

© Springer International Publishing AG 2017
K.K. Jain, *Textbook of Hyperbaric Medicine*, DOI 10.1007/978-3-319-47140-2_21

damaged brain for recovery. This must be followed by the use of agents to prevent the cyclical events of ischemia, edema, elevated intracranial pressure (ICP), cellular disruption, and the metabolic and enzymatic derangements that occur subsequent to brain injury. The enclosure of the brain in the rigid and compartmentalized skull adds an additional challenge. HBO along with other non-operative care must be considered as an adjuvant to surgery or as the primary therapy in nonsurgical cases.

Osmotic and renal diuretics continue to be used for control of cerebral edema but their use is not quite satisfactory The current emphasis on treatment of TBI involves investigation of pharmacological methods and control of intracranial pressure in an effort to produce an environment that will either allow the injured brain to heal, and/or prevent the development of progressive damage. Use of various neuroprotective agents in TBI has been reviewed elsewhere (Jain 2011). There has been experimental and clinical experience with various cerebral protective agents such as calcium channel blockers, barbiturates, glutamine antagonists, free radical scavengers, steroids, receptor antagonists, and volatile anesthetics.

On a practical and accepted level, we now have very adequate monitoring facilities for TBI patients. To support our clinical judgment, we have neuro-imaging and improved methods of measuring ICP, cerebral blood flow (CBF), and cerebral metabolism. These would facilitate the development of comprehensive approaches to deal with the complexity of brain injury. Because the traumatized brain can respond to the therapeutic effects of HBO, continued efforts to develop appropriate regimes utilizing this modality are mandatory. Virtually any trauma to the central nervous system (CNS) includes the vicious cycle of interacting ischemia, hypoxia, edema, and metabolic-enzymatic disturbances. The metabolic disturbances include the production of free radicals capable of causing vasodilatation and vascular wall damage. Hypoxia causes a shift in glycolysis with the production of lactic acid and lowering of the pH. An imbalance of energy demand and availability results in the consequent ischemia-like state with loss of ATP available to the neurons and glia. In addition to the oxygen free radicals, excitatory amino acids are released as a consequence of vascular injury. The initial or subsequent loss of cellular integrity, combined with the ionic derangements and vascular dilatation effects of free radicals, and compounded by fluid and electrolyte shifts both into the interstitial spaces and extracellular components, will result in cerebral edema and increased ICP. Thus, the main therapeutic efforts of treating the head injured patient are directed toward the above noted pathophysiological changes. Agents must be used to reduce increased ICP, ischemia, and metabolic and enzymatic derangements.

Mechanism of Action of HBO in TBI

The properties of HBO that have enabled both clinical and investigational advances in the management of TBI are well known. As we have seen in previous chapters, vasoconstriction reduces cerebral blood flow, and the increased oxygenation of the blood mitigates against ischemia. The decrease in blood flow reduces a major element of ICP. However, there are additional mechanisms involved in the therapeutic effects of HBO. Studies of CBF and damaged cerebral tissue in humans demonstrate that variations of CBF are minimized by HBO. The hypothesis is that if the reduction of ICP by HBO is the result of decreased cerebral edema, then hyperoxia causes a reduction in CBF and the damaged areas manifest an increased flow after HBO. This statement does contradict the fact that hyperoxia reduces blood flow. Rather, it supports the multiple mechanisms that are present when using hyperoxia and are necessary in the treatment of cerebral trauma, a complex and multidimensional pathological entity. Variations in CBF, cerebral autoregulation have been well investigated (Jaeger et al. 2006).

Effect of HBO on ICP in Acute TBI

HBO alone has been demonstrated to reduce ICP. Even normobaric hyperoxia, defined as treatment with 100 % oxygen, has been shown to elevate brain oxygen, improve brain oxidative metabolism, and reduce intracranial pressure in TBI. ICP continues to decrease post therapy although during baseline periods there may be no difference between the control patients and those receiving 100 % oxygen. These findings provide a strong impetus for the use of oxygen in TBI. Because O_2 is being treated as a drug, dosimetry and monitoring are necessary. The correct utilization of HBO involves documentation of the patient's neurological status, measurement of ICP, and cerebral metabolism; particularly the lactate/pyruvate ratio effects an increase in the pH by decreasing the lactate level. This facilitates the decision as to when to treat, how often to treat, and what atmospheric pressure of oxygen to use. Clearly, if the same results can be obtained with normobaric oxygen (NBO), the clinician should reserve HBO for those patients that respond better to this HBO than to NBO as assessed by multimodality monitoring and neurological status. Avoidance of oxygen toxicity is paramount. The use of continuous 100 % oxygen must be accompanied by evidence of the absence of oxygen toxicity. Because HBO is dosimetry controlled, the patient's clinical status is monitored (ICP, cerebral metabolism), and if it is used intermittently, the patient has time to recover from potential O_2 toxicity with the normal indigenous anti-oxidant mechanisms. If confirmation of ICP reduction and improved metabolism aid is obtained, a combination of HBO and "hyperoxia" should be considered for TBI. Alternate sessions of HBO and NBO can be considered. Differences in response reflect the differences and complexity of TBI. In any event, there is more than ample evidence of the need to adequately use oxygen in TBI and measure partial pressure of brain O_2 in TBI. Similarly, safety and understanding the issues of ischemia and altered metabolism continue to be stressed (Verweij et al. 2007).

The use of hyperventilation to diminish cerebral blood volume (secondary to hypocarbia causing increased pH and vasoconstriction) can be enhanced by HBO. The complexities of the use of HBO for TBI, however, must not be understated. Vasoconstriction secondary to hyperventilation can cause areas of cerebral ischemia. In addition, after 30 h of hyperventilation, the CSF pH returns to normal. Vessel diameter becomes greater than that at baseline during this time frame. It is unlikely that under hyperoxic conditions vasoconstriction itself could be deleterious. However, it has been shown that under excessive hyperoxic conditions, cerebral metabolism can be adversely affected. Thus, as in any treatment, both dosimetry and appropriate indications are essential. CBF measurements, before and after HBO, will assist in determining the efficacy of the treatment and in deciding upon dosimetry and schedules of HBO treatments. HBO is contraindicated when a stage of vasomotor paralysis has developed. In that condition, the vasoconstrictive effects of oxygen are absent and toxic hyperoxia can result. Patients receiving HBO, therefore, must show a response to hyperventilation by reduction in ICP. They must not have fixed and dilated pupils. Continuous monitoring of the neurological status when using HBO for the acute brain damaged patient is necessary. It must include jugular venous lactate and pH determinations, and periodic evaluation of cerebral blood flow. This, along with measurement of ICP and periodic neuro-imaging and clinical evaluation, will allow the appropriate application of HBO therapy. Each individual patient will require a specific dose with a specific frequency of administration during well-defined times if HBO is to be appropriately and successfully utilized.

Toxic effects of hyperoxia should be avoided (see Chap. 6). Oxygen toxicity involves metabolic production of partially reduced ROS. These oxygen free radicals include superoxide, peroxide, and hydroxyl radicals. They are produced by a univalent reduction of oxygen during aerobic metabolism. Thus, the use of HBO to reduce edema and oxygenate ischemic tissue may pose a dilemma because the original cerebral injury itself may alter cerebral metabolism, resulting in anaerobic metabolism and the production of oxygen free radicals. Free radical production in experimentally injured animals, however, has been shown to be reduced by HBO application. In spite of this observation, caution should be exercised in the use of HBO in brain injury and free radical scavengers may be used as adjuncts to HBO.

Oxygen toxicity is a dose-related phenomenon because oxygen is a drug. Dosimetry, therefore, must be appropriate. Monitoring must be continuous and accurate. HBO is administered intermittently to allow the anti-oxidant defenses to recover. Concomitant drugs that may potentiate oxygen toxicity must be avoided. These include adrenal cortical steroids which have been used in acute head injury patients. Untoward results from the use of HBO in head trauma are seen at pressures over 2 ATA. Usually HBO at 1.5–2 ATA is used in CNS disorders and is considered to be quite safe. Modifications of this will depend upon the metabolic monitoring factors and ICP measurements.

Effect of HBO Therapy in Chronic Sequelae of TBI

Most of emphasis on treatment has been in acute TBI in the past. In recent years there is increasing attention paid to chronic sequelae of TBI such as post-concussion syndrome (PCS) and possibly post-traumatic stress disorder (PTSD), which has been seen in US war veterans. Because of prevalence of PTSD in civilian population, its relation to TBI is still somewhat controversial and is the subject of ongoing investigations in war veterans. Blast-related mild TBI (mTBI) is a common injury among returning troops due to the widespread use of improvised explosive devices in the Iraq and Afghanistan Wars. Use of diffusion tensor imaging (DTI) has shown that mTBI with loss of consciousness is associated with white matter injury of the brain. The findings of a study suggest that at higher levels of PTSD symptom severity, loss of consciousness was correlated with postmortem reports of diffuse axonal injury following mTBI and that such injuries may be particularly detrimental to white matter integrity, which in turn influence neurocognitive function (Hayes et al. 2015).

In a phase I study of the safety and efficacy of HBO in 16 war veterans with chronic blast-induced mild to moderate TBI/PCS, each patient received 40 HBO sessions (1.5 ATA/60 min) in 30 days (Harch et al. 2012). Significant improvements occurred in symptoms, abnormal physical exam findings, cognitive testing, and quality-of-life measurements, with concomitant significant improvements in SPECT.

Chronic repeated trauma in sports, particularly football, is known to lead to chronic traumatic encephalopathy.

Experimental and Clinical Studies of HBO in TBI

Table 21.1 gives a brief summary of classical studies dealing with the clinical and investigative work on this topic, which indicates that HBO has an important place in the management

Table 21.1 Clinical and investigative work on HBO in traumatic brain injury: classical studies

Traumatic brain injury (TBI)
Experimental
Coe and Hayes (1966): Increased lifespan in experimentally injured rats treated with HBO
Sukoff et al. (1968): Psyllium seed-induced cerebral edema and acute epidural balloon inflation successfully treated with HBO
Wan and Sukoff (1992): Demonstrated improved neurological status and mortality in experimentally produced brain injury when HBO utilized
Clinical
Fasano et al. (1964): HBO in traumatic brain injury demonstrated to be therapeutic
Holbach et al. (1972): Acute and subacute brain injuries were demonstrated to have better results when treated with HBO. ICP and cerebral metabolism improvement documented
Mogami et al. (1969): Traumatic brain injuries and postoperative edema after brain tumor surgery successfully treated with HBO. ICP, EEG and clinical improvement most favorable in the lesser injured patients
Artru et al. (1976a): The neurological status, ICP and metabolism of certain patients with traumatic encephalopathies improved when treated with HBO. Patients under 30 without mass lesions fared better than similar control group
Országh and Simácek (1980) and Isakov et al. (1981): Positive results in patients treated with HBO for traumatic encephalopathies
Sukoff (1982): Clinical and ICP improvement seen in those patients with mid-level coma scales undergoing HBO therapy for acute head trauma
Rockswold (1992): Increased survival in acute head injury with HBO
Barrett et al. (1998): Cognitive and cerebral blood flow improvement in chronic stable traumatic brain injury by use of HBO at 1.5 ATA
Intracranial pressure (ICP)
Experimental
Miller and Ledingham (1970, 1971) and Miller (1973): HBO demonstrated to reduce ICP in experimental cerebral edema. Vasomotor changes in response to CO_2 are necessary for the vasoconstrictor effects of HBO to lower ICP. HBO and hyperventilation causes a greater reduction in ICP than hyperventilation alone. Additionally, cerebral vasoconstriction does not occur when arterial PO_2 is >1800 mmHg. Cerebral pH at 2 ATA was also shown to increase
Clinical
Mogami et al. (1969): TBI patients with the least severe symptoms had the greatest ICP reduction
Artru et al. (1976b): Improvement in patients treated with HBO for TBI
Sukoff (1982): Statistically significant reduction in ICP in all monitored TBI patients

of the severely injured but therapeutically responsive patient with TBI. A study on the effect of HBO in TBI evaluated CBF and cognitive improvement (Barrett et al. 1998). In this study five patients with TBI, at least 3 years after injury, underwent 120 HBO treatments each at 1.5 ATA for 60 min. There was a rest period of 5 months before the first set of 80 treatments and the second set of 40 treatments. Sequential studies of SPECT scanning, CBF, speech, neurological, and cognitive function were carried out. Six patients with TBI, who were not treated with HBO, served as controls. Results of SPECT scanning showed that there was no significant change over time whereas HBO-treated patients had permanent increases in penumbra area CBF. Speech fluency improved in the HBO group as well as memory and attention. The improved peaked at 80 HBO treatments. The authors concluded that HBO therapy can improve cognitive function as CBF in the penumbra in chronic stable TBI patients where no improvement would ordinarily be expected 3 years after the injury.

Increased cerebral metabolic rate of oxygen and decreased level of lactate in CSF found in TBI patients treated with HBO indicate that HBO can improve cerebral metabolism. The correlation between CBF and cerebral metabolic rate

and HBO is important in understanding why HBO may be useful in the treatment of severe TBI. Intracranial pressure is the sum total of brain blood volume, brain tissue volume, and water, and may be lowered by reducing blood volume. HBO can reduce blood volume. ICP responds better to HBO when the rate of CBF is lowered. There is no correlation between the response of ICP to HBO therapy and the level of CBF. In patients with elevated ICP, HBO tends to decrease it.

Experimental studies confirm some of the findings observed in earlier studies of TBI patients with HBO. In a rat model of chronic TBI, a 40-day series of 80 HBO treatments at 1.5 ATA produced an increase in contused hippocampus vascular density and an associated improvement in cognitive function as compared to controls and sham-treated animals (Harch et al. 2007). These findings reaffirm the favorable clinical experience of HBO-treated patients with chronic TBI.

A phase I/II open-label study (ClinicalTrials.gov Identifier: NCT01847755), which was on-going in 2016, will test the effect of HBO at 1.5 ATA (5 times/week) on cognitive function and CBF determined by SPECT in TBI patients. Each patient will have a SPECT scan, cognitive assessment, and physician evaluation prior to first treatment and after 40, 80, and 120 treatments to document progress of the treatment. Cognitive assessment will include the Trail Making Test Parts A and B. HBO treatments may be adjusted for patient comfort. If the SPECT scan, cognitive assessment, and physician evaluation show improvement after 40 treatments, another 40 HBO treatments will be administered. Treatments will be discontinued after a 40-session interval if the SPECT scan, cognitive assessment, and physician evaluation show no improvement.

Controlled Clinical Trials of HBO for TBI

In 2012, wars in the Middle East had resulted in between 10 and 20 % of US service members with mTBI. Anecdotal reports had associated HBO with improved outcomes after mTBI, but controlled clinical trials were lacking. The Department of Defense (DoD), in collaboration with the Department of Veterans Affairs (DVA), planned a compre-

hensive program to examine this issue (Weaver et al. 2012). The DoD's 4 planned randomized controlled trials were to enroll a total of 242 service members with post-concussion syndrome (PCS) and expose them to a range of control, sham, and HBO conditions for 40 sessions over a period of 8–11 weeks. Compression pressures will range from 1.2 ATA (sham) to 2.4 ATA, and oxygen concentration will range from room air (sham and control) to 100 %. Outcomes measures include both subjective and objective measures performed at baseline, at exposure completion, and at 3–12 months' follow-up. This integrated program of clinical trials investigating the efficacy of HBO in service members with persistent symptoms following mTBI exposure will be important in defining practice guidelines and, if needed, for the development of definitive clinical trials in this population. However, at the time of writing this chapter in 2016, none of these planned trials could be identified. Published as well as ongoing controlled clinical trials of TBI and its sequelae (those where information is available) are listed in Table 21.2.

Table 21.2 Controlled clinical trials of HBO for TBI and sequelae

Reference/trial #	Description	Results/comments
Lin et al. (2008)	Prospective randomized trial on 44 patients with TBI half of whom received HBO after the stabilization of condition. Evaluation before and 3–6 m after HBO with Glasgow Coma Scale (GCS) and Glasgow Outcome Scale (GOS)	GCS of the HBO group was improved from 11.1 to 13.5 in average, and from 10.4 to 11.5 for control group. Among those patients with GOS of 4 before the HBO, significant GOS improvement was observed in HBO group 6 m after HBOT
Rockswold et al. (2010)	A prospective randomized study on 69 patients with severe TBIs were treated within 24 h of injury once/day for 3 days in 3 groups: (1) HBO, 60 m 1.5 ATA; (2) NBH, 3 h of 100 % O2 at 1 ATA; and (3) control, standard care	HBO had a more robust post-treatment effect than NBH on oxidative cerebral metabolism by producing brain tissue $PO_2 \geq 200$ mmHg. However, this effect was not all or none, but graduated
Boussi-Gross et al. (2013)	A prospective, randomized, crossover trial of 1.5 ATA HBO on 56 mTBI patients 1–5 years after injury with PCS using 40 1-h sessions (5 day/week)	HBO-induced neuroplasticity led to improvement of brain functions and quality of life at a chronic stage
Cifu et al. (2014)	Randomized, double-blind 10-week trial of effect of 40 HBO treatments (1.5–2 ATA once a day) on eye movement abnormalities in 60 war veterans with at least 1 mTBI	Neither 1.5 nor 2 ATA HBO had an effect on post-concussive eye movement abnormalities after mTBI when compared with a sham-control
Wolf et al. (2015)	Randomized trial of effect of 30 exposures of HBO at 2.4 ATA on cognitive function in TBI	No significant difference between a sham and HBO treatments but subgroups with favorable response to HBO
ClinicalTrials.gov #:NCT02089594/Completion 2015, not published yet	A phase III randomized, prospective, single-blind crossover trial of 40 treatments with HBO at 1.5 ATA versus maintenance medication on 100 patients with mTBI/PCS who have been symptomatic continuously for at least 6 months	After 8 weeks the no treatment group will be crossed over to receive 40 HBO treatments

Use of HBO for TBI in Clinical Practice

When HBO is utilized as an adjunct to the treatment of TBI, the following regime should be followed:

- A neurosurgeon is involved with the patient care.
- Treatments must be initiated within 12 h of the trauma, unless there has been a recent deterioration of the patient's condition.
- An ICP monitor must be in place.
- Concurrent methods to reduce ICP include hyperventilation for the first 48 h and consideration for barbiturate coma.
- An experienced hyperbaric team.
- The protocol must consist of exposure to HBO at between 1.5 and 2 ATA on an intermittent basis.
- Treatments can be given every 4, 6, 8, or 12 h depending upon the clinical status, ICP, and results of measurement of cerebral metabolism, neuro-imaging, and CBF measurements.
- Jugular venous glucose, pH, and lactic acid determinations are necessary. The goal is to achieve a diminished lactic acid concentration and an increased pH.
- Cerebral perfusion pressure must be adequate (70 mmHg or above).
- The patient must have therapeutic levels of an anticonvulsant.

Besides dosimetry of HBO, complete monitoring is essential including frequent neurological examinations, ICP measurements as well as analysis of CSF, blood pH, and lactic acid. Each patient must be treated according to an individual schedule, and the dose should be based on response and results. Although HBO is not established as treatment of severe TBI, therapeutic effectiveness may be established when full analysis including total monitoring of further randomized clinical trials is completed. Subgroups of appropriate patients for treatment can be identified. For these patients the ideal pressure, duration, and frequency of HBO sessions can be determined.

Conclusions

HBO has been shown both experimentally and clinically to improve the outcome of TBI. Its therapeutic effects are based on the ability of the hyperoxic environment to reduce CBF by vasoconstriction, reduce ICP, and increase oxygenation. There is supportive evidence for increasing tissue pO_2 as a consequence (tissue and microcirculation). Cerebral trauma results in a cascade of events characterized by ischemia, hypoxia, edema, increased ICP, increased CBF, and metabolic and enzymatic alterations. This results in a lowering of the pH and increase in lactic acid production, and free radical release resulting in vasodilatation, impaired carbon dioxide reactivity, and damage to the cerebral vascular endothelium. The ability of HBO to modify these pathophysiological changes is postulated, and there is sufficient experimental and clinical evidence to support this.

The toxic effects of oxygen itself is explained by the free radical theory of molecular oxygen toxicity and parallels the metabolic effects initiated subsequent to head injury; the release of toxic oxygen free radicals. However, when utilized appropriately as regards dosage, patient selection, CBF, and cerebral metabolic monitoring, the vasoconstrictive effect of HBO, while enabling increased tissue oxygenation, will maintain the tissue pO_2 at a level that allows the cellular antioxidant defense mechanisms to overcome the potential of hyperoxia to induce oxygen toxicity. It appears that the most favorable patients to treat are those with midlevel Glasgow coma scales using HBO pressure between 1.5 and 2 ATA, on an intermittent short-term basis. Intriguing issues in the use of HBO to manage cerebral injury include the fact that HBO has persistent effects. Additionally, the use of HBO with pharmacological agents such as oxygen radical scavengers may potentiate their therapeutic effects.

The hemodynamic phases following TBI are well defined. Autoregulation impairment after even minor brain trauma, and the importance and manner of CBF in cerebral trauma, have been well studied and are well defined. This, along with experimental and clinical success, supports the use of HBO for TBI.

Historically, cerebral vasoconstriction and increased oxygen availability were seen as the primary mechanisms of HBO in TBI. HBO now appears to improve cerebral aerobic metabolism at a cellular level, i.e., by enhancing damaged mitochondrial recovery. HBO given at the ideal treatment paradigm, 1.5 ATA for 60 min, does not appear to produce oxygen toxicity and is relatively safe (Rockswold et al. 2007). The authors believe that, by virtue of over 40 years of experimental and clinical evidence, supported by their own experience, HBO has stood the test of time and can be considered a valuable therapeutic modality in the treatment of TBI. The importance of monitoring, clinically, analysis of the ICP and metabolism, and realization that HBO is a drug, remains important. Multicenter prospective randomized clinical trials are still needed to resolve some of the controversies and to definitively define the role of HBO in severe TBI. Such clinical trials are in progress.

Role of HBO in the Management of Spinal Cord Injury

The concept of using HBO for spinal cord injury (SCI) parallels the application of this therapy for brain injuries. The ability of HBO to reduce both edema and ischemia are the key factors. Traumatic myelopathies are characterized by ischemia and edema, which may be a consequence of vaso-paralysis and direct injury to the spinal cord and its vasculature. There is compromise of spinal cord microvasculature, resulting in decreased blood flow and oxygen supply to the gray matter with surrounding hyperemia. Anatomical or physiological cellular disruption may occur as a result of the initial injury, or consequent to the pathophysiological changes that occur over a period of 2–4 h. The evolution of SCI entails gray matter ischemia and increased spinal cord blood flow with subsequent white matter edema. There are numerous publications reporting experimental work supporting the effectiveness of HBO in TBI. Clinical studies have suggested but not substantiated the potentially beneficial effects of HBO for the TBI. Encouraging reports have been anecdotal at best. However, none of the clinical studies but ours deals with patients treated within 2–4 h post-injury. This time period represents the window of opportunity that relates to the progression of pathophysiological sequelae of SCI resulting in permanent anatomical disruption of an originally physiologically functional cord. Initially, they may be indistinguishable. In our experience, patients without definite evidence of anatomical disruption of the spinal cord treated within 2–4 h of their trauma may respond to HBO treatment. Clinical monitoring of the patient must be accompanied by somatosensory-evoked potentials (SSEPs). MRI must not show evidence of anatomical disruption of the spinal cord. CT and plain X-ray films similarly must not show evidence of anatomical disruption. It is essential to begin HBO no later than 4 h post-injury. Treatment sessions are either at 1.5 or 2 ATA, depending upon the initial and subsequent clinical evaluation and pre- and post-treatment SSEPs. If there is evidence of either clinical or electrodiagnostic improvement, it is justified to continue HBO. The patient's spine must be maintained in proper alignment with traction at all times in cervical injuries. A portable traction gurney, compatible with HBO therapy as well as ground and air ambulance transfer, initial emergency hospital care, neurodiagnostic procedures, surgery, and initial nursing care, including prone and supine positioning, is used.

Effects of Spinal Cord Injury

There are two major effects of trauma to the spinal cord:

- Anatomical disruption and secondary vascular compromise following venous stasis, edema, and hypoxia. If uncorrected, it leads to tissue necrosis.
- Functional loss and paralysis below the level of the lesion.

Various surgical and drug treatments have been advanced for SCI, with little or no cure. The role of conventional surgery is confined to removal of compressive lesions and stabilization of the bony spine. Currently, research is in progress for stem cell transplantation and regeneration of the spinal cord. Major advances in SCI research during the past quarter of a century include use of SSEP, rCBF, methods to detail the morphology and content of the spinal cord tissues, and use of HBO.

Rationale of the Use of HBO in SCI

Rationale of the use of HBO in SCI is as follows:

- Some neuronal damage, due to bruising rather than laceration, is reversible by HBO.
- HBO relieves ischemia of the gray matter of the spinal cord.
- HBO reduces edema of the white matter.
- HBO corrects biochemical disturbances at the site of injury in the spinal cord substance, e.g., lactic acidosis.

Publications about research on this topic combined with clinical experience support the conclusion that HBO holds an important place in the management of the severely injured but therapeutically responsive patient with a traumatic myelopathy.

Animal Experimental Studies of HBO in SCI

The initial experimental studies suggesting the use of HBO in SCI were published by Maeda (1965). He demonstrated tissue hypoxia resulting from injury to the spinal cords of dogs induced by clamp crushing. When the animals were subjected to HBO at 2 ATA, significant elevations in spinal cord pO_2 were observed as long as 72 h after the injury. Hartzog et al. (1969) demonstrated reversibility of the neurological deficit in cord-traumatized baboons by administration of 100 % oxygen at 3 ATA during the first 24 h after trauma. Locke et al. (1971) found that lactic acid accumulates in the injured spinal cord. This supports the concept that ischemia plays a role early in the traumatic process following SCI. The lactic acid levels remain elevated up to 18 h.

Kelly et al. (1972) studied the tissue pO_2 of the normal and the traumatized spinal cord in dogs. The tissue pO_2 of the normal spinal cord rose on breathing 100 % oxygen. After trauma the tissue pO_2 dropped to near zero and did not respond to 100 % oxygen at ambient pressure. However, at 2 ATA the tissue pO_2 rose to high levels during the period of mechanical compression of the cord. The animals rendered paraplegic and then given HBO recovered to a greater degree than the untreated animals in the control group. The beneficial effects were similar to those of glucocorticosteroids and hypothermia. The authors suggested a clinical trial of HBO in patients with acute spinal cord injury.

Yeo (1976) reported the results of use of HBO therapy (3 ATA) to control the onset of paraplegia after SCI induced in sheep. Institution of HBO within 2 h of injury resulted in improved motor recovery over the following 8 weeks. Yeo's further research into the effect of HBO on experimental paraplegia in sheep, which correlated recovery of motor power and histopathology at the level of lesion after controlled contusion to the spinal cord, confirmed his earlier findings (Yeo et al. 1977). They compared the treatments used, which were prednisolone, α-methyl-*para*-tyrosine (AMT, an inhibitor of norepinephrine synthesis that produces some recovery of motor activity in SCI), mannitol, or HBO. There was significant motor recovery in the untreated (control) animals, but none regained the ability to stand or walk. There was no significant recovery with methylprednisolone. In AMT-treated as well as HBO-treated groups there was significant motor recovery. Examination at 8 weeks showed cystic necrosis of the central portion of the spinal cord at the level of the lesion in all animals, but it was least marked in those treated by HBO.

Higgins et al. (1981) studied the spinal cord-evoked potentials in cats subjected to transdural impact injuries and treated with HBO, and demonstrated beneficial effects on the long tract neuronal function. The authors suggested that HBO may afford protection against the progression of intrinsic post-traumatic spinal cord processes destructive to long tract function if this treatment is applied early.

Sukoff (1982) reported the effects of HBO on experimental SCI. Seventeen cats were treated immediately after graded SCI by intermittent exposure to 100% oxygen at ambient pressure. No animals treated with HBO were paralyzed, whereas six of the 13 controls were. Five treated animals recovered fully and all but one could walk. Only one of the control cats could do so.

Gelderd et al. (1983) performed spinal cord transection in rats and tested the therapeutic effects of dimethyl sulfoxide (DMSO) and/or HBO at various pressures in different groups of animals. The animals were killed 60–200 days after the treatment and the spinal cord was examined with light microscopy, scanning electron microscopy, and transmission electron microscopy. Normally, the growth of axons is aborted within a few days following transection. In animals treated with DMSO and HBO, Gelderd et al. found naked axons 90–100 days post-lesion. These findings suggest that both DMSO and HBO can prolong the regeneration process for extended periods following injury. There was less cavitation in the spinal cords of animals treated with DMSO and HBO than in the controls which did not receive any treatment.

An additional study using 20 gerbils with controlled and graded spinal cord trauma caused by aneurysm clip has confirmed the therapeutic effect of HBO, and the decrease in pathological changes has been verified histologically (Sukoff 1986).

The effects of HBO have been compared with that of methylprednisolone regarding the oxidative status in experimental SCI (Kahraman et al. 2007). Clip compression method was used to produce acute SCI in rats. HBO was administered twice daily for a total of eight 90 min sessions at 2.8 ATA. Tissue levels of superoxide dismutase and glutathione peroxidase were evaluated as a measure of oxidant antioxidant status and were elevated in untreated animals. Methylprednisolone was not able to lower these levels, but HBO administration diminished all measured parameters significantly. Thus, HBO, but not methylprednisolone, seems to prevent oxidative stress associated with SCI.

Clinical Studies of HBO in SCI

Jones et al. (1978) treated seven SCI patients with HBO within 12 h of injury. Two of these patients had functional recovery, and three patients' complete lesions became incomplete (partial recovery). One of the patients had enough motor and sensory recovery after two treatments to allow the functional use of calipers.

Gamache et al. (1981) presented the results of HBO therapy in 25 of 50 patients treated during the preceding years. HBO was generally initiated 7.5 h after injury. The patients continued to receive conventional therapy for SCI, and their pre- and post-treatment motor scores were compared with those of patients not receiving HBO. Patients paralyzed for more than 24 h failed to make any significant recovery with or without HBO. The authors concluded:

The fact that HBO patients, at 4–6 months, were closer to the 1 year results of the patients treated conventionally is a reflection of the alterations in the rate of recovery rather than a difference in the overall outcome. Ideally the HBO therapy should be initiated within 4 h of the injury. Sukoff protocol for treatment of patients with traumatic myelopathy is as follows:

- Initial evaluation, including complete neurological and systemic examination, took place in the shock-trauma unit.
- Respiratory function was assisted as necessary to maintain pO$_2$ above 90 mmHg. Problems outside the nervous system were treated and BP was maintained at 100–130 mmHg systolic.
- X-rays of the spine were obtained and skeletal traction was applied to maintain the alignment in cases of fracture-dislocation.
- IV mannitol was given as long as BP was above 110 mmHg systolic.
- Cisternal myelography or metrizide-assisted CT scan was promptly obtained.

- HBO treatment was performed in a Sechrist monoplace chamber. A special traction device was used in the chamber and nursing attention was maintained.
- Treatment consisted of 100 % oxygen at 2 ATA for 45 min repeated every 4–6 h for 4 days. If no response had occurred by that time, treatment was discontinued.

Motor improvement was seen in those patients who were treated within 6 h of injury. Two patients with sensory problems obtained relief. Two patients showed significant reduction of myelographic block, although neither improved clinically. In three patients there was dramatic recovery. Sukoff felt that his clinical success with HBO therapy, as well as that reported by others to date, was anecdotal. He suggested that clinical trials using double-blind techniques should be initiated on patients within 4 h of SCI. Yeo (2009) reviewed his experience with the use of HBO therapy in 45 patients with SCI over the period 1978–1982. Patients were given one, two, or three treatments, usually 90 min in duration at 2.5 ATA. Thirty-five of the patients had upper motion neuron lesions. Twenty-seven of these could tolerate two or three treatments, and 15 (56 %) of them recovered functionally. During the same period of time, 29 (46 %) of the 63 patients who did not receive HBO also recovered. The difference in the recovery rate is significant, considering that the average delay from the time of injury to the commencement of treatment was 9 h. All patients who showed recovery had incomplete lesions with some preservation of function below the level of the lesion.

Role of HBO in Rehabilitation of SCI Patients

Rehabilitation is the most important part of the management of SCI patients. The role of HBO in physical therapy and rehabilitation is discussed in Chap. 36. HBO can be a useful aid in the rehabilitation of paraplegics in the following ways:

- Capacity for physical exercise can be increased in neurologically disabled persons by using HBO at 1.5 ATA (see Chap. 4).
- Metabolic complications associated with fatigue are reduced. Quadriplegics have a reduced vital capacity. Hart and Strauss (1984) tested the effect of HBO on 22 quadriplegics with an average vital capacity of 2.38 L, as compared with the expected normal of 5.10 L for that age group. HBO at 2 ATA for 2 h per day for 3 weeks did not impair pulmonary function, vital capacity, or inspiratory and expiratory forces. The vital capacity of 41 % of the patients was improved by more than 10 %.
- Spasticity is a major hindrance in rehabilitation, but it can be reduced by HBO, particularly when combined with physical therapy.

Treatment should be instituted in the first 4 h following injury, but in practice this is difficult to achieve. Perhaps the treatment of acute spinal cord injuries in a mobile hyperbaric chamber could resolve the time factor. Such a mobile facility should have all the standard emergency equipment and a physician competent to deal with spinal injuries. Sensory-evoked potentials should be used to monitor the progress of the patient, and eventually the patient should be transferred to an SCI center where further treatment should be given, along with any surgery and rehabilitation measures deemed necessary. In the first few hours of SCI, it may be difficult to sort out the serious damage to the spinal cord from spinal cord concussion and contusions. Because time is such an important factor, we suggest that all SCI patients with any degree of neurological involvement (minor or major) be treated with HBO prophylactically during the first few hours following injury. This may possibly prevent edema at the site of contusion with spinal cord compression.

Role of HBO in Compressive and Ischemic Lesions of the Spinal Cord

Compressive Lesions of the Spinal Cord

Holbach et al. (1978) reported three patients with compressive lesions of the spinal cord: one with a protruded cervical disc, one due to arachnoidal adhesions of the spinal cord, and one due to an arachnoid cyst of the lower thoracic cord. There was no improvement of the neurological deficits of these patients in spite of surgical correction of the lesions. HBO therapy was given in the hope of correcting the ischemic process associated with the compressive lesions. The first patient improved after the first HBO session but regressed afterward. Fifteen sessions at 1.5 ATA, each lasting 35–40 min, were then given on a daily basis to all three patients, who all improved. CSF oxygen was monitored and showed a significant increase during HBO. EMG was used to obtain an insight into the mode of action of HBO on the spinal cord lesions. Recordings were taken from many muscles corresponding to the level of the lesion in the spinal cord. In all three cases there was a marked increase in the density of the muscular action potentials after each course of HBO. The improvement reverted to some extent in the new few hours but never dropped to the pretreatment level. The cumulative result of a series of treatments was progressively increased action potentials, and the record had the appearance of an ascending step-like curve.

Holbach et al. (1975) reported use of HBO in the treatment of 13 patients with compressive spinal cord lesions. The therapy was administered postoperatively when neurological deficit persisted. Six of the 13 patients improved markedly, particularly in motor function, while the others showed slight changes. There were no adverse effects.

Neretin et al. (1985) used HBO for treatment of 43 patients with dyscirculatory myelopathy in developmental anomalies and spondylosis. Regression of neurological deficits was observed in patients with spastic tetraparesis within 5–6 days, in contrast to the control group, which was given only vasodilators. There was little improvement in patients with syringomyelia.

Cervical Myelopathy

The effectiveness of HBO in predicting the recovery after surgery in patients with cervical compression myelopathy was evaluated by Ishihara et al. (1997). This is the first paper to utilize HBO as a diagnostic tool to evaluate the functional integrity of the spinal cord. The study group consisted of 41 cervical myelopathy patients aged 32–78 years. Before surgery, the effect of HBO was evaluated and was graded. The severity of the myelopathy and the recovery after surgery were evaluated by the score proposed by the Japanese Orthopedic Association (JOA score). The correlation between many clinical parameters including the HBO effect and the recovery rate of JOA score was evaluated. The recovery rate of JOA score was found to be $75.2 \pm 20.8\%$ in the excellent group, $78.1 \pm 17.0\%$ in the good group, $66.7 \pm 21.9\%$ in the fair group, and $31.7 \pm 16.4\%$ in the poor group. There was a statistically significant correlation between the HBO effect and the recovery rate of the JOA score after surgery. The effect of HBO showed a high correlation with the recovery rate after surgery as compared to the other investigated parameters. HBO can be employed to assess the chance of recovery of spinal cord function after surgical decompression.

Spinal Epidural Abscess

Ravicovitch and Spalline (1982) obtained good results with HBO as an adjunct to laminectomy for drainage of epidural spinal abscesses and to antibiotic therapy. Some of these cases are associated with osteomyelitis of the vertebrae, for which HBO has proven to be very useful.

Conclusions About Use of HBO in SCI

From the available evidence in the literature, it appears that HBO has beneficial effects in some patients with SCI. Because it is difficult to distinguish between anatomical and physiological disruption during the initial stages of spinal cord trauma, all patients should be treated in a hyperbaric chamber if seen within 4 h after a spinal cord injury, unless otherwise contraindicated (MRI, CT, or plain films). Pressures of 1.5–2 ATA are utilized. Monitoring of these patients must include SSEPs and neuro-imaging studies. Determination of spinal fluid glucose metabolism utilizing ventricular CSF samples may significantly advance the treat-

ment of traumatic myelopathies with HBO. As in brain injury, dosimetry and periodicity of treatment will depend upon the results of clinical, electrodiagnostic, and metabolic monitoring.

Experimental studies showing positive effect of HBO on SCI continue to be published and these combined with clinical experience support the role of HBO in acute SCI.

HBO as an Adjunct to Radiotherapy of Brain Tumors

HBO has been used as an adjunct to radiotherapy (Chap. 38) of brain tumors. Chang (1977) carried out a clinical trial on the radiotherapy of glioblastomas with and without HBO. Eighty previously untreated patients with histologically proven glioblastoma were evaluated. Thirty-eight were irradiated under HBO and 42 (controls) in atmospheric air. At the end of 18 months the survival rate appeared considerably higher in the HBO group (28%) than in the controls (10%). After 36 months no patients in the control group survived, whereas two patients in the HBO group were alive beyond 45 and 48 months, respectively. The median survival time was 38 weeks for the HBO group and 31 weeks for the controls. Owing to the small population samples and the pilot nature of the study, the difference in the survival rate between the two groups was not statistically significant. The quality of survival in the HBO group was equal to or slightly better than that of the control group.

A study of preconditioned experimental TBI under 3 ATA HBO found a protective effect of the HBO and suggested it may be a method of limiting brain injury during invasive neurosurgery (Zhiyong et al. 2007). Experimental extradural hematoma produced in a hyperbaric chamber causes no adverse effects. However, when the same mass lesion is produced under normobaric conditions, the animal suffers seizures and does not survive.

The results of radiotherapy combined with HBO in 9 patients with malignant glioma were compared with those of radiotherapy without HBO in 12 patients (Kohshi et al. 1996). This is the first report of a pilot study of irradiation immediately after exposure to HBO in humans. All patients receiving this treatment showed more than 50% regression of the tumor, and in 4 of them, the tumors disappeared completely. Only 4 out of 12 patients without HBO showed decreases in tumor size, and all 12 patients died within 36 months. So far, this new regimen seems to be a useful form of radiotherapy for malignant gliomas. Radiotherapy, within 15 min following HBO exposure, has been studied at several institutes and has demonstrated promising clinical results for malignant gliomas of the brain (Kohshi et al. 2013).

Role of HBO in the Management of CNS Infections

Two types of infections are of particular concern to the neurosurgeon: postoperative infections and brain abscess. HBO has a proven value in the management of infections (Chap. 14). Role of HBO in the management of these will be discussed in this section.

HBO for Postoperative Infections

A study was conducted to evaluate the clinical usefulness of HBO therapy for neurosurgical infections after craniotomy or laminectomy (Larsson et al. 2002). The study involved the review of medical records, office visits, and telephone contacts for 39 consecutive patients who were referred to a neurosurgical department in 1996–2000. Infection control and healing without removal of bone flaps or foreign material, with a minimum of 6 months of follow-up monitoring, were considered to represent success. Successful results were achieved for 27 of 36 patients; one patient discontinued HBO therapy because of claustrophobia, and two could not be evaluated because of death resulting from tumor recurrence. In Group 1 (uncomplicated cranial wound infections), 12 of 15 patients achieved healing with retention of bone flaps. In Group 2 (complicated cranial wound infections, with risk factors such as malignancy, radiation injury, repeated surgery, or implants), all except one infection resolved; three of four bone flaps and three of six acrylic cranioplasties could be retained. In Group 3 (spinal wound infections), all infections resolved, five of seven without removal of fixation systems. There were no major side effects of HBO treatment. The study concluded that HBO treatment is an alternative to standard surgical removal of infected bone flaps and is particularly useful in complex situations. It can improve outcomes, reduce the need for reoperations, and enable infection control without mandatory removal of foreign material such as that used for the reconstruction of cranial operative defects. HBO therapy is a safe, powerful treatment for postoperative cranial and spinal wound infections, it seems cost-effective, and it should be included in the neurosurgical armamentarium.

The prevalence of postoperative wound infection in patients with neuromuscular scoliosis surgery is significantly higher than that in patients with other spinal surgery. A review of six high-risk pediatric patients with neuromuscular spine deformity who received HBO therapy for postoperative infections 2003–2005 revealed that infection resolved in all cases and healing occurred without removal of implants or major revision surgery (Larsson et al. 2011). A retrospective review of effect of effect of HBO on postoperative infections involved 42 neuromuscular scoliosis cases in addition to cerebral palsy or myelomeningocele, operated between 2006 and 2011 (Inanmaz et al. 2014). HBO prophylaxis (30 sessions, 2.4 ATA for 90 min/day) was used in 18 patients and 24 formed the control group. All patients received standard antibiotic prophylaxis. The overall incidence of infection in the whole study group was 11.9% (5/42). The infection rate in the HBO and the control group were 5.5% (1/18) and 16.6% (4/24), respectively. The use of HBO was found to significantly decrease the incidence of postoperative infections.

A retrospective clinical study included 19 cases of iatrogenic spinal infection between 2008 and 2013 where adjuvant HBO therapy was applied because there was no improvement in clinical and laboratory findings despite medical treatment for at least 3 weeks (Onen et al. 2015). Iatrogenic spinal infections were most frequent in the lumbar region and occurred after spine instrumentation in 12 cases and after microdiscectomy in 7 cases. The average number of HBO therapy sessions applied was 20 (range: 10–40). Wound discharge and clinical and laboratory findings recovered in all cases at the end of the therapy course. HBO therapy is considered to be a safe and efficient as an adjuvant therapy in the treatment of infections. It was found to be effective in the prevention of revision procedures and instrumentation failures in iatrogenic osteomyelitis cases, which had occurred following spinal instrumentation.

HBO for Brain Abscess

Brain abscesses may stem from a variety of infective organisms, but anaerobic organisms predominate, which make the abscess difficult to treat by antibiotics, normally the first mode of treatment. Surgical drainage is reserved for encapsulated abscesses that do not resolve and situations where increased intracranial pressure occurs. Brain abscesses are associated with a high mortality and the survivors have severe neurological sequelae. Lampl et al. (1989) treated a series of ten unselected consecutive patients with brain abscess using HBO as an adjunct. All the patients recovered and only one had residual neurological disability. HBO therapy in children with brain abscesses seems to be safe and effective, even when they are associated with subdural or epidural empyemas (Kurschel et al. 2006). It provides a helpful adjuvant tool in the usual multimodal treatment of cerebral infections and may reduce the intravenous course of antibiotics and, consequently, the duration of hospitalization. The rationale of the use of HBO for treatment of brain abscesses is based on the following:

- HBO has a bactericidal effect on predominantly anaerobic organisms.
- HBO has a synergistic effect with the antibiotics used for the treatment of the brain abscess.
- Intermittent opening of the blood–brain barrier (BBB) as an effect of HBO facilitates entry of the antibiotics into the abscess cavity.

- HBO reduces cerebral edema surrounding the abscess and reduces the intracranial pressure.

Experimental studies in the rat have shown that BBB is damaged in staphylococcal cerebritis and that there is surrounding edema in the early stage of the formation of the brain abscess (Lo et al. 1994). This would provide an additional rationale for the use of HBO in the early stages of human brain abscesses, because oxygen entry into the area of cerebritis would be facilitated and brain edema would also be reduced.

In an experimental study, 80 female Wistar rats with brain abscess induced by inoculation of *Staphylococcus aureus* were randomized into groups and treated either with antibiotics, HBO, or with a combination of both (Bilic et al. 2012). Beneficial effect of HBO was evident in groups treated with HBO or with a combination of antibiotic + HBO, which was mainly manifested on days 3 and 5 of the experiment and was evident as statistically significant increase of a number of newly formed blood vessels, increase in mean vascular density, and smaller abscess necrotic core.

Although patients with supratentorial listerial brain abscesses showed a longer survival with surgical drainage, the standard therapy for patients with subtentorial lesions has not been established. In a patient with supra- and subtentorial brain abscesses caused by *L. monocytogenes* infection, which did not respond to antibiotics and the symptoms gradually worsened, HBO treatment was used along with antibiotics, because drainage was not indicated for subtentorial lesions (Nakahara et al. 2014). HBO dramatically reduced the volume of abscesses and improved the symptoms. In a rare case of cerebellar abscess produced by anaerobic bacteria where CT and MRI showed the presence of a multiloculated cerebellar abscess and *Fusobacterium nucleatum* was cultured on aspiration of the abscess (Shimogawa et al. 2015). The patient was administered antibiotic treatment combined with HBO. The symptoms were briefly relieved but the cerebellar abscess recurred, which required a second aspiration. The combined treatment with antibiotics and HBO was maintained after the second operation. After 6 weeks of treatment, the cerebellar abscess was completely controlled. It was concluded that antibiotic treatment combined with HBO is useful for treatment of cerebellar abscesses caused by infection with anaerobic bacteria.

A population-based, comparative cohort study included 40 consecutive adult patients with spontaneous brain abscess treated with surgery and antibiotics between 2003 and 2014; 20 of them received adjuvant HBO, while the remaining patients received only standard therapy (Bartek et al. 2016). Resolution of brain abscesses and infection was seen in all patients. Two patients had reoperations after HBO initiation (10%), while nine patients (45%) in the non-HBO group underwent reoperations. Of the 26 patients who did not receive HBO after the first surgery, 15 (58%) had one or several recurrences that lead to a new treatment: surgery, surgery + HBO or just HBO. In contrast, recurrences occurred in only 2 of 14 (14%) who did receive HBO after the first surgery. A good outcome (Glasgow Outcome Score [GOS] of 5) was achieved in 16 patients (80%) in the HBO cohort versus 9 patients (45%) in the non-HBOT group. Prospective studies are warranted to establish the role of HBOT in the treatment of brain abscesses.

Role of HBO in Cerebrovascular Surgery

The use of HBO for primary cerebral ischemia remains controversial in spite of many clinical and experimental demonstrations of its effectiveness. The rationale for increased tissue and microcirculatory oxygenation has been presented in previous chapters. Role of HBO for acute ischemic stroke is described in Chap. 19. Potential of combination of HBO with thrombolysis by tPA has been discussed. Direct thrombolysis of the clot by intraarterial administration of streptokinase and urokinase is also under clinical investigation. This involves manipulation of the clot and has the advantage of a lesser dose of the thrombolytic and less risk of intracerebral hemorrhage. HBO may be used as an adjunct during the preparation of the patient for the procedure which may be performed by a neuroradiologist/neurosurgeon and also in the postoperative period to reduce cerebral edema and possible reperfusion injury. This chapter deals with neurosurgical aspects of cerebral ischemia. HBO has a role as an adjunct in the following situations in cerebrovascular surgery:

- As a measure for cerebral protection during cerebral vascular procedures requiring vascular occlusion. Complicated neurosurgical procedures requiring lasers and electrocoagulation cannot be performed in a hyperbaric operating room; simpler procedures such as endarterectomy of the cervical portion of the carotid artery can be carried out.
- HBO should be particularly considered in the high-risk carotid endarterectomy patients to afford cerebral protection from stroke during preoperative waiting period.
- Postoperative complications of cerebrovascular surgery; particularly those associated with surgery of intracranial aneurysms.
- As a decision-making measure to select patients for carotid endarterectomy and extracranial/intracranial (EC/IC) bypass operation.
- For cerebral protection during the preoperative waiting period for patients with cerebrovascular occlusive disease.

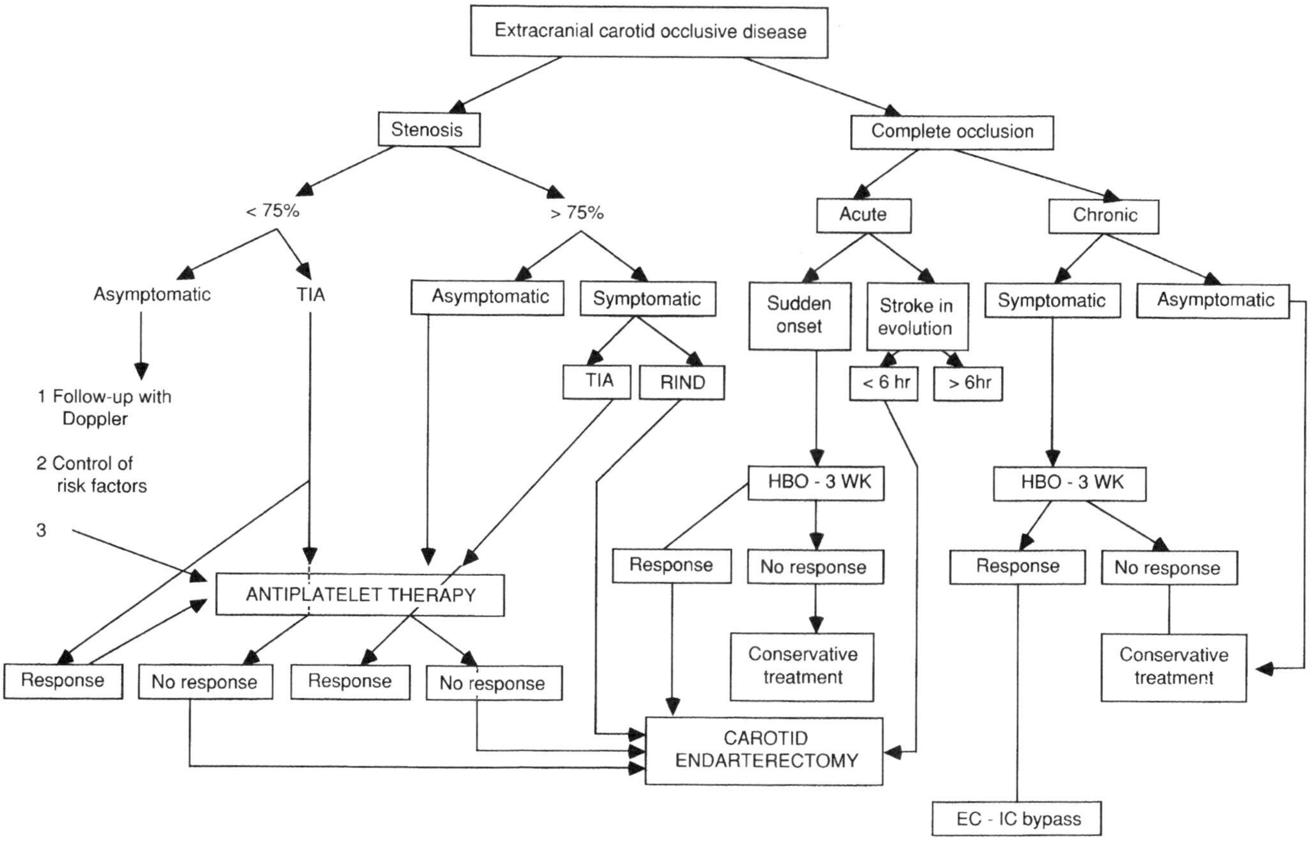

Fig. 21.1 Decision-making for conservative versus surgical management of extracranial carotid occlusive disease. *HBO* hyperbaric oxygen, *EC/IC* extracranial–intracranial bypass, *TIA* transient ischemic attack, *RIND* reversible ischemic neurological deficit, *TPA* tissue plasminogen activator, *asterisk* not eligible for TPA cerebral oxygenation

Use of HBO in Relation to Carotid Endarterectomy

Early attempts to employ HBO as an adjunct to cerebrovascular surgery were made by Illingworth (1962) and Jacobson et al. (1963a). Oxygen at 2 ATA was used during carotid endarterectomy, but it did not afford protection against temporary carotid occlusion, and an intraluminal bypass had to be used. There was, however, an increase in cerebral oxygenation. McDowall et al. (1966) believed that Jacobson's failure was due to cerebral vasoconstriction from HBO and halothane anesthesia, and they subsequently performed a carotid endarterectomy under HBO using chloroform anesthesia, which had a vasodilating effect on cerebral vessels. The procedure was successful.

Lepoire et al. (1972) described the beneficial effect of HBO in six cases of post-traumatic thrombosis of the terminal part of the internal carotid artery. Those lesions are amenable to surgical procedures—direct or bypass—but it is important to give supportive treatment to prevent brain damage from infarction and edema in the acute stage before the surgery can be performed.

Carotid endarterectomy is the most commonly performed surgical procedure for stroke. HBO can be included in the decision tree for the management of a patient with carotid occlusion, as shown in Fig. 21.1. Reversibility of neurological deficit can be determined by response to HBO and improvement seen on SPECT scan. As an alternative to carotid endarterectomy, a less invasive procedure—percutaneous angioplasty with stenting—is being carried out. An incidence of 5% of minor strokes and 1% major strokes has been reported to be associated with this procedure. It is feasible to reduce this complication rate by the use of HBO which has a beneficial effect in cerebral ischemia (see Chap. 18).

Use of HBO for Postoperative Complications of Surgery for Intracranial Aneurysms

Neurological deficits after aneurysm surgery stem from a number of causes, including vasospasm, vascular occlusion, and cerebral edema. Holbach and Gött (1969a) used HBO in a patient with a large middle cerebral artery aneurysm who developed hemiplegia and seizures after surgical repair of the aneurysm. The patient recovered. Several surgeons have used HBO in managing the postoperative complications of intracranial aneurysm surgery and found that HBO prevented the development of severe and fixed neurological deficits in many cases.

Kitaoka et al. (1983) tried HBO treatment in 25 patients with postoperative mental signs after direct operations on anterior communicating aneurysms. Ischemia and edema of the frontal lobes occurred due to spasm of the anterior cerebral arteries. The HBO treatments were started in the "chronic phase" after cerebral edema had subsided. The effects of HBO were marked in three cases, moderate in six cases, slight in 11 cases, and insignificant in four cases. Generally, the results were favorable. The degree of efficacy of HBO was closely related to the previous condition of the patient. HBO was distinctly effective in patients who did not have marked spasm of the anterior cerebral arteries or infarction of the frontal lobes before or after the operation. In contrast, the treatment was ineffective in patients who were in a poor condition (grade) before surgery, e.g., coma. Many patients improved mentally, although EEG, rCBF, and CT scan showed no changes. The authors recommended the use of HBO therapy for postoperative mental signs as soon as cerebral edema disappears.

Isakov and Romasenko (1985) also used HBO in the postoperative care of patients with complications of aneurysm surgery. They used oxygen at 1.6–2.0 ATA. The course of 47 patients treated with HBO was compared with that of 30 patients not subjected to HBO (control group). The conclusions were that in patients with HBO therapy:

1. The serious phase was less prolonged
2. The duration of meningeal syndrome (fever, headache) was shorter by 6 days
3. The number of patients with good results from surgery increased by 18 %
4. Mental disorders were prevented in patients who had no frontal lobe hematoma
5. There was a decrease of postoperative wound infections

HBO to be useful in the management of patients with neurological deficits resulting from vasospasm associated with subarachnoid hemorrhage. HBO is a useful adjunct in moderate cerebral edema, but it is not as effective in severe edema with midline shifts seen on CT scan. Kohshi et al. (1993) evaluated the usefulness of HBO in 43 patients who developed vasospasm following surgery in the acute stage following rupture of intracranial aneurysms. They found that HBO was a useful adjunct to mild hypertensive hypervolumia for the treatment of mild symptomatic vasospasm.

HBO has been shown to ameliorate disturbances following experimental subarachnoid hemorrhage in rats: decreased Na+, K+, and ATPase activity and impaired function of cerebrocortical cell membrane proteins (Yufu et al. 1993). This may be one basis of useful effect of HBO in patients with subarachnoid hemorrhage.

HBO as an Adjunct to Surgery for Intracerebral Hematoma

Holbach and Gött (1969b) reported the use of HBO in a patient with a massive intracerebral hematoma (caused by an angioma) who was comatose and did not regain consciousness after surgery. HBO at 2 ATA was started on the seventh postoperative day, and the patient showed improvement in EEG and in level of consciousness. Sugawa et al. (1988) used HBO therapy on a patient who did not recover from coma after evacuation of an intracerebellar hematoma. The patient regained consciousness but motor recovery was incomplete in spite of continuation of HBO treatments.

A favorable response to HBO is useful in deciding on surgery in patients with hypertensive putaminal hemorrhage. These patients are more likely to continue to improve with the use of HBO following surgery. Patients who do not respond to HBO show a poor outcome regardless of subsequent surgery. Kanno and Nonomura (1996) reviewed 81 patients with hypertensive putaminal hemorrhage treated with HBO after an initial CT scan. The surgical technique used was mostly stereotactic aspiration of the clot. Open craniotomy was used only in three cases. The patients were divided into four groups: (1) patients who showed improvement with HBO and underwent surgery ($n = 21$); (2) patients who showed improvement with HBO but did not undergo surgery; (3) patients who showed no improvement with HBO but underwent surgery; and (4) patients who showed no improvement with HBO and did not undergo surgery. Of all the groups, patients who had shown clinical improvement with HBO had significantly better outcomes that those who did not respond to HBO. The number of surgical procedures for intracerebral hemorrhage has declined considerably at the authors' institution following the adoption of the policy that only responders to HBO are operated on. The authors have not tried to maintain the patients only on HBO stating that the effects of HBO are not durable. It is conceivable that HBO alone may be able to sustain clinical improvement in these patients in the acute phase and it may not be necessary to operate on these patients at all. This approach has not been tested in any clinical study.

Role of HBO in Extracranial/Intracranial Bypass Surgery

The EC/IC bypass operation was devised to bypass the obstruction in a major cranial artery by anastomosis of an extracranial branch with an intracranial branch, using microsurgical techniques. The most common type of operation was an anastomosis between the superficial temporal and the middle artery branches. The usual indications for this procedure in the past were:

• TIA or RIND (reversible ischemic neurological deficit) or a slowly evolving stroke

- Bilateral carotid occlusion
- Unilateral carotid occlusion with contralateral carotid stenosis (prior to endarterectomy of the stenosed artery)
- Occlusive disease of the intracranial arteries: internal carotid, middle cerebral, or basilar
- Generalized cerebrovascular insufficiency
- Moyamoya disease
- Generalized (primary orthostatic) cerebral insufficiency usually associated with multiple occlusions of intracranial vessels
- As a preoperative adjunctive measure for the treatment of giant intracranial aneurysms requiring carotid occlusion, or vertebral artery aneurysms requiring vertebral artery occlusion.

The Cooperative Study of IC/EC bypass (1985) conducted a multicenter review of more than 1400 patients, and compared the medical versus the surgical treatment. The study concluded that the operation had no advantage over medical management, and that it was useless in preventing TIA and stroke. The 30-day mortality of the surgically treated patients was 0.6% and the morbidity 2.5%. A decrease of TIA was noted in 77% of the surgically treated patients, as compared with a decrease in 80% of the medically treated patients.

The shortcomings of the EC/IC bypass operation are as follows:

- The operation aims at increasing blood flow to the brain, but this alone may not be effective in preventing stroke and limiting the size of the infarct. Large vessel occlusion is not the only cause of stroke, and the problem may lie at the EC/IC bypass may not prevent strokes due to atherosclerosis.
  - EC/IC bypass does not prevent embolization from the stump of the occluded extracranial carotid artery, which may be the cause of the TIA. A patent bypass may even increase the possibility of passage of emboli through it.
  - Many studies have reported the short-term benefits of EC/IC bypass on rCBF, neurological, and psychological function, but the long-term effects are debatable. Di Piero et al. (1987) monitored the rCBF using SPECT in 14 patients before and after EC/IC bypass operation performed because of carotid occlusion. Preoperatively, all patients showed hypoperfusion in the affected cerebral hemisphere. Shortly after surgery rCBF was shown to improve in six of the patients, but studies repeated at the 6- and 12-month postoperative follow-ups did not show any difference from the preoperative status.

The health technology assessment report of the United States Department of Health and Human Services (Holohan 1990) admits the shortcomings of the cooperative study of 1985, but maintains that no objective evidence has come up since this study to alter its conclusions. The burden of the proof rests on those who advocate the prophylactic value of this surgery for stroke.

Selection of Patients for EC/IC Bypass Operation

Most of the bypass operations reviewed in the cooperative study were carried out on the basis of angiographic studies. CT scan was not available in some of the centers during the earlier part of the study. Many methods of investigation have evolved during the past decade. They are shown in Table 21.3. Of all the methods used for evaluation of patients who are considered for an EC/IC bypass operation, EEG analysis and the SPECT scan are the most practical and most useful when combined with response to HBO.

Holbach et al. (1977) treated 35 patients in the chronic poststroke stage with HBO. These patients had had internal carotid occlusion for an average of 10 weeks, and their neurological deficits were fixed. The treatments were given at 1.5 ATA for 40 min daily and continued for 10–15 days. Fifteen of these patients improved neurologically; when subsequent EC/IC arterial bypass was carried out, the improvement was maintained. Fifteen patients who did not improve were not operated on. A small group of five patients who did not improve with HBO nevertheless underwent EC/IC bypass, but still did not improve. The authors therefore suggested that the response to HBO be used as a guideline to selection of patients for EC/IC bypass. Response of the patients to HBO was considered a sign of reversibility of the brain lesion, and hence an indicator of a good chance of continuing improvement after a cerebral revascularization procedure. Therefore, EC/IC bypass is useful not only for transient ischemic attacks but also for completed strokes if there is a response to HBO and thus neuronal viability in the penumbra zone. Kapp (1979) reported two cases to illustrate the use of HBO as an adjunct to revascularization of the brain. In both these patients—one with embolism of the middle cerebral artery and the other with occlusion of the left internal carotid artery—circulation was restored to the ischemic areas by surgical means. Both of these patients recovered. In the first case, HBO was used to reverse the patient's neurological deficits while the operating room was being prepared for surgery. A successful embolectomy then restored the patency of the middle cerebral artery. In the second case, HBO treatment stabilized the patient during occlusion of the blood supply to the left hemisphere while the operation was developing enough flow to nourish this hemisphere.

Ohta et al. (1985) elaborated on Holbach's technique and described a method of choosing EC/IC bypass candidates by topographic evaluation of EEG and SSEP with concomitant rCBF studies under HBO.

Table 21.3 Investigation of patients for EC/IC bypass operation

Preoperative

1. Methods for detection of cerebral infarction CT scan and MRI

2. Assessment of vasodilatory capacity of the intracranial arteries
   - Acetazolamide response with rCBF
   - CO_2 response by transcranial Doppler

3. rCBF measurement
   - Xenon 133
   - PET
   - Xenon and CT blood flow mapping
   - SPECT (single photon emission computerized tomography

4. Cerebral blood volume
   - C11 carboxyhemoglobin and PET

5. Cerebral metabolism
   - Radioactive markers for glucose and oxygen
   - PET

6. Electrophysiological
   - SSEP
   - EEG analysis
   - Power spectrum

7. Neuropsychological testing

8. Methods to show reversibility of the cerebral ischemic effects
   - HBO therapy
   - HBO and EEG analysis
   - HBO + EEG + rCBF
   - SPECT

Intraoperative

1. Measurement of blood flow through bypass using Doppler and electromagnetic flowmeter

2. Fluorescein angiography

3. pO_2 measurement over the cerebral cortex

Postoperative

1. Angiography

2. rCBF

3. EEG analysis

4. Psychometric tests

5. PET response to HBO may be of use in selecting patients with neurological deficits who could benefit from surgical revascularization

Kapp (1980) reported on the treatment by HBO at 1.5 ATA of 22 patients with cerebral infarction secondary to occlusion of the carotid or the middle cerebral arteries. Ten patients demonstrated motor improvement during HBO. Seven of these had successful surgical revascularization and no recurrence of neurological deficits. In three patients who were not successfully revascularized, the neurological deficits recurred. It was concluded that the response to HBO may be of use in selecting patients with neurological deficits who could benefit from surgical revascularization. The author confirmed the views of Holbach, and agreed that HBO is useful in about 40 % of patients in the chronic stroke stage. Sukoff (1984) also found the response to HBO and improvement of EEG to be good selection criteria for EC/IC bypass operation. Rossi et al. (1987) performed the EC/IC

bypass operation on 50 patients using the response to HBO and EEG analysis. Neurological improvement was observed in 43 patients, and in 40 of these the improvement persisted.

The EC/IC bypass study failed to take into consideration any subgroups such as those patients selected by response to HBO. The lack of a favorable response to HBO in a stroke patient can help to exclude those who are unlikely to benefit from surgery, who are then spared the expense and risk of unnecessary surgery. This operation should now be reevaluated critically. It is known that the clinical improvement of the patient may be independent of the improvement of CBF. An increase in CBF is not necessarily accompanied by improved oxygenation of the brain tissue. A response to HBO means that the "idling" cerebral neurons show improved function when their hypoxic environments are corrected by raising the tissue oxygen tension. This does not mean that restoring the blood flow to the infarcted area will provide an equivalent effect by carrying only normal amounts of oxygen dissolved in the blood. Although the HBO response test can show the viability of the neurons affected by stroke, its effects cannot be compared quantitatively with those of cerebral revascularization.

In an effort to better define the indications for cerebral revascularization in patients with carotid artery occlusion or middle cerebral artery stenosis, a group of 29 patients was examined. Exposure to HBO (1.5 and 2 ATA) for 30 min each with computer analysis of the EEG was utilized. It proved to be confirmatory for denying surgery in patients with large infarctions or diffused intracranial vascular disease. In clinically stable or transient ischemic episode patients, an improved EEG (increase in alpha activity) supported the indications for EC/IC bypass. The EC/IC bypass operation is contraindicated in the following situations:

1. Stroke patients who show no response to HBO therapy: They are unlikely to benefit from EC/IC bypass.
2. Patients with completed cerebral infarcts who have shown no neurological recovery and have no further ischemic episodes.
3. Patients with single TIA and recovery: Even though these patients may have carotid occlusion, the risk of stroke is not high enough to justify an operation.
4. TIA with marginal circulation and no fixed neurological deficit (EC/IC Bypass Study 1985).
5. Stroke due to thromboembolism.
6. In the acute phase of a stroke in the presence of edema and hemorrhagic infarct: The operation should not be performed within 3 weeks of the onset of infarction.
7. Patients with infarcts located in a strategic location, such as internal capsule with dense hemiplegia are not candidates for EC/IC bypass.
8. Elderly patients with cerebral atrophy and mental impairment associated with chronic cerebrovascular ischemia are not candidates for this operation.

Redefinition of the Indications for EC/IC Bypass Operation in Cerebral Ischemia

The EC/IC bypass is a useful and safe operation. It has been technically refined using sutureless laser microvascular anastomosis (Jain 1984). Its use as a planned supplement to permanent occlusion of the internal carotid artery for the treatment of a giant intracranial aneurysm is justified in some circumstances. HBO may be useful for identifying patients with viable yet nonfunctional ischemic brain, who may benefit from cerebral revascularization. There is need for a controlled study to compare the effect of the EC/IC bypass operation in responders to HBO, where the control group would be maintained on long-term HBO treatments. The objective of such a study would be to determine if long-term

HBO treatment may make the use of an EC/IC bypass operations unnecessary. Redefinition of the indications of the EC/IC bypass operation would involve further separation of the HBO responders into those who should be maintained on long-term HBO therapy and those who should have the operation. Stroke patients who do not respond to HBO therapy are unlikely to benefit from an EC/IC bypass operation.

Neuroprotection During Neurosurgery

Neurosurgical procedures that carry a risk of stroke are most those on the cerebrovascular system and most of these are carried out to prevent a stroke. These complications have been reduced to extremely low figures with the introduction of modern monitoring during surgery and refinement of surgical techniques such as microsurgery. Several methods for neuroprotection have been described (Jain 2011; Jain 2016). Refinements of neurosurgical technique have reduced the need for vascular interruption during neurosurgery but cerebral edema as well as cerebral ischemia are still encountered as complications of some neurosurgical procedures.

HBO preconditioning (PC), described in Chap. 19, may be useful for neuroprotection in procedures where ischemia is anticipated. A study has explored the role of osteopontin (OPN) in HBO-PC-induced neuroprotection (Hu et al. 2015). In a randomized comparative study on rat models, neurological outcome in HBO-PC group was better than that of stroke group. After OPN siRNA was administered, neurological function aggravated compared with control siRNA group. Brain morphology and structure seen by light microscopy was diminished in stroke group and OPN siRNA group, while fewer pathological injuries occurred in HBO-PC and control siRNA group. The infarct volume in HBO-PC group was the lowest, followed by OPN siRNA group and stroke group, respectively. OPN reduced the expression of IL-1β/ nuclear factor-k-gene binding (NFkB) and augmented protein kinase B. OPN siRNA reversed these changes. OPN plays an important role in the neuroprotection elicited by HBO-PC. Pretreatment with HBO may be beneficial for patients prior to brain surgery.

Conclusion

The most important application of HBO appears to be in the management of acute TBI. The bulk of the evidence available indicates the effectiveness of HBO in reducing cerebral edema and intracranial pressure. Sufficient experimental and clinical studies have demonstrated the effectiveness of HBO as a part of comprehensive multimodality management of survivors of TBI to improve the outcome. HBO is increasingly under clinical investigation in the treatment of sequelae of less severe TBI such as posttraumatic stress syndrome.

Pressures used for treatment of patients with brain injury are usually less than those for other systems of the body. Dosimetry and monitoring are the essence of success with HBO in TBI. In most cases it is safe to start with 1.5 ATA.

Postoperative cerebral edema is still a problem in neurosurgery, and the use of HBO in reducing this is well documented and should be utilized. There is still no satisfactory treatment for acute spinal cord injury. Experimentally and anecdotally HBO has proven more effective in the acute stages than any pharmacological method. Its potential is high.

A decision regarding the removal of intracerebral hematomas can be facilitated by response to HBO. Additionally, it will afford protection to the patient during the period that the decision to operate or not to operate is being deliberated. Parallel to the potential of HBO in redefining the indications for extracranial/intracranial bypass operation based on favorable response to HBO is the usefulness of this therapy in the treatment of acute vascular occlusive disease. TBI had received the most support and investigation and has arrived at a stage, in our opinion, of acceptance.

References

Artru F, Chacornac R, Deleuze R. Hyperbaric oxygenation for severe head injuries. Eur Neurol. 1976a;14:310.

Artru F, Philippon B, Gauf F, Berger M, Deleuze R. Cerebral blood flow, cerebral metabolism and cerebrospinal fluid biochemistry in brain-injured patients after exposure to hyperbaric oxygen. Eur Neurol. 1976b;14:351–64.

Barrett K, Harch P, Masel B, et al. Cognitive and cerebral blood flow improvements in chronic stable traumatic brain injury induced by 1.5 ATA hyperbaric oxygen. Undersea Hyperbaric Med. 1998;25:9 (abstract).

Bartek Jr J, Jakola AS, Skyrman S. Hyperbaric oxygen therapy in spontaneous brain abscess patients: a population-based comparative cohort study. Acta Neurochir (Wien). 2016;25 [Epub ahead of print].

Bilic I, Petri NM, Krstulja M, Vuckovic M, Salamunic I, Kraljevic KS, et al. Hyperbaric oxygen is effective in early stage of healing of experimental brain abscess in rats. Neurol Res. 2012;34:931–6.

Boussi-Gross R, Golan H, Fishlev G, Bechor Y, Volkov O, Bergan J, et al. Hyperbaric oxygen therapy can improve post concussion syndrome years after mild traumatic brain injury — randomized prospective trial. PLoS One. 2013;8, e79995.

Calvert JW, Cahill J, Zhang JH. Hyperbaric oxygen and cerebral physiology. Neurol Res. 2007;29:132–41.

Chang CH. Hyperbaric oxygen and radiation therapy in the management of glioblastoma. NCI Monogr. 1977;47:163–9.

Cifu DX, Hoke KW, Wetzel PA, Wares JR, Gitchel G, Carne W. Effects of hyperbaric oxygen on eye tracking abnormalities in males after mild traumatic brain injury. J Rehabil Res Dev. 2014;51:1047–56.

Coe JE, Hayes TM. Treatment of experimental brain injury by hyperbaric oxygenation. A preliminary report. Am Surg. 1966;32: 493–5.

Di Piero V, Lenzi G, Collice M, et al. Long term non-invasive single photon emission computed tomography monitoring of perfusional changes after EC/IC bypass surgery. J Neurol Neurosurg Psychiatry. 1987;50:988–96.

Fasano VA, Nunno T, Urciuoli R, et al. First observations on the use of oxygen under high atmospheric pressure for treatment of traumatic coma. In: Boerema I, Brummelkamp WH, Meijne NG, Editors. Clinical applications of hyperharic oxygen. Proceedings of the first international congress on hyperbaric medicine. Amsterdam: Elsevier; 1964. p. 168–73.

Gamache FW, Myers RAM, Ducker TB, Cowley RA. The clinical application of hyperbaric oxygen therapy in spinal cord injury: a preliminary report. Surg Neurol. 1981;15:85–7.

Gelderd JB, Fife WP, Bowers DE, Deschner SH, Welch DW. Spinal cord transection in rats: the therapeutic effects of dimethyl sulfoxide and hyperbaric oxygen. Ann N Y Acad Sci. 1983;911:218–33.

Harch PG, Kriedt C, Van Meter KW, Sutherland RJ. Hyperbaric oxygen therapy improves spatial learning and memory in a rat model of chronic traumatic brain injury. Brain Res. 2007;1174:120–9.

Harch PG, Andrews SR, Fogarty EF, Amen D, Pezzullo JC, Lucarini J, et al. A phase I study of low-pressure hyperbaric oxygen therapy for blast-induced post-concussion syndrome and post-traumatic stress disorder. J Neurotrauma. 2012;29:168–85.

Hart GB, Strauss MB. Vital capacity of quadriplegic patients treated with hyperbaric oxygenation. J Am Paraplegia Soc. 1984;7:113–4.

Hartzog JI, Fisher RG, Snow C. Spinal cord trauma: effect of hyperbaric oxygen therapy. Proc Ann Clin Spinal Cord Injury Conf. 1969;17:70–1.

Hayes JP, Miller DR, Lafleche G, Salat DH, Verfaellie M. The nature of white matter abnormalities in blast-related mild traumatic brain injury. Neuroimage Clin. 2015;8:148–56.

Higgins AC, Pearlstein RD, Mullen JB, Nashold Jr BS. Effect of hyperbaric therapy on long tract neuronal conduction in acute phase of spinal cord injury. J Neurosurg. 1981;55:501–10.

Holbach KH, Gött U. Cerebrale Durchblutungsstörungen und hyperbare Sauerstoff Therapie. Radiologie. 1969a;9:453–8.

Holbach KH, Gött U. Beobachtungen und Erfahrungen mit der hyperbaren Sauerstofftherapie bei Hirngeschädigten. DVL Research Report 69–78, Bad Godesberg, 1969b. p. 91–109.

Holbach KH, Schröder FK, Köster S. Alterations of cerebral metabolism in cases with acute brain injuries during spontaneous respiration of air, oxygen and hyperbaric oxygen. Eur Neurol. 1972;8:158–60.

Holbach KH, Wassmann H, Hoheluchter KL, Linke D, Ziemann B. Clinical course of spinal lesions treated with hyperbaric oxygenation (HO). Acta Neurochir (Wien). 1975;31(3–4):297–8.

Holbach KH, Wassmann H, Hohelochter KL, Jain KK. Differentiation between reversible and irreversible poststroke changes in brain tissue. Surg Neurol. 1977;7:325.

Holbach KH, Wassmann H, Linke D. The use of hyperbaric oxygenation in the treatment of spinal cord lesions. Eur Neurol. 1978;16:213–21.

Holohan TV. Extracranial-intracranial bypass to reduce the risk of ischemic stroke. AHCPR Health Technology Assessment Report Publ No. 91-3473. Washington, DC: U.S. Department of Health & Human Services; 1990.

Hu SL, Huang YX, Hu R, Li F, Feng H. Osteopontin mediates hyperbaric oxygen preconditioning-induced neuroprotection against ischemic stroke. Mol Neurobiol. 2015;52:236–43.

Illingworth CF. Treatment of arterial occlusion under oxygen at two atmospheres pressure. Br Med J. 1962;2:1272.

Inanmaz ME, Kose KC, Isik C, Atmaca H, Basar H. Can hyperbaric oxygen be used to prevent deep infections in neuro-muscular scoliosis surgery? BMC Surg. 2014;14:85.

Isakov IV, Romasenko MV. Effect of hyperbaric oxygenation on the water content of brain tissue in experimental toxic cerebral edema. Zh Nevropatol Psikhiatr. 1985;85:1786–9.

Isakov IV, Ananev GV, Romasensko MV, Ajde K. Hyperbaric oxygenation in the acute period of craniocerebral injuries. Zh Nevropatol Psikhiatr. 1981;82:7–12.

Ishihara H, Matsui H, Kitagawa H, Yonezawa T, Tsuji H. Prediction of the surgical outcome for the treatment of cervical myelopathy by using hyperbaric oxygen therapy. Spinal Cord. 1997;35:763–7.

Jacobson I, Bloor K, McDowell DG, Norman JN. Internal carotid endarterectomy at two atmospheres of pressure. Lancet. 1963;1:546–9.

Jaeger M, Schuhmann MU, Soehle M, Meixensberger J. Continuous assessment of cerebrovascular autoregulation after traumatic brain injury using brain tissue oxygen pressure reactivity. Crit Care Med. 2006;34:1783–8.

Jain KK. Sutureless extra-intracranial anastomosis using Nd: YAG laser-clinical application. Lancet. 1984;2:816–7.

Jain KK. Handbook of neuroprotection. New York: Springer; 2011.

Jain KK. Neuroprotection. Basel: Jain PharmaBiotech Publications; 2016.

Jones RF, Unsworth IP, Marosszeky JE. Hyperbaric oxygen and acute spinal cord injuries in humans. Med J Aust. 1978;2:573–5.

Kahraman S, Düz B, Kayali H, Korkmaz A, Oter S, Aydin A. Effects of methylprednisolone and hyperbaric oxygen on oxidative status after experimental spinal cord injury: a comparative study in rats. Neurochem Res. 2007;32:1547–51.

Kanno T, Nonomura K. Hyperbaric oxygen therapy to determine the surgical indication for moderate hypertensive intracerebral hemorrhage. Min Invas Neurosurg. 1996;39:56–9.

Kapp JP. Hyperbaric oxygen as an adjunct to acute revascularization of the brain. Surg Neurol. 1979;12:457–62.

Kapp JP. Neurological response to hyperbaric oxygen—criterion for cerebral revascularization. Surg Neurol. 1980;15:43.

Kelly DL, Lassiter KRL, Vongsvivut A, Smith JM. Effects of hyperbaric oxygenation and tissue oxygen studies in experimental paraplegia. Neurosurgery. 1972;36:425–9.

Kitaoka K, Nakagawa Y, Abe H, et al. Hyperbaric oxygen treatment in patients with the postoperative mental signs after direct operations of ruptured anterior communicating aneurysms. Hokkaido Igaku Zasshi. 1983;58:154–61.

Kohshi K, Yokota A, Konda N, Munaka M, Yasukouchi H. Hyperbaric oxygen therapy adjunctive to mild hypertensive hypervolumia for symptomatic vasospasm. Neurol Med Chir (Tokyo). 1993;33:92–9.

Kohshi K, Kinoshita Y, Terashima H, Konda N, Yokota A, Soejima T. Radiotherapy after hyperbaric oxygenation for malignant gliomas: a pilot study. J Cancer Res Clin Oncol. 1996;122:676–8.

Kohshi K, Beppu T, Tanaka K, Ogawa K, Inoue O, Kukita I, et al. Potential roles of hyperbaric oxygenation in the treatments of brain tumors. Undersea Hyperb Med. 2013;40:351–62.

Kurschel S, Mohia A, Weigl V, Eder HG. Hyperbaric oxygen therapy for the treatment of brain abscess in children. Childs Nerv Syst. 2006;22:38–42.

Lampl LA, Frey G, Dietze T, et al. Hyperbaric oxygen in intracranial abscesses. J Hyperb Med. 1989;4:111–26.

Larsson A, Engstrom M, Uusijarvi J, Kihlström L, Lind F, Mathiesen T. Hyperbaric oxygen treatment of postoperative neurosurgical infections. Neurosurgery. 2002;50:287–96.

Larsson A, Uusijärvi J, Lind F, Gustavsson B, Saraste H. Hyperbaric oxygen in the treatment of postoperative infections in paediatric patients with neuromuscular spine deformity. Eur Spine J. 2011; 20:2217–22.

Lepoire J, Larcan A, Fiévé G, Frisch R, Picard L. Acute post-traumatic carotid occlusions. Diagnosis and treatment (value of hyperbaric oxygenation. J Chir (Paris). 1972;104:129–42.

Lin JW, Tsai JT, Lee LM, Lin CM, Hung CC, Hung KS, et al. Effect of hyperbaric oxygen on patients with traumatic brain injury. Acta Neurochir Suppl. 2008;101:145–9.

Lo WD, Wolny A, Boesel C. Blood-brain barrier permeability in the staphylococcal cerebritis and early brain abscess. J Neurosurg. 1994;80:897–905.

Locke GE, Yashon D, Feldman RA, Hunt WE. Ischemia in primate spinal cord injury. J Neurosurg. 1971;34:614.

Maeda N. Experimental studies on the effect of decompression procedures and hyperbaric oxygenation for the treatment of spinal cord injury. J Natl Med Assoc. 1965;16:429–47.

McDowall DG, Jennett WB, Bloor K, Ledingham IM. The effect of hyperbaric oxygen on the oxygen tension of the brain during chloroform anesthesia. Surg Gynecol Obstet. 1966;122:545–9.

Miller JD. The effects of hyperbaric oxygen at 2 and 3 atmospheres: absolute and intravenous mannitol on experimentally increased intracranial pressure. Eur Neurol. 1973;10:1–10.

Miller JD, Ledingham IM. The effect of hyperbaric oxygen on intracranial pressure in experimental cerebral edema. In: Wada J, Takashi IWA, editors. Proceedings of the fourth international congress on hyperbaric medicine. Baltimore: Williams and Wilkins; 1970. p. 543–56.

Miller JD, Ledingham IM. Reduction of increased intracranial pressure: comparison between hyperbaric oxygen and hyperventilation. Arch Neurol. 1971;24:210.

Mogami H, Hayakawa T, Kanai N, Kuroda R, Yamada R, Ikeda T, et al. Clinical application of hyperbaric oxygenation in the treatment of acute cerebral damage. J Neurosurg. 1969;31:636–43.

Nakahara K, Yamashita S, Ideo K, et al. Drastic therapy for listerial brain abscess involving combined hyperbaric oxygen therapy and antimicrobial agents. J Clin Neurol. 2014;10:358–62.

Neretin VI, Kirjakov VA, Lobov MA, Kiselev SO. Hyperbaric oxygenation in dyscirculatory myelopathies. Sov Med. 1985;3:42–4.

Ohta H, Yasui N, Kawamura S, et al. Choice of EIAB operation candidates by topographic evaluation of EEG and SSEP with concomitant RCBF studies under hyperbaric oxygenation. In: Spetzier RF, Carter LP, Selman WR, Martin NA, editors. Cerebral revascularization for stroke. New York: Thieme Stratton; 1985. p. 208–16.

Onen MR, Yuvruk E, Karagoz G, Naderi S. Efficiency of hyperbaric oxygen therapy in iatrogenic spinal infections. Spine (Phila Pa 1976). 2015;40:1743–8.

Országh J, Simácek P. Hyperbaroxia in neurologic patients. Cesk Neurol Neurochir. 1980;43:185–91.

Ravicovitch MA, Spalline A. Spinal epidural abscesses. Surgical and parasurgical management. Eur Neurol. 1982;21:347–57.

Rockswold SB, Rockswold GL, Defillo A. Hyperbaric oxygen in traumatic brain injury. Neurol Res. 2007;29:162–72.

Rockswold GL, Ford SE, Anderson DC, et al. Results of a prospective randomized trial for the treatment of severely brain-injured patients with hyperbaric oxygen. J Neurosurg. 1992;6:929–34.

Rockswold SB, Rockswold GL, Zaun DA, Zhang X, Cerra CE, Bergman TA, et al. A prospective, randomized clinical trial to compare the effect of hyperbaric to normobaric hyperoxia on cerebral metabolism, intracranial pressure, and oxygen toxicity in severe traumatic brain injury. J Neurosurg. 2010;112:1080–94.

Rockwell S, Kelley M, Irvin CG, Hughes CS, Yabuki H, Porter E, et al. Biotechnol preclinical evaluation of oxydent as an adjuvant to radiotherapy. Biomater Artif Cells Immobil Biotechnol. 1992;20:883–93.

Rossi GF, Maira G, Vignati A, Puca A. Neurological improvement in chronic ischemic stroke following surgical brain revascularization. Ital J Neurol Sci. 1987;8:464–75.

Shimogawa T, Sayama T, Haga S, Akiyama T, Morioka T. Cerebellar abscess due to infection with the anaerobic bacteria fusobacterium nucleatum: a case report. No Shinkei Geka. 2015;43: 137–42.

Sugawa N, Sekimoto T, Ueda S. Oxygenation under hyperbaric pressure (OHP) therapy for the patient with deep coma caused by cerebellar hemorrhage: a case report. J Kyoto Perfect Univ Med. 1988;97:1091–6.

Sukoff MH. Use of hyperbaric oxygenation for spinal cord injury. Neurochirurgia. 1982;24:19.

Sukoff MH. Update on the use of HBO for diseases of the central nervous system. Hyperb Oxygen Rev. 1984;5:35–47.

Sukoff MH. Use of hyperbaric oxygenation in spinal injury. Presented at the fifth Chinese conference on hyperbaric medicine, Fuzhow, China 26–29 Sept. (Abstract); 1986.

Sukoff MH, Hollin SA, Espinosa OE, Jacobson JH. The protective effect of hyperbaric oxygenation in experimental cerebral edema. J Neurosurg. 1968;29:236–41.

The EC/IC Bypass Study Group. Failure of extracranial-intracranial arterial bypass to reduce the risk of ischemic stroke. Results of an international randomized trial. N Engl J Med. 1985;313:1191–200.

Verweij BH, Amelink GJ, Muizelaar JP. Current concepts of cerebral oxygen transport and energy metabolism after severe traumatic brain injury. Prog Brain Res. 2007;161:111–24.

Wan J, Sukoff MH. The use of HBO in experimental brain injury and its metabolic sequela. Regional HBO conference, Shanghai Hosp No. 5, Shanghai, China; 1992.

Weaver LK, Cifu D, Hart B, Wolf G, Miller S. Hyperbaric oxygen for post-concussion syndrome: design of Department of Defense clinical trials. Undersea Hyperb Med. 2012;39:807–14.

Wolf EG, Baugh LM, Kabban CM, Richards MF, Prye J. Cognitive function in a traumatic brain injury hyperbaric oxygen randomized trial. Undersea Hyperb Med. 2015;42:313–32.

Yeo JD. Treatment of paraplegic sheep with hyperbaric oxygen. Med J Aust. 1976;1:538–40.

Yeo JD, Stabbach S, McKenzie B. A study of the effects of HBO on experimental spinal cord injury. Med J Aust. 1977;2:145–7.

Yeo JD. The use of hyperbaric oxygen to modify the effects of recent contusion injury to the spinal cord. Cent Nerv Syst Trauma. 2009;1(2):161–5.

Yufu K, Itoh T, Edamatsu R, Mori A, Hirakawa M. Effect of hyperbaric oxygenation on the Na+, K+, ATPase and membrane fluidity of cerebrocortical membranes after experimental subarachnoid hemorrhage. Neurochem Res. 1993;18:1033–9.

Zhiyong Q, Shuijiang S, Guohua X, Silbergleit R, Keep RF, Hoff JT, et al. Preconditioning with hyperbaric oxygen attenuates brain edema after experimental intracerebral hemorrhage. Neurosurg Focus. 2007;22, E13.

Oxygen Treatment for Multiple Sclerosis Patients

22

Philip B. James

Abstract

No treatment has yet been established for the acute attacks, such as optic neuritis, and transverse myelitis, that often precede the development of multiple sclerosis. They are referred to as "clinically isolated syndromes" although magnetic resonance imaging has shown that in most such patients multiple areas are affected. This is consistent with a micro-embolic mechanism which would also account for the multifocal blood–brain barrier disruption demonstrated by several imaging systems. Magnetic resonance spectroscopy has demonstrated lactate in lesions indicating focal hypoxia, which may signal the recruitment of neutrophils resulting in inflammation and cause tissue damage from the release of free radicals. Imaging has shown that mildly affected areas often resolve indicating that the concentration of oxygen in air may be sufficient to ensure remission. Scarring may involve adjacent neural tissue leading to progression of disability over many years. The prompt use of oxygen even at ambient pressure may restore acute blood–brain barrier disruption and resolve disability. Benefit has been demonstrated under controlled conditions from a course of hyperbaric oxygen treatment in patients with advanced chronic disease.

Keywords

Multiple sclerosis • Optic neuritis • Transverse myelitis • Mono sclerosis • Clinically isolated syndromes • Magnetic resonance imaging • Magnetic resonance spectroscopy • Micro-embolism • Blood–brain barrier • Oedema • Neutrophils • Inflammation • Hypoxia • Hyperoxia • Hyperbaric oxygen treatment

Introduction

Multiple sclerosis (MS) is defined as a chronic degenerative disease of the nervous system. However, the terms "multiple" and "sclerosis" are a pathological label, not a diagnosis and describe the presence of more than one area of reactive sclerosis, or more correctly, gliosis, in the nervous system. Although the descriptive criteria, have undergone several revisions since the first was published in the 1970s (Schumacher 1974) they remain unique in medicine by arbitrarily requiring clinical

P.B. James, MB, ChB, DIH, PhD, FFOM (✉)
Department of Surgery, Ninewells Hospital and Medical School, Ninewells Avenue, Dundee, Angus DD1 9SY, UK
e-mail: pbjames@talktalk.net

evidence of more than one lesion and also dissemination over time. The minimum interval specified is a lunar month although the interval may be as long as 45 years. Although symptoms may resolve spontaneously, in many and probably most instances attacks leave residual damage, especially to myelin sheaths, evident on T2 weighted magnetic resonance imaging (MRI) (Young et al. 1981). The affected areas are often referred to as white matter hyperintensities (WHMs) or unidentified bright objects (UBOs) on MRI because MRI has yet to demonstrate the grey matter lesions evident on microscopy (Kidd et al. 1999). Unfortunately, this form of imaging is not able to distinguish between oedema, which is treatable, and sclerosis which is not. Although some damage is usually sustained in attacks, it may be compatible with the return of normal function at least on clinical examination. Evoked response studies, however, usually indicate conduction delays as, for example, in visual evoked responses in patients who have suffered an episode of optic neuritis.

Pathophysiology

The recognition of the presence of discrete lesions in the nervous system, visible as hardened "plaques" in the white matter and first described as "Disseminated Sclerosis" dates back to the early nineteenth century. Despite the development of computerised imaging systems, the certain identification of the disease still awaits post-mortem examination in order to exclude a wide range of conditions: in the absence of any diagnostic test attribution of the label still requires "no better explanation" (Chari et al. 2006). Many accounts describe the disease as simply involving the white matter, but cortical lesions often occur in the brain and in the spinal cord grey and white matter are affected equally. Demyelination has been emphasised because it has been necessary to postulate an antigen derived from myelin to support the theory of autoimmunity. However, despite the lapse of over 50 years no antigen has been demonstrated indicating that the immune changes are secondary, that is, an innate immune response. This would explain the occurrence of the same immunological changes and at the same levels in stroke patients (Wang et al. 1992). In the spinal cord, there is a minimum axonal loss of 20 % (Putnam and Alexander 1947), and similar quantification has been found in lesions in the brain (Kidd et al. 1999). This accounts for the changes in cognitive function often experienced by patients that are usually not apparent clinically.

Magnetic resonance spectroscopy (MRS) has shown that lactate, the hallmark of hypoxia, is present in acute lesions (Miller et al. 1991). Focal hypoxia signals the recruitment of neutrophils resulting in inflammation and tissue damage from the release of free radicals (Weiss 1989). The local disturbance of the blood–brain barrier and inflammation in attacks has been demonstrated by five imaging systems, including CT with contrast enhancement, which has even demonstrated that blood–brain barrier disturbance precedes the symptoms. Although rarely discussed, the vascular changes can be seen in the retina as a periphlebitis indicating dysfunction of the blood–retinal barrier. As there is no myelin in the retina, this indicates the primary nature of the blood–brain barrier changes in MS (McDonald 1986). The prevalence of chronic MS is between 100 and 150 patients per 100,000 of the population of Western countries, but MRI has demonstrated that asymptomatic lesions are common in up to 40 % of the population (James 1997).

The disease typically runs an intermittent course, but it is important to recognise that following damage to the blood–brain barrier subsequent attacks may not involve the primary disease mechanism. This has been demonstrated by neurolo-gists by the use of the hot bath test. The deterioration provoked by this test may result in permanent disability (Berger and Sheremater 1983). There is poor correlation between the patient's disability and the pathology found in the brain at post-mortem but, for obvious reasons, even small lesions in the optic nerves, brain stem and spinal cord are usually associated with clinical signs and symptoms. The clinical course is extremely unpredictable. Patients who satisfy the criteria for multiple sclerosis are described, after several attacks and often with increasing disability, as having "relapsing remitting disease". In a much smaller number, the disease may be "chronic progressive" from the onset. Sometimes, the patient stabilises but with disability and is then described as having "chronic stable" disease. Evidence from MRI indicates that MS is far from being a progressively disabling disease for the majority of patients, as only 25 % of patients so labelled become wheelchair dependent.

The abrupt onset of symptoms, dissemination in time, the affected sites, and the blood–brain barrier dysfunction all point to a vascular mechanism. There is strong circumstantial evidence that the common cause of the disease is micro-embolic due to failure of the pulmonary filtration of circulating debris, especially fat which may release toxic fatty acids (James 1982). A micro-embolic mechanism due to failure of pulmonary entrapment can account for the well-established perivenous nature of lesions (Zulch and Tzonos 1965; Lumsden 1970a, b). Many neuropathologists have observed that the late lesion of acute fat embolism is indistinguishable from the acute lesions of MS (Scheinker 1943; Courville 1959; Sevitt 1962; Lumsden 1970a, b). The same focal lesions result from microbubble damage to the blood–brain barrier in decompression sickness (Hills and James 1991) accounting for the pathological similarities with the sites affected, that is the optic nerves, brain stem and spinal cord (James 2007).

Although the term "clinically isolated syndrome" (CIS) is frequently used to describe conditions such as optic neuritis and transverse myelitis, MRI has shown that in most such patients multiple areas are already affected (Ormerod et al. 1987). The use of the term "clinically isolated" emphasises the continuing problem posed by the requirement for objective evidence and dissemination over time, but it is still central to the practice of neurology. Logically, these patients could be described as suffering from mono sclerosis (James 2002) although this term has yet to be adopted.

Rationale for Hyperbaric Oxygen Treatment

The attacks that typify the development of multiple areas of sclerosis have not been regarded as constituting an emergency. Intravenous high-dosage methylprednisolone is the only intervention shown to reduce the severity and duration of an attack of optic neuritis under controlled conditions (Beck et al. 1991). The trial required symptoms to have been present for days to avoid spontaneous remission masking a treatment effect. The same logic was used in the recruitment of multiple sclerosis patients for studies of hyperbaric oxygen treatment: the stipulation was that patients should have chronic stable disease and disease durations of 10 or more years (Fischer et al. 1983).

The discovery of the hypoxia-inducible factor transcription proteins has provided an explanation for the complex changes caused by lack of oxygen, (Cramer et al. 2003) especially the role of hypoxia and inflammation (Eltszhig and Carmeliet 2011). The role of changes in cellular oxygen levels in signalling has also been comprehensively reviewed (Semenza 2011). The focal oedema that characterises lesions typical of MS inevitably increases the diffusion distance for oxygen and provides a sound rationale for increasing the gradient for oxygen transfer from plasma by delivering oxygen under hyperbaric conditions. Also the calibre of the cerebral vasculature is related to the oxygen tension of the perfusing blood and the active transfer of substances, for example glucose, across the blood–brain barrier is oxygen dependent. In human diving experiments, vasoconstriction produced by hyperbaric oxygenation caused transient unilateral visual loss in a patient with a history of optic neuritis (Nichols et al. 1969).

With the recognition that at the time isolated attacks characteristic of the eventual development of chronic multiple sclerosis multiple sites in the nervous system are involved attention should clearly be focused on the hyperbaric oxygen treatment of such attacks. Hyperbaric oxygen treatment has been used successfully in ischaemic optic neuritis (Beiran et al. 1995; Bojic et al. 2002; Borruat et al. 1993; Boschetti et al. 2006) and in optic neuritis associated with decompression sickness (Butler 1991) and radiotherapy (Guy and Schatz 1986) where oedema is a major component. The author has treated an attack of optic neuritis in a patient with multiple sclerosis in which there was complete loss of vision in the affected eye. It responded to treatment with return of light perception at 2.8 ATA on US Navy Table 5 and full vision was restored by a course of five sessions of 1 h at 2 ATA. A male patient who developed focal neurological signs and visual disturbance after soft tissue bruising and a blow to the head in a car accident also responded to the use of 2.8 ATA in the same procedure despite a delay of 2 days (James 1982). The effectiveness of HBO in the reduction of global cerebral oedema has been demonstrated by direct measurement in man (Sukoff and Ragatz 1982). Rockswold et al. (1992) have shown that HBO reduces the mortality of severe head injury by 50 %.

The effect of HBO on the oedema associated with MS is has been demonstrated by MRI (Fig. 22.1) (Neubauer 1986). One or more lesions shown on MRI disappeared in 11 of 35 patients (31.4 %) after 1 h of treatment, which suggests that it is the resolution of focal oedema that accounts for the improvement. Administering oxygen under hyperbaric conditions allows a substantial increase of plasma oxygen tension despite paradoxically reducing blood flow (Jacobson et al. 1963). This improves the gradient for oxygen transport to tissue enabling the relief of severe tissue hypoxia and resumption of normal aerobic metabolism in acute areas affected by the disease process. Hyperbaric conditions are needed to significantly increase the venous oxygen tension— at 2 ATA breathing 100 % oxygen at an arterial oxygen tension of 1100 mmHg the venous oxygen tension is only of the order of 70 mmHg. Increasing cellular oxygen availability in hypoxia reduces inflammation by down-regulating the transcriptional protein hypoxia-inducible factor 1α (HIF-1α) (Semenza 2011). This protein, which is continually produced by every cell is normally destroyed by the action of the Von Hippel Landau protein (VHL). Falling oxygen levels reduces the production of VHL leading to an increase in the level of HIF-1α. A second, recently described, mechanism likely to contribute to the repair of focal areas of damage in the nervous system is the release of stem cells by HBO treatment. A course of 20 sessions at 2.4 ATA 5 days a week for a month in patients undergoing HBOT for complications of treatment for head and neck cancer has been found to increase circulating stem cells eightfold (Thom et al. 2008).

Although not yet acknowledged, the critical factor in barrier and tissue repair in the CNS is the availability of oxygen in affected tissue and the driving force increasing the delivery to cells is solely the plasma oxygen tension (James 1983). A mild disturbance of the barrier may simply increase the water content of the nervous tissue, but more severe failure is associated with the extravasation of plasma constituents, including proteins into the extracellular space and thence to neural tissue. This degree of barrier failure primarily causes damage to the most vulnerable cell in the nervous system, the oligodendrocyte and its associated myelin sheaths. The most severe form of barrier failure is associated with perivenular extravasation of red blood cells, the phenomenon being known as diapedesis. The release of free iron from the breakdown of haemoglobin results in hydroxyl radical formation and tissue necrosis.

In the 1970s, studies indicated that oxygen delivered under hyperbaric conditions ameliorated symptoms in the experimental disease Experimental Allergic Encephalomyelitis (EAE) the putative model of multiple sclerosis also induces blood–brain barrier disruption (Prockop and Grasso 1978; Warren et al. 1978). HBO has been found to be immunosuppressive in mice (Hansbrough et al. 1980). EAE involves the remote injection of brain tissue derived from a healthy animal in an emulsion with Freund's adjuvant. This adjuvant is a mixture of mineral oils and tubercle bacilli and it causes blood–brain barrier disruption probably by a micro-embolic mechanism. (James 1983) The inflammation produced by the

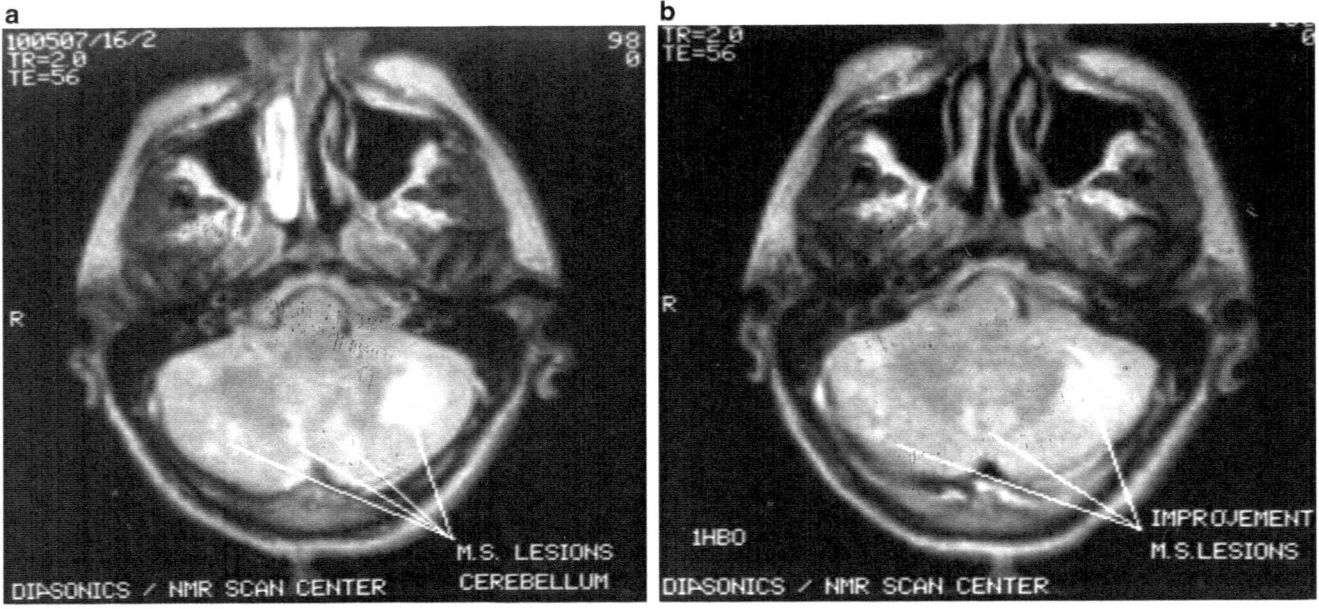

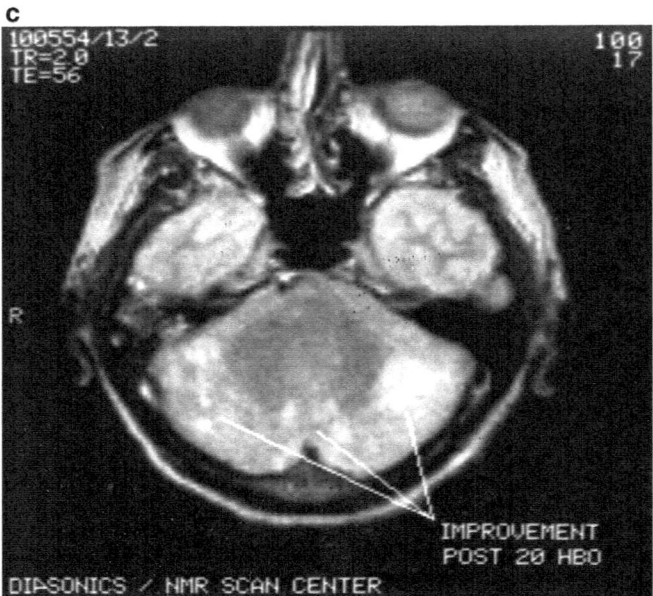

Fig. 22.1 (a) Magnetic resonance image of a 58-year-old multiple sclerosis patient with cerebellar ataxia before treatment showing oedematous lesion. (b) Image after one session of HBO at 1.5 ATA showing improvement. (c) Image after 20 sessions of HBO at 1.5 ATA showing reduction of oedema. The patient showed marked clinical improvement. Courtesy of the late Dr. Richard A. Neubauer, Lauderdale-by-the-Sea, Florida

tuberculin reaction in man can be associated with a developing tissue hypoxia that results from oedema limiting the rate of oxygen flux at a time when the area is being invaded by highly metabolically active cells (Abbot et al. 1994). Reduction of oedema in the spinal cord by hyperbaric oxygenation has been demonstrated in an animal model in which tissue oxygen measurements were recorded (Kelly et al. 1972).

In some studies of EAE, measurements of tissue oxygen levels were made using indwelling electrodes, which demon-strated that the lesions in EAE are also associated with focal hypoxia, and this was confirmed using metabolic markers of hypoxia. The neurological deficits observed were found to be quantitatively, temporally and spatially correlated with hypoxia and resolved by oxygen administration at ambient pressure. Further studies undertaken on this topic (Desai et al. 2016) used the direct injection of lipopolysaccharide and *Salmonella abortus* into the spinal cord to provoke local-ised inflammation. Oxygen delivered in a chamber at 80 % for 2 days was able to resolve the disabilities induced and prevent the development of demyelination. This clearly supports the emergency use of oxygen at ambient pressure in the clinical management of the isolated attacks typical of multiple sclerosis.

Clinical Trials of HBO in Multiple Sclerosis

The first report of the use of oxygen treatment under hyperbaric conditions for MS patients was in 1970 (Boschetty and Cernoch 1970). They used two 30 min sessions at 2 ATA daily for 10–20 days in 26 patients. Symptomatic improvement occurred in 15 but was of limited duration and no follow on treatment was given. Baixe (1978) compared the symptoms of MS to those of decompression sickness and reported favourable results in 11 patients. These effects were confirmed independently in the USA (Neubauer 1978, 1986) following his use of HBO for a patient with osteomyelitis who was also suffering from MS and the course of HBO markedly improved the patient's neurological symptoms. Italian reports (Pallota et al. 1980; Formai et al. 1980) also described a beneficial effect and some longer term studies were undertaken.

These clinical reports influenced the design and execution of the first randomised, placebo-controlled, double-blind study in New York University Medical Center (Fischer et al. 1983). Only patients with a low Kurtzke disability score (KDS) (Kurtzke 1983) were studied and uniquely patients were matched in pairs in the experimental and control groups according to age, sex, age at onset of the disease, duration and type of disease, and disability before randomisation. It was shown that at 2 ATA once a day for 90 min, 5 days a week to a total of 20 treatments, objective improvement in mobility, fatigue, balance and bladder function occurred in 12 of 17 patients ($p < 0.0001$). Those patients having a less severe form of the disease had a more favourable and long lasting response. In contrast, only 1 out of 20 placebo-treated patients showed a positive change. After 1 year, with no further treatment the treated patients had deteriorated less than the controls ($p < 0.0008$). The authors appreciated the necessity for further studies, particularly in the treatment of acute attacks and the effect of long-term treatment.

This was the first double-blind controlled study using matched pairs of patients and has provided a standard against which other studies should be compared: No other trial has been undertaken in this way. However, it also set several unfortunate precedents by using a fixed pressure (2 ATA) and limiting the number of sessions to 20. Although patients were followed for 1 year after the completion of the course of treatment no continuation treatment was provided. The arterial blood-gas measurements ranged from 1.11 to 1.59 ATA. With the special mask used (Acme Scotoramic no. 707) most of the difference can be accounted for by ventilation/perfusion abnormalities in the lung rather than by mask leakage. However, leakage did occur as shown by a value of 145 mmHg recorded in a control patient which indicated that chamber air was entrained. Most subsequent trials were undertaken at 2.0 ATA, but no account was taken in the type of equipment with both pure oxygen monoplace chambers and multiplace units with mask breathing also being used. There is good evidence that the reduction in vessel calibre in the lesions of chronic MS will make patients more sensitive to the vasoconstriction induced by oxygen (Nichols et al. 1969). Evidence has been produced (Holbach et al. 1977) indicating that the optimal inspired partial pressure of oxygen in the injured brain of stroke patients is about 1.75 ATA.

Subsequent trials have been of variable quality and have used patients with very long disease durations usually with stable disabilities. After dismissing HBO therapy on the basis of their preliminary findings despite overall significance ($p < 0.01$), the Newcastle group (Barnes et al. 1985a, b) called for further studies in their final report (Barnes et al. 1987). Their follow-up of patients who received HBO showed that the bladder improvement present after 1 month of treatment ($p < 0.03$) was maintained for 6 months without additional treatment. After a year, there was less deterioration in cerebellar function compared to controls ($p < 0.05$). In the second UK study based in London, (Wiles et al. 1986), recorded objective improvement in bladder function in their most severely affected patients under controlled conditions ($p < 0.03$) using cystometry.

Two further studies have reported sustained benefit with follow-on treatment. In Italy, Oriani et al. (1990) used patients with a low KDS disability score and compared 22 controls with 22 patients treated each week for a year. They detected an appreciable difference in outcome ($p < 0.01$) and also found improvement in visual evoked responses. Pallota et al. (1986) followed 22 patients for 8 years. All received an initial course of 20 HBO treatments, and 11 were treated thereafter with two exposures every 20 days. The frequency of relapses decreased dramatically in the prolonged treatment group whereas they gradually increased in the group which received only an initial course of treatment (Fig. 22.2).

Following the New York Medical Center study, patients in the United Kingdom established a charity now known as *The MS National Therapy Centres* began installing a network of multiplace HBO facilities (Fig. 22.3). The problems associated with the evaluation of any treatment for MS are widely appreciated, indeed, Dr. George Schumacher (1974), a former chairman of the International Federation of Multiple Sclerosis Societies, considered that MS does not readily lend itself to double-blind studies because of the unpredictable fluctuation of signs and symptoms. He suggested that the best experimental design for investigating the effectiveness of a therapeutic regime is a longitudinal one involving large numbers of patients who serve as their own controls. The

Fig. 22.2 Incidence of relapses in 22 multiple sclerosis patients with and without regular HBO treatment, followed for 8 years. Redrawn and modified from Pallotta (1982)

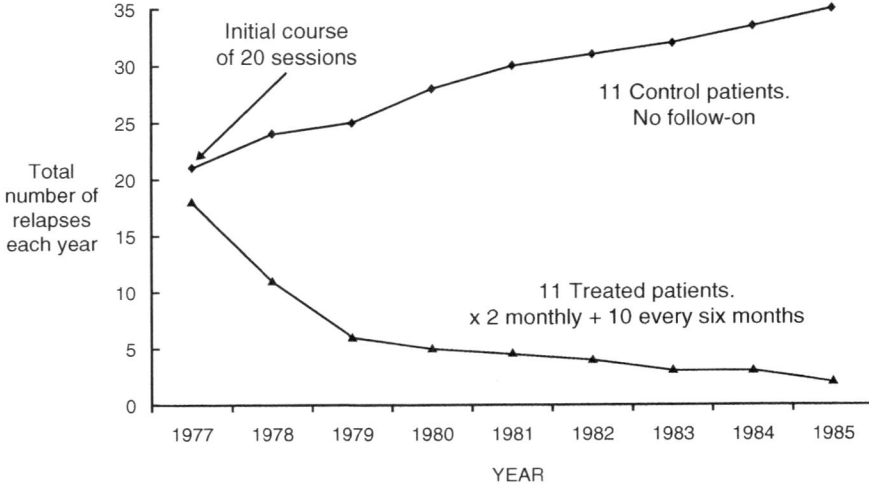

Fig. 22.3 The location of the centres for HBO therapy of multiple sclerosis in the United Kingdom

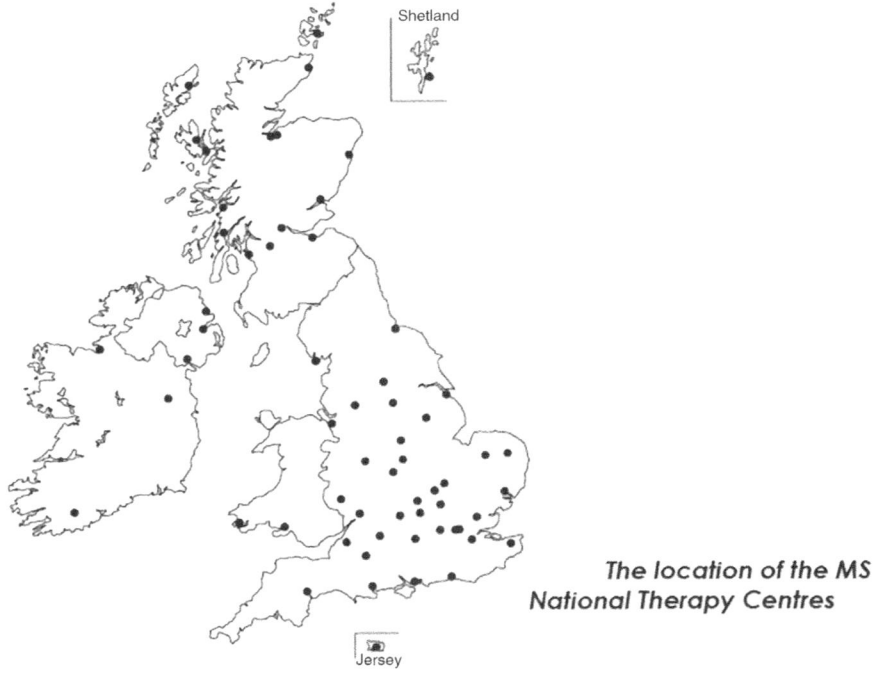

The location of the MS National Therapy Centres

sole criterion of efficacy should be the arrest of further downhill progression in an overwhelming majority of patients over a 2-year period, a view now supported by the fact that only hyperbaric oxygen treatment has shown persistent benefits in long-term studies. Since 1982 the MS Therapy Centres movement has treated over 25,000 patients and more than 3,000,000 individual exposures have been administered without a significant incident. They are therefore in a unique position to evaluate the effectiveness of prolonged courses of HBO in a considerable number of patients over 10 or more years. In 2008, the centres were deregulated by an Act of Parliament.

Seven hundred and three patients were followed in detail (Table 22.1) since first receiving treatment (Perrins and

James 2005). They breathed oxygen from a face mask in a chamber compressed with air. Five daily treatments of 1 hour were given at 1.25 or 1.5 ATA. If two or more symptoms improved, a course of 20 treatments in 4 weeks was completed at this pressure. Otherwise, the pressure was raised in weekly increments of 0.25 ATA until a response was obtained or five treatments at 2.0 ATA had no effect. Thereafter, the patients were invited to return for a "follow-on" treatment on a weekly basis, or failing that, as often as they felt the need or found it possible.

Patients were interviewed and assessed immediately before the initial course when the MS Type and the KDS were determined. A further assessment was made immediately after the initial course of 20 daily treatments. About

70% of patients obtained relief of two or more symptoms (Table 22.2). The bladder improvements observed in other studies were confirmed (Tables 22.2 and 22.3). In general, the response was better in patients with less advanced disease. Lower pressures than those used by others were found to be effective, while the initial response was found to be an unreliable guide to the outcome of prolonged treatment. Further assessments were made between 2 and 4 years, and again between 6 and 8 years after the initial course. They suggested that the initial improvements were being maintained by regular treatment (Table 22.4).

A third survey was conducted between 10 and 14 years. By now 126 patients had died (8% were over 60 years old when first treated), 99 had become "lost to follow up", 29 had suffered injuries that affected their Kurtzke value and 2 had had their original diagnosis revised; 447 patients there-

Table 22.1   Patients recruited to the study

	Females	Males	Total
	464=66%	239=34%	703
Mean age years (range)	47 (20–70)	14 (0–54)	
Average duration of MS	47 (19–73)	15 (0–50)	
Diagnosis confirmed by a neurologist	670=95%		
MS type			
Relapsing/remitting	126=18%	41=6%	167
Chronic progressive	262=37%	155=22%	417
Relapsing/remitting	76=11%	43=6%	119

Table 22.2   The patients' assessment of symptomatic response to the initial course

	n	Improved %	No change %	Worse %
Fatigue	567	70	22	8
Speech	187	64	34	1
Balance	562	59	37	4
Bladder	523	68	30	0
Walking	638	77	19	4

Table 22.3   Urinary frequency of 523 patients—before and after the initial course

	Sum total of times voided					
	Before initial course		After initial course		Improvement
Frequency	x	x			
– At night	1232	2.4	651	1.2	47%
– During the day	3873	7.4	2960	5.7	24%

Table 22.4   Specific abilities regained after initial course and maintained 2 or 4 years later

	After the initial course	With 0–27 treatments in 2 years	With 1–104 treatments in fourth year
		After the initial course	
n=703	%	%	%
Brushing teeth	39	26	20
Doing up buttons	81	54	40
Threading a needle	50	34	29
Holding a cup	54	46	23
Brushing hair	48	33	26
Fastening brassiere	25	22	11
Cutting up food	36	11	18
Shaving	30	11	18
		Abilities	
		Regained	Maintained
		67% of 410	73% of 276

fore remained for an assessment (Table 22.5). This shows that 103 (23 %) were no worse after regular treatment for 10–14 years. Even more remarkable are the 30 patients (7 %) who have actually improved. An analysis reveals that about 300 treatments in 10+ years (about one treatment a fortnight) are required to retard the progression of relapsing/remitting patients, while more than 500 treatments (say, once a week) are more effective (Fig. 22.4).

Very long-term double-blind controlled studies of oxygen treatment are not possible as patients do not comply with their allocation. However, it is possible to compare groups of patients who have received different treatment regimes (Fig. 22.5). The importance of regular treatment is shown at all points examined.

Although there is wide variation in the rate and pattern of decline, the majority of MS patients deteriorate over a 2-year period of observation (Schumacher 1974). In this study, the five relapsing/remitting patients who had less than ten follow-on treatments had deteriorated by 2.0 on the KDS after 10+ years, while the 31 who received more than 400 had only deteriorated by 1.1 ($p \leq 0.001$). This

represents a difference of being able to walk without assistance and the need to use two sticks, or the ability to walk 200 m and being confined to a wheelchair. A search of the records has revealed 1384 patients who were first treated 17 or more years ago and 104 (11 %) are still attending for regular treatment. The fate of 117 patients who have been attending regularly without interruption for 5–17 years are shown in Table 22.6. It is noteworthy that between and 15 years the Kurtzke value has not increased by more than 1 point.

The treatment, as administered by the UK MS Therapy Centres, has been shown to be practicable and cost-effective in community centres. After 10 or more years, 38 % of the 447 patients were still attending regularly. There were no side effects recorded other than ear discomfort from the change in pressure. The cost of each HBO treatment is about the same as for a haircut, so that relief may be obtained for less than £300 ($US 450) a year. Many patients continue to attend as their symptoms, especially frequency of micturition, are only controlled by regular attendance. Some arrange their holidays so as to be near a centre. Some patients have

Table 22.5 Patients who were no worse after regular treatment for 10–14 years

447 Patients	112 Relapsing/remitting	259 Chronic progressive	76 Chronic static	Total
Improved	14 (13 %)	12 (5 %)	4 (5 %)	30 (7 %)
Unchanged	23 (21 %)	31 (12 %)	19 (25 %)	73 (16 %)
No worse	37 = 33 %	43 = 17 %	23 = 30 %	103 = 23 %
Mean no. of treatments	*338*	*257*	*266*	

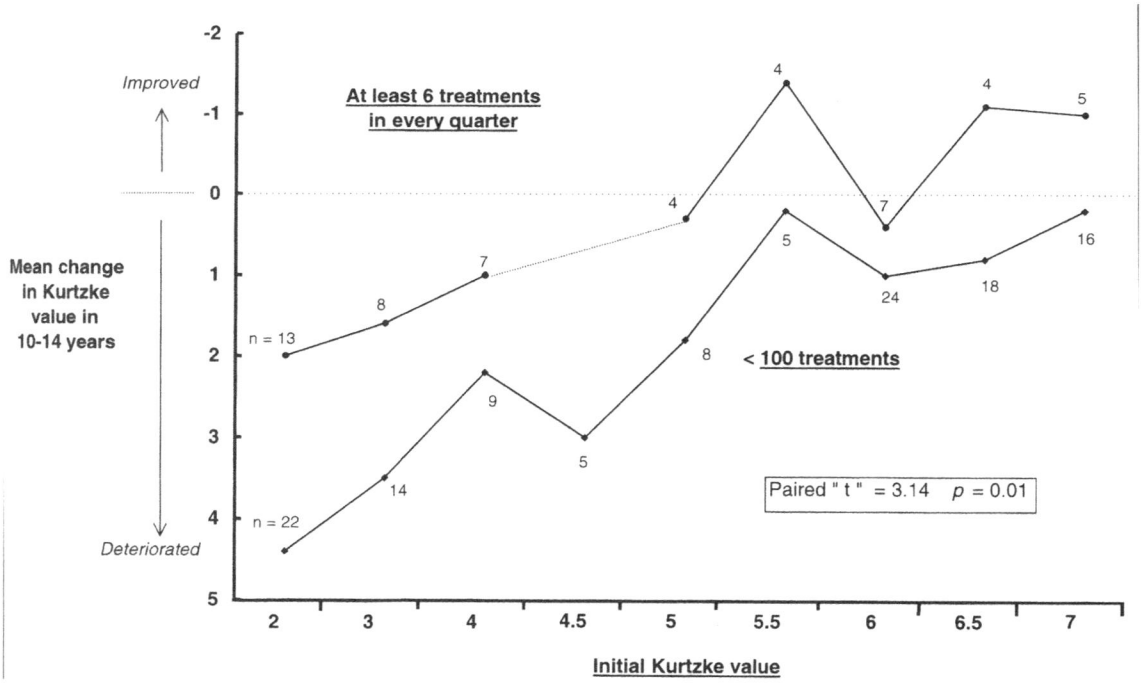

Fig. 22.4 The mean change in Kurtzke value related to the number of treatments in 10–14 years during the course of multiple sclerosis

Fig. 22.5 Multiple sclerosis patients, of all types, who received at least six treatments in every quarter versus those with less than 100 in 10–14 years

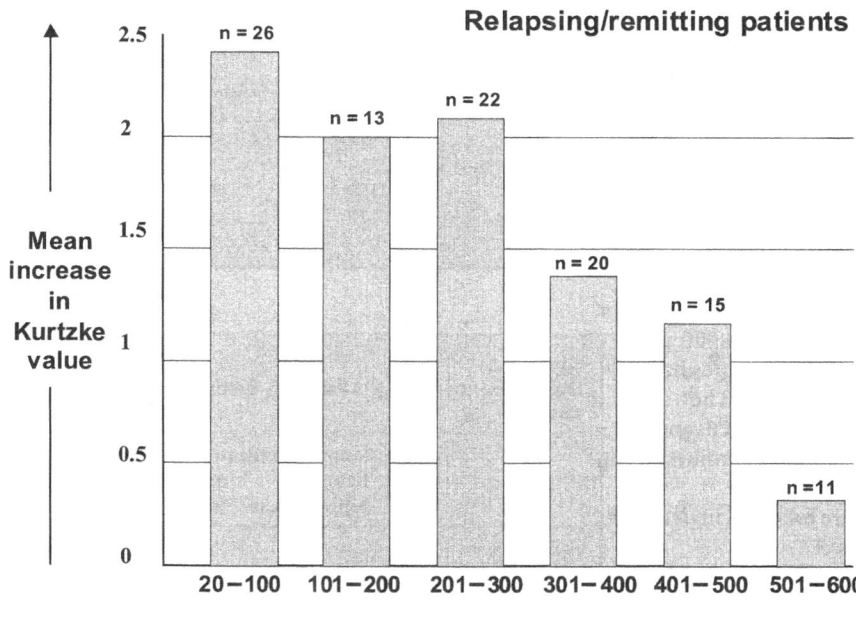

Table 22.6 117 Patients who have attended regularly for 5–17 years

Years attended	No. of patients	MS type	Average difference in Kurtzke value	Average no. of treatments
5–10	13	Relapsing/remitting	.6	351
	19	Chronic progressive	1	323
	2	Chronic static	.75	248
10–15	17	Relapsing/remitting	1	464
	24	Chronic progressive	.8	523
	8	Chronic static	.5	488
>14	12	Relapsing/remitting	0	466
	16	Chronic progressive	1	494
	6	Chronic static	2	664
Total	**117**			

difficulty in reaching a centre and are so dependent on regular treatment that they have installed monoplace chambers in their own homes.

Conclusion

The demonstration of hypoxia in acute lesions by MRS and of the control of the inflammatory response by the hypoxia-inducible factor proteins argues strongly for the emergency use of oxygen treatment of the attacks that lead to multiple areas of scarring. The findings of all the long-term studies of established chronic MS patients suggest that a course of hyperbaric oxygen treatment followed by regular HBO favourably influences the course of the disease. As should be expected, the response has been shown to be better in patients with less advanced disease and is related to the frequency and continuity of treatment. The social and economic advantages to be gained from regular and prolonged treatment are obvious. There are no side effects.

References

Abbot NC, Beck JS, Carnochan FMT, Gibbs JH, Harrison DK, James PB, et al. Effect of hyperoxia at 1 and 2 ATA on hypoxia and hypercapnia in human skin during experimental inflammation. J Appl Physiol. 1994;77:767–73.

Baixe JH. Bilan de onze annees d'activite en medicine hyperbare. Med Aer Spatiale Med Subaquatique Hyperbare. 1978;17:90–2.

Barnes MP, Bates D, Cartlidge NEF, French JM, Shaw DA. Hyperbaric oxygen and multiple sclerosis: short term results of a placebo-controlled, double-blind trial. Lancet. 1985a;1:297–300.

Barnes MP, Bates D, Cartlidge NEF, French JM, Shaw DA. Hyperbaric oxygen and multiple sclerosis: final results of a placebo-controlled, double-blind study. J Neurol Neurosurg Psychiatry. 1985b;50:1402–6.

Barnes MP, Bates D, Cartlidge NE, et al. Hyperbaric oxygen and multiple sclerosis: final results of a placebo-controlled, double-blind study. J Neurol Neurosurg Psychiatry. 1987;50:1402–6.

Beck RW, Cleary PA, Anderson MM, Keltner JL, Shults WT, Kaufman DI, et al. A randomised controlled trial of corticosteroids in the treatment of acute optic neuritis. N Engl J Med. 1991;326:581–8.

Beiran I, Rimon I, Weiss G, Pikkel J, Miller B. Hyperbaric oxygenation therapy for ischemic optic neuropathy. Eur J Ophthalmol. 1995;5:285–6.

Berger JR, Sheremater WA. Persistent neurological deficit precipitated by hot bath test in multiple sclerosis. JAMA. 1983;249:1751–3.

Bojic L, Ivanisevic M, Gosovic G. Hyperbaric oxygen therapy in two patients with non-arteritic anterior optic neuropathy who did not respond to prednisone. Undersea Hyperb Med. 2002;29:86–92.

Borruat FX, Schatz NJ, Glass JS, Feun LG, Matos L. Visual recovery from radiation-induced optic neuropathy: role of hyperbaric oxygenation. J Clin Neuroophthalmol. 1993;13:98–101.

Boschetti M, De Lucchi M, Giusti M, Spena C, Corallo G, Goglia U, et al. Partial visual recovery from radiation-induced optic neuropathy after hyperbaric oxygen therapy in a patient with Cushing disease. Eur J Endocrinol. 2006;154:813–8.

Boschetty V, Cernoch J. Aplikace Kysliku za pretlaku u nekterych neurlogickych onemocnemi. Bratisl Lek Listy. 1970;53:298–302.

Butler FK. Decompression sickness presenting as optic neuropathy. Aviat Space Environ Med. 1991;62:346–50.

Chari A, Yousry TA, Rowaris M, Barkhof F, Barkhof F, De Stefano N, Fazekas F, et al. MRI and the diagnosis of multiple sclerosis: expanding the concept of "no better explanation". Lancet Neurol. 2006;5:841–52.

Courville CB. Multiple sclerosis as an incidental complication of a disorder of lipid metabolism: close resemblance of the lesions resulting from fat embolism to the plaques of multiple sclerosis. Bull Los Angel Neuro Soc. 1959;24:60–75.

Cramer T, Yamanishi Y, Clausen B, et al. Hypoxia-inducible factors as essential regulators of inflammation. Cell. 2003;112:645–57.

Desai RA, Davies AL, Tachrount M, Kasti M, Laulund F, Golay X, et al. Cause and prevention of demyelination in a model multiple sclerosis lesion. Ann Neurol. 2016;79:591–604.

Eltszhig HK, Carmeliet P. Hypoxia and inflammation. N Engl J Med. 2011;364:656–65.

Fischer BH, Marks M, Reich T. Hyperbaric oxygen treatment of multiple sclerosis. A randomised placebo-controlled double-blind study. N Engl J Med. 1983;308:181–6.

Formai C, Sereni G, Zannini D. L'ossigenterapia iperbarica nel trattamento della sclerosi multipla. Presented at the 4th Congresso Nazionale di medicina subacqua ed iperbarica, Naples, Italy, 24–26 Oct 1980.

Guy J, Schatz NJ. Hyperbaric oxygen in the treatment of radiation-induced optic neuropathy. Ophthalmology. 1986;93:1083–8.

Hansbrough JF, Piacentine JG, Eisman B. Immunosuppression by hyperbaric oxygenation. Surgery. 1980;87:662–7.

Hills BA, James PB. Microbubble damage to the blood–brain barrier. Undersea Biomed Res. 1991;18:185–201.

Holbach KH, Caroli A, Wassmann ZH. Cerebral energy metabolism in patients with brain lesions at normo- and hyperbaric oxygen pressure. J Neurol. 1977;217:17–30.

Jacobson I, Harper AM, McDowall DG. The effects of oxygen under pressure on cerebral blood flow and cerebral venous oxygen tension. Lancet. 1963;2:549.

James PB. Evidence for subacute fat embolism as the cause of multiple sclerosis. Lancet. 1982;1:380–6.

James PB. Oxygen for multiple sclerosis. Lancet. 1983;1:1161.

James PB. Multiple sclerosis as a "diagnosis". Lancet. 1997;350:1178.

James PB. MRI monosclerosis and multiple sclerosis. Lancet. 2002;359:1436.

James PB. Hyperbaric oxygenation in fluid microembolism. Neurol Res. 2007;29:156–61.

Kelly DL, Lassiter KRL, Vongsvivut A, Smith JM. Effects of hyperbaric oxygenation and tissue oxygen studies in experimental paraplegia. J Neurosurg. 1972;36:425–9.

Kidd D, Barkoff F, McConnell R, Algra PR, Allen IV, Revesz T. Cortical lesions in multiple sclerosis. Brain. 1999;122:17–26.

Kurtzke JF. Rating neurologic impairment in multiple sclerosis: an expanded disability scale. Neurology. 1983;33:1444–52.

Lumsden CE. The neuropathology of multiple sclerosis. In: Vinken PJ, Bruyn GW, editors. Handbook of clinical neurology. Amsterdam: Elsevier; 1970a. p. 296–8.

Lumsden CE. Pathogenetic mechanisms in the leucoencephalopathies in anooxic-ischaemic processes in disorders of the blood and in intoxications. In: Vinken PJ, Bruyn GW, editors. Handbook of clinical neurology. Amsterdam: Elsevier; 1970b. p. 570–663.

McDonald WI. Pathogenesis of optic neuritis. In: Hess RF, Plant GT, editors. Optic neuritis. Cambridge, UK: Cambridge University Press; 1986.

Miller DH, Austin SJ, Connelly A, Youl BD, Gadian DG, McDonald WI. Proton magnetic resonance spectroscopy of an acute and chronic lesion in multiple sclerosis. Lancet. 1991;337:58–9.

Neubauer RA. Treatment of multiple sclerosis with monoplace hyperbaric chamber. JFl Med Soc. 1978;65:101.

Neubauer RA. Hyperbaric oxygen therapy in multiple sclerosis—a multimodal evaluation. First Swiss Symposium on Hyperbaric Medicine, Foundation for Hyperbaric Medicine, Basel, 1986. p. 103–114.

Nichols CW, Lambertsen CJ, Clark JM. Transient unilateral loss of vision associated with oxygen at high pressure. Arch Ophthalmol. 1969;81:548–52.

Oriani G, Barbieri S, Cislaghi G, et al. Long-term hyperbaric oxygen in multiple sclerosis. J Hyperb Med. 1990;5:239–45.

Ormerod IEC, Miller DH, McDonald WI, du Boulay EP, Rudge P, Kendall BE, et al. The role of NMR imaging in the assessment of multiple sclerosis and isolated neurological lesions. Brain. 1987;110:1579–616.

Pallota R, Anceschi S, Costilgliola N, et al. Prospettive di terapia iperbarica nella sclerosi a placche. Ann Med Nav. 1980;85:57–62.

Pallotta R. La terapia iperbarica nella sclerosi multipla. Minerva Med. 1982;73:2947–54.

Pallota R, Longobardi G, Fabbrocini G. Experience in protracted follow-up on a group of multiple sclerosis patients treated with hyperbaric oxygen therapy. In: Baixe JH, editor. Symposium sur le traitment de la sclerose multiple par l'oxyene hyperbare, Paris, 1986.

Perrins DJD, James PB. Long-term hyperbaric oxygenation retards progression in multiple sclerosis patients. IJNN. 2005;2:45–8.

Prockop LD, Grasso RJ. Ameliorating effects of HBO on experimental allergic encephalomyelitis. Brain Res Bull. 1978;3:221–5.

Putnam T, Alexander L. Loss of axis cylinders in sclerotic plaques and similar lesions. Arch Neurol. 1947;57:661–72.

Rockswold GL, Ford SE, Anderson DC, Bergman TA, Sherman RE. Results of a prospective randomized trial for the treatment of severely brain-injured patients with hyperbaric oxygen. J Neurosurg. 1992;76:929–34.

Scheinker M. Formation of demyelinated plaques associated with cerebral fat embolism in man. Arch Neurol Psychiatry. 1943;49:754–64.

Schumacher GA. Critique of experimental trials in multiple sclerosis. Neurology. 1974;24:1010–4.

Semenza GL. Oxygen sensing homeostasis and disease. N Engl J Med. 2011;365:537–47.

Sevitt S. Fat embolism. London: Butterworths; 1962. p. 59.

Sukoff MH, Ragatz RE. Hyperbaric oxygenation for the treatment of acute cerebral edema. Neurosurgery. 1982;10:29–38.

Thom SR, Bhopale VM, Velazquez OC, Goldstein LJ, Thom LH, Buerk DG. Stem cell mobilization by hyperbaric oxygen. Am J Physiol Heart Circ Physiol. 2008;290:H1378–86.

Wang WZ, Olsson T, Kostulas V, et al. Myelin antigen reactive T cells in cerebrovascular diseases. Clin Exp Immunol. 1992;88:157–62.

Warren J, Sacksteder MR, Thuning CA. Oxygen immunosuppression: modification of experimental allergic encephalomyelitis in rodents. J Immunol. 1978;121:315–20.

Weiss SJ. Tissue destruction by neutrophils. N Engl J Med. 1989;320:365–76.

Wiles CM, Clarke CRA, Irwin HP, et al. Hyperbaric oxygen in multiple sclerosis: a double-blind study. Br Med J. 1986;292:367–71.

Young IR, Hall AS, Pallis CA, et al. Nuclear magnetic resonance imaging of the brain in multiple sclerosis. Lancet. 1981;2:1063–6.

Zulch RJ, Tzonos T. Transudation phenomena at the deep veins after blockage of arterioles and capillaries by micro-emboli. Bibl Anat. 1965;7:279–84.

Paul G. Harch

Abstract

Cerebral palsy is a chronic neurological disorder that can be due to several causes of brain damage in utero, in the perinatal period, or postnatally. Hyperbaric oxygen has been shown to be useful in treating children with cerebral palsy. This topic is discussed under the following headings.

Keywords

Birth injury • Brain injury • Cerebral palsy • GMFM • HBO • Hyperbaric oxygen • Oxygen toxicity • Retinopathy of prematurity • Retrolental fibroplasia • Spasticity • SPECT

Introduction: Causes of Cerebral Palsy

The term *cerebral palsy* (CP) covers a group of nonprogressive, but often changing, motor impairment syndromes secondary to lesions or anomalies of the brain arising in the early stages of development. It is the most common physical disability of childhood. Worldwide prevalence is 2.1 per 1000 live births (Oskoui et al. 2013). Problems may occur in utero, perinatal, and postnatal. Infections, traumatic brain injury, near-drowning, and strokes in children suffering from neurological problems come under the heading of cerebral palsy. Diagnosis of cerebral palsy resulting from in utero or early perinatal causes may be made immediately after birth, but more commonly occurs between 15 and 24 months. It is possible that CP may be misdiagnosed for years because specific symptoms may show up very late in childhood. Some of the possible causes of CP are listed in Table 23.1.

Although several antepartum causes have been described for CP, the role of intrapartum asphyxia in neonatal encephalopathy and seizures in term infants is not clear. There is no evidence that brain damage occurs before birth. A study using brain MRI or post-mortem examination was conducted in 351 full-term infants with neonatal encephalopathy, early seizures, or both to distinguish between lesions acquired antenatally and those that developed in the intrapartum and early postpartum period (Cowan et al. 2003). Infants with major congenital malformations or obvious chromosomal disorders were excluded. Brain images showed evidence of an acute insult without established injury or atrophy in 80% of infants with neonatal encephalopathy and evidence of perinatal asphyxia. Although the results cannot exclude the possibility that antenatal or genetic factors might predispose some infants to perinatal brain injury, the data strongly suggest that events in the immediate perinatal period are most important in neonatal brain injury. These findings are important from management point of view as HBO therapy in the perinatal period (Chap. 21) may be of value in preventing the evolution of cerebral palsy.

Oxygen Therapy in the Neonatal Period

Following World War II, oxygen tents and incubators were introduced, and premature infants were given supplementary oxygen to improve their chances of survival, with levels up to 70% being given for extended periods. Epidemics of blindness due to retrolental fibroplasia (retinopathy of

P.G. Harch (✉)
Louisiana State University School of Medicine, New Orleans, LA, USA

Department of Hyperbaric Medicine, Emergency Medicine, University Medical Center, Louisiana Children's Medical Center, 2000 Canal Boulevard, New Orleans, LA 70112, USA
e-mail: paulharchmd@gmail.com

K.K. Jain, *Textbook of Hyperbaric Medicine*, DOI 10.1007/978-3-319-47140-2_23

Table 23.1 Causes of cerebral palsy

Prenatal causes
Amniotic fluid embolus
Anoxia due to cord strangulation
Cerebrovascular accident in utero
Inadequate prenatal care
Maternal abdominal injury during pregnancy
Maternal cardiovascular disorders complicating pregnancy
Maternal drug or alcohol abuse or other toxicity (thalidomide, carbon monoxide)
Maternal infections, i.e., rubella, toxoplasmosis, herpes simplex, syphilis, cytomegalovirus
Maternal metabolic and endocrine disorders, i.e., diabetes, hyperthyroidism
Mitochondrial disruptions
Premature placental separation
Rh sensitization
Underdeveloped (low weight) fetus
Perinatal causes
Cerebrovascular accident at birth
Mechanical respiratory obstruction
Premature delivery, complications of delivery, low birth weight, respiratory distress
Trauma during labor/delivery, hemorrhage, use of forceps, breech delivery
Acquired cerebral palsy as a sequel of:
Anoxic ischemic encephalopathy resultant from near-drowning, near hanging, near-electrocution, cardiac arrest, etc.
Brain tumors
Infections of the nervous system: meningitis, encephalitis, brain abscess
Neurological complications of vaccination
Thrombosis or hemorrhage of the brain
Traumatic brain injury including shaken baby syndrome
Uncontrolled high fever

prematurity—ROP) ensued in the 1950s, which led to a restriction of the level of supplemental oxygen to 40 %. A reduction in the incidence of blindness followed, which appeared to confirm the involvement of oxygen in the development of the retinopathy. The link between the use of recurrent supplemental oxygen and the rise of retinopathy was rapidly accepted, even though it was suggested that retrolental fibroplasia was produced by initially preconditioning a child to an enriched oxygen environment and then suddenly withdrawing the same: the disease occurred only after the child's removal from the high oxygen environment (Szewczyk 1951). It was also noted that a more gradual weaning of the oxygen resulted in a lesser incidence of ROP (Bedrossian et al. 1954). Forrester (1964) found that the best course of action was to return the child to the oxygen environment. Under these circumstances, in many of the patients, the results were encouraging, and vision returned to normal. A slow reduction of oxygen and final return to the atmospheric concentration for several weeks was all that was needed to restore the vision. Thus, there is no rational basis for withholding oxygen therapy in the neonatal period.

The rapid withdrawal of oxygen as the etiology of ROP was reinforced decades later by work implicating the altered regulation of vascular endothelial growth factor (VEGF) in the retina. Pierce et al. (1996) postulated that repeated cycles of hyperoxia and hypoxia in the neonatal period for premature infants may stimulate an increase in VEGF (Saito et al. 1993; Penn et al. 1995). Multiple successful studies on anti-VEGF ocular treatment for ROP (Shah et al. 2016) support this VEGF hypothesis. To prevent ROP, however, Bedrossian's and Forrester's approach has been validated by careful management of oxygen administration and withdrawal that minimizes the cycles of hyperoxia/hypoxia (Chow et al. 2003).

As mentioned in other chapters of this textbook, retrolental fibroplasia is not associated with HBO, either short or prolonged exposures or abrupt cessation of the hyperbaric exposure. Ricci and Calogero (1988) demonstrated that rats continuously exposed to 5 or 10 days of 80 % oxygen developed retinopathy with the 10d rats additionally showing extraretinal neovascularization and total or subtotal retinal detachment. Rats continuously exposed to 1.8 ATA oxygen, however showed no signs of retinopathy and were equivalent to control rats. Using both normal rats and a rat model of cerebral palsy, Calvert showed that doses of HBO as high as 3.0 ATA for 1 h had no structural effect on the retina and showed no evidence of retinal neovascularization (Calvert et al. 2004). In 60 neonates with hypoxic–ischemic encephalopathy a daily exposure to 1.4, 1.5, or 1.6 ATA HBO improved serum antioxidant levels, neurobehavioral scores, and decreased lipid peroxidation, while causing no retinal damage (Zhou et al. 2008).

It is unfortunate that affected newborns today are deprived of appropriate oxygen therapy because of the fear that it will cause retrolental fibroplasia (see Chap. 32). Some observations indicate that an increased incidence of cerebral palsy has occurred since perinatal high level oxygen administration has been abandoned. Regardless of the controversy about supplemental 1ATA 100 % oxygen usage, there is no evidence that hyperbaric oxygen therapy induces ROP.

Treatment of Cerebral Palsy with HBO

The use of hyperbaric oxygenation in the pediatric patient was relatively common in Russia (see Chap. 56). HBO has been used in Russia for resuscitation in respiratory failure, for cranial birth injuries, and for hemolytic disease of the newborn. HBO was reported to reduce high serum bilirubin levels and prevent development of neurological disorders. In cases of respiratory distress, delayed use of HBO (12–48 h after birth) was considered useless. However, early use (1–3 h after birth) led to recovery in 75 % of cases. This was similar to Hutchison's experience in England with newborn respiratory failure (Hutchison et al. 1963; see Chapter 20, Table 20.2, Human Studies, Hyper Acute Period). Italian physicians began treating the small fetus in utero in 1988 demonstrating a reduction of cerebral damage. Patients were hospitalized before the 35th week and hyperbaric treatments were given every 2 weeks for 40 min at 1.5. The fetal biophysical profile showed a remarkable improvement as soon as the second treatment. Chinese physicians have had extensive experience with HBOT in neonatal resuscitation. A recent review of 20 randomized or quasi-randomized controlled trials for HBO in HIE revealed a near uniformity of results (Liu et al. 2006). While the trials did not use rigorous methodology the reproducible findings were a reduction in mortality and improvement in neurological sequelae, which was consistent with the results of animal studies (Chap. 21).

In the chronic phase, the preponderance of literature suggests a benefit of hyperbaric oxygen therapy in CP. To understand the CP HBOT studies, one must embrace the definition of hyperbaric oxygen therapy stated in Chap. 21 where HBOT is defined as a combination therapy of increased pressure and increased oxygen. As discussed in Chap. 21, both hyperoxia and increased ambient pressure in the hyperbaric chamber are bioactive independently and in combination across the entire phylogenetic spectrum (Harch 2013). In other words, homo sapiens along with all other living organisms is sensitive to changes in both oxy-

gen and ambient pressure. The clinical and clinical experimental difficulty is that no operational method has been devised to separate the effects of pressure from those of hyperoxia. In some of the clinical trials discussed below (e.g., Lacey et al. 2012), the children were exposed to air during the compression and decompression phases of the experiment and then a treatment gas at depth for some period of time. The potential biological effects of oxygen and increased pressure during compression and decompression are mixed with those of pressure, hyperoxia, or both during the time spent during the plateau phase of the treatment. The same is true for the experiments performed in a monoplace chamber with 100 % oxygen; it has been shown that it takes 11 min or more to convert the air in the chamber to greater than 95 % oxygen concentration at 1.5 ATA (Churchill et al. 2013). Therefore, the compression phase is a mixture of increasing pressure and oxygen effects combined with hyperoxic and pressure effects during the plateau phase of treatment and decreasing oxygen and pressure effects during decompression. Importantly, the effects of pressure and hyperoxia begin within 30–60 s of compression (Harch 2013). The sum of these facts converge on the conclusion that all of the purportedly "controlled" CP studies are multi-dosing studies except for the (Packard 2000; Sethi and Mukherjee 2003; Mukherjee et al. 2014) studies where the comparison control group was not subjected to pressurization or hyperoxia.

Awareness of potential for HBOT in CP began at the conference "New Horizons for Hyperbaric Oxygenation" in Orlando, Florida, in 1989. Data were presented on 230 HBO-treated young CP patients from 1985 to 1989 in Sao Paulo, Brazil (Machado 1989). Treatment consisted of twenty 1.5 ATA/1 h HBOTs, once or twice/day (100 % oxygen), in a Vickers monoplace chamber. The results showed significant reduction of spasticity: 50 % reduction in spasticity was reported in 94.78 % of the patients. Twelve patients (5.21 %) remained unchanged. Four patients (1.73 %) experienced "convulsions during the course of treatment, but not in the chamber." Follow-up at 6 months or more included only 82 patients, but 62 of these (75.6 %) had lasting improvement in spasticity and improved motor control. The parents reported positive changes in balance, attention, and "intelligence with reduced frequency of convulsions and episodes of bronchitis." Twenty patients were unchanged. Zerbini (2002) presented results of a continuation of this work at the 2nd International Symposium on Hyperbaric Oxygenation and the Brain Injured Child held in Boca Raton, Florida. Two thousand and thirty patients with chronic childhood encephalopathy were treated from 1976 to 2001. Two hundred and thirty-two children were evaluated with long-term follow-up, age range from 1 to 34 years. Improvements were noted in spasticity (41.8 %), global motor coordination (18 %), attention (40.1 %), memory (10.8 %), comprehension (13.3 %), reasoning (5.60 %), visual perception (12.9 %), and sphincter control (6.5 %). It was concluded from this study that HBO therapy should be instituted as early as possible in such cases.

At the same conference (Chavdarov 2002), Director of the Specialized Hospital for Residential Treatment of Prolonged Therapy and Rehabilitation of Children with Cerebral Palsy in Sofia, Bulgaria, presented a study on 50 CP children: 30 spastic, 8 ataxic/hypotonic, and 12 mixed. Measurements included nine tests of motor ability, mental ability, functional development, and speech. Overall psycho-motor function (single or combined) improved in 60 % of the patients following 20 consecutive days of 1.5–1.7 ATA/40–50 min once daily HBOTs. Motor ability improved in 41 %, mental abilities in 35 %, and speech in 43 % of children with abnormalities of each of these functions. Four experienced "unwanted effects, including seizures, oral automatic movements, hyperesthesia of right face-part, extreme pulse-rate increasing (between 7 and 10 treatments). All unwanted effects disappeared immediately after the stopping of HBO."

The first North American case of CP treated with HBO was in 1992 (Harch et al. 1994). The child was a non-ambulatory 4.5-year-old boy with hypotonic CP secondary to a traumatic precipitous birth. After eighty 1.5 ATA/90 min HBOTs the child acquired gait with fingertip support for balance, improved coordination, increased awareness, and increased alertness. Dr. Richard Neubauer began treating CP in 1995 and a number of cases were treated at freestanding sites in the U.K. by 1998. Based on a small positive case experience in the U.K. a charity to treat CP and brain-injured children, Hyperbaric Oxygen Trust, was established in the late 1990s. Through 2003 the Trust, renamed Advance, had treated over 350 unpublished cases. This positive experience included a few patients from Montreal who were influential in raising money for the first formal pilot trial of HBOT in cerebral palsy (Montgomery et al. 1999).

Published Clinical Trials

Montgomery et al. (1999) involved 23 children (10 female, 15 male; age range 3.1–8.2 years) with spastic diplegia who had an absence of previous surgical or medical therapy for spasticity, and a 12-month clinical physiotherapy plateau. The study was performed at McGill University Hospital's Cleghorn Hyperbaric Laboratory in a monoplace chamber at 1.75 ATA (95 % oxygen) for 60 min daily and at the Rimouski Regional Hospital in a multiplace chamber (1.75 ATA/60 min, twice daily) for 20 treatments in total. The Gross Motor Function Measure (GMFM), fine motor function assessment (Jebsen's Hand Test), spasticity assessment (Modified Ashworth Spasticity Scale), parent questionnaire, and video analysis were performed pre and post HBOT. Results were

an average of 5.3 % improvement in GMFM and a notable absence of complications or clinical deterioration in any of the children. "Cognitive changes" were observed, but these were nonspecific. Video analysis was also positive. The obvious flaws of this study were the lack of placebo control and the application of two different HBO protocols. The assessment tools utilized also had inherent variations. Montgomery et al. achieved improvement in CP children using 20 treatments at 1.66 ATA oxygen ((1.75 ATA 95 % O_2)/60 min), but the children experienced rapid regression of neurological gains after cessation of treatment (personal communication from the authors). The number of treatments was inadequate as the authors of this chapter had recommended 40 treatments at 1.5 ATA/60 min; consolidation of gains does not occur until 30–35 treatments. This first study, however, provided useful data regarding the potential efficacy of HBO therapy and provided the justification for a larger controlled, randomized study.

That larger "controlled" trial was performed by the same and additional investigators in 2001 "with intriguing results" (Collet et al. 2001). It was the first multi-dosing study of HBOT in CP and was not a true controlled study. The study included 111 CP children (ages 3–12 years) that were randomized into two groups who received forty 1 h treatments of either 1.75 ATA 100 % oxygen or 1.3 ATA room air (the equivalent of 28 % oxygen at 1 ATA). Half of the children were treated in a monoplace chamber by themselves and half in a multiplace chamber where the parents accompanied the children. Gross and fine-motor function, memory, speech, and language were assessed. Statistically significant improvement in global motor function occurred in both groups (3 % in the hyperbaric air group and 2.9 % in the hyperbaric-oxygen group). Although the results were statistically similar in both groups, the HBO-treated group had a more rapid response rate in the more severely disabled children. Cognitive testing was performed on 75 of the 111 children who could comply with testing (Hardy et al. 2002). Children in both the oxygen and air groups showed better self-control and significant improvements in auditory attention and visual working memory compared with the baseline. However, no statistical difference was found between the two groups. Furthermore, the purported "sham" group improved significantly on eight dimensions of the Conners' Parent Rating Scale, whereas the oxygen group improved only on one dimension. Most of these positive changes persisted for 3 months. No improvements were observed in either group for verbal span, visual attention, or processing speed.

Unfortunately, the Collet study used both a higher dose than what had previously been used 1.75 ATA of 100 % oxygen for 60 min (40 treatments), and a lower dose, 1.3 ATA air for 60 min and 40 treatments, i.e., a 30 % increase in oxygen for the controls. These doses of HBO had not been used previously in CP patients. The oxygen dose was possibly an overdose (Harch 2002) and likely inhibited the HBO group' gains. Evidence for this was seen in the GMFM data where five of the six scores increased in the HBO group from immediate post HBO testing to the 3-month retest versus 3 of 6 scores in the controls. Possibly, some of the negative effects of 1.75 ATA had worn off in the 3 months before final testing. The serendipitous flaw in the study was the 1.3 ATA air control group which was not a control group, but another dose of hyperbaric therapy. This underscored the fact that the ideal dose of HBO is unknown in chronic pediatric brain injury, but it suggested that oxygen signaling may occur at very low pressures since biological effects of very slight increases in pressure have been documented across the entire phylogenetic spectrum (Macdonald and Fraser 1999). The equivalent Collet air dose of hyperbaric therapy has been demonstrated to be effective in improving SPECT as well as attention and reaction times in toxic brain injury (Heuser et al. 2002). Collet explained the beneficial effect in the air group as a parent participation effect, an explanation that was refuted by the 50 % of children who underwent HBOT in the monoplace chambers without the accompaniment of their parents. The beneficial effect in the Collet air group could only be explained by the beneficial effects of slightly pressurized air rather than the act of participating in the study. This was also the leading explanation of the U.S. Agency for Healthcare Research and Quality in their review of HBOT in stroke, traumatic brain injury, and CP (AHRQ 2003).

The controversy regarding this study is unresolved, but the study has raised some very important issues and questions about the validity of "mild" HBO (1.3–1.35 ATA air or oxygen-enriched air). The first issue is that 1.3 ATA ambient air was not an inert or true placebo, but had a real effect on the partial pressure of blood gases and perhaps other physiological effects as well (Macdonald and Fraser 1999; Harch 2013). Compressed air at 1.3 ATA increases the plasma oxygen tension by 50 % from 12.7 kPa (95 mmHg) to 19.7 kPa (148 mmHg), a notable increase for a reactive substrate. Rather than answer the question of effectiveness of HBO in CP, the Collet study and its offspring (Hardy et al. 2002) substudy confused the hyperbaric and non-hyperbaric scientific communities and prompted a review of longstanding overlooked scientific literature on the effects of "micropressure" (Macdonald and Fraser 1999; Harch 2013). The unequivocal finding of these studies is that both pressure protocols achieved statistically significant objective durable neurocognitive and motor gains, a phenomenon that cannot be attributed to placebo. This reinforced the findings of the other noncontrolled studies in the chronic category (Chap. 21), and was strengthened by the studies using functional brain imaging as surrogate markers (Harch et al. 1994; Neubauer 2002; Golden et al. 2002).

The United States Army Study on Adjunctive HBO Treatment of Children with Cerebral Anoxic Injury

Shortly after the previous studies were begun, physicians at the US Army base in Fort Augusta, Georgia conducted a small study on functional outcomes in children with anoxic brain injury (Waalkes et al. 2002). Eight volunteer (parental) subjects with varying degrees of CP and one near-drowning victim were included in this investigation. Of the CP cases studied, the mean age was 6.4 years (range 1.0–16.5 years), and the near drowning patient was 5.6 years of age seen 1 year post incident. Pretreatment evaluation included the GMFM, the Modified Ashworth Scale (MAS) for spasticity, rigidity, flexion/extension, the Functional Independence Measure for Children (WeeFIM) regarding self-care, sphincter control, transfers, locomotion, communication and social cognition, video, 24-h time measure, parental questionnaire, and single photon emission computerized tomography (SPECT) scanning. Testing was conducted every 20 treatments with the exception of SPECT and parental questionnaire which were completed at 40 and 80 sessions. Importantly, all children continued existing physical and occupational therapy during the study.

The study tested the 80 HBOT protocol underway in the IRB-approved Perfusion/Metabolism Encephalopathies Study of Harch, Gottlieb, and Van Meter in New Orleans (Harch 2010) (1.5 ATA/60 min in blocks of 40 treatments with SPECT and video exams), but at a higher pressure of oxygen (1.7 ATA). All subjects received 80 HBO treatments in a multiplace chamber (100 % oxygen) at 1.70 ATA (60 min for each session) daily (Monday–Friday) for 4 months. Each patient served as his or her own control as compared to the baseline scores. Baseline and serial evaluations showed improvement in gross motor function and total time necessary for custodial care in eight children with CP. Improvements in GMFM in the categories of lying and rolling, crawling and walking, sitting and walking, running and jumping were statistically significant ($p < 0.05$). The total time necessary for parental care was statistically less ($p < 0.03 \%$). On the parental questionnaire, overall improvement was indicated through the end of the study. Three children demonstrated improved swallowing function and were able to ingest a variety of liquids and foods; there was reduction in strabismus in two subjects, nystagmus was resolved in one participant, and one patient experienced complete resolution of a grade 3 vesicoureteral reflux, obviating the need for surgery. Unfortunately, the SPECT scan results were omitted due to multiple technical and procedural problems.

Overall improvement was 26.7 % at 30 treatments, up to 58.1 % at 80 treatments. These improvements were nearly an order of magnitude higher than the (Montgomery et al. 1999) study and any subsequent study. Explanations include non-blinded evaluators, small sample size, combined HBOT and other therapies, and other unexplained factors. Their conclusions were that HBO therapy seemed to effect overall improvement in CP (with little response in the near-drowning case), although the optimum number of treatments remained undetermined, since the improvements were noted at the end of the study. They advised further research and follow-up studies to determine the true potential of HBO for children with anoxic injury and CP.

The New Delhi Study of HBOT in CP

Based on the above experience Drs. Sethi and Mukherjee in New Delhi conducted a randomized prospective controlled trial of HBOT in CP (Sethi and Mukherjee 2003). Thirty subjects were randomly assigned to either standard occupational (OT) and physical therapy (PT) or HBO plus OT/PT. Children also underwent home physical therapy. Children 2–5 years old with all types of CP were included and had a SPECT scan showing presence of recoverable penumbra. HBO patients received 40 HBO treatments at 1.75 ATA/60 min 6 days/week. Gross motor ability was measured using Norton's Basic Motor Evaluation Scale before HBOT and after 6 months of OT/PT or 6 months of OT/PT and HBOT. Both groups improved significantly, but the improvement in the HBO group was significantly greater (87 % vs. 73 %).

Unpublished Studies

The Cornell Study

Upon the urging of interested parents, Dr. Maureen Packard of Cornell University in New York City agreed to perform a randomized prospective controlled study (Packard 2000). Children were randomized to immediate or delayed (6 months later) treatment with HBO (the delayed treatment group served as a crossover control group). Age range was 15 months to 5 years (average 30 months) with moderate to severe CP and patients were given forty 1-h sessions at 1.5 ATA, once a day, 5 days a week for 4 weeks. The study population included 26 children with cerebral palsy secondary to prenatal insults, premature birth, birth asphyxia, and postnatal hemorrhage. Nine patients presented with cortical visual impairment. Assessments were the Bayley II (cognitive), Preschool Language Scale, Peabody Motor Scale, and Pediatric Evaluation of Disabilities Inventory (PEDI), a parental report of specific skills including mobility, self-care, and social interaction. Final assessments were available on 20 subjects. The only side effects of the study were barotrauma in nine children, requiring placement of ventilation tubes or myringotomies. One child in the immediate HBOT group "developed complex febrile seizures and was dropped from the study." Two of 14 subjects in the delayed group developed seizures "and could not participate." Apparently, the seizures developed during the control wait period pre-HBOT.

Assessments were performed at four time points: enrollment (T1), after the immediate group had received treatment (T2), prior to the delayed groups" HBO therapy 5 months after enrollment (T3), and after the delayed groups' treatment (T4). There was a significant difference ($p < 0.05$) in the improvement of scores on the mobility sub-domains for the time period T2 minus T1 in favor of the immediately treated group. For the period T4 minus T3 there was a trend favoring the recently treated delayed group and a trend in the social function subdomain in the more recent treated group. Parental diaries over the month of treatments demonstrated 83 % improvement in mobility, 43 % increase in attention, and 39 % increase in language skills. Overall, 91 % experienced some improvement in mobility, 78 % in attention, 87 % in language, and 52 % in play. One family saw no improvement and six families minimal improvement (30 %). Five families (22 %) reported major gains in skills, and 11 families reported modest gains (48 %). Four of the nine children with cortical visual impairment had improvement in vision noted by families, vision therapists, and ophthalmologists. There was no statistical difference in Peabody or Bayley II scores on blinded assessment.

Conclusions at 6-month post-interview were that changes in spasticity may diminish over time after HBOT while improvements in attention, language, and play were sustained. "This increase in attention is particularly important for children must be aware' in order to learn. This represents a direct impact on cognitive functioning. The main differences between HBO and traditional therapies are the rapid gains over time and the impact on cognitive skills, which, in general are not improved by physical, occupational and speech therapies." Results of this study have only been published on a website after presentation at an HBO conference in Graz, Yugoslavia (Packard 2000).

Comparative Effectiveness Studies

Studies of the use of mild HBO, hyperbaric air, supplemental oxygen, and higher pressures of HBO continued despite the seemingly controversial results of the Collet study. At the 2003 3rd International Symposium on Hyperbaric Oxygenation and the Brain Injured Child, a variety of these studies were presented from around the world. While the studies were of varied design rigor, the results were similar, showing benefit of HBOT in CP, regardless of the lower dose of HBOT employed. The most significant study to date, however, reviewed both published and unpublished studies of

HBO in CP and compared published studies using the Gross Motor Function Measure (GMFM) in HBO to traditional accepted therapies that used the GMFM (Senechal et al. 2007). Compared to intensive physical therapy, dorsal rhizotomy, strength training, electrical stimulation, intrathecal baclofen, family-centered functional therapy, equine therapy, Bobath physical therapy, and other types of physical therapy HBO showed faster and more impressive improvements. Moreover, HBO was the only therapy to improve cognition and language. This study alone refutes the errant conclusion of the Collet study that the improvement in both groups of children was due to a parent-participation effect. The parent-participation effect as well as other "placebo"-type effects, such as surgery, is clearly present in every one of the studies and therapies reviewed by Senechal. Such a dramatic effect with HBOT that simultaneously improved cognition and language is consistent only with a biological cause–effect relationship of HBO on CP and the entire brain.

Recent Studies (Since 2007)

In 2012, Lacey et al. conducted a randomized prospective "controlled" trial of HBOT in CP children which was prematurely terminated for "futility." The study was similar to the Collet trial in that it was another multi-dosing study (not a true controlled study), but used hyperbaric oxygen versus hyperbaric hypoxic air (14 % oxygen at 1.5 ATA). Both groups received forty 1 h treatments at depth, once/day, 5days/week with compression and decompression on air. It employed an aggressive primary endpoint of a 5 % increase in GMFM-88 or 66, as well as secondary endpoints of improvement in the PEDI and Test of Variables of Attention (TOVA). A stopping rule for efficacy was set in advance, but not one for futility. At the second interim analysis that included 46 patients "the conditional probability of obtaining a difference between groups if the study continued to the end was only between 0.5 % and 1.6 %" so the study was stopped. The results at that point showed no change between groups, but a 1.5 % absolute increase (3.8 % of baseline score) in the HBO group and 0.6 % increase (1.5 % of baseline score) in the HBA group on the GMFM-88. In other words, the effect in the HBO group was more than double the effect in the "control" group.

Simultaneously, there were significant improvements in both groups on the PEDI that were similar in magnitude to the Collet PEDI results. In addition, the GMFM-66 increases were 1.2 points absolute (3.0 % of baseline) and 1.1 points absolute (2.7 % of baseline) in the two groups, respectively, with p values that approached significance (0.057 oxygen group, 0.074 hypoxic air group). Both the GMFM-88 and 66 improvements in Lacey et al. (2012) were less than those achieved in Collet et al. (2001), but very similar to the effect

of other therapies used for CP (Senechal et al. 2007). This muted response in Lacey et al. (2012) may be explained by inclusion of dissimilar CP patients in the two studies: subjects in Collet et al. (2001) had to have evidence of perinatal hypoxia and excluded subjects with postneonatal onset CP, while subjects in Lacey et al. (2012) did not have to have neonatal hypoxia and did not exclude subjects with postneonatal onset CP. It appears the futility of stopping decision was based partly on a design flaw that was looking for a large and unrealistic difference between two doses of HBO, a pseudo-control group and a second dose of HBOT. Mukherjee et al. (2014) extended the findings in their earlier study (Sethi and Mukherjee 2003) with a non-randomized unblinded controlled study comparing standard intensive rehabilitation versus three different doses of hyperbaric oxygen therapy: 1.3 ATA air, 1.5 ATA oxygen, or 1.75 ATA oxygen, each for 1 h/day (90 min total treatment time), 6 days/week, for 40 treatments. GMFM-66 was measured pre and 2, 4, 6, and 8 months after beginning treatments. Forty percent of the children had "minor to moderate epilepsy" and 50 % of them were on anticonvulsants which were increased "marginally" during HBOT. The results showed that all four groups significantly improved over the course of the study, but the hyperbaric groups improved significantly greater and faster, consistent with the results of Collet. All three hyperbaric groups increased nearly one-half of a GMFM level on the longitudinal GMFM curves, uncharacteristic of and inconsistent with the natural history of CP. There was a slight dose–response effect (greater effect with increasing doses of oxygen and pressure), yet there was no significant difference between the three hyperbaric groups. The hyperbaric groups showed continued significant increases through the follow-up period with overall improvement rates from the beginning of the study equivalent to those HBOT rates published in Senechal's review and greater than other therapies for CP using the GMFM. No side effects were recorded in the study except for three patients with middle ear barotrauma. This was surprising given that 40 % of the subjects had epilepsy.

The final study, Asl et al. (2015), is a SPECT brain imaging study on 11 CP patients with perinatal asphyxia, four of whom were administered HBOT. HBOT was delivered at 1.75 ATA/60 min, once/day, 5 days/week for 40 treatments. Two of the four patients experienced significant improvement in SPECT, ages 7 and 12, while the 24- and 27-year-old patients did not. No other outcomes were measured.

Side Effects

The most common side effect in all of the above studies was middle ear barotrauma with rates as high as 50 % in one study (Collet et al. 2001). Pressure equalization tubes were inserted in 58 % of the Collet study children (Muller-

Bolla et al. 2006). The second most common side effect in the Collet study was pharyngitis which was seen in 22 % of the children. New onset seizures or exacerbation of seizures were seen in one treated patient in the Packard study ("complex febrile seizures"), at least one patient in Chavdarov's study and some of the patients in the Machado study. However, on follow-up in Machado's study parents reported "reduced frequency of seizure activity." Seizures were not reported in any of the more detailed and rigorous studies. While there does not appear to be an ability to predict sensitivity to oxygen (seizures) middle ear barotrauma is a largely avoidable side effect that is dependent on technique. In our very early experience treating CP, 1992–1998, middle ear barotrauma was common, but as our experience accrued with treating children with neurological disorders this has become a rare occurrence. The summary experience from the above studies is that HBOT in CP is a low-risk treatment.

The exception to this experience is the report of two purported complications of HBOT by Nuthall et al. (2000). The report consists of a child with an episode of vomiting and aspiration while in a hyperbaric chamber during treatment. Following the acute episode he was found to have "free gastroesophageal reflux with aspiration" on a feeding study. The second case involved a child undergoing HBOT who contracted a rapidly progressive parainfluenza type 3 infection with respiratory failure, seizures, and idiopathic thrombocytopenic purpura. During his critical illness, he suffered an acute middle cerebral artery stroke. Echocardiogram documented a patent foramen ovale with bidirectional flow. As pointed out in a rebuttal letter to the editor by Harch et al. (2001), the scientific explanations provided by Nuthall et al. were insufficient to attribute the complications to the HBOT. Harch et al. pointed out that their three authors had over 35,000 HBO treatments of brain injured children without any such complications. Moreover, they are complications never before seen in hyperbaric medicine. They recommended that proper medical evaluation and attendance of treatment was an important factor in delivering safe HBOT to children with neurological disorders.

To date, countless numbers of children with CP have been successfully treated with HBO worldwide. The studies with "negative" results, no difference between groups, are studies that compared multiple doses of HBOT. Neither of these (Collet et al. 2001; Lacey et al. 2012) have had true control groups. Both are multi-dose HBOT studies. In Collet et al. (2001) both groups improved significantly and at a greater rate than has been achieved by multiple other therapies for CP, and in Lacey et al. (2012) both groups achieved results equivalent to other therapies for CP. The Lacey et al. (2012) study was confounded by having studied a pathologically different group of CP children than Collet. Regardless, the net effect is one of benefit of HBOT for CP children using multiple different doses of HBOT.

The medical and scientific community, however, continues to be misled by a misunderstanding of the science of HBO and its effects on chronic brain injury. In 2007, the scientific underpinning of HBO in chronic brain injury was partially elucidated in a study that represents the first ever improvement of chronic brain injury in animals (Harch et al. 2007). This study demonstrated in a model of chronic traumatic brain injury that HBO could improve cognition and blood vessel density in a damaged hippocampus with a low-pressure HBO protocol originally employed on chronic trauma, stroke, CP, and toxic brain injury patients in the early 1990s. The unusual nature of the study was its retrograde proofing of concept in animals after 18 years of application of low-pressure HBO to chronic human brain injury. Since HBO's effects on acute and chronic pathophysiology documented in this text and the scientific literature are generic effects that cross species boundaries, they apply to patients with other types of chronic brain injury such as CP. What is most important is that these beneficial effects have been extended to children with cerebral palsy at both the doses used in the animal study (1.5 ATA) and in a wide range of adult neurological disorders (1.5 ATA) as well as at much lower doses, including compressed air. Examples of the effect of HBO on brain blood flow and metabolism that is responsible for the observed clinical effects can be seen in the cases below treated in New Orleans by this author over the past three decades.

Case Reports

Patient 1: Cerebral Palsy

The patient is a 2-year-old boy whose twin died in utero at 14 weeks. He was delivered at term by vacuum extraction and developmental delay was detected at the age of 4–5 months. He was diagnosed as a case of cerebral palsy. At 2 years of age SPECT brain imaging was performed and showed a heterogeneous pattern of cerebral blood flow. The patient underwent a course of twice daily, 5 days/week HBO treatments in blocks of 50 and 30 treatments. At the conclusion of treatments he showed improvement in spasticity, speech, chewing/swallowing, cognition, and ability to sit in his car seat and stroller for prolonged periods. Repeat SPECT brain imaging showed a global improvement in flow and smoothing to a more normal pattern consistent with the patient's overall clinical improvement. The two SPECT scans are shown side by side in Fig. 23.1. Three-dimensional reconstructions of the two scans are shown in Figs. 23.2 and 23.3.

Fig. 23.1 SPECT brain imaging transverse images of baseline pre-HBOT study on the left and after 80 HBO treatments on the right. Note the global increase in flow and change from heterogeneous to the more normal homogeneous pattern. Slices begin at the top of the head in the upper left corner and proceed to the base of the brain in the lower right corner of each study. Orientation is standard CT: the patient's left is on the viewer's right and vice versa with the patient's face at the top and the back of the head at the bottom of each image. Color scheme is white, yellow, orange, purple, blue, and black from highest to lowest brain blood flow.

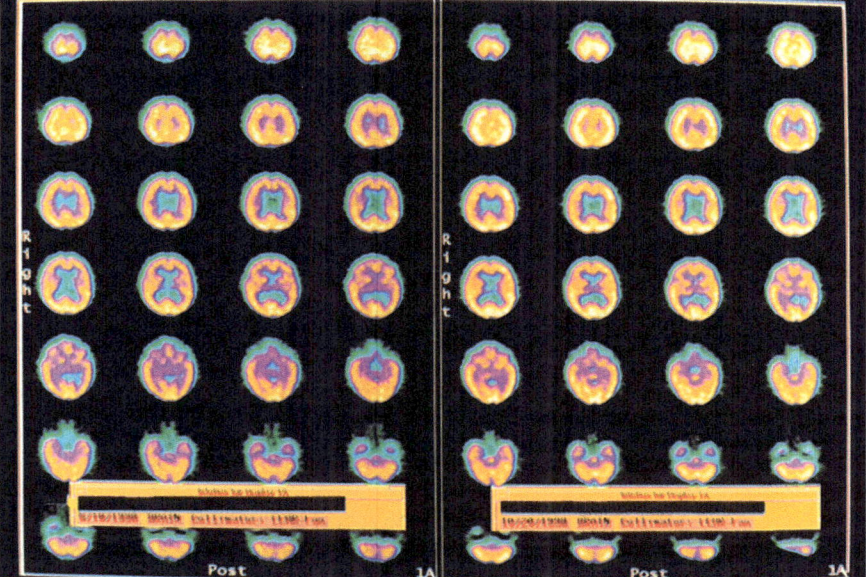

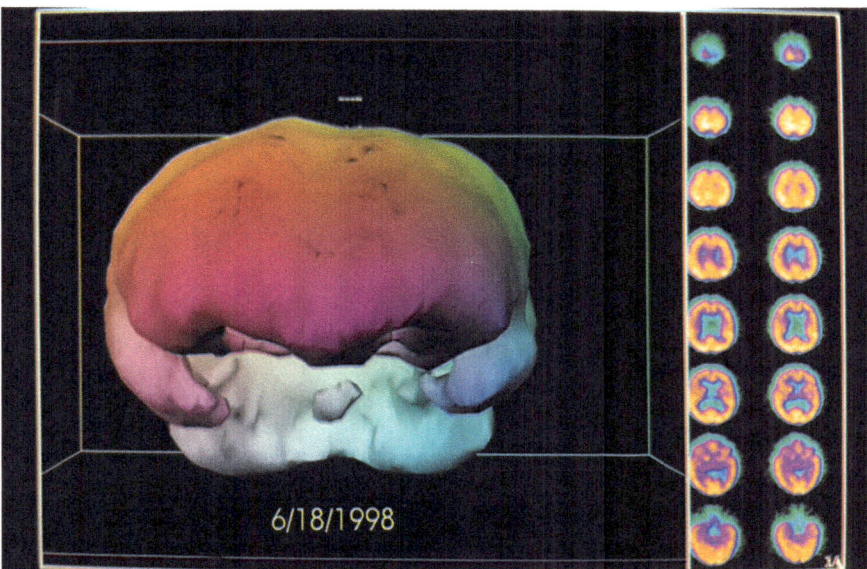

Fig. 23.2 Three-dimensional surface reconstruction of baseline SPECT study on left side in Fig. 23.1. Part of the transverse slices of the Fig. 23.1 baseline study are reproduced on the right side of this figure. The three-dimensional figure is reconstructed from the circumferential edge of each transverse slice. The three-dimensional figure is the face view of the patient. The large purple colored area in the middle of the figure represents the frontal lobes. The two inferior and lateral "bucket handles" are the temporal lobes. The eyes sit just below the frontal lobes and between the temporal lobes. The cerebellar lobes are the two rounded blue-white structures at the bottom of the figure in the back of the brain. The coloring is purely aesthetic/artistic and does not represent blood flow levels as do the colors on the slice images. Note reduction in flow to both temporal lobes, inferior frontal lobes, and the brainstem (central round white blue structure that appears to be "floating" between the temporal lobes below the purple frontal lobes).

Patient 2: Cerebral Palsy

The patient is an 8-year-old boy with a history of cerebral palsy. He had spastic diplegia secondary to premature birth from a mother with eclampsia. Patient was delivered by emergency Cesarean section at 27 weeks when his mother developed seizures. APGARS scores were 7 and 8. The patient spent 5 months in the hospital primarily because of feeding problems. The patient did not achieve normal milestones and developed infantile spasms at 2 years of age. Baseline SPECT brain imaging (Fig. 23.4) showed a mildly/moderately heterogeneous pattern and reduction of blood

Fig. 23.3 Three-dimensional surface reconstruction of SPECT after 80 HBO treatments (right hand study in Fig. 23.1). Note the increased flow to the temporal lobes, inferior frontal lobes, and brainstem.

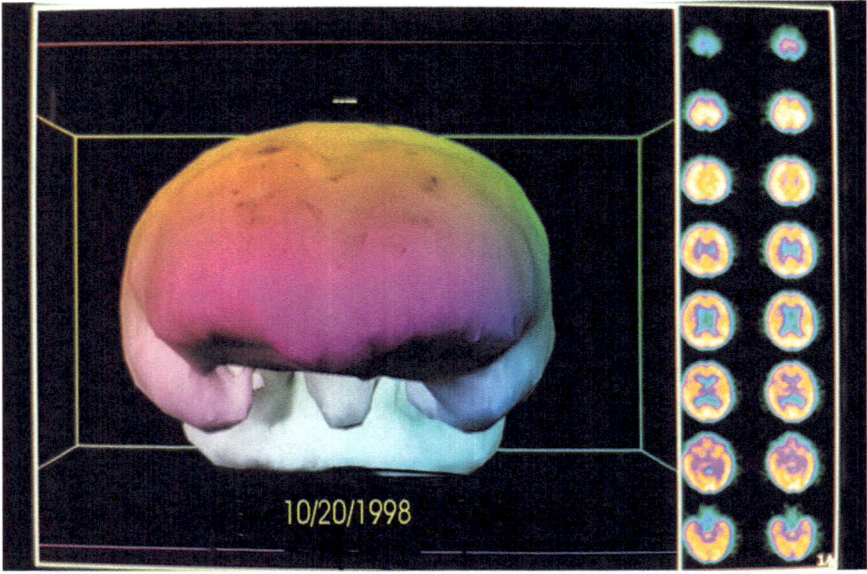

Fig. 23.4 Sagittal slices of baseline pre-HBOT SPECT brain imaging through the center of the brain. Note the heterogeneous pattern of blood flow. Slices proceed from the right side of the head in the upper left corner to the left side of the head in the lower right corner. The front of the brain (face) is on the left side and the back of the brain (back of the head) is on the right side of each slice.

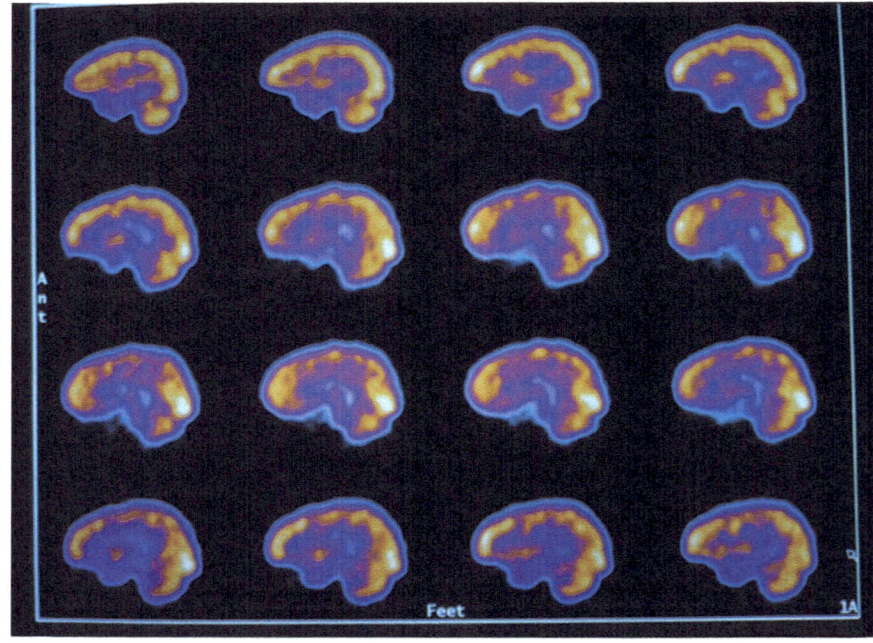

flow. Three hours after a single HBO session at 1.5 ATA for 60 min, repeat SPECT showed global improvement and smoothing to a more normal pattern in Fig. 23.5. The patient underwent a course of 80 HBO sessions (1.5 ATA/60 min) over the next 6 months in two blocks of treatment (twice daily, 5 days/week × 40, then once-daily 5 days/week × 40), and showed improvement in his impulsive inappropriate behavior, motor function, vision, and constipation. Repeat SPECT brain imaging reflected these neurological gains (Fig. 23.6), showing generalized improvement in cerebral blood flow and pattern. Three-dimensional surface recon-

struction of Figs. 23.4, 23.5, and 23.6 are presented in Figs. 23.7, 23.8, and 23.9, respectively. While there is a global increase in blood flow, the most significant relative increase in flow is to the temporal lobes as shown in the three-dimensional figures.

All SPECT brain imaging was performed on a Picker Prism 3000 at West Jefferson Medical Center, Marrero, Louisiana. All scans were identically processed and three-dimensional thresholds obtained by Phillip Tranchina. Pictures of the scans in the above figures were produced by 35 mm single frame photography under identical lighting and exposure conditions.

Fig. 23.5 Sagittal slices of SPECT three hours after a single 1.5ATA/60 min HBO treatment. Note the generalized increase in flow and smoothing to a more normal pattern.

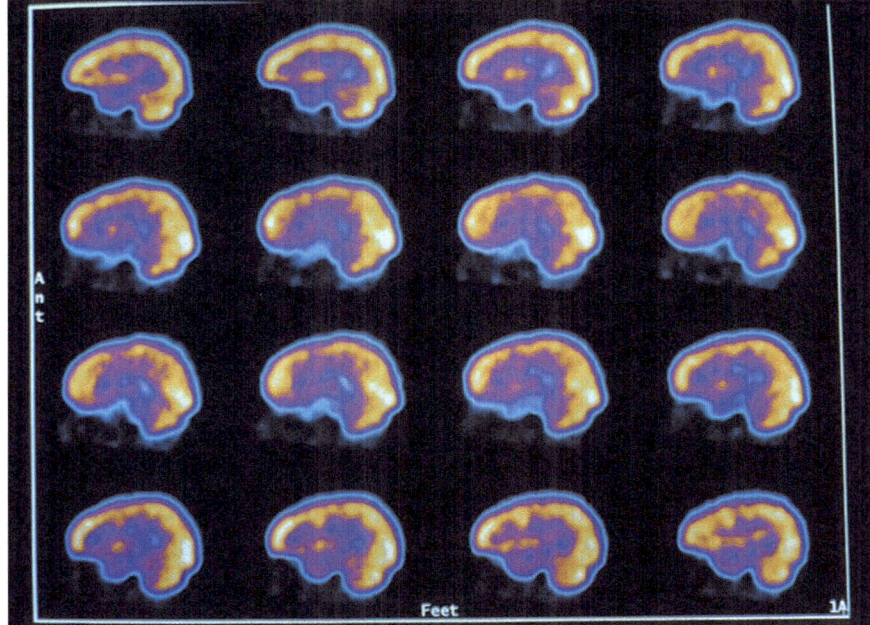

Fig. 23.6 Sagittal slices of SPECT after 80 HBO treatments. Note the marked increase in flow and smoothing of the pattern compared to the baseline in Fig. 23.4.

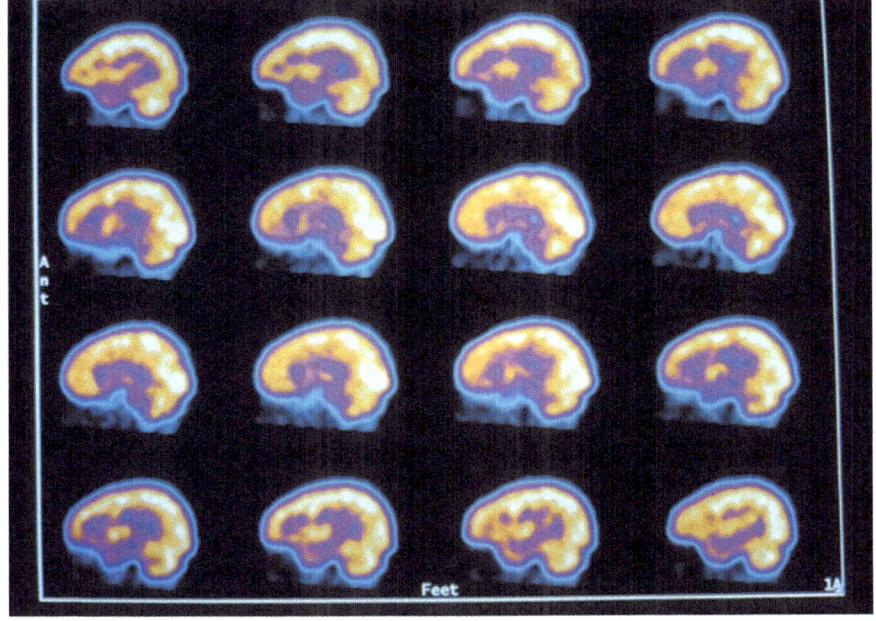

Conclusions

Cerebral palsy is a neurological disorder of diverse etiology. As a result, it is difficult to design trials with subgroups of patients with similar pathomechanisms. Regardless, the results of multiple studies on CP patients have been presented, including three controlled studies, and two rigorous multi-dosing studies mischaracterized as sham or placebo-controlled. Collectively, the data are showing faster, greater, and more durable improvements with a variety of doses of hyperbaric oxygen therapy, including compressed air, compared to therapies that are the standard of care for cerebral palsy. Some studies feature follow-up for as long as 6 months post-treatment and some have also documented sustained cognitive improvements. Positive outcomes have been demonstrated with as few as 20 treatments, but generally 40 or more treatments are recommended.

Controlled studies of HBO in CP should continue to refine and personalize the dosing of hyperbaric therapy for CP patients. However, it will likely take generations of

Fig. 23.7 Three-dimensional surface reconstruction of SPECT in Fig. 23.4. Note reduction in flow to the temporal lobes and coarse appearance of flow to the surface of the brain.

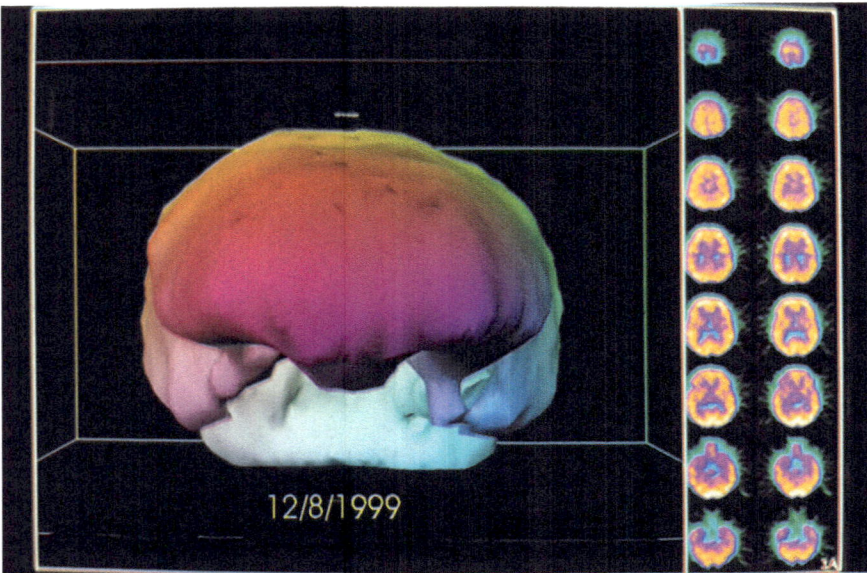

Fig. 23.8 Three-dimensional surface reconstruction of SPECT in Fig. 23.5. Note improvement in flow to the temporal lobes and slight smoothing of flow to the surface of the brain

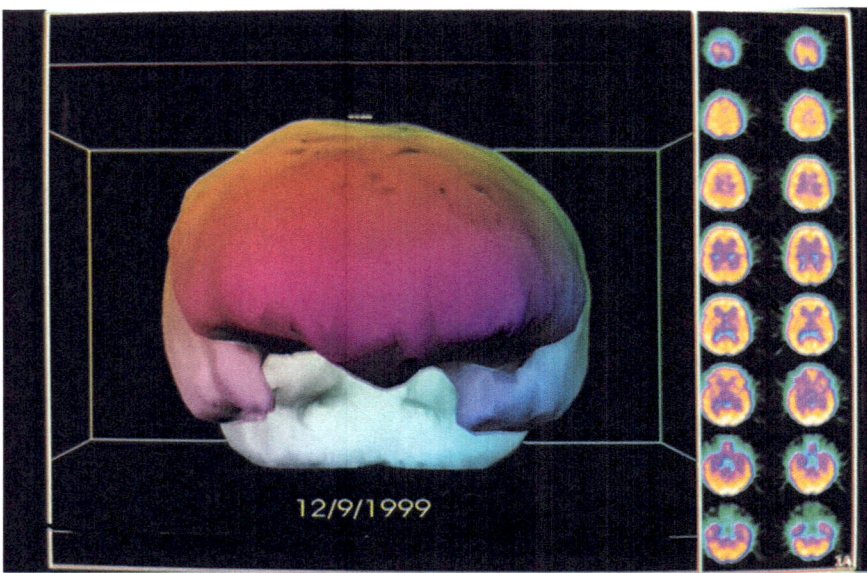

properly conducted studies that incorporate the pressure and hyperoxic dosing concepts discussed above to reverse the imbedded negative sentiment in the pediatric neurology community (Novak and Badawi 2012; invited editorial to the Lacey 2012 study) toward hyperbaric oxygen therapy for CP. The likelihood of securing funding for such clinical trials is extremely low. The extensive positive data generated in the above clinical studies is sufficient to recommend hyperbaric oxygen therapy for CP. In a condition where there is no therapy to offer than can generate permanent improvements, HBO therapy is worth a trial. However, caution should be used in patients with seizure disorders and the patients watched carefully for manifestations of oxygen sensitivity/overdosing.

The concept of personalized medicine as described in Chap. 48 should be applied to HBO treatments in CP. One cannot recommend a standard protocol based on the above data, but the ideal treatment schedule should be determined for each patient including the pressure, dose, and duration of treatment. It may be possible to identify responders early on in the treatment. While molecular diagnostic procedures, genotyping, and gene expression studies may contribute to the evaluation and HBOT treatment of CP children in the future (Jain 2015), dosing of HBOT in CP still remains a clinical practice of medicine issue.

Fig. 23.9 Three-dimensional surface reconstruction of SPECT in Fig. 23.6. Note improvement in flow to the temporal lobes and slight smoothing of flow to the surface of the brain

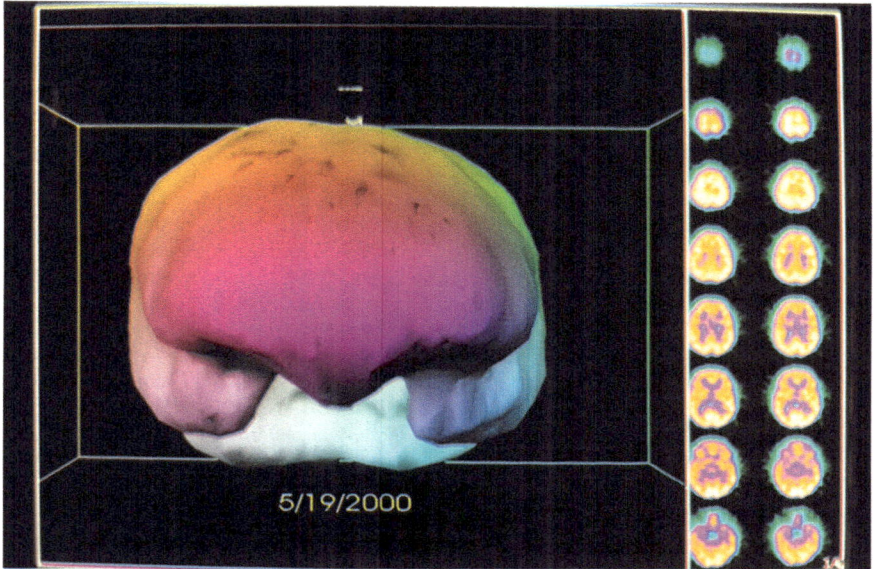

5/19/2000

References

AHRQ. Systems to rate the strength of scientific evidence. Evidence report. Technology Assessment no. 47. Rockville, MD: AHRQ; 2003.

Asl MT, Yousefi F, Nemati R, Assadi M. 99mTc-ECD brain perfusion SPECT imaging for the assessment of brain perfusion in cerebral palsy (CP) patients with evaluation of the effect of hyperbaric oxygen therapy. Int J Clin Exp Med. 2015;8(1):1101–7.

Bedrossian RH, Carmichael P, Ritter J. Retinopathy of prematurity (retrolental fibroplasia) and oxygen. I. Clinical study. II. Further observations on the disease. Am J Ophthalmol. 1954;37:78–86. doi:10.1016/0002-9394(54)92034-6 [PMID: 13114325].

Calvert JW, Zhou C, Zhang JH. Transient exposure of rat pups to hyperoxia at normobaric and hyperbaric pressures does not cause retinopathy of prematurity. Exp Neurol. 2004;189:150–61.

Chavdarov I. The effects of hyperbaric oxygenation on psycho-motor functions by children. In: Joiner JT, editor. Hyperbaric oxygenation for cerebral palsy and the brain-injured child, the proceedings of the 2nd international symposium. Flagstaff: Best Publishing; 2002. p. 91–6.

Chow LC, Wright KW, Sola A, CSMC Oxygen Administration Study Group. Can changes in clinical practice decrease the incidence of severe retinopathy of prematurity in very low birth weight infants? Pediatrics. 2003;111(2):339–45.

Churchill S, Weaver LK, Deru K, Russo AA, Handrahan D, Orrison WW, et al. A prospective trial of hyperbaric oxygen for chronic sequelae after brain injury (HYBOBI). Undersea Hyperb Med. 2013;40(2):165–93.

Collet JP, Vanasse M, Marois P, Amar M, Goldberg J, Lambert J, et al. Hyperbaric oxygen for children with cerebral palsy: a randomized multicentre trial. Lancet. 2001;357:582–6.

Cowan F, Rutherford M, Groenendaal F, Eken P, Mercuri E, Bydder GM, et al. Origin and timing of brain lesions in term infants with neonatal encephalopathy. Lancet. 2003;361(9359):736–42.

Forrester RM. Oxygen, cerebral palsy and retrolental fibroplasias. Dev Med Child Neurol. 1964;186:648–50.

Golden ZL, Neubauer R, Golden CJ, Greene L, Marsh J, Mleko A. Improvement in cerebral metabolism in chronic brain injury after hyperbaric oxygen therapy. Int J Neurosci. 2002;112:119–31.

Harch PG. The dosage of hyperbaric oxygen in chronic brain injury. In: Joiner JT, editor. The proceedings of the 2nd international symposium on hyperbaric oxygenation for cerebral palsy and the brain-injured child. Flagstaff: Best Publishing; 2002. p. 31–56.

Harch PG. Hyperbaric oxygen therapy in the treatment of chronic traumatic brain injury: from Louisiana boxers to U.S. veterans, an American chronology. Wound Care Hyperb Med. 2010;1(4):26–34. ISSN: 2157-9148.

Harch PG. Hyperbaric oxygen therapy for post-concussion syndrome: contradictory conclusions from a study mischaracterized as sham-controlled. J Neurotrauma. 2013;30:1995–9.

Harch PG, Deckoff-Jones J, Neubauer RA. Low pressure hyperbaric oxygen therapy for pediatric brain injury, a minimal risk medical treatment. Pediatrics Online.12 Fb 2001 (P3R Response):1–3. Pediatrics (ISSN: 0031 4005). Copyright C2000 by the American Academy of Pediatrics.

Harch PG, Kriedt C, Van Meter KW, Sutherland RJ. Hyperbaric oxygen therapy improves spatial learning and memory in a rat model of chronic traumatic brain injury. Brain Res. 2007;1174:120–9. Epub Aug 2007.

Harch PG, Van Meter KW, Gottlieb SF, Staab P. HMPAO SPECT brain imaging and low pressure HBOT in the diagnosis and treatment of chronic traumatic, ischemic, hypoxic, and anoxic encephalopathies. Undersea Hyperb Med. 1994;21(Suppl):30.

Hardy P, Collet JP, Goldberg J, Ducruet T, Vanasse M, Lambert J, et al. Neuropsychological effects of hyperbaric oxygen therapy in cerebral palsy. Dev Med Child Neurol. 2002;44(7):436–46.

Heuser G, Heuser SA, Rodelander D, Aguilera O, Uszler M. Treatment of neurologically impaired adults and children with "mild" hyperbaric oxygen (1.3ATA and 24% oxygen). In: Joiner JT, editor. The proceedings of the 2nd international symposium on hyperbaric oxygenation for cerebral palsy and the brain-injured child. Flagstaff: Best Publishing; 2002. p. 109–16.

Hutchison JH, Kerr MM, Williams KG, Hopkinson WI. Hyperbaric oxygen in the resuscitation of the newborn. Lancet. 1963;2(7316):1019–22.

Jain KK. Textbook of personalized medicine. 2nd ed Springer: New York; 2015.

Lacey DJ, Stolfi A, Pilati LE. Effects of hyperbaric oxygen on motor function in children with cerebral palsy. Ann Neurol. 2012;72:695–703.

Liu Z, Xiong T, Meads C. Clinical effectiveness of treatment with hyperbaric oxygen for neonatal hypoxic-ischaemic encephalopathy: systematic review of Chinese literature. BMJ. 2006;333(7564):374. Epub 11 May 2006.

Macdonald AG, Fraser PJ. The transduction of very small hydrostatic pressures. Comp Biochem Physiol A Mol Integr Physiol. 1999;122(1):13–36.

Machado J. Clinically observed reduction of spasticity in patients with neurological diseases and in children with cerebral palsy from hyperbaric oxygen therapy. Proceedings of "New Horizons in Hyperbaric Medicine." American College of Hyperbaric Medicine; 1989.

Montgomery D, Goldberg J, Amar M, Lacroix V, Lecomte J, Lambert J, et al. Effects of hyperbaric oxygen therapy o children with spastic diplegic cerebral palsy: a pilot project. Undersea Hyperb Med. 1999;26(4):235–42.

Mukherjee A, Raison M, Sahni T, Arya A, Lambert J, Marois P, et al. Intensive rehabilitation combined with HBO₂ therapy in children with cerebral palsy: a controlled longitudinal study. Undersea Hyperb Med. 2014;41(2):77–85.

Muller-Bolla M, Collet J-P, Ducruet T, Robinson A. Side effects of hyperbaric oxygen therapy in children with cerebral palsy. Undersea Hyperb Med. 2006;33(4):237–44.

Neubauer RA. New hope for the neurologically damaged child, cerebral palsy, anoxic ischemic encephalopathy, and traumatic brain injury. In: Joiner JT, editor. The proceedings of the 2nd international symposium on hyperbaric oxygenation for cerebral palsy and the brain-injured child. Flagstaff: Best Publishing; 2002. p. 3–8.

Novak I, Badawi N. Last breath; effectiveness of oxygen hyperbaric treatment for cerebral palsy. Ann Neurol. 2012;72:633–4.

Nuthall G, Seear M, Lepawsky M, Wensley D, Skippen P, Hukin J. Hyperbaric oxygen therapy for cerebral palsy: two complications of treatment. Pediatrics. 2000;106:80. doi:10.1542/peds.106.6.e80.

Oskoui M, Coutinho F, Dykeman J, Jette N, Pringsheim T. An update on the prevalence of cerebral palsy: a systematic review and meta-analysis. Dev Med Child Neurol. 2013;55:509–19.

Packard M. The Cornell study. Presented at the University of Graz 18th November 2000; 2000. http://www.netnet.net/mums/Cornell.htm. Accessed 5 Mar 2016.

Penn JS, Henry MM, Wall PT, Tolman BL. The range of PaO₂ variation determines the severity of oxygen-induced retinopathy in newborn rats. Invest Ophthalmol Vis Sci. 1995;36:2063–70.

Pierce EA, Foley ED, Smith LE. Regulation of vascular endothelial growth factor by oxygen in a model of retinopathy of prematurity. Arch Ophthalmol. 1996;114:1219–28.

Ricci B, Calogero G. Oxygen-induced retinopathy in newborn rats: effects of prolonged normobaric and hyperbaric oxygen supplementation. Pediatrics. 1988;82:193–8.

Saito Y, Omoto T, Cho Y, Hatsukawa Y, Fujimura M, Takeuchi T. The progression of retinopathy of prematurity and fluctuation in blood gas tension. Graefes Arch Clin Exp Ophthalmol. 1993;231:151–6.

Senechal C, Larivee S, Richard E, Marois P. Hyperbaric oxygenation therapy in the treatment of cerebral palsy: a review and comparison to currently accepted therapies. J Am Phys Surg. 2007;12(4):109–13.

Sethi A, Mukherjee A. To see the efficacy of hyperbaric oxygen therapy in gross motor abilities of cerebral palsy children of 2–5 years, given initially as an adjunct to occupational therapy. Indian J Occup Ther. 2003;35(1):1–11.

Shah PK, Prabhu V, Karandikar SS, Ranjan R, Narendran V, Kalpana N. Retinopathy of prematurity: past, present and future. World J Clin Pediatr. 2016;5(1):35–46.

Szewczyk TS. Retrolental fibroplasia: etiology and prophylaxis; a preliminary report. Am J Ophthalmol. 1951;34(12):1649–50.

Waalkes P, Fitzpatrick D, Stankus S, Topolski R. Adjunctive HBO treatment of children with cerebral anoxic injury. Army Med Dept J. 2002:13–21. PB. 8-2002.

Zerbini S. The use of hyperbaric oxygenation in the treatment of chronic childhood encephalopathy. In: Joiner JT, editor. The proceedings of the 2nd international symposium on hyperbaric oxygenation for cerebral palsy and the brain-injured child. Flagstaff: Best Publishing; 2002. p. 3–8. Boca Raton Symposium. p. 189–98.

Zhou BY, Lu GJ, Huang YQ, Ye ZZ, Han YK. Efficacy of hyperbaric oxygen therapy under different pressures on neonatal hypoxic-ischemic encephalopathy. Zhongguo Dang Dai Er Ke Za Zhi. 2008;10(2):133–5.

K.K. Jain

Abstract

This chapter deals with the role of HBO in miscellaneous disorders not covered in other chapters. Some of these, such as vascular headaches, are common but HBO has a limited role. HBO has been found useful in some peripheral neuropathies, which has led to further investigation of its role in relief of neuropathic pain. HBO has been tried in degenerative neurological disorders such as Alzheimer's disease with no proof of its efficacy, whereas it is effective in dementia due to vascular insufficiency. Conditions where HBO has not been found to be effective include muscular dystrophy and myasthenia gravis.

Keywords

Autism spectrum disorder • Benign intracranial hypertension • Cerebral malaria • Dementia • Hyperbaric oxygen (HBO) • Muscular dystrophy • Myasthenia gravis • Peripheral neuropathic pain • Peripheral neuropathy • Susac's syndrome • Vascular headaches

Introduction

The use of HBO in significant neurological disorders is described in separate chapters. A few miscellaneous indications, particularly cerebral malaria, peripheral neuropathy, and vascular headaches, that do not fit into these are described here.

HBO in the Treatment of Benign Intracranial Hypertension

Benign intracranial hypertension (BIH) is characterized by prolonged raised intracranial pressure without ventricular enlargement, focal neurological signs, or disturbances of consciousness and intellect. The most frequent symptoms are headaches, diplopia, and impairment of visual acuity. It occurs most frequently in obese women in the childbearing period. The cause is not known, but the following explanations have been considered for the pathophysiology of BIH:

1. An increased rate of CSF formation
2. Sustained increase in intracranial venous pressure.
3. A decreased rate of CSF absorption by arachnoid villi apart from venous occlusive disease.
4. Increase in brain volume because of an increase in cerebral blood volume or interstitial fluid. There is histological evidence for cerebral edema.

Diagnostic criteria of BIH are as follows:

1. Signs and symptoms of raised intracranial pressure
2. No localizing neurological signs in an awake and alert patient except for abducent palsy
3. Documented elevation of intracranial pressure (250 mmH$_2$O)
4. Normal CSF composition
5. Normal neuroimaging studies except for small ventricles and empty sella turcica

Various methods are used for lowering the intracranial pressure, including lumbar punctures, dehydrating agents such as mannitol, diuretics, and corticosteroids. Ventriculoperitoneal shunts have been performed frequently

K.K. Jain, MD, FRACS, FFPM (✉)
1 Blaesiring 7, Basel 4057, Switzerland
e-mail: jain@pharmabiotech.ch

and afford good relief from headaches, but the small ventricles present a technical difficulty in inserting catheters into this space. The main concern is preservation of vision and the preferred operation is fenestration of the sheath of the optic nerve.

Luongo et al. (1992) treated various groups among 53 patients with BIH by several methods. Eight of the patients were treated only by HBO at 2 ATA, daily for 15 days. In all patients a gradual disappearance of signs and symptoms of elevated intracranial pressure was observed. However, the intracranial pressure was elevated again after discontinuation of HBO. The mechanism of this effect is not clear, but reduction of CSF production and an anti-edema effect of HBO are possible explanations. Further studies are required to assess this therapy for BIH but to date there have been no further publications on this topic.

Peripheral Neuropathy

Peripheral neuropathy is a general term referring to any disorder that affects the peripheral nervous system, including infections, toxins, metabolic disturbances, and trauma. Drug-induced peripheral neuropathy can be due to a large number of drugs and various methods of management are described elsewhere (Jain 2011).

Clioquinol-induced damage to the peripheral nerves has been shown to be decreased in animals treated using HBO as compared with controls (Mukoyama et al. 1975). The authors speculated that oxygenation might prevent the death of intoxicated neurons in the spinal root ganglia and resuscitate them, as well as accelerate the sprouting and regeneration of nerve fibers in the peripheral part. They indicated that HBO may be useful in the treatment of peripheral nerve lesions.

Peripheral neuropathy in streptozotocin-induced diabetic rats has been shown to be partially reversed by HBO treatment (2 ATA, 2 h, 5 days/week) for 4 weeks (Low et al. 1988). There was enhancement of nerve energy metabolism in the HBO-treated animals as compared with the control animals with similar lesions, not treated by HBO.

Neretin et al. (1988), after a review of their experience in treating polyradiculoneuritis with HBO, have concluded that: "The results of clinico-electromyographic examinations point to a sufficiently high effectiveness of hyperbaric oxygenation in polyradiculoneuritis and permit its inclusion into the multimodality treatment of the latter. HBO accelerates regression of neurological disorders, with the predominant effect on the severity of motor and autonomic-trophic disturbances. HBO makes it possible to reduce the doses of glucocorticoids and the period of treatment and hospitalization of patients."

HBO for the Treatment of Peripheral Neuropathic Pain

Studies in rats have investigated the effect of HBO treatment at various stages following chronic constriction injury (CCI)-induced neuropathic pain in rats, to explore the mechanisms of effect of HBO treatment. In one such study, methane dicarboxylic aldehyde (MDA) and superoxide dismutase (SOD) parameters were used as indices of oxidative stress response and tested before and after the treatment (Zhao et al. 2014). The inflammatory cytokines IL-1β and IL-10 were assayed in the sciatic nerve with enzyme-linked immunoassay. Glial fibrillary acidic protein activation in the spinal cord was evaluated immunohistochemically. The rats exhibited temporary allodynia immediately after HBO treatment completion. This transient allodynia was closely associated with changes in MDA and SOD levels. A single HBO treatment caused a short-acting antinociceptive response phase. Repetitive HBO treatment led to a long-acting antinociceptive response phase and inhibited astrocyte activation. These results indicated that HBO treatment played a dual role in the aggravation and alleviation of neuropathic pain, though the aggravated pain effect (transient allodynia) is far less pronounced than the antinociceptive phase. Astrocyte inhibition and anti-inflammatory effect may contribute to the relief of neuropathic pain by HBO treatment after nerve injury.

In another study on CCI-induced neuropathic pain model, early HBO treatment beginning on postoperative day 1 produced a persistent antinociceptive effect and inhibited the CCI-induced increase in the expression of P2X4R without changing CCI-induced apoptosis (Zhao et al. 2015). In contrast, late HBO treatment beginning on postoperative day 11 produced a persistent antinociceptive effect and inhibited CCI-induced apoptosis and upregulation of caspase-3 without changing the expression of P2X4R. In addition, late HBO treatment reduced CCI-induced ultrastructural damage. However, HBO treatment beginning on postoperative day 6 produced a transient antinociceptive effect without changing the expression of P2X4R or CCI-induced apoptosis.

HBO for Treatment of Drug-Induced Neuropathy

A 3-month study evaluated the effects of HBO (2-h sessions at 2 ATA twice weekly) on drug-induced neuropathies in 22 patients with HIV (Jordan 1998). All patients included in the study had been taking an antiretroviral medication for at least 12 months and had subjective symptoms of numbness or tingling, lethargy, and a decrease in deep tendon reflexes. Of the 20 patients who completed the study, 17 had significant improvement, 2 had a demyelinating disorder that may have affected the outcome, and 1 had no change.

HBO for the Treatment of Trigeminal Neuralgia

In clinical trials, one course of HBO therapy (10 consecutive days) produced a rapid-onset, dose-dependent, and long-lasting analgesic effects evidenced by the decreased doses of carbamazepine required for keeping patient pain at a minimum and decreased scores of visual analog scales, which was used for patient's self-evaluation (Gu et al. 2012). These findings support that HBO therapy is an effective approach for treating not only peripheral neuropathies but also cranial neuropathies in human beings. Neuroprotection, anti-inflammatory effect, and inhibition of altered neural activity may contribute to the analgesic effect of HBO therapy.

HBO in Susac's Syndrome

The Susac's syndrome consists of a clinical triad of encephalopathy, loss of vision, and hearing defects (Jain 2016). It is caused by microangiopathy of unknown origin affecting the small arteries of the brain, retina, and cochlea. This rare disorder, with 75 cases documented in the literature, affects mainly young women. The course of the illness is self-limiting. The deficit of visual acuity is caused by occlusion of tributaries of the retinal artery. The auditory defect is bilateral and symmetrical and particularly affects medium and low frequencies. MRI is of great diagnostic value, showing multiple lesions in the gray and white matter. Li et al. (1996) were the first to report HBO treatment with favorable outcome in a young woman with Susac's syndrome who presented on two separate occasions with visual acuity loss from a recurrent branch retinal artery occlusion. Meca-Lallana et al. (1999) reported the case of a young woman who presented with psychiatric symptoms and migraine followed by clinical encephalopathy and acute/subacute coma. There were also visual and auditory deficits. The patient responded to systemic treatment with corticosteroids and HBO. The encephalopathy resolved in a few days, and 2 months later, she had resumed her former daily activities. Treatment with HBO was considered to have definitely reduced visual sequelae in this case. In another similar case, combination of intravenous steroids and HBO reduced the ischemic lesions (Cubillana Herrero et al. 2002).

Cerebral Malaria

Over 200 million people worldwide suffer from malaria every year, a disease that causes 584,000 deaths annually. In recent years, significant improvements have been achieved on the treatment of severe malaria, but mortality remains high, at 8% in children and 15% in adults in clinical trials, and even worse in the case of cerebral malaria (18% and 30%, respectively). Cerebral malaria (CM) is a syndrome characterized by neurological signs, seizures, and coma. Some individuals who do not succumb to cerebral malaria present long-term cognitive deficits. These observations indicate that strategies focused only on parasite killing fail to prevent neurological complications and deaths associated with severe malaria, possibly because clinical complications are associated in part with a cerebrovascular dysfunction.

Despite the fact that CM presents similarities with cerebral stroke, few studies have focused on new supportive therapies for the disease.

An experimental study has explored the use of HBO for CM. Mice infected with *Plasmodium berghei* ANKA (PbA) were exposed to daily doses of HBO (100% oxygen at 3 ATA for 1–2 h per day) before or after parasite establishment (Blanco et al. 2008). Cumulative survival analyses demonstrated that HBO therapy protected 50% of PbA-infected mice and delayed CM-specific neurological signs when administrated after patent parasitemia. HBO reduced peripheral parasitemia; expression of TNF-α, IFN-γ, and IL-10 mRNA levels; and percentage of $\gamma\Delta$ and $\alpha\beta$ CD4+ and CD8+ T lymphocytes sequestered in mice brains, thus resulting in a reduction of BBB dysfunction and hypothermia. These data indicate that HBO treatment could be used as supportive therapy, perhaps in association with neuroprotective drugs, to prevent CM clinical outcomes, including death. Gaseous therapies including HBO alter vascular endothelium dysfunction and modulate the host immune response to infection (Kayano et al. 2016). Other experimental studies support the use of HBO as a rational and effective adjunct therapy for CM (Bruce-Hickman 2011).

Vascular Headaches

Vascular headaches include migraine headaches with and without aura as well as cluster headaches. Migraine affects up to 18% of women, while cluster headaches are much less common (0.2% of the population). A number of acute and prophylactic therapies are available. HBO is a potential treatment for drug-resistant migraines and in patients who cannot tolerate conventional antimigraine therapies. Logistic problems of availability of hyperbaric chambers at the time of onset of an attack have limited the use of HBO.

Rationale for the Use of HBO in Vascular Headaches

Vasodilatation is a well-known phenomenon in vascular headaches. Even 100% NBO is effective against vascular headaches because of its vasoconstricting effect (Jain 1989). HBO is more effective as a vasoconstrictor and has the added advantage of preventing symptoms due to cerebral ischemia improving cerebral oxygenation.

Current Status of Use of HBO in Vascular Headaches

A number of open studies have reported the effectiveness of HBO in vascular headaches. A systematic review of 11 randomized controlled trials on 209 patients compared HBO or NBO with one another, other active therapies, placebo (sham) interventions, or no treatment in participants with migraine or cluster headache (Bennett et al. 2015). There was some evidence that HBO was effective for the termination of acute migraine in an unselected population and some evidence that NBO was similarly effective in cluster headache. In the author's opinion, in view of the cost and poor availability of HBO, more research should be done on patients unresponsive to standard therapy. NBO is cheap, safe, and easy to apply, so it will probably continue to be used despite the limited evidence in this review.

HBO for Autism Spectrum Disorder

Autism spectrum disorder (ASD) is a neurodevelopment disorder characterized by social communication impairment, restricted interests, repetitive behaviors, and hyper- or hyporeactivity to sensory input. Estimated prevalence in the United States is 1 in 68 children. ASD is a complex disorder with multiple etiological factors. Treatment is primarily behavioral analysis and therapy. Pharmacotherapy is used for control of certain symptoms such as irritability and hyperactivity.

HBO is currently lumped with list of therapies with minimal or no efficacy for ASD. However, rationale of proposing HBO for ASD is based on demonstration of hypoperfusion to several areas of the autistic brain by SPECT and PET studies, most notably the temporal regions as well as areas specifically related to language comprehension and auditory processing, which correlate with many of the clinical features associated with ASD (Rossignol and Rossignol 2006). HBO has been shown to be effective in other cerebral hypoperfusion syndromes. In a study on seven Thai autistic children, who received HBO (100 % oxygen, 1.3 ATA, ten sessions), assessment was done before and after treatment in five domains: social development, fine motor and eye-hand coordination, language development, gross motor development, and self-help skills (Chungpaibulpatana et al. 2008). Significant improvement was shown in 75 % of children, whereas 25 % did not seem to respond to the treatment. The

first controlled clinical trial in the United States examined the effects of 40 HBO sessions using 24 % oxygen at 1.3 ATA on 11 topographies of directly observed behavior in ASD (Jepson et al. 2011). Five replications of multiple baselines were completed across a total of 16 participants, but no consistent effects were observed across any group or within any individual participant, demonstrating that HBO was not an effective treatment for the participants in this study. This study represents the first relatively large-scale controlled study evaluating the effects of HBO at the level of the individual participant, on a wide array of behaviors. The results of this study are not valid because 24 % oxygen at 1.3 ATA does not meet the definition of HBO. There is a need for properly designed studies to settle the issue of effectiveness of HBO in ASD.

Neurological Disorders in Which HBO Has Not Been Found to Be Useful

This section presents historical information on several diseases where HBO has been used. Dementia and neuromuscular diseases are two examples. There have been no further studies done to prove the efficacy of HBO in these areas, and at present HBO cannot be recommended for these conditions.

Dementia Due to Degenerative Disorders of the Brain

Dementia is defined as "a global impairment of higher cortical function, including memory, the capacity to solve problems of everyday living, the performance of learned motor skills, the correct use of social skills and the control of emotional reactions, in the absence of gross clouding of consciousness."

The causes of dementia are varied, and no single mode of treatment is applicable uniformly to the varied causes. HBO has been used as a treatment for dementia. As described in other chapters, HBO is useful in the treatment of vascular dementia and dementia as a manifestation of delayed neurological sequelae of CO poisoning. However, it is not useful for dementia due to degenerative disorders of the brain, e.g., Alzheimer's disease. Anecdotal cases of improvement with HBO in patients diagnosed as "Alzheimer's disease" may be due to role of vascular insufficiency in multifactorial dementia, which responds to HBO.

Interest in the use of hyperbaric environments for central nervous system pathology has existed since the report by Corning (1891). McFarland (1963) theorized that sensory and mental impairments in the elderly are due to diminished availability or utilization of oxygen in the nervous system.

Considerable criticism followed publication of the study by Jacobs et al. (1972), some of which can be summarized as follows:

1. Lack of oxygen supply to the brain was the main reason for using hyperoxygenation therapy. According to Sokoloff (1966), however, the proportional relationship between oxygen supply and oxygen consumption is near normal in patients with chronic brain syndrome.
2. The study failed to sort out the various reversible psychotic states that need to be differentiated from senility.
3. The validity of some of the psychological tests used was questioned by discussants of the paper. There was paucity of measurement.
4. There was no randomization regarding inclusion in the study or division into groups.
5. A wide variety of symptoms and signs were manifested by the patients and they belonged to a large number of diagnostic categories. Such a heterogeneous group would make the interpretation of the most precise and the most concrete results difficult.
6. The treatment is time-consuming and expensive. Elderly patients may dislike it or refuse it. The results are short-lived.
7. The placebo treatment of 5 patients with $10\% O_2 + 90\% N_2$ is dangerous in elderly patients. Thomas et al. (1976) studied the interaction of hyperbaric nitrogen and oxygen mixtures on behavior in rats. Raised oxygen pressure modulated and interacted with the narcotic effect of nitrogen on behavior—an initial increase in response rate was followed by decline.

Raskin et al. (1978) assigned 82 elderly subjects with significant cognitive impairment to treatment with HBO, hyperbaric air, normobaric air, or normobaric oxygen. Treatment consisted of two 90-min sessions per day for 15 days. Psychological evaluation immediately after treatment and 1, 2, 3, and 8 weeks later did not reveal any enhanced cognitive function in experimental subjects (who received NBO or HBO) as compared with controls (who received normobaric or hyperbaric air). Kron et al. (1981) reviewed the published literature on the application of HBO in senile dementia and their own experience. They made a number of observations about the difficulties encountered in evaluating this therapy's usefulness in treating mental dysfunction and came to the following conclusions:

1. The definitive study on the efficacy of HBO in the treatment of senile dementia has yet to be performed.
2. The gross discrepancies in the published reports may be attributed to inadequate design of experiments, poor research methodologies, and great variability in the clinical research populations. They noted that many of the psychological test instruments used in these studies lack the precision and reliability necessary to demonstrate small changes in mental capacity in response to therapeutic intervention. Further, because of logistical and safety considerations, the administration of HBO does not lend itself to well-controlled double-blind studies. Also, there is lack of agreement on the etiology and diagnosis of mental dysfunction in the aged, contributing to the difficulty in determining which patients may benefit from HBO therapy.

Schmitz (1977, 1981) evaluated HBO therapy for senility and concluded:

"At the present time, there is no basis for claiming that HBO is beneficial in reversing senility or any other central nervous system deficit that occurs in the aged … the only indication for HBO therapy in senility would be as a part of research study … Subjecting older people to hyperbaric environments, even if the risks are minimal, is contraindicated."

HBO in the Management of Neuromuscular Disorders

Muscular Dystrophy

The muscular dystrophies are hereditary degenerative disorders of the muscles. Most of the theories of the etiology of muscular dystrophy relate to the neuromuscular system. According to other theories, however, the primary disturbance is in the vascular supply to the skeletal muscles; blood flow is reduced to the exercising muscles. Biochemical abnormalities in the muscles may either be the cause or the effect of muscle degeneration.

Hirotani and Kuyama (1974) treated 10 patients with muscular dystrophy using HBO. Five were of the Duchenne type and five of the limb-girdle type; 100% oxygen was used at 2 ATA daily and 19 sessions were completed in 3 weeks. Along with this an intravenous infusion of fructose + adenosine triphosphate (cytidine phosphatase choline), reduced glutathione, and sodium carbazochrome sulfonate was given. As controls, 3 patients with muscular dystrophy of the Duchenne type were subjected to HBO without the intravenous medications. There was improvement in muscle strength in the group given HBO plus medications but none in the group given HBO alone. The effect, however, was transient, and 5 years later there was no difference in condition between the controls and the treated group. The authors concluded that HBO in combination with ATP and CDP-choline may be effective in the symptomatic relief of muscular dystrophy.

Badalian et al. (1975) of Russia summarized their experience in treating 306 patients with muscular dystrophy during different phases of the disease. The treatment was carried out keeping in mind the disturbance of protein metabolism and decreased permeability of the cell membranes. The treatment consisted of HBO with anabolic hormones, amino acids, vitamins, muscle electrostimulation, and so forth. There was no clinical progression of symptoms in 3 years of follow-up.

There has been no further progress in this area during the past 40 years and there appears to be no rational basis for the use of HBO for this indication. Considerable advances are taking place in molecular genetics and gene therapy for muscular dystrophy is a reasonable possibility.

Myasthenia Gravis

Myasthenia gravis is an autoimmune disease. A specific antibody against the acetylcholine receptor is found in 85% of the patients, and the major component of this antibody is IgG.

Li et al. (1987) carried out a controlled trial of HBO in 40 patients with myasthenia gravis; one group was treated with HBO alone and the other with HBO plus steroids. The rate of improvement with HBO alone was 88.9%; with HBO plus steroids, it was 86.5%; and in the control group treated by steroids alone, it was 45%. IgA and IgM were reduced in the HBO group, indicating an immunosuppressive effect.

There has been no further work done in this area during the past three decades. The immunosuppressive effect of HBO has not been demonstrated conclusively. There appears to be no justification for using HBO in myasthenia gravis at present.

References

Badalian LO, Dunaevskaya GN, Sitnikov VF. The treatment of patients with progressive dystrophy. Zh Nevropatol Psikhiatr. 1975;75:1317–23.

Bennett MH, French C, Schnabel A. Normobaric and hyperbaric oxygen therapy for the treatment and prevention of migraine and cluster headache. Cochrane Database Syst Rev. 2015;12, CD005219.

Blanco YC, Farias AS, Goelnitz U, Lopes SC, Arrais-Silva WW, Carvalho BO, et al. Hyperbaric oxygen prevents early death caused by experimental cerebral malaria. PLoS One. 2008;3, e3126.

Bruce-Hickman D. Oxygen therapy for cerebral malaria. Travel Med Infect Dis. 2011;9:223–30.

Chungpaibulpatana J, Sumpatanarax T, Thadakul N, Chantharatreerat C, Konkaew M, Aroonlimsawas M. Hyperbaric oxygen therapy in Thai autistic children. J Med Assoc Thai. 2008;91:1232–8.

Corning JL. The use of compressed air in conjunction with medical solutions in treatment of nervous and mental affections. Medical Records. 1891;40:225.

Cubillana Herrero JD, Soler Valcarcel A, Albaladejo Devis I, Rodríguez González-Herrero B, Minguez Merlos N, Jiménez Cervantes-Nicolás JA. Susac syndrome as a cause of sensorineural hearing loss. Acta Otorrinolaringol Esp. 2002;53:379–83.

Gu N, Niu JY, Liu WT, Sun YY, Liu S, Lv Y, et al. Hyperbaric oxygen therapy attenuates neuropathic hyperalgesia in rats and idiopathic trigeminal neuralgia in patients. Eur J Pain. 2012;16:1094–105.

Hirotani H, Kuyama T. Hyperbaric oxygen therapy for muscular dystrophy. Arch Jpn Chir. 1974;43:161–7.

Jacobs EA, Alvis HJ, Small SM. Hyperoxygenation: a central nervous system activator? J Geriatr Psychiatry. 1972;5:107–21.

Jain KK. Oxygen in physiology and medicine. Springfield: Charles C. Thomas; 1989.

Jain KK. Drug-induced peripheral neuropathies. In: Jain KK, editor. Drug-induced neurological disorders. 3rd ed. Göttingen: Hogrefe; 2011.

Jain KK. Susac syndrome. In: Greenamyre JT, editor. Medlink neurology. California: San Diego; 2016.

Jepson B, Granpeesheh D, Tarbox J, Olive ML, Stott C, Braud S, et al. Controlled evaluation of the effects of hyperbaric oxygen therapy on the behavior of 16 children with autism spectrum disorders. J Autism Dev Disord. 2011;41:575–88.

Jordan WC. The effectiveness of intermittent hyperbaric oxygen in relieving drug-induced HIV-associated neuropathy. J Natl Med Assoc. 1998;90:355–8.

Kayano AC, Dos-Santos JC, Bastos MF, Carvalho LJ, Aliberti J, Costa FT. Pathophysiological mechanisms in gaseous therapies for severe malaria. Infect Immun. 2016;84:874–82.

Kron RER, Garfinkel SL, Pfeffer SL, et al. Hyperbaric oxygen therapy in senile dementia: a review. In: Yefuni SN, editor. Abstracts of the 7th International Congress of HBO medicine. Moscow: USSR Academy of Sciences; 1981. p. 301–2.

Li W. Myasthenia gravis treated by hyperbaric oxygenation. A report of 40 cases. Presented at the 9th International Congress on Hyperbaric Medicine. Sydney, Australia, 1987 March 1–4.

Li HK, Dejean BJ, Tang RA. Reversal of visual loss with hyperbaric oxygen treatment in a patient with Susac syndrome. Ophthalmology. 1996;103:2091–8.

Low PA, Schmelzer JD, Ward KK, Curran GL, Poduslo JF. Effect of hyperbaric oxygenation on normal and chronic streptozotocin diabetic peripheral nerves. Exp Neurol. 1988;99:201–12.

Luongo C, Mignini R, Vicario C, Sammartino A. Hyperbaric oxygen therapy in the treatment of benign intracranial hypertension. Follow-up of a preliminary study. Minerva Anestesiol. 1992;58 suppl 1:97–8.

McFarland RA. Experimental evidence of relationship between aging and oxygen want. Ergonomics. 1963;6:339–66.

Meca-Lallana JE, Martin JJ, Lucas C, Marín J, Gomariz J, Valenti JA, et al. Susac syndrome: clinical and diagnostic approach. A new case report. Rev Neurol. 1999;29:1027–32.

Mukoyama M, Tida M, Sobve I. Hyperbaric oxygen therapy. Exp Neurol. 1975;47:371–80.

Neretin VI, Va K, Kotov SV, Lobov MA, Agafonov BV. Hyperbaric oxygenation in the combined treatment of patients with polyradiculoneuritis. Zh Nevropatol Psikhiatr Im S S Korsakova. 1988;88:61–4.

Raskin A, Genshon S, Crook TH, Sathananthan G, Ferris S. Effects of hyperbaric and normobaric oxygen on cognitive impairment in the elderly. Arch Gen Psychiatry. 1978;35:50–6.

Rossignol DA, Rossignol LW. Hyperbaric oxygen therapy may improve symptoms in autistic children. Med Hypotheses. 2006;67:216–28.

Schmitz G. Cognitive function: a review of the problems of research on senility. In: Davis JC, Hunt TK, editors. Hyperbaric oxygen therapy. Bethesda: Undersea Medical Society; 1977. p. 329–41.

Schmitz G. Evaluation of hyperbaric oxygen therapy for senility. HBO Rev. 1981;2:231.

Sokoloff L. Cerebral circulation and metabolic changes associated with aging. Assoc Res Nerv Ment Dis. 1966;41:237–54.

Thomas JR, Burch LS, Brandvard RA. Interaction of hyperbaric nitrogen and oxygen effects on behavior. Aviat Space Environ Med. 1976;47:965–8.

Zhao BS, Meng LX, Ding YY, Cao YY. Hyperbaric oxygen treatment produces an antinociceptive response phase and inhibits astrocyte activation and inflammatory response in a rat model of neuropathic pain. J Mol Neurosci. 2014;53:251–61.

Zhao BS, Song XR, Hu PY, Meng LX, Tan YH, She YJ, et al. Hyperbaric oxygen treatment at various stages following chronic constriction injury produces different antinociceptive effects via regulation of P2X4R expression and apoptosis. PLoS One. 2015;10, e0120122.

K.K. Jain

Abstract

Hyperbaric oxygen (HBO) has been found to be useful in the management of myocardial ischemia, as an adjunct to cardiac surgery, and for improving the walking distance in ischemic limb pain. The role of HBO in various cardiovascular disorders is described. Experimental studies as well as clinical experience are reviewed. HBO can be used for the emergency management of cardiogenic shock. A rational basis is provided for the effectiveness of HBO.

Keywords

Acute coronary syndrome • Cardiac surgery • Cardioprotection • HBO and cardiology • HBO as adjunct to exercise therapy • HBO in shock • Heart failure • Hyperbaric oxygen (HBO) • Myocardial infarction • Myocardial ischemia • Neuroprotection • Peripheral vascular disease (PVD) • Peripheral vascular surgery

Introduction

Normobaric oxygen (NBO) therapy has been in use for many years in the management of ischemic heart disease (Jain 1989). It is well known that cardiovascular diseases are the leading cause of death in Western countries, causing, for example, about one million deaths every year in the USA (half of the deaths due to all causes). About half of the deaths from cardiovascular diseases are due to coronary artery disease. This chapter deals with the role of HBO in treating cardiovascular disorders. Some aspects of the pathogenesis of cardiovascular disease relevant to HBO will also be mentioned briefly. Some of the pioneer work in this area was done in Russia and several Russian studies are cited in this chapter.

Pathophysiology

Risk Factors

The important risk factors for the cardiovascular diseases are arteriosclerosis, hypertension, hypercholesterolemia, diabetes, and smoking.

Hypoxia, Hyperoxia, and Atherosclerosis

The major factor in coronary artery stenosis and occlusion is atherosclerosis. Hypoxia is a cause of atherosclerosis. Experimental studies have shown an enhancing effect of hypoxia (achieved by inhalation of low-percentage oxygen) on the development of aortic atherosclerosis in cholesterol-fed rabbits and reversal of this with the application of HBO. This occurs by direct action on the vessel wall and not by changes in the blood lipid concentration. Inhibition of diet-induced atherosclerosis in New Zealand White rabbits by HBO treatment is accompanied by a significant reduction of autoantibodies against oxidatively modified LDL

K.K. Jain, MD, FRACS, FFPM (✉)
1 Blaesiring 7, Basel 4057, Switzerland
e-mail: jain@pharmabiotech.ch

cholesterol and profound changes in the redox state of the liver and aortic tissues (Kudchodkar et al. 2007). This anti-oxidant response may be the key to the anti-atherogenic effect of HBO treatment.

Stillman (1983) carried out experiments on rabbits to assess the effects of changes in the inspired oxygen concentration on intimal healing. The aorta was stripped and the animals were kept in various NBO concentrations (14–40%) for up to 10 days. After 6 months nearly all the animals showed normal healing, but the progress of healing was different. Hypoxia appeared to cause more platelet adhesions, exaggerated media proliferation, and aberrant migration. This finding explains the unfavorable results of surgery if there is hypoxia. Formation of platelet mass on the surface of the intima of the traumatized vessel will cause local hypoxia that affects the cells beneath the thrombus. Intimal hyperplasia at the site of vascular anastomosis is suppressed by steroids. HBO also has an immunosuppressive effect, and this may lead to a more orderly intimization.

There are two distinct oxygen-sensitive mechanisms in peripheral arteries, both of which regulate vascular tone. One mechanism is activated at high pO_2 values (10–40%), and vasoconstriction induced by this mechanism is mediated by vascular prostaglandin synthesis. The other comes into effect at low pO_2 levels and is related to limitation of oxidative energy metabolism.

In addition to relieving the effects of tissue anoxia, attention has been directed to the pathogenesis and possible reversal of atherosclerotic lesions. Hypoxia induced by CO is an accepted risk factor in atherogenesis. It seemed likely that the reverse process, hyperoxia induced by HBO, may be of benefit in animals with induced atherosclerosis.

Alpha-tocopherol (vitamin E) decreases systemic oxidant stress. Concentration of free cholesterol in rabbits with experimentally induced hypercholesteremia has been shown to be reduced one and a half times by a combination of HBO and alpha-tocopherol effect.

Hyperbaric Oxygenation in Cardiology

Effect of Hypoxia, Hyperoxia, and Hyperbaric Environments on Cardiovascular Function

Schraibman and Ledingham (1969) investigated the effect of hypoxia and hyperoxia on the left chamber systole and contractility of the heart in 20 young healthy male volunteers. ECG, carotid sphygmogram, phonocardiogram, and acceleration ballistocardiogram techniques were used to record the changes. The authors concluded that acute hypoxia (8% oxygen) augments contractility, probably through an adrenergic mechanism. Under the influence of hyperoxygenation

(100% oxygen), a vagotonic effect was observed. Both direct and indirect mechanisms are involved in these changes.

Experimental studies on cardiovascular changes in anesthetized dogs under hyperbaric conditions show that breathing air at 3 ATA has little effect on the physiological parameters, whereas breathing oxygen at 3 ATA depresses the heart rate and diminished the iliac blood flow as determined by the Doppler flowmeter. There is little effect on mean blood pressure. Breathing air at 5 ATA increases the blood pressure in all the animals and diminished the iliac artery flow as well as the heart rate.

With exercise under hyperoxia, the peripheral vasoconstriction does not seem to play a role, as increased blood flow is required for the skeletal muscles. Exercise heart rate is markedly depressed in hyperbaric environments. This is due to the effect of raised oxygen partial pressure on the heart, both directly and also via parasympathetic stimulation of the heart. The cardiodepressive influences may be of importance in limiting the tolerance for heavy exercise in hyperbaric environments, particularly with normoxia. Review of the literature on hyperoxia and human performance does not provide evidence of difference in cardiac output during heavy exercise under HBO, although there are reports of elevations of mean blood pressure (BP) and reduction of heart rate during exercise under hyperoxia.

Studies of the effects of hypoxia as well as hyperoxia on healthy male volunteers in hypobaric as well as in a hyperbaric chambers show that there is a decrease of minute cardiac force while breathing 100% oxygen at 1, 2, and 3 ATA due to decrease of heart rate and systolic force. In hypoxia there is an increase in minute cardiac force mainly due to an increase of heart rate. Further studies of the hemodynamic effects of oxygen at 2 ATA on healthy human subjects breathing 100% oxygen at rest show a 10% fall in cardiac index (mostly due to fall of heart rate). There is a 15% increase in systolic vascular resistance and an 8% decrease in left ventricular work. There is also a 3% rise in the mean arterial pressure.

The effect of 100% oxygen on the cardiovascular response to vasoactive compounds in the dog demonstrates a significant increase in the mean arterial pressure responsiveness to both angiotensin I and II. The control dogs breathing ambient air show no significant changes for any of the compounds tested. These data indicate that hyperoxia augments the renin-angiotensin system's ability to influence cardiovascular function.

Metabolic Effects of HBO on the Heart

Mitochondrial respiratory rate is an essential component of myocardial function because it influences production of adenosine triphosphate (ATP) during oxidative phosphorylation.

Mitochondrial phosphorylation depends upon oxygen tension. This is the key to understanding the pathophysiological processes that appear in the heart, such has hypoxia, ischemia, and the changes in the oxygen-carrying capacity. Cardiac energy metabolism depends on the oxygen-carrying capacity of the blood. Oxygen supply becomes a limiting factor of mitochondrial respiratory rate in the absence of hemoglobin in the perfusate. The use of reconstituted blood allows normal arterial oxygen pressure and enables the maintenance of the physiological capacity of the cardiac energy metabolism. It may be possible to obtain the same effect using HBO instead of blood. HBO at 3 ATA decreases the hemoglobin concentration of pigs to <1.0 % but results in no ECG evidence of myocardial anoxia (Boerema et al. 1959).

Miroshnichenko et al. (1983) studied the effect of guanine nucleotides and HBO on cardiac adenine cyclase activity in rabbits with myocardial hypertrophy. They believe that this hypertrophy is the result of the reduction of sensitivity of the adenylate cyclase system to hormonal action. This disturbance is normalized by HBO. Under HBO, guanine nucleotides participate in both the desensitization of adenosine cyclase to hormonal action and resensitization of this during HBO.

The metabolic effects of HBO in patients with acute cardiac insufficiency are not secondary to changes of systemic circulation, but precede them due to direct action of hyperoxia on metabolic processes in the peripheral tissues. Moreover, improvement of regional blood flow and metabolism of peripheral tissues by HBO also exerts a beneficial effect on the systemic circulation, thus breaking the vicious circle: circulatory hypoxia → myocardial hypoxia → circulatory hypoxia. These findings are confirmed by a decrease of both lactate level and metabolic acidosis, with an unchanged cardiac output. Further improvement in the hemodynamics of these patients is conditioned by a mechanism of compensation, including myocardial hypofunction, with removal of peripheral oxygen debt.

Role of HBO in Experimental Myocardial Infarction

Various studies of the effect of HBO on experimental myocardial infarction are shown in Table 25.1, which is reproduced from previous editions of the book. A more recent study evaluated the effect of a single session of HBO on the size of risk, ischemic, and necrotic zones in the rat model of MI produced by irreversible occlusion of the coronary artery (Dotsenko et al. 2015). The size of the risk, ischemic, and necrotic zones were evaluated. HBO (60-min session) was performed 3 h after artery occlusion at excessive oxygen pressure of 0.02 and 0.1 MPa. In rats not exposed to HBO, the risk zone median was 31.7 % of the left ventricle weight,

while after the session it did not exceed 25 %. In spontaneous course of MI, the ischemia to necrosis zone ratio was 1.7:1, while under conditions of HBO at oxygen pressure of 0.1 and 0.02 MPa, these values were 0.6:1 and 2:1, respectively. Excessive oxygen pressure of 0.02 mPa (2 ATA) was considered to be better than traditionally used 0.1 MPa, because it promotes redistribution of the ischemic and necrotic areas in the risk zone: the area of necrotic zone decreased at the expense of the ischemic zone. It was concluded that HBO produces a positive effect on the myocardium under conditions of total occlusion of the coronary artery.

Literature cited gives a somewhat favorable view concerning the role of HBO in MI; other reports have been published that indicate no beneficial effect of HBO. This conflict can be resolved by analysis of the volume of tissue necrotized by vascular occlusion. This is considered in relation to the radius of the tissue supplied by the vessel before the occlusion. The volume of necrosis increases rapidly, as the cube of the original radius. The volume of tissue saved by breathing 100 % oxygen at 3 ATA increases more slowly, as the square of the original radius. The percentage of the tissue thus saved varies according to the reciprocal of the original radius. Any phenomenon that produces multiple small infarcts will respond more favorably to HBO therapy than one large area of necrosis. This might possibly explain the variations in the results of different experiments where different sizes of infarcts were produced in different species of animals. In a clinical situation, it can be predicted that HBO is more likely to be beneficial in a small vessel embolus, or in a thrombosis with multiple small infarcts, than in a single massive infarct.

Animal studies show that combination of thrombolytic therapy and HBO would be more effective in reducing the size of MI than either of these modalities alone. These studies provide encouraging evidence for the validity of the hypothesis that both of these methods have a synergistic effect.

Clinical Applications of HBO in Cardiology

Acute Myocardial Infarction

The term acute coronary syndrome (ACS) includes acute myocardial infarction (MI) and unstable angina. Stable angina pectoris is a manifestation of chronic ischemic heart disease and is dealt with under that section.

Clinical Features and Principles of Management
MI is one of the most common diagnoses in hospitalized patients in developed countries. Characteristic features are chest pain, ECG abnormalities, and enzyme changes.

Table 25.1 Experimental studies of the effect of HBO in myocardial infarction

Authors and year	Experimental model	Results	Conclusions or comments
Smith and Lawson (1958)	Ligation of anterior descending coronary artery	Mortality in dogs breathing O_2 at 2 ATA was 10 % compared with 50–60 % mortality of dogs breathing air	HBO may reduce the mortality by protecting from ventricular fibrillation following myocardial infarction
Chardack et al. (1964) Trapp and Creighton (1964)	Coronary artery ligation	Reduction of infarct size and reduction of ventricular fibrillation in HBO-treated animals	
Kline et al. (1979)	Infarction	Excess lactate associated with ischemia disappeared with 100 % oxygen at 3 ATA. Animals breathing room air continued to produce excess lactate	Return to oxidative (aerobic) metabolism with HBO and reduction of myocardial ischemia
Kleep (1977)	Occlusion of the circumflex branch of the left coronary artery in sheep	Mortality of this procedure greatly reduced	
Demurov et al. (1981)	Left coronary artery ligation in rabbits	HBO at 2 ATA for 1 H starting 30 min after occlusion	Partial restoration of myocardial contractility Improvement of energy metabolism of the heart Decrease of cAMP in ischemic areas Increase of guanosine monophosphate in intact areas
Efuni et al. (1984)	Experimental myocardial infarction in rabbits	Combined use of HBO and antioxidants	Improvement of cardiac function
Thomas et al. (1990)	Dogs. Occlusion of left anterior descending coronary artery for 2 h. Myocardial injury was measured by histochemical staining	Four groups: (i) control, no treatment, (ii) HBO 2 ATA for 90 min, (iii) rtPA only, and (iv) HBO + rtPA simultaneously	Although HBO and recombinant tissue plasminogen activator (rtPA) caused 35.9 % and 48.9 % restoration of enzyme activity, maximal effect was obtained by combining both which reduces the extent of infarction
Sterling et al. (1993)	Open-chest rabbit model of myocardial ischemia. A branch of left coronary artery was occluded for 30 min followed by 3 h of reperfusion. Infarction measured by triphenyl tetrazolium staining	Control group ventilated with 100 % oxygen at 1 ATA. Treated animals with HBO at 2 ATA	Animals exposed to HBO had smaller infarcts than controls. HBO given after 30 min of reperfusion had no protective effect
Kim et al. (2001)	Rats were intermittently exposed to 100 % O_2 at 3 ATA for 1 h daily and then sacrificed after 24 h of recovery in room air. Isolated hearts were subjected to 40 min of ischemia and 90 min of reperfusion	HBO pretreatment enhanced enzymatic activity and gene expression of catalase, thereby significantly reducing infarct size after reperfusion	HBO preconditioning may be developed as a new preventive measure for reperfusion injury in the heart
Spears et al. (2002)	60-min balloon occlusion of the left anterior descending coronary artery in swine. Control groups consisted of autoreperfusion alone	Intracoronary aqueous oxygen (AO) hyperoxemic perfusion for 90 min. Significant improvement in left ventricular ejection fraction at 105 min of reperfusion	Intracoronary hyperbaric reperfusion with AO attenuates myocardial ischemia/reperfusion injury
Xuejun et al. (2008)	Rats with occlusion of the left anterior descending coronary artery. HBO pretreatment at 2.5 ATA for 60 min, twice daily for 2 days followed by 12 h of recovery in room air prior to the myocardial ischemic insult	The infarct size of the HBO group was smaller than that of the control normoxic group. Capillary density, VEGF levels, and cell proliferation higher in HBO group	HBO pretreatment accelerates angiogenesis and alleviates myocardial ischemia

Approximately 1.5 million myocardial infarctions occur each year in the USA. The mortality rate in acute infarction is about 30 % with half of these occurring before the stricken individual can reach the hospital. Death usually occurs due to ventricular fibrillation. Silent myocardial infarctions may occur in 20–40 % of cases who later develop clinically manifest MI.

Diagnostic procedures are treadmill stress testing, biomarkers, cardiac imaging, thallium 201 scintigraphy, radionuclide angiography, echocardiography, and ambulatory ECG monitoring (Holter). Different cardiac biomarkers have been used to evaluate patients with suspected acute MI. The cardiac-specific troponins I and T, creatine kinase (CK), MB isoenzyme of CK (CK-MB), and myoglobin have been used as surrogates for myocardial infarction.

Biomarkers and ECG are the most important tool in the initial evaluation and triage of patients in whom an acute myocardial infarction is suspected. Multidetector computed tomography (MDCT) coronary angiography should be considered as an alternative to invasive angiography to exclude coronary artery occlusion, when there is a low to intermediate likelihood of coronary artery disease and when cardiac troponin and/or ECG results are inconclusive. The use of myocardial perfusion imaging (MPI) with SPECT or PET scanning in the emergency department for low-risk patients has a low yield for detecting ischemia.

The goal for the management of patients with suspected MI is rapid identification of patients who are candidates for reperfusion therapy. Current measures employed for reperfusion are intravenous thrombolytics, angioplasty (balloon or laser), and medications. Commonly used thrombolytic is tissue plasminogen activator (tPA). Other approved thrombolytics are streptokinase (STK) and anisoylated plasminogen STK activator complex. The main goal is prompt restoration of patency of the occluded coronary artery to stop the life-threatening tachyarrhythmias. Thrombolytic therapy can reduce the inhospital death by 50 % when administered within the first hour of onset of symptoms of MI. Primary percutaneous transluminal coronary angioplasty (PTCA) is used in patients where prior angiography shows areas of narrowing or those with cardiogenic shock where immediate opening of the occluded artery is required. Pharmacologic measures are intravenous lidocaine for correction of ventricular tachyarrhythmia and potassium to correct auricular fibrillation. Other drugs used are aspirin, beta-blocker, and angiotensin-converting enzyme inhibitors. There is evidence that these agents reduce mortality. Calcium channel blockers are given to reduce the size of the infarct but results of clinical trials failed to establish this. Supplemental oxygen inhalation is given quite frequently to patients with MI. The extent of the infarct size is the major determinant of prognosis in MI. A reduction of infarct size is the major therapeutic goal.

Normobaric Oxygen in Myocardial Infarction

Arterial desaturation and hypoxemia following acute myocardial infarction has been documented for years and is worse in patients with heart failure. Traditionally inhalation of NBO has been used, and oxygen concentrations below 50 % are used for inhalation to counteract hypoxia, but some cardiologists recommend 100 % oxygen inhalation. Decision to give oxygen can be made on the basis of pulse oximetry which measures oxygen saturation reliably. Here one is talking about correction of general hypoxia which affects other organs. The issue is focal hypoxia in the myocardium where systemic oxygen cannot diffuse easily because of vascular occlusion. It is unlikely that this method of oxygen administration can counteract myocardial hypoxia in the face of vascular occlusion. Therefore, the use of HBO in the management of patients with acute myocardial infarction has been investigated.

Role of HBO in Myocardial Infarction

Since there are localized areas of lack of oxygen in MI, there is a rationale for reperfusion of these areas with high concentrations of oxygen. Cameron et al. (1966) investigated the hemodynamic and metabolic effects of HBO in 10 patients with acute myocardial infarction who breathed air, oxygen at atmospheric pressure, or oxygen at 2 ATA. Under HBO, systemic vascular resistance rose progressively, accompanied by some reduction in cardiac output and stroke volume, with little change in heart rate. In patients with raised lactic acid levels, there was a reduction of this parameter with HBO. The authors felt that HBO therapy may turn out to be of most value to patients with severe hypoxia, hypotension, and metabolic acidosis who have responded poorly to conventional therapy.

Thurston et al. (1973) carried out the first randomized controlled investigation into the effects of HBO on mortality following recent MI in 103 patients and in 105 controls treated by conventional methods in the same coronary care unit in London, England. Seventeen (16.5 %) of the patients in the HBO group died, compared with 24 (22.9 %) in the control group. Detailed analysis revealed that mortality in high-risk patients may be reduced by half by means of HBO. The only patients who survived cardiogenic shock were in the HBO group. The incidence of arrhythmias was lower in the HBO group and some of those were shown to disappear with HBO. The authors felt that the evidence in favor of HBO in the treatment of myocardial infarction was sufficiently strong to justify its use in selected patients where the facilities were available.

Efuni et al. (1984) used HBO in combined therapy of acute myocardial infarction in 30 patients. Pressure of 1.5–2 ATA was used for 60–90 min and the treatment course consisted of 5–6 sessions. All patients had acute myocardial infarction of the left ventricle with predominant damage of the anterior wall and duration of affliction ranging from 12 to

48 h. Patients with initial arterial hypoxemia ($n = 16$) showed a proven increase in arterial pO_2 from 64 ± 7 mmHg to 82 ± 5 mmHg following the first session and 86 ± 4 mmHg at the end of the course. Cardiac output and stroke volume tended to increase, the former mainly at the expense of the latter. Simultaneously there was a decrease in lactate to pyruvate ratio with fall of metabolic acidosis. The authors recommend HBO treatment in myocardial ischemia complicated by arterial hypoxemia. SPECT and thallium exercise scintigraphy have been used to document the improvement in patients following myocardial infarction treated with HBO.

A systematic review of controlled clinical trials of HBO in ACS concluded that there is some evidence from small trials to suggest that HBO is associated with a reduction in the risk of death, the volume of damaged muscle, the risk of major adverse cardiac events, and time to relief from ischemic pain (Bennett et al. 2015). The authors cautioned that, in view of the modest number of patients, methodological shortcomings, and poor reporting, this result should be interpreted cautiously, and an appropriately powered trial of high methodological rigor is justified to define those patients who can be expected to derive most benefit from HBO. The routine application of HBO to these patients cannot be justified from this review.

Combination of HBO and Thrombolysis

HBO in combination with thrombolysis has been demonstrated to salvage myocardium in acute myocardial infarction in the animal model. Therefore, a randomized pilot trial was undertaken to assess the safety and feasibility of this treatment in human beings (Shandling et al. 1997). Patients with an acute MI who received recombinant tissue plasminogen activator (rtPA) were randomized to treatment with HBO combined with rtPA or rtPA alone. Sixty-six patients were included for analysis. Forty-three patients had inferior acute MIs and the remainder had anterior acute MIs. The mean creatine phosphokinase level at 12 and 24 h was reduced in the patients given HBO by approximately 35 % ($p = 0.03$). Time to pain relief and ST segment resolution was shorter in the group given HBO. There were two deaths in the control group and none in those treated with HBO. The ejection fraction on discharge was 52.4 % in the group given HBO compared with 47.3 % in the control group (difference not significant). The authors concluded that adjunctive treatment with HBO appears to be a feasible and safe treatment for acute MI and may result in an attenuated rise in creatine phosphokinase levels and more rapid resolution of pain and ST segment changes.

A randomized multicenter trial was conducted to further assess the safety and feasibility of this treatment in human subjects (Stravinsky et al. 1998). Patients with acute MI treated with rtPA or STK were randomized to treatment with HBO combined with either rtPA or STK, or rtPA or STK alone. Results indicate that treatment with HBO in combination with thrombolysis appears to be feasible and safe for patients with AMI and may result in an attenuated CPK rise, more rapid resolution of pain, and improved ejection fractions. More studies are needed to assess the benefits of this treatment.

Chronic Ischemic Heart Disease (Angina Pectoris)

Ischemia here refers to lack of oxygen due to inadequate perfusion, which results from an imbalance between oxygen supply and demand. The most common cause of myocardial ischemia is atherosclerotic disease of the coronary arteries. Coronary artery disease is the most common, serious, chronic, life-threatening illness in the USA where there are about 11 million sufferers. Angina pectoris is due to transient myocardial ischemia. Management of ischemic heart disease starts with preventive measures such as lowering of cholesterol and treatment of hypertension. Several vasodilators are used for the treatment of angina pectoris of which nitrates are the best known. Other agents are beta-blockers and calcium channel blockers.

Smetnev et al. (1979) treated 77 patients with chronic ischemic heart disease using HBO. Fifty-two of these had angina pectoris and 25 had multifocal postinfarction cardiosclerosis with insufficiency of systemic or pulmonary circulation. HBO in combination with drug therapy alleviated or arrested the symptoms of angina and corrected the central hemodynamics in other patients.

Kuleshova et al. (1981) discussed the rehabilitation phase of 233 patients with ischemic heart disease. All patients received physical therapy, autogenic training, massage, and therapeutic walking exercises. Group I ($n = 179$) received HBO while group II ($n = 54$) served as controls. HBO treatment was started on the 5th–10th day of admission with exposure to 1.5–2 ATA for 60 min daily. There was improvement of the general condition with relief of angina pectoris. Therefore, the rehabilitation measures in group I could be applied more intensively. There was clearance of arrhythmias in 72 % of the patients in group I. Loading tests at the time of discharge from the hospital revealed that patients in group I adapted better to physical load. The range of activities in group II was limited. Therefore, physical rehabilitation with HBO enhances the functional compensatory possibilities in cardiovascular disease. Efuni et al. (1984) conducted an isometric test prior to and after HBO sessions in 31 patients with chronic myocardial ischemia. It was shown that the isometric test could assess the HBO effect objectively in this situation. There was reduction in the severity of angina pectoris after HBO. Goliakov et al. (1986b) studied the effect of HBO on thromboelastogram, platelet aggregation, and prothrombin index in 40 patients with angina pectoris. There was a decrease of fibrinogen and fibrinogen degradation products, and adequate clinical effectiveness was seen in 84 % of the patients.

The effect of HBO in reducing platelet aggregation and the serum fibrinogen content was shown to produce a favorable effect in 84 % of the 40 patients with angina pectoris (Goliakov et al. 1986a).

Cardiac Arrhythmias

Moderate sinus bradycardia is a common physiological response to HBO. This is due to marked increase in parasympathetic tone while breathing 100 % oxygen at 2.5 ATA. This level of HBO does not cause any cardiac arrhythmias. During the treatment of acute myocardial infarction with HBO, various observers have noted an improvement of arrhythmias.

Allaria et al. (1973) used HBO in a young patient with ECG abnormalities resulting from electrocution. The abnormalities cleared up. Zhivoderov et al. (1980) noted disorders of rhythm and conductivity in 85 % of 75 patients with myocardial infarction after the 15th day following the onset of the disease. HBO was used in 14 patients, and in 11 of these arrhythmias disappeared after 10–12 exposures. Isakov et al. (1981) used HBO in 31 patients with paroxysmal tachyarrhythmias in ischemic heart disease and concluded that the number and duration of paroxysms were reduced and that long-term remissions occurred. HBO also reduced the number of extrasystoles. Zhivoderov et al. (1982) applied HBO to 29 patients with ischemic heart disease (68.9 %). In 17 patients there was disappearance of extrasystoles, which allowed the physical activity of the patients to be increased. There was no change in the acid–base balance resulting from the HBO treatment. Among other 28 patients where HBO was used along with antiarrhythmic drugs, improvement was seen in 21 cases (77.8 %).

Goliakov et al. (1986b) showed that there was improvement of ventricular extrasystoles in 67 % of the coronary disease patients treated by HBO therapy. There was no change in 17 % of the patients, and in 16 % the arrhythmias increased.

Heart Failure

Acute myocardial infarction is a major contributing factor to heart failure, a chronic condition that is expected to increase in incidence along with increased life expectancy and an overall aging population. HBO has been shown to induce the production of heat shock proteins (HSPs) with a resultant protective effect. By augmenting the induction of endogenous HSPs, HBO may serve to repair and improve the function of failing hearts that have been damaged by myocardial infarction.

Cardiac Resuscitation

Effect of HBO at 2 ATA on myocardial contractility during cardiac resuscitation applying external counter pulsation has been studied in dogs. Myocardial contractility is not affected, but cardiac output and carotid blood flow are increased significantly. There is a rise of arterial pAO_2 as well. HBO has potential applications during human cardiac resuscitation.

HBO as an Adjunct to Cardiac Surgery

Experimental Studies

Boerema (1961) was the first to report the use of a hyperbaric chamber in performing cardiac surgery. HBO is indicated in palliative cardiac surgery for high-risk cases. The advantages are as follows:

- Hypoxia or hypoxic bradycardia, which occurs easily during compression of the lungs or impairment of the circulation, is much less severe.
- When flow is restored following inflow occlusion, optimal oxygenation is reached more rapidly because the low cardiac output phase is shorter.
- Cardiac resuscitation, when necessary during surgery, is markedly facilitated. Even when ventricular fibrillation occurs, defibrillation is very easy.

Bockeria and Zelenkini (1973) studied ECG changes in "dry" hearts of dogs under HBO and found that the best myocardial protection was achieved at 3.5 ATA for 60 min. Longer periods of HBO lead to oxygen intoxication. Preservation of the isolated heart for transplantation has been investigated by Todo et al. (1974). Isolated canine hearts preserved by hypothermia and HBO at 3 ATA, as well as addition of magnesium as a metabolic inhibitor, showed no significant abnormality after 18–36 h.

Kawamura et al. (1976) investigated the protective effect of HBO immediately after removal of an occluding ligation of a coronary artery in the dog. One group of dogs breathed room air and served as controls, while the other group breathed 100 % oxygen at 2 ATA before and after the release of the coronary ligature. In the HBO group, the ischemic area was markedly reduced after reinstatement of the coronary blood flow. These dogs also had more stable hemodynamic conditions during operation, and ventricular fibrillation was suppressed. The authors considered HBO a useful aid in the reconstruction of the acutely occluded coronary arteries. Richards et al. (1963) investigated the role of HBO and hypothermia for suspended animation as an aid to open-heart surgery. Anesthetized dogs were observed in a refrigerated hyperbaric chamber at 3 ATA. The authors concluded that the dogs could survive total circulatory arrest of up to 1 h with no gross evidence of central nervous system or myocardial damage. Accompanying acid–base disturbances were transient and reversible.

Ischemia–reperfusion injury (IRI) occurs frequently in revascularization procedures such as coronary artery bypass graft (CABG). Conditioning of myocardial cells to an oxidative stress prior to IRI may limit the consequences of this injury. Preconditioning (PC) the myocardium with HBO before reperfusion has been shown to have a myocardial protective effect by limiting the infarct size post ischemia and reperfusion. HBO preconditioning may partly attenuate IRI by stimulating the endogenous production of nitric oxide (NO), which has the ability to reduce neutrophil sequestration, adhesion, and associated injury and to improve blood flow (Yogaratnam et al. 2008). HBO preconditioning induced NO may play a role in providing myocardial protection during operations that involve an inevitable episode of IRI and protection of the myocardium from the effects of IRI during cardiac surgery.

Human Cardiac Surgery

Burakovsky and Bockeria (1977) reported on the resuscitative value of HBO in cardiac surgery. Deliveries have been conducted on women with cardiac disease in a hyperbaric chamber without any complications.

Bockeria et al. (1977) described extracorporeal circulation under HBO. They performed 43 operations for conditions such as atrial and ventricular septal defects and Fallot's tetralogy. During perfusion, hemodynamic and biochemical indices were quite satisfactory. At 3 ATA, performance of perfusions was possible without donor blood for the priming machine. The main danger of HBO was air emboli in the perfusate during decompression.

Bockeria et al. (1978) analyzed changes in the total activity of lactic dehydrogenase (LDH), aspartic aminotransferase, and the isoenzyme spectrum of LDH in the plasma of patients with congenital heart defects. Some were operated on under HBO; others under normobaric conditions. The elevations of these enzymes as a result of trauma to the myocardium were less pronounced under HBO.

Gadzhiev (1979) investigated the dynamics of venous pressure in 80 patients during open-heart surgery, where the heart was disconnected from the circulation (dry heart) using HBO. After occlusion of the vena cava, the blood was drained and subsequently autotransfused. HBO prevented disorders of the central nervous system in the intraoperative period. Burakovsky et al. (1981) reported their experience of operations on the heart under conditions of HBO in 170 operations. HBO of 3–3.5 ATA allowed perfusion with hemodilution of 45–55 %. Induced diuresis rapidly restored the oxygen capacity of the blood and prevented hypoxic complications in the postoperative period. The regimen of HBO for surgical treatment of patients with heart disease was based on experiments on dogs. The appropriate value of HBO for each individual patient was calculated beforehand and controlled during the surgery. Pressure of 3.5 ATA was usually found to be optimal and the period of saturation was usually 30 min. Prolongation of this period was not accompanied by an increase of blood gas parameters. HBO was found to be a highly effective method of correction of gas metabolism problems in chronic arterial hypoxemia. Drawbacks of the method include the possibility of the development of acid–base equilibrium disturbances (hyperbaric acidosis) during long periods of saturation. Trisaminol was found to be the best drug for correction of this imbalance. Friehs et al. (1977) performed 28 operations on congenital heart disease patients in a hyperbaric operating room at the University Clinic, Graz, Austria, and found this technique to be useful in:

- Heart operations like vascular ring, aortopulmonary shunt, and aortic isthmus stenosis with few collaterals
- High-risk operations on patients with coronary insufficiency
- Operations where blood transfusion is not permitted
- Operations with hypothermia and induced circulatory arrest: aortic or pulmonary valvotomy and atrioseptectomy

In open-heart surgery in adult humans, up to 1 L of blood is often withdrawn from the inferior vena cava just before the institution of extracorporeal circulation. Hemoglobin is reduced to one-third of normal values and yet there is no sign of anoxia. Such a hemodilution can be performed safely only under HBO. Most of the hearts resume beating spontaneously at the conclusion of the operation. This shows that blood can be highly diluted with no deleterious effect on the patient. Retransfusion of the withdrawn blood after surgery has the following advantages:

- Blood coagulation is hastened and postoperative oozing from the wound is reduced.
- Because of hemodilution, the internal organs are well perfused and microcirculation is improved.
- The perfusion rate can be reduced to 40–50 mL/kg/min. This reduces the damage to the blood cells during the period of extracorporeal circulation.

The advantages of HBO as an adjunct to cardiac surgery can be summarized as follows:

- HBO increases the safe time of induced cardiac arrest under normothermia.
- HBO reduces the impact of hypoxic complications and metabolic disturbances associated with cardiac surgery.
- HBO enables surgery to be performed without blood transfusion in some cases.
- HBO is the treatment of choice for air embolism as a complication of cardiac surgery.
- HBO has been found to be useful for the treatment of low cardiac output syndrome developing after cardiac surgery and associated with pulmonary hypertension.
- Pretreatment with HBO can reduce neuropsychometric dysfunction and also modulate the inflammatory response after cardiopulmonary bypass surgery. However, further multicenter randomized trials are needed to clinically evaluate this form of therapy.

Protective Effect of HBO Preconditioning in Cardiac Surgery

Accumulated data shows the benefits offered by HBO therapy as an adjunct in the treatment of CABG patients. It has been shown that ischemia–reperfusion injury is deleterious to the myocardium, causing left ventricular dysfunction, structural damage to the myocytes and endothelial cells, myocardial stunning, reperfusion arrhythmias, and potentially irreversible injury. There is substantial evidence pointing to the role of HBO in mitigating the harmful effects of ischemia–reperfusion injury. Animal experimental studies have shown that HBO preconditioning increases expression of HO-1, which is suppressed by PI3K inhibitor LY294002, Nrf2 knockout, and Akt inhibitor triciribine (Yin et al. 2015). The expression of Nrf2 is enhanced by HBO preconditioning, but decreased by LY294002 and triciribine. The Akt is also activated by HBO preconditioning but suppressed by LY294002. These data show a novel signaling mechanism by which HBO preconditioning protects myocardium ischemia–reperfusion injury via PI3K/Akt/Nrf2-dependent antioxidant defensive system.

Primary endpoint of a randomized clinical study demonstrated that HBO preconditioning consisting of two 30-min intervals of 100% oxygen at 2.4 ATA prior to CABG surgery led to an improvement in left ventricular stroke work (LVSW) 24 h following CABG as compared to routine management. Results of the exploratory secondary endpoints from that study, specifically the effects of HBO preconditioning on biomarkers of myocardial protection, have been reported (Jeysen et al. 2011). Intraoperative right atrial biopsies were assessed, via an enzyme-linked immunosorbent assay (ELISA), for the expression of eNOS and HSP72. In this study, no significant differences were observed between the groups with respect to the quantity of myocardial eNOS and HSP72. However, in the HBO group, following ischemia and reperfusion, the quantities of myocardial eNOS and HSP72 were increased. This suggests that HBO preconditioning in this group of patients may be capable of inducing endogenous cardioprotection following IRI.

Evidence from a number of studies clearly points to both clinical and cost–benefit HBO when used to precondition non-emergency patients having on-pump CABG surgery (Allen et al. 2015). Study data show that adding adjunctive HBO into the plan of care leads to improved myocardial function, reduces length of stay in the ICU, and limits postsurgical complications. Further, it has only minimal impact on the presurgical preparation, i.e., time must be allowed for the hyperbaric treatment(s), and no role in the surgery or postsurgical care of the patient. The studies pointing to clinical and cost–benefit of preconditioning have been conducted outside the USA. Given the pressure on costs in all areas of health care, it seems that a therapeutic approach, which has been shown to be of benefit in both animal and human trials over the course of many years, should attract funding for a properly structured study designed to test whether significant and simultaneous improvements in clinical outcomes and cost reductions can be achieved within the framework of a US healthcare facility.

CNS Complications of Cardiac Surgery

HBO has a potential role in the management of CNS complications of cardiovascular surgery. Some of the neurological complications of CABG are:

- Stroke: cerebral infarction
- Periventricular leukomalacia resulting in spastic diplegia
- Central retinal artery occlusion resulting in unilateral, painless visual loss
- Spinal cord infarction resulting in paraplegia

A prospective, randomized, single-blinded study, including patients scheduled for CABG surgery between 2007 and 2009, evaluated the cerebral and myocardial protective effects of HBO preconditioning (PC) in both on-pump and off-pump surgery (Li et al. 2011). Patients in the HBO groups underwent preconditioning for 5 days before surgery. On-pump CABG surgery patients preconditioned with HBO had significant decreases in S100B protein, neuron-specific enolase, and troponin I perioperative serum levels compared with the on-pump control group. Postsurgically, patients in the on-pump HBO group had a reduced length of stay in the intensive care unit and a decreased use of inotropic drugs. Serum catalase activity 24 h postoperatively was significantly increased compared with the on-pump control group. In the off-pump groups, there was no difference in any of the same parameters. It was concluded that preconditioning with HBO resulted in both cerebral and cardiac protective effects as determined by biomarkers of neuronal and myocardial injury and clinical outcomes in patients undergoing on-pump CABG surgery.

Spinal cord ischemia remains one of the most feared complications in patients undergoing thoracic endovascular aortic repair. These patients often suffer irreversible paraplegia with lifelong consequences with physical and psychological distress. Patients who develop postoperative spinal cord ischemia following aortic repair can recover after immediate HBO therapy and therapeutic hypothermia.

During the past decade, improvements in techniques of cardiovascular surgery and increase in transvascular catheter approaches and stenting have reduced complications such as thromboembolism, and HBO no longer has a critical role, but hyperbaric chambers should still be available in cardiovascular surgical centers.

HBO in Preventive Cardiology

Prevention and Rehabilitation of Coronary Artery Disease

According to the animal research reports reviewed, atherosclerosis can be reversed with hyperoxia, but there are no clinical studies. It would be worthwhile to conduct a study on patients with angiographically proven coronary atherosclerosis, using HBO treatments on a long-term basis. This could also be combined with a rehabilitation program using HBO for chronic myocardial ischemia.

Physical Training of Patients with Chronic Myocardial Insufficiency

These patients should ideally be trained in a hyperbaric chamber fitted with an ergometer. The hypothesis is that exercise leads to an increase in oxygen demand and lowers the threshold for angina. HBO increases this threshold and provides a longer duration of exercise. Exercise augments the cerebral blood flow, and the interaction of improved mental function and improved physical health leads to a longer survival for these patients.

Conclusion and Comments

The role of hypoxia in the genesis of the consequences of coronary artery occlusion and myocardial infarction is well recognized. Oxygen therapy is generally accepted to be useful. The role of HBO in myocardial infarction is controversial: the bulk of animal experimental evidence favors the view that HBO has a beneficial effect in reducing the mortality and diminishing the size of the infarct. Among the clinical reports by Thurston et al. (1973) was a randomized double-blind study, which remains the most important to date. According to this study, HBO is beneficial in acute myocardial infarction. The effect of HBO in reducing or reversing cardiac arrhythmias is not so important, as many useful drugs are available for this purpose.

The use of HBO as an adjunct to cardiac surgery remains confined to a few countries, notably Russia, where most of the papers reviewed have been published. Hyperbaric operating rooms have not become popular in the USA, where the operative mortality figures for cardiac surgery without HBO are lower than those reported with HBO in other countries.

HBO in Shock

Pathophysiology of Shock

The common denominator in shock, regardless of cause, is a failure of the circulatory system to deliver the chemical substances necessary for cell survival and to remove the waste products of cellular metabolism. This leads to cellular membrane dysfunction, abnormal cellular metabolism, and eventually cellular death. Some major causes of shock are:

- Decreased intravascular volume: acute hemorrhage, excessive fluid loss, and vasodilatation (relative hypovolemia).
- Cardiac conditions: acute myocardial infarction, myocarditis, acute valvular insufficiency, arrhythmias, and mechanical compression or obstruction.
- Microvascular endothelial injury: burns and disseminated intravascular coagulation.
- Cellular membrane injury: septic shock and anaphylaxis.
- Cardiac output is diminished in most states of shock; oxygen availability is reduced, and generally stagnant hypoxia ensues.

Oxygen Delivery by Blood

Hypoxia may reduce the rate of ATP synthesis, but it does not cause significant damage to mitochondrial membranes unless it is severe, sustained, and accompanied by ischemia, which also reduces the availability of other substrates. The mechanism by which ischemia and endotoxins have their adverse effect on mitochondrial function is not known.

There is little evidence that the shock state, except perhaps in its terminal stages, is associated with inability of the tissues to handle oxygen. Oxygen consumption of tissue cells falls in shock and the duration of anoxia is a measure of oxygen debt. There is a relationship between the duration of oxygen debt and survival.

NBO can correct arterial desaturation, but in some situations HBO is required to achieve normal oxygen saturation and even hyperoxia is necessary to reduce mortality.

Traumatic and Hypovolemic Shock

Initial investigations of the effect of HBO in shock produced disappointing results. Subsequent experimental studies (Clark and Young 1965) showed that if HBO is administered during a period of hemorrhagic shock, the most striking observation is an elevation of arterial BP, which is due to a rise in peripheral arterial resistance rather than in cardiac output.

Myocardial zonal lesions are pathognomonic of hypovolemic shock. This is a unique form of myocyte injury, which probably results from a combination of altered hemodynamics and inotropic stimulation accompanying hypovolemic shock. These lesions may have a role in the development of cardiac failure and loss of ventricular contractility. These lesions respond to HBO and are potentially reversible.

Experimental and clinical investigations show a high degree of effectiveness of auxiliary perfusions in the treatment of traumatic shock. The use of HBO in the early postperfusion period increases the efficacy of resuscitative measures and stabilizes the good results achieved. Gross et al. (Gross et al. 1983a, b; 1984) produced hemorrhagic shock in animals and divided them into different groups, which were treated under varying conditions of pressure. One group received 100 % oxygen at 1 ATA and another group 100 % oxygen at 2.8 ATA. The only common factor in the treatment was that each animal received lactated Ringer's solution in one series and a mixture of 10 % dextrose and dextran 70 in another series. The authors found no significant differences in results with the addition of HBO in any of the groups.

HBO at 3 ATA improves metabolic disturbances associated with experimental shock in animals induced by third-degree burns. The use of HBO in conjunction with oxygen-carrier blood substitutes is more promising in hemorrhagic shock.

Cardiogenic Shock

Jacobson et al. (1964) induced cardiogenic shock in dog experiments by microsphere embolization of the coronary vessels. In the control animals, mean central aortic pressure fell by 71 %, cardiac output by 79 %, and heart rate by 57 %. With HBO at 3 ATA, mean central aortic pressure fell by only 28 %, cardiac output by 43 %, and heart rate by 10 % following embolization. Survival was significantly greater in dogs exposed to HBO at 3 ATA; 65 % of them were alive 24 h after myocardial infarction, compared with 23 % of the control animals (breathing air at atmospheric pressure). Scheidt et al. (1973) studied 73 patients with shock resulting from massive myocardial infarction, which they believed had evolved over a period of hours or sometimes even over a number of days. Based on the experimental evidence that infarcts can be prevented from extending by the use of various drugs and HBO, they recommended early intervention in patients with myocardial infarcts in order to prevent shock.

In patients with cardiogenic shock, those who have a low cardiac output and falling arterial pressure can benefit from circulatory support. Various measures for this, such as left ventricle bypass via an interventricular drainage cannula, are carried out in conjunction with HBO to increase the oxygenation of the myocardium. Moderate hypothermia is added to reduce oxygen demand.

Barcal et al. (1975) studied 18 patients to evaluate the effects of HBO therapy in cardiogenic shock complicated by the acute phase of myocardial infarction. This method achieved results equal to or better than those of the intraaortic balloon counterpulsation technique or other methods. Success, according to these authors, depends upon early initiation of HBO therapy.

As far as cardiogenic shock is concerned, HBO appears to be a useful adjunct. There is, however, a paucity of well-documented clinical studies on this subject.

Peripheral Vascular Disease

Causes

The term peripheral vascular disease (PVD) usually refers to ischemic diseases of the extremities, mainly the legs. Various diseases that produce ischemia of the extremities are shown in Table 25.2.

Arteriosclerosis obliterans denotes segmented arteriosclerotic narrowing or obstruction of the lumen in the arteries supplying the limbs. It is the commonest type of PVD and becomes manifest between the ages of 50 and 70 years. The lower limbs are involved more frequently than the upper limbs. Thromboangiitis obliterans is an obstructive arterial disease caused by segmental inflammatory and proliferative lesions of the medium and small vessels of the limbs. The etiology is unknown, but there is a strong association with cigarette smoking and autoimmune factors. There may be a genetic disposition to this disease; it is most prevalent between the ages of 20 and 40 years. Sudden occlusion of an artery to a limb may result from an embolus or thrombosis in situ. It occurs in 10 % of cases of arteriosclerosis obliterans, but it is rare in thromboangiitis obliterans. The heart is the most frequent source of emboli in this syndrome; they may arise from a thrombus in the left ventricle.

Table 25.2 Diseases that produce ischemia in the extremities

1. Arteriosclerosis obliterans
2. Thromboangiitis obliterans (Buerger's disease)
3. Sudden embolic or thrombotic occlusion of the artery to the limb
4. Traumatic arterial occlusion of an extremity
5. Miscellaneous arteriopathies
    - Vasculopathy resulting from drug abuse (intra-arterial)
    - Granulomatous angiitis
    - Allergic vasculitis
    - Collagen vascular disease

Symptoms and Signs

Limb pain is the most frequent symptom of PVD. In the case of the legs, calf pain appears on walking a certain distance and disappears on rest. This is referred to as intermittent claudication. Pain at rest is a sign of severe PVD and occurs when there is a profound reduction in the resting blood flow to the limb. In sudden arterial occlusion, there may be numbness and weakness of the affected limb as well.

The arterial pulses distal to the site of obstruction are lost or reduced. The skin temperature is low and there may be pallor or reddish blue discoloration. There may be ulceration or gangrene of the affected extremity.

Critical limb ischemia (CLI) is a severe form of peripheral arterial disease that often causes disabling symptoms of pain and can lead to loss of the affected limb. It is also associated with increased risk of myocardial infarction, stroke, and death from cardiovascular disease.

Pathophysiology of Limb Ischemia

Reduction of blood flow to a limb is due to stenosis of the arteries. Stenosis that decreases the cross-sectional area of an artery by less than 75 % usually does not affect the resting blood flow to the limb; lesser degrees of stenosis may induce muscle ischemia during exercise. The presence or absence of ischemia in the presence of obstruction is also determined by the degree of collateral circulation. Some collateral vessels that are normally present do not open up until the obstruction occurs and may take several weeks or months to be fully developed. Vasodilatation in response to ischemia is the result of several mechanisms such as the release of vasodilating metabolites.

Biochemical Changes in Skeletal Muscle in Ischemia and Response to Exercise

A simple schematic overview of the energy metabolism of the skeletal muscles is shown in Fig. 25.1. The fatty acids are introduced into the citric acid cycle and the mitochondrial

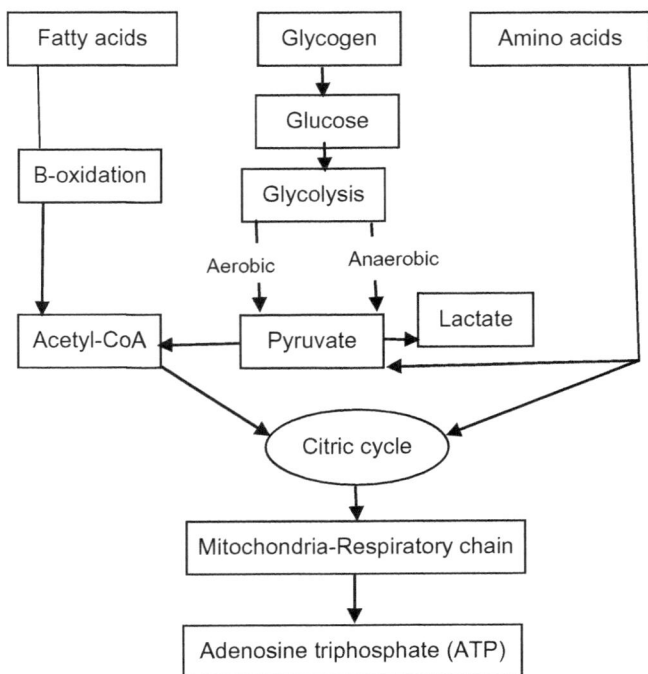

Fig. 25.1 An overview of energy metabolism in skeletal muscles

respiratory chain by ß-oxidation. Decrease of glycogen content and succinic dehydrogenase activity has been observed in the muscles of the lower extremities in patients with circulatory disturbances.

Study of enzyme activity, fiber types, and capillarity in the calf muscles of patients with intermittent claudication shows that the low oxidation potential of the muscle is related to the low level of physical activity. Frequent episodes of ischemia are not considered to be stimuli for the glycolytic enzymes to adapt. A study on leg muscle metabolism in patients with intermittent claudication led to somewhat different results (Bylund-Fellenius et al. 1987). These authors found that patients with stable intermittent claudication had a spontaneous increase of inactivity of enzymes in the β-oxidation pathway for fatty acids, the citric acid cycle, and the respiratory chain in the gastrocnemius muscle tissue, as compared with matched controls.

During leg exercise, when the blood flow to the exercising muscles is limited and claudication develops, there was a more pronounced increase in the lactate content per unit of power in the patients compared with the controls. The fractional extraction of oxygen was higher in the patients, while the extraction of free fatty acids and glucose was similar to that in controls. A lower RQ during exercise in patients indicates that the endogenous fat was an important energy substrate. The results support the hypothesis that there is a beneficial effect of enzyme adaptation in maintaining an oxidative metabolism and that pain develops from hypoxia in certain fiber types.

Acute occlusion of a limb artery does not lead to complete ischemia due to collateral circulation. Sjöström et al. (1982) studied human skeletal muscle metabolism and morphology after temporary incomplete ischemia resulting from aortic clamping during surgery for atherosclerotic occlusive disease of the aortic bifurcation. During the ischemic state, there were no significant changes in the muscle metabolism. After restoration of the blood flow, extensive morphological and metabolic changes were observed in the muscle biopsy tissue. The adenylate (ATP + ADP + AMP) and creatinine (Pcr + Cr) pools declined by 30–40 % and the energy charge of the adenine nucleotides dropped significantly. The metabolic pool changes were closely related to the changes in lactate to pyruvate ratios. Signs of membrane disturbances such as fiber edema and swelling of mitochondria were seen in many muscle fibers. Type 2 fibers seemed to be selectively damaged.

An increased mitochondrial enzyme capacity in the skeletal muscle tissue is a well-documented adaptation to endurance training in humans, but the mechanism triggering this enzyme induction is not known. There is a parallel increase of key enzymes in the citric acid cycle and respiratory chain with physical training. The skeletal muscle of patients with PVD adapts in a similar way to endurance training by an increase in the activity of mitochondrial enzymes. Reduced blood supply to the muscle during exercise might generate the trigger for the induction of mitochondrial enzyme activity. Elander et al. (1985) have demonstrated that, in a rat model, reduced blood flow induced by arterial ligation leads to an adaptive increase of citrate synthesis and cytochrome c oxidase, when intermittent muscle contractions were induced by electrical stimulation.

Lundgren et al. (1988) have studied the exchange of amino acids in leg muscles during exercise in patients with arterial insufficiency. They demonstrated that a higher glutamine efflux and a correspondingly lower efflux of asparagine occur in hypoxic leg muscles during exercise, compared with leg muscles during normal blood flow. This suggests an increase in the rate of amino acid oxidation in hypoxic muscles during exercise. Their results confirm that a normal resting balance of amino acids is restored within 10–20 min following interruption of exercise because of intermittent claudication. The membrane integrity, therefore, is not seriously affected by hypoxia due to arterial insufficiency.

Clinical and Laboratory Assessment of Patients with Peripheral Vascular Disease

During assessment of a PVD patient, it is important to rule out nonvascular causes of extremity pain such as intermittent claudication due to spinal cord stenosis. Clinical examination of the cardiovascular system with evaluation of the peripheral pulses and pressures in the distal arteries is an important part of clinical evaluation. Special laboratory diagnostic procedures are listed in Table 24.3.

Transcutaneous oxygen tension (tcpO$_2$) is a noninvasive method of measuring the tissue oxygen tension: the technique has been described in detail elsewhere (Jain 1989). This test has been used to detect the presence or absence of peripheral arterial insufficiency. Bakay-Csorba et al. (1987) compared the tcpO$_2$ measurements with changes in arteriograms of PVD patients. The results are shown in Table 25.4. These results show that tcpO$_2$ is more useful for the detection of femoral artery disease (below the knee) than iliac artery disease (above the knee).

Lusiani et al. (1988) measured tcpO$_2$ on the dorsum of the foot in healthy subjects and found an average value of 71.2 ± 14.26 mmHg. In patients with PVD, these values were an average of 51.56 ± 26.38 mmHg; the deviations from the average were more marked than in normal subjects. Hence, the accuracy of this test is limited: it can, however, be useful in assessing the response of a patient with PVD to exercise

Table 25.3 Laboratory procedures for the evaluation of peripheral vascular disease

1.	Doppler flowmetry: detection of location of obstruction to blood flow
2.	Duplex ultrasonography: noninvasive evaluation of a patient's vascular hemodynamics
3.	Venous occlusion plethysmography: measurement of rate of volume of arterial inflow into a limb after occlusion of the venous outflow
4.	Transcutaneous oxygen tension (tcpO$_2$) measurement
5.	Response to physical exercise; measurement of limits of performance
6.	Angiography: definite diagnosis and localization of pathology
7.	Magnetic resonance angiography (MRA): useful for imaging large and small vessels

Table 25.4 Transcutaneous oxygen tension measured with changes in arteriograms of patients with peripheral vascular disease

	Above knee (%)	Below knee (%)
Sensitivity	86	91
Specificity	20	33
Accuracy	69	76

and HBO therapy. A more accurate method of measuring muscle tissue oxygen tension is a pO_2 histogram. A staging system usually followed to evaluate the progress and the results of treatment of PVD patients is shown in Table 24.5.

General Management of PVD Patients

The various methods that have been used for the management of PVD patients are listed in Table 25.6.

Drug Therapy

Most of the vasodilator drugs are no longer approved for use in PVD patients. The diseased vessels do not dilate; thus, these medications dilate the vessels in the healthy areas and cause a "steal" effect from the ischemic area.

The role of platelet-inhibiting drugs in PVD has not been defined. These drugs, of which aspirin is an example, remain the most widely used drugs in cardiovascular disorders.

Pentoxifylline and cilostazol are the only two approved drug for ischemic pain due to PVD. The postulated mecha-

nism of action is rheological. In a double-blinded, controlled study, pentoxifylline combined with exercise led to an increase in pO_2 of the muscle as shown in a pO_2 histogram; there was no change in muscle pO_2 in the control subjects given normal saline and exercise (Ehrly and Saeger-Lorenz 1988).

CLI is a special category in management, and the aim is to relieve ischemic pain, heal ulcers, prevent limb loss, improve function and quality of life, and prolong survival. A review of recent evidence regarding the medical management of CLI indicates that antiplatelet agents (either aspirin or clopidogrel) are recommended to reduce the risk of arterial occlusion (Lambert and Belch 2013). There is insufficient evidence to support the use of cilostazol, and pentoxifylline is not beneficial. Clinical trials show promising results of cell therapy. Thrombolysis may be an alternative for patients who develop acute limb ischemia and are unsuitable for surgical intervention. Although benefits of HBO have not been proven by controlled clinical trials, it can alleviate ischemic symptoms and improve limb salvage (Mangiafico and Mangiafico 2011).

Table 24.5 Staging of patients with peripheral vascular disease

Stage I:	Free from symptoms
Stage II:	Intermittent claudication
Stage IIa:	Walking distance over 200 m
Stage IIb:	Walking distance less than 200 m
Stage III:	Pain at rest
Stage IV:	Ulceration and gangrene

Table 25.6 Management of patients with peripheral vascular disease

Medical management
Vasodilator drugs
Platelet inhibitors: aspirin, dipyridamole, sulfapyrazine
Drugs to improve hemorheology: pentoxifylline
Exercise therapy
Gradual intermittently increasing exercise
Exercise with supplemental oxygen: normobaric or hyperbaric
Biological therapies
Stem cells
Gene therapy
Surgery
Angioplasty; balloon catheter or laser
Endarterectomy of the occluded vessel
Vein bypass
Teflon grafts
Sympathectomy
Prevention
Smoking cessation
Control of risk factors for atherosclerosis

Exercise Therapy

Exercise training appears to be an effective treatment for claudication, the primary symptom of peripheral arterial disease. Exercise-induced increases in functional capacity and lessening of claudication symptoms may be explained by several mechanisms, including measurable improvements in endothelial vasodilator function, skeletal muscle metabolism, blood viscosity, and inflammatory responses. This is currently the method of choice for managing patients with intermittent claudication who do not have surgically correctable lesions. Some patients, however, are not able to increase the walking distance by this approach alone, and supplemental oxygen has been found to be helpful in these cases.

Surgery

Several surgical procedures are available. Endarterectomy, where the thrombus is removed, is usually done in acute occlusion. This procedure is less successful in small vessel occlusion. Where the stenotic lesion cannot be corrected, vein bypass or excision and replacement with a synthetic graft may be tried. Percutaneous balloon angioplasty is quite popular although the long-term results are controversial. Laser angioplasty and radiofrequency angioplasty are promising new techniques. Lumbar sympathectomy has been performed to release the alpha-adrenergic vasoconstriction. This procedure is performed rarely these days.

Role of HBO in the Management of Peripheral Vascular Disease

The various reasons given to explain the usefulness of HBO in PVD are summarized in Table 25.7. Tissue ischemia has two primary effects—reduction of oxygen supply to the part and retention of CO_2 and other products of tissue metabolism. It is difficult to modify the retention of toxic products, but the lack of oxygen can be compensated by HBO.

The most important of the beneficial effects of HBO in intermittent claudication treatment is the role in increasing walking capacity in patients who have reached a limit with simple gradually increasing exercise. This effect will be examined later in this chapter.

Experimental Studies

Bird and Telfer (1965) tested the effect of 100 % oxygen on the blood flow to the arms of healthy young volunteers. At 1 ATA the reduction was 11.2 %. At 2 ATA the reduction was 18.9 %. After the HBO, the amount of available oxygen was increased even though the blood flow remained unchanged. The authors suggested that there was a homeostatic mechanism to keep the oxygen tensions constant.

This mechanism does not apply to the ischemic limb, where the oxygen tension is much below normal. The rate at which the oxygen diffuses from the blood through the capillary wall to the tissue fluids and the cells depends upon the gradient of the partial pressures between the plasma and the tissue cells.

Ackerman and Brinkley (1966) showed that under HBO, pO_2 tensions rise more than 5.6 times in the ischemic tissues compared with the normal tissues (Fig. 25.2). NBO was shown to lead to a slight rise of pO_2 in the normal limb, but

not in the ischemic limb. Stalker and Ledingham (1973) produced acute hind limb ischemia in anesthetized dogs. Oxygen extraction and consumption rose initially, but then fell below the normal levels. HBO at 2 ATA did not influence the blood flow or the metabolic exchange. Kawamura et al. (1978) conducted similar experiments to test the effects of HBO on hind limb ischemia in dogs and concluded that oxygen does not act as a vasoconstrictor in hypoxic tissues until oxygen deficit is improved.

Schraibman and Ledingham (1969) studied the effect of HBO and regional vasodilation in foot ischemia. They stated that the problem of the ischemia had not been solved by reconstructive surgery or sympathectomy, which benefits just over 50 % of the patients. They measured foot blood flow in healthy volunteers and patients by means of strain gauge plethysmography. The resting blood flow was similar in normal subjects and patients with claudication and showed a significant decrease with HBO. Resting blood flow was low in those with skin ischemia, but showed a significant increase with HBO when this was given in combination with an intravenous infusion of tolazoline hydrochloride (vasodilator). After sympathectomy neither HBO nor vasodilator produced any change in blood flow.

Kawamura et al. (1978) investigated the effect of HBO on normal tissues and hypoxic tissues. Acute temporary ischemia was produced in the right hind limbs of dogs, while the left hind limbs served as a control. HBO at 2 ATA produced vasoconstriction in the normal limbs (control), whereas there was no vasoconstriction in the ischemic limbs until after the hypoxia had been corrected.

Following acute ischemia of a limb, there are changes in microcirculation and interference with flow and transport. The integrity of membranes separating intravascular and

Table 25.7 Rationale for the use of HBO in peripheral vascular disease

1. Relief of hypoxia
–HBO raises the low $tcpO_2$ in the marginally perfused ischemic/hypoxic tissues
–HBO improves the cellular metabolism which has been impaired by hypoxia
2. Relief of effects of ischemia: HBO is not a vasoconstrictor in ischemic tissues
–HBO reduces the incidence and extent of gangrene in the limbs
–HBO helps in demarcating the line between viable and nonviable tissues as a guide to amputation where it is unavoidable
–HBO promotes healing of ulcers due to vascular insufficiency
–HBO helps the limb salvage in arterial trauma in patients who are (a) waiting for a surgical procedure or those in whom (b) the surgical procedures have failed
3. Relief of pain; the various mechanisms are:
–Improved local circulation with decreased accumulation of algogenesic polypeptides
–Secondary to relief of hypoxia
–Secondary to antiedema effect of HBO
–HBO increases the affinity of endorphins for receptor sites
4. Increase of exercise capacity in combined HBO and exercise therapy
–HBO and exercise both improve hemorheology and contribute to better perfusion of the ischemic limb
–HBO improves the biochemical disturbances due to exercise and thus permits better physical performance
–Exercise with resulting vasodilatation may prevent the vasoconstricting effect of HBO on arterioles in the non-affected areas of the limbs

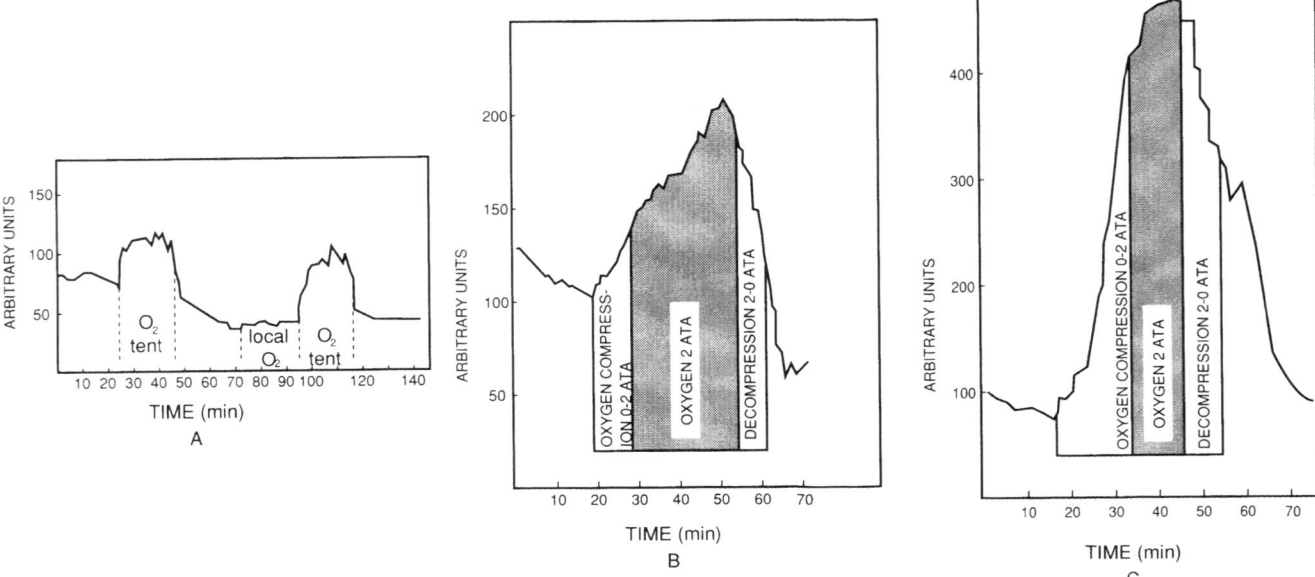

Fig. 25.2 Oxygen tension in normal and ischemic tissues during hyperbaric therapy. (**a**) Response of tissue pO_2 in normal limb to inhalation of oxygen at atmospheric pressure and to a local oxygen-rich environment. (**b**) Response of tissue pO_2 in normal limb to hyperbaric oxygen at 15 psig. (**c**) Response of tissue pO_2 in ischemic limb to hyperbaric oxygen at 15 psig. Modified and redrawn from Ackerman and Brinkley 1966

extravascular spaces is impaired, and edema may result in ischemic muscle. Even when the circulation is restored, edema may persist or get worse. This can cause compression of capillaries and aggravation of ischemia, thus starting a vicious circle. Nylander et al. (1985) produced edema in rats using a limb tourniquet to interrupt the circulation. HBO caused a significant reduction of postischemic edema, and this effect persisted 40 h after the last treatment. The authors considered HBO to be a useful adjunct to the treatment of acute ischemic conditions where surgical repair alone fails or is not adequate to reverse the condition.

Repeated HBO treatments in the postischemic phase have been shown to stimulate aerobic metabolism. Reduction of phosphorylase activity, which is a sensitive marker of muscle damage, is improved by HBO in the postischemic phase.

Review of Clinical Applications of HBO for PVD

Illingworth (1962) was the first to use HBO for PVD and was able to salvage a few limbs after acute arterial injuries. He was the first to notice relief of pain in patients with thrombo-angiitis obliterans while undergoing HBO therapy. There was healing of skin ulcerations. In the 1960s, other surgeons reported the effect of HBO in patients with atherosclerosis and incipient early gangrene of the lower extremities. It was noted that the gangrenous tissue was consistently rendered dry and the margins sharp and clear-cut. The level of amputation required was usually lower than that necessary without the use of HBO.

Gorman et al. (1965) described their experiences in the end stage of occlusive arterial disease in the lower extremities. In contrast to occlusion of proximal major vessels, these patients had involvement of small arteries and arterioles supplying the skin and subcutaneous tissues, where development of the collateral network is at a minimum. Forty-eight such patients were treated with HBO at 3 ATA for 1 h daily. All of them had potential or incipient gangrene and all had undergone lumbar sympathectomy. The overall limb salvage and progression of ischemic process were not significantly altered by HBO in these cases. Microscopic examination of tissues at the margin of necrosis revealed less inflammatory reaction in HBO-treated patients than in controls, indicating an important relationship between hyperoxia and cellular response to injury.

During HBO in patients with chronic thrombo-obliterating disease of the extremities, there is normalization of metabolic processes in ischemic tissues together with elimination of oxygen deficits and deviations in acid–base balance. Sakakibara (1986), from Japan, presented their experience with the use of HBO in 159 patients with chronic PVD seen over a period of 18 years. These included 109 cases of thromboangiitis obliterans, which has a high incidence in Japan. Of these cases, 69 % had healing of their sores. Of the 43 patients with atherosclerotic occlusive disease, 70 % had healing of their skin ulcers. The incidence of amputation required was decreased in all the patients.

Kostiunin et al. (1985) analyzed the HBO treatment of 122 patients with advanced arterial occlusive disease of the lower extremities and showed that the effectiveness of HBO can be enhanced by a combination with continuous intra-arterial infusions and lumbar sympathectomy. An important factor, according to them, is an increase of low cardiac output. Rosenthal et al. (1985) presented three cases of infants with disseminated intravascular clotting involving peripheral arterial occlusions and gangrene of parts of the arms and legs. They were able, with HBO, to affect regression of the demarcation line of gangrene, and the amputations were minimized.

HBO treatments reduce gangrene and the amputation rate in patients with diabetic gangrene. Fredenucci (1985) used HBO in treating arteriopathies of the limbs in 2021 patients between 1966 and 1983. Plethysmographic studies showed that blood flowed from the healthy areas (with vasoconstriction) to nonresponding hypoxic territories in 40 % of the patients. The author felt that HBO is an important method of treatment of patients with asymptomatic arteriopathies.

Efuni et al. (1984) believe that reduction of regional blood flow to 1.5 mL/min/100 g muscle tissue is the limit of HBO effectiveness. According to them, the primary reaction of ischemic tissues to HBO treatment is higher blood flow volume, which is due to opening of nonfunctioning capillaries, thus leading to a considerably larger oxygen diffusion area. HBO also improves the rheological properties of blood: fibrinogen concentration and plasma tolerance to heparin decrease, while fibrinolytic activity increases. Efuni et al. evaluated the degree of effectiveness of HBO treatment by polarography. In 70 % of cases, tissue pO_2 does not return to baseline for 1 h or more, as compared with a drop to normal values in the blood within 0.5 h. This "after effect" is due to the reduction of tissue oxygen consumption after HBO treatment. There is some interrelationship between the duration of the after effect and the therapeutic effect of HBO, and this makes a fair prediction of the effects of HBO possible. The treatment is supplemented by vasodilators. The authors' 7-year experience with over 3000 cases is summarized in Table 25.8. The best results were obtained in patients with chronic arterial insufficiency.

Visona et al. (1989) treated patients in various stages of PVD and reported long-term improvement in more than 50 % of the cases. Urayama et al. (1992) studied the therapeutic effect of HBO in patients with chronic occlusive disease of the lower extremities in 50 patients. These patients had a variety of sequelae of limb ischemia: pain at rest, ulceration, etc. HBO was used at 2 ATA for 60 min and the number of sessions varied from 3 to 40. Five out of 6 patients with pain at rest were relieved. Necrosis or ulceration healed in 16 out of 30 patients. Transcutaneous oxygen tension was markedly increased during HBO sessions and remained so for some time afterwards. Lipid peroxide and SOD levels were not changed significantly by HBO treatments.

Kovacevic (1992) carried out a prospective placebo-controlled, double-blind study of the effect of HBO on atherosclerotic occlusive disease of the lower extremities in 65 patients. Treatment group (35 patients) was given HBO at 2.8 ATA, twice a day, for a total of 20 treatments during 2 weeks. The control group (30 patients) was given normoxic mixture (nitrox 7.5) to breathe in the hyperbaric chamber. Both groups maintained the conservative medical therapy and were advised to quit smoking. The treatment group showed improvement during the first 3 months as manifested by an increase of pain-free walking distance. The improvement persisted during the 6-month follow-up period.

HBO as an Adjunct to Exercise Therapy for Ischemic Leg Pain

Prior to 1989 there was no publication describing the use of ergometry under HBO for the rehabilitation of patients with ischemic leg pain. At first, NBO supplementation was used (Jain 1989). Those patients who could not make any further progress with bicycle ergometry breathing room air or 100 % NBO were selected for a pilot study using HBO at Fachklinik

Table 25.8 HBO treatment results in some types of vascular pathologies

Type of pathology	Patients (n)	Treatment results		
		Good	Satisfactory	No effect
Obliterative endarteritis	1684 100 %	1297 77 %	236 14 %	151 9 %
Obliterative atherosclerosis	1537 100 %	1061 69 %	384 25 %	92 6 %
Total	3221 100 %	2358 73.2 %	620 19.3 %	243 7.5 %
Acute arterial insufficiency	18 % 100 %	11 61 %	– 39 %	7
Chronic venous insufficiency	163 100 %	72 44 %	48 29.5 %	43 26.5 %
Trophic ulcers of vascular genesis	370 100 %	192 52 %	113 30.5 %	65 17.5 %

Klausenbach in Germany. Four male patients, with varying degrees of limitation of walking due to ischemic leg pain, were treated with a combination of ergometry and HBO during the past 2 years. All of them had angiographic confirmation of arterial occlusion and of hemodynamic disturbance by plethysmography. All had been treated medically and all were in stable condition. None of them had had surgical treatment. Various medications including pentoxifylline were maintained during our treatment.

All the patients underwent ergometric training on a treadmill installed in the hyperbaric chamber, with a computerized control outside. The speed, distance traveled, and time were recorded. The pressure used was 1.5 ATA for a 45-min session (10 min compression+30 min of 100% oxygen at full pressure+5 min decompression). The exercise was started at the completion of the compression phase and stopped at the onset of leg pain, when the patient rested in the chamber until the session was completed. The control studies were ergometry in the chamber under normobaric air, hyperbaric air (1.5

ATA), and NBO (100%). Laboratory studies included blood ammonia, lactate glucose, free fatty acids (FFA), and glycerin both before and after exertion during the first 4 days and last 4 days of the treatment (Fig. 25.3). No treatments were done on weekends. No transcutaneous pO_2 measurements were taken, but arterial and venous pO_2 tensions were measured during the laboratory sessions. Clinical results of training in 4 patients are shown in Table 25.9.

One of the selection criteria of the patients was the ability to do ergometry. This excluded the stroke patients with hemiplegia, who were treated in the chamber and showed improvement of the ischemic leg pain and improved capacity for walking. They performed leg exercises, but were not considered fit to proceed with the ergometry program. All the treatments were given on an outpatient basis. The first 2 patients were treated once a week and the last two on a daily basis except on weekends. This frequency was determined by the availability of the patients (retired or working) and the distance of their residence from the clinic. The protocol

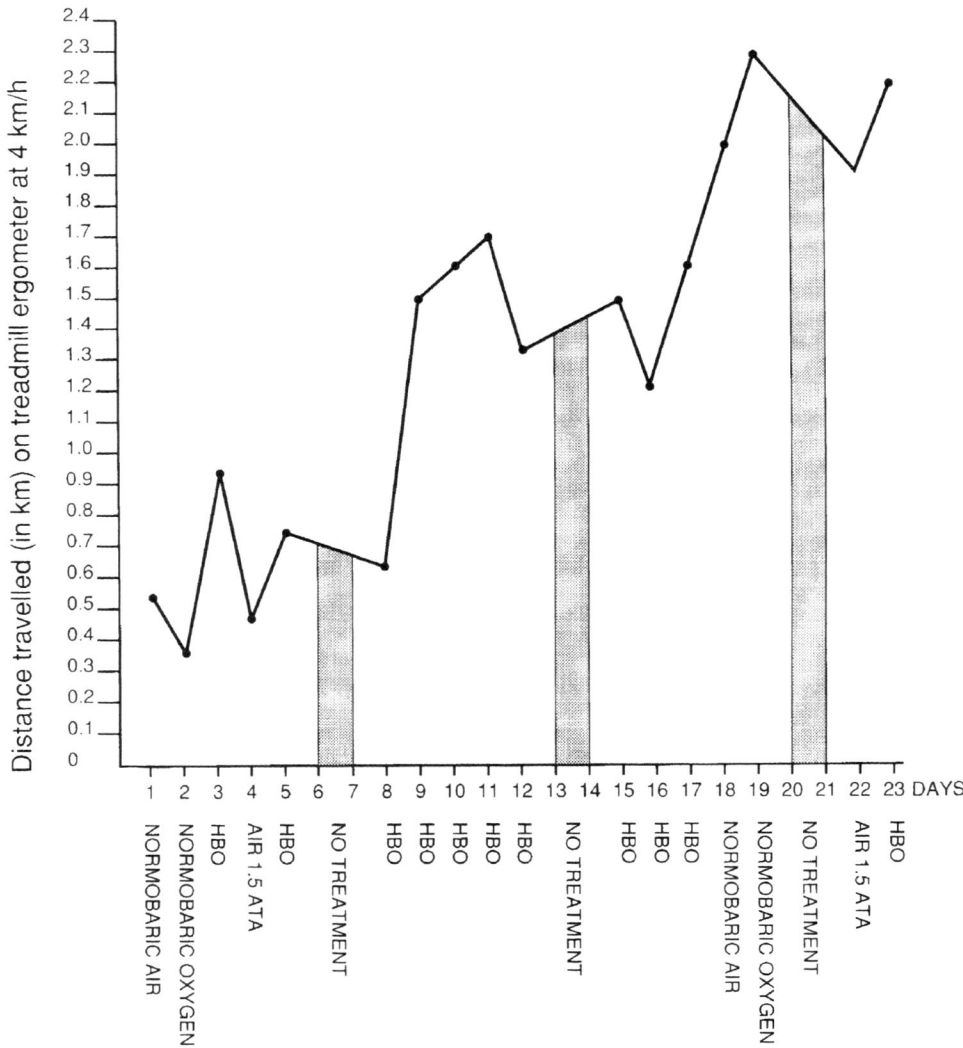

Fig. 25.3 Treatment schedule of case no. 4 (Table 25.9). Pretreatment, days 1–4; posttreatment, days 18, 19, 22, and 23: HBO, 100% hyperbaric oxygen, 1.5 ATA

Table 25.9 Summary of the results of training in 4 patients with PVD using ergometry plus HBO

No.	Age Stage	Diagnosis walking range	Before HBO treatment Normobaric O_2	Maximum distance under HBO	Maximum distance sessions	No. of current condition	Remarks
1	70	Bilateral stenosis femorals, stage III; rest pains	150 m/3 min level 10 m at 25 W on 15° upgrade	Not done 400 m level	150 m with 15° upgrade	10	Relief of pain walks 3–4 km
2	51	Left femoral occlusion; stage IIa	605 m in 6 min	1074 m in 14 min	3166 m in 33 min	14	Ergometry in room air: 2285/24 min; 7 km mountain hike
3	66	Bilateral occlusive disease; stage IIa; myocardial and cerebrovascular insufficiency	529 m in 6 min	685 m in 9 min	1258 m in 20 min	10	Maintains improvement
4	49	Right femoral occlusion; stage IIa	526 m in 8 min	2358 m in 35 min	2250 m in 34 min	11	Maintains improvement (see Fig. 25.3)

is still being modified. In patient no. 2, HBO sessions followed on the same days as sessions with room air. The protocol for patient no. 4 is shown in Fig. 25.3. All 4 patients showed improvement of the distance they could walk on the treadmill ergometer. In spite of fluctuations in performance, there was overall improvement, as shown in Table 25.9. The laboratory results conformed to the pattern previously observed in healthy volunteers. Lactate and ammonia accumulation was less during exertion under HBO than under NBO or in room air.

It is likely that HBO helped these patients to cross the "barrier" of limitation of walking, even though the vascular pathology was not reversed. The improvement in these patients was adequate to carry out the daily activities required for their jobs.

The number of HBO sessions (with exercise) should be guided by the "ceiling effect," i.e., when the performance under HBO is not significantly different from that while breathing NBO or ambient air. At that point, HBO treatments serve no purpose and should be discontinued, and the patient should continue to exercise daily in room air.

Role of HBO in Miscellaneous Arteriopathies

Monies-Chass et al. (1976) described the case of a child with allergic vasculitis due to penicillin affecting the limbs and abdominal wall. HBO was used successfully after failure of conventional treatment. The authors' explanation was that ischemia of the vessel wall leads to increased permeability with exudation of electrolytes, fluids, and proteins into the extracellular space, causing edema, which further aggravates ischemia. Fasciotomy does not help in this situation. HBO interrupted the circle of ischemia of vessel wall exudation compression of vessel aggravation of vessel wall ischemia. De

Myttenaere et al. (1977) described a case of self-administration by injection of methylphenidate into the brachial artery by an addict. Intensive treatment started within 12 h and a combination of HBO, vasodilators, and stellate ganglion block saved the arm, with limited loss of the fingertips.

Ergotism can result from prolonged use of ergot-derived alkaloids in migraine. There is arterial constriction leading to peripheral ischemia and gangrene. Ergotamine may also cause toxic endothelial damage, either acute or chronic. Some cases recover after discontinuation of ergot and others improve with vasodilators. Merrick et al. (1978) saw 8 patients with ergotism after unsuccessful treatment using other methods. They were given HBO at 3 ATA for 1 h two to three times a day along with an epidural block for relief of pain due to ischemia of the limb. The treatment was successful in all cases.

Livedoid vasculopathy is a painful, ulcerating condition of the legs, ankles, and feet with typical histological feature of hyalinizing vascular change of dermal blood vessels with minimal inflammation. Diverse treatments have been varyingly successful. A biopsy-proven case of livedoid vasculopathy was reported to respond rapidly and completely to HBO therapy (Banham 2013).

HBO as an Adjunct to Peripheral Vascular Surgery

Eisterer and Staudacher (1971) found backflow during surgery on 7 patients with severe vascular disease of the lower extremities. These patients were treated with multiple sessions of HBO after surgery, and the surgeons believed that this method saved the limbs in these patients. The authors pointed out that a single exposure to HBO without surgery is useless.

Monies-Chass et al. (1976) presented a series of seven young men suffering from severe vascular trauma and acute ischemia of the limbs. Standard repair, though technically successful, failed to achieve satisfactory restoration of the circulation. HBO treatment of 2.8 ATA prevented the development of gangrene in all cases. The authors considered HBO a useful adjunct to reconstructive surgery in cases needing repair long after the injury.

The role of HBO in the treatment of skin ulcers caused by arterial insufficiency is reviewed in Chap. 16, and its use in limb edema in trauma and compartment syndrome is reviewed in Chap. 30.

Conclusions Regarding the Role of HBO in Peripheral Vascular Disease

Since the first observation by Illingworth (1962) on the effect of HBO in relieving pain due to limb ischemia, there has been no study to evaluate the effectiveness of HBO in patients where pain is the only symptom. Most of the reports in the literature deal with more serious cases, where there is gangrene or skin ulceration. HBO therapy is generally considered useful in the treatment of occlusive peripheral arterial disease and its role should be investigated further.

References

Ackerman NB, Brinkley FB. Oxygen tensions in normal and ischemic tissues during hyperbaric therapy. JAMA. 1966;98:142–5.

Allaria B, Decio B, Libutti M. Electrocution and hyperbaric oxygen therapy: a case with electrocardiographic changes from electrocution cured by hyperbaric oxygen therapy. Anesteziol Reanimatol. 1973;14:167–72.

Allen MW, Golembe E, Gorenstein S, Butler GJ. Protective effects of hyperbaric oxygen therapy (HBO₂) in cardiac care—a proposal to conduct a study into the effects of hyperbaric pre-conditioning in elective coronary artery bypass graft surgery (CABG). Undersea Hyperb Med. 2015;42:107–14.

Bakay-Csorba PA, Provan JL, Ameli FM. Transcutaneous oxygen tension measurements in the detection of iliac and femoral arterial disease. Surg Gynecol Obstet. 1987;164:102–4.

Banham ND. Livedoid vasculopathy successfully treated with hyperbaric oxygen. Diving Hyperb Med. 2013;43:35–6.

Barcal R, Emmerova M, Sova J, Topinka I, Hadravský M. Hyperbaric oxygen therapy of cardiogenic shock in the acute stage of myocardial infarction. Cas Lek Cesk. 1975;114:259–62.

Bennett MH, Lehm JP, Jepson N. Hyperbaric oxygen therapy for acute coronary syndrome. Cochrane Database Syst Rev. 2015;7, CD004818.

Bird AD, Telfer ABM. Effect of hyperbaric oxygen on limb circulation. Lancet. 1965;13:355–6.

Bockeria LA, Khapy KH, Gazhiev AA, et al. Extracorporeal circulation under hyperbaric oxygenation. In: Smith G, editor. 5th international congress on hyperbaric medicine. Aberdeen: University of Aberdeen Press; 1977. p. 189–97.

Bockeria LA, Sokolova NA, Ladynima EA, Gadzhiev AA. Enzyme determinants as a check on adequacy of body defences during heart operations under hyperbaric oxygenation. Anesteziol Reanimatol. 1978;3:45–9.

Bockeria LA, Zelenkini MA. Electrocardiographic changes during exclusion of the heart from the circulation under hyperbaric oxygenation and hypothermia (in Russian). Eksp Khir Anestesiol. 1973;18:80–4.

Boerema I, Meyne NG, Brummelkamp WH, Bouma S, Mensch MH, Kamermans F, et al. Life without blood. Arch Chir Neer. 1959;11:70–83.

Boerema I. An operating room for high oxygen pressure. Surgery. 1961;47:291–8.

Burakovsky VI, Bockeria LA. Experience of operating on the heart under conditions of hyperbaric oxygen. In: Proceedings of the 7th international congress on hyperbaric medicine, Moscow, Sept. 2–6, 1981.

Burakovsky VI, Bockeria LA. The resuscitative value of HBO in cardiac surgery and cardiology. In: Smith G, editor. 6th international congress on hyperbaric medicine. Aberdeen: University of Aberdeen Press; 1977. p. 184–8.

Bylund-Fellenius AC, Elander A, Lundgren F. Effects of reduced blood flow on human muscle metabolism. In: OkyayuzBaklonti I, Hudlicka O, editors. Muscle ischemia – functional and metabolic aspects. Wolff: Munich; 1987. p. 75–88.

Cameron AJV, Hutton I, Kenmure ACF, Murdoch WR. Haemodynamic and metabolic effects of hyperbaric oxygen in myocardial infarction. Lancet. 1966;i:833–7.

Chardack WM, Gage AA, Frederico AJ, Cusick JK, Matsumoto PJ, Lanphier EH. Reduction by hyperbaric oxygenation of the mortality from ventricular fibrillation following coronary artery ligation. Circ Res. 1964;15:497–502.

Clark RG, Young DG. Effects of hyperoxygenation and sodium bicarbonate in hemorrhagic hypotension. Br J Surg. 1965;52:704.

De Myttenaere S, Heifetz M, Shilansky H, Monies I, Shramek A. Different treatments used in a case of gangrene due to accidental intraarterial injection of methylphenidate (Ritalin). Anesth Analg. 1977;34:405–10.

Demurov EA, Vesilieva NN, Kakhnovskaya VB, et al. The effect of hyperbaric oxygenation on some indices of neurohormonal regulation, metabolic and heart contractile function under conditions of acute occlusion of the coronary artery. In: Yefuny SN, editor. Proceedings of the 7th international congress on hyperbaric medicine. USSR Academy of Sciences, Moscow, 1981:273.

Dotsenko EA, Nikulina NV, Salivonchik DP, Lappo OG, Gritsuk AI, Bastron AS. Low doses of hyperbaric oxygenation effectively decrease the size of necrotic zone in rats with experimental myocardial infarction. Bull Exp Biol Med. 2015;158:732–4.

Efuni SN, Kudryashev V, Rodionov VV, et al. Significance of the isometric test in the objective assessment of the efficacy of hyperbaric oxygenation in coronary heart disease. Kardiologiia. 1984;24:77–80.

Ehrly AM, Saeger-Lorenz K. Einfluss von Pentoxifyllin auf den Muskelgewebesauerstoffdruck von Patienten mit Claudicatio intermittens vor und nach fussergometrischer Belastung. Med Welt. 1988;39:739–44.

Eisterer H, Staudacher M. Die Anwendung der hyperbaren Sauerstoffkammer in Verbindung mit gefässrekonstruktiven Massnahmen. Chirurg. 1971;42:187–90.

Elander A, Idström JP, Schersten T, Bylund-Fellenius AC. Metabolic adaptation to reduced muscle blood flow. I. Enzyme and metabolite alterations. Am J Physiol. 1985;249:E63–9.

Fredenucci P. Oxygénothérapie hyperbare et artériopathies. J Mal Vasc. 1985;10(Suppl A):166–72.

Friehs G, Klepp G, Rader W, Schalk H, Stolze A. Hyperbaric oxygenation in a large hyperbaric chamber. Med Klin. 1977;72:2013–8.

Gadzhiev AA. Prevention of venous hypertension on the dry heart under hyperbaric oxygenation. Grudn Khir. 1979;5:7–10.

Goliakov VN, Eroshina VA, Zimin YV, Semiletova VI. Hemostasis in patients with ischemic heart disease during hyperbaric oxygenation. Klin Med (Mosk). 1986a;64:92–5.

Goliakov VN, Zimin IV, Eroshina VA, Gasilin VS, Efuni SN. Effect of hyperbaric oxygenation on extrasystole in ischemic heart disease patients. Kardiologiia. 1986b;26:45–9.

Gorman JF, Stansell GB, Douglas F. Limitations of hyperbaric oxygenation in occlusive arterial disease. Circulation. 1965;32:936–9.

Gross DR, Dodd KT, Welch DW, Fife WP. Hemodynamic effects of 10 % dextrose and of dextran 70 on hemorrhagic shock during exposure to hyperbaric air and hyperbaric hyperoxia. Aviat Space Environ Med. 1984;55:1118–28.

Gross DR, Moreau RM, Chaikin BN, Welch DW, Jabor M, Fife WP. Hemodynamic effects of lactated Ringer's solution on hemorrhagic shock during exposure to hyperbaric air and hyperbaric hyperoxia. Aviat Space Environ Med. 1983a;54:701–8.

Gross DR, Moreau RM, Jabor M, Welch DW, Fife WP. Hemodynamic effects of dextran 40 on hemorrhagic shock during hyperbaria and hyperbaric hyperoxia. Aviat Space Environ Med. 1983b;54:413–9.

Illingworth CFW. Treatment of arterial occlusion under oxygen at two atmospheres pressure. Br Med J. 1962;2:1271–5.

Isakov IV, Golikov AP, Ustinova EZ, Tret'iakova NG. Hyperbaric oxygenation in the combined treatment of paroxysmal tachyarrhythmias in ischemic heart disease. Kardiologiia. 1981;21:42–5.

Jacobson JH, Wang MCH, Yamaki T, Kline HJ, Kark AE, Kuhn LA. Hyperbaric oxygenation in diffuse myocardial infarction. Arch Surg. 1964;89:905.

Jain KK. Oxygen in Physiology and Medicine. Charles C Thomas: Springfield, IL; 1989.

Jeysen ZY, Gerard L, Levant G, Cowen M, Cale A, Griffin S. Research report: the effects of hyperbaric oxygen preconditioning on myocardial biomarkers of cardioprotection in patients having coronary artery bypass graft surgery. Undersea Hyperb Med. 2011;38:175–85.

Kawamura MK, Sakakibara K, Sasakibara B. Protective effect of hyperbaric oxygen for the temporary ischemic myocardium. Macroscopic and histologic data. Cardiovasc Res. 1976;10:599–601.

Kawamura MK, Sakakibara K, Yusa T. Effect of increased oxygen on peripheral circulation in acute, temporary limb hypoxia. J Cardiovasc Surg. 1978;19:161–8.

Kim CH, Choi H, Chun YS, Kim GT, Park JW, Kim MS. Hyperbaric oxygenation pretreatment induces catalase and reduces infarct size in ischemic rat myocardium. Pflugers Arch. 2001;442:519–25.

Kleep G. Additive Wirkung von hyperbarem Sauerstoff und intraaortaler Ballonpumpe bei der Therapie des akuten Koronarverschlusses im Experiment. Wien Med Wochenschr. 1977;127:35.

Kline HJ, Marano AJ, Johnson CD, Goodman P, Jacobson 2nd JH, Kuhn LA. Hemodynamics and metabolic effects of hyperbaric oxygenation in myocardial infarction. J Appl Physiol. 1979;28:256–63.

Kostiunin VN, Pahkomov VI, Feoktistov PL, Petrova EA. Increasing the effectiveness of hyperbaric oxygenation in the treatment of patients with stage IV arterial occlusive disease of the lower limbs. Vestn Khir. 1985;135:48–51.

Kovacevic H. The Investigation of Hyperbaric Oxygen Influence in the Patients with Second Degree of Atherosclerotic Insufficiency of Lower Extremities. Doctoral Dissertation: University of Rijeka, Croatia; 1992.

Kudchodkar BJ, Pierce A, Dory L. Chronic hyperbaric oxygen treatment elicits an anti-oxidant response and attenuates atherosclerosis in apoE knockout mice. Atherosclerosis. 2007;193:28–35.

Kuleshova MP, Flora AA. Physical rehabilitation of patients with ischemic heart disease using hyperbaric oxygen. In: Yefuny SN, editor. Proceedings of the 7th international congress of hyperbaric medicine, USSR Academy of Sciences, Moscow, 1981:p 268.

Lambert MA, Belch JJ. Medical management of critical limb ischaemia: where do we stand today? J Intern Med. 2013;274:295–307.

Li Y, Dong H, Chen M, Liu J, Yang L, Chen S, et al. Preconditioning with repeated hyperbaric oxygen induces myocardial and cerebral protection in patients undergoing coronary artery bypass graft surgery: a prospective, randomized, controlled clinical trial. J Cardiothorac Vasc Anesth. 2011;25:908–16.

Lundgren F, Zachrisson H, Emery P, Bylund-Fellenius AC, Elander A, Bennegård K, et al. Less exchange of amino acids during exercise in patients with arterial insufficiency. Clin Physiol. 1988;8:227–41.

Lusiani L, Visona A, Nicolin P, Papesso B, Pagnan A. Transcutaneous oxygen tension (TcPO$_2$) measurement as a diagnostic tool in patients with peripheral vascular disease. Angiology. 1988;39:873–80.

Mangiafico RA, Mangiafico M. Medical treatment of critical limb ischemia: current state and future directions. Curr Vasc Pharmacol. 2011;9:658–76.

Merrick J, Gufler K, Jacobsen E. Ergotism treated with hyperbaric oxygen and continuous epidural analgesia. Acta Anaesthesiol Scand. 1978;Suppl 67: 87–90.

Miroshnichenko VP, Demurov EA, Koloskow YB, Zubovskaia AM. Effect of guanine nucleotides and hyperbaric oxygenation on cardiac adenylate cyclase activity in rabbits with myocardial hypertrophy. Bull Exp Biol Med. 1983;95:179–81.

Monies-Chass I, Herer D, Alon U, Birkhahn HJ. Hyperbaric oxygen in acute ischaemia due to allergic vasculitis. Anaesthesia. 1976;31:1221–4.

Nylander G, Lewis D, Nordstrom H, Larsson J. Reduction of postischemic edema with hyperbaric oxygen. Plast Reconstr Surg. 1985;76:596–603.

Richards V, Pinto D, Coombs P. Studies in suspended animation by hypothermia combined with hyperbaric oxygenation. Ann Surg. 1963;58:349–62.

Rosenthal E, Benderly A, Monies-Chass I, Fishman J, Levy J, Bialik V. Hyperbaric oxygenation in peripheral ischaemic lesions in infants. Arch Dis Child. 1985;60:372–4.

Sakakibara K. The history and future prospects of hyperbaric oxygen therapy in japan. Jpn J Hyperbaric Med. 1986;21:21–40.

Scheidt S, Wilner G, Fillmore S, Shapiro M, Killip T. Objective haemodynamic assessment after acute myocardial infarction. Br Heart J. 1973;35:908–16.

Schraibman IG, Ledingham IM. Hyperbaric oxygen and local vasodilatation in peripheral vascular disease. Brit J Surg. 1969;56:295–9.

Shandling AH, Ellestad MH, Hart GB, Crump R, Marlow D, Van Natta B, et al. Hyperbaric oxygen and thrombolysis in myocardial infarction: the "hot MI" pilot study. Am Heart J. 1997;134:544–50.

Sjöström M, Neglen P, Friden J, Eklof B. Human skeletal muscle metabolism and morphology after temporary incomplete ischaemia. Eur J Clin Invest. 1982;12:69–79.

Smetnev AS, Efuni SN, Rodionov VV, Ashurova LD, Aslibekian IS. Hyperbaric oxygenation in the overall therapy of chronic ischemic heart disease. Kardiologiia. 1979;19:41–6.

Smith G, Lawson DA. Experimental coronary arterial occlusion: effects of the administration of oxygen under pressure. Scott Med J. 1958;3:346–50.

Spears JR, Henney C, Prcevski P, Xu R, Li L, Brereton GJ, et al. Aqueous oxygen hyperbaric reperfusion in a porcine model of myocardial infarction. J Invasive Cardiol. 2002;14:160–6.

Stalker CG, Ledingham IM. The effect of increased oxygen in prolonged acute on limb ischaemia. Br J Surg. 1973;60:959–63.

Sterling DL, Thornton JD, Swafford A, Gottlieb SF, Bishop SP, Stanley AW, et al. Hyperbaric oxygen limits infarct size in ischemic rabbit myocardium in vivo. Circulation. 1993;88:1931–6.

Stillman RM. Effects of hypoxia and hyperoxia on progression of intimal healing. Arch Surg. 1983;118:732–7.

Stravinsky Y, Shandling AH, Ellestad MH, Hart GB, Van Natta B, Messenger JC, et al. Hyperbaric oxygen and thrombolysis in myocardial infarction: the 'HOT MI' randomized multicenter study. Cardiology. 1998;90:131–6.

Thomas MP, Brown LA, Sponseller DR, Williamson SE, Diaz JA, Guyton DP. Myocardial infarct size reduction by the synergistic effect of hyperbaric oxygen and recombinant tissue plasminogen activator. Am Heart J. 1990;120:791–800.

Thurston JG, Greenwood TW, Bending MR, Connor H, Curwen MP. A controlled investigation into the effects of hyperbaric oxygen on mortality following acute myocardial infarction. Q J Med. 1973;42:751–70.

Todo K, Nakae S, Wada J. Heart preservation with metabolic inhibitor, hypothermia, and hyperbaric oxygenation. Jpn J Surg. 1974;4:29–36.

Trapp WG, Creighton R. Experimental studies of increased atmospheric pressure on myocardial ischemia after coronary ligation. J Thorac Cardiovasc Surg. 1964;47:687–92.

Urayama H, Takemura H, Kasajima F, Tsuchida K, Katada S, Watanabe Y. Hyperbaric oxygen therapy for chronic occlusive disease of the extremities. Nippon Geka Gakkai Zasshi. 1992;93:429–33.

Visona A, Lusiani L, Rusca F, Barbiero D, Ursini F, Pagnan A. Therapeutic, hemodynamic, and metabolic effects of hyperbaric oxygenation in peripheral vascular disease. Angiology. 1989;40:994–1000.

Yin X, Wang X, Fan Z, Peng C, Ren Z, Huang L, et al. Hyperbaric Oxygen Preconditioning Attenuates Myocardium Ischemia-Reperfusion Injury Through Upregulation of Heme Oxygenase 1 Expression: PI3K/Akt/Nrf2 Pathway Involved. J Cardiovasc Pharmacol Ther. 2015;20:428–38.

Yogaratnam JZ, Laden G, Guvendik L, Cowen M, Cale A, Griffin S. Pharmacological preconditioning with hyperbaric oxygen: can this therapy attenuate myocardial ischemic reperfusion injury and induce myocardial protection via nitric oxide? J Surg Res. 2008;149:155–64.

Zhivoderov VM, Doshchitsin VL, Dunaeva ZI, Kolomeĭtseva SP, Nazarova VI. Late arrhythmias in myocardial infarct. Kardiologiia. 1980;20:22–5.

Zhivoderov VM, Zakharov VN, Doshchitsin VL, Kolomeĭtseva SP, Aksenova TN. Use of hyperbaric oxygenation for treating arrhythmias in ischemic heart disease. Klin Med (Mosk). 1982;60:51–5.

HBO Therapy in Hematology and Immunology

26

K.K. Jain

Abstract

This chapter examines the effect of HBO on various elements of the blood: red blood cells (RBCs), white blood cells (WBCs), platelets, and hemoglobin. Particular attention is paid to the effect of HBO on stem cells. Effects on hemorheology and hematology parameters are considered in view of the role of HBO in the management of coagulation disorders as well as plasma and blood volume depletion. HBO has clinical applications in certain hematological and immunological disorders.

Keywords

HBO and platelets • Hematology • Hemorheology • Hyperbaric oxygen (HBO) • Immunology • Red blood cells (RBCs)

Introduction

This chapter will examine the important effects of hyperbaric oxygenation on the elements of the blood. The overall effect is improvement of hemorheology, which is useful in many microcirculation disorders. The effect of HBO in lowering hematocrit and whole blood viscosity and increasing the RBC elasticity has been used in treating disorders of the inner ear. The effect of HBO on constituents of the blood and its applications in hematological disorders, which are rather limited, will be discussed in this chapter. Immunological effects of HBO are also considered as they involve the leukocytes.

Effect of HBO on Red Blood Cells

The major function of red blood cells (RBCs) is to transport hemoglobin, which in turn carries oxygen from the lungs to the tissues. They also contain carbonic anhydrase, which catalyzes the reaction between CO_2 and H_2O, and the product is transported in the form of bicarbonate ion (HCO_2) to the lungs.

K.K. Jain, MD, FRACS, FFPM (✉)
1 Blaesiring 7, Basel 4057, Switzerland
e-mail: jain@pharmabiotech.ch

Deformability

RBCs are concave discs with a mean diameter of 8 μm and a maximum thickness of 2 μm at the periphery and 1 μm or less at the center. The average volume of the RBC is 83 μm³. As the RBC passes through the capillaries, it can be deformed into any shape. This deformability is an important determinant of whole blood viscosity, particularly in the microcirculation, where capillary diameter is smaller than the RBC diameter. This contributes to the inversion phenomenon—increased viscosity at the capillary level compared with larger vessels. The RBC can traverse a channel 14 μm long and 2.8 μm wide and can squeeze through a 0.5 μm opening between cells. The deformability of the RBC depends upon the normal hemoglobin structure, as well as adenosine triphosphate (ATP) stores. A normal RBC can undergo deformation without stretching the membrane or rupturing it. This ability of the RBC is an important factor in the microcirculation and tissue oxygen exchange.

Animal experimental studies of the effect of HBO on RBC deformability give conflicting results. Higher pressures usually transiently decrease the deformability. Pressures below 2 ATA usually increase the deformability. Erythrocyte elasticity increases, and hematocrit drops in healthy volunteers exercising under HBO at 1.5 ATA. This improves the ability of the

RBC to navigate the capillaries and improve oxygenation of the tissues. The maximum oxygen delivery to the tissues is at a hematocrit level of 30–33 % (Fig. 26.1), which is significantly lower than the normal hematocrit range of 36–47 % at sea level.

Oxygen Exchange

Oxygen transport requires diffusion of oxygen into the RBC and chemical combination with intracellular hemoglobin. Oxygen does not combine with the two positive valences of the ferrous iron in the hemoglobin molecule (Fig. 26.2). Instead, it binds loosely with one of the six "coordination" valences of the iron atom. This is an extremely loose bond so that the combination is easily reversible. Furthermore, the oxygen does not become ionic oxygen, but is carried on to the tissues as molecular oxygen. There, because of the loose, readily reversible combination, it is released into the tissue fluids in the form of dissolved molecular oxygen rather than ionic oxygen.

Several factors, including RBC morphology and physiology, influence the rate of these processes. Cell size and shape define the surface area available for oxygen influx into the cytoplasm. Intracellular hemoglobin concentration determines the maximum amount of oxygen that can diffuse in and out of the cell, and changes in intracellular pH or organic phosphate concentration shift the rate of chemical reaction between oxygen and hemoglobin.

Studies of the kinetics of oxygen uptake of RBCs reveal that:

- The rate of oxygen uptake roughly depends on the second power of the surface area to volume ratio of the RBC, whereas the rate of release is much less dependent on these factors.
- The rate of RBC oxygenation is independent of the pH and internal 2,3-diphosphoglycerate (DPG) concentration, whereas the deoxygenation depends markedly on these conditions.

As pH is lowered or DPG concentration is raised, the overall oxygen affinity of the cell decreases sevenfold and oxygen release increased by the same extent. Under hyperoxic conditions, oxygen release reaches its maximum value at a partial pressure of 300 mmHg in resting cells and 100–200 mmHg in flowing cells. The efficient release of oxygen from RBCs depends upon oxygen and oxyhemoglobin diffusion, as well as intracellular convection as a result of deformation of RBCs during flow.

Fig. 26.1 Relation of hematocrit, hemoglobin, and viscosity to relative oxygen transport capacity

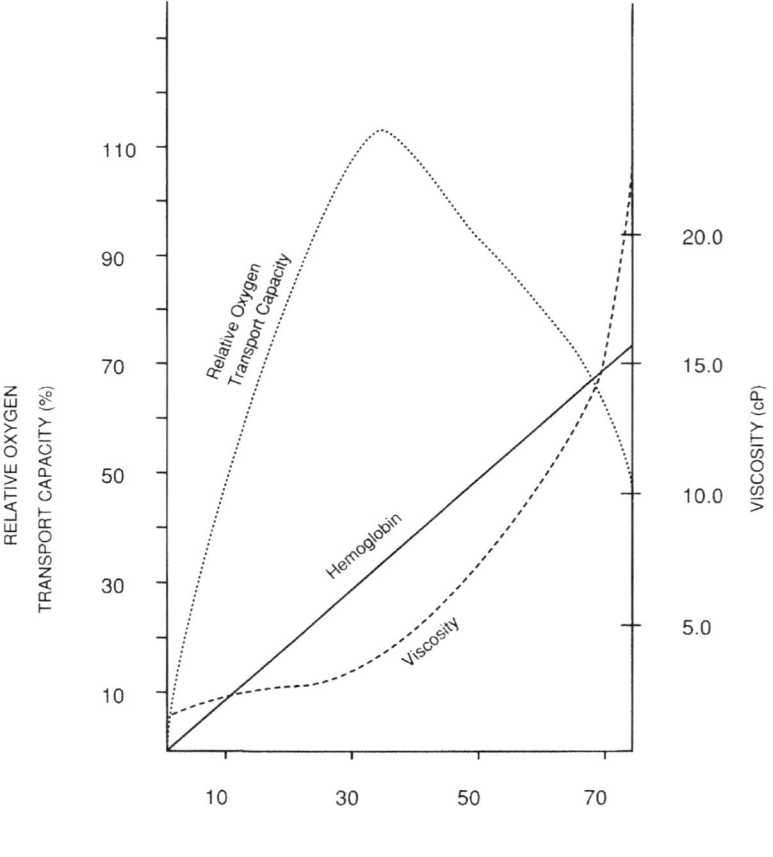

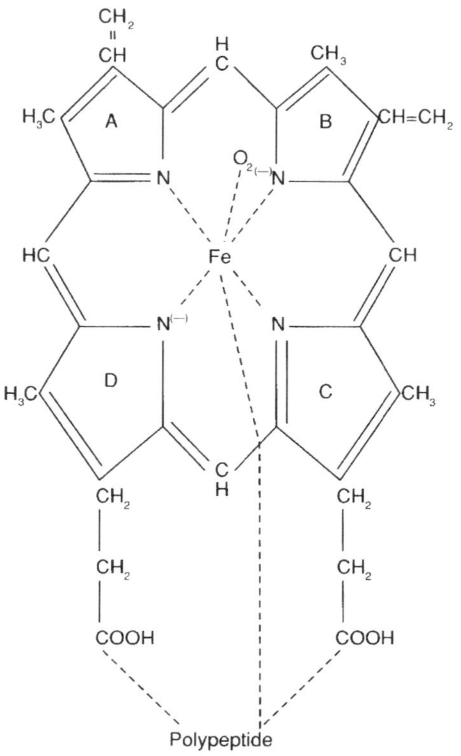

Fig. 26.2 Basic structure of the hemoglobin molecule

The normal oxygen tension difference between RBCs and plasma is small, 6 mmHg or less. In anemia larger differences may exist between RBC pO_2 and plasma pO_2 because the diffusion of oxygen from the RBC lags behind tissue demand. Hemoglobin, which is outside the red cells (3 %), enhances transfer and diminishes these differences.

Structure and Biochemistry

There are several changes in RBCs after exposure to HBO. Hemolysis and reduction of hematocrit may occur. Effects such as these may be related to alterations of membrane structures, which are largely composed of phospholipids and may undergo peroxidation. The levels of several phospholipids in plasma and RBCs are reduced following hyperoxygenation. Under hyperoxia there is a decrease in the RBC levels of ATP and DPG. This is accompanied by a decrease in the active RBC K^+ flux. It has already been mentioned (Chap. 5) that under hypoxic conditions, the level of organic phosphates, particularly DPG, is increased. The decrease of ATP with hyperoxia may be due to inhibition of glycolytic enzymes. It may also be pointed out that it is the combined level of both DPG and ATP that are significant in determining the oxygen affinity of the hemoglobin.

Rats continually exposed to 100 % oxygen at sea level for a few months show no changes in RBC mass, plasma vol-ume, or plasma iron turnover, but prolonged exposure to high pressures of oxygen (>3.5 ATA) may lead to deformity of RBCs due to toxic effect, and rupture may occur. Rarely, hemolytic anemia has been reported after exposure to HBO (2 ATA). Experimental studies on vitamin E-deficient mice indicate that hemolysis may occur due to sensitivity to hydrogen peroxide demonstrated in vitro. RBC hemolysis may manifest as drop in hemoglobin and hematocrit levels with a transient rise in bilirubin and reticulocyte percentage.

The reduced glutathione (GSH) content of the intact erythrocytes is increased by 15 % after HBO exposure and remains so for 24 h after the cessation of therapy. The erythrocyte phospholipid fatty acid turnover is inhibited, and this may be an early biomarker of oxygen toxicity. HBO at 3 ATA for 2 h does not affect the GSH content of the RBC. In oxygen-induced seizures, morphological changes have been observed in RBC, which are likely the result of a decrease in the quantity of SOD. There are changes in the membrane that are likely due to free radical formation. These changes are not found in RBCs during epileptic seizures.

Effect of HBO on Stored Blood

Human RBCs stored at 4 °C for 3 weeks at 2 ATA are more resistant to hemolysis caused by osmotic fragility than are RBCs stored at sea level for the same period. The increased viability of the cellular membranes at depth is due to diminution of the metabolic rate and reduced binding of ATP and DPG to hemoglobin resulting in conservation of energy metabolism with a more viable glucose transport and lipid synthesis mechanism. HBO exposure has positive effects on pH, stability of RBCs, and energy source (glucose) of the medium, which may be a useful application for life and quality of stored blood (Ay et al. 2015).

Hemoglobin

Hemoglobin is a respiratory pigment and enables blood to carry high levels of nascent, molecular oxygen at 1 ATA in chemical solution to capillary beds that supply cells of all organ systems in the body. If hemoglobin drops below critical levels, e.g., by severe loss of blood, adequate oxygen delivery is not possible, and HBO may be used for temporary supply of urgently needed oxygen.

Exposure to hyperoxia in individuals with normal hemoglobin can reduce hemoglobin and increased ferritin concentrations. The changes may reflect a shift of iron from synthesis of hemoglobin in the bone marrow to storage in macrophages caused by a downregulation of hemoglobin synthesis or an increased oxidative stress. The changes are too small to be of clinical significance with respect to HBO treatment.

Erythropoiesis

The principal factor that stimulates RBC production is a circulating hormone called erythropoietin, most of which is formed in the kidneys. Tissue oxygen is the basic regulator of RBC production. Any condition that causes the quantity of oxygen transported to the tissues to decrease increases the rate of RBC production. Increase of oxygen tension in the blood inhibits erythropoiesis and diminishes RBC production.

The erythropoietin content of the plasma of the peripheral blood has been investigated in volunteers exposed for the first time to the action of hyperbaric hyperoxia simulating diving (Voitkevich et al. 1979). The pressure was 7 ATA and the breathing mixture was $25\% \ O_2 + 15\% \ He + 60\% \ N_2$, so that the pO_2 rose to 1400 mmHg. After 10 min the pressure was lowered to 2.5 ATA, and decompression was continued so that the total procedure took 40 min. The concentration of erythropoietic factor in the plasma was markedly reduced 24 h after exposure, but no erythropoiesis-inhibiting factors were detected in the plasma.

Erythropoiesis is suppressed in mice exposed to HBO at 4 ATA for 24 h, and it cannot be stimulated by administration of exogenous erythropoietin. The fact is that the RBC count does not increase in response to hypoxia or decrease in response to hyperoxia within 24 h. Therefore, hyperbaric exposures should not result in a drop in the count of RBC unless the pressure is maintained for prolonged periods, which is not the case in clinical applications.

Effect of HBO on Hemorheology in Human Patients

Hemorheological and hematological parameters such as RBC deformability and aggregation, blood and plasma viscosity, and superoxide dismutase activity were investigated in patients who underwent HBO treatment using an electronic hematology analyzer (Sinan et al 2015). Results of the study revealed a significant decrease of the hematocrit and the RBC count after the 20th session of HBO compared to the baseline, but none of the hemorheological parameters changed significantly. These results show that HBO did not cause any significant changes in hemorheology that might pose any problems for the patients.

Effect of HBO on Leukocytes

Some experimental studies in rats indicate that HBO causes a metabolic derangement in polymorphonuclear leukocytes that impaired the function of B2-integrins. HBO inhibits B2-integrin-dependent adherence because it impairs cGMP synthesis by activated neutrophils. In contrast to experimental data, repetitive exposure of human patients to hyperoxia does not influence human monocyte and lymphocyte functions.

Effect of HBO on Platelets and Coagulation

Exposure to hyperbaric conditions influences the coagulation system; thromboembolic events and disseminated intravascular coagulation have been observed. Previously reported fibrinolysis has not been confirmed.

A single exposure of isolated horse platelets to 100 % oxygen at 2.2 ATA showed no detrimental effect on platelet biochemistry, and it does not cause overt oxidative stress in vitro (Shaw et al. 2005). In a study on human patients exposed to 90 min of HBO intermittently at 2.4 ATA as in a wound-healing protocol, point-of-care coagulation analyzers were used (Monaca et al 2014). Multiplate showed a platelet activation mediated by thrombin (AU TRAP test) and by arachidonic acid (AUC ASPI test). Standard laboratory assays revealed a lower activated partial thromboplastin time and a higher leukocyte count. These indicate activation of platelets after HBO therapy via thrombin and arachidonic acid pathways.

There are concerns about the cytotoxicity of oxygen to platelet function during prolonged HBO therapy. A study was conducted on patients scheduled for multiple HBO treatments in order to evaluate oxidative metabolism in platelets and platelet aggregation (Handy et al 2005). The capacity for oxidative metabolism (lactate ratio) in platelets was not affected by HBO, except in smokers, where it increased by the 20th HBO treatment. There was also a 23 % increase in platelet protein content and a 24 % increase in arachidonic acid-dependent platelet activation. Collagen-dependent platelet aggregation was unaffected. Overall, there was no evidence that 20 HBO sessions caused adverse effects on platelet aggregation or oxidative metabolism in platelets or total antioxidant status of the plasma.

Effect of HBO on Stem Cells

Stem cells have two important characteristics that distinguish them from other types of cells. First, they are unspecialized cells that renew themselves for long periods through cell division. The second is that, under certain physiological or experimental conditions, they can be induced to become cells with special functions such as myocytes (cells of the heart muscle) or the insulin-producing cells of the pancreas. In the embryo, these cells are the starting point for the development of the complete human being. In the adult body, stem cells are one of the mechanisms for the repair and renewal of some cells and tissues.

Embryonic stem cells (ESCs) are continuously growing stem cell lines of embryonic origin derived from the pluripo-

Table 26.1 Combination of stem cells and HBO in models of neurological disorders

Type of stem cell	Experimental model/reference	Effect and mechanism
Neural stem cells (NSCs)	NSCs, isolated from rat cortex, exposed to HBO at 2 ATA for 60 min (Chen et al. 2010)	HBO promotes differentiation of NSCs into neurons
Endogenous NSCs	Neonatal rat with hypoxic-ischemic brain damage given HBO at 2 ATA once daily for 1 week (Wang et al. 2009)	NSCs migrate to the cortex and differentiate into mature neurocytes
	Similar study with focus on NSCs in the subventricular zone (Feng et al. 2013)	Proliferation of NSCs in the subventricular zone with potential clinical application in neonatal hypoxic-ischemic encephalopathy
Amniotic fluid mesenchymal stem cells (MSCs)	Rat sciatic nerve injury model treated with local application of MSCs in combination with HBO at 2 ATA once daily for 1 h (Pan et al. 2009)	Peripheral nerve regeneration was enhanced by suppression of apoptosis in implanted cells and the attenuation of an inflammatory response
Circulating stem cells	In a mouse model of ischemia, exposure to HBO 2.8 ATA for 90 min combined with lactate as an oxidative stressor (Milovanova et al. 2009)	HBO plus lactate activates a physiological redox-active autocrine loop in stem cell, which stimulates vasculogenic growth and differentiation of SCs in vivo

tent cells of the inner cell mass or epiblast of the mammalian embryo. They may give rise to any cell type but not to an independent organism. Embryonic germ cell lines, established from primitive reproductive cells of the embryo, are functionally equivalent to ESCs. The distinguishing features of ESCs are their capacity to be maintained in an undifferentiated state indefinitely in culture and their potential to develop into every cell of the body. Their ability to develop into a wide range of cell types makes ESCs as a useful basic research tool and a novel source of cell populations for new therapies. Human embryonic stem cell (hESC) is a type of pluripotent stem cell derived from the inner cell mass of the preimplantation blastocyst produced by sperm–egg fertilization.

Further details of stem cells are described elsewhere (Jain 2016). This chapter includes a brief description of role of stem cells in hematology and effect of HBO on stem cells. Autologous transplantation of hematopoietic stem cells (HSCs) from patients with genetic hematological disorders and immunodeficiencies could provide the same benefits as allogeneic HSC transplantation, without the attendant immunological complications. Autologous HSCs have been used as targets of gene transfer, with applications in inherited disorders, cell therapy, and acquired immunodeficiency. The types of cells include hematopoietic progenitor cells, lymphocytes, and mesenchymal stem cells (MSCs). Preclinical studies have been conducted in thalassemia, sickle cell anemia, Wiskott–Aldrich syndrome, and Fanconi anemia.

The bone marrow is home to MSCs that are able to differentiate into many different cell types. The effect of HBO on MSCs is poorly understood. Placental growth factor (PlGF) is an attractive therapeutic agent for stimulating revascularization of ischemic tissue. HBO has been shown to improve diabetic wound healing by increasing circulating stem cells. HBO mobilizes stem/progenitor cells by stimulating NO synthesis (Thom et al. 2006). HBO induces PlGF expression in bone

marrow-derived MSCs at least through the oxidative stress-related pathways, which may play an important role in HBO-induced vasculogenesis (Shyu et al 2008).

Ability of HBO to mobilize stem cells as well as synergistic effect in treatment of animal models of neurological disorders is shown in Table 26.1. These findings indicate potential clinical applications that would be worth investigating further.

Effect of HBO Treatment on the Immune System

HBO has been reported to have both a stimulant and a depressant effect on the immune system, depending upon the pressure used and the experimental model.

De Graeve et al. (1976) studied the effect of HBO (2 ATA, 5 h) on the thymus of adult rats. There was hyperplasia of the cortex after a transient depression. The newly formed thymic cells migrated and were stored in the red pulp of the spleen. The authors concluded that HBO has a stimulating effect on thymic cells and that this can be considered to belong to the general phenomenon of immune defense. Lotovin et al. (1981) reported a study of the problem of cellular and humoral activity under hyperoxia. They found that six sessions of HBO at 2.5 ATA resulted in an increase of T lymphocytes in guinea pigs. When pressure was raised to 5 ATA for 30 min, a form of oxygen toxicity occurred with depression of the functional activity of the T lymphocytes and a decrease in the cellular indices of immunity in the blood. The animals recovered from this 10 days after the exposure. In patients who were given 15 daily sessions of HBO at 2.5 ATA (60 min), the number of T lymphocytes increased 1.4-fold and that of B lymphocytes 2.8-fold. There was also an increase in all the immunoglobulins.

Feldmeier and Boswell (1987) analyzed a broad range of immune responses in nine healthy human volunteers exposed to 20 treatments of HBO at 2.4 ATA over 4 weeks. They found no effect on the immune system of these subjects.

Bitterman and Melamud (1993) studied the effect of a single exposure to HBO (2.8 ATA for 90 min) on blood mononuclear subset in healthy volunteers. Immediately after the exposure, a significant increase was observed in the percentage and absolute number of CD8 (suppressor/cytotoxic) T cells, with a concomitant decrease in the CD4 (helper/inducer) T cells as compared with controls. The result was a decreased CD4:CD8 ratio. A rise was also observed in the number of HLA-DR antigen-bearing cells with a transient increase in monocytes. These changes were only partially reversed 24 h following HBO exposure and suggest specific HBO-induced shifts and sequestration of T cell subpopulations.

Biriukov et al. (1988) observed that the number of lymphocytes is diminished after surgery and that HBO stimulates lymphocyte production and improves the patient's resistance against infections in the postoperative period.

Published evidence supports the beneficial effect of HBO on type I hypersensitivity reactions, i.e., anaphylactic reaction, by reducing the level of immunoglobulins IgE and IgG. This may also explain the beneficial effect of HBO observed in asthma. Reported increase of complement activity in the serum following HBO exposure may be of benefit in counteracting hypersensitivity reactions of types II and III. There is evidence also for the benefit of HBO on type IV hypersensitivity reactions.

HBO has been found to mitigate immune reactions, many of which are involved in rejection of allograft transplants, and thus offers a rationale for its possible use as an adjunct to help preserve and protect transplanted tissues (see Chap. 37). Rejection may involve both immunological reactions of the lymphoid system or lymphoid-independent damage from trauma or other factors, including reperfusion injury. Lymphoid-induced damage involves cellular elements such as CD4 and macrophage cell types, as well as both proinflammatory and inhibitory cytokines. Cytokines such as TNFs and interleukins activate T cells and macrophages, resulting in endothelial damage and its consequences. The immunosuppressive effects of HBO include suppression of autoimmune symptoms, decreased production of IL-1 and CD4 cells, and increased percentage and absolute number of CD8 cells (Al-Waili et al. 2006). HBO improves engraftment of ex vivo expanded and gene transduced human CD34+ cells in a murine model of umbilical cord blood transplantation (Aljitawi et al. 2014). HBO normalizes cell-bound immunity and decreases the serum concentration of immune complexes. Studies have shown MHC class I expression to be altered when cultures were exposed to HBO, so as to become undetectable by monoclonal antibodies or cytotoxic T lymphocytes. In addition to its specific effects on the immune system, HBO improves tissue oxygenation, reduces free radical damage during reperfusion, maintains marginally ischemic tissue, and accelerates wound healing.

In conclusion, a great deal of work still needs to be done on the immunological aspects of HBO, but it is important as it may explain the beneficial effect of HBO in infections, disorders of the immune system, and transplantation.

Effect of HBO Treatment on Plasma and Blood Volume

It has already been mentioned in Chap. 2 that enough oxygen (6 vol.%) can be dissolved in plasma to support life. The classical study on the subject of life without blood was made by Boerema et al. (1959). The authors lowered the level of hemoglobin in young pigs to 0.4 % by exchanging the blood for plasma by venesection. The animals breathing oxygen at a pressure of 3 ATA in the hyperbaric chamber lived for 45 min with a level of hemoglobin that would be incompatible with life at atmospheric pressure. These animals were kept alive virtually without any hemoglobin. ECG showed no changes, and the circulation and the blood pressure remained spontaneously normal. Recovery was uneventful after reinfusion of blood prior to decompression to the surface. Bokeria et al. (1979) reported the use of hemodilution up to 55 %. HBO was able to provide adequate oxygenation during open-heart surgery. Koziner et al. (1981) replaced 94–98 % of the blood volume with dextran in cats and kept them alive for 8–9 h, breathing 100 % oxygen.

The effect of hyperoxia on oxygen uptake (VO_2) during acute anemia is being reexamined experimentally. Chapler et al. (1984) anesthetized dogs and ventilated them for 20-min periods with room air (normoxia), 100 % oxygen (hyperoxia), and then normoxia again. Anemia was then induced by isovolemic dextran-for-blood exchange, and the sequence of normoxia–hyperoxia–normoxia was repeated. Whole-body VO_2 and cardiac output rose following hypoxia during anemia. Both of these values fell following hyperoxia. The authors postulated that this could result from redistribution of the capillary blood flow away from exchange vessels in response to elevated pO_2. It was mentioned previously that hematocrit falls after exposure to HBO. Buxton et al. (1964) reported that anesthetized dogs exposed to 3 ATA at 100 % oxygen showed a marked elevation of hematocrit. This effect did not occur in controls kept at 1 ATA, splenectomized, or given buffering agents. The authors postulated that rise of hematocrit was due to splenic contracture. In evaluating this report, it must be borne in mind that dogs under pentobarbital anesthesia sequester up to 30 % of blood volume in the spleen and release it into the circulation in response to catecholamines, which could result from the stress of HBO and/or anesthesia.

The Use of HBO in Conjunction with Oxygen Carriers

In recently reported studies, rats, subjected to loss of about half their blood volume causing respiratory arrest, were resuscitated by the intravenous infusion of 6% hetastarch in lactated electrolyte injection and HBO (Segal 2003). In the experiments, six of nine rats resuscitated with the plasma expander and treated with 100% oxygen at 2 ATA survived long term in comparison to survival of only 1 of the 11 rats given the same intravenous infusion but ventilated with 100% oxygen at atmospheric pressure. The results were statistically significant and confirmed previous experiments in which HBO had been shown to be advantageous in reviving rats following hemorrhagic shock causing a near-death condition. While hemorrhaging, and in the following period of respiratory arrest, all the animals' body temperatures declined. Restoring body temperature to normal by externally warming the animal was also an important feature of the resuscitation process.

Clinical Applications of HBO in Disorders of the Blood

Hypovolemia and Acute Anemia Due to Blood Loss

The average blood volume of a normal adult is approximately 5000 mL (3000 mL plasma + 2000 mL RBC). After an acute hemorrhage, the body replaces plasma within 1–3 days, but a low concentration of RBCs persists. In chronic blood loss, a person cannot compensate, and the hemoglobin can fall to dangerously low levels (severe anemia). The decrease in viscosity of the blood lowers the resistance to blood flow in the peripheral vessels. The peripheral vessels may dilate further due to the effect of hypoxia. The major impact is an increased workload on the heart and increased cardiac output. This may be able to sustain the individual at rest, but during exercise, which greatly increases the tissue demands on oxygen, it can lead to extreme tissue hypoxia with acute cardiac failure. The conventional treatment consists of whole blood or packed RBC transfusion and, if possible, correction of the cause.

There are problems with blood transfusion because of fear of contamination with HIV. There are difficulties in administering blood in some situations, particularly in patients who are Jehovah's Witnesses, since they do not accept any blood or blood component because of their religious beliefs. An alternative method for oxygenation of the blood is by oxygen carriers or blood substitutes.

HBO can temporarily meet the oxygen needs of the body in the absence of blood and has been termed "bloodless transfusion." Amonic et al. (1969) reported the case of a Jehovah's Witness with gastric bleeding and a hemoglobin level of 2.2 g/100 mL who refused blood transfusion, but survived with HBO treatment.

Hart (1974) reported 3 patients who were dying of acute blood loss anemia and whom he treated successfully with HBO. All three had very low hemoglobin levels (2–3 g/100 mL), hematocrit of 10–11.5%, and falling blood pressure, as well as a rising pulse rate. The treatment in all cases was limited to intravenous fluids, intramuscular iron dextran, and HBO at 2 ATA for 60–90 min. HBO was repeated whenever the pulse rate rose above 120. All the patients improved dramatically, and in one case the hemoglobin rose from 2 to 8 g in 1 week of treatment. Adjunctive HBO therapy should be considered in the management of patients with exceptional severe blood loss anemia who refuse the use of blood products (Graffeo and Dishong 2013). HBO can be used as an interim measure to save patients and improve their condition for more definite measures, such as surgical correction of the primary pathology or the cause of bleeding.

After this experience, Hart et al. (1987) further treated 23 patients using HBO. Of the 26 patients, 6 patients who arrived in a decerebrate state with Hb of 3.8 g/dL and Hct of 10.5% died. The survivors had somewhat higher Hb (4.79 g/dL) and Hct (13.6%) on admission. Treatment was discontinued in the survivors when they no longer suffered from hypoxic sprue, postural hypotension, and when Hct was >22% and Hb >7 g/dL. The authors concluded that HBO may be useful in the treatment of acute blood loss anemia if applied early.

Treatment with HBO favorably affects recovery from adverse effects moderate acute blood loss in experimental animals and hastens recovery to baseline hemoglobin levels. These observations support the successful use of HBO treating extreme blood loss in humans. HBO enables oxygen to be dissolved in higher concentration in RBC-deficient or crystalloid/colloid-diluted intravascular fluids in a volume-resuscitated patient. Pulsed, intermittent NBO or HBO induces an increase in RBC/hemoglobin mass in subacute as well as chronic anemic patients (Van Meter 2012). Although search for an ideal blood substitute or artificial blood continues, physically dissolved oxygen has advantages over chemically bound oxygen under some circumstances. Besides the necessary volume effects (isoosmotic) and physiological bicarbonate concentration (prevention of dilutional acidosis), the solution should be shear-rate independent (having Newtonian behavior). Oxygen concentration at the given oxygen partial pressure should be at least 6 mL/dL. Such a blood substitute should be evaluated by means of the oxygen supply index:

$$\frac{(\text{oxygen concentration}) \times (\text{mean capillary oxygen pressure in mmHg})}{\text{viscosity}}$$

HBO can reliably reduce oxygen debt in exsanguination with cardiopulmonary arrest as well as in severely anemic patient who cannot be transfused with blood if it is not available or because of immunologic problems or religious beliefs. One HBO treatment is equivalent in cost to a unit of packed RBCs in the Western world. Thus HBO provides a low-technology, cost-competitive means of pharmacologically reducing accumulated oxygen debt in the anemic, injured, or critically ill patient with low risk of adverse effects. Potential applications of HBO include battlefield casualties and trauma centers. In the hospital setting, HBO will be useful in emergency departments, operation/recovery rooms, and intensive care units.

Hemolytic Anemia

Hemolysis of RBC may occur from a variety of causes, some of which are hereditary and others acquired. One example is sickle cell anemia. It is present in 0.3–1.0 % of West Africans and American blacks. RBCs in this condition contain an abnormal hemoglobin called hemoglobin S. When this hemoglobin is exposed to a low concentration of oxygen, it is precipitated into long crystals inside the RBC. The crystals elongate the cell and give it the appearance of a sickle rather than a biconcave disc. The precipitated hemoglobin also damages the cell membrane so that the cells become highly fragile, leading to severe anemia. Such patients suffer a phenomenon called sickle cell disease crisis with a sequence of events as follows:

Low oxygen tension in tissues → sickling → impairment of blood flow through the tissues → further decrease of oxygen tension

Once the process starts, it progresses rapidly, leading to a severe decrease of RBC mass and possible death. Oxygen has been used at the crisis stage to combat hypoxia, and the potential of HBO should be investigated. Patients with sickling hemoglobinopathies, including sickle cell trait, have an increased risk of permanent loss of vision following hyperemia caused by blunt trauma. RBCs with hemoglobin S sickle more readily in the aqueous humor of the eye than in the venous blood, become trapped, and lead to secondary glaucoma. HBO at 2 ATA for 2 h was successful in reducing the number of sickle cells injected into the anterior chamber of the eyes in rabbits (Wallyn et al. 1985).

There are anecdotal reports of the successful use of HBO for complications of sickle cell disease. Vaso-occlusive crisis (VOC) is the most frequent complication of sickle cell disease and is associated with significant acute bone pain. Effect of HBO on bone pain was tested in a retrospective study of HBO in VOC in 9 patients who had received appropriate conventional treatment prior to 15 sessions of HBO (Stirnemann et al. 2012). Pain scores using a visual analog scale (0–10) are determined whether HBO was effective or not in improving symptoms. Pain scores fell significantly from 3.3 prior to HBO to 1.9 24 h after HBO. The median

morphine dose 1 day after HBO tended to be lower than the day before and decreased to zero 2 days after HBO.

The central retinal artery was diagnosed by fluorescein angiography in a young man with a history of sickle cell disease who developed sudden painless loss of vision in the left eye (Canan et al. 2014). He underwent exchange transfusion and HBO therapy, and in the following 3 months, his visual acuity improved to 20/30.

Priapism affects up to 50 % of all males with sickle cell disease, and there is no standard treatment. Delayed and unsuccessful treatment leads to corporal fibrosis and impotence. An 11-year-old patient with sickle cell disease was presented with priapism 72 h after onset and was successfully treated with automated red cell exchange and HBO following unsuccessful surgical and conventional interventions (Azık et al. 2012).

Mismatched blood or cell transfusion can also cause hemolytic anemia. HBO has also been used for hemolysis due to mismatched transfusion.

Potential Benefits of HBO in Cerebrovascular Diseases Due to Blood Disorders

The relationship of the blood to the brain is quite apparent in cerebrovascular diseases. Primary RBC disorders cause cerebral ischemia by adversely affecting oxygen delivery or CBF. Hemoglobinopathies limit the binding and delivery of oxygen and cause altered erythrocyte shape and increased viscosity, as well as anemia. This moves oxygen delivery away from the apex of the parabolic curve (see Fig. 26.1). Therapy of cerebral ischemia may be aimed at altering the viscosity or the properties of RBC in order to improve oxygen delivery. HBO, in addition to providing oxygenation, also improves blood rheology parameters such as Hct and RBC deformability. These may prove to be additional benefits to the useful role of HBO in combating cerebral ischemic and metabolic sequelae of stroke.

Li et al. (1986) studied the hemorheology of patients with cerebrovascular disease treated by HBO (2.5 ATA, 100 % oxygen for 45 min, air break for 15 min, twice daily). They found that there was decrease of Hct and blood viscosity as well as of platelet aggregation. The oxygenation of the brain was improved in these cases without increasing the Hct.

Contraindication: Congenital Spherocytosis

In congenital spherocytosis, the RBCs are rigid and less deformable than normal. HBO is considered to be contraindicated because of the risk of increased hemolysis. Even though no reports were found in literature about this complication, the following precautions are recommended in patients with congenital spherocytosis who need HBO treatment for another medical condition:

- Close monitoring of the hemogram, hemolysis parameters, and vitamin E levels
- Supplementary vitamin E
- Cessation of HBO therapy if there is any evidence of hemolysis

References

Aljitawi OS, Xiao Y, Eskew JD, Parelkar NK, Swink M, Radel J, et al. Hyperbaric oxygen improves engraftment of ex-vivo expanded and gene transduced human CD34+ cells in a murine model of umbilical cord blood transplantation. Blood Cells Mol Dis. 2014;52:59–67.

Al-Waili NS, Butler GJ, Petrillo RL, et al. Hyperbaric oxygen and lymphoid system function: a review supporting possible intervention in tissue transplantation. Technol Health Care. 2006;14:489–98.

Amonic RS, Cockett AT, Lorhan PH, Thompson JC. Hyperbaric oxygen therapy in chronic hemorrhagic shock. JAMA. 1969;208:2051–4.

Ay H, Yüksel R, Şimşek K, Topal T, Yeşilyurt Ö, Öter Ş, et al. A new utilization area for hyperbaric oxygen? Improving quality of stored blood. Turk J Med Sci. 2015;45:105–11.

Azık FM, Atay A, Kürekçi AE, Ay H, Kibar Y, Ozcan O. Treatment of priapism with automated red cell exchange and hyperbaric oxygen in an 11-year-old patient with sickle cell disease. Turk J Haematol. 2012;29:270–3.

Biriukov IB, Tsygankova ST, Bronskaia LK, Namazbekov BK, Akimova NI. Immunological indicators as the criteria of prognosis and treatment of nonspecific diseases of the lungs and pleura. Vestn Khir. 1988;140:10–3.

Bitterman H, Melamud Y. Delayed hyperbaric treatment of cerebral air embolism. Israel J Med Sci. 1993;29:22–6.

Boerema I, Meyne NG, Brummelkamp WH, Bouma S, Mensch MH, Kamermans F, et al. Life without blood. Arch Chir Neer. 1959;11:70–83.

Bokeria LA, Krutik IG, Khapyi KK, Gadzhiev AA. The characteristics of EEG, ECG and hemodynamics in artificial circulation with hemodilution under hyperbaric oxygenation. Anesteziol Reanimatol. 1979;4:23–8.

Buxton JT, Stallworth JM, Bradham GB. Hematocrit changes under hyperbaric oxygen. Am Surg. 1964;30:18–22.

Canan H, Ulas B, Altan-Yaycioglu R. Hyperbaric oxygen therapy in combination with systemic treatment of sickle cell disease presenting as central retinal artery occlusion: a case report. J Med Case Rep. 2014;8:370.

Chapler CK, Cain SM, Stainsby WN. The effects of hyperoxia on oxygen uptake during acute anemia. Can J Physiol Pharmacol. 1984;62:809–12.

Chen CF, Yang YJ, Wang QH, Yao Y, Li M. Effect of hyperbaric oxygen administered at different pressures and different exposure time on differentiation of neural stem cells in vitro. Zhongguo Dang Dai Er Ke Za Zhi. 2010;12:368–72.

De Graeve PH, Bimes C, Barthelemy R, et al. Histological modifications of the guinea pig thymus subjected to hyperbaric oxygen. Bull Assoc Anat (Nancy). 1976;60:663–7.

Feldmeier JJ, Boswell RN. The effect of hyperbaric oxygen on the immunologic status of healthy human subjects. In: Kindwall EP, editor. Proceedings of the 8th international congress on hyperbaric medicine. San Pedro: Best; 1987. p. 41–6.

Feng Z, Liu J, Ju R. Hyperbaric oxygen promotes neural stem cell proliferation in subventricular zone of neonatal rats with hypoxic-ischemic brain damage. Neural Regen Res. 2013;8:120–7.

Graffeo C, Dishong W. Severe blood loss anemia in a Jehovah's Witness treated with adjunctive hyperbaric oxygen therapy. Am J Emerg Med. 2013;31:756, e3–4.

Handy RD, Bryson P, Moody AJ, Handy LM, Sneyd JR. Oxidative metabolism in platelets, platelet aggregation, and hematology in patients undergoing multiple hyperbaric oxygen exposures. Undersea Hyperb Med. 2005;32:327–40.

Hart GB. Exceptional blood loss anemia. Treatment with hyperbaric oxygen. JAMA. 1974;288:1028–9.

Hart GB, Lennon PA, Strauss MB. Hyperbaric oxygen in exceptional acute blood-loss anemia. J Hyperbaric Med. 1987;2:205–10.

Jain KK. Cell therapy. Basel: Jain PharmaBiotech; 2016.

Koziner VB, Yarochkin VS, Fedorov NA, Kolonina IR. Life support by oxygen breathing after total blood replacement by dextran. Exp Biol Med. 1981;91:444–6.

Li XL, Li WR, Lin HY. Effect of hyperbaric oxygen therapy on the patients' blood rheology. In: Presented at the 5th Chinese conference on hyperbaric medicine, Fuzhow, China, 26–29 Sept 1986.

Lotovin AP, Morozov VG, Khavinson VK, et al. On the problem of cellular and humoral activity under conditions of hyperoxia. In: Yefuni SN (Ed.). Proceedings of the 7th international congress on hyperbaric medicine. USSR Academy of Sciences, Moscow, 1981, p. 399.

Milovanova TN, Bhopale VM, Sorokina EM, Moore JS, Hunt TK, Hauer-Jensen M, et al. Hyperbaric oxygen stimulates vasculogenic stem cell growth and differentiation in vivo. J Appl Physiol. 2009;106:711–28.

Monaca E, Strelow H, Jüttner T, Hoffmann T, Potempa T, Windolf J, et al. Assessment of hemostaseologic alterations induced by hyperbaric oxygen therapy using point-of-care analyzers. Undersea Hyperb Med. 2014;41:17–26.

Pan HC, Chin CS, Yang DY, Ho SP, Chen CJ, Hwang SM, et al. Human amniotic fluid mesenchymal stem cells in combination with hyperbaric oxygen augment peripheral nerve regeneration. Neurochem Res. 2009;34:1304–16.

Segal P. Hyperbaric oxygen and hypothermia improves revival of Hextend-resuscitated hemorrhagic, apneic rats. In: Presented at the Experimental Biology 2003 conference in San Diego, 15 April 2003.

Shaw FL, Handy RD, Bryson P, Sneyd JR, Moody AJ. A single exposure to hyperbaric oxygen does not cause oxidative stress in isolated platelets: no effect on superoxide dismutase, catalase, or cellular ATP. Clin Biochem. 2005;38:722–6.

Shyu KG, Hung HF, Wang BW, Chang H. Hyperbaric oxygen induces placental growth factor expression in bone marrow-derived mesenchymal stem cells. Life Sci. 2008;83:65–73.

Sinan M, Ertan NZ, Mirasoglu B. Acute and long-term effects of hyperbaric oxygen therapy on hemorheological parameters in patients with various disorders. Clin Hemorheol Microcirc. 2015;62:79–88.

Stirnemann J, Letellier E, Aras N, Borne M, Brinquin L, Fain O. Hyperbaric oxygen therapy for vaso-occlusive crises in nine patients with sickle-cell disease. Diving Hyperb Med. 2012;42:82–4.

Thom SR, Bhopale VM, Velazquez OC, Goldstein LJ, Thom LH, Buerk DG. Stem cell mobilization by hyperbaric oxygen. Am J Physiol Circ Physiol. 2006;290:H1378–86.

Van Meter KW. The effect of hyperbaric oxygen on severe anemia. Undersea Hyperb Med. 2012;39:937–42.

Voitkevich VI, Volzhskaya AM, Korchinskii LA. Effect of hyperbaric hyperoxia on human plasma erythropoiesis inhibitors. Biull Eksp Biol Med. 1979;87:96–8.

Wallyn CR, Jampol LM, Goldberg MF, Zanetti CL. The use of hyperbaric oxygen therapy in the treatment of sickle cell hyphema. Invest Ophthalmol Vis Sci. 1985;26:1155–8.

Wang XL, Yang YJ, Xie M, Yu XH, Wang QH. Hyperbaric oxygen promotes the migration and differentiation of endogenous neural stem cells in neonatal rats with hypoxic-ischemic brain damage. Zhongguo Dang Dai Er Ke Za Zhi. 2009;11:749–52.

K.K. Jain

Abstract

This chapter deals with a wide variety of HBO applications involving the gastrointestinal tract, including its use in dealing with peptic ulceration, intestinal obstruction, adynamic ileus, adhesive intestinal obstruction, infections, ischemic disorders, acute pancreatitis, and diseases of the liver. An important application is in irritable bowel syndrome. Pneumatosis intestinalis is an interesting application with a sound rationale as the trapped air is resolved with high pressure. Experimental studies in animals as well as clinical applications are described.

Keywords

Acute pancreatitis • Adhesive intestinal obstruction • Adynamic ileus • Diseases of the liver • Gastrointestinal disorders • Hyperbaric oxygen (HBO) • Infections • Intestinal obstruction • Irritable bowel syndrome • Ischemic disorders • Peptic ulceration • Pneumatosis intestinalis

Introduction

Hyperbaric oxygen (HBO) therapy has an important role in the management of gastrointestinal disorders. There are, however, few controlled studies. The rationale is the same as for the application of HBO in disorders of other systems: it counteracts ischemia and hypoxia, and it promotes resistance to infections and healing of ulcers. An additional effect is the compression and reduction of volume of gases.

HBO in Peptic Ulceration

Pathophysiology and Rationale of HBO Therapy

A peptic ulcer is a mucosal lesion of the stomach or duodenum in which acid and pepsin play major pathogenic roles.

The major forms of peptic ulceration are duodenal ulcer and gastric ulcer, both of which are chronic diseases caused by the bacterium *Heliobacter pylori*. In addition to the known causes, a few additional factors play a role in progression of ulceration. The gastric epithelium has mainly an aerobic metabolism and is dependent on a constant supply of oxygen for oxidative metabolism. Gastric mucosal ischemia is believed to be a factor in the pathogenesis of acute mucosal injury as occurs in patients with general medical or surgical illnesses (stress ulcers). It is not known whether reduction in blood flow contributes to the development of chronic gastric or duodenal ulcers. Most gastric ulcers occur on the lesser curvature, where there are fewer collateral vessels than on the greater curvature. Whether this anatomical difference leads to reduced blood flow at the lesser curvature has not been proven. Reduced blood flow, venous stasis, or disturbances of microcirculation can lead to hypoxia. It has been shown experimentally that necrosis of the surface epithelium of the gastric mucosa starts at a pO_2 value of 9 mmHg in the dog (Efuni et al. 1986). Studies on patients with gastric ulcers using endoscopic polarography show low pO_2 values near the ulcer margins. These values rise during the initial

K.K. Jain, MD, FRACS, FFPM (✉)
1 Blaesiring 7, Basel 4057, Switzerland
e-mail: jain@pharmabiotech.ch

© Springer International Publishing AG 2017
K.K. Jain, *Textbook of Hyperbaric Medicine*, DOI 10.1007/978-3-319-47140-2_27

stage of healing or regeneration ("red scar" phase) and fall again later in the healing process ("white scar" phase).

Studies of Bowen et al. (1984) point to perturbations in the subepithelial microcirculation concomitant with cellular hypoxia and inhibition of oxidative metabolism as common denominators of cellular injury. Due to functional arteriovenous shunting, there are focal areas of cellular hypoxia even when the total blood flow to the organ is normal or even increased. It is the more severely hypoxic areas in the fundus of the stomach that are susceptible to ulceration when exposed to gastric irritants such as acid and bile. Efuni et al. (1986) concluded that a hypoxic disorder with a fall of energy supply underlies ulcer formation and gave this as a rationale for the use of HBO therapy in patients with gastric ulcers. Earlier attempts to treat local hypoxia of the stomach ulcers by ingesting oxygen foams and oxygen cocktails given by gastric tube were not successful in raising the oxygen tension in the ulcerated areas.

HBO has an antibacterial effect (see Chap. 14). Part of the efficacy of HBO in peptic ulceration may be due to an antibacterial effect against *H. pylori*, although no studies have been done to demonstrate this. This is an area for further investigation. HBO promotes the healing of ulcers of the skin, and there is reason to believe that it will promote healing of mucosal ulcers as well. There is no evidence that HBO affects gastric acid secretion.

Experimental Studies in Animals

Koloskow and Dumurow (1986) induced gastric ulcers in rats using acetic acid (Okabe model). These lesions were morphologically similar to human gastric ulcers. After 10 days, HBO treatment was started at 2 ATA. One 45-min session was given daily for 10 days. In 3 of the 15 animals, there was healing of the ulcer, and in the other 12, the appearance of the ulcer differed from that in controls. There was no necrotic material on the surface, but granular tissue appeared instead, and the ulcer margins showed signs of regeneration. In a second series, HBO was given for 16 sessions. The ulcers healed, with formation of an overlying mucous membrane, in 60% of the animals in this group. The unhealed ulcers in the remaining animals were much smaller than those in the controls and were slit-like with no necrotic material at the base. Only 20% of the ulcers in the control animals healed spontaneously.

Clinical Assessment of HBO in Gastric and Duodenal Ulcer Patients

Perrins (1977) treated one gastric ulcer patient with ten daily 1-h sessions of HBO at 2 ATA. The ulcer healed completely.

The case was never formally reported, and there are no clinical reports on this subject in the Western literature. All the studies quoted below are from Russia.

Lukich et al. (1981) reported 92 patients with peptic ulcer in whom the lesions measured 0.2–2.0 cm in diameter. The progress was checked gastroscopically after 10–12 sessions of HBO treatment, and healing was complete in 65 patients with 10–12 treatments.

Komarov et al. (1985) reported 132 patients, and in 127 of these (94.9%), healing of the ulcer was confirmed by endoscopy. The average duration of the healing process was 21.7 ± 1.2 days in gastric ulcers and 20.2 ± 0.7 days in duodenal ulcers. Usually 10–15 treatments at 2 ATA sufficed, but in a few exceptional cases, 30 treatments were required. The authors studied the gastrin content of the blood in 25 patients: it was 80.11 pg/mL before the treatment and 88.5 pg/mL afterward. Also, they observed increased mucous secretion and free hydrochloric acid secretion in the healing phase. This was interpreted as an increase in the basic function of the gastric mucous membrane. The ulcers healed in spite of this.

Efuni et al. (1986) used HBO for treatment of peptic ulcer in 217 patients. The only drug therapy used as an adjunct was antacid, and this was stopped after the first week of daily HBO treatments. The number of HBO sessions ranged from 9 to 17, each given at 2 ATA for 45 min. The healing time for the gastric ulcers was 19.7 ± 7 days and for the duodenal ulcers 19.3 ± 7 days. The healing was accompanied by improvement of symptoms such as pain. There was healing of 89.2% of the stomach ulcers and 95.8% of the duodenal ulcers. The results were compared with those of a control group of 350 patients who had been treated with medications such as H2-receptor blockers. The HBO treatment shortened the healing of the ulcers by 7–28 days. Further HBO treatment helped the 39.2% of patients in the control group in whom ulcers persisted in spite of medical treatment.

HBO in the Treatment of Intestinal Obstruction

Basic Considerations and Rationale of HBO Therapy

Intestinal obstruction can be divided into two categories:

1. Paralytic ileus, where obstruction results from neural, humoral, or metabolic inhibition of bowel mobility. The most common causes are abdominal surgery, peritonitis, trauma, and intestinal ischemia.
2. Mechanical ileus, where there is intestinal obstruction secondary to mechanical causes such as:
   (a) Intrinsic, including tumors and inflammatory disease
   (b) Extrinsic, including adhesions, tumors, and volvulus

(c) Lumen obstruction, including foreign bodies and intussusceptions

Obstruction may be partial or complete, and the obstructed bowel may be viable or strangulated. The composition of the gas in the nonobstructed human intestine is 64 % nitrogen, 0.69 % oxygen, 19 % hydrogen, 8.8 % methane, and 4 % carbon dioxide.

After experimental intestinal obstruction, the factors that govern the diffusion rates of intestinal gases are:

1. The partial pressure gradient of the gases across the intestinal mucous membrane separating the bowel lumen and the blood
2. The absorption coefficient of the gases in the blood
3. The molecular weight (density) of the gases involved
4. The area of surface contact between the gases and the permeable membrane
5. The thickness of the membrane
6. The diffusion velocity, which is inversely proportional to the square root of the molecular weight and directly proportional to its absorption coefficient in the medium in which it is diffusing

The origin of intestinal gases in clinical and experimental bowel obstruction is shown in Fig. 27.1. Nitrogen leaves the bowel slowly because of its low diffusion velocity, based on its molecular weight and low absorption coefficient, and because blood and alveolar air are already saturated with nitrogen. Once nitrogen enters the bowel as swallowed air, it cannot be readily absorbed in significant amounts under the existing conditions. Since it is impossible to change the absorption coefficient of nitrogen, the only logical way to get rid of it is by changing its partial pressure gradient. This can be achieved by breathing 100 % oxygen or even more effectively by HBO.

The application of HBO therapy to bowel obstruction is based on the gas laws of Dalton and Boyle (see Chap. 2). It is the internal diameter of the distended bowel rather than the actual volume of the enclosed gas that determines the pathological effects of overdistension, which lead to loss of contractility and jeopardize viability by ischemia/hypoxia. There is a risk of peritonitis by transmural leakage or perforation. Boyle's law, as applied to bowel obstruction or paralytic ileus, means that there will be a 50 % reduction of the intestinal gas volume and the diameter of the intestinal lumen (a cylinder) will be decreased by 29 % when the pressure is doubled from 1 to 2 ATA.

Experimental Studies in Animals

Cross described a series of experiments that demonstrated the efficacy of HBO therapy in dogs with mechanical closed loop obstruction (Cross 1965). In experiments involving the pressure/volume relationship, he studied the effects of increased atmospheric pressure on intestinal viability. In animals breathing air at ambient pressure, there was loss of viability in 70 % of the obstructed loops, whereas, in animals breathing air at 2–4 ATA, only 10 % of the obstructed loops lost their viability. This suggests that pressure, plus the 80 % oxygen derived from the increased partial pressure, resulted in increased intestinal viability and survival in animals with closed loop obstructions. Although pressure alone reduced the volume of gas and luminal diameter within closed intestinal loops, addition of oxygen leads to the combined effect of diffusion and gas volume reduction. Hopkinson and Schenk (1969) used HBO therapy at 2 ATA in long-term animal

Fig. 27.1 Intestinal gas origin in bowel obstruction

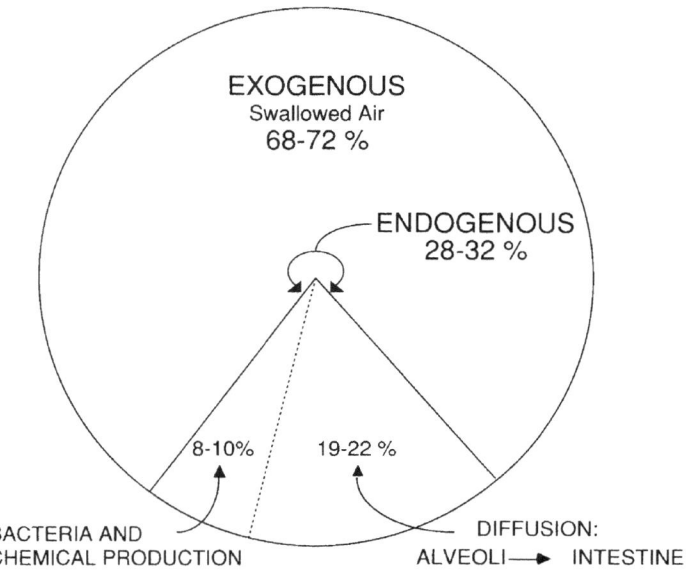

experiments and showed that it reduced mortality in animals with colon obstruction (17% vs. 55% in controls).

In the rat model of acute small bowel obstruction, the maximum fall of cytochrome oxidase and succinate dehydrogenase in the liver, kidney, and intestinal loops occurs after 72 h of obstruction. Removal of obstruction alone fails to return the enzyme levels to normal, but HBO therapy can restore normal enzyme levels regardless of the time elapsed following obstruction. The clinical implications of this observation are not as yet clear.

Secondary infection following intestinal obstruction increases morbidity. HBO has a beneficial effect as an antibacterial agent. In Wistar albino rats, HBO treatment at 2.5 ATA for 90 min daily for 2 days significantly reduces the endogenous bacterial overgrowth in the small intestine of rats following obstruction and prevents the bacterial translocation almost completely.

HBO Therapy in Adynamic Ileus

Adynamic ileus is the most common cause of intestinal obstruction. It usually follows abdominal surgery but may occur after any peritoneal insult such as peritonitis and retroperitoneal hematoma. Other diseases such as pneumonia, myocardial infarction, and electrolyte disturbances (potassium depletion) are associated with adynamic ileus. Intestinal ischemia, whether due to intestinal distension or as a result of vascular occlusion, perpetuates this condition. Stewart et al. (1974) using the rationale based on the work of Cross (1965) treated two critically ill patients with severe adynamic ileus with HBO at 2–2.5 ATA. Both improved but died later from their underlying illness. Watanuki et al. (1970) reported excellent results after treating 10 patients with postoperative paralytic ileus, using HBO for 60 min at 1–2 ATA. Ratner et al. (1978) reported the results of HBO treatment of 216 patients with postoperative adynamic ileus. The duration of each treatment was 45–60 min at a pressure of 1.8–2.0 ATA, and this treatment was repeated 3–5 times. Sixty-four patients with adynamic ileus who were not treated with HBO served as controls and received only conventional therapy. There was a mortality of 30% in this group, compared with 16% mortality in the group treated by additional HBO therapy.

Grokhovsky et al. (1978) treated 418 pediatric surgical patients with HBO. The pressures used were 1.8–2.2 ATA in younger children and 2.5–3 ATA in older children. Of these patients, 293 had peritonitis, and the results were excellent in this group; postoperative morbidity was reduced from 50 to 10% and mortality from 14 to 7%, and the average hospital stay was reduced by 5 days. HBO was highly effective in 94% of the patients, less than optimal in 6%, and ineffective in 0.7%. For HBO therapy to be most effective, it should be instituted as soon as possible after surgery; it was ineffective if delayed by more than 5 days after surgery. This study failed to include controls, making an objective evaluation of the results difficult.

Loder (1977) treated 12 patients with adynamic ileus, 10 of whom had this associated with infection. HBO was given from the second to the eighth postoperative days at 2.5 ATA for 1 h twice daily. Eleven patients recovered after 4–10 h of compression. Loder recommended that if there is no improvement with nasogastric decompression and intravenous fluids, a course of HBO should be tried. Perrins (1977) reported similar results and attributed the improved circulation in the bowel wall and return of peristalsis to the rapid reduction in intestinal distension.

Belokurov and Medvedev (1976) investigated the effectiveness of HBO in 92 patients with diffuse peritonitis and adynamic ileus. They found that HBO promoted restoration of the motor emptying junction of the gastrointestinal tract and increased the peristalsis of the small intestine, as evidenced by electroenterographic data. Mamistov and Dildin (1976) treated 50 patients with peritonitis on the rationale that HBO controls intestinal paresis, metabolic disorders, and hypoxia. Recovery was achieved in 41 patients.

Saito et al. (1977) used HBO (2–12 2-h sessions at 2 ATA) in 24 patients with postoperative adynamic ileus, some of whom had lysis of adhesions of the intestines as a result of previous surgery. Twenty-four (75%) of these patients improved. The authors also investigated the effect of HBO on experimental paralytic ileus in dogs. They noted a reduction of the diameter of the distended intestine to half at 2 ATA. The pO_2 of the intestinal wall at 2 ATA rose to 13 times the preexposure value.

A retrospective review of postoperative paralytic ileus associated with abdominal surgery that underwent HBO therapy was undertaken to examine the efficacy of HBO therapy (Ambiru et al. 2007). The overall resolution rate for patients receiving HBO was 92%. Among patients who were more than 75 years old, the therapies resolved 97% of cases of postoperative paralytic ileus. The mortality rate was 1.2% overall. Complications related to HBO therapy occurred in 3.8% of the admissions, and most of them were not serious. These results suggest that HBO therapy deserves further assessment for use in management of postoperative paralytic ileus.

HBO in Adhesive Intestinal Obstruction

Intestinal obstruction may occur because of adhesions formed as a result of abdominal surgery. Further surgery to relieve adhesions leads to the formation of more adhesions. HBO therapy is still a controversial treatment for adhesive postoperative small bowel obstruction, and only a few studies have been reported.

A clinical trial was conducted to investigate the effects of HBO therapy on patients with adhesive intestinal obstruction who had failed to respond to more than 7 days of conservative treatment (Ambiru et al. 2008). Patients were divided into groups according to the treatment and interval between the first day of the therapy and clinical symptoms of obstruction: tube decompression therapy within 7 days after appearance of clinical symptoms (Group I) and clinical symptoms that have persisted for less than 7 days before the start of HBO therapy (Group II) and for more than 7 days (Group III). Results showed that the overall resolution and mortality rates in the cases of adhesive intestinal obstruction were 79.8 % and 2.2 % in Group I, 85.9 % and 1.4 % in Group II, and 81.7 % and 1.6 % in Group III, respectively. Group II had significantly better resolution rates than Group I. It is concluded that HBO therapy may be useful in management of adhesive intestinal obstruction associated with abdominal surgery, even in patients who fail to respond to other conservative treatments. HBO therapy may be a preferred option for treatment of patients for whom surgery should be avoided.

In another study between 2006 and 2012, 305 patients with adhesive postoperative small bowel obstruction were treated using either decompression therapy or HBO (Fukami et al. 2014). Of these 142 underwent tube decompression therapy during the first 3 years, and the remaining 163 had HBO therapy during the last 3 years. Patients undergoing HBO therapy were treated once a day at a pressure of 2 ATA and 100 % oxygen. Patients showing no clinical and radiological improvement with HBO therapy were switched to decompression therapy by means of a long tube. Success rate with HBO without long-tube decompression was 87×7 %. HBO therapy was associated with earlier resumption of oral intake and a shorter hospital stay. The rate of operation was 7×4 % in the HBO group and 14×8 % in the group treated by decompression alone. In this study, HBO therapy was safe for the treatment of adhesive postoperative small bowel obstruction. It reduced the need for surgery and time to recovery as well as the hospital stay.

Repeated episodes of acute bowel obstruction are a potential complication following pelvic radiation therapy. It has been previously thought that hyperbaric oxygen therapy (HBOT) may not be useful for treatment of such obstructive episodes. We report our experience with the use of HBOT for recurrent radiation-induced acute bowel obstruction.

Methods

In a retrospective study during 2007–2010, 5 patients with recurrent episodes of acute obstructive bowel symptoms following previous therapeutic pelvic irradiation were evaluated for results of HBO therapy (Abu-Asi and Andreyev 2013). Patients received 100 % oxygen in a multiplace hyper-

baric chamber at a pressure of 2.4 ATA for up to 90 min once a day, 5–7 days weekly. Although 40 sessions of HBO were planned, 3 patients required a further extra 20 sessions for complete resolution of bowel symptoms. HBOT was well tolerated with no side effects. Patients have remained well after 6–24 months of follow-up. It was concluded that HBOT may be an effective treatment of radiation-induced bowel obstruction and deserves prospective evaluation.

HBO in Chronic Idiopathic Intestinal Pseudo-obstruction

Chronic idiopathic intestinal pseudo-obstruction is a syndrome in which symptoms of intestinal obstruction are present in the absence of mechanical obstruction. It is one of the disorders that is most refractory to medical and surgical treatment. Even when patients are given nutritional support, including total parenteral nutrition, obstructive symptoms seldom disappear. A case is reported of chronic idiopathic intestinal pseudo-obstruction, due to myopathy, in which HBO therapy was strikingly effective (Yokota et al. 2000). HBO resulted not only in relief of the patient's obstructive symptoms but also in a rapid decrease of abnormally accumulated intestinal gas. This case suggests that HBO can be an effective therapy in the management of chronic idiopathic intestinal pseudo-obstruction.

HBO in Inflammatory Bowel Disease

Inflammatory bowel disease (IBD) is a general term for a group of inflammatory disorders of unknown cause involving the gastrointestinal tract. A typical example is ulcerative colitis and a variant of it called Crohn's disease. Various factors (genetic, immunologic, and infectious) play a role in the pathogenesis even though the cause is unknown.

Ulcerative Colitis and Crohn's Disease

HBO was shown to be as effective as dexamethasone therapy as treatment for trinitrobenzenesulfonic acid–ethanol (TNBS-E)-induced distal colitis in rats, which is an animal model of IBD (Atug et al. 2008). HBO has been combined with conventional medical management in patients with chronic ulcerative colitis. HBO has also been used in the treatment of a patient with ulcerative colitis, refractory to conventional therapies (Buchman et al. 2001). Therapy consisted of 30 courses of 100 % oxygen at a pressure of 2 ATA. Clinical remission was achieved, and corticosteroids were successfully tapered off. Two pediatric patients with exacerbations of Crohn's disease without improvement despite prolonged medical therapy underwent cycles of HBO therapy (Green et al. 2013). Following treatment with HBO, both patients showed resolution of the inflammatory lesions and improvement in conditions, enabling them to reduce drug therapy. Although the mechanism by which HBO reduces inflammation in Crohn's disease is poorly defined, this therapy seems to have offered a safe adjunct in the treatment of refractory exacerbations.

In a systematic review, 13 studies of HBO therapy in Crohn's disease and six studies in ulcerative colitis were identified (Rossignol 2012). In all studies, participants had severe disease refractory to standard medical treatments, including corticosteroids, immunomodulators, and anti-inflammatory medications. In patients with Crohn's disease, 31/40 (78 %) had clinical improvements with HBO, while all 39 patients with ulcerative colitis improved. One study in Crohn's disease reported a significant decrease in proinflammatory cytokines (IL-1, IL-6, and TNF-α), and one study in ulcerative colitis reported a decrease in IL-6 with HBO. Adverse events were minimal. Twelve publications reported using HBO in animal models of experimentally induced IBD, including several studies reporting decreased biomarkers of inflammation or immune dysregulation, including TNF-α (three studies), IL-1β (two studies), neopterin (one study), and myeloperoxidase activity (five studies). HBO also decreased oxidative stress biomarkers including malondialdehyde (three studies) and plasma carbonyl content (two studies), except for one study that reported increased plasma carbonyl content. Several studies reported HBO lowered nitric oxide (three studies) and nitric oxide synthase (three studies), and one study reported a decrease in prostaglandin E2 levels. Four animal studies reported decreased edema or colonic tissue weight with HBO, and eight studies reported microscopic improvements on histopathological examination. Although most publications reported improvements with HBO, some studies suffered from limitations, including possible publication and referral biases, the lack of a control group, the retrospective nature, and a small number of participants.

The review concluded that HBO lowered biomarkers of inflammation and oxidative stress and ameliorated IBD in both human and animal studies. Most treated patients were refractory to standard medical treatments. Additional studies are warranted to investigate the effects of HBO on biomarkers of oxidative stress and inflammation as well as clinical outcomes in individuals with IBD.

Another systematic review of the effect of HBO was based on 17 studies involving 613 patients with IBD of which 286 were diagnosed as Crohn's disease and 327 as ulcerative colitis (Dulai et al. 2014). The overall response rate in Crohn's disease patients was 86 % and in ulcerative colitis 88 %. Of the 40 ulcerative colitis patients with endoscopic follow-up reported, the overall response rate to HBO was 100 %. The conclusion was that HBO is a relatively safe and potentially effective treatment option for IBD patients. To understand the true benefit of HBO in IBD, well-controlled, blinded, randomized trials are needed for both Crohn's disease and ulcerative colitis.

Although there are several reports of success of HBO therapy in ulcerative colitis, a prospective randomized open-label study, which compared HBO in addition to conventional medical treatment with conventional treatment alone, found no statistically significant differences between the treatment groups in any of the assessed variables (Pagoldh et al. 2013).

Mechanism of Effectiveness of HBO in Ulcerative Colitis

A review of records of patients with refractory ulcerative colitis who received HBO showed that all patients clinically improved by the 40th cycle of HBO therapy based on clinical and histopathological scoring, and none of the patients manifested persistent blood passage (Bekheit et al. 2016). Histologically, a significant reduction of the scores of activity was recorded accompanied by a significant increase in the proliferating cell nuclear antigen labeling index of the CD44 cells of the colonic mucosa. The conclusion of the study was that effectiveness of HBO is due to stimulation of colonic stem cell HBO which promotes healing.

HBO in Infections of the Gastrointestinal Tract

Infectious diseases are also included in this section, and the examples are toxic megacolon (TM), pseudomembranous colitis, and necrotizing enterocolitis.

Toxic Megacolon

Toxic megacolon (TM) is a rare but potentially lethal complication of idiopathic IBD characterized by total or segmental nonobstructive colonic dilatation of at least 6 cm associated with toxicity. The mechanisms involved in development of TM are not clearly delineated, but chemical mediators such as nitric oxide and interleukins may play a pivotal role in the pathogenesis. New evidence suggests that TM and its associated morbidity may be predicted by the extent of small bowel and gastric distension in patients with colitis.

Initial treatment is medical with intravenous corticosteroids and colonic decompression via tube drainage or positional techniques. Surgery is done in emergency cases involving subtotal colectomy with end ileostomy. There is some rationale for trying HBO therapy in this condition as some of the antecedent conditions are amenable to HBO. HBO shows strong anti-inflammatory effect in TM due to ulcerative colitis. It is considered to be the safest and most reliable nonsurgical method of treatment for patients with toxic colitis (Kuroki et al 1998).

Pseudomembranous Colitis

Pseudomembranous colitis (induced by antimicrobial agents) is caused by a toxin-producing anaerobic organism, *Clostridium difficile*. The presence of the organisms and toxins upon assay is suggestive of the diagnosis that can be confirmed by proctoscopy and colonoscopy. Most of the cases of this disease are self-limiting. Vancomycin has produced symptomatic improvement in some cases. HBO therapy has been shown to be useful in the management of this disease, but further research is required.

Necrotizing Enterocolitis

"Necrotizing enterocolitis" is the English translation of the term "entérocolite nécrosante," from the French literature, which refers to necrosis of the intestine, usually following surgery. There are infective factors in the etiology, but mesenteric artery occlusion is excluded. In the English language literature, the term "necrotizing enteritis" refers to involvement of the bowel with gas gangrene.

Chevrel et al. (1979) reported three cases of postoperative necrotizing enterocolitis; only one of these patients was treated by HBO and was the only survivor. The cause of this disease was considered to be prolonged distension of the intestine and anaerobic bacterial overgrowth resulting in mucosal ischemia. HBO not only reduced the volume of the distension but also improved the blood circulation of the intestine. The control of the anaerobic infection was also an important factor in the favorable outcome with HBO treatment. Michaud et al. (1989) used HBO in six cases of acute neonatal necrotizing enterocolitis. The rationale was to control the aerobic and anaerobic infection and to reduce the volume of intraperitoneal and intraluminal gases. HBO was administered via a helmet at 2 ATA for 1 h daily. Four of the six patients recovered in 6–9 days.

Radiation Enterocolitis

Delayed effects of radiation lead to ischemia and necrosis of the soft tissues due to obliterative endarteritis (see Chap. 17). In case of lesions of the mucous membranes, there is secondary infection as well. HBO has been shown to be beneficial in radiation-induced enteritis, colitis, and proctitis and should be initiated in the ischemic, rather than the necrotic phase of the disease.

A double-blind, sham-controlled, phase III randomized study to test the effect of HBO was conducted on patients with chronic gastrointestinal symptoms for 12 months or more after radiotherapy and which persisted despite at least 3 months of optimal medical therapy and no evidence of cancer recurrence (Glover et al. 2016). Participants in the active treatment group breathed 100 % oxygen at 2×4 ATA, and the control group breathed 21 % oxygen at 1×3 ATA; both treatment groups received 90-min air pressure exposures once daily for 5 days per week for a total of 8 weeks (total of 40 exposures). Results showed no evidence that patients with radiation-induced chronic gastrointestinal symptoms, including those patients with rectal bleeding, benefit from HBO therapy.

HBO in Pneumatosis Intestinalis

Pneumatosis intestinalis is a rare condition of air in the bowel wall, which is most often secondary to another medical condition. One type is pneumatosis cystoides intestinalis (PCI).

Pathophysiology of Pneumatosis Cystoides Intestinalis

PCI is a rare disease characterized by the presence of multiple intramural gas-filled cysts in the gastrointestinal tract. The cause is uncertain, but the condition is most commonly diagnosed in patients who have chronic obstructive pulmonary disease, IBD, or collagen disease. The patients present with profound disturbances of bowel function. The choice of therapy depends upon the pathophysiology of the cyst.

The cysts vary in size from a few millimeters to 2 cm and may obliterate the bowel lumen. There are three theories of pathogenesis of this lesion. The mechanical theory states that the cyst is due to distortion of the intestinal mucosal barrier. Healing of the underlying disorder as well as the epithelial break could thus result in obliteration of the cyst. According to the bacterial theory, bacterial fermentation and hydrogen gas buildup lead to cyst formation. Antibiotics and/or HBO would be recommended here. Finally, the pulmonary hypothesis postulated that severe coughing produced alveolar rupture and pneumomediastinum with gas dissecting down to the retroperitoneal space and then along the perivascular spaces to the bowel wall.

The diagnosis of pneumatosis intestinalis is most often made radiologically. A simple X-ray of the digestive tract shows a change in the characteristics of the intestinal wall in two-thirds of these patients. However, one-third of the patients do not have a diagnostic X-ray and require a CT scan or MRI that may reveal a thickened bowel wall containing gas to confirm the diagnosis and distinguish PCI from intraluminal air or submucosal fat. CT also enables detection of additional findings that may suggest an underlying, potentially worrisome cause of PCI such as bowel wall thickening, altered contrast mucosal enhancement, dilated bowel, soft tissue stranding, ascites, and the presence of portal air.

The disease severity ranges from benign to life-threatening. Early recognition of life-threatening signs and symptoms is critical. Treatment options include bowel rest, antibiotics, surgery, and the use of HBO therapy.

Rationale for HBO Therapy

The earlier treatment for this condition was normobaric oxygen therapy. There was some success, and this led to the hypothesis that the cysts were created and maintained by anaerobic organisms which produce gas at a rate that exceeds the rate of absorption. The high tissue oxygen tension was supposed to kill the organisms. This theory has not been substantiated. Disadvantages of normobaric oxygen are that excessive amounts of 100% oxygen are required to be inhaled for prolonged periods, and this may produce oxygen toxicity. In contrast to this, HBO treatments are of shorter duration and more effective and lower the total pressure of gases in the surrounding tissues thus increasing the pressure gradient between the cysts and the tissues. The balance of pressure then favors diffusion, and cysts will deflate. HBO represented a significant advance in the treatment of PCI. When surgery is not emergently needed, symptomatic pneumatosis intestinalis can be safely treated with HBO with a high likelihood of success without any considerable adverse effects (Feuerstein et al. 2014).

Clinical Experience

Mathus-Vliegen et al. (1983) treated 2 patients with this condition by HBO, with rapid relief of symptoms and disappearance of the cysts. Iitsuka et al. (1993) presented a case of PCI associated with nephrotic syndrome and long-term use of steroids. The patient improved with HBO treatment. Grieve and Unsworth (1991) presented 8 patients with PCI who underwent 11 courses of HBO treatment. All patients responded with symptomatic relief. This was followed by seven recurrences and four long-term cures. The authors concluded that HBO is effective for PCI provided it is continued until the cyst has resolved and not just for symptomatic relief.

Paw and Reed (1996) presented another case of PCI involving the small intestine which was diagnosed by barium meal and treated with HBO. The patient received HBO at 2 ATA for 1 h/day/5 days a week for 2 weeks with improvement. The frequency of treatments was reduced to twice a week and then once a week. Relief was noted at the first treatment, and the patient recovered completely with no recurrence. Repeat barium meal examination showed no evidence of recurrence of the lesions.

Several cases have been reported in the literature from Japan where HBO was used successfully for the treatment of PCI (Tomiyama et al. 2003; Takada et al. 2002; Shimada et al. 2001; Iimura et al. 2000; Togawa et al. 2004). A case of systemic lupus erythematosus with enteritis and peritonitis which later developed PCI was treated successfully with a combination of intravenous cyclophosphamide, antibiotics, and HBO (Mizoguchi et al. 2008).

HBO in Ischemic Disorders of the Intestine

Vascular accidents are rare in the intestine, but when they occur, they have serious consequences because of the toxic and infective nature of the bowel contents. Splenic ischemia can injure other organs such as the liver and pancreas. Restoration of the blood supply to the ischemic tissue leads to reperfusion injury mediated by free radical generation. Many of these patients are not candidates for surgical resection of the bowel, and there is no satisfactory medical treatment. The mortality is high in these cases.

Experimental intestinal ischemia produced in dogs by vascular interruption has been treated by exposing animals to normobaric pressures (controls) and hyperbaric pressures (treated groups). Breathing of oxygen and administration of gases by intestinal or respiratory routes have also been tried. All these modalities, including HBO, fail to preserve ischemic intestine without perfusion. Bowel death occurs in all animals. Takahashi et al. (1987) presented the effect of HBO on experimental thrombosis of the mesenteric artery in dogs. HBO was given at 2 ATA for 75 min and repeated for 3 days following the arterial ligation. Animals were sacrificed on the third and the seventh postoperative days, and changes in the infarcted intestine were observed. Hemorrhage, edema, and multiple ulcers were characteristic of the control animals but were less marked in the animals treated by HBO; as well, evidence of the repair process was seen in these animals. Microangiography revealed rich revascularization around the margins of infarction in HBO-treated animals. The authors concluded that HBO has the following benefits in mesenteric artery thrombosis:

- It minimizes the hemorrhagic and edematous changes of the infarcted intestine.
- It promotes revascularization and the repair process.

In a rat model, HBO therapy has been shown to limit tissue damage due to ischemia/reperfusion (I/R) injury, by inducing reparative signaling pathways (Daniel et al. 2011). In rats were subjected to 60-min ischemia by clamping the superior mesenteric artery and 60-min reperfusion by removal of clamping, association between HBO, small intestinal I/R injury, and mucosa apoptosis was observed (Zhou et al. 2012). HBO maintains ATP and aerobic metabolism, inhibits TNF-α production, and thus prevents intestinal mucosa from apoptosis. Best results are expected when HBO is administered to patients in the period of ischemia, and no side effects are produced when HBO is given during the period of reperfusion. However, there is no report of the use of HBO in human patients with acute occlusion of the superior mesenteric artery.

Another potential use of HBO is to facilitate healing of colonic anastomosis as anastomotic leakage is the major cause of morbidity and mortality in colorectal surgery. A common factor in several cases of leaking or dehiscence in patients with tension sutures and excessive devascularization of the ends is hypoperfusion of the anastomosis leading to hypoxia–ischemia. The results of an experimental study in rats suggest that HBO increases neovascularization and bursting pressures in ischemic colon anastomosis, and best results were obtained in combination with the antithrombic agent enoxaparin (Kemik et al. 2013).

Use of Hyperbaric Therapy in Removal of Entrapped Intestinal Balloons

Intestinal tube balloons may get entrapped in the intestine and become markedly distended. The balloons can be punctured by passing needles percutaneously under radiographic control, but this technique is not always successful. Hyperbaric therapy facilitates removal of the balloons by decompressing them. Increasingly, the procedure of "gastric bubble" for obesity is being used. Some of these balloons may pass through the pylorus and become entrapped in the intestine.

Kulak et al. (1978) reported four cases where a Kaslow gastrointestinal tube balloon was successfully removed with hyperbaric pressure to 4 ATA. Peloso (1982) reported the successful removal of a trapped Kaslow tube balloon that became distended and led to recurrence of intestinal obstruction. Following a single compression at 2.5 ATA for 60 min, the tube could be pulled out. Another successful removal of a gas distended tube balloon has been reported (Lautin and Scheinbaum 1987). D'Hemecourt and Stem (1987) reported the use of hyperbaric treatment (2 ATA, two sessions) to aid the successful passage through the intestine of a gastric bubble that had become entrapped in the proximal jejunum.

HBO in Acute Pancreatitis

Acute pancreatitis is thought to be due to autodigestion of the pancreas by activated enzymes. The commonest causes are chronic alcoholism and gallstones, and the most frequent symptom is abdominal pain. The main feature of this condition is pancreatic necrosis leading to sepsis, with both localized and systemic inflammatory response syndromes. Early pathophysiological changes of the pancreas include alterations in microcirculation, ischemia reperfusion injury, and leukocyte and cytokine activation. In about 50 % of cases, the attack is mild and the patients recover without any treatment; in 40 % the attack is severe and they are quite ill, and 10 % die. The use of HBO has been explored in severely ill patients.

Animal Experimental Studies of HBO in Acute Pancreatitis

Daily HBO therapy at 2.5 ATA in a rat model of acute pancreatitis, induced by pancreatic duct ligation, was effective in reducing the hemorrhage and acinar necrosis but was not sufficient to reduce edema and leukocyte infiltration (Festugato et al. 2008). HBO and N-acetylcysteine combination was shown to markedly reduce the development of L-arginine-induced acute necrotic pancreatitis in rats as assessed by decreases in oxidative stress parameters, serum amylase, calcium, and LDH levels, as well as histopathologic score (Onur et al. 2012). In another study, poly(ADP-ribose) polymerase inhibition by combination of 3-aminobenzamide and HBO treatment was effective in the course of severe AP, because of the improved cascades of inflammatory process in rat model of severe acute pancreatitis (Inal et al. 2015). Apoptosis of peripheral blood lymphocytes (PBLs) promoted by HBO treatment was shown to attenuate the severity of acute pancreatitis in rats (Bai et al. 2014). This study demonstrated that the HBO treatment can promote the apoptosis of PBLs via a mitochondrial-dependent pathway and inhibit the inflammatory response. These immunoregulatory effects may play an important role in attenuating the severity of early stage of the disease. Repeated administration of HBO or its use in combination with other approaches may further improve outcomes.

Clinical Applications of HBO in Acute Pancreatitis

Pallota et al. (1980) treated 9 patients with acute pancreatitis, of whom had associated paralytic ileus. HBO resulted in improvement in all cases. Serum amylase fell on average from about 88 U/L initially to slightly less than half this level after the first treatment and was down to about 11 U/L in 72 h. A case of severe acute pancreatitis was treated by HBO therapy at a pressure of 2.5 ATA for 90 min given twice daily for a total of 5 days with improvement (Christophi et al. 2007). Pancreatic abscess is a late complication of severe acute pancreatitis, and peripancreatic abscess may follow surgical exploration. Izawa et al. (1993) treated 5 such patients with HBO which was effective in reducing fever, leukocytosis, serum amylase levels, and size of the abscess.

HBO in Diseases of the Liver

Effect of HBO on the Normal Liver

A number of investigators have studied the effect of HBO on the normal liver. Trytyshnikov (1986) noted that exposure of rats to HBO at 3 ATA for 60 min immediately after acute massive loss of blood prevented the depression of RNA and protein synthesis in the liver. Subsequent daily use of HBO at 0.5–3 ATA had a stimulating effect on the reparative plastic processes in the liver and increased survival. Mattle (1963) showed that exposure of rats to 3 ATA did not influence significantly the rate of ethanol elimination. Incubation of liver slices in vitro (under oxygen) showed a significant correlation between oxygen uptake and ethanol elimination.

Effect of HBO on Experimentally Induced Hepatic Disorders in Animals

HBO offers no protection against hepatic artery ligation in the dog in experimental studies. HBO leads to slight improvement in the appearance of arterioportal shunt causes lesions in the walls of the liver sinusoids in experimental animals as seen on electron microscopy. Hill (1976) evaluated HBO in the treatment of abscesses produced by intraperitoneal injection of *Fusobacterium necrophorum* plus *F. nucleatum* or *Bacteroides fragilis* in mice. A group of animals were exposed to HBO at 2 ATA for 3 h daily. Autopsy revealed that the number of abscesses was significantly lower in the HBO-treated group than in the controls. This study has practical implications for the treatment of hepatic abscesses in patients.

Mininberg and Kvetnoy (1974) studied the effect of HBO on rats with hepatotoxicity induced by carbon tetrachloride. The liver tissue in treated animals showed a reparative process: necrosis was absent, and the activity of succinic dehydrogenase was increased, as was the quantity of glucagon. The functional activity of the liver chromaffin cells containing melatonin and serotonin was enhanced. Belokurov et al. (1981) used HBO on 380 rats with mechanical jaundice. The

basis for the favorable effect appeared to be elimination of oxygen insufficiency in the liver tissues with subsequent regeneration. Korkhov et al. (1981) noted that in animals with induced hepatic insufficiency, the morphological changes in the liver were characterized by mild dystrophy of the hepatocytes, insignificant accumulation of glycogen, and transient manifestations of fatty degeneration. Under the effect of HBO, oxygen tensions in the liver tissues were rapidly restored, with recovery from the changes.

In contrast to the beneficial effect of HBO in hepatic insufficiency, the regeneration of the liver after hepatectomy is delayed at day 15 in rats exposed to oxygen at 2 ATA for 90 min daily (Di Guilio et al. 1989).

Clinical Applications

Most of the clinical applications of HBO in liver disease are in the more severe forms, such as acute hepatic failure with encephalopathy. This condition usually results from viral hepatitis but may also follow exposure to hepatotoxic drugs.

Hepatic Encephalopathy

Hepatic encephalopathy is a complex syndrome that occurs due to diverse liver disease and spontaneous or iatrogenic portosystemic venous shunting (Jain 2016). It may be due to hepatotoxicity of drugs. Clinical manifestations range from subtle neuropsychiatric abnormalities to deep coma. Various pathomechanisms have been proposed for hepatic encephalopathy. The best known of these hypotheses concern hyperammonemia, neuroinflammation, false neurotransmitters, and increased GABA neurotransmission. Ammonia-induced changes in the nervous system include depletion of glutamic acid, aspartic acid, and adenosine triphosphate. While often present in increased amounts in the blood, the absolute concentrations of ammonia; ammonia metabolites, including glutamine; and mercaptans correlate only roughly with the presence or severity of encephalopathy. Low values of cerebral metabolic rate of oxygen and cerebral blood flow observed during hepatic encephalopathy increase after recovery and are thus associated with encephalopathy rather than the liver disease (Dam et al. 2013). These are not linked to blood ammonia concentration. MRI may also be useful in monitoring cerebral edema and response to treatment. Multimodality MRI is a useful tool for early diagnosis, prognosis, and monitoring of hepatic encephalopathy, particularly the combination of fMRI and diffusion tensor imaging (Zhang et al. 2014).

Treatment is aimed at reduction of production or absorption of ammonia, increasing metabolism of ammonia in the tissues, reduction of false neurotransmitters (aromatic amino acids), inhibition of GABA–benzodiazepine receptors, and correction of manganese deposits in basal ganglia. Orthotopic liver transplantation is increasingly used in treatment of patients with end-stage liver cirrhosis. As an interim measure, cell therapy by transplantation of genetically modified hepatocytes or hematopoietic stem cells may reduce disease and extend survival until a donor becomes available for liver transplant or the patient's own liver recovers function.

Reports of the use of HBO in disorders of the liver are reviewed against this background. Aubert et al. (1967) treated 2 patients in hepatic coma with HBO. The patients improved, but the author drew no conclusions, and suggested further research in this area was necessary. Dordain et al. (1968) found HBO to be successful in treating a case of hepatic coma due to viral hepatitis. Goulon et al. (1971) found HBO useful in treating 16 patients with viral hepatitis associated with hepatic encephalopathy, and Tacquet et al. (1970) found it useful in a case of acute hepatic failure with hepatic coma.

Blum et al. (1972) treated four children in acute hepatic failure with exchange transfusion and in three of them also gave HBO. The neurological status and EEG improved with exchange transfusion, but HBO had no effect and produced some complications, including death of one of the patients. Laverdant et al. (1971, 1973) treated patients with viral hepatitis by a variety of methods, including HBO, and concluded that no special treatment beyond basic resuscitation and correction of electrolyte and acid–base balance made any difference to the outcome of the disease.

Novikova and Klyavinsh (1981) considered improvement of oxygen delivery to the liver and the brain in viral hepatitis A and B to be of great importance. They used HBO at 1.8 ATA for 30 min, and the number of sessions required was 3–24. Fourteen patients with severe viral hepatitis, hyperbilirubinemia exceeding 10 mg%, and impairment of liver function were treated. Three of the patients were in hepatic coma. After 3–4 treatments, hyperbilirubinemia was reduced, liver function tests improved, and the patients started to recover. In hepatic coma, the signs disappeared with 5–7 treatments. Eventually all the patients recovered.

Orynbaev and Myrzaliev (1981) used HBO in the treatment of 96 children with viral hepatitis. A study of the long-term results showed residual symptoms of viral hepatitis in only 7% of the patients (a frequency four times lower than in the controls). Belokurov et al. (1985) analyzed the causes of endogenous intoxication in 39 patients with acute hepatic insufficiency and identified 11 toxic compounds. They discussed the role of hemadsorption and HBO in eliminating the toxic products and found this approach to be useful.

Tsygankova et al. (1986) treated 30 patients with acute hepatitis that developed with renal failure or after renal transplant. One-half of these patients were treated by conventional therapy and the other half by HBO. In the HBO group, 8–10 treatments at 1.5 ATA proved to be effective in reducing the pathological process as shown by immune homeostasis recovery.

Okihama et al. (1987) used HBO in treating a patient with liver cirrhosis who developed hyperbilirubinemia after percutaneous transhepatic variceal obliteration and splenic artery embolization. HBO therapy was performed 33 times during 54 days, and the level of serum bilirubin was successfully reduced to 1.2 mg/dL, and other clinical findings also improved. This result suggests that HBO therapy may be worth trying in cirrhotic patients who have hyperbilirubinemia and liver failure.

HBO has been used in combination with plasma exchange and hemodialysis in a 3-year-old girl suffering from acute hepatic failure and coma (Ponikvar et al. 1998). She received nine HBO sessions each with 100% oxygen at 2.5 ATA for 90 min over a course of 1 month. Throughout the treatment, the patient was in good clinical, physical, and mental condition, but she was dependent on blood purification procedures. She was referred to a liver transplant center and successfully transplanted.

In conclusion, we may state that the reports of the use of HBO in liver disease are all anecdotal and thus difficult to evaluate. There are several reports of the use of HBO in acute viral hepatitis, but practically no information on the effect of HBO on viruses. Most of the described effects of HBO are on the biochemical sequelae of liver disease. HBO has been found to be useful in hepatic encephalopathy. This may possibly be due to an ammonia lowering effect of HBO. There are no reports of the use of HBO in drug-induced hepatitis. It would be worthwhile to explore the use of HBO in this condition.

Conclusions Regarding the Use of HBO in Gastroenterology

The use of HBO in peptic ulcers appears to be a logical extension of its successful application in skin ulcers. Counteracting ischemia and hypoxia appears to be a reasonable rationale for using HBO to promote healing of peptic ulcers. A controlled study, however, is required. Antibacterial effect of HBO against *H. pylori* needs to be examined in the laboratory. Although there are no double-blind randomized studies, the sheer number of cases with peptic ulcer reported from Russia (over 500) with good clinical and laboratory documentation presents in favor of prescribing HBO for cases of refractory peptic ulcer.

The role of HBO in intestinal ischemia needs to be investigated further. HBO accelerates new vessel growth in ischemia by angiogenesis, but the mechanism has not been defined. Role of HBO treatments done more frequent and for longer periods needs to be determined. Combination of HBO with free radical scavengers to avoid reperfusion injury also needs to be investigated. Observations may have to be made on human patients, but controlled clinical trials are not practical for this condition.

Another area where the use of HBO is promising is intestinal obstruction. Although controlled studies of the treatment of patients with adynamic ileus are inadequate, clinical experience is extensive and is well documented. In patients who have adynamic ileus or bowel obstruction associated with adhesions, HBO may be considered appropriate as an adjunctive treatment along with nasogastric decompression and intravenous fluid therapy. If there is complete bowel obstruction with strangulation or impending perforation, surgery should not be delayed in order to use HBO therapy. Rather, such patients may be given supplemental HBO in the postoperative period. HBO be a useful adjunct to nonoperative therapy for intestinal obstruction when a patient's overall condition does not allow operative intervention.

References

Abu-Asi MJ, Andreyev HJ. The utility of hyperbaric oxygen therapy to treat recurrent acute bowel obstruction after previous pelvic radiotherapy: a case series. Support Care Cancer. 2013;21:1797–800.

Ambiru S, Furuyama N, Aono M, Kimura F, Shimizu H, Yoshidome H, et al. Hyperbaric oxygen therapy for the treatment of postoperative paralytic ileus and adhesive intestinal obstruction associated with abdominal surgery: experience with 626 patients. Hepatogastroenterology. 2007;54:1925–9.

Ambiru S, Furuyama N, Kimura F, Shimizu H, Yoshidome H, Miyazaki M, et al. Effect of hyperbaric oxygen therapy on patients with adhesive intestinal obstruction associated with abdominal surgery who have failed to respond to more than 7 days of conservative treatment. Hepatogastroenterology. 2008;55:491–5.

Atug O, Hamzaoglu H, Tahan V, Alican I, Kurtkaya O, Elbuken E, et al. Hyperbaric oxygen therapy is as effective as dexamethasone in the treatment of TNBS-E-induced experimental colitis. Dig Dis Sci. 2008;53:481–5.

Aubert L, Arroyo H, Malavaud A. Note sur le traitement du coma hépatique par l'hyperoxie hyperbarique. Marseille Med. 1967;104:357–62.

Bai X, Song Z, Zhou Y, Pan S, Wang F, Guo Z, et al. The apoptosis of peripheral blood lymphocytes promoted by hyperbaric oxygen treatment contributes to attenuate the severity of early stage acute pancreatitis in rats. Apoptosis. 2014;19:58–75.

Bekheit M, Baddour N, Katri K, Taher Y, El Tobgy K, Mousa E. Hyperbaric oxygen therapy stimulates colonic stem cells and induces mucosal healing in patients with refractory ulcerative colitis: a prospective case series. BMJ Open Gastroenterol. 2016;3(1), e000082.

Belokurov YN, Medvedev VF. Restoration of gastro-intestinal motility in patients with diffuse peritonitis in conditions of hyperbaric oxygenation. Klin Khir. 1976;5:22–5.

Belokurov YN, Rybachkov VV. Possibilities of hyperbaric oxygen treatment under conditions of hepatic insufficiency. In: Proceedings of the 7th international congress on hyperbaric medicine, Moscow, 2–6 Sept 1981.

Belokurov YN, Rybachkov VV, Pankov AG. Endogenous toxicity on acute hepatic failure and ways of eliminating it. Vestn Khir. 1985;134:60–4.

Blum D, Viart P, Szliwowski HB, Thys JP, Dubois J. Exchange transfusion and hyperbaric oxygen in the treatment of children with acute hepatic failure. Helv Paediatr Acta. 1972;27:425–36.

Bowen JC, Fairchild RB. Oxygen in gastric mucosal protection. In: Allen A et al., editors. Mechanisms of mucosal protection in the upper gastrointestinal tract. New York: Raven; 1984. p. 259–66.

Buchman AL, Fife C, Torres C, Smith L, Aristizibal J. Hyperbaric oxygen therapy for severe ulcerative colitis. J Clin Gastroenterol. 2001;33:337–9.

Chevrel JP, Guterman R, Rathat C, Gatt MT, Kemeny J. Entérocolites aigues nécrosantes: à propos de trois observations. Sem Hop. 1979;55:897–904.

Christophi C, Millar I, Nikfarjam M, Muralidharan V, Malcontenti-Wilson C. Hyperbaric oxygen therapy for severe acute pancreatitis. J Gastroenterol Hepatol. 2007;22:2042–6.

Cross FS. Hyperoxic treatment of experimental intestinal obstruction. Dis Chest. 1965;47:374–81.

D'Hemecourt PA, Stem W. Dislodged gastric bubble. J Hyperbaric Med. 1987;2:233–4.

Dam G, Keiding S, Munk OL, Ott P, Vilstrup H, Bak LK, et al. Hepatic encephalopathy is associated with decreased cerebral oxygen metabolism and blood flow, not increased ammonia uptake. Hepatology. 2013;57:258–65.

Daniel RA, Cardoso VK, Góis Jr E, Parra RS, Garcia SB, Rocha JJ, et al. Effect of hyperbaric oxygen therapy on the intestinal ischemia reperfusion injury. Acta Cir Bras. 2011;26:463–9.

Di Guilio C, Innocenti P, Loffredo B, et al. Hyperbaric hyperoxia and rat's hepatic regeneration. J Hyperbaric Med. 1989;4:27–31.

Dordain M, Humbert G, Robert M, Leroy J, Delaunay P. Coma hépatique par hépatite virale avec succès par l'oxygène hyperbare. Sem Hop. 1968;44:1617–2622.

Dulai PS, Gleeson MW, Taylor D, Holubar SD, Buckey JC, Siegel CA. Systematic review: The safety and efficacy of hyperbaric oxygen therapy for inflammatory bowel disease. Aliment Pharmacol Ther. 2014;39:1266–75.

Efuni SN, Pogromov AP, Jegorov AP. The use of hyperbaric oxygen in the treatment of gastric and duodenal ulcers. In: Schmutz J, editor. Proceedings of the 1st Swiss symposium on hyperbaric medicine. Basel: Foundation for Hyperbaric Medicine; 1986. p. 212–21.

Festugato M, Coelho CP, Fiedler G, Machado FP, Gonçalves MC, Bassani FR, et al. Hyperbaric oxygen therapy effects on tissue lesions in acute pancreatitis. Experimental study in rats. JOP. 2008;9:275–82.

Feuerstein JD, White N, Berzin TM. Pneumatosis intestinalis with a focus on hyperbaric oxygen therapy. Mayo Clin Proc. 2014;89:697–703.

Fukami Y, Kurumiya Y, Mizuno K, Sekoguchi E, Kobayashi S. Clinical effect of hyperbaric oxygen therapy in adhesive postoperative small bowel obstruction. Br J Surg. 2014;101:433–7.

Glover M, Smerdon GR, Andreyev HJ, Benton BE, Bothma P, Firth O, et al. Hyperbaric oxygen for patients with chronic bowel dysfunction after pelvic radiotherapy (HOT2): a randomised, double-blind, sham-controlled phase 3 trial. Lancet Oncol. 2016;17:224–33.

Goulon M, Rapin M, Barois A. Trial treatment of severe viral hepatitis with hyperbaric oxygenation (apropos of 16 cases). Ann Med Interne (Paris). 1971;122:93–8.

Green MS, Purohi M, Sadacharam K, Mychaskiw G. Efficacy of hyperbaric oxygen in patients with Crohn's disease: two case reports. Undersea Hyperb Med. 2013;40:201–4.

Grieve DA, Unsworth IP. Pneumatosis cystoides intestinalis: an experience with hyperbaric oxygenation. Aust N Z J Surg. 1991;61:423–6.

Grokhovsky VI, Mogiliak OL, Bonovik PI. Five-year experience using hyperbaric oxygenation in pediatric surgery. Klin Khir. 1978;6:66–70.

Hill GB. Hyperbaric oxygen exposures for intrahepatic abscesses produced in mice by nonsporeforming anaerobic bacteria. Antimicrob Agents Chemother. 1976;9:312–7.

Hopkinson BR, Schenk WG. Effect of hyperbaric oxygen on experimental intestinal obstruction. Arch Surg. 1969;98:228–32.

Iimura M, Iizuka B, Kishino M, Shinozaki S, Yamagishi N, Honma N, et al. A case of chronic idiopathic intestinal pseudo-obstruction and pneumatosis cystoides intestinalis with pneumatoperitoneum, improved by the hyperbaric oxygen therapy. Nippon Shokakibyo Gakkai Zasshi. 2000;97:199–203.

Iitsuka T, Kobayashi M, Izumi Y, Koyama A. Pneumatosis cystoides intestinalis following steroid treatment in a nephrotic syndrome patient: report of a case. Nippon Jiinzo Gakkai Shi. 1993;35:293–7.

Inal V, Mas MR, Isik AT, Comert B, Aydn S, Mas N, et al. A new combination therapy in severe acute pancreatitis—hyperbaric oxygen plus 3-aminobenzamide: an experimental study. Pancreas. 2015;44:326–30.

Izawa K, Tsunoda T, Ura K, Yamaguchi T, Ito T, Kanematsu T, et al. Hyperbaric oxygen therapy in the treatment of refractory peripancreatic abscess associated with severe acute pancreatitis. Gastroenterol Jpn. 1993;28:284–91.

Jain KK. Hepatic encephalopathy. In: Greenamyre JT, editor. Medlink Neurology. California: San Diego; 2016.

Kemik O, Adas G, Arikan S, Gurluler E, Dogan Y, Toklu AS, et al. Evaluation of the effects of hyperbaric oxygen treatment and enoxaparin on left colon anastomosis. An experimental study. Eur Rev Med Pharmacol Sci. 2013;17:2286–92.

Koloskow JB, Dumurow JA. The influence of hyperbaric oxygen in the treatment of gastric and duodenal ulcers. In: Schmutz J, editor. Proceedings of the 1st Swiss symposium on hyperbaric medicine. Basel: Foundation for Hyperbaric Medicine; 1986. p. 212–21.

Komarov FI, Pogronov AP, Egorov AP, et al. Treatment of gastric and intestinal ulcers by hyperbaric oxygen. Hyperb Oxygen Rev. 1985;6:227–30.

Korkhov SI, Kilchevsky GS, Shiryaev II, et al. Hyperbaric oxygenation in complex treatment of hypoxic status of the liver. In: Yefuny SN, editor. Proceedings of the 7th international congress on hyperbaric medicine. Moscow: USSR Academy of Sciences; 1981. p. 354.

Kulak RG, Friedman B, Gelernt IM, Jacobson JH. The entrapped intestinal balloon colon deflation by hyperbaric therapy. Ann Surg. 1978;187:309–12.

Kuroki K, Masuda A, Uehara H, Kuroki A. A new treatment for toxic megacolon. Lancet. 1998;352:782.

Lautin EM, Scheinbaum KR. Hyperbaric therapy for the removal of an obstructing intestinal tube balloon. Gastrointest Radio. 1987;12:243–4.

Laverdant C, Molinie C, Poujol C, Contant A, Lombard J. Résultats comparés du traitement de deux groupes l'hepatites virales graves. Ann Med Interne. 1971;122:85–91.

Laverdant C, Poujol C, Lombard E, et al. A further comparative study of the treatment of two groups of patients suffering from malignant viral hepatitis. Lyon Med. 1973;230(20):767–71.

Loder R. Use of hyperbaric oxygen in paralytic ileus. Br Med J. 1977;1:1448–9.

Lukich VL, Shirokova KI, Matrinitskaya NA, et al. The results of the use of hyperbaric oxygen in the treatment of peptic ulcer. In: Yefuny SN, editor. Proceedings of the 7th international congress on hyperbaric medicine. Moscow: USSR Academy of Sciences; 1981. p. 357.

Mamistov VA, Dildin AS. Employment of hyperbaric oxygenation in the treatment of patients with acute generalized peritonitis. Khirurgiia (Mosk). 1976;2:89–92.

Mathus-Vliegen L, Tijtgat GNJ, Bakker DJ. Pneumatosis cystoides intestinalis and HBO therapy. In: Paper presented at the 1st European conference on hyperbaric medicine, Amsterdam, 7–9 Sept 1983.

Mattle H. Elimination of ethanol in rats and in vitro at different oxygen pressures. Acta Physiol Pharmacol. 1963;12:1–11.

Michaud A, Mongredien-Taburet H, Barthelemy L, et al. Traitment par oxygenotherapie Hyperbare (OHB). Medsubhyp. 1989;8:139–49.

Mininberg ES, Kvetnoy IM. Hyperbaric oxygenation in the prophylaxis and treatment of acute hepatic insufficiency. Anesteziol Reanimatol. 1974;4:46–9.

Mizoguchi F, Nanki T, Miyasaka N. Pneumatosis cystoides intestinalis following lupus enteritis and peritonitis. Intern Med. 2008;47:1267–71.

Novikova OA, Klyavinsh YA. Effectiveness of hyperbaric oxygen in severe forms of virus hepatitis of hepatic coma in children. In: Yefuny SN, editor. Proceedings of the 7th international congress of hyperbaric medicine. Moscow: USSR Academy of Sciences; 1981. p. 350–1.

Okihama Y, Umehara M, Naitoh Z, et al. A successful treatment with hyperbaric oxygenation therapy for a cirrhotic patient with hyperbilirubinemia. Jpn J Hyperbaric Med. 1987;22:77–82.

Onur E, Paksoy M, Baca B, Akoglu H. Hyperbaric oxygen and N-acetylcysteine treatment in L-arginine-induced acute pancreatitis in rats. J Invest Surg. 2012;25:20–8.

Orynbaev TO, Myrzaliev VA. Hyperbaric oxygenation in the therapy of viral hepatitis in children. In: Yefuny SN, editor. Proceedings of the 7th international congress of hyperbaric medicine. Moscow: USSR Academy of Sciences; 1981. p. 35.

Pagoldh M, Hultgren E, Arnell P, Eriksson A. Hyperbaric oxygen therapy does not improve the effects of standardized treatment in a severe attack of ulcerative colitis: a prospective randomized study. Scand J Gastroenterol. 2013;48:1033–40.

Pallota R, Anceschi S, Costagliola N. Therapy with hyperbaric oxygen of acute pancreatitis. Ann Med Nav. 1980;85:27–34.

Paw HGW, Reed PN. Pneumatosis cystoides intestinalis confined to the small intestine treated with hyperbaric oxygen. Undersea Hyperbaric Med. 1996;23:115–7.

Peloso OA. Hyperbaric oxygen treatment of intestinal obstruction and other related conditions. Hyperbaric Oxygen Rev. 1982;3:103–19.

Perrins D. Hyperbaric oxygenation in paralytic ileus. Br Med J. 1977;1:1602.

Ponikvar R, Buturovic J, Cizman M, Mekjavić I, Kandus A, Premru V, et al. Hyperbaric oxygenation, plasma exchange, and hemodialysis for treatment of acute liver failure in a 3-year-old child. Artif Organs. 1998;22:952–7.

Ratner GL, Kaluzhskikh VN, Dildin AS, et al. Hyperbaric oxygenation in intensive therapy of automotor disorders of intestinal function. Anesteziol Reanimatol. 1978;4:64–8.

Rossignol DA. Hyperbaric oxygen treatment for inflammatory bowel disease: a systematic review and analysis. Med Gas Res. 2012;2(1):6.

Saito H, Ota K, Sageusa T, et al. Clinical and experimental studies of hyperbaric oxygen treatment of postoperative ileus. In: Smith G, editor. Proceedings of the 6th international congress on hyperbaric medicine. Aberdeen: University of Aberdeen Press; 1977. p. 333–7.

Shimada M, Ina K, Takahashi H, Horiuchi Y, Imada A, Nishio Y, et al. Pneumatosis cystoides intestinalis treated with hyperbaric oxygen therapy: usefulness of an endoscopic ultrasonic catheter probe for diagnosis. Intern Med. 2001;40:896–900.

Stewart JSS, Meddie NC, Middleton MD, Balestrieri GG. Gut decompression with hyperbaric oxygen (Letter to the editor). Lancet. 1974;1:669.

Tacquet A, Voisin C, Lelievre G, Mouton Y. Treatment of acute hepatic insufficiency by hyperbaric oxygen therapy. Lille Med. 1970;15:1066–9.

Takada C, Kaneko H, Tomomasa T, Tsukada S, Kanazawa T, Sotomatsu M, et al. Endosonographic diagnosis of pneumatosis cystoides intestinalis in infancy. Tech Coloproctol. 2002;6:121–3.

Takahashi H, Kobayashi S, Hayase H, et al. Effect of HBO upon experimental thrombosis of mesenteric artery. Presented at the 9th international congress on hyperbaric medicine, Sydney, Australia, March 1–4, 1987.

Togawa S, Yamami N, Nakayama H, Shibayama M, Mano Y. Evaluation of HBO$_2$ therapy in pneumatosis cystoides intestinalis. Undersea Hyperb Med. 2004;31:387–93.

Tomiyama R, Kinjo F, Hokama A, Kishimoto K, Oshiro J, Saito A. A case of pneumatosis cystoides intestinalis with diabetes mellitus successfully treated by hyperbaric oxygen therapy. Nippon Shokakibyo Gakkai Zasshi. 2003;100:212–4.

Trytyshnikov IM. Dynamics of the plastic processes in the liver during the use of hyperbaric oxygenation in the recovery period following acute massive blood loss. Biull Eksp Biol Med. 1986;101:154–6.

Tsygankova ST, Ashurova LD, Sultanova BG. Hyperbaric oxygenation in the combined therapy of acute hepatitis in patients before and after renal allotransplantation. Anesteziol Reanimatol. 1986;3:64.

Watanuki T, Istubo K, Fumoto T. Study on the effects of hyperbaric oxygenation upon intestinal peristalsis. In: Wada J, Iwa T, editors. Proceedings of the 4th international congress on hyperbaric medicine. London, Baillere, 1970 pp. 395–399.

Yokota T, Suda T, Tsukioka S, Takahashi T, Honma T, Seki K, et al. The striking effect of hyperbaric oxygenation therapy in the management of chronic idiopathic intestinal pseudo-obstruction. Am J Gastroenterol. 2000;95:285–8.

Zhang XD, Zhang LJ, Wu SY, Lu GM. Multimodality magnetic resonance imaging in hepatic encephalopathy: an update. World J Gastroenterol. 2014;20:11262–72.

Zhou SH, Sun YF, Wang G. Effects of hyperbaric oxygen on intestinal mucosa apoptosis caused by ischemia-reperfusion injury in rats. World J Emerg Med. 2012;3:135–40.

K.K. Jain

Abstract

Reports on the use of HBO in the field of endocrinology are relatively few in number. These are based mostly on animal experimental work. Effect of HBO is described on thyroid gland, adrenocortical function, epinephrine/norepinephrine, prostaglandins, and testosterone. The most significant clinical application is in management of type 2 diabetes apart from the role in promoting healing of diabetic skin ulcers.

Keywords

Adrenocortical function • Diabetes type 2 • Epinephrine/norepinephrine • HBO and endocrinology • Hyperbaric oxygen (HBO) • Prostaglandins • Testosterone • Thyroid disease

Introduction

Changes in various endocrine organs have been reported under hyperbaric oxygenation (HBO) and include adrenal hypertrophy, decrease in the weight of the thymus, and increase in the weight of the thyroid. Changes observed in the nervous and the endocrine systems have been viewed as represented nonspecific stress reactions. Several cases of hypotension in adolescents and children with a history of perinatal disturbances of the central nervous system (CNS) and functional activity of the pituitary-thyroid axis have been reported to normalize following HBO treatment. Most of the studies on this topic are based on animal experiments with few clinical applications. Effect of HBO on individual endocrines will be considered in the following sections.

Thyroid Glands

Sjöstrand (1964) exposed rats to HBO at 6 ATA for 4–5 days and sacrificed them on the 6th day. In contrast to the results of previous investigators, the thyroid weight was found to be

K.K. Jain, MD, FRACS, FFPM (✉)
1 Blaesiring 7, Basel 4057, Switzerland
e-mail: jain@pharmabiotech.ch

decreased but ^{131}I was increased. The author believed that this represented a specific effect of HBO on the thyroid.

Glucocorticoid Receptors

Golikov et al. (1986) studied the effect of a single exposure of HBO at 3 ATA for 5 h on glucocorticoid receptors in the lungs of rats. The level of these receptors was reduced to nearly half after the exposure. Twenty-four hours later the number of receptors in lungs had increased, while the blood cortisol level was reduced but was still a little higher than in the control animals.

Adrenocortical Function

HBO (2 ATA, 90 min/day) increases adrenocortical function in rats. Adrenocorticotropic hormone (ACTH) response in healthy adult male athletes after HBO exposure at 2.8 ATA for 1 h daily for 10 days has been studied (Casti et al. 1993). On day one (acute phase), ACTH level increased significantly, whereas in the chronic phase (days 5–10), the values remained stable. No significant variations were found during exposure to hyperbaric air. HBO, thus, has potential clinical application in the treatment of steroid dependency in patients with arthritis, possibly enabling withdrawal.

© Springer International Publishing AG 2017
K.K. Jain, *Textbook of Hyperbaric Medicine*, DOI 10.1007/978-3-319-47140-2_28

Rabbits exposed to HBO for 1 h after detonator-blast-induced craniocerebral injury showed significantly reduced aquaporin 4 expression and ACTH expression in the pituitary gland on immunohistochemical examination (Huo et al. 2012). Aquaporin 4 expression was positively correlated with ACTH expression. These findings indicate that early HBO therapy may suppress ACTH secretion by inhibiting aquaporin 4 expression.

Epinephrine/Norepinephrine

Hale et al. (1973) studied the endocrinological and metabolic responses of healthy young men to a range of oxygen-rich and oxygen-poor gaseous environments (varying between 15 and 100 % oxygen). The norepinephrine:epinephrine ratio (as index of catecholamine balance) varied directly with oxygen balance, ranging from 2:1 to 6:1. Norepinephrine and epinephrine act jointly in regulating regional blood flow – norepinephrine acting as a vasoconstrictor, while epinephrine acts as a vasodilator in low concentrations and as a constrictor in high concentrations.

Nakada et al. (1984) found increased adrenal epinephrine and norepinephrine in spontaneously hypertensive rats treated with HBO at 2 ATA. Catecholamines have been described as facilitating oxygen toxicity and hence the rationale for experimental adrenalectomy for protection against oxygen toxicity in experimental animals (see Chap. 6). Studies in divers have shown that HBO and hyperbaric air at 2.5 ATA do not induce a generalized hormonal stress reaction but induce an increase in endothelin-1 levels.

Epinephrine (E), norepinephrine (NE), adrenocorticotropic hormone (ACTH), and dopamine (DA) are involved in human stress response in acute exposed to high altitude. In a study on male volunteers, preconditioning with HBO prior to ascent to an altitude of 4000 m, the plasma expressions of DA, E, NE, and ACTH were elevated, speeding up the establishment of a new balance of homeostasis to adapt to the acute hypoxia at high altitude (Li et al. 2015).

Prostaglandins

Effect of hyperoxia on renal prostaglandin E2 (PGE2) excretion and diuresis in the dog has been studied (Walker et al 1980). Hypoxia caused a 13 % increase in renal blood flow, whereas hyperoxia caused a 5%–7 % decline due to vasoconstriction. HBO at 1.8 ATA and 2.8 ATA caused a decrease in urinary flow of 61 % and 70 %, respectively. The urinary PGE2 declined by 61 % at 2 ATA, 92 % at 1.8 ATA, and 99 %

at 2.8 ATA. Plasma antidiuretic hormone (ADH) remained unchanged. The authors postulated that HBO antidiuresis may be a consequence of an increased medullary osmotic gradient secondary to reduced vasa recta blood flow or may be due to a lowering of the normal functional antagonism between PGE2 and ADH, so that influence of endogenous ADH is potentiated.

Effect of HBO on prostaglandin synthesis was studied in the cortex and striatum of the rat brain; 3 groups were subjected to the following oxygen environments (Mialon and Barthelemy 1993):

1. Neurotoxic HBO at 6 ATA
2. Mild hyperoxia at 6 ATA room air
3. Normoxia

Examination of brain samples after decapitation showed that release of 6-keto-PGF1a was reduced significantly in the mild hyperoxia group.

Concentration of PGE values were restored to normal in gastric ulcer patients treated with HBO where previous treatment with H2-blockers had reduced the PGE concentration (Serebrianskaia and Masenko 1993).

The contents of PGE2 in alveolar bone and gingiva increase markedly in experimental periodontitis. The value of PGE2 in alveolar bone and gingiva reduces markedly after HBO treatments at 2.5 ATA (Chen et al. 2002).

In an experimental study, inflammation and fever was induced in rabbits by systemic administration of lipopolysaccharide, which increased hypothalamic levels of glutamate, hydroxyl radicals, and prostaglandin E2 (Niu et al. 2009). The febrile response was suppressed by HBO pretreatment or treatment. Simultaneous administration of an antioxidant (e.g., N-acetyl-L-cysteine) significantly enhanced the antipyretic effects exerted by HBO treatment. These results indicate that HBO may exert its antipyretic effect by inhibiting the glutamate–hydroxyl radicals–prostaglandin-E2 pathways in the hypothalamus.

Testosterone

Reduction of blood flow to the testes and a decrease in plasma testosterone have been observed in experimental animals under hyperbaric conditions. A reversible change in the rate of DNA synthesis can occur in the testes of rats after exposure to hyperbaric air. Human divers also show a decrease in plasma testosterone on exposure to 6 ATA. However, no changes were found in the testosterone concentration in serum or testes of rats after daily exposures to HBO under conditions similar to clinical use, e.g., at 2–3 ATA daily 90-min sessions.

Clinical Applications

The only reported clinical applications of HBO in endocrinology are in disorders of the thyroid and in diabetes mellitus. All the clinical reports are from the USSR. Little of the experimental evidence quoted above is relevant to the clinical applications.

Thyroid Disease

Shakarashvilli et al. (1981) studied the effect of HBO on thyroid function in normal subjects and in patients with thyrotoxicosis. HBO (2 ATA, 60 min) was given daily for 10–12 days. The levels of thyrotropic hormone, triiodothyronine, and thyroxine were checked daily. They became normal after the HBO treatment regardless of whether the level before exposure had been normal, decreased, or increased. The therapeutic effect lasted an average of 1–1.5 months.

Droviannikova (1981) used HBO for preoperative preparation of patients with diffuse toxic goiter. The optimal course of treatment was found to be one 45- to 60-min session per day for 6–10 days. The pressure was selected by titration according to the pulse, blood pressure, and cardiac output of each patient, but did not exceed 2 ATA. As a result, tachycardia was eliminated. The circulating blood volume decreased by 10–12 % and the contractile action of the myocardium improved. There was no increase in the level of thyroid hormones in the blood. The authors concluded that HBO in combination with conventional drug therapy improved cardiovascular hemodynamics and reduced the period of preoperative preparation by 8–10 days. Rakhmatullin et al. (1981) used HBO in the treatment of thyrotoxicosis crises in the postoperative period of patients with thyrotoxic goiter. The principal mechanism of postoperative complication was considered to be increased ejection of thyroid hormone into the circulation and emergence of hypoxia. HBO was used as preoperative preparation in 36 patients with toxic goiter. In eight of these patients, HBO was required in the postoperative period for crises. In another series of cases from Russia, in patients who underwent surgery for diffuse toxic goiter, recurrence of the disease was less in those who had undergone HBO therapy for preoperative preparation (Kariakin et al. 1992).

Diabetes Mellitus

The effect of HBO has not been studied on experimentally induced diabetes in animals but there are reports of this application in human patients. Most of the human studies are in diabetic foot (see Chap. 16). The focus of this section is on the effect of HBO on systemic manifestations of diabetes mellitus.

Kakhnovski et al. (1980 a, b, c) noted improvement of cardiovascular complications in diabetic patients on using HBO therapy and later reported HBO as an adjunct to diet and insulin in the treatment of moderately severe diabetes in 130 patients. The dosage of insulin was reduced by 4–38 units in 62.3 % of the patients after treatment. The authors concluded that the hypoglycemic effect of HBO is due to inhibition of the effect of anti-insulin hormones (somatotropic hormone and glucagon) by HBO. There was increased S-peptide secretion and tissue sensitivity to insulin due to correction of the acid-base balance. Kakhnovskii et al. (1982) also studied the indices of blood acid-base balance, glucose level, blood lactate and pyruvate concentration, and serum activity of malate dehydrogenase and lactate dehydrogenase, as well as of succinate dehydrogenase and glycerophosphate dehydrogenase in lymphocytic mitochondria. Diet and insulin therapy combined with HBO was accompanied by a rapid stabilization (within 12–18 days) of carbohydrate metabolism and good dynamics of all the tests. The results indicated a significant improvement in tissue metabolism – both glycolysis and the tricarboxylic cycle.

Ostashevskaia et al (1986) incorporated HBO in the treatment of juvenile diabetes and established high efficiency of the method for managing complications such as angiopathy, polyneuritis, and trophic changes in the tissues. Longoni et al. (1987) treated 15 diabetic patients with HBO and found that insulin requirements were reduced in 11 of them. There was a concomitant improvement in the diabetic ulcers in these patients.

Epshtein et al. (1988) treated 32 male patients with diabetes mellitus using HBO as a part of comprehensive management. They found that 10–14 sessions of HBO at 1.5–1.7 ATA for 40–50 min improved the carbohydrate metabolism, circulation in the lower extremities, and general condition of these patients. It was possible to reduce the dose of insulin and oral hypoglycemic agents in these patients. These authors recommended repetition of HBO courses every 6–8 months.

Transient hyperglycemia is common in patients with cerebrovascular accidents and is also a recognized risk factor for stroke. Hyperglycemia is more frequent in patients with an unfavorable outcome of stroke. This provides a rationale for the use of HBO in patients with stroke and high blood glucose levels. Apart from its effect on hyperglycemia, HBO has been used as an adjunct to pancreatic islet transplantation in diabetes mellitus. Peritransplant treatment of diabetic recipients by daily HBO sessions (2.4 ATA, 90 min) improves the outcome of the transplantation (Juang et al. 2002).

HBO reduces autoimmune diabetes incidence in non-obese diabetic mice via increased resting T cells and reduced activation of dendritic cells with preservation of β-cell mass resulting from decreased apoptosis and increased proliferation (Faleo et al. 2012). The safety profile and noninvasiveness makes HBO an appealing adjuvant therapy for prevention of diabetes and intervention trials.

Carotid bodies (CBs) regulate peripheral insulin sensitivity. Because CB is functionally blocked by hyperoxia and HBO improves fasting blood glucose in diabetes patients, a study to investigate the effect of HBO on glucose tolerance in type 2 diabetes patients is justified (Vera-Cruz et al. 2015). After 20 sessions of HBO, fasting, and 2-h postoral glucose tolerance test (OGTT), glycemia decreased significantly. In control group without diabetes, HBO did not modify fasting glycemia and post-OGTT glycemia. These results showed that HBO ameliorates glucose tolerance in diabetic patients and supports the use of HBO as treatment for type 2 diabetes.

Conclusion

In contrast to other areas of hyperbaric medicine, studies on the endocrinological aspect are scant. In view of the controversy regarding the effect of HBO on thyroid function, further experimental studies, as well as controlled trials on patients with thyrotoxicosis, should be carried out.

The idea of using HBO as an adjunct in the treatment of diabetes mellitus is a logical one. Fall in blood glucose has been observed in volunteers exposed to HBO. Controlled studies need to be done in diabetics to prove or disprove the beneficial effect of HBO. There is a lack of basic experimental studies assessing the effect of HBO in experimentally induced diabetes mellitus. HBO may also be a useful adjunct in reducing the transient hyperglycemia sometimes seen in cerebrovascular accidents. Diabetic patients who are given HBO for other indications should be carefully monitored for blood glucose, as the insulin requirements are usually reduced and the dosage needs to be readjusted. A calculation method enables the effect of HBO in lowering the insulin requirement in diabetics to be assessed (Dreval et al. 1988).

References

Casti A, Orlandini G, Vescovi P. Acute and chronic hyperbaric oxygen exposure in humans: effects on blood polyamines, adrenocorticotropin and beta-endorphin. Acta Endocrinol Copenh. 1993;129:436–41.

Chen T, Lin S, Liu J, Xu B, Hai J, Tang D. Effects and mechanism of hyperbaric oxygen on prostaglandins in alveolar bone and gingival of experimental periodontitis in animal. Zhonghua Kou Qiang Yi Xue Za Zhi. 2002;37:228–30.

Dreval AV, Dreval TP, Lukicheva TI. Two-dimensional parameter of the kinetics of glucose in the assessment of the efficacy and prognosis of therapy of diabetes mellitus. Ter Arkh. 1988;60:20–4.

Droviannikova IP. Hyperbaric oxygen in the complex treatment of patients with diffuse toxic goiter. In: Yefuny SN, editor. Proceedings of the 7th international congress on hyperbaric medicine. Moscow: USSR Academy of Sciences; 1981. p. 372.

Epshtein BV, Nishchenko VF, Timchenko PM. Hyperbaric oxygenation in the comprehensive treatment of patients with diabetes mellitus. Vrach Delo. 1988;1:65–6.

Faleo G, Fotino C, Bocca N, Molano RD, Zahr-Akrawi E, Molina J, et al. Prevention of autoimmune diabetes and induction of β-cell proliferation in NOD mice by hyperbaric oxygen therapy. Diabetes. 2012;61:1769–78.

Golikov PP, Rogatsky GG, Nikolaeva NY. Glucocorticoid receptors in the lungs in hyperbaric oxygenation. Patol Fiziol Eks Ter. 1986;2:32.

Hale HB, Williams EW, Ellis JP. Human endocrine-metabolic responses to graded oxygen pressures. Aerospace Med. 1973;44:33–6.

Huo J, Liu J, Wang J, Zhang Y, Wang C, Yang Y, et al. Early hyperbaric oxygen therapy inhibits aquaporin 4 and adrenocorticotropic hormone expression in the pituitary gland of rabbits with blast-induced craniocerebral injury. Neural Regen Res. 2012;7:1729–35.

Juang JH, Hsu BR, Kuo CH, Uengt SW. Beneficial effects of hyperbaric oxygen therapy on islet transplantation. Cell Transplant. 2002;11:95–101.

Kakhnovskii IM, Efuni SN, Gitel EP. Effects of hyperbaric oxygenation on the dynamics of the phase structure of right ventricular systole in diabetics. Ter Arkh. 1980a;52:88–91.

Kakhnovskii IM, Efuni SN, Grishina I. Electrocardiographic changes during hyperbaric oxygenation in diabetes mellitus. Kardiologii. 1980b;20:90–4.

Kakhnovskii IM, Efuni SN, Sokolovskaya MV. Correlation of respiratory and pulmonary circulatory oxygenation on the enzyme activity of tissue metabolism in diabetes mellitus. Probl Endokrinol (Mosk). 1982;28:11–7.

Kakhnovskii IM, Pgosbekian LM, Bokaneva IA, Novikova LL, Fedorova EV. Biochemical indices in diabetes mellitus patients undergoing hyperbaric oxygenation. Sov Med. 1980c;10:33–7.

Kariakin AM, Kucher VV, Kirienko IV. The pathogenetic and clinical grounds for the advantages of nondrug procedures in the preoperative preparation of patients with diffuse toxic goiter. Vestn Khir Im I I Grek. 1992;148:216–20.

Li Y, Shi L, Wu N, Liu J, Zhang Y, Zhang M, et al. Effects of hyperbaric oxygen preconditioning on human stress responses during acute exposure to high altitude. Zhonghua Lao Dong Wei Sheng Zhi Ye Bing Za Zhi. 2015;33:731–4.

Longoni C, Ferani R, Agliati G, et al. Hyperbaric oxygen therapy and glucose metabolism in patients with diabetic vasculopathic lesions. Presented at the European Undersea and Biomedical Society meeting, Palermo, Italy, Sept. 1987;9–12.

Mialon P, Barthelemy L. Effect of hyperbaric oxygenation on prostaglandin and thromboxane synthesis in the cortex and the striatum of rat brain. Mol Chem Neuropathol. 1993;20:181–9.

Nakada T, Koike H, Katayama T, Watanabe H, Yamori Y. Increased adrenal epinephrine and norepinephrine in spontaneously hypertensive rats treated with hyperbaric oxygen. Hinyokika Kiyo. 1984;30:1357–66.

Niu KC, Huang WT, Lin MT, Huang KF. Hyperbaric oxygen causes both antiinflammation and antipyresis in rabbits. Eur J Pharmacol. 2009;606:240–5.

Ostashevskaia MI, Afanas-Eva NB, Valuiskova RP, Serebriakova AD, Shirenkov IA. Experience in the use of hyperbaric oxygenation to treat diabetes mellitus in children. Probl Endokrinol. 1986;32:16–9.

Rakhmatullin IG, Hallev MA. Hyperbaric oxygen in pre and postoperative periods of patients with thyrotoxic goiter. In Yefuny SN

(Ed.) Proceedings of the 7th international congress on hyperbaric medicine. USSR Academy of Sciences, Moscow 1981:p 373.

Serebrianskaia MV, Masenko VP. Dynamics of prostaglandin E content in patients with duodenal ulcer during various treatment regimens. Klin Med Mosk. 1993;71:45–7.

Shakarashvilli NV, Gankin EK, Uskov IA. Normalizing effect of hyperbaric oxygen on the production of hormones by thyroid gland. In Yefuny SN (Ed.) Proceedings of the 7th International Congress on Hyperbaric Medicine. USSR Academy of Sciences, Moscow, 1981:p 371.

Sjöstrand J. The effect of oxygen at high pressure on thyroid function in the rat. Acta Physiol Scand. 1964;62:91–100.

Vera-Cruz P, Guerreiro F, Ribeiro MJ, Guarino MP, Conde SV. Hyperbaric oxygen therapy improves glucose homeostasis in Type 2 diabetes patients: a likely involvement of the carotid bodies. Adv Exp Med Biol. 2015;860:221–5.

Walker BR, Attallah AA, Lee JB, Hong SK, Mookerjee BK, Share L, et al. Antidiuresis and inhibition of PGE excretion by hyperoxia in the conscious dog. Undersea Biomed Res. 1980;7:113–26.

K.K. Jain

Abstract

This chapter reviews the modest number of applications in the area of pulmonary disorders as normobaric oxygen is more frequently used for most indications in this area. Effects of HBO on lungs include a discussion of pulmonary arterial hemodynamics as well as lung mechanics and pulmonary gas exchange. Pulmonary oxygen toxicity is also discussed although normal therapeutic uses at most pressures of HBO do not adversely affect the lungs. Clinical applications include respiratory insufficiency, bronchial asthma, bronchitis, inflammatory processes of the lungs, and pulmonary embolism. Contraindications include nitrogen dioxide poisoning, emphysema, shock lung, and pneumothorax.

Keywords

Bronchial asthma • Emphysema • HBO and lungs • HBO contraindications • Hyperbaric oxygen (HBO) • Normobaric oxygen • Oxygen toxicity • Pneumothorax • Pulmonary disorders • Pulmonary embolism

Introduction

Hyperbaric oxygen (HBO) therapy has a limited role in pulmonary disorders, which are usually treated by normobaric oxygen (Jain 1989). Nonetheless, HBO has been used for a number of pulmonary conditions, and these are reviewed in this chapter. Effects of HBO on lungs such as pulmonary hemodynamics and gas exchange are important basic aspects. Pulmonary oxygen toxicity and contraindications for the use of HBO will also be described.

Effects of HBO on Lungs

Arterial and Pulmonary Arterial Hemodynamics

Effects of exposure to hyperbaric air and HBO have been studied on healthy volunteers using arterial and pulmonary

K.K. Jain, MD, FRACS, FFPM (✉)
1 Blaesiring 7, Basel 4057, Switzerland
e-mail: jain@pharmabiotech.ch

arterial (PA) catheters breathing air at 0.85, 3.0, 2.5, 2.0, 1.3 (decompression stop), 1.12 (decompression stop), and 0.85 ATA (lab altitude) and then at identical pressures breathing oxygen followed by atmospheric pressure air, while measurements were made of arterial and PA pressures (PAP), cardiac output (Q), and blood gas measurements from both arterial and PA catheters (Weaver et al. 2009). Although hemodynamic changes occurred during exposure to both hyperbaric air and HBO, the magnitude of change under HBO conditions was greater: heart rate changes ranged from −9 to −19 % (air to oxygen), respiratory rate from −12 to −17 %, Q from −7 to −18 %, PAP from −18 to −19 %, pulmonary vascular resistance from −38 to −48 %, and right-to-left shunt fraction from −87 to −107 %. Mixed venous CO_2 fell 8 % from baseline during HBO despite mixed venous oxygen tensions of several hundred Torr. The stroke volume, oxygen delivery, and oxygen consumption did not change across exposures. The arterial and mixed venous partial pressures of oxygen and contents were elevated, as predicted. Oxygen extraction increased 37 % during HBO. The data presented in this study are in agreement with other studies which show that heart rate and Q decrease with HBO exposure.

Lung Mechanics and Pulmonary Gas Exchange

The physical and physiological aspects of gas exchange in the lungs under HBO have been discussed in Chap. 2. Respiratory compliance is not changed when pressure is increased to 2 ATA on breathing air. Lung dynamics, however, fall by 15 % in individuals breathing oxygen at a pressure of 2 ATA for 6–11 h. Respiratory effects of 90 min long HBO sessions at 2.4 ATA repeated 2–3 times a week for 3 months during treatment of patients with peripheral vascular disease are increased airway resistance, increased pulmonary elasticity, decreased vital capacity, and respiratory rate. These changes are completely reversible within 2 h of completion of the treatment. Pulmonary function studies on subjects breathing oxygen at 3 ATA for 90 min show a decrease of pulmonary compliance, which is attributed to absorption atelectasis, pulmonary vascular congestion, and edema. The oxygen diffusion capacity and diffusion pressure ratios are markedly reduced. Most of the respiratory changes are observed in treatments using >2 ATA pressure. Disparity in some of these findings may also be due to individual variations in tolerance of HBO. Most HBO treatments are carried out at 1.5–2 ATA, and the duration usually does not exceed 1 h. Within these limits no adverse effects have been observed on pulmonary function. If there are any adverse effects, they certainly clear up within 24 h, which is the usual interval between treatments. The changes observed in the mechanics of respiration can be early signs of oxygen toxicity.

Pulmonary Oxygen Toxicity

Pulmonary oxygen toxicity is more commonly seen with prolonged exposure to 100 % normobaric oxygen (Jain 1989). It is less of a problem during short exposures to HBO. Oxygen exposures at high pressures are limited by CNS rather than pulmonary intoxication because no pulmonary symptoms are reported by subjects who breathe oxygen at pressures ranging from 2.4 to 4 ATA until occurrence of neurological manifestations. Experimental observations regarding the toxicity of oxygen under normobaric and hyperbaric conditions are not comparable. Although the structural changes in the lungs produced by oxygen inhalation under normobaric and hyperbaric conditions are the same, the degree of change depends on the magnitude and duration of oxygenation.

Hyperoxia induced by breathing 95 % oxygen for >12 h causes a significant alveolar-capillary leak. These changes were reversible, but such alterations may induce processes that can result in fibrosis. One popular theory of the mechanism of lung toxicity suggests that high concentrations of oxygen are directly toxic to lung parenchyma, probably via toxic oxygen radicals. Although the metabolism of lung connective tissue is unaffected by short-term exposure to HBO,

the mechanism of toxicity is due, at least in part, to the effect of oxygen on surfactant synthesis. Oxygen inhibits enzymes involved in synthesis of surfactant and may also inhibit transport of surfactant to the alveoli. An important causal mechanism involved in the development of lung injury is an initial increase in minimal surface tension due to increased intra-alveolar cholesterol. Hyperoxia induced by breathing a concentration of oxygen higher than 95 % for 48 h impairs phosphatidylcholine synthesis, secretion, and uptake in the newborn rabbit lung. This is consistent with the existence of multiple sites of action of hyperoxia on the pulmonary surfactant system in the newborn. This has serious implications for the premature infant with respiratory distress syndrome, for which oxygen may be administered. The pathological changes occurring in the lungs in response to hyperbaric oxygen are shown in Fig. 29.1.

Symptoms and signs of pulmonary function changes consistent with early pulmonary oxygen toxicity (POT) occurred in 12 subjects exposed to 5 ATA air for 48 h, while none occurred in six subjects exposed to 5 ATA normoxic nitrogen-oxygen (6 % oxygen) for a similar period (Eckenhoff et al. 1986). All subjects eventually recovered completely. Morphological changes in the lungs have been shown to depend on the degree and duration of oxygen pressure. Daily exposure to 2 ATA for 60 min for 2 weeks or 2.5 ATA for 1 week is considered to be the safe limits of HBO (Kharchenko et al. 1986). Alterations in pulmonary function that were observed in subjects breathing oxygen at 3.5 ATA for 3.5 h include small but significant decreases in several indices of both inspiratory and expiratory function (Clark et al. 1991).

At higher inspired O_2 pressures, 2–3 ATA, pulmonary injury is greatly accelerated but less inflammatory in character, and events in the brain are a prelude to a distinct lung pathology. The CNS-mediated component of this lung injury can be attenuated by selective inhibition of neuronal nitric oxide synthase (nNOS) or by unilateral transection of the vagus nerve. Extrapulmonary, neurogenic events predominate in the pathogenesis of acute pulmonary oxygen toxicity in HBO, as nNOS activity drives lung injury by modulating the output of central autonomic pathways.

Hyperoxic acute lung injury (HALI) is a clinical syndrome resulting from prolonged administration of high concentrations of oxygen. HBO preconditioning (HBO-PC) has a protective effect on oxidative injury, and this effect of HBO-PC on HALI was tested in rats (Feng et al. 2015). The results demonstrated that HBO-PC ameliorated biochemical and histological alterations in the lung induced by hyperoxia, decreased oxidative products, but increased antioxidant enzymes. Furthermore, HBO-PC upregulated heme oxygenase-1 (HO-1) mRNA and activity in lung tissues. The administration of HO-1 inhibitor, zinc protoporphyrin IX, abolished its protective effects. Thus HBO-PC could protect rats against HALI, and the anti-oxidative effect may be related to the upregulation of HO-1.

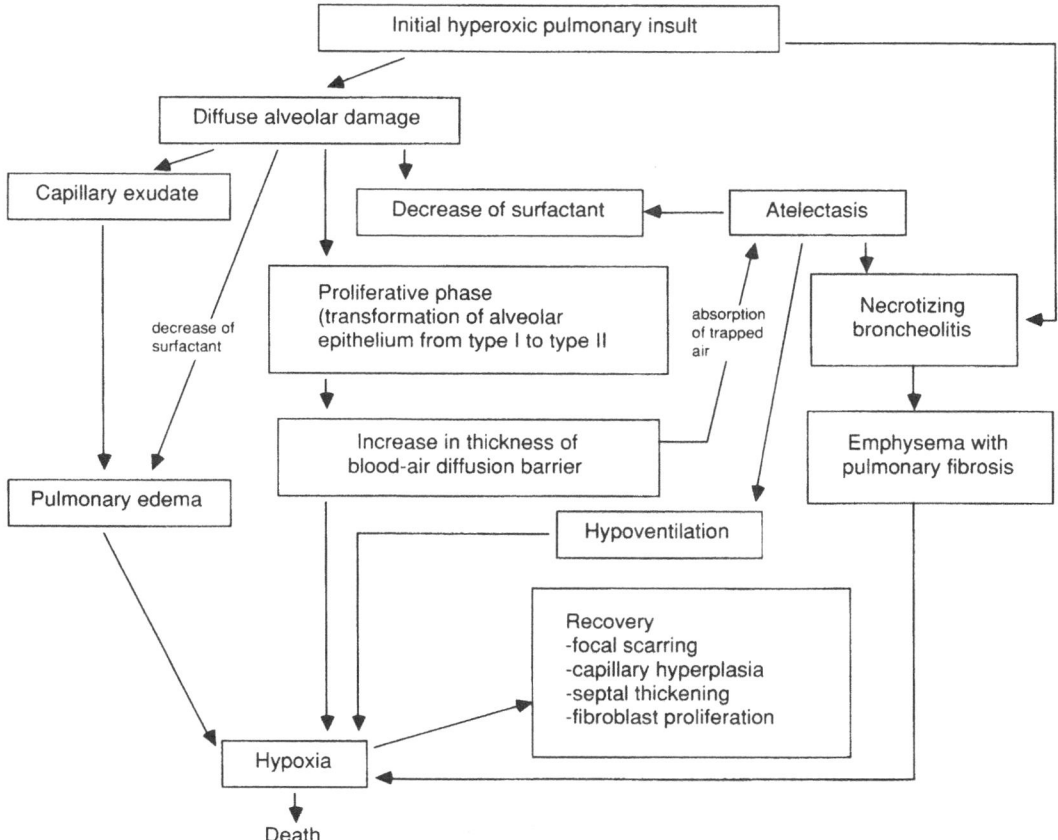

Fig. 29.1 Sequence of events in pulmonary edema due to oxygen toxicity

Methods of prevention of oxygen toxicity have been discussed in Chap. 6. Lung toxicity can be prevented or minimized by alternation of HBO (2 ATA) and air breathing.

Clinical Applications

Respiratory Insufficiency

Lukich et al. (1978) treated by means 16 patients with restrictive and obstructive disease of the lungs and respiratory insufficiency with HBO at 1.3–1.5 ATA for 40–60 min. Arterial hypoxemia was eliminated, the acid-base balance became normal, and respiratory acidosis disappeared in all the patients. The use of HBO in more severe forms of respiratory in sufficiency has been investigated experimentally. Rogatsky et al. (1988) showed that in Wistar rats with induced respiratory insufficiency HBO at 3 ATA for 2 h reduced the mortality and prevented the structural changes peculiar to the "wet lung" syndrome.

Jansen et al. (1987) performed lung lavage under HBO conditions in two patients suffering from severe respiratory insufficiency in pulmonary alveolar proteinosis. Under these conditions, gas exchange was maintained, and mixed venous partial pressure of oxygen and oxygen saturation showed increases to acceptable levels. This enabled the authors to limit the FiO_2 in order to extend the oxygen tolerance and to perform the lavage procedures more effectively. Both patients improved significantly, and the authors concluded that the use of HBO in unilateral lung lavages is a useful procedure.

Most patients with chronic obstructive pulmonary disease (COPD) are treated with normobaric oxygen than HBO (Jain 1989). Miller et al (1987) reassessed the role of hyperbaric air in the treatment of COPD. Patients with this condition were placed in a hyperbaric chamber of 1.25 ATA (air). Their arterial oxygen saturations were comparable to when they were breathing oxygen by nasal prongs at 2 L/min. The ability to exercise was improved under compressed air. The authors suggested hyperbaric air as an alternative to long-term oxygen therapy. No adverse effects were observed in their patients. It should be borne in mind that emphysema is a contraindication for HBO therapy. The pressure of 1.25 ATA may be safe for these patients, but those with emphysematous bullae should not go into a hyperbaric chamber.

Bronchial Asthma

Acute exacerbation of asthma is challenging as both severity and response to therapy varies. High-dose, frequent, or continuous nebulized short-acting beta2 agonist (SABA) therapy that can be combined with a short-acting muscarinic antagonist (SAMA) is the backbone of treatment. When patients do not rapidly clinically respond to SABA/SAMA inhalation, the early use of oral or parenteral corticosteroids should be considered and has been shown to impact the immediate need for ICU admission or even the need for hospital admission. Adjunctive therapies such as the use of intravenous magnesium and helium/oxygen combination gas for inhalation should be considered and are best used early in the treatment plan if they are likely to impact the patients' clinical course (Albertson et al. 2015). Physicians should be prepared to use the entire spectrum of therapies available for the treatment of acute asthma exacerbations and the agents that should be initiated to prevent worsening or additional exacerbations.

Korotaev et al. (1981) used HBO in 16 adult patients with bronchial asthma of infectious-allergic etiology. The medical management was supplemented by 5–9 daily sessions of HBO at 1.5 ATA lasting 30–50 min each. Improvement was noted in half of the patients. The rest had been on steroids for long periods; attempts to wean them off steroid dependence by means of HBO treatment were not successful. The authors also treated four children with acute bronchospasm. Dyspnea was relieved during the HBO sessions. Mikhailov (1982) stated that HBO was used in asthma in order to normalize various types of glucocorticoid metabolic disturbances associated both with the decreased synthesis of adrenocortical hormones and inactivation of glucocorticoids by blood transcortin and their reduced utilization. Normalization of glucocorticoid metabolism was maximal in patients with milder forms of asthma, and the best results were obtained in these cases.

Liu and Zhi (1986) treated 387 patients with bronchial asthma who were resistant to conventional treatment, using HBO at 2 ATA (80- to 90-min sessions with an air break of 10 min in the middle) for an average of 24 sessions. Good results (decrease in the frequency of asthma attacks and discontinuance of drug therapy) were obtained in 182 (47%) of the patients; satisfactory results (decrease in the dosage and frequency of the use of medications) were observed in 163 patients (42%); and no effect was seen in 41 patients (11%).

Bronchitis

Efuni (1984) used HBO therapy in 92 patients with dust-induced bronchitis. There was improvement in 88.9% of the patients as determined by tolerance to physical exercise and blood gas measurements.

Inflammatory Processes of the Lungs

Ermakov and Barksy (1981) investigated the effect of HBO on acute and chronic pneumonia. Three to five sessions at 1.5 ATA were used. The authors concluded that HBO had no adverse effects on the acute inflammatory processes and actually had some benefit in the chronic cases. They cautioned against the use of HBO in cases of hypercapnia. A pCO_2 value of 60 mmHg or above is considered to be a contraindication for the use of HBO unless the patient is on artificial ventilation.

A combination of HBO and antioxidants (unithiol and alpha-tocopherol) was used in a complex intensive therapy of 194 children, aged 3 days to 3 years, with severe pneumonias (Zhdanov et al. 1991). HBO yielded excellent and good results in 75.8% of patients, was ineffective in 17% of cases, and produced signs of oxygen toxicity in 7.2% of patients.

There is a significant reduction in the activity of inducible nitric oxide synthase and a rise in the expression of surfactant protein D in lung tissue of different pulmonary aspiration models with the use of HBO therapy (Sahin et al. 2011). The study concluded that HBO treatment might be beneficial in lung injury and has potential for clinical use.

Pulmonary Embolism

Pulmonary air embolism occurs in inappropriate decompressions or clinical complications. Sudden lodging of air bubbles in the pulmonary circulation results in pulmonary hypertension, pulmonary edema, and deficiency in cardiopulmonary functions, which are often fatal without timely intervention. There are cases of massive pulmonary embolism that underwent successful embolectomy with HBO support and recovered.

Pulmonary Edema

Iazzetti and Maciel (1988) induced neurogenic pulmonary edema in rats by bilateral cervical vagotomy. The group of animals exposed to HBO at 1.8 ATA had less pulmonary edema than the controls breathing room air. High-altitude pulmonary edema (HAPE) is a noncardiogenic pulmonary edema which usually occurs in inhabitants at sea level who ascend rapidly to altitudes greater than 2500–3000 m. Treatment of HAPE consists of immediate rapid descent to sea level or improvement of oxygenation either by supplemental oxygen or by HBO (Paralikar 2012). HBO preconditioning was shown to attenuate HAPE in rats by preinduction of lung heat shock protein 70 (Tsai et al. 2014).

Although pulmonary edema is a feature of oxygen toxicity, it appears that some types, such as neurogenic and cardiogenic pulmonary edema, may be reduced by HBO therapy. Some smoke inhalation victims who are treated by HBO may experience relief through the beneficial effect on pulmonary edema. Administration of HBO (2.8 ATA for 45 min) inhibited adhesion of circulating neutrophils subsequent to smoke inhalation in rats (Thom et al. 2001). HBO reduced pulmonary neutrophil accumulation whether used in a prophylactic manner, 24 h before smoke inhalation, or as treatment immediately after the smoke insult. The beneficial effect appears related to inhibition of neutrophil adhesion to the vasculature. Clinical studies are required to assess the effect of HBO in pulmonary edema in humans.

Mechanism of Action of HBO in Type II Decompression Syndrome

Decompression syndrome (DCS) was described in Chap. 11 and most of discussion centers on tape I DCS affecting the central nervous system. An experimental study has investigated ultrastructural changes in rabbits with type II DCS and the therapeutic effects of HBO (Geng et al. 2015). Histological examination revealed severe and rapid damage to lung tissue, and air bubbles could be seen in the blood vessels. Ultrastructural examination showed exudation of RBCs in the alveolar space. Type I alveolar epithelia cells and endothelial cells of the capillaries illustrated slight shortening of cells, swollen cytoplasm, and decreased cell processes. Type II alveolar epithelial cells showed slight swelling of the mitochondria, decreased vacuolar degeneration of lamellar bodies, and increase in the number of free ribosomes. In the HBO treatment group, the findings were somewhat similar to those in the DCS group, but the extent of damage was less. Only a small amount of tiny bubbles could be seen in the blood vessels . This study confirms the benefits of HBO treatment in DCS.

Contraindications for the Use of HBO

Nitrogen Dioxide Poisoning

Experimental nitrogen dioxide poisoning in dogs carries high mortality due to lung edema and respiratory failure. The mortality and the pathological effects on the lungs are increased in animals treated with HBO compared with the controls. On this basis, the use of HBO in cases of human nitrogen dioxide poisoning is contraindicated.

Paraquat Poisoning

Locket (1973) indicated that HBO may be useful in cases of poisoning due to paraquat, which is a highly toxic herbicide. A study of lungs in 11 cases of death from paraquat poisoning in comparison with lungs in cases of oxygen poisoning led to the hypothesis that paraquat exerts its toxic action by sensitizing the lungs to oxygen at atmospheric pressure (Rebello and Mason 1978). Experimental studies in rats have shown that lung damage in paraquat poisoning and HBO exposure both involve superoxide-mediated inhibition of phospholipase A2 (Giulivi et al. 1995). HBO would thus be contraindicated in paraquat poisoning.

Emphysema

Emphysema is a long-term, progressive disease of the lungs that primarily causes shortness of breath due to overinflation of the alveoli. Emphysema is a COPD and is often associated with chronic bronchitis. Supplemental oxygen is frequently used for patients with COPD. HBO has been suggested as a treatment adjunct in emphysema to lessen the trapped air, to oxygenate the blood without causing hypercapnia, and to alter the pulmonary perfusion. Past anecdotal reports of subjective improvement in such cases by the use of HBO have not been supported by objective data. More recent studies have thoroughly investigated pre- and post-HBO respiratory status by objective investigations and found no improvement. Emphysema is listed as a contraindication for HBO therapy.

Shock Lung

Although HBO is useful in the treatment of shock, it has been reported that serious respiratory distress, the so-called shock lung, can be aggravated by HBO. Ouda et al. (1977) induced shock lung in rats by injection of endotoxins. They showed that the decrease of mucopolysaccharide of the alveolar epithelium and the decrease of phospholipid of the alveolar lining layer observed in endotoxic shock were prevented after 2 h of HBO at 3 ATA, but not after 4 h of HBO at the same pressure, which induces lung damage independent of endotoxin. They concluded that HBO treatment may be effective in endotoxin-induced damage if one observes the proper precautions. The authors did not spell out the proper conditions for treatment of a human patient. There are no clinical reports of HBO use for shock lung, and it remains on the contraindication list.

Pneumothorax

Pneumothorax (PTX) is rare complication in patients receiving HBO therapy. Patients with air-trapping lesions in the lungs and those with a history of spontaneous PTX, lung disease, mechanical ventilation, or chest trauma are at an increased risk for PTX during HBO therapy. A case of PTX is reported in a young male earthquake survivor with multiple wounds who had been intubated and put on mechanical ventilation because of adult respiratory distress syndrome and given HBO treatments (Cakmak et al. 2015). At initial presentation, he was conscious, well-oriented, and hemodynamically stable. The initial six HBO treatments were uneventful, but during the seventh session, the patient lost consciousness and developed cardiopulmonary arrest near the end of decompression. A diagnosis of tension PTX was made, the patient was removed from the chamber, and a chest tube was inserted, which improved the symptoms. Patients with PTX will have problems during decompression and should not be placed in the hyperbaric chamber until a chest tube is placed by closed thoracotomy.

Conclusion

HBO therapy has no advantages over the normobaric oxygen therapy widely used in respiratory insufficiency. The main concern in the use of HBO for pulmonary disorders is the fear of aggravation of lung pathology by oxygen-induced pulmonary toxicity. Pulmonary toxicity is not a problem in patients with healthy lungs who receive HBO at up to 3 ATA for periods as long as 90 min once or twice daily.

There is no absolute or ideal indication for HBO in pulmonary disorders. Further research and controlled trials are required to assess the reported beneficial effect in asthma and bronchitis. It is worth noting that most of these treatments have been carried out at 1.5 ATA. Patients undergoing HBO treatment for other indications should be subjected to a thorough examination of the lungs supplemented by chest X-rays and pulmonary function studies. It must be remembered, of course, that PTX and silent lung lesions are contraindications for HBO therapy.

References

Albertson TE, Sutter ME, Chan AL. The acute management of asthma. Clin Rev Allergy Immunol. 2015;48:114–25.

Cakmak T, Battal B, Kara K, Metin S, Demirbas S, Yildiz S, et al. A case of tension pneumothorax during hyperbaric oxygen therapy in an earthquake survivor with crush injury complicated by ARDS (adult respiratory distress syndrome). Undersea Hyperb Med. 2015;42:9–13.

Clark JM, Jackson RM, Lambertson CJ, Gelfand R, Hiller WD, Unger M. Pulmonary function in men after oxygen breathing at 3.0 ATA for 3.5 h. J Appl Physiol. 1991;71:8788–885.

Eckenhoff RG, Osborne SF, Parker JW, Bondi KR. Direct ascent from shallow air saturation exposures. Undersea Biomed Res. 1986;13:305–16.

Efuni SM. Effect of combined treatment including hyperbaric oxygenation on bronchitis. Sov Med. 1984;9:8–12.

Ermakov EV, Barksy RL. Hyperbaric oxygen in cases of inflammatory diseases of the lungs. In: Yefuny SN, editor. Proceedings of the 7th international congress on hyperbaric medicine. Moscow: USSR Academy of Sciences; 1981. p. 290.

Feng Y, Zhang Z, Li Q, Li W, Xu J, Cao H. Hyperbaric oxygen preconditioning protects lung against hyperoxic acute lung injury in rats

via heme oxygenase-1 induction. Biochem Biophys Res Commun. 2015;456:549–54.

Geng M, Zhou L, Liu X, Li P. Hyperbaric oxygen treatment reduced the lung injury of type II decompression sickness. Int J Clin Exp Pathol. 2015;8:1797–803.

Giulivi C, Lavagno CC, Lucesoli F, Bermúdez MJ, Boveris A. Lung damage in paraquat poisoning and hyperbaric oxygen exposure: superoxide-mediated inhibition of phospholipase A2. Free Radic Biol Med. 1995;18:203–13.

Iazzetti PE, Maciel RE. Effects of hyperbaric oxygen on the rat neurogenic pulmonary edema. Braz J Med Biol Res. 1988;21:153–6.

Jain KK. Oxygen in Physiology and Medicine. Charles C. Thomas: Springfield, IL; 1989.

Jansen HM, Zuurmond WW, Roos CM, Schreuder JJ, Bakker DJ. Whole-lung lavage under hyperbaric oxygen conditions for alveolar proteinosis with respiratory failure. Chest. 1987;91:829–32.

Kharchenko NM, Boikova SP, Drozdova GA, Demurov EA. Structural changes in the lungs induced by different levels of hyperbaric oxygenation. Biull Eksp Biol Med. 1986;102:604–6.

Korotaev GM, Zavarzin YA, Mamorov SD. Hyperbaric treatment of patients with bronchial asthma. In: Yefuni SN, editor. Proceedings of the 7th international congress on hyperbaric medicine. Moscow: USSR Academy of Sciences; 1981. p. 291.

Liu ZF, Zhi Y. Application of HBO in the treatment of 387 cases of bronchial asthma. Presented at the 5th Chinese congress on hyperbaric medicine. Fuzhow, China, Sept 26–29, 1986.

Locket S. Clinical toxicology. IV. The treatment of poisoning. What do I do first? Part 2. Practitioner. 1973;210:575–9.

Lukich VL, Filimonova MV, Bazarova VS. Gas exchange in patients with chronic cardiac and pulmonary insufficiency in hyperbaric oxygenation. Klin Med (Mosk). 1978;56:74–83.

Mikhailov AM. Correction of glucocorticoid metabolism disorders in patients with bronchial asthma treated by hyperbaric oxygenation. Klin Med. 1982;60:52–6.

Miller WC, Suich DM, Unger KM. Hyperbaric environment for chronic hypoxemia. J Hyperbaric Med. 1987;2:211–4.

Ouda M, Moriyama Y, Haibara T, et al. The therapeutic effect of hyperbaric oxygen in the "shock lung.". In: Smith G, editor. Proceedings of the 6th International Congress on Hyperbaric Medicine. Aberdeen: University of Aberdeen Press; 1977. p. 82–3.

Paralikar SJ. High altitude pulmonary edema-clinical features, pathophysiology, prevention and treatment. Indian J Occup Environ Med. 2012;16:59–62.

Rebello G, Mason KJ. Pulmonary histological appearances in fatal paraquat poisoning. Histopathology. 1978;2:53–66.

Rogatsky GG, Vainshtein MB, Sevostianova TV. Use of hyperbaric oxygenation to correct an acute experimental respiratory insufficiency syndrome. Biull Eksp Biol Med. 1988;105:410–1.

Sahin SH, Kanter M, Ayvaz S, Colak A, Aksu B, Guzel A, et al. The effect of hyperbaric oxygen treatment on aspiration pneumonia. J Mol Histol. 2011;42:301–10.

Thom SR, Mendiguren I, Fisher D. Smoke inhalation-induced alveolar lung injury is inhibited by hyperbaric oxygen. Undersea Hyperb Med. 2001;28:175–9.

Tsai MC, Lin HJ, Lin MT, Niu KC, Chang CP, Tsao TC. High-altitude pulmonary edema can be prevented by heat shock protein 70-mediated hyperbaric oxygen preconditioning. J Trauma Acute Care Surg. 2014;77:585–91.

Weaver LK, Howe S, Snow GL, Deru K. Arterial and pulmonary arterial hemodynamics and oxygen delivery/extraction in normal humans exposed to hyperbaric air and oxygen. J Appl Physiol 2009;107:336-45.

Zhdanov GG, Nechaev VN, Alipov PA. Hyperbaric oxygenation and antioxidants in the complex intensive therapy of severe forms of pneumonia in children. Anesteziol Reanimatol. 1991;2:54–8.

Hyperbaric Oxygenation in Traumatology and Orthopedics

30

K.K. Jain

Abstract

HBO has several applications in traumatology and orthopedics. HBO has been shown to be useful in crush injuries, and its complications such as skeletal muscle compartment syndrome and traumatic ischemia where it may enable limb salvage. These uses are relevant to management of battlefield injuries. HBO also facilitates healing of fractures and reimplantation of limbs as well as other body parts. Long-term HBO is an effective treatment of osteonecrosis. There is some evidence of usefulness for treatment of rheumatoid arthritis. Although there are some favorable reports of HBO as an adjunct to repair of peripheral nerve injuries, this indication has not been established.

Keywords

Amputations • Compartment syndrome • Crush injuries • Fractures • Hyperbaric oxygen (HBO) • Limb reimplantation • Military medicine • Osteonecrosis • Peripheral nerve injuries • Rheumatoid arthritis

Introduction

Traumatology, by definition, has a multidisciplinary character and includes injuries of various systems of the body. In this chapter the focus is principally on musculoskeletal injuries and related orthopedic problems where hyperbaric oxygen (HBO) has been used. Injuries to specific organs are discussed under the appropriate system, e.g., head injuries in Chap. 21 and traumatic shock in Chap. 25. Complications of trauma such as gas gangrene and osteomyelitis are described in Chap. 14.

The major role of HBO is considered to be in combating hypoxia—both local and general—that develops as a result of trauma. Therefore, HBO is an important auxiliary therapeutic measure in traumatology.

Crush Injuries

Crush injuries resulting from trauma vary in presentations from minor contusions to limb-threatening damage. Crush injuries involve multiple tissues, from the skin and subcutaneous to the muscle and tendons to the bone and joints and those involving limbs present frequently in emergency departments. They may not be as apparent as open fracture dislocations or neurovascular injuries. If treatment of these lesions is delayed, irreversible changes may occur in the tissues. Late complications of severe crush injuries include osteomyelitis, nonunion of fractures, and amputations, and failed flaps occur in approximately 50% of cases. The following criteria are used to define a crush injury:

- Two or more tissues (muscle, bone, other connective tissue, skin, nerve) must be involved.
- The injury must be severe enough to render the viability of the tissues questionable. If the tissues recover, functional deficits are likely.
- Severity of injury varies from minimal to irreversible with a partially viable gray zone between the two. Enhancing survival from injuries in the gray zone is the object of therapy.

K.K. Jain, MD, FRACS, FFPM (✉)
1 Blaesiring 7, Basel 4057, Switzerland
e-mail: jain@pharmabiotech.ch

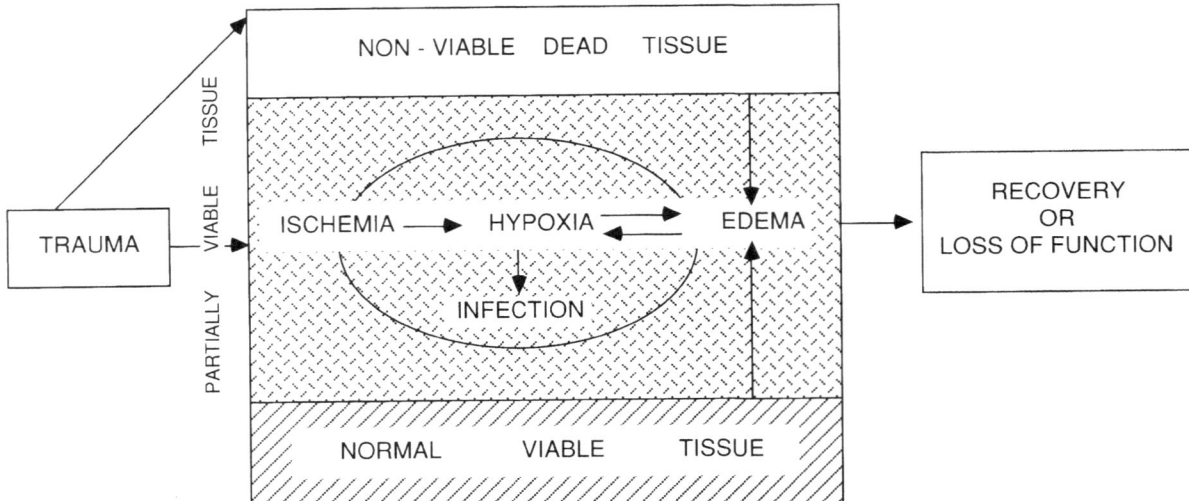

Fig. 30.1 Pathophysiology of crush injury

Pathophysiology

The pathophysiology of crush injuries is illustrated in Fig. 30.1. Trauma leads to death of tissue, which swells up (edema) and contributes to ischemia of the partially viable tissue. Ischemia is also a result of direct vascular injury. Ischemia and edema are parts of a vicious circle where hypoxia plays a central role. The partially viable tissue may recover if this circle is interrupted; otherwise, there is loss of function due to tissue damage. Edema of partially viable tissue may also affect the function of the adjacent normal tissue. Edema compounds the problem of ischemia, as it increases the diffusion distance from the capillary to the cell. With hypoxia, the tissues lose their ability to resist infection and repair themselves.

In a closed compartment, fluid pressure can rise higher than the capillary perfusion pressure, leading to ischemia of the tissues within the compartment. There is red cell clumping at the site of injury and this interferes with the microcirculation. Plasma may still go through the capillaries (no red cells), but normally it does not contain enough oxygen to sustain the tissues. Trauma may be direct or indirect. Direct trauma or crush injury may result from one of many causes. Indirect or closed trauma may occur from staying in one posture for a long time, such as in suicidal overdose, or may be exercise induced. Indirect trauma is also referred to as compartment syndrome.

Diagnosis

History and physical examination are important for making a diagnosis. During the examination five Ps should be kept in mind: pain, paralysis, paresthesia, pallor, and pulselessness. The most useful laboratory investigations are those measuring serum myoglobin, creatinine, potassium, and BUN. Urine may show myoglobinuria. Special investigations comprise the following:

- Measurement of compartment tissue fluid pressure
- X-rays to detect fractures, cavitation, or air in soft tissues
- Angiography, electromyography, and thermography for neurovascular assessment

Treatment

Crush injury must be recognized immediately and treated aggressively. The basic therapy consists of management of the wound if present, treatment of any fracture, prophylactic antibiotics, and surgical debridement if required.

Role of HBO in Treatment

HBO is usually administered at 2–3 ATA and is an ideal adjuvant to the basic treatment for the following reasons:

- It counteracts the tissue hypoxia by elevating tissue pO_2.
- It reduces edema by vasoconstriction and reduction of blood flow. The latter is more than compensated by hyperoxia. By raising the oxygen dissolved in plasma tenfold, HBO creates a favorable diffusion gradient through the edema fluid and other barriers, such as blood, to the hypoxic cells. It breaks the vicious circle referred to in Fig. 30.1 and allows the compromised tissues to survive in spite of deficient hemoglobin–oxygen delivery in low-flow states.
- It promotes wound healing.
- It prevents infection.

Most publications on this topic are uncontrolled studies and indicate that patients with crush injuries do better with HBO than they would have done without HBO under similar conditions. About 60 % of the patients are reported to have a good response to HBO treatment. Controlled studies are difficult to perform under such condition.

Bouachour et al. (1996) carried out a controlled study on 36 patients with crush injuries who were assigned in a blinded randomized fashion, within 24 h after surgery, to treatment with HBO (session of 100 % O_2 at 2.5 ATA for 90 min, twice daily, over 6 days) or placebo (session of 21 % O_2 at 1.1 ATA for 90 min, twice daily, over 6 days). All the patients received the same standard therapies (anticoagulant, antibiotics, wound dressings). Transcutaneous oxygen tension ($PtcO_2$) measurements were done before (patient breathing normal air) and during treatment (HBO or placebo) at the first, fourth, eighth, and twelfth sessions. The two groups (HBO group, $n = 18$; placebo group, $n = 18$) were similar in terms of age; risk factors; number, type or location of vascular injuries, neurologic injuries, or fractures; and type, location, or timing of surgical procedures. Complete healing was obtained for 17 patients in the HBO group vs. 10 patients in the placebo group ($p < 0.01$). New surgical procedures (such as skin flaps and grafts, vascular surgery, or even amputation) were performed on 1 patient in the HBO group vs. 6 patients in the placebo group ($p < 0.05$). Analysis of groups of patients matched for age and severity of injury showed that in the subgroup of patients older than 40 with grade III soft tissue injury, wound healing was obtained for 7 patients (87.5 %) in the HBO group vs. 3 patients (30 %) in the placebo group. No significant differences were found in the length of hospital stay and number of wound dressings between groups. For the patients with complete healing, the $PtcO_2$ values of the traumatized limb, measured in normal air, rose significantly between the first and the twelfth sessions. No significant change in $PtcO_2$ value was found for the patients in whom healing failed. The bilateral perfusion index (BPI = $PtcO_2$ of the injured limb/$PtcO_2$ of the uninjured limb) at the first session increased significantly from 1 ATA air to 2.5 ATA O_2. In patients with complete healing, the BPI was constantly greater than 0.9–2.5 ATA O_2 during the following sessions, whereas the BPI in air progressively rose between the first and the 12th sessions, reaching normal values at the end of the treatment. The authors concluded that HBO was effective in improving wound healing and reducing repeat surgery and is a useful adjunct in the management of severe (grade III) crush injuries of the limbs in patients >40 years old.

In a systematic review of the literature, eight of nine studies showed a beneficial effect of HBO crush injury with only one major complication (Garcia-Covarrubias et al. 2005). It was concluded that adjunctive HBO is not likely to be harmful and could be beneficial if administered early. A cohort study included patients with crush injuries and open fractures with severities greater than or equal to Gustilo class III and compared the control group which received conventional treatment with the group that received conventional treatment plus HBO (Yamada et al. 2014). HBO was found to be effective in the management of crush injuries from the viewpoint of reducing complications and reoperations. Well-designed clinical studies on larger number of patients are warranted.

Promptness in treatment is important in case of crush injury. If there is delay of more than 5–6 h and the extremity remains blue and swollen during this time, the prognosis for limb survival becomes poorer. Since oxygen tension remains elevated for only 1 h in the muscles and 3 h in the subcutaneous tissues following each HBO treatment, frequent treatments are necessary until the patient's condition is stabilized. The treatments can then be reduced in frequency, e.g., to once a week, until the patient is fully recovered.

Traumatic Ischemia

Various causes of acute peripheral traumatic ischemia are listed in Table 30.1.

Vascular disease as a cause of limb ischemia is discussed in Chap. 25. The causes relevant to this chapter are direct compression, trauma, and compartment syndromes. Posttraumatic ischemic disturbances in the limbs are:

- Edema
- Disturbances of microcirculation
  - Reduction of capillary perfusion
  - Loss of endothelial integrity
  - Plugging of capillaries by leukocytes
- Reperfusion injury
  - Formation of oxygen-derived free radicals
  - Generation of leukotrienes
- Decreased level of adenosine triphosphate and creatine phosphate within muscle cells

Animal experimental studies have shown the beneficial effect of HBO on some of the disturbances listed above. Nylander et al. (1985) used a tourniquet model of limb ischemia in the rat. In a group treated with HBO at 2.5 ATA for 45 min, the edema was reduced significantly, and this reduction persisted for 40 h after the treatment. The authors recommended the use of HBO as an adjuvant in treatment of acute ischemic conditions where surgical repair alone fails or is not sufficient to reverse the ischemic process. HBO treatments have been shown to enhance aerobic metabolism in the postischemic muscle. Reduction of phosphorylase activity, a sensitive marker for muscle cell damage, is prevented to a great extent by HBO treatment (Nylander et al. 1988).

Table 30.1 Causes of acute peripheral vascular ischemia

Cause	Comment and therapy suggestions
1. Allergic vasculitis	Adverse reaction to medicines. Discontinue offending agent
2. Compartment syndrome	A vicious circle with acute muscle and nerve ischemia. HBO is beneficial
3. Direct compression	Positional (secondary to overdose, stroke) fractures, tumors, or tourniquets. Removal of compression and treatment of the cause
4. Direct traumas	Lacerations, vascular injury during surgery on limbs, gunshot wounds, and crush injuries. HBO is useful
	Profound vasoconstriction, usually at the extremities
5. Ergot poisoning	Oxygenation of frostbitten tissues essential during rewarming process
6. Frostbite	Usually flow problems or diffusion problems. HBO is useful
7. Postvascular surgery	Latent effect seen with radiation. HBO is useful
8. Radiation vasculitis	Usually a chemical irritation rather than an ischemic problem
9. Snakebite	Arterial, immediate ischemia, venous congestion, and delayed ischemia. HBO is useful
10. Thromboembolism	Arteriosclerosis
11. Vascular diseases	Buerger's disease
	Diabetes mellitus
	Precipitating causes
	Acute ischemias may be precipitated by injury, infection, or systemic problems

HBO treatments have been shown to enhance the recovery of blood flow and functional capillary density in pressure-induced postischemic muscle tissue in the dorsal skinfold chamber in hamsters (Sirsjo et al. 1993). Experiments in rats by Zamboni et al. (1993) have shown that adherence of leucocytes in the ischemic venules following reperfusion is reduced by HBO at 2.5 ATA.

There is some concern that HBO may cause increase of free radical formation and aggravate reperfusion tissue injury. Nylander et al. (1989) studied the effect of HBO on the formation of free radicals in the tourniquet model of ischemia of the rat hind limb and used muscle biopsies with measurement of thiobarbituric acid-reactive material which includes lipid peroxides and alkyds including malondialdehyde, a key intermediate in the formation of peroxides. Their results showed that HBO treatment at 2.5 ATA for 45 min had a favorable effect on the muscle tissue and did not cause increased lipid peroxidation in the skeletal muscle of rats.

Transcutaneous oxygen monitoring was shown to reflect tissue perfusion and advocated to predict the final outcome of major vascular trauma of the limb. Transcutaneous oxygen measurement at 2.5 ATA is a valuable, noninvasive adjunctive method for prediction of final outcome of major vascular trauma of the limbs.

Schramek and Hashmonai (1978) reported HBO treatment of seven soldiers with gunshot wounds of limb arteries in whom arterial repair did not reverse the ischemia. There was improvement in these patients and they were spared amputation. Shupak et al. (1987) reported the use of HBO in 13 patients suffering from acute posttraumatic ischemia of the lower extremities. The average delay from the moment of injury to the institution of HBO therapy was 11 h and 53 min.

Complete limb salvage was accomplished in eight cases (61.5 %), and there was some improvement in four cases (30.7 %). Only one case did not show any improvement.

Patients with preexisting vascular disease are more susceptible to ischemia and more likely to suffer gangrene. Kuyama et al. (1988) have treated such cases by a combination of repeated HBO treatments, sympathetic blocks, and anticoagulation in combination with reconstructive surgery. These authors found this combined approach to be quite effective in salvaging limbs.

Isakov et al. (1979) explained the good results of HBO in severe trauma of the extremities on the basis of improved cardiac and respiratory functions, which further contribute to improved tissue oxygenation. This factor may be of importance in a victim of severe multiple injuries with cardiac and respiratory disturbances.

Cases continue to be reported where badly crushed limbs have been spared amputation because of the use of HBO. An amputation was suggested when hypoxia/ischemia persisted despite surgical intervention crush injury of the right foot (Gustillo IIIC) due to severe vessel injury, and 72 h later the patient was referred HBO treatment to define the limits of viable tissues prior to amputation (Stefanidou et al. 2014). After six sessions, clinical improvement was so obvious the decision to amputate was rejected. After a total of 32 HBO sessions, in addition to frequent debridement and administration of antibiotics, surgical reconstruction with a vascularized cutaneous flap was performed successfully. Full healing was achieved. HBO should be considered not only for the definition of viable tissue limits in ischemic crush injuries but also for enhancing tissue viability even in the most serious situations.

Compartment Syndromes

Compartment syndromes develop when pressures in the skeletal muscle compartments in the extremities are elevated enough to reduce capillary perfusion, resulting in ischemia, nonfunction, and necrosis of the tissues. Direct measurement of the compartment pressure enables quantitative assessment of the severity and outcome of this complication. A single pressure measurement, however, is not enough to indicate progression or resolution of the compartment syndrome. Fasciotomy is the accepted surgical treatment. The circulation is improved after fasciotomy, but the tissue damage is not always reversed. Controversy still exists regarding the pressure at which fasciotomy should be performed. HBO is expected to correct ischemia and edema which are important components of the pathophysiology of the compartment syndrome. HBO reduces the muscle damage significantly in experimentally produced compartment syndrome in dogs. HBO (three 1-h sessions at 3 ATA) should be used in human compartment syndromes under the following conditions:

- If the patient has an elevated intracompartmental pressure in a range that borders on surgical decompression. Instead of just observing the patient for progression of symptoms, as is done conventionally, HBO may be used to prevent the progression. However, HBO is not a substitute for decompression.
- As provisional treatment of compartment syndrome where surgery is indicated but there is delay in performing it. HBO may prevent further damage until surgery can be undertaken.
- In postoperative management of patients after surgical decompression if there is residual neurological deficit or muscle necrosis. HBO may improve the chances of recovery of marginally viable tissues.

Studies in experimental animal models have shown that HBO reduces edema and necrosis of skeletal muscle associated with hemorrhagic hypotension. Even if HBO therapy in the compartment syndrome is delayed, there is still significant reduction of edema and muscle necrosis once treatment by HBO is started.

Strauss et al. (1987) reported a prospective study of 38 patients who were given HBO as an adjunct to the management of posttraumatic and iatrogenic skeletal muscle compartment syndromes (SMCS). In two-thirds of the patients, HBO was started after surgical decompression of the compartment because of threatened necrosis of the flaps and intracompartment tissues or the presence of a neuropathy. The results were resolution of the neuropathies, arrest of tissue necrosis, and absence of secondary infections. In the remaining one-third of patients, HBO was started for symptoms and signs including elevated intracompartment pressure. No one in this group required surgical decompression and all recovered fully. SMCS, particularly in incipient stages before a fasciotomy is required, is a therapeutic challenge since no means to arrest its progression exist other than HBO. Unfortunately, the use of HBO as an adjunct for managing SMCS is often ignored although there is evidence-based information about its usefulness and how it mitigates the pathology of SMCS (Strauss 2012).

Fasciotomies performed for compartment syndrome and ischemic vascular disease often require closure in 2–4 weeks by skin graft. This leaves the patient with an unsightly scar and a limb with reduced strength. The use of vacuum-assisted closure (VAC) and HBO therapy quickly reduces the edema and permits earlier closure with adjacent skin. In three trauma patients with SMCS, fasciotomies, and the use of HBO and VAC of the fasciotomy wounds with adjacent skin led to closure of the fasciotomy wounds in 3–18 days (Weiland 2007). The simultaneous use of HBO and VAC accelerates the reduction of edema in a synergistic fashion, permitting early closure of fasciotomy wounds.

HBO for High Pressure Water Gun Injection Injury

Accidental injection with a high pressure water gun in workers can cause extensive soft tissue injury with empyema. This is a painful condition and resolves slowly and sometimes with residual disability. Excellent results are described with the use of HBO in such patients with immediate resolution of subcutaneous empyema, edema, and pain. Two possible explanations have been offered for the effectiveness of this treatment:

1. Oxygen and carbon dioxide in the injected air are absorbed leaving nitrogen in the tissues which is similar to the situation in decompression sickness. HBO helps in the elimination of nitrogen.
2. HBO helps to alleviate ischemic limb pain.

Peripheral Nerve Injuries

Injuries of peripheral nerves are common. These are usually a part of traumatic injuries of extremities. Peripheral nerves may be crushed or severed. Injured nerves may have impairment of blood supply, oxygenation, and edema which may set in a vicious cycle of further edema and hypoxia. Surgical techniques particularly with microsurgical refinements have improved the rate of recovery in peripheral nerve injuries, but some problems still remain. Nerve regeneration is slow and sometimes erratic. The search continues for techniques to improve nerve regeneration and recovery after injury.

Rationale for the Use of HBO

In vitro fast axonal transport can be restored by administration of 95% normobaric oxygen to an anoxic nerve. It has been speculated that HBO can provide optimal tissue pO_2 tension to restore axonal transport and enable the necessary delivery of materials to the site of injury for regeneration to occur. Restoration of transportation would obviate the need for the natural compensatory response to nerve injury by increased neurofilament concentration and eventual formation of neuroma. HBO also reduced edema in traumatized tissues and is expected to break the vicious circle of edema leading to hypoxia and further aggravation of edema with compression of the nerve fibers and ischemia. HBO counteracts tissue ischemia as well.

Peripheral nerve injury induces persistent vascular dysfunction and endoneurial hypoxia, which contributes to the development of neuropathic pain as a complication (Lim et al. 2015). This provides a rationale for the use of HBO as the most effective methods to counteract hypoxia of peripheral nerves.

Experimental Studies

HBO has shown some promise to aid healing of mechanically damaged peripheral nerves where axonotmesis was induced either by nerve transection or nerve crush. Nerve regeneration has been documented by electrophysiological studies. Bradshaw et al. (1996) used oxygen environments to study the regenerative effects of HBO on crushed sciatic nerves in 30 adult male rabbits. Treatments were initiated 4 days post injury and six different oxygen environments were used. Transmission electron microscopy and light microscopy were used to evaluate the regenerative morphology of crushed nerves. The morphology of crushed nerves after 7 weeks of treatment with compressed oxygen at 202, 242, and 303 kPa resembled normal uncrushed nerves, with nerve fibers uniformly distributed throughout the section. The treatment groups receiving 202 kPa compressed air, 100% normobaric oxygen, or ambient air did not display morphologies similar to normal uncrushed nerve. The nerves in these animals were edematous and contained disarrayed nerve fibers. Myelination in the animals receiving 100% O_2 at high pressures resembled undamaged nerves. Collagen and blood vessels were more evident in the lower pressure/oxygen tension treatments than in the animals receiving 100% O_2 at higher pressures. The neurofilamentous material inside the crushed control axons was dense, whereas in the axons of animals treated with compressed O_2, it was loosely packed. These differences in morphology suggest that treatments consisting of 100% O_2 under pressure can accelerate a peripheral nerve's recovery from a crush injury.

In contrast to the study of Bradshaw et al. (1996), Santos et al. (1996) found no effect of HBO in accelerating regeneration of peripheral nerves. In their study, rat peroneal nerves were transected and entubulated with a Silastic channel. The experimental group was treated with HBO to evaluate changes in acute edema, functional recovery, and histology. HBO was administered with 100% O_2 at 2.5 ATA for 90 min twice a day for 1 week and then four times a day for 1 week. Acute edema changes based on nerve water weight, and transfascicular area measurements were greater in injured than in uninjured nerves but demonstrated no differences between HBO-treated and HBO-untreated groups 2, 8, and 16 days after surgery. Functional evaluation with gait analysis demonstrated significant changes between injured and uninjured group 1, 3, 7, and 13 weeks after injury, but no differences between HBO-treated and HBO-untreated groups. Thirteen weeks after the initial injury, elicited muscle force measurements demonstrated no significant improvement from HBO treatment of injured nerves. Histologic evaluation of the nerve area, myelinated axon number, myelinated axon area, myelin thickness, and blood vessel number and area revealed no significant differences between HBO-treated and HBO-untreated groups. HBO was not associated with improvement of nerve regeneration with any of the outcome variables in this model. One explanation of this may be the technique of entubulation with which might have prevented access of HBO to the site of injury.

The effect of HBO treatment on regeneration of the rat sciatic nerve was studied by Haapaniemi et al. (1998). The sciatic nerve was crushed with a pair of pliers, and the animals were either left untreated or subjected to a series of 45-min exposures to 100% O_2 at 3.3 ATA pressure at 0, 4, and 8 h postoperatively and then every 8 h. Regeneration was evaluated using the pinch-reflex test at 3, 4, or 5 days following surgery and with neurofilament staining at 4 days. The regeneration distances at all time points were significantly longer in animals exposed to HBO treatment independent of the evaluation procedure. A short initial period of the same HBO treatment schedule, with no more treatments after 25 h, appeared as effective as when treatments were maintained being given every 8 h until evaluation. The authors concluded that HBO treatment stimulates axonal outgrowth following a nerve crush lesion. A further study by the same authors, however, has shown that HBO does not promote regeneration in traumatic peripheral nerve lesions. In standardized models of nerve crush injury as well as transection and repair, the animals were treated postoperatively with 100% oxygen at 2.5 ATA pressure for 90 min, and the treatment was employed twice daily for 7 days (Haapaniemi et al. 2002). The treatment was not effective in the restoration of gait or the muscular strength after 90 days. In another study using a similar model, exposure to 2.5 ATA HBO moderately enhanced early regeneration of the fastest sensory axons, but it decreased the number of regenerating axons in the injured nerves with compromised blood perfusion of the distal nerve stump (Bajrovic et al. 2002). Results of a study in rats suggest that functional recovery in transected peripheral nerves may be improved and accelerated by HBO following microsurgical repair (Eguiluz-Ordoñez et al. 2006).

Clinical Applications

The use of HBO as an adjunct to peripheral nerve repair has also been explored clinically. Zhao (1991) obtained good results in 89.2% of the 54 patients with 65 nerve injuries repaired using HBO as a supplementary treatment. In 60 patients with similar injuries where HBO was not used, good results were seen in only 73.2% ($p > 0.05$). In subgroups of patients with fresh injuries, the results were not different in the two groups, but HBO was significantly more beneficial in older cases.

In clinical practice, primary end-to-end repair is considered to be the preferred approach tension that occurs frequently at the site of repair. HBO facilitates primary repair even when nerve tension is foreseen (Oroglu et al. 2011).

Concluding Remarks

Although nerve crush injury or nerve transection and repair are not listed as recognized indications for HBO treatment, animal experimental studies and clinical case reports have shown benefits of HBO in inducing neurological recovery following nerve trauma and preventing complications such as neuropathic pain. Since there is a rational basis for the use of HBO in peripheral nerve injuries, further clinical studies are warranted.

Fractures

Basic and Experimental Considerations

Most bone fractures heal spontaneously, but 3–5% of them have delayed union or nonunion. This proportion may rise markedly in certain locations with compound comminuted fractures. The major cause of nonunion is interruption of blood supply at the ends of the fractures.

Lack of oxygen is considered to be a limiting factor in the healing of fractures. Multipotential precursors of fibroblastic origin form bone when exposed to increased oxygen tensions and compressive forces. If, instead, oxygen tensions are low, cartilage is formed. The cartilage is a relatively avascular tissue and its presence is noted at fracture sites in cases of nonunion. Low oxygen tensions are observed in healing fractures until the medullary canal is reformed. This is secondary to increased oxygen utilization associated with the fracture repair process.

Yablon and Cruess (1968) studied healing of fractured femurs in rats treated with 100% oxygen at 3 ATA for 1 h twice a day. By the 40th day, the fractures treated with HBO had completely remodeled, while healing was just completed in the control animals. Microradiography showed abundant medullary canal and subperiosteal new bone in HBO-treated animals at a time when there was incomplete bony union in the control animals.

Coulson et al. (1966) showed that rats treated at 3 ATA oxygen displayed a greater calcium ion uptake and lower fragility than air-breathing controls. Niinikoski et al. (1970) demonstrated that 100% oxygen at 2.5 ATA for 2 h twice daily produced an increased callus formation in experimental fractures. There was increased accumulation of calcium, magnesium, phosphorus, sodium, potassium, and zinc, as well as accelerated collagen production compared with air-breathing controls.

Gray and Hamblin (1976) studied the effects of hyperoxia on the bone in organ culture and noted that bone resorption was inhibited by exposure to 95% O_2 or HBO at 2 ATA. Hyperoxia also depressed new bone formation by osteoclasts. This finding contradicts the studies already quoted and may stem from the absence of vital factors in the culture media. Karapetian et al. (1985) demonstrated that HBO at 2 ATA stimulates the repair of noninflamed mandibular fractures in rats, whereas HBO at 2.5 ATA hinders it. If, however, the bone wound is inflamed, HBO at 2.5 ATA is more effective for healing.

Tkachenko et al. (1988) have shown that, in rabbits with experimental defects of the radius, HBO therapy results in the greatest activation of bone repair in the early period after trauma with the formation of osseous matrix. They recommended reduction of HBO exposure intensity at this stage. Nilsson (1989) studied the effect of HBO on bone regeneration by inserting a bone harvest chamber in the rat tibia and rat mandible. Their results showed that HBO treatments caused a significant increase of bone mineralization in the implant and that the lamellar bone had invaded the implant as quantified by microradiography and microdensitometry.

Experimental studies in rats that have shown once-daily HBO treatments (2 ATA for 90 min) appeared to accelerate bone repair with vessel ingrowth, whereas twice-daily treatments retarded these processes (Barth et al. 1990).

One serious obstacle to bone regeneration is migration of connective tissue from the surrounding soft tissues into the bony defect. Porous expanding membranes have been used to prevent the fibroblasts from entering the defect. Combination of this technique with HBO has been shown to produce better healing of mandibular defects in experimental animals as compared with HBO or membrane technique alone. Ueng et al. (1998) investigated the effect of intermittent hyperbaric oxygen (HBO) therapy on the bone healing of tibial lengthening in rabbits. Twelve male rabbits were divided into two groups of six animals each. The first group went through 2.5 atm absolute of HBO for 2 h daily, and the second group did not receive HBO. Each animal's right tibia was lengthened 5 mm using a uniplanar lengthening device. Bone mineral density (BMD) study was performed for all of the animals at 1 day before operation and at 3, 4, 5, and 6 weeks after operation. All of the animals were killed at 6 weeks postoperatively for biomechanical testing. Using the preoperative BMD as an internal control, the authors found that the BMD of the HBO group was increased significantly compared with the non-HBO group. The mean %BMD at 3, 4, 5, and 6 weeks were 69.5%, 80.1%, 87.8%, and 96.9%, respectively, in HBO group, whereas the mean %BMD were 51.6%, 67.7%, 70.5%, and 79.2%, respectively, in non-HBO group (two tailed t-test, $p<0.01$, $p<0.01$, $p<0.01$, and $p<0.01$ at 3, 4, 5, and 6 weeks, respectively). Using the contralateral nonoperated tibia as an internal control, they found that the torsional strength of the lengthened tibia of the HBO group was increased significantly compared with the non-HBO group. The mean percent of maximal torque was 88.6% in HBO group at 6 weeks, whereas the mean percent of maximal torque was 76.0% in non-HBO group (two-tailed t-test, $p<0.01$). The results of this study suggest that the bone healing of tibial lengthening is enhanced by intermittent HBO therapy.

Clinical Experience

Strauss and Hart (1977) presented 20 patients with 24 long bone fractures treated by HBO. Primary healing occurred in 15 (75%) of the patients. The healing was 100% in cases where HBO was started within 10 days of the fracture. These are good results: the incidence of nonunion can be as high as 75% in displaced tibial fractures. The authors recommended the use of HBO when there is a significant risk of delayed union or nonunion.

Kolontai et al. (1976) treated 295 patients with compound fractures of the long bones with a combination of local antibiotics, HBO (2–3 ATA), hypothermia, and surgery. They were able to reduce the complications, such as infections and nonunion, considerably. Halva et al. (1978) reported 142 cases of fracture dislocations in the region of the ankle where HBO was used as an adjunct to open or closed reduction and immobilization. Where treatment was started within 8 h of injury, good results were obtained in 90% of cases. This figure dropped to 60% when the treatment was started after a delay of between 8 h and 24 h. With a delay of more than 24 h, the circulatory disturbances were not reversible.

Pseudoarthrosis is a pathological fracture with inadequate healing and false joint formation, which requires surgery such as bone grafting to correct it. HBO is a useful adjunct to surgery both preoperatively and postoperatively in such cases, as well as in other nonhealing fractures. HBO therapy in patients with defects of the long tubular bones contributes to shortening the period of rehabilitation. Based on the clinical evidence and cost analysis, medical institutions that treat open fracture and crush injuries are justified in incorporating HBO as a standard of care.

Bone Fractures with Arterial Injuries

Blunt arterial injuries secondary to bone fractures are frequently associated with nerve, vein, and soft tissue lesions. A delayed diagnosis or treatment is the main cause of high amputation rate. Porcellini et al. (1997) described 34 patients who presented with acute arterial occlusion (15 cases), false aneurysms (13 cases), or arteriovenous fistulas (6 cases) of the extremity. Various procedures were performed to repair injured arteries; associated venous lesions were treated. External fixation of long bone fractures was made in 29 patients, before vascular reconstruction, to prevent further injury during orthopedic stabilization. Fasciotomies were made to treat compartmental where necessary. Hyperbaric oxygen therapy was applied in 7 patients to control bacterial contamination and improve wound healing. The authors emphasized that a multidisciplinary diagnostic and management strategy is required to improve limb and patient survival. HBO is an important component of such multidisciplinary strategies.

Traumatic Amputations and Reimplantations of Body Parts

Reimplantation of Limbs

After the establishment of blood circulation following reimplantation of a severed limb, the tissues of the implanted limb are apt to develop varying degrees of edema and degenerative changes due to anoxia. If these changes are not reversed, necrosis develops. The time limit of reimplantation at room temperature is 12 h and can be prolonged if the severed limb is preserved by hypothermia. HBO can help in reducing edema, improving microcirculation, reversing degenerative changes, and salvaging limbs reimplanted as long as 36 h after traumatic amputation. Smith (1961) reported a case of near-avulsion of a foot treated by replacement and subsequent repeated exposures to HBO at 2 ATA. Although the foot had to be eventually amputated, a segment below the ankle survived. There are few reports in the literature about the use of HBO in reimplantation surgery. Bao (1987) used HBO in reimplantation of severed limbs in 34 cases. The indications were:

- Prolonged anoxia or ischemia of the severed limb before reimplantation
- Failure of arterial anastomosis: vasospasm or thrombosis
- Microcirculatory disturbances with patent vessels

Seventy percent of their reimplants survived with the use of intermittent hyperbaric therapy at 2.5 ATA. These are good results considering that many of their implants were severed as long as 36 h prior to implantation and kept at room temperature.

The most extensive experience in this area is that of Colignon et al. (1987) who have used HBO in 371 cases with crush injuries and amputation of the limbs. Not only were the results of reimplantation by microsurgery good in terms of recovery of function, but the rate of complications such as infections and nonhealing was markedly reduced. Only one of their patients developed gas gangrene.

Reimplantation of Other Body Parts

The results of reanastomosis of some severed body parts are usually poor. The reconstruction of a severed ear is a difficult procedure and the cosmetic results are poor. Neubauer et al. (1988) have reported the use of HBO in successful reanastomosis of the severed ear in three cases. After the ear was sutured, HBO was used at 2.5 ATA for 90 min twice daily for 8–15 days.

Penile amputation and successful replantation is rare, and there are no routine standard procedures for this procedure. HBO has even been used as an aid to penile reimplantation (McGough et al. 1989). There is a case reported of microsurgical penile replantation with postoperative *Pseudomonas* wound infection that was treated with HBO to prevent potential replant loss (Landström et al. 2004). In another case, the use of HBO accelerates the healing process following microsurgical procedure, which led to successful engraftment and function of penile implant (Zhong et al. 2007).

Role of HBO in Battle Casualties

The use of HBO for decompression sickness was pioneered in the US Navy. The role of the Italian Navy in conflict regions is described in Chap. 43. HBO therapy is a recognized form of treatment for certain emergencies in the US Air Force. The potential of HBO therapy for the injured soldier has been recognized (Workman and Calcote 1989), but hyperbaric chambers have not been used by the US Armed Forces in the battlefield so far although these facilities were available on board US Navy ships during the Gulf Wars of 1991 and 2003. The Soviet Armed Forces used mobile field hyperbaric chambers for combat and chemical warfare casu-

alties during the Afghanistan war (Gatagov 1982). A mobile multiplace chamber can be adapted for military use. During the war in Croatia from 1991 to 1995, 67 patients with war injuries of the femoral vein and/or artery were treated at the Surgical Clinic of Split Clinical Hospital (Radonic et al. 1997). Vascular repair was carried out of 70 arterial (28 isolated) and 49 venous injuries (six isolated). Intermittent HBO therapy was given to 18 of these patients with beneficial effect. The injured soldier can be transported in a mobile hyperbaric chamber while receiving the emergency care. It is technically possible to install such a chamber in an airplane, helicopter, or motorboat. The Indian Armed Forces have a battlefield experience with the use of HBO where it is being evaluated for a variety of illnesses such as posttraumatic stress disorder (PTSD) and high-altitude cerebral edema (Verghese et al. 2013). Some injuries seen in the battlefield for which adjunctive HBO would be useful in an emergency are shown in Table 30.2.

The use of HBO in treating the victims of nuclear fallout would be contraindicated as the effect of radiation would be enhanced (see Chap. 38) although HBO is useful in treating the late sequelae of radiation such as radionecrosis (see Chap. 17).

Effect of HBO on Osteogenesis

Various studies showing the effect of HBO in enhancing osteogenesis are quoted in the section of fractures. Makihara et al. (1996) have shown a beneficial effect of intermittent HBO on osteogenesis in the rachitic bone. The authors used 4-week-old rats which were rendered rachitic by 1-hydroxyethylidene-1, 1-bisphosphonic acid disodium that exerts an inhibitory effect on deposition of calcium phosphate in bone. Radiologic and histologic findings indicated marked calcification in the center of the growth plate in rats treated with HBO.

HBO for Treatment of Osteonecrosis (Aseptic Necrosis)

Osteonecrosis is synonymous with aseptic or avascular necrosis of the bone. These terms describe infarction of bone, presumably resulting from ischemia. Several factors play a role in the pathogenesis of dysbaric osteonecrosis: intraosseous vessel obstruction by bubbles, platelet aggregation, fat embolism, and narrowing of the arterial lumen by bubble-induced myointimal thickening. The bone is vulnerable because of gas supersaturation of the fatty marrow and poor vascularization. Ischemia leads to hypoxia and impaired nutrition of bone, which leads to necrosis. The various causes of osteonecrosis are listed in Table 30.3.

Table 30.2 Indications for the emergency use of HBO in the battlefield

1. Crush injury
2. Air embolism
3. Decompression sickness—aviators and divers
4. Gunshot wounds of the limbs: vascular injuries with limb ischemia
5. Hemorrhagic shock and acute blood loss anemia
6. Thermal burns
7. Acute spinal cord injury
8. Acute head injury with cerebral edema (gunshot wounds)
9. Chemical weapon-induced injury
10. Radiation exposure injury
11. Cold injury: frostbite

Table 30.3 Causes of osteonecrosis (aseptic avascular necrosis)

1. Repeated exposure to compressed gases
2. Decompression sickness: intraosseous vessel obstruction by bubbles
3. Fat embolism
4. Work at high altitudes
5. Medical conditions
– Alcoholism
– Arteriosclerosis
– Alkaptonuria
– Cirrhosis of the liver
– Cushing's syndrome
– Diabetes mellitus
– Gaucher's disease
– Gout
– Hemoglobinopathies
– Hepatitis
– Rheumatic arthritis
– Sickle cell disease
6. Prolonged steroid therapy
7. Trauma to the hip, with or without fracture dislocation
8. Ionizing radiation injury
9. Idiopathic osteonecrosis

Although osteonecrosis is an occupational hazard of commercial and navy divers, it is also a growing problem in recreational divers. It is found in individuals with no history of exposure to compressed gas environments. The bones usually involved are the humerus, femur, and tibia, the femoral head being the most common. The delay in onset of symptoms may be months to years following a decompression exposure. An idiopathic form of aseptic necrosis of the femoral head has also been described. Lesions of the bone shaft are painless, but pain and disability are associated with juxta-articular lesions. Fracture and collapse of the head of the femur may occur.

There is no satisfactory conservative treatment. The affected joints are immobilized. Surgical procedures consist of removal of the necrotic tissue, replacement with bone graft, and immobilization. These measures have only a limited success. Therefore, HBO has been investigated as a treatment for this condition.

HBO Therapy of Osteonecrosis

HBO therapy has been used in this condition with good results. The role of HBO in osteoradionecrosis is described in Chap. 17. HBO restores tissue oxygenation of the femoral head, reduces edema, and induces angiogenesis. By reducing intraosseous pressure, venous drainage is restored and the microcirculation is improved.

The diagnosis and progress of this disease can be followed up with MRI (Fig. 30.2). X-rays of the hip in another

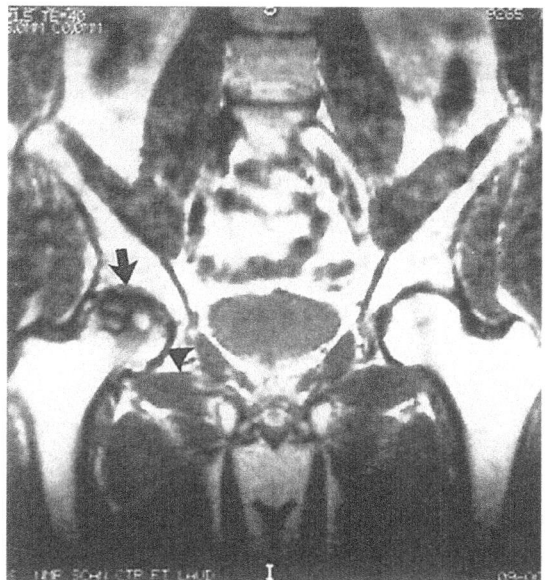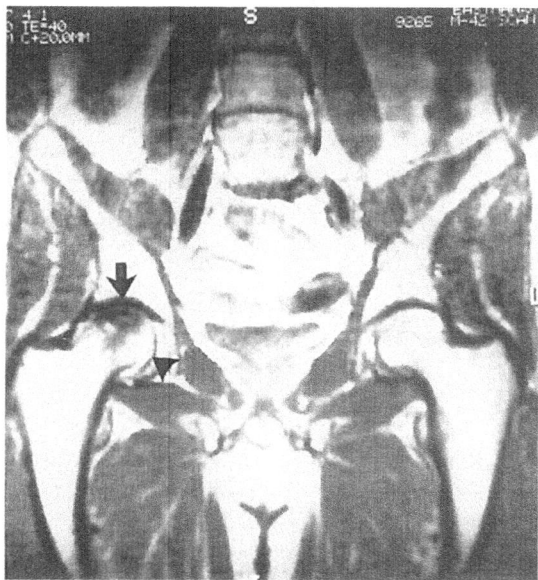

Fig. 30.2 *Left*: Pre-HBO treatment MRI of the right femur of a 41-year-old male with diagnosis of aseptic necrosis. The intact hyaline articular cartilage (*arrow*) shows no evidence of femoral head collapse. Small medial area of high signal (*arrowhead*) shows normal fatty mar- row. *Right*: Post-HBO treatment. The intact hyaline cartilage (*arrow*) overlies a small ringlike zone of aseptic necrosis. Also, normal area of fatty marrow (*arrowhead*) is now larger. Photo courtesy of the late Dr. Richard Neubauer, Ft. Lauderdale, FL

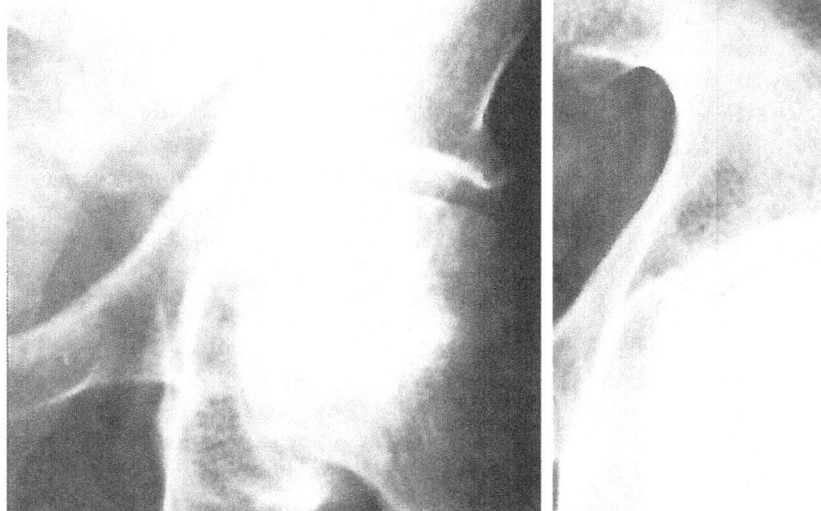

Fig. 30.3 *Left*: Pretreatment X-ray of the left femoral head showing aseptic osteonecrosis. *Right*: Post-HBO treatment (100 sessions) X-ray show- ing reossification. Photo courtesy of the late Dr. J H Baixe, Toulon, France

case of osteonecrosis of the hip are shown in Fig. 30.3. There was reossification after HBO treatments.

HBO therapy is usually given at 2.0–2.5 ATA and several treatment sessions may be required, even as many as 100. It is important that the treatment be adequate. Relief of symp- toms alone is not a guide to cure. There must be radiological evidence of increase of bone density.

Cases treated by HBO for osteonecrosis due to other causes in older studies are listed in Table 30.4. Strauss and Winant (1998) have carried out a meta-analysis of survivor- ship in femoral head necrosis from previous studies and com- pared them with results from HBO treatment. Survivability of 8567 hips was determined from meta-analysis of 86 studies. Treatment interventions that were analyzed were core decom-

Table 30.4 Reported cases of osteonecrosis treated by hyperbaric oxygen therapy (HBO)

Authors and year	Cases (n)	Diagnosis	HBO schedule	Results and comments
Baixe et al. (1969)	41	Aseptic necrosis, various bones	2.8 ATA, (90 min)/day; average of 120 treatments	Improvement in all cases clinically as well as by X-rays
Sainty et al. (1980)	9	Aseptic necrosis	2 ATA, 10–30 exposures	Pain relief in all cases but later recurrences; no X-ray improvement
Lepawsky et al. (1983)	1	Aseptic necrosis, both femoral heads; wheelchairbound	2.5 ATA; (90 min)/day; number of treatments?	Improvement both clinical and radiological; patient became ambulatory and remained so to follow-up 2 years later
Mao (1986)	44	Aseptic necrosis, various bones	2.8 ATA, (90 min); extended therapy?	Final results described as satisfactory
Neubauer et al. (1989)	1	Idiopathic aseptic necrosis, right femoral head	2–2.5 ATA, 90 min/day; total of 108 treatments	Full functional recovery with increase of bone density demonstrated on MRI (see Fig. 30.2); best documented case in literature
Scherer et al. (2000)	12	Aseptic osteonecrosis following chemotherapy	HBO (2.4 ATA for 100 min, 38 sessions)	Retrospective study with evaluation by MRI. No beneficial effect in those treated by HBO

pression (CD), osteotomy, bone graft, HBO, HBO and CD, and no intervention. Survivability of hips with femoral head necrosis treated with HBO was as good as any other treatment intervention, but combination therapies gave better results. Since then the largest study has reviewed the files of 68 patients with 78 symptomatic joints with Steinberg stage I and II osteonecrosis of the femoral head of effect of HBO (Koren et al. 2015). There was posttreatment improvement in 88 % of joints and on follow-up at a mean of 11.1 ± 5.1 years, 93 % of the joints survived. The authors concluded that HBO treatment is effective in preserving the hip joint in stage I and II osteonecrosis of the femoral head.

Prospective randomized studies and cost-benefit analyses are required for a more definite opinion regarding the suitability of HBO as a treatment for this condition.

Rheumatoid Arthritis

Basic Considerations

Rheumatoid arthritis is a systemic inflammatory disease of a chronic nature that is characterized primarily by a pattern of involvement of the synovial joints. The inflammatory process may involve soft tissues such as tendons, ligaments, and muscle and may invade the bone. The etiology of the disease remains uncertain; suspected causes include immunological disturbances and infectious agents. Hypoxia of the arthritic patient is evidenced by low synovial pO_2 levels but these are not specific to rheumatoid arthritis. The causes of hypoxia are:

- Increased metabolic demand for oxygen by an inflamed joint
- Decrease of blood flow to the joint by raised intra-articular pressure

There is a fall in the synovial fluid of a rheumatoid knee joint after exercise. The hypoxic condition of many inflamed joints may be responsible for microinfarction of particulate collagens in joint fluid that are qualitatively and quantitatively identical to the collagens of the synovial membrane.

Rationale of Use of HBO in Rheumatoid Arthritis

HBO can suppress sterile inflammation due either to immunologic factors or microbial infection. Thus, arthritis induced in rats by injections of adjuvant is suppressed if HBO is started within 2 days after injection. Moreover, daily HBO therapy suppresses the inflammatory response even if given when the arthritis is fully developed. Shakhbazyan et al. (1988) studied the effect of HBO (1.5 ATA and 3 ATA) on the development of clinical, immunological, and morphological manifestations of adjuvant arthritis in C57BL/6 mice. In comparison with the control group, HBO was found to inhibit the development of clinico-morphological manifestations of adjuvant arthritis and hindered the development of the process. The treatment was more effective in the early stages of the disease. Pressure of 3 ATA was more effective than 1.5 ATA, but toxic manifestations were seen with 3 ATA in the pulmonary vessels.

Clinical Applications

Kamada (1985) carried out laboratory examination of patients with rheumatoid arthritis undergoing HBO therapy. Under HBO therapy, serum superoxide dismutase values increased and lipid peroxidase activity decreased. At the same time, ESR and Lansbury's index showed a remarkable recovery. From these results, the authors suggested that HBO therapy may be an effective treatment for patients with rheumatoid arthritis.

Saikovsky et al. (1986) have used HBO in treatment of 20 patients with rheumatoid arthritis and recommend it as an appropriate therapy when systemic symptoms such as ischemic neuropathy, arteritis, or Raynaud's phenomenon are present.

Davis et al. (1988) conducted a pilot study in 10 patients with rheumatoid arthritis of which 8 received HBO treatments (100 % oxygen at 2.5 ATA, ten 90-min sessions once a day on alternate days) and 2 sham treatments (breathing air at normal pressure). There was no remission of the disease during treatment period, and authors concluded that further large-scale double-blind trials to assess efficacy of HBO in rheumatoid arthritis were not worthwhile.

Lukich et al. (1991) treated 35 patients with rheumatoid arthritis by HBO. Each patient received 21 sessions of HBO under 1.7 ATA for 40 min. Good clinical results, both immediate and late, were obtained. The effect of HBO on the immune system of the patients intensified the suppressive function of T lymphocytes (especially in those with systemic manifestations of the disease), normalized cell-bound immunity, and decreased the serum concentration in immune complexes.

Rui-Chang (1994) reported on the results of HBO treatment of 37 patients with rheumatoid arthritis using relief of pain and swelling with improved mobility as criteria of success. Nine patients (24.3 %) recovered completely, 19 (51.4 %) improved markedly, and 6 (16.2 %) showed slight improvement. Only 3 (8.1 %) patients failed to respond.

Rheumatological disorders are among the causes of skin ulcers. The role of HBO in the management of skin ulcers is described in Chap. 16. The management of chronic leg ulcers in rheumatological patients is challenging, and the importance of careful clinicopathological correlation and treatment of the underlying cause is important (Chia and Tang 2014).

Conclusion

HBO has proven to be a useful adjunct to surgery in the treatment of trauma to the extremities, particularly crush injuries. Most of the benefit is obtained by counteracting the effects of ischemia and anoxia commonly found in such injuries. Plainly HBO would have an even more important role to play in patients with multiple trauma. There is already evidence for the beneficial effects of HBO in head injuries (cerebral edema) and acute spinal cord injuries.

Every large trauma center should have a hyperbaric facility, as it is vital to institute HBO therapy as soon as possible.

References

Baixe JH, Bidart J, Nicolini JC. Treatment of osteonecrosis of the femoral head by hyperbaric oxygen. Bull Med Subhyp. 1969;1:2.

Bajrovic FF, Sketelj J, Jug M, Gril I, Mekjavić IB. The effect of hyperbaric oxygen treatment on early regeneration of sensory axons after nerve crush in the rat. J Peripher Nerv Syst. 2002;7:141–8.

Bao JYS. Hyperbaric oxygen therapy in re-implantation of several limbs. In: Kindwall EP, editor. Proceedings of the 8th international congress on hyperbaric medicine. San Pedro, CA: Best Publishing; 1987. p. 182–6.

Barth E, Sullivan T, Berg E. Animal model for evaluating one repair with and without adjunctive hyperbaric oxygen therapy: comparing dose schedules. J Invest Surg. 1990;3:387–92.

Bouachour G, Cronier P, Gouello JP, Toulemonde JL, Talha A, Alquier P. Hyperbaric oxygen therapy in the management of crush injuries: A randomized double-blind placebo-controlled clinical trial. J Trauma. 1996;41(2):333–9.

Bradshaw PO, Nelson AG, Fanton JW. Effect of hyperbaric oxygenation on peripheral nerve regeneration in adult male rabbits. Undersea Hyperbaric Med. 1996;23:107–13.

Chia HY, Tang MB. Chronic leg ulcers in adult patients with rheumatological diseases—a 7-year retrospective review. Int Wound J. 2014;11(6):601–4. doi:10.1111/iwj.12012. Epub 2012 Dec 12.

Colignon M, Carlier A, Khuc T, et al. Hyperbaric oxygen therapy in acute ischemia and crush injuries. In: Marroni A, Oriani G, editors. Proceedings of the 13th annual meeting of the European Undersea Biomedical Society, Palermo, Italy, Sept 9–12, 1987.

Coulson DB, Ferguson AB, Diehl RC. Effect of hyperbaric oxygen on healing femur of the rat. Surg Forum. 1966;17:449.

Davis TRC, Griffiths ID, Stevens J. Hyperbaric oxygen treatment for rheumatoid arthritis: failure to show worthwhile benefit. Br J Rheumatol. 1988;27:72 (Letter).

Eguiluz-Ordoñez R, Sánchez CE, Venegas A, Figueroa-Granados V, Hernández-Pando R. Effects of hyperbaric oxygen on peripheral nerves. Plast Reconstr Surg. 2006;118:350–7.

Garcia-Covarrubias L, McSwain Jr NE, Van Meter K, Bell RM. Adjuvant hyperbaric oxygen therapy in the management of crush injury and traumatic ischemia: an evidence-based approach. Am Surg. 2005;71:144–151.5.

Gray DH, Hamblin DL. The effects of hyperoxia upon bone organ culture. Clin Orthop Relat Res. 1976;119:225–30.

Gatagov B. Possibility of hyperbaric oxygen at medical evacuation. Slages Mosk Vogenno-Med Zh. 1982;5:16–9.

Haapaniemi T, Nylander G, Kanje M. Hyperbaric oxygen treatment enhances regeneration of the rat sciatic nerve. Exp Neurol. 1998;149:433–8.

Haapaniemi T, Nishiura Y, Dahlin LB. Functional evaluation after rat sciatic nerve injury followed by hyperbaric oxygen treatment. J Peripher Nerv Syst. 2002;7:149–54.

Halva ZD, Koziel M, Zoch V. Die Anwendung der Hyperbaroxie bei Sprunggelenksverletzungen. Application of hyperbaric oxygen in ankle joint injuries (English abstracts). Beitr Orthop Traumatol. 1978;25:324–7.

Isakov YV, Atroschenko ZB, Yufit IS, Bialik IF. Hyperbaric oxygenation in the severe compound trauma of the extremities. Ortop Traumatol Protez. 1979;9:34–6.

Kamada T. Superoxide dismutase and hyperbaric oxygen therapy of the patient with rheumatoid arthritis. Nippon-Seikeigaka Gakkai Zasshi. 1985;59:17–26.

Karapetian TS, Volozhin AT, Oleinik NN. Treatment of mandibular fractures using hyperbaric oxygenation. Stomatologiia (Mosk). 1985;64:33–8.

Kolontai YU, Smirnova LA, Kondrashov AN. Treatment of open fractures in long tubular bones. Sov Med. 1976;39:94–100.

Koren L, Ginesin E, Melamed Y, Norman D, Levin D, Peled E. Hyperbaric oxygen for stage I and II femoral head osteonecrosis. Orthopedics. 2015;38:e200–5.

Kuyama T, Umemura H, Sudo T, Kawamura M, Shobu R, Tsubakimoto R, et al. Clinical studies on various therapy for the intractable trauma of toes and fingers in cases of diabetes mellitus and peripheral ischemic diseases. Nippon Geka Gakkai Zasshi. 1988;89:763–70.

Landström JT, Schuyler RW, Macris GP. Microsurgical penile replantation facilitated by postoperative HBO treatment. Microsurgery. 2004;24:49–55.

Lepawsky M, Tredwall SJ, Kirenman DS. Avascular osteonecrosis ameliorated by hyperbaric oxygen. In: Paper presented at the 1st European conference on hyperbaric medicine. Amsterdam, Sept 7–9, 1983.

Lim TK, Shi XQ, Johnson JM, Rone MB, Antel JP, David S, et al. Peripheral nerve injury induces persistent vascular dysfunction and endoneurial hypoxia, contributing to the genesis of neuropathic pain. J Neurosci. 2015;35:3346–59.

Lukich VL, Poliakova LV, Sotnikova TI, Belokrinitskii DV. Hyperbaric oxygenation in the comprehensive therapy of patients with rheumatoid arthritis (clinico-immunologic study). Fiziol Zh. 1991;37:55–60.

Makhihara N, Hasegawa Y, Sakano S, Matsuda T, Kataoka Y, Iwata H, et al. Effect of hyperbaric oxygenation on bone in HEBP-induced rachitic rats. Undersea Hyperbaric Med. 1996;23:1–4.

McGough EK, Gallagher TJ, Hart J, et al. Hyperbaric oxygen as an adjuvant in penile re-implantation: a case report. In: Paper presented at the annual meeting of the Undersea and Hyperbaric Medical Society, Honolulu, June 10, 1989.

Neubauer RA, Pinella J, Hill RK, et al. The use of hyperbaric oxygen in the successful reanastomosis of the severed ear: three cases. In: Presented at the 14th annual meeting of the European Undersea Biomedical Society, Aberdeen, Scotland, Sept 5–9, 1988.

Neubauer RA, Kagan RL, Gottleib SF. Use of hyperbaric oxygen for the treatment of aseptic bone necrosis: a case study. J Hyperbaric Med. 1989;4:69–76.

Niinikoski JR, Pentinnen R, Kulonen E. Effects of hyperbaric oxygen on fracture healing in the rat: a biochemical study. Calcif Tissues Res. 1970;4:115–6.

Nilsson LP. Effects of hyperbaric oxygen treatment on bone repair. Swedish Dental J. 1989;64(suppl):1–33.

Nylander G, Lewis D, Nordstrom H, Larsson J. Reduction of postischemic edema with hyperbaric oxygen. Plast Reconstr Surg. 1985;76:596–603.

Nylander G, Nordstrom H, Franzen L, Henriksson KG, Larsson J. Effects of hyperbaric oxygen treatment in post-ischemic muscle. Scand J Plast Reconstr Surg. 1988;22:31–9.

Nylander G, Otamiri DH, Larsson J. Lipid products in postischemic skeletal muscle and after treatment with hyperbaric oxygen. Scand J Plast Reconstr Surg. 1989;23:97–103.

Oroglu B, Turker T, Aktas S, Olgac V, Alp M. Effect of hyperbaric oxygen therapy on tense repair of the peripheral nerves. Undersea Hyperb Med. 2011;38:367–73.

Porcellini M, Bernardo B, Capasso R. Combined vascular injuries and limb fractures. Minerva Cardioangiol. 1997;45:131–8.

Radonic V, Baric D, Giunio L, et al. War injuries of the femoral artery and vein: a report on 67 cases. Cardiovasc Surg. 1997;5:641–7.

Rui-Chang Y. Rhematoid arthritis treated with hyperbaric oxygen. In: Proceedings of the XI International Congress of Hyperbaric Medicine. Best, San Pedro,1994.

Saikovsky RS, Alekberova ZS, Dmitriev AA. The role of hemocarboperfusion and hyperbaric oxygenation in the treatment of patients with rheumatoid arthritis with systemic symptoms. Ter Arkh. 1986;58:105–9.

Sainty JM, Aubert L, Conti V, Allessandrini G. Place de l'oxygénothérapie hyperbare dans le traitement de l'ostéonécrose aseptique de la hanche. Med Aeronaut Spat Med Subaquat Hyperbare. 1980;19:215–7.

Santos PM, Zamboni WA, Williams SL. Hyperbaric oxygen treatment after rat peroneal nerve transection and entubulation. Otolaryngol Head Neck Surg. 1996;114:424–34.

Scherer A, Engelbrecht V, Bernbeck B, May P, Willers R, Göbel U, et al. MRI evaluation of aseptic osteonecrosis in children over the course of hyperbaric oxygen therapy. Rofo. 2000;172:798–801.

Schramek A, Hashmonai M. Vascular injuries in the extremities in battle injuries. Br J Surg. 1978;64:644–8.

Shakhbazyan IE, Lukich VL, Madzhidov VV. Effect of hyperbaric oxygenation on the development of adjuvant arthritis in C57BL/6 strain mice. Rheumatology (USSR). 1988;3:44–50.

Shupak A, Gozal D, Ariel A. Hyperbaric oxygenation in acute peripheral posttraumatic ischemia. J Hyperbaric Med. 1987;2:7–14.

Sirsjo A, Lehr HA, Nolte D, Haapaniemi T, Lewis DH, Nylander G, et al. Hyperbaric oxygen treatment enhances the recovery of blood flow in the postischemic striated muscle. Circ Shock. 1993;40:9–13.

Smith G. Near avulsion of fort treated by replacement and subsequent prolonged exposure of patient to oxygen at two atmospheres pressure. Lancet. 1961;2:1122.

Stefanidou S, Kotsiou M, Mesimeris T. Severe lower limb crush injury and the role of hyperbaric oxygen treatment: a case report. Diving Hyperb Med. 2014;44:243–5.

Strauss MB. The effect of hyperbaric oxygen in crush injuries and skeletal muscle-compartment syndromes. Undersea Hyperb Med. 2012;39:847–55.

Strauss MB, Hart GB. Clinical experiences with HBO in fracture healing. In: Smith G, editor. Proceedings of the 7th international congress on hyperbaric medicine. Aberdeen: University of Aberdeen Press; 1977. p. 329–32.

Strauss MB, Winant DM. Femoral head necrosis: a meta-analysis comparing HBO with other interventions. Undersea Hyperbaric Med. 1998;25: 16 (abstract).

Strauss MB, Snow K, Greenberg D, et al. Hyperbaric oxygen in the managementof skeletal muscle compartment syndrome. In: Presented at the 9th international congress on hyperbaric medicine, Sydney, Australia, March 1–4, 1987.

Tkachenko SS, Ruskii VV, Tikhilov RM, Vovchenko VI. Normalization of bone regeneration by oxygen barotherapy. Vestn Khir. 1988;140:97–100.

Ueng SW, Lee SS, Lin SS, Wang CR, Liu SJ, Yang HF, et al. Bone healing of tibial lengthening is enhanced by hyperbaric oxygen therapy: a study of bone mineral density and torsional strength on rabbits. J Trauma. 1998;44:676–81.

Verghese G, Verma R, Bhutani S. Hyperbaric oxygen therapy in the battlefield. Med J Armed Forces India. 2013;69:94–6.

Weiland DE. Fasciotomy closure using simultaneous vacuumassisted closure and hyperbaric oxygen. Am Surg. 2007;73:261–6.

Workman WT, Calcote RD. Hyperbaric oxygen therapy and combat casualty care: a viable potential. Milit Med. 1989;154:111–5.

Yablon IG, Cruess RL. The effect of hyperbaric oxygen on fracture healing in rats. J Trauma. 1968;8:186.

Yamada N, Toyoda I, Doi T, Kumada K, Kato H, Yoshida S, et al. Hyperbaric oxygenation therapy for crush injuries reduces the risk of complications: research report. Undersea Hyperb Med. 2014;41:283–9.

Zamboni WA, Roth AC, Russel RC, Graham B, Suchy H, Kucan JO. Morphologic analysis of the microcirculation during reperfusion of ischemic skeletal muscle and the effect of hyperbaric oxygen. Plast Reconstr Surg. 1993;91:1110–23.

Zhao DW. Therapeutic effect of hyperbaric oxygen on recovery of surgically repaired peripheral nerve injury. Chung Hua Wai Ko Tsa Chih. 1991;29:118–20.

Zhong Z, Dong Z, Lu Q, Li Y, Lv C, Zhu X, et al. Successful penile replantation with adjuvant hyperbaric oxygen treatment. Urology. 2007;69:983, e3–5.

K.K. Jain

Abstract

This chapter deals with applications of HBO in otolaryngology. Sudden deafness and acute acoustic trauma are good indications for HBO therapy, and there is improvement of these conditions if the treatment is carried out soon after the onset of symptoms. However, HBO therapy is an adjunctive to conventional treatments and not an alternative. HBO is effective in relieving tinnitus as a component of inner ear disorders, but its use for tinnitus alone as a symptom is questionable. HBO is usually ineffective in chronic conditions encountered in otolaryngology where chronic anoxic is a factor in pathogenesis, e.g., its use in Meniere's syndrome is controversial. In symptoms secondary to ischemia, e.g., of the acoustic nerve, its HBO may be effective in the chronic stages, as the situation is comparable to that of ischemia in the brain. Effectiveness in facial palsy (Bell's palsy) has not been proven, although good results have been obtained in several series of patients. Malignant otitis externa is a good indication for the use of HBO as the effect of HBO in enhancing the effect of antibiotics is well documented.

Keywords

Acute acoustic trauma • Chronic hearing loss • Disturbances of the inner ear • Facial palsy (Bell's palsy) • Hyperbaric oxygen (HBO) • Meniere's disease • Neuro-otology • Otolaryngology • Sudden deafness • Tinnitus

Introduction

The role of hyperbaric oxygenation (HBO) therapy in otolaryngology has mostly been investigational in the past, but its clinical applications in diseases of the inner ear are being increasingly recognized by physicians in the Federal Republic of Germany, Japan, and China. HBO has also proven to be useful in some diseases of the head and neck that partially overlap the domain of the otolaryngologist. The application of HBO in the treatment of infections such as malignant otitis externa and osteomyelitis of the jaw is well recognized in the United States. Indications for the use of HBO are shown in Table 31.1.

K.K. Jain, MD, FRACS, FFPM (✉)
1 Blaesiring 7, Basel 4057, Switzerland
e-mail: jain@pharmabiotech.ch

Tinnitus

Tinnitus is the most common symptom associated with inner ear damage, and it is estimated that more than 1 % of the population of the Federal Republic of Germany (i.e., about 800,000 cases) suffers from disabling tinnitus and impairment of hearing. The yearly incidence of new cases is about 15,000.

Tinnitus may be acute or chronic. Chronic tinnitus is of more than a year's duration and is responsible for most of the cases. It is often part of a triad of hearing loss, vertigo, and tinnitus because of the involvement of both the cochlea and the vestibular apparatus in many of the disease processes. Various causes of tinnitus are shown in Table 31.2. Because of the subjective nature of the complaints, it is not possible to evaluate the symptom objectively but various scales are sued. In the visual analog scale, the patient depicts the loudness of the tinnitus.

Table 31.1 Indications for HBO therapy in ear, nose, and throat disorders as well as relevant areas of the head and neck (as practiced in Germany)

- Barotrauma
    - Labyrinthine contusions
    - Decompression sickness of inner ear
- Bone involvement in ear nose throat area
    - Osteomyelitis
    - Osteonecrosis
- Hearing loss
    - Acute acoustic trauma
    - Drug-induced hearing loss
    - Noise-induced hearing loss
    - Postoperative hearing loss
    - Retrocochlear hearing loss of unknown origin
    - Sudden deafness
- Meniere's disease
- Otitis externa maligna
- Tinnitus
- Vertigo

Table 31.2 Causes of tinnitus

- Barotrauma
- Hypotension
- Ototoxic drugs
- Stress
- Vasculopathies of inner ear
- Vasomotor disorders
- Viral infections of the inner ear

Medical therapy of tinnitus is not satisfactory and HBO has been used. Using this method in patients who had suffered from tinnitus for <3 months, excellent improvement was seen in 6.7 % and noticeable improvement in 44.3 % expressed by means of a visual analog scale (Kau et al. 1997). In 44.3 % the tinnitus was described as unchanged. Patients who had had tinnitus for more than 3 months before HBO therapy showed a less favorable response to HBO. In none of the patients did the tinnitus disappear; 34.4 % of the patients described a noticeable improvement in their complaints. A study from Germany reported an improvement rate of 60–65 % with HBO treatment in patients with tinnitus (Bohmer 1997). In another study from Germany, a total of 193 patients, having undergone primary intravenous hemorheologic therapy, were treated with HBO (Delb et al. 1999). Tinnitus was evaluated before, after 10 sessions and after 15 sessions using a tinnitus questionnaire. Additionally, an audiometric examination was performed. Measurable improvements of the tinnitus occurred in 22 % of the patients. The improvement rate decreased in those cases where the time from onset of tinnitus exceeded 40 days. It was concluded that HBO is a moderately effective additional treatment in the therapy of tinnitus after primary hemorheologic therapy, provided the time from onset of tinnitus is less than

1 month. In another study, HBO was prescribed to 20 patients who had had severe tinnitus for more than 1 year and who had already had other forms of tinnitus therapy with unsatisfactory results (Tan et al. 1999). Four patients could not cope with hyperbaric pressure gradient. The effect of HBO was assessed using subjective evaluation and VAS scores before and after HBO. Follow-up continued until 1 year after treatment. Six patients had a reduction of tinnitus and accompanying symptoms, 8 patients did not notice any change and 2 patients experienced an adverse effect. Any outcome persisted with minor changes until 1 year after treatment. The authors concluded that HBO may contribute to the treatment of severe tinnitus, but the negative effect on tinnitus should be weighed carefully.

Most of the studies which have shown the beneficial effect of HBO on tinnitus are uncontrolled. However, the improvement of tinnitus has been documented in patients recovering from acute acoustic trauma following HBO treatment. A MEDLINE search from 2000 to 2007, yielding 22 studies of the effect of HBO on tinnitus, showed no significant effect in four prospective studies, but retrospective studies indicated greater improvement in tinnitus in acute cases compared with tinnitus episodes exceeding 3 months (Desloovere 2007). One study, however, showed significantly more improvement in patients with positive expectations before therapy (60.3 %) compared with those with negative expectations (19 %). Although there are indications of a better effect in acute cases, a major psychological component and a low risk of enhancement of the tinnitus should be considered.

Review of MEDLINE from 2007 to 2016 showed 46 further studies of the use of HBO in tinnitus patients. In most of the cases, tinnitus was associated with impairment of sensory neural hearing. Noteworthy studies were as follows:

- One publication has indicated that HBO therapy may improve tinnitus and suggested large randomized trials of high methodological rigor in order to define the true extent of the benefit because of a need for relief of high prevalence of tinnitus in war veterans (Baldwin 2009).
- A systematic review of clinical trials of HBO for idiopathic sudden sensorineural hearing loss (ISSHL) concluded that it significantly improved hearing but there was no evidence of a beneficial effect on chronic ISSHL or tinnitus (Bennett et al. 2012).
- One study that claimed beneficial effect of HBO on tinnitus had no control group without HBO, and several patients had psychosocial disturbances, making conclusions about the results unjustified (Hesse et al. 2012).
- Repetitive transcranial magnetic stimulation (rTMS) therapy administered in addition to standard cortisone treatment (SCT) and HBO therapy resulted in significantly greater recovery of hearing function and improvement of tinnitus perception compared to SCT and HBO therapy without rTMS therapy (Zhang and Ma 2015).

Sudden Deafness

Sudden hearing loss is a sensorineural hearing impairment, which develops over a period of few hours to a few days. The incidence of sudden sensorineural hearing loss has been reported to range from 5 to 20 per 100,000 persons per year. The most common forms of recent ear damage are sudden deafness and acute acoustic trauma. The conventional treatment of these conditions involves (1) infusions to improve microcirculation and (2) vasodilators. The effectiveness of these measures, however, remains unproven and there are indications that these measures may be more harmful than beneficial. Experimental animal studies, for example, show that the cortilymph pO_2 decreases during exposure to infusions. Some of the pioneering work referred in this chapter has been done by Pilgramm in Germany and described originally in his habilitation thesis (Pilgramm 1991).

The causes of sudden deafness are listed in Table 31.3. The pathogenesis of sudden deafness is not well understood: the oldest explanation of the disorder is that it is due to vascular insufficiency such as that resulting from occlusion of the labyrinthine artery; however, conclusive proof has never been provided. Animal experimental studies show that the hair cells of the inner ear react in a uniform way to damage caused by different agents such as noise, viruses, ototoxic substances, and hypoxia. The hair cells first swell and lose their function. This effect is reversible in case of minor damage. In cases of severe damage or if the swelling persists for more than 1 year, the hair cells degenerate and are replaced by nonfunctioning endothelial cells.

The pathophysiology of ear damage in diving is described in Chap. 3. Clinically, one should differentiate between the hearing loss secondary to lesions such as an acoustic neuroma (an intracranial tumor) and that due to idiopathic disturbances of the inner ear.

Role of HBO in the Management of Sudden Deafness

Pioneer work on the role of HBO in disorders of the inner ear was done by Lamm in 1969 and reported in various publications. Lamm and Klimpel (1971) reported 33 patients with diagnosis of hypoxia of the inner ear who improved after HBO therapy. Lamm and Gerstmann (1974) treated many inner ear disorders with HBO, but obtained the best results in 45 cases of sudden deafness. More than 90 % of these patients showed an improvement of hearing, and in 40 % of these, a normal hearing was achieved. The therapeutic usefulness of HBO in sudden deafness was confirmed by several other authors. Most of the studies on this subject are uncontrolled. A summary of the controlled studies is shown in Table 31.4. From these studies it is concluded that HBO improves the results of the conventional treatment for sudden deafness, and best results are achieved if the treatment is started early after the onset of deafness. The spontaneous recovery rate, which is as high as 90 %, makes the selection of patients for therapy and the evaluation of the results particularly difficult. This enthusiasm is not shared by other authors. If oxygen tension in the cochlea is reduced, restoration of oxygen tension by HBO would be effective for the treatment of sudden deafness. HBO has been used successfully in the management of sudden deafness based on the concept that pathogenesis may involve a reduction in cochlear blood flow and perilymph oxygenation (Domachevsky et al. 2007).

Rationale for HBO Therapy in Sudden Deafness

The rationale for this therapy is based on the following effects:

- HBO increases the pO_2 in the inner ear. The experimental evidence for this has been provided by Lamm et al. (1988). The insertion of oxygen-sensitive microelectrodes into the inner ears of guinea pigs led to a drop of pO_2 in the scala tympani. The animals were placed in the hyperbaric chamber, and, after it was flooded with oxygen at normal pressure, pO_2 was noted to increase by 204 %; when pressure was raised to 1.6 bar, pO_2 increased by 563 % as compared with the original value. The increased oxygen supply corrects the hypoxia.

Table 31.3 Causes of sudden deafness

1. Vascular
Thromboembolic disease
Labile hypertension or hypotension
Microcirculatory disturbances
2. Viral infections and their sequelae
3. Autoimmunological disorders, e.g., Cogan's syndrome
4. Metabolic disorders
Hyperlipidemia
Diabetes
5. Toxic
Exposure to ototoxic drugs
Carbon monoxide poisoning
6. Neoplastic
Tumors of the auditory nerve
7. Inner ear problem such as Meniere's disease
8. Diving injuries
Barotrauma
Decompression sickness of the inner ear
8. Miscellaneous
Rupture of the membrane of the round window
Intra-labyrinthine membrane rupture
Stress

- HBO lowers hematocrit, whole blood viscosity, and improves erythrocyte elasticity, which lead to better hemorrheology as well as microcirculation.

Acute Acoustic Trauma

Acute acoustic trauma is defined as an acute impairment of hearing caused by sharp sounds like that of a gun going off near an unprotected ear. Sounds of moderate intensity as encountered in everyday life usually do not affect the oxygen tension within the cochlea, but high-intensity sounds can reduce it. Important sequelae of acute acoustic trauma are:

- Failure of outside hair cells and then inside hair cells
- Rupture of cell membranes and decreased cochlear blood flow
- Decrease of hearing potentials corresponding to decrease of oxygen tension in the inner ear

Experimental Studies

Lamm et al. (1977, 1982) as well as Lamm and Lamm (1987), in experimental studies in guinea pigs, investigated the effects of HBO on cochlear microphonics, action potentials of the auditory nerve, and brainstem responses that had been damaged by short exposures to noise. The beneficial effect was variable and was seen in only 14 of 26 animals. Testing of postmortem cochlear microphonics after HBO treatment showed that oxygen can diffuse through the round window. Pilgramm et al. (1986) wrote that the impact of high levels of sound energy on an inadequately protected inner ear always results in the failure of the outside hair cells and the corresponding Deiters' supporting cells from the end of the first spiral to the middle of the second spiral. If the damage is pronounced, the inner hair cells will also fail. The damaged sensory cells will then be maintained in a transitional phase between regeneration and cell death. It is in this transitional phase that therapy has a chance. It was shown histologically that the alterations in the sensory cells, such as formation of cavernous nuclei, are the same as those resulting from anoxia. It was also shown in experimental animals that HBO has a beneficial effect in such a situation.

Lamm et al. (1989a) exposed guinea pigs to a broadband of noise as well as impulse noise from gunfire. Some of the animals were treated with HBO at 1.5 ATA for 30 min after exposure to the noise. Hearing potentials (cochlear microphonics or CM) and compound action potentials (CAP) of the auditory nerve were registered via the microaxial needle electrode for the polarographic measurements of pO_2 directly in the inner ear (scale tympani). In all of the animals, pO_2 decreased during the first 24 min of noise (broadband) exposure by more than one-third of the original values. Amplitudes of CM and CAP decreased by more than 20–25 % of the original values. Treatment with HBO increased the pO_2 in the inner ear by 70 % of the original values and hearing potentials recovered during the therapy.

After exposure to the noise of the first 6–12 gunshots (G3 of the German Army, 150–160 dB), the pO_2 in the inner ear

Table 31.4 Controlled studies of the use of HBO in the treatment of sudden deafness

Authors and year	Method	Patients (n)	Results
Goto et al. (1979)	1. Standard treatment (vasodilators + steroids + vitamins) 2. Stellate ganglion block + HBO 3. Treatments 1 and 2 combined	22 49 20	Best results were obtained in group 3 where treatments were combined; those treated within 2 weeks showed an improvement of over 10 dB in hearing loss
Dauman et al. (1985)	1. Steroids + vasodilators Total 2. HBO + hemodilution	43	First randomized controlled study; better results in the second group using HBO
Pilgramm et al. (1985)	1. Hemodilution + vasodilators 2. Hemodilution + HBO	80	Statistically better results in group 2 in cases of acute sudden deafness
Takahashi et al. (1989)	1. Standard, e.g., vasodilators 2. HBO (2 ATA, 1 h twice daily for 14–20 sessions added to the standard treatment)	316 ears 591 ears (900 cases)	No difference between the two groups in week of treatment, but improvement greater in the second group (with HBO) during the second week
Nakashima et al. (1998)[a]	1. Standard, e.g., vasodilators 2. HBO (2 ATA, 1 h twice daily for 14–20 sessions added to the standard treatment)	254 546	There were some cases where the hearing improved significantly after initiation of the HBO therapy. Because most of the patient in this series had poor outcome after basic treatment, the authors did not consider that it was worthwhile to compare the two groups
Shiraishi et al. (1998)	1. HBO 2. Stellate ganglion block 3. Oral vasodilator and vitamins	119	Therapeutic outcome in the HBO group was better than in the control group of 107 patients treated with various other therapies. Recovery rate of hearing in the HBO group was superior to that in the control group for those cases which had severe hearing loss at onset, had been seen more than 2 weeks after onset, and were resistant to other treatments
Murakawa et al. (2000)	1. HBO (2.5 ATA for 80 min daily) from 10 to 15 times 2. Intravenous steroid, vitamin B12, prostaglandin E1, adenosine triphosphate, and low-molecular weight dextran	522	Definite improvement in 34.9% (complete in 19.7%) and slight improvement in 58.1% of the patients. HBO given within 14 days from onset of SD was able to achieve hearing improvement in many cases unresponsive to the initial medical therapy even if given very early
Fattori et al. (2001a)	1. Once-daily administration of HOB for 10 days in treatment group 2. Other group was treated for 10 days with an intravenous vasodilator	50	Within 48 h of the onset of SD, 30 patients were randomly assigned to HBO or intravenous vasodilator treatment. Patients in the HBO group experienced a significantly greater response to treatment than did those in the vasodilator group, regardless of age and sex variables
Kestler et al. (2001)	Primary HBO therapy compared to primary infusion therapy and no treatment in patients with SD of up to 3 weeks' duration	49	Neither the results of the infusion therapy nor those of the hyperbaric oxygenation surpass the rate of complete spontaneous remission
Racic et al. (2001)	100% oxygen at 2.8 ATA, for 60 min twice day, either until recovered or for a maximum of 30 sessions	17	The average hearing level for all patients and for all five basic frequencies was 67.8 dB before therapy, in comparison with 21.6 dB after HBO therapy
Aslan et al. (2002)	1. Betahistine hydrochloride, prednisone, and daily stellate ganglion block 2. HBO (4 ATA, 90 min) four treatments	25	Addition of HBO therapy to the conventional treatment significantly improved the outcome of SD compared to the control group of 25 patients who received the same basic treatment. HBO therapy is most useful in patients younger than 50 years, provides limited benefit in patients older than 50 years and no benefit in patients older than 60 years
Inci et al. (2002)	Patients unresponsive to medical treatment (steroids, vasodilators, vit B) were given HBO (2.4 ATA), two sessions daily for the first 3 days, followed by a single daily session, to make 20 sessions of 90 min Medications were continued during HBO treatment	51	The mean hearing thresholds were 75.3 dB and 65.6 dB before and after treatment, respectively. Recovery was rated as complete in 3.9%, moderate in 3.9%, mild in 37.25%, and as no recovery in 54.9%

(continued)

Table 31.4 (continued)

Authors and year	Method	Patients (n)	Results
Muminov et al. (2002)	1. Antioxidants 2. HBO (1.4 ATA for 40 min) ten sessions	36 children	Improvement of sound perception at 5–25 dB in 72.2 % patients The highest effectiveness was seen in acute neurosensory hypoacusis
Narozny et al. (2004)	Retrospective analysis of patients treated with HBO + corticosteroids, vasodilators, etc. vs. those treated with drugs alone (81 subjects)	52	HBO at 2.5 ATA for 1 h daily for 5 days/week. Improvement of hearing loss was statistically significantly better for HBO group
Yan et al. (2006)	Retrospective study of medical records of patients with sudden deafness treated by HBO vs. non-HBO methods. Logistic regression was used in multivariate analysis	236	Efficacy (hearing threshold elevated above 15 dB) ratio of HBO group comparing to the control group (non-HBO group) showed significant difference. It was concluded that HBO is effective for sudden deafness
Dundar et al. (2007)	Prospective study of combined HBO and medical treatment vs. medical treatment alone in 25 subjects	52	In the HBO and medical treatment group, patients with tinnitus showed the highest hearing improvement but not in the medical treatment only group

[a]Since this study is from Nagoya University, some of the patients in the study may be the same as in the previous report by Takahashi et al. (1989)

initially increased slightly and then decreased by 20 %–25 % of the original values. The CM and CAP amplitudes were reduced by 40 % and by a further 20 % of the original values after six extra shots. HBO increased the pO_2 to 3.5-fold of the postexposure values. Hearing also recovered.

Broadband noise increases the K+ permeability in the transduction tissues of the inner ear, which have to be repolarized again by Na+/K+ pumps, which are dependent upon oxygen and energy. These pumps decompensate for lack of oxygen, which leads to an ion imbalance within the inner ear, which leads to structural changes reflected in decreased hearing potentials, as shown in Fig. 31.1 (Lamm et al. 1989b). In the case of impulse gunfire shots, these ion pumps decompensate for lack of oxygen while restoring the ion imbalance within the inner ear fluids, which had been disturbed by rupture of the cell membrane, as in Fig. 31.2.

Cochlear blood flow, perilymphatic partial pressure of oxygen, cochlear microphonics, compound action potentials of the auditory nerve, and auditory brainstem responses were studied in noise-exposed guinea pigs during and after the several treatments (Lamm and Arnold 1999). A sustained therapeutic effect on noise-induced cochlear ischemia was achieved only by hydroxyethyl starch (HES), HBO + HES, and pentoxifylline. However, the best therapeutic effect on noise-induced hearing loss was achieved with a combination of HBO and prednisolone, followed by monotherapy with prednisolone or HES with the result that not only did the compound action potentials and auditory brainstem responses completely recover, but the cochlear microphonics also showed significant improvement, although full recovery did not occur. All other therapies were significantly less effective or did not improve noise-induced reduction of auditory evoked potentials.

In acute acoustic trauma, excessive noise exposure causes rupture of cell membranes and decreased cochlear blood flow. This leads to decreased oxygen tension in inner ear fluids and reduction of a variety of different oxygen-dependent cellular activities. HBO may help the cells suffering from hypoxia to survive. Kuokkanen et al. (2000) exposed male Wistar rats to 60 impulses of 162-dB SPL from a 7.62-mm assault rifle equipped with a blank adaptor. After the exposure, 15 animals were given HBO treatment for 90 min daily for 10 consecutive days at 0.25 MPa. After a survival time of 4 weeks, auditory brainstem responses were measured and the left cochleae processed for light microscopy. The impulse noise caused permanent damage to the cochlea of all animals, with the most severe lesions in the lower middle coil, where a significantly smaller number of hair cells were missing in the HBO-treated group. The morphological damage was also reflected in function, as measured by auditory brainstem responses, which showed the greatest threshold shifts at 6.0, 8.0, and 10.0 kHz.

In another study guinea pigs were exposed to noise in the 4-kHz range with intensity of 110-dB sound level pressure HBO at 2 ATA for 1 h. The electrophysiological data did not demonstrate effectiveness of HBO against acute acoustic trauma damage, but there was improvement of the anatomical pattern of damage detected by scanning electron microscopy, with a significant reduction of the number of injured cochlear outer hair cells and their functionality (Colombari et al. 2011).

Clinical Studies

Lamm (1969) was the first to use HBO in vestibular disorders. Clinical studies of the use of HBO in acute acoustic trauma are summarized in Table 31.5. Most of the studies show that HBO therapy is useful in relieving tinnitus accompanying acute acoustic trauma, provided it is started within a few days following trauma. The only clinical study with negative effects is

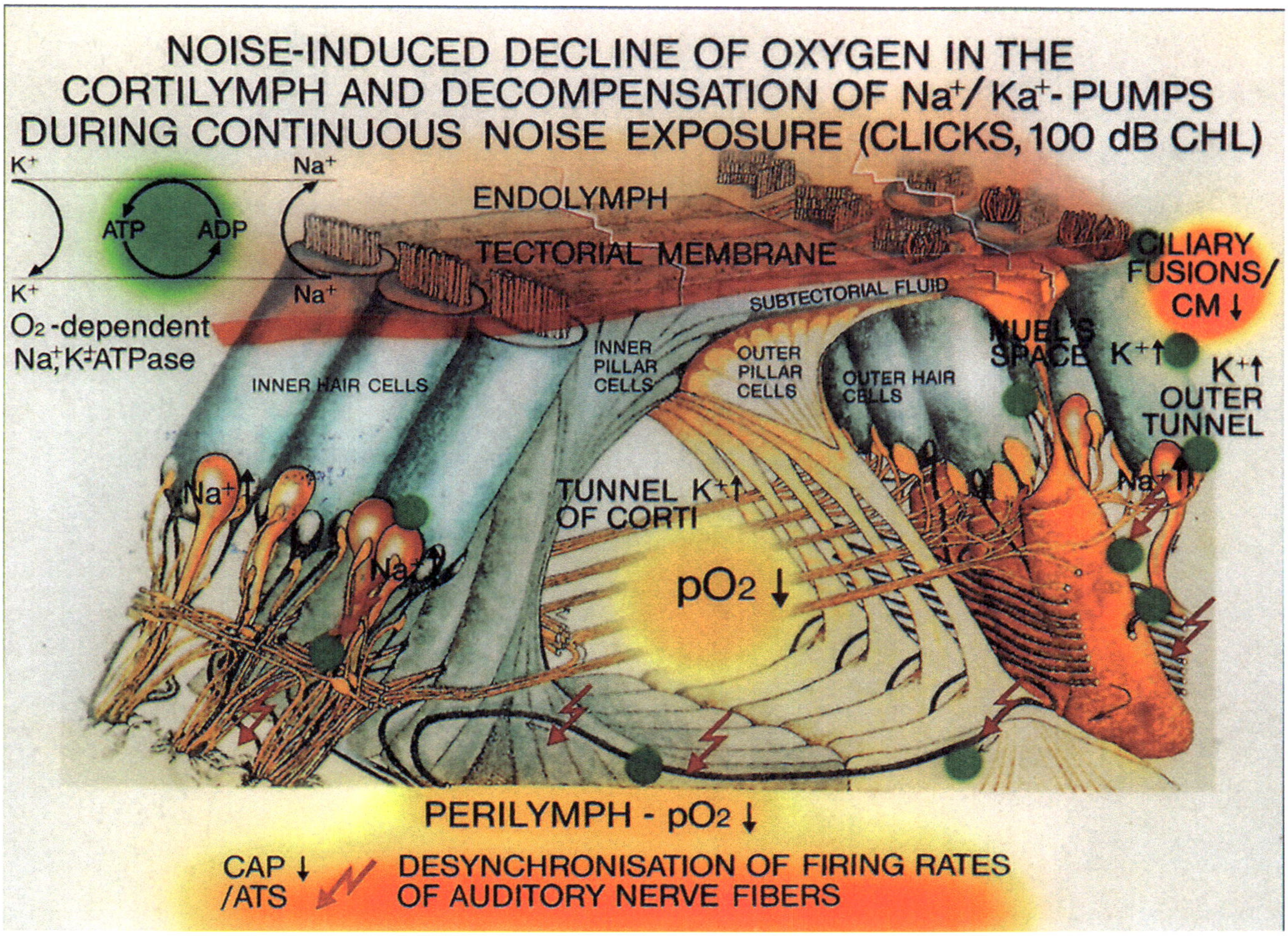

Fig. 31.1 Noise-induced decline of pO_2 in the fluid spaces of the inner ear, i.e., the perilymph and cortilymph. Based on photos from Bild-Atlas Innenohr, edition Duphar Pharma, redrawn by Dr. K. Lamm

that of Kestler et al. (2001) where the HBO was compared with infusion therapy but the two were not combined. Moreover, the authors included patients with onset of sudden deafness up to 3 weeks prior to start of treatment. Perhaps the lesson from that study was to avoid the approaches followed by the authors. The following protocol was recommended:

- Institution of treatment within the first 3 days after the episode
- Ten exposures on 10 consecutive days at 2.5 ATA using 100 % oxygen for 1 h

A systematic review of clinical studies about the effect of HBO therapy on hearing thresholds in patients found that the mean dB of hearing recovery in these studies ranged from 17 to 47 dB in the groups treated with HBO versus 5–46 dB in the groups who did not receive HBO therapy (van der Veen et al. 2014). The authors concluded that the effect of HBO therapy on hearing thresholds in patients with hearing loss caused by a recent acute acoustic trauma

remains unclear. A well-designed randomized controlled trial with enough power was advised to answer this clinical question.

Concluding Remarks About the Use of HBO in Hearing Loss

The published clinical data on this subject that were reviewed by conclusions are as follows (Lamm et al. 1998):

- In the case of patients with idiopathic sudden hearing loss, acoustic trauma, or noise-induced hearing loss, 65 % of those treated by multiple methods demonstrated a hearing improvement of 19 ± 4 dB. In 35 % of the cases, no hearing improvement was detected independent of the drugs administered. This corresponds to the results obtained from placebo-treated patients who demonstrated a hearing improvement of 20 ± 2 dB in 61 % of cases and no hearing gain in 39 % of cases.

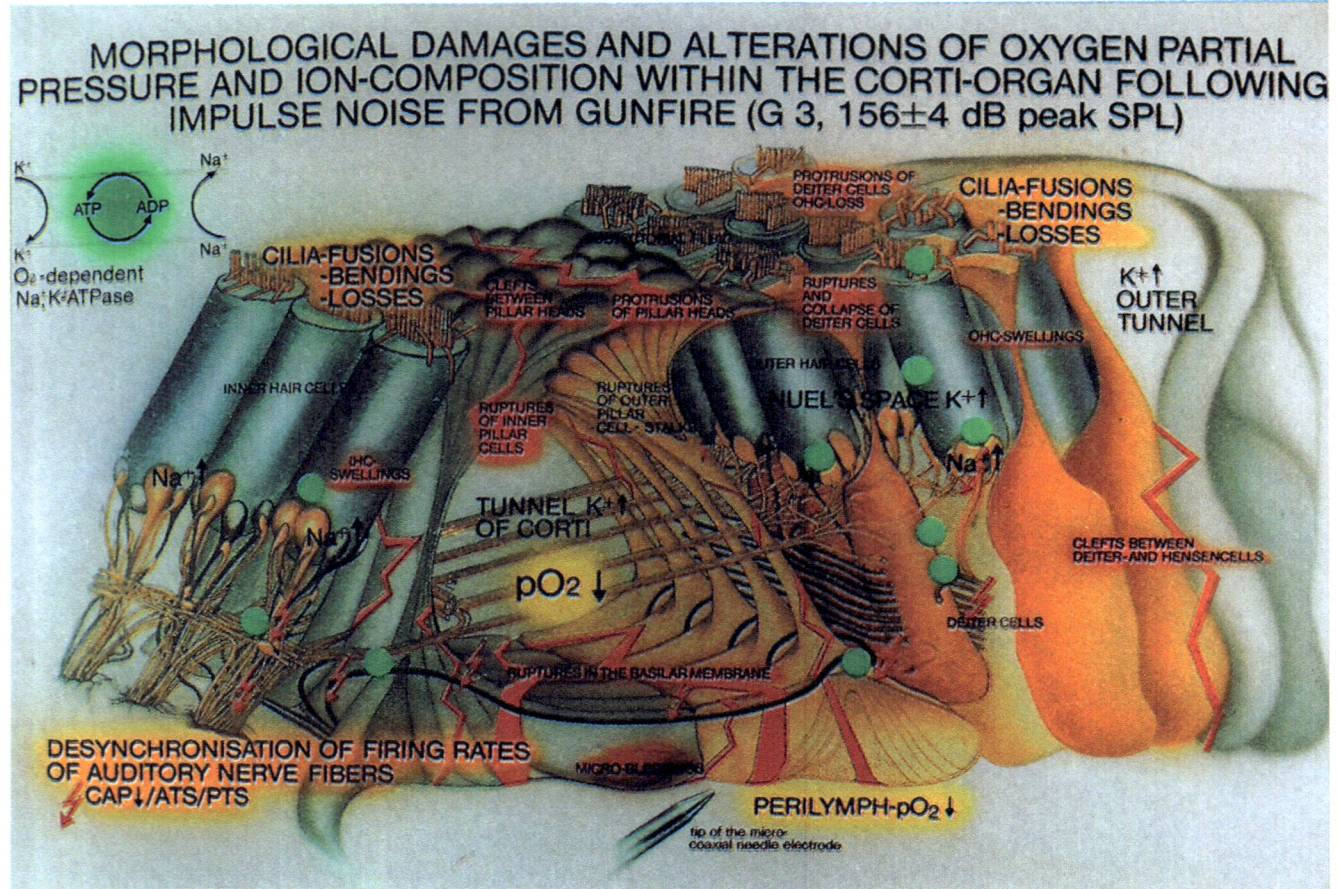

Fig. 31.2 Morphological damage resulting from noise of gunfire, leading to intra- and extracellular ion imbalances, hearing damage, and decline of pO₂ in the fluid spaces of the inner ear. Based on photos from Bild-Atlas Innenohr, edition Duphar Pharma, redrawn by Dr. K. Lamm

Table 31.5 Clinical studies of the use of HBO in acute acoustic trauma

Authors and year	Patients (n)	Cause	Results and comments
Lamm and Gerstmann (1974)	7	Noise damage	Only four obtained relief (two complete and two partial); in three cases that did not improve, treatment was started more than 8 weeks after onset
Demaertelaere and Van Opstal (1981)	50	Gunshot noise	HBO combined with vasodilators and explosion and antiinflammatory drugs; better results with early treatment
Le Mouel et al. (1981)	30	Diving accidents	Good results
Pilgramm and Schumann (1985)	22	Gunshot noise	Random allocation to four groups: therapy 1, 10 % dextran-40 + 5 % sorbitol; therapy 2, therapy 1 + 24 mg betahistine; therapy 3, therapy 1 + 10 HBO treatments; therapy 4, therapy 2 + 10 HBO treatments Best results in groups 3 and 4. Patients with spontaneous recovery (48) excluded from the study. HBO shortens course of recovery and reduces relapse rate after improvement of hearing and tinnitus
Vavrina and Muller (1995)	78	Acute acoustic trauma from various causes	All subjects received saline or dextran (Rheomacrodex) infusions with *Ginkgo biloba* extracts and prednisone. Thirty-six patients underwent additional HBO 2 ATA for 60 min once daily. Both treatment groups were comparable as far as age, gender, initial hearing loss, and prednisone dose are concerned. Treatment was started within 72 h in all cases The average hearing gain in the group without HBO was 74.3 dB and in the group treated additionally with HBO 121.3 dB
Ylikoski et al. (2008)	60	Acute acoustic trauma	HBO, given daily for 1–8 days, led to recovery of normal hearing at the end of the follow-up period in 42/60 compared with 24/60 in controls treated with normobaric oxygen

- A different set of results were obtained in placebo-controlled studies on patients with a hearing loss who were treated either with prednisolone or nonsteroidal antiinflammatory drugs, which concluded that the percentage of patients who regained normal hearing were not significantly different from those with placebo. Problems arise when comparing non-treated patients since information on spontaneous remission rates differs greatly in the references, i.e., between 25 and 68% for spontaneous full remissions and 47–89% for spontaneous partial remissions. From a statistical point of view, 35% and 39% of patients experienced no success with drugs or placebo, respectively. These patients can still be helped with HBO therapy.
- In only 18 studies, the patients underwent primary HBO therapy. In all other 50 studies evaluated by the authors, with a total of 4, 109 patients suffering from idiopathic sudden hearing loss, acoustic trauma, or noise-induced hearing loss and/or tinnitus, HBO therapy was administered as a secondary therapy, i.e., following unsuccessful conventional therapy. If the onset of affliction was more than 2 weeks but no longer than 6 weeks, one-half of the cases showed a marked hearing gain (in at least three frequencies of more than 20 dB), one-third showed a moderate improvement (10–20 dB), and 13% showed no hearing improvement at all. Four percent no longer experienced tinnitus, 81.3% observed an intensity decrease, 1.2% experienced an intensity increase of their tinnitus condition, and 13.5% remained unchanged.
- If HBO therapy was administered at a later stage, but still within 3 months following onset of affliction, 13% showed a definite improvement in hearing, 25% a moderate improvement, and 62% no improvement at all. If the onset of affliction was longer than 3 months up to several years, no hearing improvement can be expected in the majority of patients; however, one-third of the cases reported a decrease in intensity of tinnitus, 60–62% reported no change, and 4–7% noticed a temporary intensity increase.

In conclusion, HBO therapy is recommended and warranted in patients with idiopathic sudden deafness, acoustic trauma, or noise-induced hearing loss within 3 months after onset of disorder. In a recent clinical study, the success rate of combined HBO and steroid therapy was rather low, but early initiation of treatment resulted in better outcomes (Salihoğlu et al. 2015).

Effect of HBO in Preventing Hearing Impairment from Chronic Noise Exposure

Hu et al. (1991) carried out a series of experiments on guinea pigs to study the protective effect of HBO on hearing during chronic repeated noise exposure. A one-third octave band of noise centered at 1000 Hz was used for 1 h daily for 4 weeks. Groups of animals were exposed too to HBO at 2–3 ATA for 1 h on alternate days. HBO was shown to markedly reduce the threshold shift and relieve cochlear damage. Further studies need to be done on this topic.

Miscellaneous Disturbances of the Inner Ear

Lamm et al. (1977) studied the effect of HBO on CO-intoxicated guinea pigs. The microphonics recovered significantly faster from hypoxia than in animals treated by air alone (controls). When HBO was applied before CO exposure, the microphonics decreased less than under normal air breathing. Hyperoxia has also been shown to reduce the damage induced by combined carbon monoxide and noise exposure (Fechter et al. 1988).

Lamm and Klimpel (1971) indicated that HBO should be given within 8 weeks of the onset of inner ear ailments due to vascular causes. They believed that the mechanism of effectiveness was oxygenation of the cochlea through increased partial pressure of oxygen in the blood.

Rzayev (1981) tested the oxygenation of arterial blood in 100 caisson workers to ascertain the pathogenesis of work-related hearing disturbances. These workers were exposed to increased atmospheric pressures and vibration. There was decreased blood oxygenation and occult hypoxia, which could be correlated with the extent of hypoacusis. HBO produced more rapid normalization of hearing than did oxygen inhalation at normal pressure.

Patients with chronic (more than 1 year) impairment due to a variety of causes, such as ototoxicity of antibiotics, infections, and traumatic or occupational diseases, usually show poor results with HBO.

Neuro-otological Vascular Disturbances

Efuni et al. (1980) used HBO in treating 10 patients with cochleovestibular syndromes due to circulatory disturbances in the vertebrobasilar system. The results of treatment with HBO were compared with those of other methods and found to be superior. The effect of HBO was characterized by disappearance of vertigo and tinnitus. Eight of the patients showed improvement of hearing on audiograms.

Lyskin and Lebshova (1981) observed that disorders of the vertebrobasilar circulation give rise to diseases characterized by cochleovestibular syndromes due to impairment of the receptor inner ear. This may arise from impairment of the internal auditory artery or its branches, or as a "symptom at a distance" when vessels such as the anterior inferior cerebellar artery or the vertebral artery are occluded. Chronic or acute ischemia may give rise to impairment of the labyrinth, which responds to HBO. There was a considerable improvement of vertigo and hearing in 12 patients.

Kozyro and Matskevich (1981) obtained good results with HBO in 107 patients with transient ischemia of the vertebrobasilar territory and of the artery to the labyrinth. Their schedule was HBO at 1.5–2 ATA for 35–40 min with daily sessions for 8–10 days.

Guseinov et al. (1989) treated 40 patients suffering from acute neurosensory hypoacusis of vascular etiology using combined HBO and drug therapy to improve microcirculation. One group was given HBO before drug therapy and the other group was given this treatment after drug therapy.

Beneficial effects were more marked in the latter group, and the explanation given was that drug therapy produced vasodilatation, improved metabolism, and counteracted the vasoconstricting effect of HBO.

Meniere's Disease

Meniere's disease is recognized as a clinical entity. The classical triad of symptoms is roaring tinnitus, episodic vertigo, and fluctuating hearing loss. A typical acute attack is followed by nausea, vomiting, and other vegetative symptoms. The classical triad is not always present. Characteristic histopathological lesion is endolymphatic hydrops. Disturbance of the quantitative relationship between the endo- and the perilymph is relevant to the pathogenesis. Further, a disturbance of the electrolyte composition of these two fluids leads to damage to the osmotic pressure regulation inside the membranous labyrinth. An endolymphatic hydrops results.

HBO reduces the hydrops both by increasing the hydrostatic pressure and by mechanically stimulating the flow of endolymph toward the duct and endolymphatic sac. In addition, an increase is seen in the amount of oxygen dissolved in the labyrinthine fluids, and this contributes to recovering cell metabolism and restoring normal cochlear electrophysiological functions. Clinical studies of the use of HBO in Meniere's syndrome and vertigo are summarized in Table 31.6. Although most of the authors have

reported benefit from this therapy, the largest study failed to support this. One of the studies used controls but there has been no randomized study evaluating the use of HBO in Meniere's disease.

Fattori et al. (1996) investigated 45 patients suffering from Meniere's disease by submitting them to pressure chamber therapy: 20 with constant pressure (2.2 ATA, hyperbaric treatment) and 25 with continuous variations in pressure levels (from 1.7 to 2.2 ATA, alternating pressure treatment). HBO therapy consisted of one session per day lasting 90 min for 15 days during the acute attacks followed by five consecutive sessions per month during a follow-up of 2 years. For a control group, the authors treated 18 patients with 10 % intravenous glycerol during the acute episode and 8 mg betahistine three times a day thereafter. They compared hearing loss, vertigo, and tinnitus in the three groups 15 days after starting treatment and at the end of the follow-up, according to the criteria suggested by the 1995 Committee on Hearing and Equilibrium. They found no statistically significant differences in recovery from the cochleovestibular symptoms in the three groups at the end of the first 15 days of therapy, whereas hyperbaric and, in particular, alternating pressure treatment permitted a significant control of the principal attacks of vertigo during the follow-up period. Hearing loss also showed a more significant and more persistent improvement in the patients treated with alternating pressure oxygenation compared to the patients in the other two groups. At the end of a 4-year follow-up of these patients, hyperbaric treatment, and in particular alternating pressure therapy, enabled a significant reduction in the episodes of dizziness as compared to the control group (Fattori et al. 2001).

Cochrane's systematic review found no randomized controlled trials or quasi-randomized controlled trials of HBO for Bell's palsy that met the eligibility criteria. Very-low-quality evidence from one trial suggests that HBO therapy may be an effective treatment for moderate to severe Bell's palsy, but this study was excluded as the outcome assessor was not blinded to treatment allocation (Holland et al. 2012). Further randomized controlled trials are needed.

Table 31.6 Clinical studies of use of HBO in Meniere's disease

Authors and year	Patients (n)	Results and comments
Nair et al. (1973)	7	Remission of nausea, dizziness, and inability to walk
Pavlik (1976)	42	Symptomatic relief with long-term use of HBO
Tjernström et al. (1980)	46	Improvement of hearing in 21 patients
Kozyro and Matskevich (1981)	35	Good results
Qu Zhan-Kui (1986)	1000	No significant improvement
Fattori et al. (1996)	45	More improvement in patients treated under varying conditions

Facial Palsy

Bell's palsy (idiopathic facial palsy) is unilateral facial paralysis of sudden onset. This term does not include lesions of the facial nerve caused by injury such as fractures of the base of the skull, infiltration by tumors, and complication of surgical procedures. The cause is not known, but there is disturbance of the facial nerve with swelling during its course in the facial canal leading to compression and ischemia of the nerve. It resolves spontaneously in 70–80% of cases, but the recovery may be prolonged and residual disability and disfigurement may persist. The outcome of the disease cannot be predicted during the first week, and electrophysiological tests such as the nerve excitability test and electromyography show abnormalities only after this period. Various treatments used include corticosteroids and surgical decompression of the facial nerve. A less frequent cause of facial palsy is Ramsay Hunt syndrome which is believed to be caused by reactivation of varicella zoster virus, and the treatment for this condition has not explored as yet.

Treatment of Bell's palsy remains controversial. Surgical decompression has not produced any better outcome than spontaneous resolution of the palsy. Several prospective and retrospective studies suggest strongly that corticosteroids are beneficial but no definitive study has been done to prove the value of corticosteroids. Ramsay Hunt syndrome responds somewhat better to corticosteroids and also to acyclovir but the benefits have not been proven. The use of HBO has been explored in these conditions.

Litavrin et al. (1985) reported on HBO as a part of multimodal therapy for Bell's palsy in 42 patients. A further 29 patients with a similar clinical picture were treated by conventional methods and served as controls. The authors concluded that the addition of HBO to other methods increases the efficacy of the treatment and reduces the period needed for restoration of the function of the damaged nerve.

Nakata (1976) treated 66 patients with Bell's palsy using HBO. In 54 patients for whom the treatment was started within 2 weeks after onset, 45 (83%) recovered completely, 7 recovered partially, and 2 did not recover. All the patients whose EMG showed evidence of neuropraxia recovered completely. Those with incomplete denervation also recovered, but their recovery period was much longer. This pattern of recovery is better than could be predicted from the natural history of the disease or as a result of other treatments such as steroids and surgical decompression.

Racic et al. (1997) compared the therapeutic effects of HBO with those of prednisone treatment in 79 patients with Bell's palsy who were randomly assigned either to the HBO-treated group ($n = 42$) or to the prednisone-treated group ($n = 37$). The HBO group was exposed to 2.8 ATA of 100% oxygen for 60 min, twice a day, and 5 days a week and was given a placebo orally. The prednisone group was exposed to 2.8 ATA of 7% O_2 (equivalent to 21% O_2 in air at normal pressure) following the same schedule as the HBO group; prednisone was given orally (total of 450 mg in 8 days). Subjects from both groups were treated in the hyperbaric chamber for up to 30 sessions or to complete recovery and were followed up for 9 months. At the end of the follow-up period, 95.2% of subjects treated with HBO and 75.7% of subjects treated with prednisone recovered completely. The average time to complete the recovery in the HBO group was 22 days as compared to 34.4 days in the control group ($p < 0.001$). These results suggest that HBO is more effective than prednisone in treatment of Bell's palsy.

Makishima et al. (1998) treated 12 patients with facial palsy and 11 patients with Ramsey Hunt syndrome by a combination therapy consisting of HBO, stellate ganglion block, as well as oral administration of a vasodilator (this combination therapy has also been used for sudden deafness). The period between the onset and start of treatment was longer than 3 days in most of the patients. Results were evaluated by a special grading system and showed satisfactory clinical results in 83.5% of Bell's palsy patients and 63.6% of Ramsay Hunt patients. The total number of patients in this study is too small for statistical analysis and comparison with other studies. A definitive study on this topic remains to be done.

Otological Complications of HBO Therapy

These have been described in Chap. 8, but a brief mention will be made in this chapter of complications of HBO related to treatment for ENT indications. As in case of other indications, barotrauma, especially to the middle ear, remains the most common complication in this area with the reported rates varying between 5 and 82%. Ueda et al. (1998) have evaluated the incidence of complications in 898 patients who received HBO therapy at the University of Nagoya, Japan, for various indications related to ENT. There was no evidence of barotrauma to the inner ear in any case. The overall incidence of barotrauma was 33.2% (577 of 1737 ears). Patients who developed barotrauma usually had poor Eustachian tube function. This observation can be used to predict barotrauma. The incidence of barotrauma was found to be unrelated to the extent of mastoid pneumatization.

Miscellaneous Conditions in Head and Neck Area

Malignant Otitis Externa

This syndrome was first described by Chandler (1968) and consists of an antibiotic-resistant *Pseudomonas aeruginosa* infection of the external auditory meatus with osteomyelitis of the temporal bone. It usually affects patients with long-standing diabetes mellitus and a weakened immune system. Over 100 cases have been described in the literature. The overall mortality is 35 %.

Lucente et al. (1983) reviewed 16 patients and found that the spread of infection beyond the external auditory meatus can produce lethal invasive osteomyelitis. They recommend investigation of such patients by using radiological procedures such as tomography of the temporal bone and intensive management with antibiotics, surgery, and HBO. HBO has been recommended for this condition by other authors (Mader and Love 1982; Shupak et al. 1989). In 1986, Pilgramm et al. reviewed the literature on this subject and presented three cases with successful management using HBO. Davis et al. (1992) treated 16 patients with malignant otitis externa with addition of a 30-day HBO course to antibiotic regimen. All of the patients recovered and remained free from infection and neurological sequelae during the follow-up from 1 to 4 years.

Advances in the diagnosis and treatment of malignant otitis externa during the past 20 years have improved substantially the prognosis of the disease. HBO potentiates the effect of antibiotic therapy. This condition should no longer be malignant for the majority of the patients where the disease is diagnosed early and treated adequately (Hlozek et al. 1989).

Bath et al. (1998) reported a case of malignant otitis externa with optic neuritis that remained refractory to standard treatment but was cured by adjuvant HBO therapy. This is the only reported case that has survived this disease with optic neuritis.

Martel et al. (2000) treated 22 patients over a period of 4 years; the causal organism was *Pseudomonas aeruginosa* in 87 % of cases. The diagnostic work-up included a computed tomography scan and a technetium scintigraphy to confirm the diagnosis and assess extension of the disease. Medical treatment was used in most cases with parenteral antibiotic therapy with a third-generation cephalosporin (ceftazidime or ceftriaxone) and a fluoroquinolone (ciprofloxacin or ofloxacin) and, if there was no contraindication, HBO. A case has been reported of *Aspergillus flavus* malignant otitis externa, successfully treated with antifungal agents, surgical debridement, and HBO (Ling and Sader 2008). Adjunctive therapies, such as aggressive debridement and HBO, are reserved for extensive or unresponsive cases (Carfrae and Kesser 2008).

Aphonia Due to Chronic Laryngitis

James (1987) presented a case of aphonia due to chronic laryngitis, which resolved following a 4-day course of HBO at 2 ATA. The course of laryngeal edema was followed by laryngoscopy. The author pointed out that this case provided visual evidence that oxygen-induced vasoconstriction can be beneficial in long-standing edema by breaking the cycle of hypoxic edema and microcirculatory insufficiency.

Conclusion

The literature on the use of HBO in otorhinolaryngology is not very extensive. There is agreement that sudden deafness and acute acoustic trauma are good indications for HBO therapy and that there is improvement of these conditions if the treatment is carried out soon after the onset of symptoms. HBO therapy does not displace but is adjunctive to conventional treatments. HBO has been used on a large scale for the treatment of tinnitus in Germany. It is effective in relieving tinnitus as a component of inner ear disorders, but whether this large-scale use for tinnitus alone as a symptom is justified is questionable.

Most authors indicate lack of effectiveness of HBO in chronic anoxic conditions, and its use in Meniere's syndrome is controversial. In symptoms secondary to ischemia, for example, of the acoustic nerve, it is reasonable to suppose that HBO may be effective in the chronic stages, as the situation is comparable to that of ischemia in the brain.

Effectiveness in Bell's palsy has not been proven, although good results have been obtained in several series of patients. Malignant otitis externa is a good indication for the use of HBO as the effect of HBO in enhancing the effect of antibiotics is well documented. This therapy is well tolerated with minor complications and its use continues to be explored in several conditions of the head and neck.

References

Aslan I, Oysu C, Veyseller B, Baserer N. Does the addition of hyperbaric oxygen therapy to the conventional treatment modalities influence the outcome of sudden deafness? Otolaryngol Head Neck Surg. 2002;126:121–6.

Baldwin TM. Tinnitus, a military epidemic: is hyperbaric oxygen therapy the answer? J Spec Oper Med. 2009;9:33–43.

Bath AP, Rowe JR, Innes AJ. Malignant otitis externa with optic neuritis. J Laryngol Otol. 1998;112:274–7.

Bennett MH, Kertesz T, Perleth M, Yeung P, Lehm JP. Hyperbaric oxygen for idiopathic sudden sensorineural hearing loss and tinnitus. Cochrane Database Syst Rev. 2012;10, CD004739.

Bohmer D. Treating tinnitus with hyperbaric oxygenation. Int Tinnitus J. 1997;3:137–40.

Carfrae MJ, Kesser BW. Alignant otitis externa. Otolaryngol Clin North Am. 2008;41:537–49.

Chandler JR. Malignant external otitis. Laryngoscope. 1968;78:1257.

Colombari GC, Rossato M, Feres O, Hyppolito MA. Effects of hyperbaric oxygen treatment on auditory hair cells after acute noise damage. Eur Arch Otorhinolaryngol. 2011;268:49–56.

Dauman R, Cros AM, Poisot D. Treatment of sudden deafness: first results of a comparative study. J Otolaryngol. 1985;14:49–56.

Davis JC, Gates GA, Lerner C, et al. Adjuvant hyperbaric oxygen in malignant external otitis. Arch Otolaryngol Head Neck Surg. 1992;118:89–93.

Delb W, Muth CM, Hoppe U, Iro H. Outcome of hyperbaric oxygen therapy in therapy refractory tinnitus. HNO. 1999;47:1038–45.

Demaertelaere L, Van Opstal M. Treatment of acoustic trauma with hyperbaric oxygen. Acta Oto Rhino Laryngol Belg. 1981;5:303–14.

Desloovere C. Hyperbaric oxygen therapy for tinnitus. B-ENT. 2007;3 Suppl 7:71–4.

Domachevsky L, Keynan Y, Shupak A, Adir Y. Hyperbaric oxygen in the treatment of sudden deafness. Eur Arch Otorhinolaryngol. 2007;264:951–3.

Dundar K, Gumus T, Ay H, Yetiser S, Ertugrul E. Effectiveness of hyperbaric oxygen on sudden sensorineural hearing loss: prospective clinical research. J Otolaryngol. 2007;36:32–7.

Efuni SN, Levashova AS, Lyskin GI. Hyperbaric oxygenation in the treatment of the cochleovestibular system. Sov Med. 1980;5:45–9.

Fattori B, De-Iaco G, Vannucci G, Casani A, Ghilardi PL. Alternobaric and hyperbaric oxygen therapy in the immediate and long-term treatment of Meniere's disease. Audiology. 1996;35:322–34.

Fattori B, Nacci A, Casani A, et al. Oxygen therapy in the long term treatment of Meniere's disease. Acta Otorhinolaryngol Ital. 2001;21:1–9.

Fechter LD, Young JS, Carlisle L. Potentiation of noise induced threshold shifts and hair cell loss by carbon monoxide. Hear Res. 1988;34:39–48.

Goto F, Fujita T, Kitani Y, Kanno M, Kamei T, Ishii H. Hyperbaric oxygen and stellate ganglion blocks for idiopathic sudden hearing loss. Acta Otolaryngol. 1979;88:335–42.

Guseinov NM, Konstantinova NP, Lukich VL, et al. Our experience in the hyperbaric oxygenation treatment of patients with acute sensorineural hearing disorders of vascular etiology. Vestn Otorinolaringol. 1989;4:76–9.

Hesse S, Meyer A, Singer S, Hinz A. Mental distress and quality of life in tinnitus patients. Laryngorhinootologie. 2012;91:774–81.

Hlozek J, Slapak I, Kucera P. Rational treatment of external otitis. Cas Lek Cesk. 1989;128:1594–6.

Holland NJ, Bernstein JM, Hamilton JW. Hyperbaric oxygen therapy for Bell's palsy. Cochrane Database Syst Rev. 2012;2, CD007288.

Inci E, Erisir F, Ada M, Oztürk O, Güçlü E, Oktem F, et al. Hyperbaric oxygen treatment in sudden hearing loss after unsuccessful medical treatment. Kulak Burun Bogaz Ihtis Derg. 2002;9:337–41.

James PB. Hyperbaric oxygen in the therapy of aphonia associated with chronic laryngitis. Presented at the 9th international congress on hyperbaric medicine, Sydney, Australia, 1–4 March 1987.

Kau RJ, Sendtner-Gress K, Ganzer U, Arnold W. Effectiveness of hyperbaric oxygen therapy in patients with acute and chronic cochlear disorders. ORL J Otorhinolaryngol Relat Spec. 1997;59:79–83.

Kestler M, Strutz J, Heiden C. Hyperbaric oxygenation in early treatment of sudden deafness. HNO. 2001;49:719–23.

Kozyro VI, Matskevich MV. Clinical aspects of using hyperbaric oxygenation in the treatment of different forms of neurosensory hypoacusis. In: Yefuny SN, editor. Abstracts of the 7th International Congress on HBO Medicine. Moscow: USSR Academy of Sciences; 1981. p. 306–7.

Kuokkanen J, Aarnisalo AA, Ylikoski J. Efficiency of hyperbaric oxygen therapy in experimental acute acoustic trauma from firearms. Acta Otolaryngol Suppl. 2000;543:132–4.

Lamm H. Klinische Ergebnisse nach Behandlung von Innenohrschwerhörigkeiten mit hyperbarem Sauerstoff. Halle/Saale: Contribution at the HNO Annual Congress of the DDR; 1969.

Lamm K, Arnold W. Successful treatment of noise-induced cochlear ischemia, hypoxia, and hearing loss. Ann N Y Acad Sci. 1999;884:233–48.

Lamm H, Gerstmann W. Erste Erfahrungen mit der hyperbaren Oxygenation in der Otologie. Wochenschr Ohrenheilk (Wien). 1974;108:6–11.

Lamm H, Klimpel L. Hyperbare Sauerstofftherapie bei Innenohr und Vestibularisstörungen. HNO. 1971;19:363–9.

Lamm H, Dahl D, Gerstmann W. Die Wirkung von hyperbarem Sauerstoff (OHP) auf die hypoxisch geschädigte Cochlea des Meerschweinchens. Arch Otorhinolaryngol. 1977;217:415–21.

Lamm H, Lamm K, Zimmermann W. The effects of hyperbaric oxygen on experimental noise damage to the ears. Arch Otorhinolaryngol. 1982;236:237–44.

Lamm H, Lamm K. The effect of hyperbaric oxygen on the inner ear. In: Kindwall EP (ed.) Proceedings of the 8th International Congress on Hyperbaric Medicine. San Pedro, CA: Best Publishing; 1987:35.

Lamm CH, Walliser U, Schumann K, Lamm K. Sauerstoffpartialdruck-Messungen in der Perilymphe der Scala tympani unter normound hyperbaren Bedingungen. HNO. 1988;36:363–6.

Lamm K, Lamm CH, Lamm H, Schumann K. The effect of hyperbaric oxygen on noise-induced hearing loss. An experimental study using simultaneous measurements of oxygen partial pressure in the inner ear, hearing potentials, arterial blood pressure and blood gas analyses. In: Schmutz J, Bakker D (Eds.) Proceedings of the joint meeting: 2nd Swiss symposium on hyperbaric medicine and 2nd European conference on hyperbaric medicine, Basel, Switzerland, Sept 22–24, 1989a.

Lamm K, Lamm CH, Lamm H, Schumann K. Simultane Laser-Doppler-Flow Metrie zur Bestimmung des kochleären Blutflusses, Sauerstoffpartialdruckmessungen und Elektrokochleographie während Hämootilution. 60th annual meeting, Deutsche Gesellschaft HNO Heilkunde, Kiel, 1989b.

Lamm K, Lamm H, Arnold W. Effect of hyperbaric oxygen therapy in comparison to conventional or placebo therapy or no treatment in idiopathic sudden hearing loss, acoustic trauma, noise-induced hearing loss and tinnitus. A literature survey. Adv Otorhinolaryngol. 1998;54:86–99.

Le Mouel C, Renon P, Asperge SUC, Asperge A. Hyperbaric treatment of dive-induced inner ear accidents. Med Subaquat Hyperbare. 1981;79:242–6.

Ling SS, Sader C. Fungal malignant otitis externa treated with hyperbaric oxygen. Int J Infect Dis. 2008;12:550–2.

Litavrin AF, Platonova GB, Gribanov VA. Hyperbaric oxygenation in the treatment of facial neuritis. Zh Nevropatol Psikhiatr. 1985;85:528–31.

Lucente RG, Parisier SC. Sone PM Complications of the treatment of malignant external otitis. Laryngoscope. 1983;93:279.

Lyskin GI, Lebshova AS. Hyperbaric oxygenation in the treatment of labyrinthopathies of vascular genesis. In Yefuny SN (Ed.) Abstracts of the 7th International Congress on Hyperbaric Medicine. USSR Academy of Sciences, Moscow, 1981. p 307.

Mader JT, Love JT. Malignant external otitis. Cure with adjunctive hyperbaric oxygen therapy. Arch Otolaryngol. 1982;108:38–40.

Makishima K, Yoshida M, Kuroda Y, et al. Hyperbaric oxygenation as a treatment for facial palsy. Adv Otorhinolaryngol. 1998;54:110–8.

Martel J, Duclos JY, Darrouzet V, et al. Malignant or necrotizing otitis externa: experience in 22 cases. Ann Otolaryngol Chir Cervicofac. 2000;117:291.

Muminov AI, Khatamov ZA, Masharipov RR. Antioxidants and hyperbaric oxygenation in the treatment of sensorineural hearing loss in children. Vestn Otorinolaringol. 2002;5:33–4.

Murakawa T, Kosaka M, Mori Y, Fukazawa M, Misaki K. Treatment of 522 patients with sudden deafness performed oxygenation at high pressure. Nippon Jibiinkoka Gakkai Kaiho. 2000;103:506–15.

Nakashima T, Fukuta S, Yanagita N. Hyperbaric oxygen therapy for sudden deafness. Acta Otorhinolaryngol (Basel). 1998;54:100–9.

Narozny W, Sicko Z, Przewozny T, Stankiewicz C, Kot J, Kuczkowski J. Sudden sensorineural hearing loss: a treatment protocol including glucocorticoids and hyperbaric oxygen therapy. Otolaryngol Pol. 2004;58:821–30.

Nakata M. Hyperbaric oxygen therapy for facial palsy. Jpn J Hyperb Med. 1976;10:99–103.

Pavlik L. Hyperbaric oxygen therapy in Meniere's disease. Cesk Otolaryngol. 1976;25:160–3.

Pilgramm H. Klinische, hämoreologische und tierexperimentelle Untersuchungen zur Therapieoptierung des akuten Knalltraumas. Certificate of Habilitation (Thesis): University of Greifswald, Germany; 1991.

Pilgramm M, Schumann K. Hyperbaric oxygen therapy for acute acoustic trauma. Arch Otorhinolaryngol. 1985;241:246–57.

Pilgramm M, Lamm H, Schumann K. Zur hyperbaren Sauerstofftherapie beim Hörsturz. Larngologie Rhinol Otol. 1985;64:351–4.

Pilgramm M, Fischer B, Frey G, Roth M. Change in rheological parameters under hyperbaric oxygen therapy in patients with inner ear damage. Kobe, Japan: Ninth international symposium on underwater and hyperbaric physiology; 1986.

Qu Zhan-Kui. A brief introduction to the HBO Dept. In Hospital of YangShang petrochemical corporation paper presented at the 5th congress of hyperbaric medicine, Fuzhow, China, 1986.

Racic G, Denoble PJ, Sprem N, et al. Hyperbaric oxygen as a therapy of Bell's palsy. Undersea Hyperb Med. 1997;24:35–8.

Racic G, Petri NM, Andric D. Hyperbaric oxygen as a method of therapy of sudden sensorineural hearing loss. Int Marit Health. 2001;52:74–84.

Rzayev RM. Role of hypoxia in pathogenesis of occupational hypoacusis and normalizing action of hyperbaric oxygenation on saturation of arterial blood with oxygen. Zh Ushn Nos Gorl Bolez. 1981;41:22–5.

Salihoğlu M, Ay H, Cincik H, Cekin E, Cesmeci E, Memis A, et al. Efficiency of hyperbaric oxygen and steroid therapy in treatment of hearing loss following acoustic trauma. Undersea Hyperb Med. 2015;42:539–46.

Shiraishi T, Satou Y, Makishima K. Hyperbaric oxygenation therapy in idiopathic sudden sensory neural hearing loss. Nippon Jibiinkoka Gakkai Kaiho. 1998;101:1380–4.

Shupak A, Greenberg E, Hardoff R, et al. Hyperbaric oxygenation for necrotizing (malignant) otitis externa. Arch Otolaryngol Head Neck Surg. 1989;115:1470–5.

Takahashi H, Sakakibara K, Murahashi K, Yanagita N. HBO for sudden deafness – a statistical survey over 907 ears. In: Schmutz J, Bakker D, editors. Proceedings of the 2nd Swiss Symposium on Hyperbaric Medicine. Basel: Foundation for Hyperbaric Medicine; 1989.

Tan J, Tange RA, Dreschler WA, vd Kleij A, Tromp EC. Long-term effect of hyperbaric oxygenation treatment on chronic distressing tinnitus. Scand Audiol 1999;28: 91–6.

Ueda H, Shien CW, Miyazawa T, et al. Otological complications of hyperbaric oxygen therapy. Adv Otorhinolaryngol. 1998;54:119–26.

Tjernström Ö, Casselbrant M, Harris S, Ivarsson A. Current status of pressure chamber treatment. Otolaryngol Clin North Am. 1980;13:723–9.

van der Veen EL, van Hulst RA, de Ru JA. Hyperbaric oxygen therapy in acute acoustic trauma: a rapid systematic review. Otolaryngol Head Neck Surg. 2014;151:42–5.

Vavrina J, Muller W. Therapeutic effect of hyperbaric oxygenation in acute acoustic trauma. Rev Laryngol Otol Rhinol (Bord). 1995;116:377–80.

Yan B, Kong W, Shi H, Wang J, Sun D. Idiopathic sudden deafness: the therapeutic evaluation of hyperbaric oxygen treatment. Lin Chuang Er Bi Yan Hou Ke Za Zhi. 2006;20:309–11.

Ylikoski J, Mrena R, Makitie A, Kuokkanen J, Pirvola U, Savolainen S. Hyperbaric oxygen therapy seems to enhance recovery from acute acoustic trauma. Acta Otolaryngol. 2008;128:1110–5.

Zhang D, Ma Y. Repetitive transcranial magnetic stimulation improves both hearing function and tinnitus perception in sudden sensorineural hearing loss patients. Sci Rep. 2015;5:14796.

Heather Murphy-Lavoie, Tracy LeGros, Frank K. Butler Jr. , and K.K. Jain

Abstract

Hyperbaric oxygen therapy (HBOT) can be a useful primary or adjunctive therapy for a variety of medical disorders, many of which involve the eye. This chapter will review the effects of oxygen on eye, the literature describing use of HBOT for a variety of conditions and the potential complications of HBOT affecting the eye. The authors recommend the following as ocular indications for HBOT: decompression sickness or arterial gas embolism (AGE) with visual signs or symptoms, central retinal artery occlusion, ocular and periocular gas gangrene, cerebro-rhino-orbital mucor mycosis, periocular necrotizing fasciitis, carbonmonoxide poisoning with visual sequelae, radiation optic neuropathy, radiation or mitomycin C-induced scleral necrosis, and periorbital reconstructive surgery. Other ocular disorders that may benefit from HBOT include selected cases of ischemic optic neuropathy, ischemic central retinal vein occlusion, branch retinalartery occlusion with central vision loss, ischemic branch retinal vein occlusion, cystoid macular edema associated with retinal venous occlusion, post-surgical inflammation, or intrinsic inflammatory disorders, periocular brown recluse spider envenomation, ocular quinine toxicity, Purtscher's retinopathy, radiation retinopathy, anterior segment ischemia, retinal detachment in sickle cell disease, refractory actinomycoticlacrimal canaliculitis, pyoderma gangrenosum of the orbit, and refractory pseudomonas keratitis. Visual function should be monitored as clinically indicated before, during, and after therapy when HBOT is undertaken to treat vision loss. Visual acuity alone is not an adequate measure of visual function to monitor the efficacy of HBOT in this setting. Because some ocular disorders require rapid administration of HBOT to restore vision, patients with acute vision loss should be considered emergent when they present and treatment with supplemental oxygen should be initiated.

Keywords

Eye diseases • Ocular blood supply • Central retinal artery • Central retinal vein • Ocular hypoxia • Ocular injury • Ocular blood flow occlusion • VGEF • Vision loss • Painless vision loss • Hyperbaric oxygen therapy (HBOT) • Retinal injury

H. Murphy-Lavoie, MD (✉) • T. LeGros, MD, PhD
Department of Emergency Medicine, Undersea and Hyperbaric Medicine, University Medical Center,
2000 Canal St., New Orleans, LA 70112, USA
e-mail: hmurph@cox.net1

F.K. Butler Jr. , MD, CAPT MC USN (Ret)
Committee on Tactical Combat Casualty Care, Joint Trauma System, Committee on Tactical Combat Casualty Care, Pensacola, FL, USA

K.K. Jain, MD, FRACS, FFPM
1 Blaesiring 7, Basel 4057, Switzerland

Introduction

Ocular and periocular tissues may benefit from hyperbaric oxygen therapy (HBOT) for certain injuries or disease states. Several uses of HBOT in diseases of the eye have been reported over the years. Pertinent anatomy and physiology of the eye and the effects of hyperbaric hyperoxia on these will be reviewed. Following this will be a

© Springer International Publishing AG 2017
K.K. Jain, *Textbook of Hyperbaric Medicine*, DOI 10.1007/978-3-319-47140-2_32

discussion of the ocular contraindications to HBOT and the reported clinical uses of HBO in ophthalmology.

Review of Pertinent Anatomy and Physiology of the Eye

The Process of Vision

In the process of producing the sensory experience of vision, light passes through the cornea, anterior chamber, pupil, posterior chamber, crystalline lens, and the vitreous body prior to reaching the retina. The cornea provides approximately two thirds of the refracting power required to focus light on the retina; the lens provides the other one third. The anterior chamber, posterior chamber, and vitreous body are filled with non-compressible fluid, providing protection from barotrauma, unless a gas space exists adjacent to the eye (as with a facemask) or within the eye (secondary to surgical procedures or trauma). The retina is comprised of nine distinct layers. The photoreceptor cells compose the outermost layer; the internal limiting membrane delineates the innermost layers. Light reaching the retina stimulates the photoreceptor cells, resulting in stimulation of the ganglion cells. The confluence of the afferent portions of the ganglion cells (the nerve fiber layer) forms the optic disk. These cells then exit the eye as the optic nerve to carry visual stimuli back to the occipital cortex of the brain via the optic chiasm and the optic tract (Regillo et al. 2007; Butler et al. 2008; Murphy-Lavoie et al. 2012; 2014).

Factors Affecting Vision

Vision may be adversely affected by any factor that prevents light from reaching the retina or being sharply focused in the retinal plane. These factors include injury to the retina, occipital cortex, or the afferent neural tissues carrying visual stimuli between these areas. The arterial supply to the eye is provided by the ophthalmic artery, a branch of the internal carotid artery. The branches of the ophthalmic artery supply various orbital structures, while other arterial branches (central retinal, posterior ciliaries, and anterior ciliaries) supply the globe (Cibis et al. 2006; Murphy-Lavoie et al. 2012). The optic nerve receives its blood supply from the branches of several vessels, including the central retinal artery, posterior ciliary arteries, and the ophthalmic artery. In approximately 15–30 % of individuals, collateral circulation via a cilioretinal artery is also present. This artery is part of the ciliary arterial supply, but supplies the macular region of the retina, which preserves central vision (Murphy-Lavoie et al. 2012).

Retinal Blood Supply

The retina in the human eye has a dual blood supply. The retinal circulation supplies the inner retinal layers; the choroidal circulation supplies the outer layers. Under normoxic conditions, approximately 60 % of the retina's oxygen supply comes from the choroidal circulation. However, animal models reveal that oxygen from the choroidal circulation diffuses in adequate quantity to the inner retinal layers under hyperoxic conditions, which maintains ganglion cell viability and retinal function even when retinal blood flow has been interrupted (Li et al. 1996; Landers 1978; Patz 1955; Butler et al. 2008; Murphy-Lavoie et al. 2012). Even with adequate ocular blood flow, if oxygen delivery to the eye is impaired, as occurs with hypobaric hypoxia, retinal vessels respond by dilating and ocular blood flow is markedly increased (Butler et al. 1992). The retinal vessels respond similarly to the hypoxia of CO poisoning (Resch et al. 2005).

Ocular Oxygen Tension

Most of the information regarding normal ocular oxygen tensions is based on animal studies. Oxygen tension in the vitreous humor (80–90 mmHg) is higher than in the anterior chamber (50 mmHg). The cornea, the lens, and the vitreous humor are mostly avascular. Pertinent findings include:

1. The corneal epithelium utilizes atmospheric oxygen.
2. Oxygen can diffuse across the cornea at a rate that is equal both inward and outward.
3. The lens consume 0.2–0.5 mL oxygen/min.
4. The retina carries out its oxygen exchange exclusively through the retinal and the choroidal vessels.
5. The ratio of tissue pO_2 when breathing 100 % oxygen to tissue pO_2 when breathing air is 2.6:3.4 for both the vitreous and the aqueous humors. This is much higher than the similar ratio for other tissues (2.1:2.3) and accounts for the increased susceptibility of the eye to the effects of hyperoxia.

Physiology of the Eye in Hyperoxic Conditions

As the retina has a dual blood supply, hyperoxygenation may enable the choroidal circulation to supply the oxygen needs of the entire retina. Since central retinal artery obstructions (CRAOs) are often transient, this phenomenon may enable the retina to survive the period of occluded blood flow. The studies published by Landers demonstrate this is a possibility in feline and rhesus monkey models. The authors induced CRAO and ventilated the animals with 100 % oxygen at 1 ATA. Normal or increased PO_2 was produced in the inner layers of the retina. They noted that a PaO_2 of 375–475 mmHg provided a normal or increased inner retinal oxygen tension, even with the CRAO (Landers 1978). Breathing 100 % oxygen at 1 ATA was shown to restore visual-evoked response (VER) to normal in CRAO models. A normal VER requires that all layers of the retina are functioning normally and indicates the inner retinal layers were adequately oxygenated (Landers 1978).

Hyperbaric oxygen is well-known to cause vasoconstriction of the retinal vessels (Yu and Cringle 2005; Vucetic et al. 2004; Polkinghorne et al. 1989; Nichols et al. 1969; Frayser et al. 1967; Anderson et al. 1965a; Saltzman et al. 1965; Haddad and Leopold 1965; Jacobson et al. 1963). As the partial pressure of oxygen is increased to 2.36 and 3.70 ATA, the retinal vessels become progressively smaller (Frayser et al. 1967). Both retinal arterioles and venules are affected (Saltzman et al. 1965). Ten minutes after the hyperoxic exposure, the vessels return to 94.5 % and 89.0 % of their primary size, respectively (Vucetic et al. 2004).

Hyperoxic retinal vasoconstriction has led some authors to theorize that there is a decrease in retinal oxygenation under hyperoxic conditions (Herbstein and Murchland 1984). This is not the case. Retinal venous hemoglobin oxygen saturation has been shown to increase from 58 % (room air) to 94 % (2.36 ATA), indicating that the hyperoxygenated choriocapillaris is supplying enough oxygen to offset any decrease in oxygen supply caused by retinal vasoconstriction at elevated partial pressures of oxygen (James 1985; Frayser et al. 1967). Jampol demonstrated that HBOT at 2 ATA (primate monkey model) markedly increased the preretinal oxygen tension, indicating higher inner retinal oxygen levels under hyperoxic conditions (Jampol 1987). Dollery confirmed that a hyperoxygenated choroid can supply the oxygen requirements of the whole retina (Dollery et al. 1969).

Laterally directed fingertip pressure on a closed eye will raise intraocular pressure (IOP) and typically cause a dimming of vision in less than 5 s. This phenomenon is thought to be due to retinal ischemia induced by the elevated IOP. HBOT at 4 ATA extends the interval from pressure application to dimming of vision to 50 s or more. Jampol found that normobaric oxygen delivered to the corneal surface of rabbits increased the pO_2 in the anterior chamber from 63.5 to 139.5 mmHg. Additionally, he found that HBOT at 2 ATA presented to the corneal surface of air breathing rabbits further raised the anterior chamber pO_2 to 295.2 mmHg (Jampol et al. 1988; Jampol 1987). Interestingly, hyperoxia (air at 3 ATA) has been shown to cause a decrease in IOP from 15.3 to 12.3 mmHg in 14 volunteers over a mean time of 38 min. Hundred percent oxygen administered at 1 ATA also produced a significant decrease in IOP from 14.8 to 12.7 mmHg. The exact mechanism of the IOP reduction is not clear (Gallin-Cohen et al. 1980). Hyperoxic vasoconstriction is one potential mechanism for the observed decrease. Note

that IOP measurements in hyperbaric environments typically describe the difference between the intraocular tissues and the external environment, not the absolute pressure which increases with the ambient environment (Butler et al. 2008).

Hyperbaric oxygen has a very mild effect on corneal thickness. A single exposure to HBO treatment reduces the central corneal thickness in non-diabetic subjects, but not in diabetic subjects. However, the change in central corneal thickness is minor (Ayata et al. 2012).

Adverse Effects of Hyperoxia

Retinal Oxygen Toxicity

Oxygen can be directly toxic to the tissues of the eye (Clark and Thom 2003). However, oxygen at 1 ATA has not been shown to produce adverse ocular effects in adult humans. Breathing oxygen at high pressures typically results in pulmonary toxicity before the eye is affected (Kinney 1985). As early as 1935, Behnke reported a reversible decrease in peripheral vision after oxygen breathing at 3ATA (Behnke et al. 1936). Lambertsen, Nichols, and their colleagues also observed a progressive decrease in peripheral vision associated with hyperoxic exposures (Lambertsen et al. 1987; Nichols et al. 1969). A decrease in peripheral vision was noted after ~2.5 h of oxygen breathing at 3.0 ATA in a dry chamber. This decrease was progressive until oxygen breathing was discontinued. The average decrement in visual field was 50 %. Recovery was complete in all subjects after 45 min of air breathing (Lambertsen et al. 1987). A decrease in ERG amplitude was noted as well, but did not correlate directly with the size of the visual field defect and returned to normal more slowly after the termination of the hyperoxic exposure (Lambertsen et al. 1987). Visual acuity and visual cortical-evoked responses remained normal in all subjects. A 4-h exposure to 1 ATA of oxygen, in contrast, produced no change in visual acuity or visual fields (Miller 1958). These changes in visual fields may represent a form of retinal oxygen toxicity rather than CNS oxygen toxicity, as they are predictable, evolve slowly, and resolve slowly after the discontinuation of the hyperoxic exposure. Retinal oxygen toxicity is not commonly reported as a complication of HBOT. However, the incidence may be underreported, as visual fields are not typically performed during the course of HBOT, and any defects present would be expected to resolve shortly after a return to normoxia. Moreover, repetitive HBOT is almost always administered at 2.0–2.5 ATA and for shorter exposure times than those that have been documented to cause retinal oxygen toxicity. Retinal oxygen toxicity has been further explored in animal models. Hyperbaric oxygen administered in severe enough exposures results in photoreceptor cell death preceded by attenuation of the electroretinogram (ERG) (Bridges 1966; Noell 1962). Beehler exposed dogs to hyperoxia (680–760 mmHg of oxygen) continuously for 72 h. All animals were either dead at the end of the exposure, or died shortly thereafter due to pulmonary complications. Fifty percent of the animals were found to have ocular lesions as a result of this exposure, including bilateral retinal detachments, corneal haze, chemosis, and hyphema (Beehler et al. 1963). Four-hour exposures of rabbits to 3 ATA of oxygen, or 40–48 h of exposure to 1 ATA of oxygen, resulted in destruction of the retinal photoreceptor cells (Nichols et al. 1969; Noell 1962). Sodium-potassium ATPase has been shown to be inhibited by hyperbaric oxygen and may also be a factor in retinal oxygen toxicity (Ubels and Hoffert 1981).

Hyperoxia is especially toxic to the immature retina, causing vasoconstriction and subsequent failure of normal vascularization in the retinas of infants given high doses of supplemental oxygen (Patz 1965). Retrolental fibroplasia was first described in 1942 (Terry 1942). It became the leading cause of blindness in preschool children in the 1950s (Beehler 1964). Following the determination that hyperoxia was the major causative factor in this disorder, the incidence of retrolental fibroplasia was greatly reduced (Butler et al. 2008).

Retrolental fibroplasia or retinopathy of prematurity was considered to be a toxic effect of oxygen on the retina of the immature infant leading to blindness. This condition still occurs, although rarely, even though oxygen is not routinely administered for long periods in high concentrations in the neonatal period. Its use is guided by transcutaneous oxygen tension ($tcpO_2$) determinations. One of the explanations given for the pathogenesis of this condition was that hyperoxygenation leads to constriction of the growing vessels and degeneration of endothelium, with neovascularization around ischemic areas. Vitamin E has been shown to have some protective effect against this complication in the premature infant. Retrolental fibroplasia has not been reported as a complication of HBOT in adult humans. It is now believed that variations of $tcpO_2$ in the first two weeks of life is a significant predictor of retinopathy of prematurity (Cunningham et al. 1995).

Ricci exposed newborn Wistar rats to normobaric oxygen (80%) for 5 days after birth. They developed retinopathy with marked peripheral retinal neovascularization. Similar animals given HBOT (1.8 ATA) did not develop peripheral retinopathy. The authors concluded that, in the newborn rat, hyperbarism provides a protective action against the toxic effects of oxygen supplementation on immature retinal vessels (Ricci et al. 1989; 1995).

Lenticular Oxygen Toxicity

Hyperoxic Myopia

The partial pressure of oxygen in HBOT typically varies from 2.0 to 3.0 ATA, depending on the treatment protocol used. However, hyperoxic myopia has also been reported in a closed-circuit mixed-gas scuba diver at a PPO_2 of 1.3 ATA, a lower partial pressure of oxygen than those typically used in HBOT (Butler et al. 1999). The myopic shift noted above resolved over a 1-month period after finishing the series of hyperoxic SCUBA dives (Butler et al. 2008). Hypermetropic changes after HBOT exposures have also been reported (Evanger et al. 2006; Fledelius and Jansen 2004).

Fledelius and colleagues (2002) recorded changes in refraction and refractive parameters associated with a standard HBOT treatment protocol (95 min at >95% O_2 at 2.5 ATA daily for 30 sessions). Refraction was determined subjectively assessed by keratometry and by A-scan axial ultrasound measurement. The refractive changes associated with HBOT were found to be smaller than previously reported in the literature. No significant changes in axial eye length measurements were found, and keratometry readings reflected only minimal change, although this was statistically significant. Therefore, it is most likely that lens changes, whether in internal refractive indices or curvatures, accounted for the transitory shift toward more myopic/less hyperopic values.

Cataract

Cataract formation has been reported by Palmquist and his co-authors in patients undergoing a prolonged (150 or more exposures) course of daily HBOT therapy at 2.0–2.5 ATA (Palmquist et al. 1984; Palmquist 1986). Seven of 15 patients with clear lenses at the start of therapy developed cataracts during their course of treatment. Fourteen of these 15 patients received a total HBOT treatment time of between 300 and 850 h. All of the patients developed myopia during treatment. Seven of the 15 patients with clear lenses prior to treatment developed cataracts and reduced visual activity during the treatment. The authors considered myopic change to be an early sign of increasing nuclear cataract. The lens opacities noted were not completely reversible after HBOT was discontinued. Gesell and Trott reported de novo cataract formation in a 49-year-old woman who underwent 48 HBOT treatments for chronic refractory osteomyelitis of the sacrum and recurrent failure of a sacral flap (Gesell and Trott 2007).

Hyperoxic myopia and subsequent cataract formation may be considered to represent two points on the continuum of severity of lenticular oxygen toxicity. The high success rate of modern cataract surgery makes cataract formation an easily manageable complication of HBOT, and this side effect is not necessarily an indication to discontinue therapy if the patient's clinical indication for continuation of HBOT is needed (Butler et al. 2008).

Ocular Contraindications to Hyperbaric Oxygen Therapy

While the presence of impaired vision itself may be a contraindication to commercial or recreational diving, it is not a contraindication to receive HBOT. The prescribed convalescent period, prior to resumption of diving activity after ocular surgery, should typically not be relevant to HBOT (except as noted below), as facemask barotrauma and water intrusion into an ocular operative site is not applicable with a clinical hyperbaric chamber. Glaucoma is also not a contraindication to HBOT, despite the presence of elevated ambient and IOPs (Butler 1995). Interestingly, oxygen has actually been shown to reduce IOP slightly (Gallin-Cohen et al. 1980).

The following ocular conditions remain contraindications to HBOT:

Hollow Orbital Prosthesis: There are reports of pressure-induced collapses of hollow silicone orbital implants at depths as shallow as 10 ft (Isenberg and Diamant 1985). Most ocular implants used presently, however, are not hollow and should not be considered a contraindication to diving or HBOT. A hollow orbital prosthesis is a relative contraindication and should not prevent HBOT required to preserve life, neurological function, or vision in the fellow eye (Butler et al. 2008).

Intraocular Gas Bubble: Intraocular gas is used in selected cases by vitreoretinal surgeons as stent to maintain juxtaposition of the retina to the retinal pigment epithelium and by anterior segment surgeons to maintain juxtaposition of Descemet's membrane to the posterior corneal stroma. Gas in the eye may result in intraocular barotrauma during compression or a CRAO during decompression and is a contraindication to exposure to changes in ambient pressure (Butler 2007). Intraocular gas bubbles expand even with the relatively small decreases in ambient pressure entailed in commercial air travel (Kokame and Ing 1994; Mills et al. 2001). This expansion causes an increase in IOP (Kokame and Ing 1994; Lincoff et al. 1989) and may cause sudden blindness at altitude due to a pressure-induced closure of the central retinal artery (Kokame and Ing 1994; Polk et al. 2002). Jackman has shown that intraocular bubbles in a rabbit model result in a dramatic decrease in IOP during compression followed by a marked increase in IOP upon return to 1 ATA as the bubble expands (Jackman and Thompson 1995).

One important exception regarding intraocular gas and HBOT relates to eye bubbles that may occur as a manifestation of decompression sickness. HBOT recompression should be undertaken for treatment, with the expectation that the normal volume of the anterior chamber, posterior chamber, and vitreous prior to the formation of the gas bubble (due to inert gas supersaturation) will prevent compression barotrauma. Resolution of the intraocular bubbles and inert gas supersaturation during HBOT would be expected to prevent an expanding gas phase on decompression and a secondary rise in IOP. Intraocular gas bubbles may also be present with intraocular gas gangrene. HBOT is recommended for this disorder as well, although the bubble dynamics during HBOT might be different in this instance from those seen with inert gas supersaturation (Butler et al. 2008).

Pre-HBOT Ocular Examination

If HBOT is indicated on an emergency basis for an ocular indication, such as CRAO, DCS, or arterial gas embolism (AGE), delays for ophthalmic consultation and detailed eye examination may result in worsening of the patient's clinical condition and are not indicated. Visual function should be quantified in an expedited manner while awaiting recompression using rapidly performed measures such as emergency department visual acuity charts, color vision plates, Amsler grids, near-vision cards, ability to read printed material, and confrontation visual fields. Some of these methods may also be used to follow visual function during HBOT. If ocular signs or symptoms were part of the indication for HBOT, an eye examination by an ophthalmologist as outlined above should be conducted as soon as feasible after recompression (Butler et al. 2008).

HBO in the Treatment of Diseases of the Eye

The authors can recommend without reservation that HBOT be used for the indications listed in the primary indications section of Table 32.1. The evidence is less strong yet promising for the indications listed under secondary indications. The indications listed in the last section may have a theoretical basis for efficacy of HBOT, but have the weakest level of evidence to support their use.

Recommended Indications

Discussions of decompression sickness with ocular signs and symptoms, AGE with ocular signs and symptoms, ocular gas gangrene, necrotizing soft tissue and fungal infections

Table 32.1 Conditions in Ophthalmology

Recommended indications
• Decompression sickness with ocular signs and symptoms
• Arterial gas embolism with ocular signs and symptoms
• Central retinal artery occlusion
• Ocular gas gangrene
• Necrotizing soft tissue and fungal infections involving the orbit/ periorbital tissues
• Carbon monoxide poisoning with visual sequelae
• Radiation optic neuropathy/retinopathy
• Compromised periorbital skin grafts and flaps (incl. conjunctival graft)
• Scleral ischemia or necrosis/recurrent pterigium
Potential indications
• Anterior segment ischemia (especially post-operative)
• Ischemic optic neuropathy
• Ischemic central retinal vein occlusion
• Branch retinal artery occlusion (esp. with central visual loss)
• Cystoidmacular edema with central retinal vein occlusion
• Cystoid macular edema with post-surgical inflammation
• Cystoid macular edema with intrinsic inflammatory disorders
• Refractory Pseudomonas keratitis
• Pyoderma gangrenosum of the orbit
Other reported uses
• Toxic amylopia (e.g., quinine toxicity)
• Retinitis pigmentosa
• Macular hole surgery
• Diabetic retinopathy
• Uveitis
• Keratoendotheliosis
• Sickle cell hyphema
• Retinal detachment (incl. associated sickle cell disease)
• Glaucoma

involving the orbit/periorbital tissues, carbon monoxide poisoning with visual sequelae, radiation optic neuropathy and compromised periorbital skin grafts and flaps will be covered in those individual chapters.

Central Retinal Artery Occlusion

The visual outcome of arterial occlusive diseases of the retina depends on the vessel occluded as well as the degree and location of the occlusion. The type of occlusion (thrombosis, embolus, arteritis, or vasospasm) may also affect the outcome (Hayreh and Zimmerman 2005; Stone et al. 1977). The classic presentation of CRAO is sudden painless loss of vision in the range of light perception to counting fingers. Vision at the "no light perception" level usually indicates an occlusion at the level of the ophthalmic artery with a resulting absence of blood flow to either the retinal or the choroidal circulation (Regillo et al. 2007). On dilated fundoscopic exam, patients with CRAO will display a pale appearance of the retina due to the opaque and edematous nerve fiber and ganglion cell layers. A cherry red spot is often present in the

fovea, but this finding may be absent, especially when there is an occlusion of the ophthalmic artery. Cilioretinal arteries are part of the ciliary (not retinal) arterial supply and supply the area of the retina around the macula (central vision area.). If a cilioretinal artery is present, central vision may be preserved in the presence of a CRAO, but the peripheral visual fields are typically severely decreased (Butler et al. 2008). In the largest published series of CRAO patients, Hayreh describes the outcome of this condition without HBOT. He found that patients with cilioretinal arteries had much better visual outcomes than those who did not. In those patients without cilioretinal arteries, 80 % had a final visual outcome of count fingers or less and only 1.5 % of individuals obtained a final vision of 20/40 or better (Hayreh and Zimmerman 2005).

Natural spontaneous recanalization eventually takes place after CRAO (Duker and Brown 1988; David et al. 1967). In relatively few cases, however, does this reperfusion lead to an improvement of vision, presumably because the retinal tissue has been irreversibly damaged during the ischemic period (Duker and Brown 1988). The retina has the highest rate of oxygen consumption of any organ in the body at 13 mL/100 g/min and is therefore very sensitive to ischemia (Hertzog et al. 1992). As with oxygen administration at one ATA, HBOT must be started within the time interval that retinal tissue can still recover. There is a point beyond which ischemic tissue can no longer recover even if reperfusion occurs (Li et al. 1996). Hayreh et al. occluded the ophthalmic artery of rhesus monkeys for varying periods of time. Retinas that went more than 105 min without blood flow showed permanent damage. If the duration of occlusion was less than 97 min, the retinas recovered their normal function (Hayreh et al. 1980). Treatment of CRAO should be aimed at promptly supplying oxygen to the ischemic retina at a partial pressure sufficient to maintain inner retinal viability until restoration of central retinal artery blood flow occurs. Animal models of retinal injury have shown a reduction in apoptosis from 58 % cell loss to 30 % in animals treated with HBOT after experimental CRAO (Gaydar et al. 2011).

Traditional treatment regimens for CRAO have been aimed at promoting downstream movement of the embolus by lowering intraocular pressure and producing vasodilatation. These measures include ocular massage, anterior chamber paracentesis, intraocular pressure-lowering medications, carbogen, and aspirin (Regillo et al. 2007; Hertzog et al. 1992; Duker and Brown 1988; Stone et al. 1977). These treatment modalities have been largely unsuccessful (Neubauer et al. 2000; Duker and Brown 1988; Stone et al. 1977). The American Academy of Ophthalmology Basic and Clinical Science Course states that "the efficacy of treatment is questionable" (Regillo et al. 2007). More recently, studied treatment modalities include thrombolytic agents (Petterson et al. 2005; Weber et al. 1998) and surgical removal or the embolus or thrombus (Garcia-Arumi et al. 2006; Tang and Han 2000). Hayreh stated recently that no currently used therapy is efficacious for CRAO (Hayreh and Zimmerman 2005). Acute obstruction of the central retinal artery without HBOT typically results in severe, permanent visual loss (Hayreh and Zimmerman 2005; Duker and Brown 1988).

In order to be effective, the administration of supplemental oxygen must be continued until retinal arterial blood flow has resumed to a level sufficient to maintain inner retinal function under normoxic conditions. If ischemia and cellular hypoxia have resulted in cell death of the inner layers of the retina, vision will not return when blood flow is re-established (Mangat 1995).

Supplemental oxygen therapy need not always be provided at hyperbaric pressures to successfully reverse retinal ischemia in CRAO. Butler reported a patient who suffered acute loss of vision in his only seeing eye and presented approximately 1 h after vision loss. His vision was 20/400 and he had fundus findings of a CRAO. He was treated with oxygen administered by reservoir mask at one atmosphere in the emergency department and his vision quickly improved to 20/25. After approximately 5 min, the supplemental oxygen was discontinued, whereupon vision equally quickly returned to 20/400. This process was repeated several times to confirm the beneficial effect of the supplemental oxygen with the same results. The patient was then hospitalized, anticoagulated, and maintained on supplemental oxygen for approximately 18 h, after which time his central retinal artery presumably recanalized, because at this point removal of the supplemental oxygen no longer caused a decrease in vision. He was discharged with a visual acuity of 20/25 in his only seeing eye (Butler 2007). In similar cases, Patz reported improvement in two CRAO patients given oxygen at 1 ATA. One patient received oxygen after a 4-h delay to therapy and improvement from 4/200 to 20/70 was maintained after supplemental oxygen therapy was discontinued 4 h later. The second patient improved from no light perception to 20/200 after a delay to treatment of 90 min and maintained this improvement when oxygen was discontinued 3 h later. In both patients, early discontinuation of oxygen was followed by deterioration of vision within minutes. Improved vision was restored when oxygen breathing was resumed shortly thereafter. This phenomenon was observed several times in both patients (Patz 1955).

The study published by Augsberger and Magargal in 1980 emphasized the importance of prompt oxygen treatment to successful outcome. They used paracentesis, ocular massage, carbogen (95 % oxygen and 5 % CO_2), acetazolamide, and aspirin to treat 34 consecutive cases of CRAO. Twelve of the 34 patients were successfully treated, with 7 of the 12 having been treated within 24 h of onset of symptoms. The longest delay to treatment after which treatment was considered successful was 72 h. The average delay to therapy in the patients with successful outcomes was 21.1 h, compared to 58.6 h in those who did not improve. Carbogen inhalation was conducted for 10 min every hour during waking hours and 10 min every 4 h at night and continued for 48-72 h (Augsburger and Magargal 1980).

Stone et al. reported two patients with CRAO of duration longer than 6 h treated with intermittent carbogen at 1 ATA, retrobulbar anesthesia, and anterior chamber paracentesis. The first patient had vision loss of 6-h duration. His vision improved from hand motion to 20/20 on the above therapy, with carbogen being administered for 10 min every hour. The second patient presented 8 h after onset of visual loss and had improvement from finger counting to 20/25. Carbogen was administered 10 min every hour for 48 h (Stone et al. 1977).

Carbon dioxide is added to the oxygen in carbogen for its vasodilatory effect in an effort to counter hyperoxic vasoconstriction. If the mechanism of improved oxygenation to the retina is diffusion from the choroidal circulation, the addition of carbon dioxide should not be required to improve oxygenation. Unlike retinal blood flow, choroidal blood flow is not significantly affected by changes in oxygen tension (Yu and Cringle 2005; Li et al. 1996).

Another case report described a patient with angiographically documented obstruction of both the central retinal artery and his temporal posterior ciliary artery (Duker and Brown 1988). He presented after 5 h of visual loss with minimal light perception vision. In addition to ocular massage, anterior chamber paracentesis, timolol, and acetazolamide, he was given carbogen for 10 min every hour around the clock. His vision did not improve significantly during his 3 days of hospitalization, but improved spontaneously approximately 96 h after onset of vision loss. Vision in the affected eye was documented to be 20/30 1 week after discharge. Although the authors of this case report do not necessarily ascribe his recovery to any one of treatments used, the role of supplemental oxygen in maintaining retinal viability until spontaneous recanalization occurred must be considered, since only rarely do patients with CRAO have a spontaneous improvement in vision (Duker and Brown 1988).

Supplemental oxygen at 1 ATA may not successfully preserve retinal function in CRAO. This intervention did not reliably prevent inner retinal hypoxia in a rat model when the retinal circulation was occluded by laser photocoagulation (Yu et al. 2007). If normobaric supplemental oxygen is not successful in restoring vision in a CRAO patient, emergent HBOT should be considered.

HBOT has been successful when normobaric hyperoxia has failed to restore vision in CRAO. Phillips reported a 71-year-old White female patient with CRAO in whom surface oxygen was ineffective in reversing "total vision loss" of approximately 2-h duration (Phillips et al. 1999). The patient was then compressed to 2.8 ATA breathing 100 % oxygen on a U.S. Navy Treatment Table 6. As she passed 15 ft during her descent, light perception was restored and at the end of her first air break at 2.8 ATA, she reported full return of vision. She was discharged with a visual acuity of 20/30 in her only seeing eye. A 2+ afferent papillary defect noted prior to treatment had resolved after treatment (Phillips et al. 1999).

Treatment of CRAO should be aimed at promptly supplying oxygen to the ischemic retina at a partial pressure sufficient to maintain inner retinal viability until central retinal artery blood flow is restored. The ophthalmology literature includes cases in which patients with CRAO have regained significant vision even when treatment was delayed for periods of up to 2 months (Desola et al. 2015; Matsuo 2001) with the strongest evidence for symptomatic improvement in cases with less than 12 h of delay (Weinberger et al. 2002; Li et al. 1996; Yotsukura and Adachi-Usami 1993; Beiran et al. 1993; Hertzog et al. 1992). In the clinical setting of CRAO, residual retinal arterial blood flow may be detected by fluorescein angiogram (Menzel-Severing et al. 2012; Augsburger

and Magargal 1980; David et al. 1967). This may help to explain the great variability in visual outcome observed with different time delays until treatment. The studies by Hayreh quoted above that noted irreversible retinal damage after 105 min entailed complete occlusion of the ophthalmic artery, the most severe model of ocular vascular occlusion and one that may not be frequently encountered in the clinical setting.

According to publications that discuss treatment options for CRAO patients, those with duration of symptoms of several weeks or longer would be expected to have a minimal chance of improvement, yet there are some patients who are reported to improve even after this prolonged time interval, although details of the level of improvement were limited in one study (Desola et al. 2015; Hirayama et al. 1990). In a review of the records of 16 patients treated with HBOT for CRAO (2.0 ATA of oxygen 90 min twice daily for 2–3 days, then once daily until reaching clinical plateau), 11 showed improvement and 4 of the 5 patients who showed no improvement had a delay to presentation of >24 h (Murphy-Lavoie et al. 2004). In a reported series of 17 patients with CRAO treated with HBOT, the patients were retrospectively divided into four treatment groups based on the time from symptom onset to HBOT (Hertzog et al. 1992). Results showed that HBOT seemed most useful in preserving visual function when applied within 8 h from the onset of visual impairment. The authors point out that the phrase "time is muscle" used in management of myocardial infarctions can be changed to "time is vision" in CRAO.

In 2001, Beiran published a retrospective study of 35 patients treated with HBOT compared to 37 matched controls from another facility where hyperbaric oxygen was not available (Beiran et al. 2001). All patients were treated within 8 h of symptom onset and none of the patients included in the trial had a cilioretinal artery. The patients in the hyperbaric group received oxygen at 2.8 ATA for 90 min twice a day for the first 3 days and then once daily until no further improvement was seen for 3 consecutive days. In the hyperbaric group, 82 % of the patients improved compared to only 29.7 % of patients in the control group. Improvement was defined as reading at least three lines better on Snellen chart compared to admission. The mean visual acuity for the hyperbaric group at discharge was 20/70 (Beiran et al. 2001).

Reports that describe failure of HBOT in CRAO sometimes fail to even note the elapsed time from symptom onset to HBOT (Haddad and Leopold 1965) and HBOT in these cases may have been started well after the time window for successful treatment had passed. Miyake reported on 53 cases of CRAO and 19 branch retinal artery occlusions treated with HBOT over a 13-year period. He found no significant difference between time to treatment and response to HBOT; however, only 3 of these patients received HBOT within 24 h of symptom onset, which places most of his patients outside the time window in which improvement from HBOT is most likely to occur. Overall, 44 % of his patients showed improvement of at least two levels on the visual acuity scale after treatment with HBOT, despite this delay to treatment. Unfortunately, no distinction was made between patients with cilioretinal arteries and those without (Miyake et al. 1987).

Failure of HBOT has been reported in one case of CRAO in which there was angiographic documentation of a complete obstruction of the involved ophthalmic artery. There must be an intact choroidal circulation for HBOT to reverse the vision loss in CRAO (Mori et al. 2007).

The case series and case reports noted above document that some patients with CRAO can be treated successfully with hyperoxia, either at 1 ATA or with HBOT. Evidence that HBOT reduces apoptosis in the ischemic retina suggests there may be added benefit to the use of hyperbaric rather than simply normobaric oxygen therapy (Gaydar et al. 2011). HBOT is a low-risk therapeutic option with demonstrated good results in treating CRAO if treatment is begun prior to the retina suffering irreversible ischemic damage and there is an intact choroidal circulation. There are no alternative therapies with similarly favorable outcomes (Hayreh and Zimmerman 2005; Neubauer et al. 2000; Hayreh and Podhajsky 1982).

The devastating vision loss that CRAO entails when left untreated calls for an aggressive approach to employing HBOT for this disorder. Triage nurses should be aware that sudden painless loss of vision of less than 24-h duration is an emergency that requires immediate attention. Patients with documented or suspected CRAO of less than 24-h duration should receive supplemental oxygen at the highest fraction attainable immediately (Murphy-Lavoie et al. 2012; 2014; Butler 2007; Duker and Brown 1988; Perkins et al. 1987; Augsburger and Magargal 1980; Stone et al. 1977; Patz 1955). Emergent HBOT should be undertaken if this intervention is not rapidly effective in improving vision. Evidence that HBOT reduces apoptosis in the ischemic retina suggests there may be added benefit to the use of hyperbaric rather than simply normobaric oxygen therapy (Gaydar et al. 2011). The patient should be maintained on supplemental oxygen at the highest possible FIO_2 until HBOT is begun, and then treated with the step-wise protocol outlined in "emergent HBOT for acute vision loss" (Table 32.2). Ocular massage and topical ocular hypotensive agents may also be employed as adjuncts. While there are some case reports of patients presenting after 24 h from onset of vision loss obtaining benefit from HBOT, the majority of cases do not respond when treated beyond this point (Desola et al. 2015; Butler et al. 2008; Murphy-Lavoie et al. 2004; Yotsukura and Adachi-Usami 1993; Hertzog et al. 1992; Miyake et al. 1987; Augsburger and Magargal 1980; Anderson et al. 1965b). Overall, approximately 64 % of cases of CRAO will show improvement when treated with HBOT.

Reports of treatment of CRAO by HBO are summarized in Table 32.3.

Radiation Retinopathy

Radiation Retinopathy (RR) is a chronic, progressive ocular injury resulting from any source of radiation (external beam, brachytherapy, proton beam, helium ion radiotherapy, and gamma knife radiotherapy). It is a complication of the treatment of head and neck tumors as well as intraocular tumors (choroidal melanomas, retinoblastomas, and choroidal metastasis) (Finger et al. 2009; Krema et al. 2009; Gragoudas et al. 1987; Haas et al. 2002; Levy et al. 1991; Wen 2009).

The pathogenesis of RR is retinal vascular endothelial damage at the DNA level. Cell death stimulates the division and migration of cells to effect repair, and these cells also succumb to the radiation effects, leading to a vicious cycle that triggers the clotting cascade. These series of events lead to the formation of micro-aneurysms, telangiectasias, neovascularization, vitreous hemorrhage, macular edema, and retinal detachment. There are two types of RR, prolifera-

Table 32.2 Emergency HBO in patients with acute vision loss: selection criteria

HBOT is indicated as an emergency measure in patients who present with acute vision loss and meet the following criteria:
• Presentation within 24 h of vision loss
• Corrected visual acuity 20/200 or worse
• Visual acuity still 20/200 or worse with pin hole testing
• Age>40
• No pain associated with the vision loss
• No history of acute onset of flashes or floaters prior to vision loss
• No history of recent eye trauma

Notes: 1. HBOT should be administered in all cases if the loss of vision is associated with exposure to a hyperbaric environment or unpressurized high-altitude conditions
2. HBOT should be administered in all cases if the history is suggestive of radiation optic neuropathy or for vision loss that occurs during or immediately after hemodialysis
3. Consultation with an ophthalmologist is desirable if it can be obtained without significantly delaying HBOT
4. Acute, painless, severe vision loss should be referred as an emergency to an ophthalmologist in all cases so that additional patients may be identified for whom HBOT might be beneficial (Murphy-Lavoie et al. 2014; Butler et al. 2008)

Table 32.3 Treatment of retinal artery occlusions: literature summary

	CRAO/BRAO	Therapy	Delay to Tx	Initial VA	Final VA	Total patients (n)	Cases improved (n)
Gool and Jong (1965)	BRAO CRAO CRAO	HBOT: 3 ATA, anticoagulants, Complamin	5 days 2 days Unknown (<24 h)	1.50% nil 125%	100% nil 125% imp VF	4	2
	BRAO		10 days	1.60%	1.60%		
Haddad and Leopold (1965)	CRAO	HBOT	Unknown	NLP CF	NLP CF	2	0
Anderson et al. (1965a, 1965b)	BRAO CRAO	HBOT, Retrobulbar lidocaine, ocular massage, nicotinic acid	"several hours" 40+ hours	CF 2–3 ft 20/25	20/20 20/25 imp VF	3	2
	BRAO		6+ days	20/200	Unknown		
Takahashi et al. (1977)		HBOT: 2.5 ATA	1–6 days	Graph	Graph	9	9
		Ocular massage paracentesis vasodilator					
Pallota et al. (1978)	CRAO	HBOT: 2.8 ATA		NLP	10/10	1	1
Sasaki et al. (1978)	CRAO	HBOT, Stellate ganglion block				10	7
Szuki et al. (1980)	CRAO	HBOT				6	6
Krasnov et al. (1981)	CRAO	HBOT				39	22
Zhang et al. (1986)	CRAO	HBOT				80	49
Desola (1987)	CRAO	HBOT				20	11
Miyake et al. (1987)	CRAO (53) BRAO (19)	HBOT @ 2ATA or 3ATA, varied vasodilators, stellate ganglion block, 2% carbocaine	18 h to 15 days, all but 3 within 12 days	Graph	Graph	72	32
Kindwall and Goldmann (1988)	CRAO	HBOT				14	7
Cho et al. (1990)	CRA0	HBOT×50 Tx, steroids	15 days	HM	0.02	1	1
Hirayama et al. (1990)	CRAO	HBOT; mixtures of urokinase, steroid, bifemelane HCL	<1 month	Graph	Graph	17	12
Hertzog et al. (1992)	CRAO	HBOT: 1.5–2.0 ATA; mixtures of Timolol maleate 0.5%, acetazolamide, paracentesis, carbogen, vasodilator, steroids, ocular massage, retrobulbar anesthesia	<8 h>8, ≥24 h > 24 h All patients	Graph	Graph	19	14
Beiran et al. (1993)	CRAO	HBOT: 2.5 ATA, ocular massage, SL nifedipine, oral glycerol	2: <100 min 1: occluding 1: 6 h	LP HM CF 2 m HM	6/20 6/6 6/9 CF 60 cm	4	4
Yotsukura et al. (1993)	CRAO	HBOT, ocular massage, IV urokinase, and 2/15 with IV prostaglandin	3 h to 6 days	Graph	Graph	15	8
Li et al. (1996)	BRAO OS	HBOT: 2.32 ATA	<24 h	20/200	20/25	2	2
	BRAO OD (15 months later)	HBOT: 2.82 ATA	<24 h	CF 2 ft	20/25		

(continued)

Table 32.3 (continued)

	CRAO/BRAO	Therapy	Delay to Tx	Initial VA	Final VA	Total patients (n)	Cases improved (n)
Phillips et al. (1999)	CRAO	100 % surface O2	<2 h	NLP	20/30	1	1
		HBOT: 2.4 ATA					
Aisenbrey et al. (2000)	CRAO (8)	HBOT: 240kPa, ocular massage,paracentesis, IV acetazolamide		Graph	Graph	18	12
	BRAO (10)						
Matsuo (2001)	BRAO (OU)	HBOT, IV prostaglandin, urokinase	4 days	20/30	20/15	2	2
				20/600	20/400		
Beiran et al. (2001)	CRAO (29)	HBOT: 2.8 ATA; mixtures of ocular massage, retrobulbar block, timolol, acetazolamide, paracentesis	<8 h	Graph	Graph	35	29
	BRAO (6)						
Weinberger et al. (2002)	CRAO	HBOT, ocular massage, antiglaucoma eyed rops	4–12 h	Graph	Graph	21	13
Murphy-Lavoie et al. (2004)	CRAO BRAO	HBOT: 2.0 ATA	6 h–4 days	Graph	Graph	16	12
Imai et al. (2004)	BRAO	HBOT, stellate ganglion block	2 days	CF	0.08	1	1
Swaby et al. (2005)	CRAO	HBOT 2.0ATA, optic nerve sheath fenestration	3 weeks	20/400	Improved	1	1
Weiss (2009)	CRAO BRAO	HBOT 1.5ATA	Hours—3 weeks	Graph	Graph	4	2
Inoue et al. (2009)	CRAO BRAO	HBOT 1.8ATA	Hours—8 days	Graph	Graph	63	30
Aten et al. (2011)	CRAO	HBOT 2.4ATA	7 h	ND	20/80	1	1
Cope et al. (2011)	CRAO	HBOT 2.4 ATA	5–144 h	Graph	Graph	11	8
Telander et al. (2011)	CRAO	HBOT×1, ocular massage, pressure lowering eye drops	11 h	CF	20/160	1	1
Menzel-Severing et al. (2012)	CRAO	HBOT 2.4 ATA, hemodilution	<12 h	Graph	Graph	51	19
Canan et al. (2014)	CRAO	HBOT 2.5 ATA, exchange transfusion	<24 h	CF	20/30	1	1
Hsaio and Huang (2014)	CRAO	HBOT2.5ATA×6 Carbogen, pressure lowering eyedrops, hemodilution, corticosteroids	4 h	CF	20/200	1	1
Masters et al. (2015)	CRAO	HBOT 2.8 ATA	<24 h	Graph	Graph	29	20
Desola et al. 2015	CRAO	HBOT 2.3 ATA×15	<2 months	NR	NR	182	138
Lu et al. (2015)	CRAO	HBOT, ocular massage, anterior paracentsis, aspirin	100 min	LP	HM	1	1
Total						758	482

% Improved: 64 %

Note: see full graphs of patient results in original papers

tive and non-proliferative. Both are associated with macular edema, portending a worse visual outcome (Shields et al. 1991, 2002; Phillpotts et al. 1995; Gunduz et al. 1999a, b).

Options for the treatment of RR range from enucleation (early treatment) to more recent advances, such as plaque brachytherapy, retinal laser photocoagulation, photodynamic therapy, corticoid steroids, pentoxifylline, and VEGF therapies (Bevacizumab, Ranibizumab, and Pepagtanib sodium). Currently, treatment is focused on globe salvaging options, which increasingly includes radiation. The incidence of RR ranges from 3–20 % and is associated with retinal neovascularization (proliferative RR).RR is dependent on the total radiation dose, with 35 Gy considered the upper limit of a safe dose. However, RR has been reported at significantly lower levels (Brown et al. 1982; Chacko 1981; Web 2009).

HBOT has been reported as a supportive adjunct in the treatment of RR. The benefit of HBOT is thought to involve the improvement of oxygenation and the sensitization of hypoxic cells. However, there is currently very little published literature on the use of HBOT for those with RR. One patient was treated with 2.0 ATA for 120 min × 20 sessions over 2 months, with improvement in her visual field and fundus examination. However, another case report using HBOT with radiotherapy resulted in severe vaso-occlusion of the retinal vessels thought to be the result of synergistic vasoconstriction (Oguz and Sobaci 2008; Gall et al. 2007; Stanford 1984).

Recurrent Pterygium/Scleral Necrosis

Pteyrgiums are benign growths of the conjunctiva, usually on the nasal side in the palpebral fissure associated with fibrotic tissue extending from the conjunctiva onto the cornea. There is degeneration of collagen and fibrovascular proliferation. The exact cause is unknown, but UV light exposure, dust, and low humidity have been considered as causes. It is often progressive and may cause ocular discomfort, cosmetic issues, and visual interference with extension into the visual axis. Treatment options include radiation, auto-grafting, amniotic membrane transplantation, mitomycin, strontium plaque therapy, anti-fibrotic agents, lamellar keratoplasty, and surgical excision (Assaad and Coroneo 2008; Assaad et al. 2011). One of the most distressing complications is recurrence. Pterygium surgery has a recurrence rate, up to 46 % without preventive measures incorporated into the surgical excision (Sebban and Hirst 1991). Preventive measures include beta irradiation, cauterization, topical steroids, thiotepa, mitomycin-C, and conjunctival autograft (Bayer et al. 2002). Irradiation may result in small-vessel obliterative endarteritis with tissue ischemia and fibrosis. Scleral necrosis is also a potentially blinding complication of both beta irradiation and mitomycin-C therapy, as necrosis may lead to perforation of the globe with endophthalmitis and devastating visual consequences (Butler et al. 2008).

Adjunctive HBOT has been shown to reverse this process in a couple of case reports. One paper reported a patient who developed severe scleral necrosis following pterygium surgery and beta radiation. The patient did not respond to conventional therapy, including topical antibiotics, topical steroids, lubricants, and patching. HBOT (2 ATA for 90 min daily × 14 days) resulted in marked improvement noted after four treatments. The patient had a complete recovery (Green and Brannen 1995). Mitomycin-C may induce a similar condition, as noted in another case report regarding a patient who developed scleral necrosis after mitomycin-C. The

patient deteriorated with conventional therapy. However, following HBOT (2.5 ATA for 90 min daily × 24 days), the patient had a remarkable recovery, noted after 5 days (Bayer et al. 2002).

Assaad and colleagues assessed the utility of surgical excision, limbal conjunctival autograft, and HBOT in 39 eyes with recurrent pterygiums. HBOT was administered, on the first day of surgery, at 2.0 ATA for 90 min, and then for four treatments, with reassessments for additional treatments. They followed these patients for 23 months, with a single recurrence noted. No HBOT complications were noted. The authors surmised that HBOT may be efficacious because it mitigates graft hypoxia, thereby increasing angiogenesis, and reduces both inflammation and edema (Assaad et al. 2011).

Potential Indications for HBOT in Ophthalmology

This section reviews ocular indications for HBOT with a strong physiological basis for the usefulness. A rapid return of vision is a valuable indicator of efficacy when treating ocular disorders with HBOT. However, the failure of vision to normalize rapidly does not necessarily indicate a lack of success, especially with disorders such as central retinal vein occlusion (CRVO) and branch retinal vein occlusion (BRVO), where macular hemorrhage may prevent immediate return of vision.

Postoperative Anterior Segment Ischemia

Strabismus surgery entails detaching selected extraocular muscles from the globe and re-attaching them in a slightly different location to improve alignment of the eyes. Anterior segment ischemia (ASI) is an uncommon but potentially serious surgical complication. It occurs in ≈ 1 of every 13,000 strabismus operations (De Smet et al. 1987). Anterior segment blood supply is provided by the long posterior ciliary arteries (≈30 %) and the anterior ciliary arteries which travel anteriorly in the rectus muscles (≈70 %) (Saunders et al. 1994). ASI results from the anterior ciliary vessel disruption when the extraocular muscles are surgically detached and repositioned. ASI typically occurs with surgeries involving three or more extraocular muscles, but may occur with two-muscle surgery (Murdock and Kushner 2001). Children have virtually no risk of developing this complication, while adults with cardiovascular disease are at higher risk (Saunders et al. 1994). Patients with ASI present with pain and decreased vision several days after their surgery. Eye examination may reveal striate keratopathy, iris atrophy, immobile pupil, posterior synechiae, cataract, and anterior uveitis with cells and flare in the anterior chamber (Saunders et al. 1994; Pfister 1991).

Systemic and topical steroids are used to treat ASI, and most patients have good recovery of visual acuity with steroid therapy. Cycloplegics decrease the ciliary spasm pain that may accompany ASI (Murdock and Kushner 2001; Saunders et al. 1994). Staged strabismus surgery allows collateral circulation to develop between surgeries and may help to prevent ASI. Using botulinum toxin as an alternative or adjunct to rectus muscle strabismus surgery is also effective (Saunders et al. 1994).

HBOT increases oxygen tension in the anterior chamber (Jampol 1987) and has promise for the treatment of anterior segment ischemia. In 1987, De Smet and colleagues noted that HBOT (2.5 ATA O_2 for 90 min for 7 days) was successful in treating a patient with anterior segment ischemia without the use of systemic steroids, which were withheld due to a history of tuberculosis (De Smet et al. 1987). HBOT represents a viable option for those with severe ASI who does not respond to steroids or for those who cannot tolerate steroids (Butler et al. 2008).

Ischemic Optic Neuropathy

Nonarteritic ischemic optic neuropathy (NAION) is one of the most visually disabling diseases in the middle-aged and elderly populations (Hayreh and Zimmerman 2008; Matthews 2005; Olver et al. 1990). It typically presents as acute unilateral vision loss affecting those over 50 years of age. It is characterized by optic disk edema, disk margin hemorrhages, and an altitudinal visual field loss that usually preferentially affects the inferior field. This pattern of injury occurs because the blood supply to the laminar and retrolaminar optic nerve is derived from the short posterior ciliary arteries (Olver et al. 1990). NAION typically results from perfusion insufficiency in the short posterior ciliary arteries, leading to infarction of the retrolaminar portion of the optic nerve.

Risk factors for NAION include hypertension, diabetes, nocturnal hypotension, and a small-cup-to-disc ratio (Desai et al. 2005). It has also been associated with the use of erectile dysfunction medications (Hayreh and Zimmerman 2007). The fellow eye of NAION patients is often sequentially affected. Involvement of the second eye occurs within 3 years in approximately 43 % of NAION patients.

Treatments for NAION have included optic nerve sheath decompression, high-dose steroids, levodopa, carbidopa, and neuroprotective agents. None of these modalities has been shown to be reliably effective (Matthews 2005; Desai et al. 2005; Arnold et al. 1996). The potential for oxygenation of the optic nerve from choroidal branches of the Circle of Haller and Zinn offers a theoretical basis for the efficacy of HBOT in NAION. Reducing intra-axonal optic nerve ischemia and its resultant edema may also interrupt the cycle of microvascular compromise that is thought to occur within the structurally crowded optic disks of patients with NAION (Arnold et al. 1996).

Bojic reported successful treatment of two NAION patients treated with HBOT (2.0 ATA for 90 min daily for 18 sessions), with improvement in both vision and visual fields (Bojic et al. 2002). HBOT was utilized 3–5 months after the onset of symptoms. The same author published a case series using HBOT (2.8 ATA for 60 min BID) for 3 patients, and 2.0 ATA for 90 min daily for the remaining 6 patients. These were nine NAION patients who had been unsuccessfully treated with steroids, and then received 14–30 sessions of HBOT. Four patients with optic disc atrophy (a sign of long-standing disease) had no improvement with HBOT, while 5 other patients without optic atrophy had marked improvement in visual acuity and/or visual field at 6-month follow-up. The time between the onset of symptoms and the initial HBOT session ranged from 21 to 84 days (Bojic et al. 2002). Another case series from the same author reported on 21 patients (with some overlap from the previous papers) in which 11 control patients were treated with corticosteroids, while the study group received steroids and HBOT (2.8 ATA for 60 min BID) for the first three patients, while seven patients received HBOT (2.0 ATA for 90 min daily). The time between the onset of symptoms and the initial HBOT session ranged from 7 to 84 days. Six of the ten HBOT patients experienced a marked improvement in visual function, and all of these patients save one had continuation of this benefit at 6-month follow-up. None of the patients in the control group showed improvement. The authors note that spontaneous improvement in NAION is unusual. Patients with optic atrophy obtained no benefit from HBOT, while those in whom optic atrophy was not evident did display improvement (Bojic et al. 2002).

Beiran treated a 66-year-old woman who presented with a 4-day loss of vision OD (finger-counting). She had lost vision in her left eye 3 months previously from an episode of NAION. Fundus examination showed the disk edema and disk margin hemorrhages of NAION. She was treated with HBOT (2.5 ATA oxygen for 90 min × 5 sessions). Vision improved from finger counting to 20/80 after the second session. No further improvement in vision was observed in the three subsequent HBOT sessions, but this improvement remained stable over one year of follow-up. The author made several observations: (1) The visual acuity OD before treatment was declining and that this decline stopped and vision began to improve immediately after starting HBOT; (2) final vision was definitely better in the treated eye than in the untreated fellow eye; and (3) the patient was legally blind when she entered the chamber, but was not when she left (Beiran et al. 1995).

Arnold reported that 22 eyes of 20 patients with NAION treated with HBOT (2.0 ATA for 90 min BID × 10 days) had no beneficial effect compared to 27 untreated controls. Patients were included in this study if they presented within 21 days after their onset of visual loss. The authors' earliest treatment break-out group in these studies was 9 days or less from onset of symptoms and noted that treatment initiated within 72 h might have been more effective (Arnold and Levin 2002; Arnold et al. 1996).

Arterial hypotension associated with blood loss during surgery and hemodialysis may also cause ischemic optic neuropathy. Hemodialysis is occasionally associated with dramatic unilateral or bilateral visual loss (Keynan et al. 2006; Wells and Forooozan 2004). The etiology of the visual loss in hemodialysis is believed to be hypotension-induced NAION (Cuxart et al. 2005; Wells and Forooozan 2004; Buono et al. 2003), but other reported etiologies for visual loss in this setting include cerebral infarction (Wells and Forooozan 2004), a Purtscher's type retinopathy (Arora et al. 1991), and posterior ischemic optic neuropathy (Buono et al. 2003). HBOT has been associated with immediate and dramatic return of vision to baseline in a patient who suffered bilateral blindness during hemodialysis. The authors emphasize that early HBOT should be considered for acute visual loss during or immediately after hemodialysis (Keynan et al. 2006). Some 15 % of individuals with NAION have been reported to suffer an attack on NAION in their fellow eye during 5-year follow-up (Newman et al. 2002). Because of the significant potential for NAION to occur in the second eyes of those with vision loss in the first eye due to this disorder, these patients should be warned to be alert for any decrease in vision in the second eye so that they can seek medical attention promptly and HBOT can be employed in an effort to prevent permanent vision loss.

Arteritic ischemic optic neuropathy (AION) is a related disorder characterized by ischemic damage to the optic nerve associated with giant cell arteritis. The visual loss is typically more severe and immediate treatment, with high-dose systemic steroids required to prevent a high percentage of vision loss from occurring in the fellow eye shortly after the index eye (Hayreh and Zimmerman 2003b). Long-term tapering and maintenance steroid administration is required to prevent recurrence (Hayreh and Zimmerman 2003b). No reports were found of HBOT being employed in AION, but there is a theoretical basis for efficacy in this type of ischemic optic neuropathy as well (Butler et al. 2008).

Ischemic Central Retinal Vein Occlusion

CRVO is a relatively common cause of visual loss. Ischemic CRVO with neovascular glaucoma is the single most common cause of surgical removal of the eye in North America (Boyd et al. 2002). Risk factors for this disorder include glaucoma, older age, male gender, systemic vascular disorders, and hyperviscosity syndromes such as multiple myeloma (Glacet-Bernard et al. 1996). CRVO may also be

seen, however, in young adults with no known systemic disease or ocular problems (Fong and Schatz 1993). The hallmarks of CRVO are four-quadrant retinal hemorrhage and distended retinal veins. An afferent pupillary defect and severe vision loss are typical of the ischemic variety of CRVO.

Vision loss in CRVO may result from macular ischemia, the development of persistent macular edema, and neovascular glaucoma (Mohamed et al. 2007). The challenge in treating CRVO is determining whether the CRVO is ischemic or nonischemic, as these two entities have significantly different natural histories and outcomes. Nonischemic CRVO does not cause neovascularization and typically has a more benign course, with final visual acuity dependent primarily on the presence and degree of macular edema. Two thirds of patients with nonischemic CRVO have final visual acuities of 20/40 or better without treatment. Some eyes with nonischemic CRVO, however, may progress to ischemic CRVO (Hayreh 2003a; Glacet-Bernard et al. 1996). One paper report that 54 % of initially nonischemic CRVO eyes developed retinal ischemia (Glacet-Bernard et al. 1996). With ischemic CRVO, there is permanent ischemic damage to the macular ganglion cells, so there is little chance of improvement in visual acuity (Hayreh 2003a). There is also a significant risk of anterior segment neovascularization, with neovascular glaucoma resulting in 40–50 % of cases (Hayreh 2003a). Differentiation between ischemic and nonischemic CRVO may be more difficult than the application of the commonly used criteria of ten disk diameters of retinal nonperfusion on IVFA (Hayreh 2003a). The degree of macular ischemia has been found to be a more significant factor affecting the outcome of retinal venous occlusion than macular edema (Miyamoto et al. 1995). Additionally, it is important to differentiate ischemic from nonischemic CRVO when considering invasive therapies such as radial optic neurotomy (Bhatt 2004).

The pathophysiology of CRVO is different in several important respects from CRAO. First, the obstruction of the CRV is chronic and is not characterized by the relatively early recanalization and restoration of blood flow seen in CRAO. Hayreh notes: "In both types of CRVO, the retinopathy spontaneously resolves after a variable period. There is marked inter-individual variation in the time that it takes to resolve; it is usually faster in younger than older people" (Hayreh 2003a). Secondly, the tissue hypoxia produced by CRVO often does not lead to rapid retinal cell death, as CRAO does. This allows the ischemic retinal cells to produce the vascular endothelial growth factors (VEGFs) responsible for the neovascularization that is a feature of CRVO, but not typically of CRAO. Third, the nonischemic version of CRVO does not produce macular ganglion cell death, but causes visual loss through macular edema.

The natural history of CRVO has been described by the CRVO Study Group. Visual acuity outcome was found to be largely dependent on visual acuity at presentation, with 65 % of individuals presenting with VA 20/40 or better maintaining that level of acuity for the 3-year follow-up period. Individuals with vision 20/200 or less had an 80 % chance of having vision at that level or worse at the end of the study. Patients with intermediate levels of visual acuity on presentation had a more variable outcome (CRVO Study Group 1997). This group also noted that one third of the eyes that were initially nonischemic CRVOs converted to ischemia in the course of the study.

Multiple interventions have been proposed for CRVO. Therapy is often aimed at preventing or reversing the neovascularization that can result in glaucoma, chronic eye pain, and loss of the eye (CRVO Study Group 1997). One study postulated that CRVO constitutes a neurovascular compartment syndrome at the site of the lamina cribosa and proposed relieving this pressure by performing a radial incision at the nasal part of the optic nerve head. The authors subsequently performed 107 radial optic neurotomies and found that the majority of patients showed rapid normalization of the morphologic fundus findings with an improvement in VA. The authors noted that surgery performed more than 90 days after the occlusion produced little improvement (Hasselbach et al. 2007). Another paper studying this technique in 5 patients produced less successful results (Weizer et al. 2003).

Other reports on the therapeutic options for CRVO have been less encouraging in reversing vision loss. Treatments have included anticoagulants, fibrinolytics, intravitreal corticosteroids, acetazolamide, isovolemic hemodilution, antivascular endothelial growth and angiostatic agents, panretinal photocoagulation (PRP), grid pattern photocoagulation, laser-induced chorioretinal anastamosis, and endovascular thrombolysis (Madhusudhana and Newsom 2007; Mohamed et al. 2007; Feltgen et al. 2007; Shahid et al. 2006; The Central Vein Occlusion Study Group M Report 1995). There have been several reports of success in treating CRVO with low-molecular weight heparin (Lee et al. 2006) and the anti-VEGF agent bevacizumab (Spandau et al. 2006; Boyd et al. 2002).

None of these interventions are useful in restoring vision if the retinal cells have already been irreversibly damaged by hypoxia prior to therapeutic intervention. The primary benefit of HBOT or the treatment of ischemic CRVO would be to maintain retinal viability, while interventions to return normal retinal venous outflow are accomplished or spontaneous resumption of flow occurs. However, the longer period required for spontaneous resumption of venous flow makes waiting for spontaneous resolution of the impaired retinal blood flow a more problematic choice than in CRAO.

HBOT has also been utilized to reverse the acute retinal ischemia observed with ischemic CRVO. One report described a 43-year-old male with CRVO who presented 2 days after symptom onset. The ischemic CRVO had macular edema and retinal hemorrhages. However, the visual fields were normal. The patient was treated with HBOT at 2.4 ATA for 90 min on the day of presentation. Vision in the affected eye improved from 20/200 to 20/30 after the first two HBOT treatments. Vision gradually deteriorated following HBOT, and improved again with the next treatment. This observation is important, as it suggests that the acute administration of HBOT can reverse the retinal cell hypoxia caused by the venous occlusion of CRVO, presumably because of the ability of oxygen to diffuse from the anatomically distinct choroidal circulation that is not affected by the retinal venous occlusion. Daily HBOT treatment was continued for 30 treatments, then treatment was decreased to 2–3 treatments per week for a total of 60 treatments. Final visual acuity was 20/20 in the affected eye, a remarkable outcome for ischemic CRVO (Wright et al. 2007). Another report describes a USAF aircraft navigator who presented with a nonischemic CRVO that progressed to an ischemic CRVO. He was treated with HBOT early in the course of his disease with return of normal vision. His vision was reported as 20/17 2 years later (Johnson 1990). Less favorable results using HBOT to treat CRVO were reported by Miyamoto, but there was no information available about the time interval after onset of the CRVO before HBOT was undertaken in these two studies (Miyamoto et al. 1993, 1995). Gismondi and colleagues reported the use of HBOT to manage CRVO in 3 patients and concluded that it was a useful treatment modality for this disorder (Gismondi et al. 1981). Others have reported HBOT to be one of the major therapeutic options in managing CRVO (Greiner and Lang 1999). Kiryu and Ogura (1996) reported 12 patients with macular edema in retinal vein occlusion (RVO) who received HBO treatment and had a median visual acuity improved from 20/100 to 20/25 ($p=0.002$). Clinically significant improvement (2 lines or more) was achieved in 10 cases (83 %).

In summary, there is a strong theoretical basis for HBOT to be useful in managing ischemic CRVO and there are case reports documenting treatment success. As with CRAO, there is likely a time window beyond which HBOT is less effective, but this time window is not well-defined. HBOT may be most effective when used with other measures designed to expedite the restoration of venous outflow. The optimum HBOT treatment regimen for CRVO is not well-defined. However, the positive effects of HBOT on both reversals of acute macular ischemia and prevention of neovascular complications from chronic retinal hypoxia should be considered, as should the possible beneficial effects of HBOT on eventual outcome even if visual acuity is not improving acutely because of macular hemorrhage. Outcome measures to be used with HBOT for ischemic CRVO should include visual acuity, visual fields, and the impact of HBOT on the development of neovascularization and neovascular glaucoma. Although rapid return of vision is a valuable indicator of efficacy when treating with HBOT, the failure of vision to normalize rapidly does not necessarily indicate a lack of success. This is especially true in disorders such as CRVO, where macular hemorrhage may prevent immediate return of vision. If HBOT is effective in preventing hypoxic cell death, vision may improve when the hemorrhage resolves, as has been reported in the hypoxic vasculopathy of high-altitude retinal hemorrhages (Lang and Kuba 1997). The role of HBOT in nonischemic CRVO is less clear, considering the more favorable visual prospects in this entity even when untreated (Butler et al. 2008).

Branch Retinal Artery Occlusion with Central Vision Loss

The presentation of branch retinal artery occlusion (BRAO) is more variable than that of CRAO. If the occluded artery does not supply the central or paracentral visual areas, the occlusion may be clinically silent. One paper reported that 24 of 30 patients with BRAO had visual acuities of 20/40 or better (Yuzurihara and Ijima 2004). Another study noted that almost 90 % of 201 patients with BRAO had visual acuities of 20/40 or better (Ros et al. 1989). Even when visual acuity is not affected, there is typically a permanent visual field defect in the area served by the infarcted retina (Regillo et al. 2007). Neovascular complications of BRAO are unusual but do occur (Yamamoto et al. 2005). BRAO is seen as a localized area of whitish opacified on the retina and may develop over the course of hours to days (Regillo et al. 2007). The embolus causing the BRAO may be visible on examination. Vision loss in BRAO may occasionally be severe. Mason reported a series of 5 patients with BRAO and severe loss of central vision. He used transluminal neodymium: YAG embolysis to disrupt the embolus and restore flow. All 5 patients had visual acuities ranging from 20/25 to 20/40 the first day after the procedure (Mason et al. 2007).

If vision loss is severe, HBOT may also have a role in the management of this disorder, with many of the same considerations that applied to CRAO. HBOT must be applied before the affected retina has been irreversibly damaged to have any beneficial effect. A 67-year-old woman with rheumatoid arthritis presented with decreased vision in both eyes for 4 days. Visual acuity in the right eye was 20/30 and 20/600 in left. She was found to have an occlusion of the superotemporal branch of the retinal artery in both eyes. Arterial sheathing and large cotton-wool patches were noted around both optic discs. IVFA findings showed delayed filling of the superotemporal retinal artery in the right eye, no filling in the superotemporal artery in the left eye, and segmental absence of filling in peripheral branches of other major retinal arteries in both eyes. She was treated with HBOT, prostaglandin E1, and urokinase for 2 weeks and had improvement of her vision to the 20/15 level in the right eye and 20/300 in the left (Matsuo 2001). Another case series reported 10 patients with BRAO who were treated with HBOT (2.4 ATA for 30 min × 3 sessions on the first day, BID on the second and third day, and once daily × 4 days) in addition to ocular massage, paracentesis, and IV acetazolamide. The authors noted that HBOT seems to be beneficial for visual acuity in eyes with BRAO (Aisenbrey et al. 2000).

Cystoid Macular Edema Associated with Retinal Vein Occlusion

Cystoid macular edema (CME) is the cystic accumulation of fluid in the macula. Gass originally described CME as the leakage of fluid from perifoveal capillaries that was low in lipid and protein (Gass and Norton 1966) with secondary polycystic expansion of the extracellular spaces (Gass et al. 1985). CME frequently complicates occlusion of a central or branch retinal vein. If the edema is severe or chronic, it may cause permanent visual loss and retinal damage (Coscas and Gaudric 1984). CME rates after RVOs of between 30 and 60 % have been reported (Quinlan et al. 1990; Gutman and Zegarra 1984; Coscas and Gaudric 1984; Hayreh 1983; Greer et al. 1980). CME may result from retinal capillary engorgement in RVO with the increase in hydrostatic pressure driving fluid out of the retinal capillaries (Dick et al. 2001), or from increased capillary permeability (Vinores et al. 1997), or a combination of these two mechanisms.

CME patients typically present with decreased vision, metamorphosia (image distortion), or scotoma. Slit-lamp exam findings include loss of the foveal depression, retinal thickening, and/or multiple cystoid spaces. Fluorescein angiographic examination in CME shows early foveal leakage with expansion and coalescence over time. In later phases, a "flower-petal" pattern of hyperfluorescence is seen as a result of the accumulation of dye within the cystoid spaces. Multiple interventions have been attempted for the treatment of RVO-associated macular edema. Medical treatments have included the use of carbonic anhydrase inhibitors (CAIs), anti-VEGF agents, and topical or intravitreal steroids (Schaal et al. 2007; Rabena et al. 2007; Iturralde et al. 2006; Tamura et al. 2005; Rosenfeld et al. 2005; Antonetti et al. 2000; Gardner et al. 1999; Nauck et al. 1998a, 1998b; Cox et al. 1988; Marmor and Maack 1982).

Intravitreal triamcinolone has been shown to improve vision in CME from BRVO and nonischemic CRVO (Park et al. 2003; Jonas et al. 2002, 2005; Ozkiris et al. 2005; Avitabile et al. 2005; Williamson and O'Donnell 2005; Chen et al. 2004; Bashshur et al. 2004; Ip 2004; Greenberg et al. 2002). However, in most cases the effect was not sustained and required repeat injections for recurrent edema. Potential complications of intravitreal steroid injections include an increase in intraocular pressure, cataract formation, endophthalmitis, injection-related vitreous hemorrhage, and retinal detachment.

A surgical option for BRVO is pars plana vitrectomy (PPV) with lysis of the common adventitial sheath at the site of the affected crossing vessels, thereby relieving the venous compression and potentially reducing hydrostatic pressure and CME (Osterloh and Charles 1988). Grid argon laser photocoagulation for CME after RVO is different from previously described PPV, in that the laser spots are smaller and delivered with a lighter intensity only within the affected region. Grid laser photocoagulation is currently the only intervention for BRVO-associated macular edema that is supported by Level I evidence. Grid laser photocoagulation is not indicated for predominantly ischemic maculopathy after RVO (Tranos et al. 2004; The Central Vein Occlusion Study Group 1995).

Miyamoto noted that the severity of macular ischemia better determines visual prognosis after HBOT than the degree of macular edema (Miyamoto et al. 1995). Additionally, a number of reports have shown HBOT to be of benefit in RVO-associated CME (Jansen and Nielsen 2004; Krott et al. 2000; Kiryu and Ogura 1996; Miyamoto et al. 1993, 1995; Miyake et al. 1993; Mandai et al. 1990; Ogura et al. 1987). HBOT for BRVO-associated CME has been shown to have a more favorable outcome than for CRVO (Miyamoto et al. 1993, 1995). In many reports, visual acuity has been noted to improve rapidly upon the initiation of HBOT, even when other treatment modalities were previously attempted (Jansen and Nielsen 2004; Krott et al. 2000; Kiryu and Ogura 1996; Miyamoto et al. 1993, 1995; Miyake et al. 1993; Ogura et al. 1987). Some of these studies reported an improvement of foveal leakage on fluorescein angiogram that correlates to the visual improvement (Miyamoto et al. 1993, 1995; Roy et al. 1989; Ogura et al. 1987), whereas others show improved visual acuity despite continued macular edema by IVFA testing (Miyake et al. 1993; Xu and Huang 1991). Hyperoxic vasoconstriction may produce a decrease in RVO-associated CME through reduction of retinal blood flow and decreased retinal venous pressure. HBOT may also reduce the production of VEGF and thereby decrease retinal vascular permeability. Xu and Huang (1991) carried out a prospective study of the effect of HBO on 14 eyes with CME secondary to RVO. Visual acuity improved 2–6 lines (average 3.6) after HBO treatment while there was no improvement in the control group. There was no reduction of leakage from perifoveal capillaries or enhancement of vision prior to improvement of the fundus.

There are potential benefits of HBOT over grid laser photocoagulation. Laser treatment may cause a permanent scotomas and is not undertaken for 3 months after the RVO to avoid its potential complications in those patients who might spontaneously resolve. HBOT offers a relatively safe treatment option for the 3-month timeframe after disease onset and may be repeated if necessary without any permanent visual consequences. If no improvement has been noted with HBOT, grid laser could be added as an adjunct after three months have elapsed. As with intravitreal injections of steroids and anti-

VEGF agents, there are reports of CME recurrence after HBOT (Miyake et al. 1993; Ishida et al. 1989; Roy et al. 1989), sometimes with vision regressing back to pre-treatment levels, and at other times with only slight regression from the improved vision obtained after HBOT (Butler et al. 2008).

Cystoid Macular Edema Associated with Postsurgical Inflammation

CME may complicate surgical procedures such as cataract extraction, Nd: YAG capsulotomy, and panretinal photocoagulation. CME occurs in approximately 1% of cataract extraction patients, but the incidence may be as high as 20% if the surgery is complicated by posterior capsule rupture and vitreous loss (Tranos et al. 2004). Available therapy for postsurgical CME includes nonsteroidal anti-inflammatory agents (NSAIDs), CAIs, steroids (topical, intravitreal, and periocular), and immunomodulators (Tranos et al. 2004).

HBOT may be a valuable adjunct to the management of patients whose CME does not respond to the above measures, or in whom side effects have required discontinuation of therapy. Pfoff and Thom reported on five patients with chronic CME documented by decreased visual acuity to the 20/40 level or worse and findings consistent with CME on IVFA. All patients had undergone cataract extraction/IOL implantation 7–11 months prior to HBOT (2.2 ATA oxygen for 90 min BID × 7 days, then 120 min once a day × 14 days). All 5 patients showed significant improvement in visual acuity with only mild regression upon follow-up, whereas three control patients treated with prednisolone acetate and indomethacin drops did not improve over a 3-month treatment period (Pfoff and Thom 1987). The authors proposed that vasoconstriction of the perifoveal capillaries serves to bring the damaged endothelial junctional complexes closer together, allowing them to repair themselves and thereby prevent further leakage (Pfoff and Thom 1987). Ishida et al. reported 12 eyes of CME treated with HBOT (2.0 ATA for 60 min × 2–4 weeks). Eight of the cases resulted from BRVO and four from cataract surgery. Seven of the eyes had an improvement in vision as a result of the HBOT (Ishida et al. 1989).

Cystoid Macular Edema Associated with Intrinsic Inflammatory Disorders

Intraocular inflammation may result from localized ocular disorders as well as in association with systemic inflammatory disorders (HLA-B27-associated inflammation, sarcoid, tuberculosis, Lyme disease). Chronic CME is the most common cause of significant visual loss in patients with intraocular inflammation. The pathogenesis of CME in uveitis is not completely understood, but may result from dysfunction of either the inner or the outer blood–eye barrier. Untreated uveitic CME tends to cause progressive injury to the macula (Coma et al. 2007). Treatment options for CME associated with intrinsic inflammatory disorders include the agents noted above for post-surgical CME (Coma et al. 2007; Tranos et al. 2004). Anti-VEGF agents have been used with success in this disorder. Five of 13 patients with uveitic CME refractory to other treatments treated with intravitreal bevacizumab had an improvement of vision of 2 or more lines (Coma et al. 2007).

HBOT may be useful in this disorder as well. Miyake treated two patients with poor vision from CME; one was from a CRVO and the other from sarcoid uveitis. HBOT was administered at 2.0 ATA for 60 min, and then 3 ATA for 60 min BID × 25 days. The author noted several points: (1) both patients improved markedly with HBOT; (2) both patients had recurrence of CME when HBOT was discontinued; (3) both patients also improved on acetazolamide therapy; and (4) the pattern of macular hyperfluorescence improved with acetazolamide, but not with HBOT, suggesting that the two therapies had different mechanisms of action (Miyake et al. 1993).

HBOT (2.0 ATA for 60 min daily × 14–17 days) was found to provide little lasting benefit in 11 eyes with CME secondary to uveitis. However, one individual with uveitis of recent onset obtained a sustained visual improvement from the HBOT (Okinami et al. 1992). HBOT (3.0 ATA for 75 min five times weekly × 5 weeks) was used to treat a 46-year-old woman with bilateral posterior uveitis and vitritis. She had previously been treated with high-dose steroids, acetazolamide, cyclosporine, and grid laser therapy without success. Her vision prior to HBOT was 20/200 OD and 20/80 OS. HBOT resulted in visual improvement to 20/100 OD and 20/40 OS (Suttorp-Schulten et al. 1997). Although the HBOT had to be repeated to provide continued benefit in this patient, when one eye is legally blind and the other has impaired vision, repeated HBOT may be a very useful therapeutic option when other treatment modalities have been unsuccessful (Butler et al. 2008).

Refractory Pseudomonas Keratitis

Chong described a 30-year-old White female with culture-proven soft contact lens-associated Pseudomonas keratitis who was getting progressively worse despite topical, oral, and intravenous antibiotics. On her third day after admission, she began HBOT (2.0 ATA for 90 min daily). She improved after the addition of HBOT. Twenty-four hours after her first HBOT treatment, her vision had improved from counting fingers to 6/24. The HBOT was continued for 2 more days with progressive improvement, and the patient was discharged after 6 days with a visual acuity of 6/9. Her vision subsequently improved to 6/6 (Chong et al. 2007).

Pyoderma Gangrenosum of the Orbit

Pyoderma gangrenosum is an uncommon inflammatory skin disorder associated with inflammatory bowel disease and

arthritis. It is characterized by its bluish color, exquisite painfulness, and potential to cause extensive tissue necrosis. It is uncommon in the periocular region, but Newman reported a case in which the lower lid lesion became extremely painful and relentlessly progressive, destroying orbital tissue, perforating the cornea, and eventually requiring evisceration of the eye. Oral and intralesional steroids, improved control of underlying diabetes, and oral clofazimime all failed to produce clinical improvement. The author used four HBOT sessions before her evisceration (2.0 ATA for 90 min) and followed with ten sessions of HBOT after surgery. The patient recovered after the surgery and HBOT sessions and the author considered HBOT a valuable adjunct in the management of this challenging patient (Newman and Frank 1993).

Other Reported Uses

This section contains a number of ocular indications for HBOT for which a theoretical basis for the usefulness of HBOT exists and/or case reports have been published documenting the use of HBOT in managing these disorders. The evidence for these indications was considered to be less strong than that for the disorders listed in the previous two sections.

Toxic Amblyopia

Toxic amblyopia is a reduction in visual acuity secondary to a toxic reaction in the optic nerve. It can be caused by many toxins including: lead, methanol, chloramphenicol, digoxin, ethambutol, and quinine. In severe cases it can lead to blindness. Bilateral amaurosis (loss of vision) is a common finding in quinine toxicity, typically occurring when serum levels are over 10 mg/L (Boland et al. 1985; Dyson et al. 1985). Visual loss usually occurs within 24 h of ingestion of a toxic dose. Tissue hypoxia is thought to be a factor in this disorder, but direct retinal toxicity may be causative as well. Although the natural course is usually return of vision, permanent visual loss may occur (Wolff et al. 1997; Bacon et al. 1988).

Kern et al. (1986) treated 4 patients with toxic amblyopia using HBO at 2 ATA. Improvement in vision was obtained in 3 of the 4 patients. Ocular quinine toxicity typically involves a partial or total and often permanent loss of vision. Apart from gastric lavage and oral administration of activated charcoal, current treatment modalities are of doubtful efficacy. Two patients with quinine amaurosis were treated with HBOT in an effort to increase oxygen delivery to the retina (Wolff et al. 1997). Two patients had visual outcomes of bilateral no light perception vision and dilated, nonreactive pupils within hours of ingesting 13–15 g of quinine in addition to other drugs. Following initial oral charcoal administration, HBOT was used.

Within 17 h after quinine ingestion, both patients underwent HBOT at 2.4 ATA for 90 min. Both patients had return of visual acuity to 20/20 in both eyes less than 24 h after treatment. Follow-up visual fields revealed constriction and paracentral scotomas bilaterally. HBOT may represent an additional or alternative, and perhaps safer, method of treatment for toxic amblyopia (Butler et al. 2008).

Retinitis Pigmentosa

Retinitis pigmentosa (RP) is a heterogeneous group of retinal disorders characterized by slowly progressive degeneration of the photoreceptor cells (rods and cones). Although the majority of RP cases are inherited as X-linked or dominant, approximately 40% of cases are isolated, with no other family members affected. Metabolic factors within the retina may also contribute to the progression of cell death. The early stage of RP is often detectable only by the presence of an abnormal ERG. Loss of visual field occurs later, with the peripheral field affected first. Affected individuals lose visual field at rates of 4–18% per year (Baumgartner 2000). Symptoms progress from light/dark adaptation difficulties to progressive loss of peripheral vision until only a central tunnel of vision remains.

It has been suggested that HBOT may be useful in slowing the progress of RP. Algan et al. (1973) advocated the use of HBOT for retinitis pigmentosa and macular degeneration. Chacia et al. (1987) reported improvement of visual acuity in a patient with retinitis pigmentosa and macular edema. Another study showed a statistically significant improvement or stability in ERG in 24 patients who received HBOT (2.2 ATA for 90 min on a tapering regimen from five times a week for 1 month to 1 week a month for 11 months to one week every 3 months for the balance of 2 years) compared to controls (Vingolo et al. 1999). This improvement in retinal ERG did not correlate with an improvement in visual acuity, but this would not be expected when HBOT is performed before the disease has reached endstage, as the loss of vision moves from peripheral to central with the central island typically being the last sector of the visual field extinguished. Skogstad reported a 26-year-old man with RP treated with HBOT (2.4 ATA for 97 min 5 days a week × 4 weeks) and noted that he had improvement of his lateral vision at the conclusion of therapy (Skogstad et al. 1994). Oxidative stress, however, has been implicated as potentially contributing to the degenerative process, and antioxidant supplements proposed as one possible therapeutic approach to RP. Baumgartner believes that HBOT is likely to be associated with considerable risk of increased oxidative damage to the retina in RP patients. Additionally, HBOT, given acutely, is unlikely to arrest the process of a disease that is chronic and progressive (Baumgartner 2000).

Visual Field Defects Following Macular Hole Surgery

Macular holes are caused by traction on the retina produced by fibrous attachments to a detaching vitreous body. Vitreoretinal surgery is indicated in some cases to close these holes. One of the complications of this surgery is temporal visual field defects (TVFD). A study reported that 7 patients with TVFD following macular hole surgery were treated with HBOT, while a control group of 5 patients were not. The preoperative VF determined by kinetic perimetry was considered to be 100%, and the VF following HBOT was compared with that standard. In all 5 patients who had no HBOT, VF defects were unchanged, while the VF recovered remarkably in all patients treated with HBOT. The VF recovered to 81.7 ± 16.7% of the preoperative VF after 3 days of HBOT, and to 91.6 ± 15.8% months after HBOT. As the cause of VF defect is likely to be chorioretinal circulation disturbance during surgery, HBOT improves VF by activating the retinal cells. The authors concluded that HBOT is useful in the treatment of VF defect after macular hole surgery. Unfortunately, visual acuity itself was unchanged despite HBOT (Kurok et al. 2002).

Diabetic Retinopathy

Diabetic retinopathy (DR) is the leading cause of blindness for Americans in the 20–64-year-old age group. The underlying pathophysiology is believed to be an endothelial vasculopathy characterized by loss of pericytes and basement membrane thickening due to sustained hyperglycemia exposure (Butler et al. 2008). Vision loss in DR can be caused by retinal edema, retinal or optic nerve neovascularization, and/or ischemic macular changes. Elevated levels of VEGF have been found in both the proliferative and nonproliferative DR types (Ishida et al. 2003). Treatment options for DR and diabetic macular edema (DME) include blood sugar control, laser PRP, grid laser therapy, intravitreal triamcinolone, and intravitreal antiVEGF agents. HBOT is most likely to be of benefit early in the disease as a method of reducing edema and reversing ischemia.

Improvement of a patient with DME from 20/125 in the right eye and 20/320 in the left, to 20/63 and 20/160, respectively, was noted after HBOT. A decrease in foveal thickness from 620 μm/580 μm to 233 μm/305 μm accompanied the improvement in vision. HBOT was administered in 14 sessions over 1 month. The DME recurred several times in the succeeding months, but each time improved after HBOT. The authors attributed the success of HBOT in this patient to either the hyperoxygenation of the macular tissue or constriction of the retinal vessels (Averous et al. 2006). A total of 22 eyes of 11 patients with DME were treated with 2 ATA for 60 min BID × 14 days, and then once a day for the third week. Visual acuity improved by two lines or more in 15 eyes (68%) after HBOT. The improvement in vision diminished over time, but at the end of follow-up was still better than pre-treatment. Static visual perimetry was also noted to improve in 76 % of eyes (Ogura et al. 1988). Krott reported a series of 5 patients (seven eyes) with macular edema (3 diabetic patients, 1 with CRVO, and 1 with BRVO) treated with HBOT (2.4 ATA for 30 min per day × 10–30 treatments). At 15-month follow-up, the mean increase in visual acuity was 3.5 lines. Other treatments for macular edema were employed as well (laser, acetazolamide, hemodilution), but HBOT was used after most other approaches had failed (Krott et al. 2000).

Haddad reported no improvement in 3 patients with "advanced DR" treated with HBOT (2–3 ATA for 60 min) and noted that none of the patients demonstrated any appreciable change in visual acuity, retinal pathology, or visual fields (Haddad and Leopold 1965). Winstanley (1963) utilized 3 ATA on 3 patients with DR, but observed no changes on fundoscopy. Dudnikov et al. (1981) noted that eye tissue hypoxia is a characteristic of DR. They used HBOT on 35 DR patients. Post-treatment angiography showed reduction of venous congestion and improvement of hemodynamics. In some patients, the authors noted ischemic edema zones in areas of neovascularization. They drew no conclusions but continue with further investigations.

A major issue in treating this very common disorder with HBOT is its chronicity. HBOT would likely have to be undertaken on a long-term basis to provide a sustained benefit. HBOT likely aids in acute episodes of edema, but cannot reverse the more chronic permanent changes of necrosis, nor can it prevent edema from recurring once HBOT is stopped (Butler et al. 2008).

Uveitis

One report of a rabbit model of uveitis noted that HBOT was as effective as topical steroids used alone in treating this disorder and enhanced the efficacy of topical steroids when the modalities were used together (Ersanli et al. 2005).

Secondary Keratoendotheliosis

Corneal endothelial dysfunction, ranging from mild postoperative corneal edema to bullous keratopathy and opacification of the cornea (secondary keratoendotheliosis), may occasionally complicate cataract removal surgery, although techniques are improving. Recupero reported that HBOT produced improved visual acuity in all 12 of the study patients compared to improvement in only 33 % in the 21 control patients (Recupero et al. 1992). Vitullo et al. (1987) have reported on the treatment of 32 patients with corneal disorders using HBO at 2.8 ATA. The various corneal diseases included were keratitis, keratoconus, traumatic injuries, and ulcerations. HBOT was found to be beneficial in most of these cases. The rationale put forth by the author for the efficacy of HBOT is that the tissue edema, hypoxia, and ischemia in these conditions are improved by hyperoxygenation. The presence of a soft lens on the anterior surface of the cornea for prolonged periods interferes with the oxygenation of the cornea and leads to anoxia and edema predisposing to the formation of corneal ulcers. Polse and Mandell (1976) produced striae on the posterior surface of the cornea in volunteers; the striae were then reversed by the use of HBOT.

Complications of Sickle Cell Disease

Patients with sickle cell disease experience obliteration of retinal arterioles and venules and develop areas of retinal avascularity. This may result in proliferative vitreoretinopathy, which in many cases progresses to retinal hole formation and retinal detachment. These patients do very poorly with standard scleral buckling procedures to repair their detachments, with anterior segment ischemia nullifying what would otherwise be successful surgery (Freilich and Seelenfreund 1972, 1973). In experimental retinal detachment, retinal hypoxia caused by the separation of the retina from its normal source of nutrients is a factor in inducing the death of photoreceptor cells. Supplemental normobaric oxygen at 70 % was found to reduce cell death in a cat model of retinal detachment (Mervin et al. 1999). Oxygen in this model was also found to limit the proliferation and hypertrophy of Muller cells that is responsible for the proliferative vitreoretinopathy that may complicate retinal detachment surgery (Lewis et al. 1999).

Freilich and his colleagues performed three scleral buckling procedures in a hyperbaric chamber with the patient breathing 100 % oxygen at 2.0 ATA. The percentage of sickled red blood cells in one patient decreased, from 10 % at the start of the procedure, to 3.5 % at the end of 2 h of hyperoxia. All patients treated using this unique surgical approach had anatomical success (no recurrence of the detachment) and improvement in their vision 6–12 months after their surgery (Freilich and Seelenfreund 1972, 1973). Five additional patients reported by the same author using hyperoxic conditions for surgery similarly produced positive results (Freilich and Seelenfreund 1975). The author subsequently provided 2-year follow-up on these 8 patients and reported that their retinas had all remained completely attached and that no new retinal tears had developed. Visual acuity improved in all 6 of the patients who had had a decrease preoperatively (Freilich and Seelenfreund 1977). The author concludes that this remarkable success in these difficult surgical cases "merits the continued use of this technique in these difficult cases of detachment of the retina" (Freilich and Seelenfreund 1977).

Hyphema is another complication of sickle cell disease, and HBOT has been advocated as a treatment for this condition on the basis of experimental evidence (Wallyn et al. 1985).

Glaucoma

Glaucoma is a chronic and progressive disorder characterized by elevated intraocular pressure (IOP), damaged optic nerve heads, and lesions in the visual fields. Elevated IOP is only one of the symptoms of this disease, and although it can be lowered by medications, visual field deficits may persist. There are several theories of the etiology of glaucoma; one is that ischemia, resulting from insufficient vascularization of the pericapillary choroid and of the optic nerve head, is one of the primary causes of glaucoma lesions. Bohne et al. (1987) recorded retinal potentials to pattern-reversal stimuli, while IOP was artificially elevated. In glaucoma patients, the amplitude of potentials decreased at higher perfusion pressures than in healthy subjects. These data indicate that the dysfunction of ganglion cells is likely caused by a diminished retinal perfusion and therefore a reduced oxygen supply of the inner retinal layer. HBOT does not significantly lower IOP (Gallin-Cohen et al. 1980); however, it may be theoretically useful in decreasing edema and ischemia.

Bojic et al. (1993) conducted a double-blind, placebo controlled study on 111 subjects to test the effect of HBOT on visual fields and IOP in patients with open angle glaucoma. Two groups were formed at random: an experimental group of 91 and a control group of 20 patients. The experimental group was divided into 4 subgroups according to the number of HBOT sessions at 2.0 ATA for 90 min × 30 sessions (31 patients), 20 sessions (20 patients), 15 sessions (20 patients), and 10 sessions (20 patients). There was improvement in visual fields in all treatment groups, except the 10 treatment group. There was no improvement in the control group. There was no change in IOP in any of the patients. The authors recommend that a 20-sessions of HBOT be given initially, and if the visual fields improvement value reaches 50 %, HBOT should be repeated. Popova and Kuz'minov (1996) treated 35 patients (64 eyes) with primary open-angle glaucoma with HBOT combined with antioxidants. Repeated courses were administered during 5 years. Stabilization of the visual function was attained in 80 % patients. Follow-up of controls (34 patients—66 eyes) showed stabilization of the visual function in only 35 % cases.

Emergency HBO in Patients with Acute Vision Loss

Patients who present with acute painless loss of vision have a differential diagnosis that includes CRAO, retinal detachment, CRVO, BRVO, BRAO, vitreous hemorrhage, posterior circulation stroke, and ischemic optic neuropathy (Beran and Murphy-Lavoie 2009). It may take several hours to several days and an ophthalmology evaluation to establish a definitive diagnosis for the vision loss. In the interim,

whatever potential that may exist to restore vision with HBOT might be lost.

Considering that at least six of the relatively common ocular disorders producing acute, painless loss of vision have the potential to benefit from HBOT, the authors propose the following approach to managing patients with acute loss of vision:

1. Patients who present with acute painless loss of vision of recent onset should be triaged as "emergent."
2. Visual acuity should be checked immediately.
3. With the patient's current glasses or contact lenses 20/200 or worse, if they cannot be improved significantly with pinhole, and the patient meets the other selection criteria listed in Table 32.2, then, in addition to emergent ophthalmology consult, he or she should be considered for emergent HBOT.
4. The patient should then be started immediately on supplemental oxygen at one atmosphere at the highest possible inspired fraction of oxygen.
5. If vision is restored by normobaric oxygen within 15 min, the patient should be admitted to the hospital and given intermittent oxygen for 15 min every hour, alternating with 45 min of breathing room air. Visual acuity should be checked at the end of each breathing period. This regime should be continued until a fluorescein angiogram shows patency, ophthalmologist determines etiology other than CRAO, the patients' visual acuity remains stable on room air for 2 h, or for a maximum of 96 h on intermittent supplemental oxygen therapy has been reached.
6. Refer for emergent HBOT if no response within the first 15 min of normobaric oxygen.
7. Compress to 2.0 ATA on 100 % oxygen. If vision improves significantly at 2.0 ATA, remain at this depth for a 90-min treatment. (Air-breathing periods at this depth may not be necessary since the incidence of oxygen toxicity seizures is four times lower at 2.0 than at 2.4 ATA).
8. If no response within 15 min, compress to 2.4 ATA, if no response at 2.4 ATA compress to 2.8 ATA and if no response perform a USN Treatment Table 6; however, if vision returns significantly during the beginning of the treatment, a 90-min treatment is probably sufficient.
9. If vision returns during HBOT, inpatient monitoring and intermittent supplemental oxygen should be considered. Monitoring by a retinal specialist should continue. Cases of relapse of loss of vision and resultant blindness after discharge have been reported (Telander et al. 2011).
10. Twice daily 90-min treatments at the depth of improvement should be continued until either, no further improvement for 3 days, restoration of patency by fluorescein angiogram, or vision remains stable under normoxic conditions (Murphy-Lavoie et al. 2014; Butler et al. 2008).

Conclusion

HBOT has not traditionally been used widely as a treatment modality in the management of ocular disorders. There are a number of ocular indications, however, in which HBOT may reverse profound vision loss, treat infection, and prevent deformity. The authors recommend prompt aggressive HBOT for the indications listed when vision loss is severe and the patient presents within the appropriate time frame (Butler et al. 2008; Murphy-Lavoie et al. 2014). Further studies will help to define which ocular disorders are best treated with HBOT, the critical time window for each, and the optimal treatment dosing.

References

Aisenbrey S, Krott R, Heller R, Krauss D, Rössler G, Heimann K. Hyperbaric oxygen therapy in retinal artery occlusion. Ophthalmologe. 2000;97:461–7.

Algan B, Benichoux R, Marchal H. First personal results of the application of hyperbaric oxygen in eye diseases. Bull Soc Belge Ophthalmol. 1973;163:183–94.

Anderson B, Heyman A, Wahlen RE. Migraine like phenomenon after decompression from hyperbaric environments. Neurology. 1965a;15:1025–40.

Anderson B, Saltzman H, Heyman A. The effects of hyperbaric oxygenation on retinal artery occlusion. Arch Ophthal. 1965b;73:315–9.

Anderson B, Shelton DL. Axial length in hyperoxic myopia. In: Bove AA, Bachrach AJ, Greenbaum LJ, editors. Ninth international symposium on underwater and hyperbaric physiology. Bethesda, MD: Undersea and Hyperbaric Medical Society; 1987. p. 607–11.

Anderson B. Hyperoxic myopia. Trans Am Ophthalmol Soc. 1978;7:116–24.

Antonetti DA, Wolpert EB, DeMaio L, et al. Hydrocortisone decreases retinal endothelial cell water and solute flux coincident with increased content and decreased phosphorylation of occluding. J Neurochem. 2000;80:667–77.

Arnold AC, Hepler RS, Lieber M, Alexander JM. Hyperbaric oxygen therapy for nonarteritic anterior ischemic optic neuropathy. Am J Ophthalmol. 1996;122:535–41.

Arnold AC, Levin LA. Treatment of ischemic optic neuropathy. Semin Ophthalmol. 2002;17:39–46.

Arora N, Lambrou Jr FH, Stewart MW, et al. Sudden blindness associated with central nervous symptoms in a hemodialysis patient. Nephron. 1991;59:490–2.

Assaad NN, Chong R, Tat LT, Bennett MH, Coroneo MT. Use of adjuvant hyperbaric oxygen therapy to support limbal conjunctival graft in the management of recurrent pterygium. Clin Sci. 2011;30:7–10.

Assaad NN, Coroneo MT. Conjunctival autograft failure in eyes previously exposed to b-radiation or mitomycin. Arch Ophthalmol. 2008;126:1460–1.

Aten LA, Stone JA, Poli, T. Treatment of a patient with acute central retinal artery occlusion with hyperbaric oxygen therapy. UHMS Annual Scientific Assembly, Ft Worth, 2011. (Abstract) Attributed to Lens Index Changes. Optometry & Vision Science 2015;92: 1076-1084.

Augsburger JJ, Magargal LE. Visual prognosis following treatment of acute central retinal artery obstruction. Br J Ophthalmol. 1980;64:913–7.

Averous K, Erginay A, Timsit J, Haouchine B, Gaudric A, Massin P. Resolution of diabetic macular edema following high altitude exercise (Letter). Acta Scand Ophthalmol. 2006;84:830–1.

Avitabile T, Longo A, Reibaldi A. Intravitreal triamcinolone compared with macular laser grid photocoagulation for the treatment of cystoids macular edema. Am J Ophthalmol. 2005;140:695–702.

Ayata A, Uzun G, Mutluoglu M, Unal M, Yildiz S, Ersanli D. Influence of hyperbaric oxygen therapy on central corneal thickness. Ophthalmic Res. 2012;47:19–22.

Bacon P, Spalton DJ, Smith SE. Blindness from quinine toxicity. Br J Ophthalmol. 1988;72:219–24.

Bashshur ZF, Ma'luf RN, Allam S, Jurdi FA, Haddad RS, Noureddin BN. Intravitreal triamcinolone for the management of macular edema due to nonischemic central retinal vein occlusion. Arch Ophthalmol. 2004;122:1137–40.

Baumgartner WA. Etiology, pathogenesis, and experimental treatment of retinitis pigmentosa. Med Hypotheses. 2000;54:814–24.

Bayer A, Mutlu FM, Sobaci G. Hyperbaric oxygen therapy for mitomycin C-induced scleral necrosis. Ophthalmic Surg Lasers. 2002;33:58–61.

Beehler CC, Newton NL, Culver JF, Tredici T. Ocular hyperoxia. Aerospace Med. 1963;34:1017–20.

Beehler CC. Oxygen and the eye. Aeromed Rev. 1964;3:1–21.

Behnke AR, Forbes HS, Motley EP. Circulatory and visual effects of oxygen at 3 atmospheres pressure. Am J Physiol. 1936;114:436–42.

Beiran I, Goldenberg I, Adir Y, Tamir A, Shupak A, Miller B. Early hyperbaric oxygen therapy for retinal artery occlusion. Eur J Ophthalmol. 2001;11:345–50.

Beiran I, Reissman P, Scharf J, Nahum Z, Miller B. Hyperbaric oxygenation combined with nifedipine treatment for recent onset retinal artery occlusion. Eur J Ophthalmol. 1993;3:89–94.

Beiran I, Rimon I, Weiss G, Pikkel J, Miller B. Hyperbaric oxygenation therapy for ischemic optic neuropathy. Eur J Ophthalmol. 1995;5:285–6.

Beran DI, Murphy-Lavoie H. Acute painless vision loss. J La State Med Soc. 2009;161:214–23.

Bhatt UK. Radial optic neurotomy in retinal vein occlusion. Am J Ophthalmol. 2004;137:970–1.

Bohne BD, Klatt A, Reimann J, Kästner R. Die Sauerstoffversorgung des vorderen Sehnervenbereiches bei künstlicher Augeninnendruckerhöhung. Z Klin Med. 1987;42:1795–7.

Bojic L, Ivanisevic M, Gosovic G. Hyperbaric oxygen therapy in two patients with non-arteritic anterior optic neuropathy who did not respond to prednisone. Undersea Hyperbaric Med. 2002;29:6–92.

Bojic L, Kovacevic H, Andric D, Romanović D, Petri NM. Hyperbaric oxygen dose of choice in the treatment of glaucoma. Arh Hig Rada Toksikol. 1993;44:239–47.

Boland ME, Roper SMB, Henry JA. Complications of quinine poisoning. Lancet. 1985;1:384–5.

Boyd SR, Zachary I, Chakravarthy U, Allen GJ, Wisdom GB, Cree IA, et al. Correlation of increased vascular endothelial growth factor with neovascularization and permeability in ischemic central vein occlusion. Arch Ophthalmol. 2002;120:1644–50.

Bridges WZ. Electroretinographic manifestations of hyperbaric oxygen. Arch Ophthalmol. 1966;75:812–7.

Brown GC, Shields JA, Sanborn G, Augsburger JJ, Savino PJ, Schatz NJ. Radiation retinopathy. Ophthalmology. 1982;89:1494–501.

Buono LM, Foroozan R, Savino PJ, Danesh-Meyer HV, Stanescu D. Posterior ischemic optic neuropathy after hemodialysis. Ophthalmology. 2003;110:1216–8.

Butler FK, Hagan C, Murphy-Lavoie H. Hyperbaric oxygen therapy and the eye. UHM. 2008;35:327–81.

Butler FK, Harris DJ, Reynolds RA. Altitude retinopathy on Mount Everest 1989. Ophthalmology. 1992;99:739–46.

Butler FK, White E, Twa M. Hyperoxic myopia in a closed-circuit mixed-gas SCUBA diver. Undersea Hyperb Med. 1999;26:41–5.

Butler FK. Diving and hyperbaric ophthalmology. Surv Ophthalmol. 1995;39:347–66.

Butler FK. The eye in the wilderness. In: Auerbach PS, editor. Wilderness medicine. 5th ed. St Louis: Mosby; 2007.

Canan H, Ulas B, Altan-Yaycioglu R. Hyperbaric oxygen therapy in combination with systemic treatment of sickle cell disease presenting as central retinal artery occlusion: a case report. J Med Case Reports. 2014;8:370.

Chacia N, Combes AM, Romdane K, Bec P. Maculopathy in typical retinitis pigmentosa a propos of 33 cases. J Fr Ophthalmol. 1987;10:381–6.

Chacko DC. Considerations in the diagnosis of radiation injury. JAMA. 1981;245:1255–8.

Chen SD, Lochhead J, Patel CK, Frith P. Intravitreal triamcinolone acetonide for ischemic macular edema caused by branch retinal vein occlustion. Br J Ophthalmol. 2004;88:154–5.

Cho S, Choi MS, Lee, JY, et al. Effect of hyperbaric oxygen therapy on central retinal artery occlusion associated with systemic lupus erythematosus (a case report). Abstract of the Undersea and Hyperbaric Medical Society, Inc. Joint Annual Scientific Meeting with the International Congress for Hyperbaric Medicine and the European Undersea Biomedical Society, 1990, Amsterdam (abstract).

Chong R, Ayer CJ, Francis IC, Coroneo MT, Wolfers DL. Adjunctive hyperbaric oxygen in pseudomonas keratitis. Br J Ophthalmol. 2007;91:560–1.

Cibis GW, Beaver HA, Johns K, et al. Basic and clinical science course: fundamentals and principles of ophthalmology. San Francisco: American Academy of Ophthalmology; 2006. p. 38–40.

Clark JM, Thom S. Oxygen under pressure. In: Brubakk AO, Neuman TS, editors. Bennett and Eliott's physiology and medicine of diving. London: WB Saunders; 2003. p. 358–418.

Coma MC, Sobrin L, Onal S, Christen W, Foster CS. Intraviteal bevacizumab for treatment of uveitic macular edema. Ophthalmology. 2007;114:1574–9.

Cope A, Eggert JV, O'Brien E. Retinal artery occlusion: visual outcome after treatment with hyperbaric oxygen. Diving Hyperb Med. 2011;41:135–8.

Coscas G, Gaudric A. Natural course of nonaphakic cystoid macular edema. Surv Ophthalmol. 1984;28(Suppl):471–84.

Cox SN, Hay E, Bird AC. Treatment of chronic macular edema with acetazolamide. Arch Ophthalmol. 1988;106:1190–5.

Cunningham S, Fleck BW, Elton RA, McIntosh N. Transcutaneous oxygen levels in retinopathy of prematurity. Lancet. 1995;346:1464–5.

Cuxart M, Matas M, Picazo M, Sans R, Juvanet J, Osuna T. Acute bilateral visual loss in a hemodialysed patient (Spanish). Nefrologia. 2005;25:703–5.

David NJ, Norton EWD, Gass JD, Beauchamp J. Fluorescein angiography in central retinal artery occlusion. Arch Ophthalmol. 1967;77:619–29.

De Smet MD, Carruthers J, Lepawsky M. Anterior segment ischemia treated with hyperbaric oxygen. Can J Ophthalmol. 1987;22:381–3.

Desai N, Patel MR, Prisant LM, Thomas DA. Nonarteritic anterior ischemic optic neuropathy. J Clin Hypertens. 2005;7:130–3.

Desola J, Papoutsidakis E, Martos P. et al. Hyperbaric oxygenation in the treatment of Central Retinal Artery Occlusions: An analysis of 214 cases following a prospective protocol. UHMS Annual Scientific Assembly: Montreal; 2015 (Abstract).

Desola J. Hyperbaric oxygen therapy in acute occlusive retinopathies. In: Schmutz J (Ed.) Proceedings of the 1st Swiss symposium on hyperbaric medicine. Foundation for Hyperbaric Medicine, Basel; 1987. p. 333.

Dick JSB, Jampol LM, Haller JA. Macular edema. In: Ryan SJ, editor. Retina. St. Louis: Mosby; 2001. p. 973–85.

Dollery CT, Bulpitt CJ, Kohner EM. Oxygen supply to the retina from the retinal and choroidal circulations at normal and increased arterial oxygen tensions. Invest Ophthalmol Vis Sci. 1969;8:588–94.

Dudnikov LK, Kakhovsky IM, Molokanova SP. Hyperbaric oxygenation in complex treatment of diabetic retinopathy. In: Yefuny SN, editor. Proceedings of the 7th international congress on hyperbaric medicine. Moscow: USSR Academy of Sciences; 1981. p. 305–6.

Duker JS, Brown GC. Recovery following acute obstruction of the retinal and choroidal circulations. Retina. 1988;8:257–60.

Dyson EH, Proudfoot AT, Prescott LF, Heyworth R. Death and blindness due to overdose of quinine. Br Med J. 1985;291:31–3.

Ersanli D, Karadayi K, Toyran S, Akin T, Sönmez M, Ciftçi F, et al. The efficacy of hyperbaric oxygen for the treatment of experimental uveitis induced in rabbits. Ocul Immunol Inflamm. 2005;13:383–8.

Evanger K, Haugen OH, Aanderud L. Hypermetropia-succeeded myopia after hyperbaric oxygen therapy. Optom Vis Sci. 2006;83:195–8.

Evanger K, Pierscionek B, Vaagbo G. Myopic shift during hyperbaric oxygenation attributed to lens index changes. Optom Vis Sci. 2015;92(11):1076–84.

Feltgen N, Junker B, Agostini H, Hansen LL. Retinal endovascular lysis in ischemic central retinal vein occlusion. Ophthalmology. 2007;114:716–23.

Finger PT, Chin KJ, Duvall G, Palladium 103 for Choroidal Melanoma Study Group. Palladium-103 ophthalmic plaque radiation therapy for choroidal melanoma: 400 treated patients. Ophthalmology. 2009;116:790–6, 796.e1.

Fledelius HC, Jansen E. Hypermetropic refractive change after hyperbaric oxygen therapy. Acta Ophthalmol Scand. 2004;82:313–4.

Fledelius HC, Jansen EC, Thorn J. Refractive change during hyperbaric oxygen therapy. A clinical trial including ultrasound oculometry. Acta Ophthalmol Scand. 2002;80:188–90.

Fong AC, Schatz H. Central retinal vein occlusion in young adults. Surv Ophthalmol. 1993;37:393–417.

Frayser R, Saltzman HA, Anderson B, Hickam JB, Sieker HO. The effect of hyperbaric oxygenation on retinal circulation. Arch Ophthalmol. 1967;77:265–9.

Freilich D, Seelenfreund MH. Hyperbaric oxygen, retinal detachment, and sickle cell anemia. Arch Ophthalmol. 1973;90:90–3.

Freilich DB, Seelenfreund MH. Further studies in the use of hyperbaric oxygen in retinal detachment with sickle cell anemia. Mod Probl Ophthalmol. 1975;15:313–7.

Freilich DB, Seelenfreund MH. Long-term follow-up of scleral buckling procedures with sickle cell disease and retinal detachment treated with the use of hyperbaric oxygen. Mod Probl Ophthalmol. 1977;18:368–72.

Freilich DB, Seelenfreund MH. The use of hyperbaric oxygen in the treatment of retinal detachment in patients with sickle cell disease. Isr J Med Sci. 1972;8:1458–61.

Gall N, Leiba H, Handzel R, Pe'er J. Severe radiation retinopathy and optic neuropathy after brachytherapy for choroidal melanoma, treated by hyperbaric oxygen. Eye (Lond). 2007;21:1010–2.

Gallin-Cohen PF, Podos SM, Yabionski ME. Oxygen lowers intraocular pressure. Invest Ophthalmol Vis Sci. 1980;19:43–8.

Garcia-Arumi J, Martinez-Castillo V, Boixadera A, Fonollosa A, Corcostegui B. Surgical embolus removal in retinal artery occlusion. Br J Ophthalmol. 2006;90:1252–5.

Gardner TW, Antonetti DA, Barber AJ, Leith E, Tarbell JA. The molecular structure and function of the inner blood-retinal barrier. Pennsylvania State Retina Research Group. Doc Ophthalmol. 1999;97:229–37.

Gass JD, Anderson DR, Davis EB. A clinical, fluorescein angiographic, and electron microscopic correlation of cystoid macular edema. Am J Ophthalmol. 1985;100:82–6.

Gass JDM, Norton EDW. Cystoid macular edema and papilledema following cataract exgtraction: a fluorescein fundoscopic and angiographic study. Arch Ophthalmol. 1966;76:221–4.

Gaydar V, Ezrachi D, Dratviman-Storobinsky O, Hofstetter S, Avraham-Lubin BC, Goldenberg-Cohen N. Reduction in apoptosis in ischemic retinas of two mouse models using hyperbaric oxygen treatment. Invest Ophthalmol Vis Sci. 2011;52:7514–22.

Gesell LB, Trott A. De novo cataract development following a standard course of hyperbaric oxygen therapy. Undersea Hyperb Med. 2007;34:389–92.

Gismondi A, Micalella F, Metrangolo C, Colonna S. Treatment of cerebral ischemia with hyperbaric oxygen therapy. Minerva Med. 1981;72:1417.

Glacet-Bernard A, Coscas G, Chabanel A, Zourdani A, Lelong F, Samama MM. Prognostic factors for retinal vein occlusion. Ophthalmology. 1996;103:551–60.

Gool J, Jong H. Hyperbaric oxygen treatment in vascular insufficiency of the retina and optic nerve. In: Ledingham IM, editor. Proceedings of the 2nd international congress on clinical and applied hyperbaric medicine. Edinburgh: Livingstone; 1965. p. 447–60.

Gragoudas ES, Seddon JM, Egan K, Glynn R, Munzenrider J, Austin-Seymour M, et al. Long-term results of proton beam irradiated uveal melanomas. Ophthalmology. 1987;94:349–53.

Green MO, Brannen AL. Hyperbaric oxygen therapy for betaradiation-induced scleral necrosis. Ophthalmology. 1995;102:1038–41.

Greenberg PB, Martidis A, Rogers AH, Duker JS, Reichel E. Intravitreal triamcinolone acetonide for macular edema due to central retinal vein occlusion. Br J Ophthalmol. 2002;86:247–8.

Greer DV, Constable IJ, Cooper RL. Macular edema and retinal branch vein occlusion. Aust J Ophthalmol. 1980;8:207–9.

Greiner KH, Lang GE. Risk-adapted management of central vein occlusions. Ophthalmologe. 1999;96:736–40.

Gunduz K, Shields CL, Shields JA, Cater J, Freire JE, Brady LW. Radiation complications and tumor control after plaque radiotherapy of choroidal melanoma with macular involvement. Am J Ophthalmol. 1999a;127:579–89.

Gunduz K, Shields CL, Shields JA, Cater J, Freire JE, Brady LW. Radiation retinopathy following plaque radiotherapy for posterior uveal melanoma. Arch Ophthalmol. 1999b;117:609–14.

Gutman FA, Zegarra H. Macular edema secondary to occlusion of retinal veins. Surv Ophthalmol. 1984;26:462–70.

Haas A, Pinter O, Papaefthymiou G, Weger M, Berghold A, Schrottner O. Incidence of radiation retinopathy after high-dosage single-fraction gamma knife radiosurgery for choroidal melanoma. Ophthalmology. 2002;109:909–13.

Haddad HM, Leopold IH. Effect of hyperbaric oxygenation on microcirculation: use in therapy of retinal vascular disorders. Invest Ophthalmol. 1965;4:1141–51.

Hasselbach HC, Ruefer F, Feltgen N, Schneider U, Bopp S, Hansen LL, et al. Treatment of central retinal vein occlusion by radial optic neurotomy in 107 cases. Graefes Arch Clin Exp Ophthalmol. 2007;245:1145–56.

Hayreh SS, Kolder HE, Weingeist TA. Central retinal artery occlusion and retinal tolerance time. Ophthalmology. 1980;87:75–8.

Hayreh SS, Podhajsky P. Ocular neovascularization with retinal vascular occlusion: II. Occurrence in central retinal and branch retinal artery occlusion. Arch Ophthalmol. 1982;100:1581–96.

Hayreh SS, Zimmerman B. Management of giant cell arteritis. Our 27-year clinical study: new light on old controversies. Ophthalmologica. 2003;217:239–59.

Hayreh SS, Zimmerman B. Nonarteritic anterior ischemic optic neuropathy. Ophthalmology. 2008;115:298–305.

Hayreh SS, Zimmerman MB. Central retinal artery occlusion: Visual outcome. Am J Ophthalmol. 2005;140:376–91.

Hayreh SS, Zimmerman MB. Incipient nonarteritic anterior ischemic optic neuropathy. Ophthalmology. 2007;114:1763–72.

Hayreh SS. Management of central retinal vein occlusion. Ophthalmologica. 2003;217:167–88.

Hayreh SS. Classification of central retinal vein occlusion. Ophthalmology. 1983;90:458–74.

Herbstein K, Murchland JB. Retinal vascular changes after treatment with hyperbaric oxygen. Med J Aust. 1984;6:728–829.

Hertzog LM, Meyer GW, Carson S, Strauss MB, Hart GB. Central retinal artery occlusion treated with hyperbaric oxygen. J Hyperbaric Med. 1992;7:33–42.

Hirayama Y, Matsunaga N, Tashiro J, Amemiya T, Iwasaki M. Bifemelane in the treatment of central retinal artery or vein obstruction. Clin Ther. 1990;12:230–5.

Hsaio S, Huang Y. Partial vision recovery after iatrogenic retinal artery occlusion. Ophthalmology. 2014;14:120.

Imai E, Kunikata H, Udono T, Nakagawa Y, Abe T, Tamai M. Branch retinal artery occlusion: a complication of iron-deficiency anemia in a young adult with a rectal carcinoid. Tohuko J Exp Med. 2004;203:141–4.

Inoue O, Kajiya S, Yachimori, et al. Treatment of central retinal artery occlusion (CRAO) and branch retinal artery occlusion (BRAO) by hyperbaric oxygen therapy (HBO) – 107 eyes over 20 years. UHMS Annual Scientific Assembly, Las Vegas, 2009. (Abstract)

Ip MS. Intravitreal injection of triamcinolone: an emerging treatment for diabetic macular edema. Diabetes Care. 2004;27:1794–7.

Isenberg SJ, Diamant A. Scuba diving after enucleation. Am J Ophthalmol. 1985;100:616–7.

Ishida K, Suzuki A, Ogino N. Oxygenation under hyperbaric pressure for cystoid macular edema. Jpn J Clin Ophthalmol. 1989;43:1171–4.

Ishida S, Usui T, Yamashiro K, Kaji Y, Ahmed E, Carrasquillo KG, et al. VEGF 164 is proinflammatory in the diabetic retina. Invest Ophthalmol Vis Sci. 2003;44:2155–62.

Iturralde D, Spaide RF, Meyerle CB, Klancnik JM, Yannuzzi LA, Fisher YL, et al. Intravitreal bevacizumab (Avastin) treatment of macular edema in central retinal vein occlusion: a short-term study. Retina. 2006;26:279–84.

Jackman SV, Thompson JT. Effects of hyperbaric exposure on eyes with intraocular gas bubbles. Retina. 1995;15:160–6.

Jacobson I, Harper AM, McDowall DG. The effects of oxygen under pressure on cerebral blood flow and cerebral venous oxygen tension. Lancet. 1963;2:549.

James PB. Hyperbaric oxygen and retinal vascular changes: Hyperbaric oxygen and retinal vascular changes. Med J Aust. 1985;142:163–4.

Jampol LM, Orlin C, Cohen SB, Zanetti C, Lehman E, Goldberg MF. Hyperbaric and transcorneal delivery of oxygen to the rabbit and monkey anterior segment. Arch Ophthalmol. 1988;106:825–9.

Jampol LM. Oxygen therapy and intraocular oxygenation. Trans Am Ophthalmol Soc. 1987;85:407–37.

Jansen EC, Nielsen NV. Promising visual improvement of cystoid macular edema by hyperbaric oxygen therapy. Acta Ophthalmol Scand. 2004;82:485–6.

Johnson GP. A navigator with non-ischemic central retinal vein occlusion progressing to ischemic central retinal vein occlusion. Aviat Space Environ Med. 1990;61:962–5.

Jonas JB, Akkoyun I, Kreissig I, Degenring RF. Diffuse diabetic macular edema treated by intravitreal triamcinolone acetonide: a comparative, non-randomized study. Br J Ophthalmol. 2005;89:321–6.

Jonas JB, Kreissig I, Degenring RF. Intravitreal triamcinolone acetonide as treatment of macular edema in central retinal vein occlusion. Graefes Arch Clin Exp Ophthalmol. 2002;240:782–3.

Kern M, Sommerauer P, Wochesländer E, Schuhmann G, Kohek P, Stolze A. Application of hyperbaric oxygen therapy in patients with toxic ambyopia. Ophthalmologie. 1986;83:312–4.

Keynan Y, Yanir Y, Shupak A. Hyperbaric therapy for bilateral visual loss during hemodialysis. Clin Exp Nephrol. 2006;10:82–4.

Kindwall EP, Goldmann RW. Hyperbaric medicine procedures. Milwaukee: St. Luke's Medical Center; 1988.

Kinney JS. Human underwater vision: physiology and physics. Bethesda: Undersea and Hyperbaric Society; 1985. p. 158.

Kiryu J, Ogura Y. Hyperbaric oxygen treatment for macular edema in retinal vein occlusion: relation to severity of retinal leakage. Ophthalmologica. 1996;210:168–70.

Kokame GT, Ing MR. Intraocular gas and low-altitude air flight. Retina. 1994;14:356–8.

Krasnov MM, Kharlap SI, Pereverzina OK, et al. Hyperbaric oxygenation in the treatment of vascular diseases of retina. In: Yefuny SN, editor. Abstracts of the 7th international congress on hyperbaric medicine. Moscow: USSR Academy of Sciences; 1981. p. 304.

Krema H, Somani S, Sahgal A, Xu W, Heydarian M, Payne D, et al. Stereotactic radiotherapy for treatment of juxtapapillary choroidal melanoma: 3-year follow-up. Br J Ophthalmol. 2009;93:1172–6.

Krott R, Heller S, Aisenbrey S, Bartz-Schmidt KU. Adjunctive hyperbaric oxygenation in macular edema of vascular origin. Undersea Hyperb Med. 2000;27:195–204.

Kurok AM, Kitaoka T, Taniguchi H, Amemiya T. Hyperbaric oxygen therapy reduces visual field defect after macular hole surgery. Ophthalmic Surg Lasers. 2002;33:200–6.

Lang GE, Kuba GB. High altitude retinopathy. Am J Ophthalmol. 1997;123:418–20.

Lambertsen CJ, Clark JM, Gelfand R. Definition of tolerance in continuous hyperoxia in man: an abstract report of Predictive Studies V. In: Proceedings of the Ninth International Symposium on Underwater and Hyperbaric Physiology. Bove AA, Bachrach AJ, Greenbaum LJ, eds. Bethesda: Undersea and Hyperbaric Medical Society; 1987:717-735.

Landers MB. Retinal oxygenation via the choroidal circulation. Trans Am Ophthalmol Soc. 1978;76:528–56.

Lee YH, Lee JY, Kim YS, Kim DH, Kim J. Successful anticoagulation for bilateral central retinal vein occlusions accompanied by cerebral venous thrombosis. Arch Neurol. 2006;63:1648–51.

Levy RP, Fabrikant JI, Frankel KA, Phillips MH, Lyman JT, Lawrence JH, et al. Heavy-charged-particle radiosurgery of the pituitary gland: clinical results of 840 patients. Stereotact Funct Neurosurg. 1991;57:22–35.

Lewis G, Mervin K, Valter K, Maslim J, Kappel PJ, Stone J, et al. Limiting the proliferation and reactivity of retinal Muller cells during experimental retinal detachment: the value of oxygen supplementation. Am J Ophthalmol. 1999;128:165–72.

Li HK, Dejean BJ, Tang RA. Reversal of visual loss with hyperbaric oxygen treatment in a patient with Susac syndrome. Ophthalmology. 1996;103:2091–8.

Lincoff H, Weinburger D, Stergiu P. Air travel with intraocular gas II—clinical considerations. Arch Ophthalmol. 1989;107:907.

Lu C, Wang J, Zhou D. Central retinal artery occlusion associated with persistent truncus arteriosus and single atrium: a case report. BMC Ophthalmol. 2015;15:137.

Lyne AJ. Ocular effects of hyperbaric oxygen. Trans Ophthalmol Soc UK. 1978;98:66–8.

Madhusudhana KC, Newsom RSB. Central retinal vein occlusion: the therapeutic options. Can J Ophthalmol. 2007;42:193–5.

Mandai M, Ogura Y, Honda Y. Effects of hyperbaric oxygen treatment on macular edema. Folia Ophthalmol Jpn. 1990;41:578–83.

Mangat HS. Retinal artery occlusion. Surv Ophthalmol. 1995;40:145–56.

Marmor MF, Maack T. Enhancement of retinal adhesion and subretinal fluid resorption by acetazolamide. Invest Ophthalmol Vis Sci. 1982;23:121–4.

Mason JO, Nixon PA, Albert MA. Trans-luminal nd:YAG laser embolysis for branch retinal artery occlusion. Retina. 2007;27:573–7.

Masters T, Westgard B, Hendrikson S. Central retinal artery occulsion treated with hyperbaric oxygen: a retrospective review. UHMS Annual Scientific Assembly: Montreal; 2015 (Abstract).

Matsuo T. Multiple occlusive retinal arteritis in both eyes of a patient with rheumatoid arthritis. Jpn J Ophthalmol. 2001;45:662–4.

Matthews MK. Nonarteritic anterior ischemic optic neuropathy. Curr Opin Ophthalmol. 2005;16:341–5.

Menzel-Severing J, Siekmann U, Weinberger A, Roessler G, Walter P, Mazinani B. Early hyperbaric oxygen treatment for nonarteritic central retinal artery occlusion. Am J Ophthalmol. 2012;153:454–9.

Mervin K, Valter K, Maslim J, Lewis G, Fisher S, Stone J. Limiting photoreceptor death and deconstruction during experimental retinal detachment: the value of oxygen supplementation. Am J Ophthalmol. 1999;128:155–64.

Miller EF. Effect of breathing 100% oxygen upon visual fields and visual acuity. J Aviation Med. 1958;29:598–602.

Mills MD, Devenyi RG, Lam WC, Berger AR, Beijer CD, Lam SR. An assessment of intraocular pressure rise in patients with gas-filled eyes during simulated air flight. Ophthalmology. 2001;108:40.

Miyake Y, Awaya S, Takahashi H, Tomita N, Hirano K. Hyperbaric oxygen and acetazolamide improve visual acuity in patients with cystoid macular edema by different mechanisms. Arch Ophthalmol. 1993;111:1605–6.

Miyake Y, Horiguchi M, Matsuura M, et al. Hyperbaric oxygen therapy in 72 eyes with retinal arterial occlusion. In: Bove AA, Bachrach AJ, Greenbaum LJ, editors. Ninth International Symposium on Underwater and Hyperbaric physiology. Bethesda: Undersea and Hyperbaric Medical Society; 1987. p. 949–53.

Miyamoto H, Ogura Y, Honda Y. Hyperbaric oxygen treatment for macular edema after retinal vein occlusion – fluorescein angiographic findings and visual prognosis. Nippon Ganka Gakkai Zasshi. 1995;99:220–5.

Miyamoto H, Ogura Y, Wakano Y, Honda Y. The long term results of hyperbaric oxygen treatment for macular edema with retinal vein occlusion. Nippon Ganka Gakkai Zasshi. 1993;97:1065–9.

Mohamed Q, McIntosh RL, Saw SM, Wong TY. Interventions for central retinal vein occlusion. Ophthalmology. 2007;114:507–19.

Mori K, Ohta K, Nagano S, Toshinori M, Yago T, Ichinose Y. A case of ophthalmic artery obstruction following autologous fat injection in the glabellar area. Nippon Ganka Gakkai Zasshi. 2007;111:22–5.

Murdock TJ, Kushner BJ. Anterior segment ischemia after surgery on 2 vertical rectus muscles augmented with lateral fixation sutures. J AAPOS. 2001;5:323–4.

Murphy-Lavoie H, Butler FK, Hagan C. Arterial insufficiencies: central retinal artery occlusion. In: Hyperbaric oxygen therapy indications, 13th edn. Best Publishing, Undersea and Hyperbaric Medical Society, 2014.

Murphy-Lavoie H, Butler FK, Hagan C. Central retinal artery occlusion treated with oxygen: a literature review and treatment algorithm. UHM. 2012;39:934–53.

Murphy-Lavoie H, Harch P, VanMeter K. Effect of hyperbaric oxygen on central retinal artery occlusion. Australia: UHMS Scientific Assembly; 2004.

Nauck M, Karakiulakis S, Perruchoud A, Papakonstantinou E, Roth M. Corticosteroids inhibit the expression of the vascular endothelial growth factor gene in human vascular smooth muscle cells. Eur J Pharmacol. 1998a;341:309–15.

Nauck M, Roth M, Tamm M, Eickelberg O, Eickelberg O, Wieland H, Stulz P, et al. Induction of vascular endothelial growth factor by platelet-activating factor and platelet-derived growth factor is downregulated by corticosteroids. Am J Resp Cell Mol Biol. 1998b;16:398–406.

Neubauer AS, Mueller AJ, Schriever S, Grüterich M, Ulbig M, Kampik A. Minimally invasive therapy for clinically complete central retinal artery occlusion-results and meta-analysis of literature. Klin Monatsbl Augenheilkd. 2000;217:30–6.

Newman NJ, Scherer R, Langenberg P, Kelman S, Feldon S, Kaufman D, et al. Ischemic Optic Neuropathy Decompression Trial Study Group. Am J Ophthalmol. 2002;134:317–28.

Newman WD, Frank HJ. Pyoderma gangrenosa of the orbit. Eye. 1993;7:89–94.

Nichols CW, Lambertsen CJ, Clark JM. Transient unilateral loss of vision associated with oxygen at high pressure. Arch Ophthalmol. 1969;81:548–52.

Noell WK. Effect of high and low oxygen tension on the visual system. In: Schaeffer KE, editor. Environmental effects on consciousness. New York: Macmillan; 1962. p. 3–18.

Ogura Y, Kiryu J, Takahashi K, Honda Y. Visual improvement in diabetic macular edema by hyperbaric oxygen treatment. Nippon Ganka Gakkai Zasshi. 1988;92:1456–60.

Ogura Y, Takahashi M, Ueno S, Honda Y. Hyperbaric oxygen treatment for chronic cystoid macular edema after branch retinal vein occlusion. Am J Ophthalmol. 1987;104:301–2.

Oguz H, Sobaci G. The use of hyperbaric oxygen therapy in ophthalmology. Surv Ophthalmol. 2008;53:112–20.

Okinami S, Nihira M, Iwaki M, et al. Hyperbaric oxygen therapy for cystoid macular edema in uveitis. Jpn J Clin Ophthalmol. 1992;46:199–201.

Olver JM, Spalton DJ, McCartney ACE. Microvasculature study of the retrolaminar optic nerve in man: the possible significance in anterior ischemic optic neuropathy. Eye. 1990;4:7–24.

Osterloh MD, Charles S. Surgical decompression of branch retinal vein occlusions. Arch Ophthalmol. 1988;106:1469–71.

Ozkiris A, Evereklioglu C, Erkilic K, Ilhan O. The efficacy of intravitreal triamcinolone acetonide on macular edema in branch retinal vein occlusion. Eur J Ophthalmol. 2005;15:96–101.

Pallota R, Anceschi S, Costagliola N, et al. Recovery from blindness through hyperbaric oxygen in a case of thrombosis on the central retinal artery. Ann Med Nav. 1978;83:591–2.

Palmquist BM, Philipson B, Barr PO. Nuclear cataract and myopia during hyperbaric oxygen therapy. Br J Ophthalmol. 1984;68:113–7.

Palmquist BM. Ophthalmological effects of hyperbaric oxygen therapy in the elderly. Geriatr Med Today. 1986;5:135–7.

Park CH, Jaffe GJ, Fekrat S. Intravitreal triamcinolone acetonide in eyes with cystoid macular edema associated with retinal vein occlusion. Am J Ophthalmol. 2003;136:419–25.

Patz A. Effect of oxygen on immature retinal vessels. Invest Ophthalmol. 1965;4:988–99.

Patz A. Oxygen inhalation in retinal arterial occlusion. Am J Ophthalmol. 1955;40:789–95.

Perkins SA, Magargal LE, Augsburger JJ, Sanborn GE. The idling retina: reversible visual loss in central retinal artery obstruction. Ann Ophthalmol. 1987;19:3–6.

Petterson JA, Hill MD, Demchuk AM, Morrish W, Hudon ME, Hu W, et al. Intra-arterial thrombolysis for retinal artery occlusion: The Calgary experience. Can J Neurol Sci. 2005;32:507–11.

Pfister RR. The intraocular changes of anterior segment necrosis. Eye. 1991;5:214–21.

Pfoff DS, Thom SR. Preliminary report on the effect of hyperbaric oxygen on cystoid macular edema. J Cataract Refract Surg. 1987;13:136–40.

Phillips D, Diaz C, Atwell G, et al. Care of sudden blindness: A case report of acute central retinal artery occlusion reversed with hyperbaric oxygen therapy. Undersea Hyperbaric Med 1999;26(supp): 23–24 (abstract).

Phillpotts BA, Sanders RJ, Shields JA, Griffiths JD, Augsburger JA, Shields CL. Uveal melanomas in black patients: A case series and comparative review. J Natl Med Assoc. 1995;87:709–14.

Polk JD, Rugaber C, Kohn G, Arenstein R, Fallon Jr WF. Central retinal artery occlusion by proxy: a cause for sudden blindness in an airline passenger. Aviat Space Environ Med. 2002;73:385.

Polkinghorne PJ, Bird AC, Cross MR. Retinal vessel construction under hyperbaric conditions. Lancet. 1989;2:1099.

Polse KA, Mandell RB. Etiology of corneal striae accompanying hydrogel lens wear. Invest Ophthalmol. 1976;15:553–6.

Popova ZS, Kuz'minov OD. Treatment of primary open-angle glaucoma by the method of combined use of hyperbaric oxygenation and antioxidants. Vestn Oftalmol. 1996;112:4–6.

Quinlan PM, Elman MJ, Bhatt AK, Mardesich P, Enger C. The natural course of central retinal vein occlusion. Am J Ophthalmol. 1990;110:118–23.

Rabena MD, Pieramici DJ, Castellarin AA, Nasir MA, Avery RL. Intravitreal bevacizumab (Avastin) in the treatment of macular edema secondary to branch retinal vein occlusion. Retina. 2007;27:419–25.

Recupero SM, Cruciani F, Picardo V, Sposato PA, Tamanti N, Abdolrahimzadeh S. Hyperbaric oxygen therapy in the treatment of secondary keratoendotheliosis. Ann Opthalmol. 1992;24:448–52.

Regillo C, Chang TS, Johnson MW, et al. Retina and vitreous: American Academy of Ophthalmology Basic and Clinical Science Course—Section 12. San Francisco: American Academy of Ophthalmology; 2007.

Resch H, Zawinka C, Weigert G, Schmetterer L, Garhöfer G. Inhaled carbon monoxide increases retinal and choroidal blood flow in healthy humans. Invest Ophthalmol Vis Sci. 2005;46:4275–80.

Ricci B, Calogero G, Lepore D. Variations in the severity of retinopathy seen in newborn rats supplemented with oxygen under different conditions of hyperbarism. Exp Eye Res. 1989;49:789–97.

Ricci B, Minicucci G, Manfredi A. Oxygen-induced retinopathy in the newborn rat: effects of hyperbarism and topical administration of timolol maleate. Graefes Arch Clin Exp Ophthalmol. 1995;233: 226–30.

Ros MA, Magargal LE, Uram M. Branch retinal artery obstruction: a review of 201 eyes. Ann Ophthalmol. 1989;21:103–7.

Rosenfeld PJ, Fung AE, Puliafito CA. Optical coherence tomography findings after an intravitreal injection of bevacizumab (avastin) for macular edema from central retinal vein occlusion. Ophthalmic Surg Lasers Imaging. 2005;36:336–9.

Ross ME, Yolton DP, Yolton RL, Fauci A, Collier B, Titus J. Myopia associated with hyperbaric oxygen therapy. Optom Vis Sci. 1996;73:487–94.

Roy M, Bartow W, Ambrus J, Fauci A, Collier B, Titus J. Retinal leakage in retinal vein occlusion: reduction after hyperbaric oxygen. Ophthalmologica. 1989;198:78–83.

Saltzman HA, Hart L, Sieker HO, Duffy EJ. Retinal vascular response to hyperbaric oxygenation. JAMA. 1965;191:114–6.

Sasaki K, Fukuda M, Otani S, Yajima M, Bando M, Gotoh Y, et al. High pressure oxygen therapy in ocular diseases: with special reference to the effect of concomitantly used stellate ganglion block. Jpn J Anesth. 1978;27:170–6.

Saunders RA, Bluestein EC, Wilson ME, Berland JE. Anterior segment ischemia after strabismus surgery. Surv Ophthalmol. 1994;38: 456–66.

Schaal KB, Hoh AE, Scheuerle A, Schütt F, Dithmar S. Bevacizumab for the treatment of macular edema secondary to retinal vein occlusion. Ophthalmologe. 2007;104:285–9.

Sebban A, Hirst LW. Pterygium recurrence rate at the Princess Alexandra Hospital. Aust N Z J Ophthalmol. 1991;19:203–6.

Shahid H, Hossain P, Amoaku WM. The management of retinal vein occlusion: is interventional ophthalmology the way forward? Br J Ophthalmol. 2006;90:627–39.

Shields CL, Naseripour M, Cater J, Shields JA, Demirci H, Youseff A, et al. Plaque radiotherapy for large posterior uveal melanomas 8 mm thick) in 354 consecutive patients. Ophthalmology. 2002;109: 1838–49.

Shields CL, Shields JA, Milite J, De Potter P, Sabbagh R, Menduke H. Uveal melanoma in teenagers and children. A report of 40 cases. Ophthalmology. 1991;98:1662–6.

Skogstad M, Bast-Pettersen R, Tynes T, Bjørnsen D, Aaserud O. Treatment with hyperbaric oxygen. Illustrated by the treatment of a patient with retinitis pigmentosa. Tidsskr Nor Laegeforen. 1994;114:2480–3.

Spandau UH, Ihioff AK, Jonas JB. Intravitreal bevacizumab treatment of macular edema due to central retinal vein occlusion. Acta Ophthlamol Scand. 2006;84:555–6.

Stanford MR. Retinopathy after irradiation and hyperbaric oxygen. J R Soc Med. 1984;77:1041–3.

Stone R, Zink H, Klingele T, Burde R. Visual recovery after central retinal artery occlusion: Two cases. Ann Ophthalmol. 1977;9:445–50.

Suttorp-Schulten MS, Riemslag FC, Rothova A, van der Kley AJ, Riemslag FC. Long-term effect of repeated hyperbaric oxygen therapy on visual acuity in inflammatory cystold macular oedema. Br J Ophthalmol. 1997;81:329.

Swaby K, Valderrama O, Schiffman J. Treatment of disc edema and retinal artery occlusion with HBO during the third trimester of pregnancy. UHMS Annual Scientific Assembly: Las Vegas; 2005 (Abstract).

Szuki H, Inie J, Horiuchi T. Hyperbaric oxygenation therapy in ophthalmology. Part I: Incipient insufficiency of the retinal circulation. J Clin Ophthalmol. 1980;34:335–43.

Takahashi K, Shima T, Yamamuro M. Hyperbaric oxygenation following stellate ganglion block in patients with retinal occlusion. In: Smith G, editor. Proceedings of the 6th international congress on hyperbaric medicine. Aberdeen: University of Aberdeen Press; 1977. p. 211–5.

Tamura H, Miyamoto K, Kiryu J, Miyahara S, Katsuta H, Hirose F, et al. Intravitreal injection of corticosteroid attenuates leukostasis and vascular leakage in experimental diabetic retina. Ophthalmol Vis Sci. 2005;46:1440–4.

Tang WM, Han DP. A study of surgical approaches to retinal vascular occlusions. Arch Ophthalmol. 2000;118:138–43.

Telander G, Hielseil G, Schwartz S. Diagnostic and therapeutic challenges. Retina. 2011;31:1726–31.

Terry TL. Extreme prematurity and fibroblastic overgrowth of persistent vascular sheath behind each crystalline lens: a preliminary report. Am J Ophthalmol. 1942;25:203.

The Central Vein Occlusion Study Group M Report. Evaluation of grid pattern photocoagulation for macular edema in central vein occlusion. Ophthalmology. 1995;102:1425–33.

The Central Retinal Vein Occlusion Study Group. Natural history and clinical management of central retinal vein occlusion. Arch Ophthalmol. 1997;115:486–91.

Thom SR, Clark JM. The toxicity of oxygen, carbon monoxide, and carbon dioxide. In: Bove AA, Davis JC, editors. Diving medicine. Philadelphia: WB Saunders; 1997. p. 131–45.

Tranos PG, Wickremasinghe SS, Stangoes NT, Topouzis F, Tsinopoulos I, Pavesio CE. Macular edema. Surv Ophthalmol. 2004;49:470–90.

Ubels JL, Hoffert JR. Ocular oxygen toxicity: the effect of hyperbaric oxygen on retinal Na+-K+ ATPase. Exp Eye Res. 1981;32:77–84.

Vingolo EM, Pelaia P, Forte R, Rocco M, Giusti C, Rispoli E. Does hyperbaric oxygen (HBO) delivery rescue retinal photoreceptors in retinitis pigmentosa? Doc Ophthalmol. 1999;97:33–9.

Vinores SA, Youssri AI, Luna JD, Chen YS, Bhargave S, Vinores MA, et al. Upregulation of vascular endothelial growth factor in ischemic and non-ischemic human and experimental retinal disease. Histol Histopathol. 1997;12:99–109.

Vitullo V, Venuti P, Di Marzio GE, et al. HBO and corneal pathology: clinical evaluations. In EUBS 87, Proceedings of the 13th annual meeting of the European Undersea Biomedical Society, Palermo, Italy, Sept 9–12, 1987. p. 296–300.

Vucetic M, Jensen PK, Jansen EC. Diameter variations of retinal blood vessels during and after treatment with hyperbaric oxygen. Br J Ophthalmol. 2004;88:771–5.

Wallyn CR, Jampol LM, Goldberg MF, Zanetti CL. The use of hyperbaric oxygen therapy in the treatment of sickle cell hyphema. Invest Ophthalmol Vis Sci. 1985;26:1155–8.

Weber J, Remonda L, Mattle HP, Koerner U, Baumgartner RW, Sturzenegger M, et al. Selective intra-arterial fibrinolysis of acute central retinal artery occlusion. Stroke. 1998;29:2076–9.

Weinberger AWA, Siekmann UPF, Wolf S, Rossaint R, Kirchhof B, Schrage NF. Treatment of acute central retinal artery occlusion (CRAO) by hyperbaric oxygenation therapy (HBO)—a pilot study with 21 patients. Klin Monatsbl Augenheilkd. 2002;219:728–34.

Weiss J. Hyperbaric oxygen treatment of nonacute central retinal artery occlusion. UHM. 2009;36(6):401–5.

Weizer JS, Stinnett SS, Fekrat S. Radial optic neurotomy as treatment for central retinal vein occlusion. Am J Ophthalmol. 2003;136:814–9.

Wells M, Forooozan R. Transient visual loss may anticipate occipital infarction from hemodialysis. Am J Kidney Dis. 2004;43:29–33.

Williamson TH, O'Donnell A. Intravitreal triamcinolone acetonide for cystoid macular edema in non-ischemic central retinal vein occlusion. Am J Ophthalmol. 2005;139:860–6.

Winstanley J. Treatment of neo-vascularization with oxygen at high pressure. Br J Ophthalmol. 1963;47:542–6.

Wolff RS, Wirtschafter D, Adkinson C. Ocular quinine toxicity treated with hyperbaric oxygen. Undersea Hyperbaric Med. 1997;24:131–4.

Wright JK, Franklin B, Zant E. Clinical case report: treatment of a central retinal vein occlusion with hyperbaric oxygen. Undersea Hyperb Med. 2007;34:315–9.

Xu YN, Huang JG. Hyperbaric oxygen treatment for cystoid macular edema secondary to retinal vein occlusion. Chung Hua Yen Ko Tsa Chih. 1991;27:216–8.

Yamamoto K, Tsujikawa A, Hangai M, et al. Neovascular glaucoma after branch retinal artery occlusion. Jpn J Ophthalmol. 2005;49:388–90.

Yotsukura J, Adachi-Usami E. Correlation of electroretinographic changes with visual prognosis in central retinal artery occlusion. Ophthalmologica. 1993;207:13–8.

Yu DY, Cringle SJ, Yu PK, Su EN. Intraretinal oxygen distribution and consumption during retinal artery occlusion and graded hyperoxic ventilation in the rat. Invest Ophthalmol Vis Sci. 2007;48:2290–6.

Yu DY, Cringle SJ. Retinal degeneration and local oxygen metabolism. Exp Eye Res. 2005;80:745–51.

Yuzurihara D, Ijima H. Visual outcome in central retinal and branch retinal artery occlusion. Jpn J Ophthalmol. 2004;48:490–2.

Zhang XZ, Cao JQ. Observations on therapeutic results in 80 cases of central serous retinopathy treated with hyperbaric oxygenation. Presented at the 5th Chinese conference on hyperbaric medicine, Fuzhow, China, Sept 26–29, 1986.

Hyperbaric Oxygenation in Obstetrics and Gynecology

K.K. Jain

Abstract

This chapter deals with the role of HBO in obstetrics and gynecology. The applications are very limited in the USA and Western Europe, and most of the work has been done in Russia. HBO has been used for threatened abortion, fetal hypoxia, toxemias of pregnancy, and diabetes in pregnant women. The use of HBO during pregnancy has been shown to be safe. HBO can be used for medical disorders during pregnancy such as diabetes and carbon monoxide poisoning. Applications in gynecology are somewhat limited. Animal experimental studies show the potential application of HBO in treatment of endometriosis. Clinical studies indicate its usefulness as an adjunct in the management of infertility.

Keywords

Carbon monoxide poisoning • Diabetes • Fetal hypoxia • HBO and congenital malformations • HBO and IVF • HBO in gynecology • HBO in obstetrics • Hyperbaric oxygen (HBO) • Neonatology • Threatened abortion • Toxemias of pregnancy

Introduction

Careful consideration must be given to use of hyperbaric oxygenation (HBO) during pregnancy. Pregnant women can benefit from HBO treatment of obstetrical disorders and associated medical conditions. There is no evidence that pregnancy is a contraindication for HBO treatment of the mother but some concern has been expressed about effects on the fetus and possible congenital malformations.

HBO and Risk of Congenital Malformations

Grote and Wanger (1973) exposed pregnant rabbits on the 9th day of gestation to oxygen pressures of 1.5 or 2 ATA for 5 h. The mother rabbits were sacrificed on the 29th day. Fetuses were removed and uteri studied for resorption, and the evidence showed increases in the resorption rate and number of congenital malformations.

Bimes et al. (1973) exposed pregnant rabbits daily to HBO (2 ATA) for periods of 1–2 h. On the 27th day or the 30th day of pregnancy, cesarean sections were performed. The weight of all fetuses was found to be about half normal. The brain was the only organ not affected consistently. The dimensions of the long bones were reduced, particularly at the diaphysis. Glycogenic and lipid overload and delay of endochondral ossification of long bones were observed.

Yusa (1981) studied the effect of oxygen on chromosomes in bone marrow. No aberration was noted in chromosomes as a result of exposure to normobaric oxygen, but significant abnormalities (breakage and gap) were noted in mice exposed to HBO at 3–4 ATA. Malformations (umbilical hernia and abnormalities of the coccyx) were noted in some newborns when the mother was exposed to HBO at 2.5 ATA for 2 h on the 5th and 8th days of gestation and in all the newborns of animals exposed to HBO daily.

In a controlled experimental study, pregnant Fischer rats were exposed to HBO at 3.2 and 4.2 ATA (90 min daily) for 5 days (Sapunar et al. 1993). The embryos in the HBO group

K.K. Jain, MD, FRACS, FFPM (✉)
1 Blaesiring 7, Basel 4057, Switzerland
e-mail: jain@pharmabiotech.ch

© Springer International Publishing AG 2017
K.K. Jain, *Textbook of Hyperbaric Medicine*, DOI 10.1007/978-3-319-47140-2_33

did not show any congenital malformations but showed reduced weight as compared with sham-treated control animals.

Pregnant mothers with CO poisoning are now treated with HBO, and one of the aims of this treatment is to prevent damage to the fetal brain from CO exposure. A prospective single-center cohort study spanning 25 years (1983–2008) included all pregnant women living in the Nord-Pas-de-Calais region of France who received HBO for CO poisoning and who gave birth to a living child (Wattel et al. 2013). Psychomotor development of children was monitored up to the age of 6 years. No significant differences in psychomotor or height/weight criteria were found between the exposed children and unexposed controls. No malformations were reported. These findings support the use of HBO therapy during pregnancy. No specific follow-up of the children is necessary if their neonatal status is normal.

Role of HBO in Obstetrics

Experimental Studies

Maillot et al. (1979) tested HBO therapy in a placental insufficiency model in the rat. HBO was used at 2.5 ATA for 2 h and resulted in definite improvement.

Chaika et al. (1981) studied the effect of HBO on the functional state of the hypothalamo-hypophysio-adrenal system (HHAS) in pregnant rats and their fetuses under conditions of experimentally induced chronic hypoxia. The HHAS was found to react actively to pregnancy, to hypoxia of the mother as well as of the fetus, and to HBO action. Hypoxia during pregnancy led to deficiency of corticosteroids, which caused intense discharge of hypothalamic corticotropin and subsequent activation of the adenohypophyseal adrenocorticotropic hormone according to the feedback principle. The functional state of the HHAS varied in pregnant rats with experimental myocardial dystrophy treated by means of HBO at pressures of 3, 2, and 1 ATA.

Morin et al. (1988) exposed pregnant ewes to 100 % oxygen at 3 ATA for 20 min. This exposure increased the pulmonary oxygen tension in the fetuses from 20 ± 1 to 54 ± 9 mmHg. It increased pulmonary blood flow from the fetal to the newborn values from 31 ± 3 to 295 ± 20 mL/kg/min. Pulmonary arterial pressure did not change during hyperoxygenation.

Clinical Applications

Various conditions in which HBO has been used in pregnant women are listed in Table 33.1. Part of this list is based on practice in Russia as there is very limited use of HBO in obstetrical disorders in the Western countries.

Threatened Abortion

HBO was employed alone and in combination with drugs acting on the hypothalamo-hypophysio-ovarian system by Pobedinsky et al. (1981) in 158 women with threatened abortion and fetoplacental insufficiency. They were able to prolong the pregnancy.

Electrophoretic properties of syntrophoblast proteins are distinctly altered under conditions of fetoplacental insufficiency of endocrine origin. HBO treatments can prevent the impairment of the membrane protein composition.

Fetal Hypoxia

A cesarean section has been performed in a hyperbaric chamber (2 ATA) on a comatose female who developed generalized convulsions; death was thought to be imminent (Ledingham et al. 1968). Fetal distress was rapidly relieved at 2 ATA with the mother breathing 100 % oxygen via an endotracheal tube. Despite inspired oxygen concentration of 1500 mmHg, the arterial oxygen tension was only 430 mmHg and the uterus remained cyanosed. However, a healthy female infant with an Apgar score of 9 was delivered. Aksenova et al. (1981) used HBO for prevention of fetal hypoxia and hypotrophy in 230 pregnant women (70 with heart disease, 70 with nephropathy, 70 with fetoplacental

Table 33.1 Conditions in which HBO has been used during pregnancy

Obstetric disorders
Threatened abortion
Fetal hypoxia
Toxemias of pregnancy
Late gestation
Medical disorders complicating pregnancy
Diabetes
Heart disease
Carbon monoxide poisoning
Air embolism
Status epilepticus

insufficiency, 10 with anemia, and 10 with hypertension). HBO was used at 1.5–1.8 ATA for 40–50 min per session, and 10–12 sessions were given in the second and third trimesters of pregnancy; 120 women with similar pathology were managed without HBO and served as controls. Signs of hypoxia and hypotrophy abated or disappeared, and the condition of newborn children in the experimental group was much better than that of those in the control group.

Korobova et al. (1981) pointed out that a high content of histamine in the blood of pregnant diabetic women may play an important role in the pathogenesis of circulatory hypoxia jeopardizing the fetal life due to hypoxia. They gave HBO at 1.2–1.6 ATA for 45 min. After an initial rise, the histamine value dropped to 37 % of the original level after the seventh HBO session. This fall coincided with a considerable improvement in the patient's condition.

Toxemias of Pregnancy

Drel et al. (1981) used HBO to treat 92 pregnant women suffering from nephropathy of stages I–III. The nephropathy improved along with improvement of catecholamine metabolism.

Use of HBO for Medical Conditions in Pregnancy

Roman et al. (2002) reported the first case of a pregnant woman presenting with a paradoxical air embolism due to accidental removal of a central venous catheter. Secondary right hemiplegia associated with a confused state justified emergency HBO therapy, which was followed by complete neurological recovery. The authors assess risk situations of gas embolism during pregnancy and puerperium, as well as indications and fetal effects of hyperbaric oxygen therapy.

Acute Carbon Monoxide Poisoning During Pregnancy

If indicated, HBO can be used for the treatment of a pregnant mother (see Chap. 12). Abboud et al. (2001) reported two cases of moderate maternal poisoning during the third trimester of pregnancy. They underwent HBO therapy at 2.5 ATA for 90 min and were delivered at term. In one case the newborn presented an antenatal ischemic cerebral lesion probably due to carbon monoxide poisoning.

Review of English language publications in MEDLINE from 1971 to 2010 revealed 19 case reports of CO poisoning during pregnancy described in varying levels of detail (Friedman et al. 2015). Diagnosis in most cases was made based on initial history and physical evaluation as well as assessment of environmental CO levels as presenting car-

boxyhemoglobin levels may be poor indicators of severity of disease. HBO therapy should be used in cases of significant maternal exposure to CO. Treatment requires a longer duration for fetal CO elimination than in the nonpregnant patients.

Diabetes

Zhdanov et al. (1981) treated pregnant women with diabetes by means of HBO at 1.4–1.8 ATA. Three to four courses, each consisting of 6–10 sessions of 45–60 min, were given during the pregnancy. There was a general improvement of the condition with normalization of blood glucose and a decrease in the levels of xanthine and guanine; the rise of the latter was a characteristic of hypoxia. Control of diabetes was achieved in 92 % of cases, and all the patients progressed to full-term pregnancies and gave birth at 37–38 weeks of gestation.

Management of Pregnancy and Delivery in Women with Heart Disease

HBO has been used extensively in Russia for the management of pregnant women with congenital as well as acquired heart disease. Molzhaninov et al. (1981) used HBO in the management of 170 pregnant women with heart disease, and labor was conducted under HBO (1.5–2 ATA). The hypoxic condition of the mother as well as the fetus was counteracted in each case, and no complications were reported.

Vanina et al. (1981) used HBO during labor in 54 patients with cardiopulmonary pathology. In 28 women the delivery was vaginal, and in 26 cases cesarean section was performed. The indication for HBO was arterial hypoxia, that is, pO_2 below 70 mmHg. Pressure of 2 ATA was used. Two women died as a result of complications of cardiac disease. Three infants died, one as a result of multiple congenital anomalies and two due to prematurity. The rest were discharged home in good condition. Vanina et al. (1977) observed labor in a patient with acute myocardial infarction in the 32nd week of pregnancy. Successful delivery by cesarean section under 3 ATA of HBO was performed at the 36th–37th week of pregnancy.

Applications of HBO in Neonatology

Various techniques of oxygen administration to infants have been described elsewhere (Jain 1989). The role of HBO in neonatology based on clinical experience is described in Chap. 34. Some historical aspects and basic studies are summarized in this section. Raising the ambient oxygen concentration can raise the paO2 of premature infants by ~8.9 mmHg (Cartlidge and Rutter 1988). Transdermal oxygen can supplement oxygen delivery to premature infants with poor pulmonary gas exchange, but the absorption is not adequate in full-term infants. The first report in the English language literature on the use of HBO in neonates was published in 1963 (Hutchinson et al. 1963). These authors resuscitated apneic newborns by means of HBO (1–3 ATA) at 2–38 min after birth. The effects were described as dramatic, with improvement of skin color and of cardiovascular as well as respiratory function. A criticism of this approach was that in the neonate, the lung alveoli are not fully open and oxygen would not diffuse through the lungs. The possibility of absorption of oxygen through the skin and the mucous membranes of the respiratory tract was considered, but such absorption may not be adequate.

Direct access to an infant may be difficult in a monoplace hyperbaric chamber. Infants should be treated in a multiplace chamber with all the facilities of modern pediatric intensive care, including intubation and controlled ventilation. Intubation and ventilation with pulsed high-dose oxygen, to rapidly establish normal tissue oxygen values in the brain and cause vasoconstriction, may well prove to be the key factor in the control of periventricular hemorrhage in neonates, where the high water content inevitably poses a barrier to oxygen diffusion. Inclusion of HBO in intensive care of asphyxic infants reduces the post-hypoxic sequelae. HBO is useful for resuscitation in respiratory failure, for cranial birth injuries, and for hemolytic disease of the newborn.

HBO in Gynecology

The use of HBO in gynecology is still limited. Most of the work is experimental in animal models of diseases.

Animal Experimental Studies

Endometriosis is a painful disorder in which tissue that normally lines the inside of the uterus—the endometrium—grows outside the uterus most commonly involving the ovaries, bowel, or the tissue lining of the pelvis. It is a challenge in treatment. A prospective, randomized controlled animal study was designed to determine the effects of HBO on surgically induced endometriosis in a rat model (Aydin et al. 2011). The study group was exposed to daily 2 h HBO treatment for 6 weeks. At the end of the study, laparotomy showed that the mean volume of the endometriotic implants in the study group was significantly lower than that of the control group. The mean histopathological and immunohistochemical scores of the endometriotic implants and the TNF-α levels were significantly lower in the study group than in the control group. HBO treatment for 2 h a day for 6 weeks resulted in significant remission of endometriosis in rats.

Clinical Applications in Gynecology

There are few indications of HBO in gynecology that are in line with applications in disorders of other systems. For example, HBO can be used as an adjunct to the management of postoperative infections in gynecology. One promising application is an adjunct to treatment of infertility.

HBO for Selection of Treatment for Infertility

Implantation of ovum usually occurs only if the endometrium has reached a certain stage of vascularization and development. A prospective pilot study of HBO as an adjunct to in vitro fertilization (IVF) therapy in women with a poor prognosis for pregnancy concluded that HBO is well tolerated by women undergoing IVF treatment and that further study is required to determine whether this is an effective adjuvant therapy for women being treated by IVF (Van Voorhis et al. 2005).

Endometrial Doppler sonography can be used to predict the occurrence of pregnancy in natural or stimulated cycles. A randomized study has evaluated endometrial development, i.e., endometrial thickness and perfusion, after HBO (Mitrović et al. 2006). Women were treated in multiplace HAUX chamber during 70 min at pressure of 2.3 ATA for 7 days consecutively starting on day 5 of menstrual cycle. Effects of HBO were evaluated by transvaginal color Doppler sonography which was continuously used starting from day 8 of menstrual cycle until the ovulation in the cycles when the therapy was applied, 1 month before and 1 month after the therapy. Folliculometry in the cycles when HBO was applied indicated an excellent response of endometrium in thickness as well as desirable quality. Doppler flowmetry of the uterine arteries indicated that the uterine blood vessel resistance was slightly higher than expected. Mapping of endometrial blood vessels in the cycles covered by HBO showed the intensive capillary network of endometrium with low resistance. HBO will thus improve the outcome of pregnancy implantation by improving endometrial receptivity.

Conclusion

The potential of HBO in obstetrics is exciting. The results of the large number of deliveries conducted in the hyperbaric chamber in Russia indicate the safety of this technique. Caution should be exercised in the introduction of HBO in resuscitation of newborn infants. The role of HBO in disorders of pregnancy needs to be verified thoroughly by controlled studies. Medical conditions affecting pregnant women can be treated safely with HBO. An important example is CO poisoning. HBO is also used in gynecology with limited potential applications as adjunct to the management of infertility.

References

Abboud P, Mansour G, Lebrun JM, Zejli A, Bock S, Lepori M, et al. Acute carbon monoxide poisoning during pregnancy: 2 cases with different neonatal outcome. J Gynecol Obstet Biol Reprod (Paris). 2001;30:708–11.

Aksenova TA, Ezbov LS, Titchenko LI, et al. Hyperbaric oxygen in prevention and treatment of fetal hypoxia and hypotrophy. In: Yefuny SN, editor. Proceedings of the 7th international congress on Hyperbaric medicine. Moscow: USSR Academy of Sciences; 1981. p. 361.

Aydin Y, Atis A, Uludag S, Tezer I, Sakiz D, Acar H, et al. Remission of endometriosis by hyperbaric oxygen treatment in rats. Reprod Sci. 2011;18:941–7.

Bimes C, Guilhem A, Mansat A, et al. Modifications staturales et pondérales des foetus nés de lapines soumises à l'oxygène hyperbare durant la gestation. Bull Assoc Anat. 1973;57:443–56.

Cartlidge PH, Rutter N. Percutaneous oxygen delivery to the premature infant. Lancet. 1988;1:315.

Chaika VA, Elsky VN, Borodin AD. The effect of hyperbaric oxygen on the functional state of HHAS in pregnant rats and their fetuses. In: Yefuny SN, editor. Proceedings of the 7th international congress on hyperbaric medicine. Moscow: USSR Academy of Sciences; 1981. p. 369.

Drel IK, Molzhaninov EV, Samsonenko RA. Effect of hyperbaric oxygenation on catecholamine metabolism in the placenta in late toxemia of pregnancy. Akush Ginekol (Mosk) 1981:16–29.

Friedman P, Guo XM, Stiller RJ, Laifer SA. Carbon monoxide exposure during pregnancy. Obstet Gynecol Surv. 2015;70:705–12.

Grote W, Wanger WD. Malformations in rabbit embryos after hyperbaric oxygenation. Klin Wochenschr. 1973;51(5):248–2250.

Hutchinson JH, Ker MM, Williams KG, Hopkinson WI. Hyperbaric oxygen in the resuscitation of the newborn. Lancet. 1963;2:1019–22.

Jain KK. Oxygen in Physiology and Medicine. IL:Charles C. Thomas: Springfield; 1989.

Korobova LN, Kabakhbaseheva IK, Khodakova AA, et al. Dynamics of histamine in the blood of pregnant women receiving hyperbaric therapy for diabetes mellitus. In: Yefuny SN, editor. Proceedings of the 7th international congress for hyperbaric medicine. Moscow: USSR Academy of Sciences; 1981. p. 362.

Ledingham IM, McBride TI, Jennett WB, Adams JH. Fatal brain damage associated with cardiomyopathy of pregnancy, with notes on Caesarean section in a hyperbaric chamber. Br Med J. 1968;4:285–7.

Maillot K, Brather R, Deeg KH. Plazenta-Insuffizienz und intermittierende hyperbare Oxygenation. Ein Tierversuchsmodell Arch Gynecol. 1979;228:223–4.

Mitrović A, Nikolić B, Dragojević S, Brkić P, Ljubić A, Jovanović T. Hyperbaric oxygenation as a possible therapy of choice for infertility treatment. Bosn J Basic Med Sci. 2006;6:21–4.

Molzhaninov EV, Chaika VK, Domanova AI, et al. Experiences and prospects of using hyperbaric oxygen in obstetrics. In: Yefuny SN, editor. Proceedings of the 7th international congress on hyperbaric medicine. Moscow: USSR Academy of Sciences; 1981. p. 360.

Morin FC, Egan EA, Norfleet WT. Indomethacin does not diminish the pulmonary vascular response of the fetus to increased oxygen tension. Pediatr Res. 1988;24:696–700.

Pobedinsky ANM, Proshina IV, Fanchenko ND. Hyperbaric oxygenation in treating disorders of the reproductive function in women. In: Yefuny SN: Proceedings of the 7th international congress on hyperbaric medicine. USSR Academy of Sciences, 1981, Moscow, 359.

Roman H, Saint-Hillier S, Dick Harms J, Duquenoy A, Barau G, Verspyck E, et al. Gas embolism and hyperbaric oxygen treatment during pregnancy: a case report and a review of the literature. J Gynecol Obstet Biol Reprod (Paris). 2002;31:663–7.

Sapunar D, Saraga-Babic M, Peruzovic M, Marusić M. Effects of hyperbaric oxygen on rat embryos. Biol Neonate. 1993;63:360–9.

Van Voorhis BJ, Greensmith JE, Dokras A, Sparks AE, Simmons ST, Syrop CH. Hyperbaric oxygen and ovarian follicular stimulation for in vitro fertilization: a pilot study. Fertil Steril. 2005;83:226–8.

Vanina LV, Efuni SN, Beilin AL, Giorgobiani TN, Rodionov VV. Labour in patient with acute myocardial infarction under hyperbaric oxygenation. Anesteziol Reanimatol. 1977;5:72–6.

Vanina LV, Efuni SN, Beilin AL, et al. Obstetrics aid under conditions of hyperbaric oxygenation. In: Yefuny SN, editor. Proceedings of the 7th international congress on hyperbaric medicine. Moscow: USSR Academy of Sciences; 1981. p. 358.

Wattel F, Mathieu D, Mathieu-Nolf M. A 25-year study (1983-2008) of children's health outcomes after hyperbaric oxygen therapy for carbon monoxide poisoning in utero. Bull Acad Natl Med. 2013;197:677–94; discussion 695–7.

Yusa T. Chromosomal and teratogenic effects of oxygen in the mouse. Br J Anaesth. 1981;53:505–10.

Zhdanov GG, Rymashevsky VK, Khabakhleashevy K, et al. Hyperbaric oxygen therapy in pregnant women with diabetes mellitus. In: Yefuny SN, editor. Proceedings of the 7th international congress on hyperbaric medicine. Moscow: USSR Academy of Sciences; 1981. p. 360.

E. Cuauhtémoc Sánchez-Rodríguez

Acute neonatal hypoxia is so common and devastating that a small difference in salvaged tissue may make a big difference in quality of life.

Modified from V. Hachinski

Abstract

Objective: To describe the value of HBO in the acute management of neonatal hypoxia (hypoxic–ischemic encephalopathy) and necrotizing enterocolitis.

Materials and methods: Neonates with hypoxic–ischemic encephalopathy (HIE) and necrotizing enterocolitis were treated in a Sechrist monoplace chamber. Electroencephalograms, evoked potential, ophthalmic evaluation, ultrasound, lab exams, and X-rays were obtained before and after HBO. The treatment protocol was 1.8–2.0 atm abs/45 min. Preventive myringotomies were conducted in all patients. A follow-up was done at 3 and 6 months.

Results: Patients were ventilator dependent and required Ambu ventilation by a neonatologist during the treatment. All showed a resolution after HBO. There was also a dramatic improvement ($p < 0.05$) in hemoglobin, hematocrit, total proteins, serum sodium, triglycerides, and pH. There were favorable changes in all other studies, although they did not meet statistical significance. There was a marked reduction of the morbidity and mortality. No CNS or ophthalmic side effects were detected.

Conclusion: When used promptly, HBO can modify the local and systemic inflammatory response caused by intestinal inflammation and cerebral or systemic hypoxia. It helps preserve the marginal tissue and recover the ischemic and metabolic penumbra. This pilot study suggests that HBO could be a safe and effective treatment in the acute management of neonatal necrotizing enterocolitis or hypoxic–ischemic encephalopathy. There is a need for a prospective, randomized, controlled, and double-blinded study to determine the real use of HBO in these cases.

Keywords

Neonates • Necrotizing enterocolitis • Hypoxic–ischemic encephalopathy • Hyperbaric oxygenation

Introduction

The use of hyperbaric oxygenation (HBO) is well accepted in adults within the approved conditions by the Undersea and Hyperbaric Medical Society (UHMS) (Gessell 2008). Historically, there has been certain resistance to treat pediatric and neonatal patients inside a hyperbaric chamber. Nevertheless, there have been published reports since the early 1960s (Hutchinson and Kerr 1963; Hutchison et al. 1964). In the last 50 years, there were several anecdotal publications; by 1981 the former USSR had already published reports of 1868 neonatal patients treated with HBO (Beryland 1981; Pilinoga 1981; Kiselev 1981; Bayboradov 1981; Babyboradov and Dodkhoev 1981; James 1988; Vazquez and Spahr 1990). In the last decade, a meta-analysis was published (Liu et al. 2006). Lately, there have been more publications on basic and clinical research of HBO for central nervous system (CNS) lesions (Barrett et al. 2004; Bennett et al. 2005; Calvert and Cahill 2007; Davidson et al. 2012; Jacobson et al. 2005; Küppers-Tiedt et al. 2011; Liu et al. 2006; McCormick et al. 2011; Namazi 2008; Nemoto

E.C. Sánchez-Rodríguez, MD, MSc, MPH (✉)
Department of Hyperbaric Medicine, Agustín O'Horan, SSY,
Mérida, Yucatán 97000, Mexico
e-mail: cuau57@hotmail.com

© Springer International Publishing AG 2017
K.K. Jain, *Textbook of Hyperbaric Medicine*, DOI 10.1007/978-3-319-47140-2_34

and Betterman 2007; Niatsetskaya et al. 2012; Nicholls and Budd 2000; Penittilia and Trump 1974; Rockswold et al. 2006; Rockswold et al. 2007; Rossignol et al. 2012; Sánchez 2007; Sánchez et al. 2003, 2004, 2005a, b; Sánchez and Elizondo, 2009; Smith et al. 2012). The experience has proven that it is a safe treatment that has the same low side effects in the adult and pediatric populations (Sánchez et al. 2002, 2003, 2005a, b). Nevertheless, specific areas require special attention (Rossignol et al. 2012). The management of neonates in hyperbaric chambers needs special equipment and trained personnel (Sánchez et al. 2002, 2005a, b).

The incidence of mortality and morbidity due to neonatal hypoxic–ischemic encephalopathy (HIE) has not been substantially modified in the last 40 years. It is estimated that close to 25 % of the neonatal deaths and 8 % of all deaths at 5 years of age throughout the world each year are associated with signs of asphyxia at birth (Lawn et al. 2005; Gonzalez de Dios and Moya 1996). Death or moderate to severe disability can occur in 50–60 % of infants diagnosed as having moderate to severe HIE (Lawn et al. 2005b; Bryce et al. 2005).

Hypoxic–Ischemic Encephalopathy of the Newborn

HIE is such a devastating pathology that any gain, no matter how little, can make a great difference in the quality of life of these children and their families. The prompt treatment should be orientated to restore adequate perfusion and correct the metabolic or cellular alterations. The amount of damage depends on the duration, extension, localization, and metabolic changes of the lesion. Few of the tested early neuroprotectors have made a real difference. Hypothermia is one of them, but it has many and frequent side effects (Shakaran et al. 2005).

When there is an interruption of the cerebral blood flow or oxygen supply to the central nervous system (CNS), several changes occur depending on the degree of hypoxia; this could be reversible or irreversible (Penittilia and Trump 1974). The reversibility depends on the ability of the mitochondrial to maintain ATP production. Once it stops, there is a dysfunction of the ion pumps (Na–K and K–Ca) that eventually will create cytotoxic edema. When the mitochondrial dysfunction is severe, calcium is freed into the cytoplasm. Calcium then becomes the first inflammatory mediator (Davidson et al. 2012; Carbonell 2007).

The principal pathophysiology of the HIE is the cellular energy failure, loss of cellular ion homeostasis, acidosis, increase of cellular calcium, excitatory toxicity, and damage by reactive oxygen species (ROS) (Carbonell 2007; Nicholls and Budd 2000; Smith et al. 2012). Other factors involved are activation of a calcium protease that promotes the conversion of xanthine dehydrogenase into xanthine oxidase, enzyme that is responsible for the production of ROS during the primary

reperfusion phase of the ischemia–reperfusion injury (IRI) (Ali-Wali et al. 2005; Rockswold et al. 2006; Sakuma et al. 2012). Activation of the phospholipase A2 cascade through the lipoxygenase and cyclooxygenase will enhance the production of prostaglandins, thromboxanes, and leukotrienes (Adibhatla et al. 2003; Muralikrishna Adibhatla and Hatcher 2006). Activation of nuclear transcription factor kappa B (NFkB) is responsible for the production of many pro-inflammatory cytokines (IL-1, IL-6, IL-8, TNFα, IFNγ, PAF) and also of anti-inflammatory cytokines (IL-10). NFkB may be the central event for the development of multi-organ failure (MOF), sepsis, and ischemia–reperfusion injury (IR) (Li et al. 2013; Nicholls et al. 2007; Pan et al. 2013; Schwaninger et al. 2006; Yang et al. 2010; Zeng et al. 2012a).

During the CNS energy crisis, there is an increased production of glutamate. There is also promotion of the production of neural (nNOS) and inducible (iNOS) nitric oxide synthase, which participate in the systemic inflammatory response syndrome (SIRS) and shock (Li et al. 2013; Pan et al. 2013).

The endothelium is an important organ in the inflammatory response. Hypoxia and hypoglycemia stimulate the expression of endothelial adhesion molecules (selectins, VCAM, and ICAM) (Blum et al. 2006; Kunz et al. 2012; Supanc et al. 2011; Wang et al. 2006) and that of neutrophils (integrin β_2) (Caimi et al. 2001). In the latter phase (reperfusion) of the IR, the expression of endothelial and neutrophil adhesion molecules is responsible for the migration of neutrophils into the affected areas. Ischemia–reperfusion injury may be the pathophysiology of all acute injuries in the first 72 h, including IHE (Caimi et al. 2001; Wang et al. 2006). Thus, it appears that maintaining adequate perfusion and the cellular metabolic needs may be the cornerstone to reduce CNS damage and promote early neuroprotection (Hermann et al. 2013).

Uses of Hyperbaric Oxygenation in Hypoxic–Ischemic Encephalopathy and Necrotizing Enterocolitis of the Neonate

Hyperoxygenation promotes the viability of marginal tissue (penumbra) (Calzia et al. 2010; McCormick et al. 2011). It is an accepted treatment for several IRIs and could be an efficient early neuroprotector for the neonatal HIE and NE, with very few side effects (Sánchez 2007).

In HIE, HBO reduces the fall of cellular ATP, phosphocreatine kinase, and uridine, thus maintaining aerobic metabolism in the tissue (Haapanemi et al. 1995; Sun et al. 2011); reduces the liberation of calcium and the activation of phospholipase A_2, thus preventing the production of leukotrienes, thromboxanes, and prostaglandins (Cheng et al. 2011; Gois et al. 2012; Smith et al. 2012; Zeng et al. 2012b); and blocks the nuclear transcription factor NFkB and prevents the production of inflammatory cytokine and of inducible nitric oxide synthase (iNOS) (Sakoda et al. 2004; Weisz et al. 1997).

HBO prevents the conversion of xanthine dehydrogenase to xanthine oxidase and the production of reactive oxygen species (ROS), which reduces endothelial damage, thus preventing loss of intravascular fluid into the interstitial tissue (Sánchez 2007). It also prevents the expression of intracellular adhesion molecules (ICAM-1) and neutrophil integrin β2, reducing the late phase of IR (Buras 2000; Buras and Reenstra 2007; Jones et al. 2010; Khiabani et al. 2008; Tsai et al. 2005; Thom 1993); it is both a local and systemic effect (Godman et al. 2010a).

HBO modifies apoptosis by the elevation of the BCL-2 system and heme oxygenase 1 (HO-1) and by enhancing the production of heat shock proteins (70, 72, and 90). It also reduces the expression of Nogo A, NG-R, and RhoA systems and of hypoxia-induced factor (HIF-1α) (Calvert et al. 2002; Godman et al. 2010b; Rothfuss and Speit 2002a, b; Shyu et al. 2004; Wada et al. 2000; Zhou et al. 2003).

In the case of NE, HBO, besides increasing the oxygen tension in the intestine, blocking NFkB, cytokines, NO, thromboxanes, and leukotrienes, also blocks platelet activation factor (PAF), which is a key inflammatory mediator. It also helps the sepsis and shock effects by blocking iNOS (Caplan and MacKendrick 1994; Claud 2009). Lately, HBO has proven to modify the expression of miRNA (Peng et al. 2014).

We must stress here that the beneficial effects of HBO in NE and HIE are not only obtained by the restoration of oxygen at the tissue and cellular levels but also through very important antioxidant effects. The antioxidant response to HBO might be as important as the oxygenation effects of HBO, especially in the ischemia–reperfusion injury (IR). There is a very thin "balance" between the beneficial effects caused by oxygenation and the damage caused by and excessive production of ROS (oxidative damage). The small oxidative stress caused by HBO appears to have a beneficiary antioxidant effect, as long as the patient's antioxidant capability is functional. HBO promotes the production of glutathione (most important nonenzymatic antioxidant defense) (Sánchez

2007) and also of antioxidant enzymes (SOD, catalase, and peroxidase) (Philip 2012; Tan et al. 2013; Visser et al. 2012). The antioxidant protective effect of HBO starts after the first hour of treatment and is maintained up to 72 h of the last one. It is also known that preconditioning with HBO can prevent IR (Visser et al. 2012; Philip 2012).

Use of Hyperbaric Oxygenation in Neonates

HBO use in neonates was almost completely discontinued after Hutchinson's and the USRR's experiences. We developed a pilot study for HIE and NE. Presently, the largest experience was published by China (Shi et al. 2003). The justification for the use of HBO in neonates was the little modification in morbidity and mortality rates in the last four decades and the increasing published experience of its possible effects as an early neuroprotector. The mayor controversy was the possible side effects of HBO, especially neonatal retinopathy (Sánchez 2013).

It is recommended that neonates treated with HBO should be older than 34.5 and weight above 1.2 kg. Younger neonates with lower weight have a higher possibility of developing complications due to prematurity by itself. The most important would be pulmonary and retinopathy (Bhaskaran et al. 2012; Speer 2011). In the USSR they only treated term neonates reducing the possibility of HBO side effects related to prematurity.

Normally, HIE is more frequent in neonates with Apgar score below 3 at 1 min and below 5 at 5 min of life, when the resuscitation efforts last longer than 8 min and when the pH is lower than 7.2. Neonates with these conditions will require management in a neonatal intensive care unit (NICU). Normally they will present cerebral edema at 4 h and convulsions at 6 h, thus aggravating their already critical cerebral condition (Ferrari et al. 2010; Thornton et al. 1998; Zhang 2002).

The evaluation of neonates with HIE should include electroencephalogram (EEG), visual and auditory evoked potential (EP), transfontanel Doppler, fundoscopic evaluation, and laboratory tests. The test should be repeated 4 h after the first HBO treatment and after 24 h (Table 34.1).

Table 34.1 HBO protocol for neonates

Gestation > 34.5 weeks of pregnancy	EEG
Weight > 1.2 kg	ECG
Resuscitation > 8 min	Evoked potentials
Apgar < 3 at 1 min and < 5 at 5 min	Transfontanel US
pH < 7.2	Funduscopic study
Availability of NICU care inside chamber	Labs
HBO < 6 h of delivery	Transcutaneous oxygen and/or BIS
HBO 1.8–2.0 ATA / 45 min (20 min O_2 + 5 min air + 20 min O_2)	

The HBO treatment should start as early as possible, the sooner the better. It should be within the first 6 h to guarantee better results. Nevertheless, if there is a good coordination between the neonatologist and the hyperbaric oxygen department, the treatment can start once the patient has been stabilized (first hour). The standard of care inside the hyperbaric chamber requires an inside attendant (neonatologist) and should be the same as in the NICU.

There are several special considerations for the treatment of a neonate patient inside a hyperbaric chamber. One of the main problems Hutchinson encountered was the lack of appropriate neonatal medical equipment for hyperbaric use. This has not changed in the last 40 years. There is no neonatal hyperbaric ventilator, although there is a manufacturer that has a hyperbaric ventilator and a neonatal one, but does not see a market for a neonatal hyperbaric ventilator. Also, there are no hyperbaric IV pumps available that can deliver the reduced flows needed by neonatal patients (½ mL per hour) (Sánchez 2013).

To cope with these technical deficiencies, we trained a neonatologist to go inside the hyperbaric chamber and ventilate the patient with an Ambu bag. To deal with the low IV volumes required, we had to turn on and off the IV pump to be able to deliver the required IV flow. The patient was monitored with ECG and with a transcutaneous oxygen monitor (TCOM). TCOM is used routinely for our ICU patients treated inside the hyperbaric chamber, because it is very sensitive for any changes in patient's ventilation. A bispectral index monitor (BIS) can be used to monitor frontal EEG during HBO treatment; it also helps in evaluating patient's sedation and can be a useful tool to detect early abnormal EEG activity related to oxygen toxicity to the CNS.

We developed a transfer protocol in coordination with the NICU and the hyperbaric department, to refer the patient as soon as possible (<4 h). The treatment profile is 2.0 atm absolute for 45 min (20 min oxygen, 5 min air brake, 20 min oxygen), QD or BID. The air brake was included to reduce the pulmonary oxygen side effects of HBO. To avoid hypothermia, the chamber linen was warmed to 40 °C in water vapor. The recommended pressurizing and depressurizing rate was 1 psi per minute. We performed myringotomies before starting the treatment. The patient was monitored during the entire procedure. All of our patients (six the HIE and two with NE) were ventilated and dependent of cardiotonic medication. The range of delay to treatment after resuscitation was 28 min to 24 h.

Results

During the HBO treatments, the neonates were very stable and actually required a reduction in the dose of cardiotonic medication. All the patients were extubated and required no further cardiotonic medication within the next 6 h after the HBO therapy. There was a dramatic change in the overall general condition of the patients, especially in their vital signs and skin coloration. After the HBO treatment, the patient was then transferred back to NICU, according to our protocol.

In the NE patients, sepsis and DIC disappeared after the first treatment. One patient that was referred late (24 h) required two HBO treatments but developed pulmonary toxicity that was successfully resolved with inhaled steroids and surfactant (Survanta).

In the IAE, there was complete resolution of the cerebral edema measured by transfontanel Doppler. The disorganization, suppression, and flat line showed a marked improvement in the EEG and recovery of EP after the treatment. There were no signs of CNS oxygen toxicity. There were no modifications in the fundoscopic examination, and the pre and post lab values are posted in Table 34.2. There were no cases of hypothermia during the treatment.

At the 3- and 6-month follow-up, all the patients had a normal neurological exam, and there was no regression in

Table 34.2 Laboratory studies pre- and post-HBO in neonates

Test	Basal	Control	P value
Hemoglobin	14.1 ± 1.47	16.2 ± 0.29[a]	0.02
Hematocrit	42.48 ± 4	47.86 ± 2[a]	0.05
Total proteins	4.94 ± 0.92	5.6 ± 4.1[a]	0.05
Sodium	1332.2 ± 8.31	141.2 ± 3.56[a]	0.04
Triglycerides	108 ± 60	88.4 ± 47[a]	0.03
pH	7.3 ± 0.35	7.39 ± 0.03[a]	0.05
Neutrophils	62.6 ± 17.42	60.8 ± 14.68[a]	0.81
TP	37.78 ± 22.85	27.62 ± 17.8	0.19
TPT	69.7 ± 26.48	48.3 ± 15.9[a]	0.22
TT	85 ± 48.6	67.2 ± 45.38	0.08
Fibrinogen	370 ± 108	317 ± 107[a]	0.13
Creatinine	2.36 ± 1.83	1.64 ± 1.25	0.20

[a]Normal reference values

the patients' status. We were able to conduct a 5-year follow-up in 2 patients of HIE: one was normal and the other had a slight attention deficit.

Discussion

HBO is an accepted treatment for several conditions including ischemia–reperfusion injuries. The use of HBO in neurological conditions is growing by the day.

Hypoxic–ischemic encephalopathy and necrotizing enterocolitis in neonates are devastating lesions; its morbidity and mortality have not been modified significantly in the last 40 years (Lawn et al. 2005a, b; Bryce et al. 2005). Any beneficial effects in salvaged tissue will make a great difference in the quality of life of patients, their families, and society. There is no treatment that has shown definitive early neuroprotection. Lately there have been several reports on hypothermia and its beneficial effects (Gluckman et al. 2005). Nevertheless, it has not been able to show a statistical significant effect. HBO has shown beneficial effects on IR, including the CNS (Bozok et al. 2012; Caldeira et al. 2013; Daniel et al. 2011; Ramalho et al. 2012; Thom 2011; Zhao et al. 2011). It could be an effective treatment for neonatal HIE and NE.

Pediatric patients are no different than adults, nevertheless, neonates are. We do not recommend HBO treatment in neonates before 34.5 weeks of pregnancy and below 1.2 kg of weight. The fear of oxygen toxicity in neonates has hindered its use in neonates.

In general, term neonates have a good antioxidant defenses, but younger than 34.5 weeks of pregnancy and 1.2 kg of weight may be at risk due to their immature antioxidant defense system (Table 34.2). Although neonatologists have great concern with respect of premature retinopathy, there are several publications that refer to it as an IR (it occurs after long exposures to oxygen at FiO_2 of 0.45 or higher and only after oxygen is discontinued). HBO seams to protect them, instead of suffering side effects from it (Calvert et al. 2004; Ricci and Calogero 1988; Ricci et al. 1989, 1995).

Special care should be taken during treatment to avoid hypothermia and oxygen toxicity, especially pulmonary, in the neonates with risk factors for bronchodysplasia and/or hyaline membrane. Pulmonary surfactant should be readily available in the event the patient presents pulmonary oxygen toxicity.

CNS oxygen toxicity is also a possibility that should be taken in account when treating neonates. The use of BIS could show early signs of it and could be promptly and adequately treated. No other types of hyperbaric oxygen toxicity have been reported so far in neonates (Sánchez 2013).

In our experience and in the one conducted in China, HBO appears to be a safe and very cost-effective treatment for the HIE and NE of the neonate (Liu et al. 2006; Sánchez 2013; Zhou et al. 2008). It promotes survival of marginal tissue (pen-

umbra), reduces cerebral edema, restores the mitochondrial dysfunction, brakes the vicious cycle of edema–hypoxia–edema, and improves microcirculation. It also enhances healing, promotes upregulation of growth factors, and reduces, inhibits, or prevents IR. It reduces sepsis and shock mediated by iNOS. Besides the beneficial effects caused by cellular and tissue oxygenation, it also has a very important antioxidant and anti-apoptotic effect (Sánchez 2007; 2013). HBO reduces neurologic sequelae and mortality, in a very significant way (Liu et al. 2006).

If we can overcome the fear of treating neonates inside a hyperbaric chamber, develop better and adequate equipment for the management of these patients during HBO, and produce a multicenter, multinational, prospective, randomized, and controlled study, HBO will undoubtedly show its beneficial effects in hypoxic–ischemic encephalopathy and necrotizing enterocolitis of the newborn. This would modify dramatically the morbidity and mortality of the newborn and could reduce the burden of disease and become a very cost-effective treatment.

References

Adibhatla RM, Hatcher JF, Dempsev RJ. Phospholipase A2, hydroxyl radicals, and lipid peroxidation in transient cerebral ischemia. Antioxid Redox Signal. 2003;5(5):647–54.

Ali-Wali NS, Butler GJ, Beale J, Abdullah MS, Hamilton RW, Lee BY, et al. Hyperbaric oxygen in the treatment of patients with cerebral stroke, brain trauma, and neurologic disease. Adv Ther. 2005; 22(6):659–78.

Barrett KF, Masel B, Petterson J, Scheibel RS, Corson KP, Mader JT. Regional CBF in chronic stable TBI treated with hyperbaric oxygen. Undersea Hyperb Med. 2004;31(4):395–406.

Bayboradov BD. Some features of the use of hyperbaric oxygenation to treat acute respiratory insufficiency in newborn children. In: Proceedings of VIIth International Congress on Hyperbaric Medicine, editor. Petrovsky BV, Yefuni SN. USSR Academy of Sciences 1981, pp. 99–305.

Bennett MH, Wasiak J, Schnabel A, Kranke P, French C. Hyperbaric oxygen therapy for acute ischaemic stroke. Cochrane Database Syst Rev. 2005;20(3), CD004954.

Beryland W. Hyperbaric oxygenation as a supporting procedure and treatment of respiratory insufficiency in neonates. In: Petrovsky BV, Yefuni SN, eds. Proceedings of VIIth International Congress on Hyperbaric Medicine. USSR Academy of Sciences 1981:289–291.

Bhaskaran M, Xi D, Wang Y, Huang C, Narasaraju T, Shu W, et al. Identification of microRNAs changed in the neonatal lungs in response to hyperoxia exposure. Physiol Genomics. 2012;44(20):970–80.

Blum A, Khazim K, Merei M, Peleg A, Blum N, Vaispapir V. The stroke trial – can we predict clinical outcome of patients with ischemic stroke by measuring soluble cell adhesion molecules (CAM)? Eur Cytokines Netw. 2006;17(4):295–8.

Bozok S, Ilhan G, Yilmaz Y, Dökümcü Z, Tumkaya L, Karamustafa H, et al. Protective effects of hyperbaric oxygen and iloprost on ischemia/reperfusion-induced lung injury in a rabbit model. Eur J Med Res. 2012;17:14. doi:10.1186/2047-783X-17-14.

Bryce J, Boschi-Pinto C, Shibuya K, Black RE. WHO Child Heath Epidemiology Reference Group: WHO estimates of the causes of death in children. Lancet. 2005;365:1147–52.

Buras JA. HBO regulation of ICAM 1 in an edothelial cell model of ischemia/reperfusion injury. Am J Physiol Cell Physiol. 2000;278:C292–302.

Buras JA, Reenstra WR. Endothelial neutrophil interactions during ischemia and reperfusion injury: basic mechanisms of hyperbaric oxygen. Nuerol Res. 2007;29(2):127–31.

Caimi G, Canino B, Ferrara F, Montana M, Musso M, Porreto F, et al. Granulocyte integrins before and after activation in acute ischaemic stroke. J Neurol Sci. 2001;186(1-2):23–6.

Caldeira DE, Souza ME, Gomes MC, Picinato MA, Fina CF, Feres O, et al. Effects of hyperbaric oxygen (HBO) as preconditioning in liver of rats submitted to periodic liver ischemia/reperfusion. Acta Cir Bras. 2013;28 Suppl 1:66–71.

Calvert JW, Cahill J, Zhang JH. Hyperbaric oxygen and cerebral physiology. J Neurol Res. 2007;29(2):132–41.

Calvert JW, Yin W, Patel M, Badr A, Mychaskiw G, Parent AD, et al. Hyperbaric oxygenation prevented brain injury induced by hypoxia in a neonatal rat model. Brain Res. 2002;951(1):1–8.

Calvert JW, Zhou C, Zhang JH. Transient exposure of rat pups to hyperoxia at normobaric and hyperbaric pressure does not cause retinopathy of prematurity. Exp Neurol. 2004;189(1):150–61.

Calzia E, Asfar P, Hauser B, Matejovic M, Ballestra C, Radermacher P, et al. Hyperoxia may be beneficial. Crit Care Med. 2010;38(10 Suppl):S559–68.

Caplan MS, MacKendrick W. Inflammatory mediators and intestinal injury. Clin Perinat. 1994;21(2):235–46.

Carbonell T. Iron, oxidative stress and early neurological deterioration in ischemic stroke. Curr Med Chem. 2007;14(8):857–74.

Cheng O, Ostrowski RP, Wu B, Liu W, Cheng C, Zhang JH. Cyclooxygenase-2 mediates hyperbaric oxygen preconditioning in the rat model of transient global cerebral ischemia. Stroke. 2011;42(2):484–90.

Claud EC. Neonatal necrotizing enterocolitis-inflammation and intestinal immaturity. Antinflamm Antiallergy Agents Med Chem. 2009;8(3):248–59.

Daniel RA, Cardoso VK, Gois Jr E, Parra RS, Garcían SB, Rocha JJ, et al. Effect of hyperbaric oxygen on the intestinal ischemia reperfusion injury. Acta Cir Bras. 2011;26(6):463–9.

Davidson SM, Yellon DM, Murphy MP, Duchen MR. Slow calcium waves and redox changes precede mitochondrial permeability transition pore opening in the intact heart during hypoxia and reoxygenation. Cardiovasc Res. 2012;19(3):445–53.

Ferrari DC, Nesic O, Perez-Polo JR. Perspective on neonatal hypoxia/ischemia-induced edema formation. Neurochem Res. 2010;35(12):1957–65.

Gessell LB. Hyperbaric Oxygen Therapy Indications. Undersea and Hyperbaric Medical Society: Durham, NC; 2008.

Gluckman PD, Wyatt JS, Azzopardi D, Ballard R, Edwards AD, Ferriero DM, et al. Selective head cooling with mild systemic hypothermia after neonatal encephalopathy: multicenter randomized trial. Lancet. 2005;365:663–70.

Godman CA, Cheda KP, Hightower LE, Perdrizet G, Shin DG, Giardina C. Hyperbaric oxygen induces a cytoprotective and angiogénico response in human microvascular endothelial cells. Cell Stress Chaperones. 2010a;15(4):431–42.

Godman CA, Joshi R, Giardina C, Perdrizet G, Hightower LE. Hyperbaric oxygen treatment induces antioxidant gene expression. Ann N Y Acad Sci. 2010b;1197:178–83.

Gois Jr E, Daniel RA, Parra RS, Almeida AL, Rocha JJ, García SB, et al. Hyperbaric oxygen therapy reduces COX-2 expression in a dimethylhydrazine-induced rat model of colorectal carcinogenesis. Undersea Hyperb Med. 2012;39(3):693–8.

Gonzalez de Dios J, Moya M. Perinatal asphyxia, hypoxic-ischemic encephalopathy and neurological sequelae in full term newborns: an epidemiological study. Rev Neurol. 1996;24(131):812–9.

Haapanemi T, Sirsjo A, Nylander G, Larsson J. Hyperbaric oxygen attenuates glutathione depletion and improves metabolic restitution of post-ischemic skeletal muscle. Free Radic Res. 1995;31:91–101.

Hermann AG, Deighton RF, Le Bihan T, McCulloch MC, Searcy JL, Kerr LE, et al. Adaptive changes in the neuronal proteome: mitochondrial energy production, endoplasmic reticulum stress, and ribosomal dysfunction in the cellular response to metabolic stress. J Cereb Blood Flow Metab. 2013. doi:10.1038/jcfm.2012.204.

Hutchison JH, Kerr MM, Williams WG, Hopkinson WI. Hyperbaric oxygen in the resuscitation of the newborn. Lancet. 1963;2:1019–22.

Hutchison JH, Kerr MM, Williams WG, Hopkinson WI. Hyperbaric oxygen in resuscitation of the newborn. Lancet. 1964;2:691–2.

James PB. Hyperbaric oxygen in neonatal care. Lancet. 1988;764–765.

Jacobson J, Duchen MR, Hotherscall J, Clark JB, Heales SJ. Induction of mitochondrial oxidative stress in astrocytes by nitric oxide precedes disruption of energy metabolism. J Neurochem. 2005;95(2):388–95.

Jones SR, Carpin KM, Woodward SM, Khiabani KT, Stephenson LL, Wang WZ, et al. Plast Reconstr Surg. 2010;126(2):403–11.

Kiselev BO, Ageyenko VF, Merkulova YY. The use of HBO to treat hemolytic diseases in neonates. In: Petrovsky BV, Yefuni SN, eds. Proceedings of VIIth International Congress on Hyperbaric Medicine. USSR Academy of Sciences 1981:295–298.

Khiabani KT, Bellister SA, Skaggs SS, Stephenson LL, Nataraj C, Wang WZ, et al. Reperfusion-induced neutrophil CD18 polarization: effect of hyperbaric oxygen. J Surg Res. 2008;150(1):11–6.

Kunz AB, Kraus J, Young P, Reuss R, Wipfler P, Oschmann P, et al. Biomarkers of inflammation and endothelial dysfunction in stroke with and without sleep apnea. Cerebrovasc Dis. 2012;33(5):453–60.

Küppers-Tiedt L, Manaenko A, Michalski D, Guenther A, Hobohm C, Wagner A, et al. Combined systemic thrombolysis with alteplase and early hyperbaric oxygen therapy in experimental embolic stroke in rats: relationship to functional outcome and reduction of structural damage. Acta Neurochir Suppl. 2011;111:167–72.

Lawn JE, Cousens S, Zupan J. 4 million neonatal deaths: when? where? why? Lancet. 2005a;365(9462):891–900.

Lawn J, Shibuya K, Stein C. No cry at birth: global estimates of intrapartum stillbirths and intrapartum-related neonatal deaths. Bull World Heath Organ. 2005b;83:409–17.

Li G, Wang X, Huang LH, Wang Y, Hao JJ, Ge X, et al. Cytotoxic function of CD8+ Y lymphocytes isolated from patients with acute severe cerebral infarction: an assessment of stroke-induced immunosuppression. BMC Immunol. 2013;14:1. doi:10.1186/1471-2172-14-1.

Liu Z, Xiong T, Meads C. Clinical effectiveness of treatment with hyperbaric oxygen for neonatal hypoxic-ischemic encephalopathy: systematic review of Chinese literature. BMJ. 2006; 333(7564):374–82.

McCormick JG, Houle TT, Saltzman HA, Whaley RC, Roy RC. Treatment of acute stroke with hyperbaric oxygen: time window of efficacy. Undersea Hyperb Med. 2011;38(5):321–34.

Muralikrishna Adibhatla R, Hatcher JF. Phospholipase A2, reactive oxygen species, and lipid peroxidation in cerebral ischemia. Free Radical Biol Med. 2006;40(3):376–87.

Namazi H. Decreasing the expression of LFA-1 and ICAM-1 as the major mechanism for the protective effect of hyperbaric oxygen on ischemia-reperfusion injury. Microsurgery. 2008;28(4):300. doi:10.1002/micr.20479.

Nemoto EM, Betterman K. Basic physiology of hyperbaric oxygen in brain. Neurol Res. 2007;29(2):116–26.

Niatsetskaya ZV, Sosunov SA, Matsiukevich D, Utkina-Sosunova IV, Ratner VI, Starkov AA, et al. The oxygen free radical originating from mitochondrial complex 1 contributes to oxidative brain injury following hypoxia-ischemia in neonatal mice. J Neurosci. 2012;32(9):3235–44.

Nicholls DG, Budd SL. Mitochondria and neuronal survival. Physiol Rev. 2000;80(1):315–60.

Nicholls DG, Johnson-Cadwell L, Vesce S, Jekabsons M, Yadava N. Bioenergetics of mitochondria in cultured neurons and their role in glutamate excitotoxicity. J Neurosci Res. 2007;85(15):3206–12.

Pan JA, Fan Y, Gandhirajan RK, Madesh M, Zong WX. Hyperactivation of mammalian degenerin MDEG promotes caspase-8 activation and apoptosis. J Biol Chem. 2013;288(5):2952–63.

Penittilia A, Trump BF. The role of cellular membrane systems in shock. Science. 1974;185:277.

Peng HS, Liao MB, Zhang MY, Xie Y, Xu L, Zhang YJ, et al. Synergistic inhibitory effect of hyperbaric oxygen combined with sorafenib on hepatoma cells. PLoS One. 2014;9(6), e100814. doi:10.1371/journal.pone.0100814. eCollection 2014.

Philip AG. Bronchopulmonary dysplasia: then and now. Neonatology. 2012;102(1):1–8.

Pilinoga VG, Kondratenko VI, Timoshenko NA. The use of hyperbaric oxygenation in neonates with intracranial birth trauma. In: Petrovsky BV, Yefuni SN, eds. Proceedings of VIIth International Congress on Hyperbaric Medicine. USSR Academy of Sciences. 1981:22–294.

Ramalho RJ, de Oliveira PS, Cavaglieri RC, Medeiros PR, Filho DM, Poli-de-Figuereido LF, et al. Hyperbaric oxygen therapy induces kidney protection in an ischemia/reperfusión model in rats. Transplant Proc. 2012;44(8):233–6.

Ricci B, Calogero G. Oxygen induced retinopathy in newborn rats: effects of prolonged normobaric and hyperbaric oxygen supplementation. Pediatrics. 1988;82:193–8.

Ricci B, Calogero G, Lepore D. Variations in the severity of retinopathy seen in newborn rats supplemented with oxygen under different conditions of hyperbarism. Exp Eye Res. 1989;49:789–97.

Ricci B, Minucucci G, Manfredi A, Santo A. Oxygen-induced retinopathy in the newborn rat: effects of hyperbarism and topical administration of timolol maleate. Graefes Arch Clin Exp Opthalmol. 1995;233(4):226–30.

Rockswold GL, Quickel RR, Rockswold SB. Hypoxia and traumatic brain injury. J Neurosurg. 2006;104(1):170–1.

Rockswold SB, Rockswold GL, Delfillo A. Hyperbaric oxygen in traumatic brain injury. Neurol Res. 2007;29(2):167–71.

Rossignol DA, Bradstreet JJ, Van Dyke K, Schneider C, Freedenfeld SH, O'Hara N, et al. Hyperbaric oxygen therapy in autism spectrum disorders. Med Gas Res. 2012;2(1):16–28.

Rothfuss A, Speit G. Investigations on the mechanisms of hyperbaric oxygen (HBO)-induced adaptive protection against oxidative stress. Mutat Res. 2002a;508(1-2):157–65.

Rothfuss A, Speit G. Overexpression of heme oxygenase-1 (HO-1) in v79 cells results in increased resistance to hyperbaric oxygen (HBO)-induced DNA damage. Environ Mol Mutagen. 2002b;40(4):258–65.

Sakoda M, Ueno S, Kihara K, Arikawa K, Dogomori H, Nuruki K, et al. A potential role of hyperbaric oxygen exposure through intestinal nuclear factor-kappaB. Crit Care Med. 2004;32:1722–9.

Sakuma S, Kitamura T, Chihiro K, Kanami T, Sayaka N, Hamashima T, et al. All-trans arachidonic acid generates reactive oxygen species via xanthine dehydrogenase/oxidase interconversion in the rat liver cytosol. J Clin Biochem. 2012;51(1):55–60.

Sanchez EC. Hyperbaric oxygenation in peripheral nerve repair and regeneration. Neurol Res. 2007;29(2):184–98.

Sánchez EC. Use of hyperbaric oxygenation in neonatal patients: a pilot study. Crit Care Nurs Q. 2013;36(3):280–9.

Sánchez EC, Chávez A, Uribe R. Mitochondrial dysfunction: possible protective role of hyperbaric oxygenation. Undersea Hyperb Med 2005;32 (Abstract)

Sánchez EC, Chávez A, Uribe R. Pathophysiology of acute hypoxic brain injury: role of HBO as a neuroprotector. Undersea Hyperb Med 2005;32 (Abstract)

Sánchez EC, Elizondo C, Medina A, Nochetto M, Schmitz G. Emergency life saving use of high oxygen in neonates. Euro J Neurol. 2002;9 Suppl 2:243.

Sánchez EC, Schmitz G, Nochetto M, Medina A, Suarez A, Gómez D, et al. Hyperbaric oxygen therapy in the treatment of acute ischemic anoxic encephalopathies. Euro J Neurol. 2003;10 Suppl 1:223.

Sánchez EC, Suárez A, Gómez D, Uribe R, Medina A, Nochetto M, et al. Effect of hyperbaric oxygenation (HBO) in the management of subacute hypoxic encephalopathy: Report of a Case. Undersea Hyperb Med 2004;31 (Abstract)

Shi XY, Tang ZQ, Xiong B, Bao JX, Sun D, Zhang YQ, et al. Cerebral perfusion SPECT imaging for assessment of the effect of hyperbaric oxygen therapy on patients with postbrain injury neural status. Chin J Traumatol. 2003;6(6):346–9.

Schwaninger M, Inta I, Herrmann O. NF-kappaB signaling in cerebral ischemia. Biochem Soc Trans. 2006;34(6):1291–4.

Shakaran S, Laptook AR, Ehrenkranz RA, Tyson JE, McDonald SA, Donovan EF, et al. Whole-body hypothermia for neonates with hypoxic-ischemic encephalopathy. N Engl J Med. 2005;353:1574–84.

Shyu WC, Lin SZ, Saeki K, Kubosaki A, Matsumoto Y, Onodera T, et al. Hyperbaric oxygen enhances the expression of prion protein and heat shock protein 70 in a mouse neuroblastoma cell line. Cell Mol Neurobiol. 2004;24:257–68.

Smith RA, Hartley RC, Cocheme HM, Murphy MP. Mitochondrial pharmacology. Trends Pharmacol Sci. 2012;33(6):341–52.

Speer CP. Neonatal respiratory distress syndrome: an inflammatory disease. Neonatology. 2011;99(4):316–9.

Sun L, Strelow H, Miles G, Veltkamp R. Oxygen therapy improves energy metabolism in focal cerebral ischemia. Brain Res. 2011;1415:103–8.

Supanc V, Biloglav Z, Kes VB, Demarin V. Role of cell adhesion molecules in acute ischemic stroke. Ann Saudi Med. 2011;31(4):365–70.

Tan SM, Stefanovic N, Tan G, Wilkinson-Berka JL, de Haan JB. Lack of the antioxidant glutathione peroxidase-1 (GPx1) exacerbates retinopathy of prematurity in mice. Invest Ophthalmol Vis Sci. 2013;54(1):555–62.

Thom SR. Functional inhibition of leukocyte B_2 integrins by hyperbaric oxygen in carbon monoxide-mediated brain injury of the rats. Toxico Appl Pharmacol. 1993;123:248–56.

Thom SR. Hyperbaric oxygen: its mechanisms and efficacy. Plast Reconstr Surg. 2011;127 Suppl 1:131S–41. doi:10.1097/PRS.0b013e318fbe2bf.review.

Thornton JS, Ordidge RJ, Penrice J, Cady EB, Amess PN, Punwani S, et al. Temporal and anatomical cariations of brain water apparent diffusion coefficient in perinatal cerebral hypoxic-ischemic injury: relationships to cerebral energy metabolism. Magn Reson Med. 1998;39(6):920–7.

Tsai HM, Gao CJ, Li WX, Lin MT, Niu KC. Resuscitation from heatstroke by hyperbaric oxygen therapy. Crit Care Med. 2005;33:813–8.

Vazquez RL, Spahr RC. Hyperbaric oxygen use in neonates: a report of four patients. AJDC. 1990;144:1022–4.

Visser L, Singh R, Young M, Lewis H, McKerrow N. Guideline for the prevention, screening and treatment of retinopathy of prematurity (ROP). S Afr Med J. 2012;103(2):116–25.

Wada K, Miyasawa T, Nomura N, Yano A, Tsuzuki N, Nawashiro H, et al. Mn-SOD and BCL-2 expression after repeated hyperbaric oxygenation. Acta Neurochir Suppl. 2000;76:285–90.

Wang JY, Zhou DH, Li J, Zhang M, Deng J, Gao C, et al. Association of soluble intercellular adhesion molecule 1 with neurological deterioration of ischemic stroke: The Chongqing Stroke Study. Cerebrovasc Dis. 2006;21(1-2):67–73.

Weisz G, Lavy A, Adir Y, Melamed Y, Rubin D, Eidelman S, et al. Modification of in vivo and in vitro TNF-alpha, IL-1, an IL-6 secretion by circulating monocytes during hyperbaric oxygen treatment in patients with perianal Crohn's disease. J Clin Immunol. 1997;17(2):154–9.

Yang ZJ, Xie Y, Bosco GM, Chen C, Camporesi EM. Hyperbaric oxygenation alleviates MCAO-induced brain injury and reduces hydroxyl radical formation and glutamate release. Eur J Appl Physiol. 2010;108(3):513–22.

Zeng L, Liu J, Wang Y, Wang L, Weng S, Chen S, et al. Cocktail blood biomarkers: prediction of clinical outcomes in patients with acute ischemic stroke. Eur Neurol. 2012a;69(2):68–75.

Zeng Y, Xie K, Dong H, Zhang H, Wang F, Li Y, et al. Hyperbaric oxygen preconditioning protects cortical neurons against oxygen-glucose deprivation injury: role of peroxisome proliferator-activated receptor-gamma. Brain Res. 2012b;1452:140–50.

Zhang N. L H, Lu L. Pathogenic factors of convulsions in neonates with hypoxic-ischemic encephalopathy. Di Yi Jun Yi Da Xue Xue Bao. 2002;22(11):1039–41.

Zhao H, Zhang Q, Xue Y, Chen X, Haun RS. Effects of hyperbaric oxygen on the expression of claudins after cerebral ischemia-reperfusion in rats. Exp Brain Res. 2011;212(1):109–17.

Zhou C, Li Y, Nanda A, Zhang JH. HBO supresses Nogo-A, NG-R or RhoA expression in the cerebral cortex after global ischemia. Biochem Biophys Res Commun. 2003;309:368–76.

Zhou BY, Lu GJ, Huang YQ, Ye ZZ, Han YK. Efficacy of hyperbaric oxygen therapy under different pressures on neonatal hypoxic-ischemic encephalopathy. Zhongguo Dang Dai Er Ke Za Zhi. 2008;10(2):133–5.

K.K. Jain

Abstract

This chapter deals with role of HBO in the management of diseases that are common in the elderly. Some of these have been described in other chapters. Theories of aging are mentioned, particularly free radical theory and role of hypoxia, which is a rationale for use of HBO. Particular emphasis is placed on the aging brain and role of HBO in the management of neurological disorders where chronic ischemia/hypoxia plays a role. HBO has also been found useful for treating photoaging of the skin. There is no proof of effect of HBO in rejuvenation.

Keywords

Hyperbaric oxygenation (HBO) • Geriatrics • Aging and HBO • Rehabilitation in elderly • Aging brain • Vascular dementia • Photoaging of skin • Decline of mental function in aging

Introduction

Geriatrics has now become a recognized medical specialty as the number of elderly in Western societies has grown and the life span has continued to increase. The older population—persons 65 years or older—numbered 46.2 million in 2014 and represented 14.5 % of the US population, about 1 in every 7 Americans. The number of elderly will rise to over 70 million by 2030, and of these almost 10 million will be 85 years and older. By 2060, there will be about 98 million older persons in the US, more than twice their number in 2014.

Aging is not a disease but certain diseases are associated with aging. Hyperbaric oxygenation (HBO) has an important role to play in the practice of geriatric medicine, as many of the indications for the use of this therapy in various diseases that have already been discussed in other chapters of this book are more common in the elderly.

Physiology of Aging

Theories of Aging

Multiple factors, including the inborn aging process, genetic defects, and environmental agents, participate in the aging process, and sequence of changes with aging is shown in Fig. 35.1. There are >300 theories to explain the aging phenomenon. The most well-known of these states is that aging may be due to deleterious, irreversible changes produced by free radical reactions. This theory will be described here.

Free Radicals and Aging

The free radical theory of aging, postulated first by Harman in 1954, remains the most popular and widely tested theory of aging. It is based on the chemical nature and ubiquitous presence of free radicals. Despite the actions of antioxidant nutrients, some oxidative damage will occur, and accumulation of this damage throughout life is believed to be a major contributing factor to aging and disease. Oxidative stress and production of free radicals tend to increase with aging, whereas the body's natural antioxidant defenses decline.

The free radical theory of aging postulates that a single common process, modified by genetic and environmental factors, is responsible for the aging and death of all living

K.K. Jain, MD, FRACS, FFPM (✉)
1 Blaesiring 7, Basel 4057, Switzerland
e-mail: jain@pharmabiotech.ch

© Springer International Publishing AG 2017
K.K. Jain, *Textbook of Hyperbaric Medicine*, DOI 10.1007/978-3-319-47140-2_35

Fig. 35.1 Sequence of changes with aging

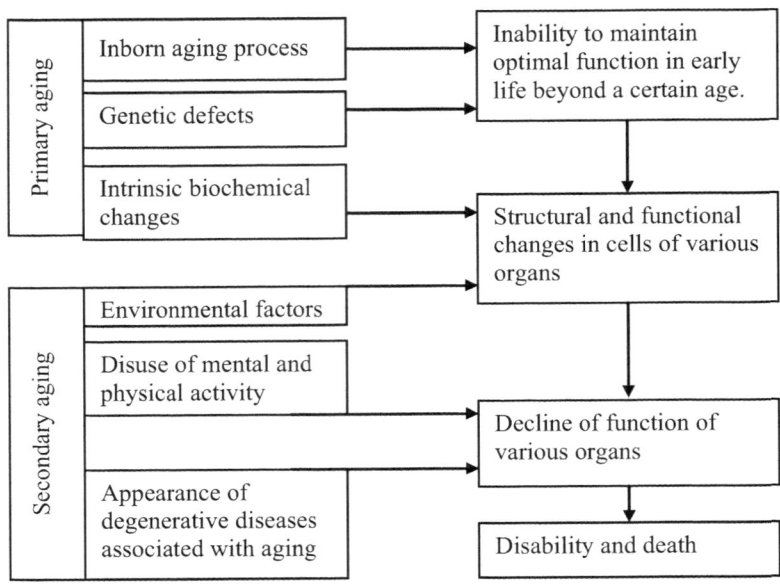

© JainPharmaBiotech

cells. The theory was extended in 1972 with the suggestion that life span was largely determined by the rate of free radical damage to the mitochondria (Harman 1999). This theory suggests the possibility that measures to decrease the rate of initiation or the chain length of free radicals may decrease the aging changes. Supporting evidence for the free radical theory of aging is as follows:

1. Studies on the origin of life and evolution indicate that free radical reactions were involved in these processes.
2. Studies of the effect of ionizing radiation on living things where the damage occurs through generation of free radicals.
3. Life span experiments in which endogenous free radical reactions were counteracted by dietary manipulations.
4. Studies on several organisms as diverse as yeast, the roundworm *Caenorhabditis elegans* and the fly *Drosophila melanogaster*, show a strong link between genetic defects in the body's oxidative stress response mechanisms and dramatic life span extensions.
5. Mammalian species with a higher rate of formation of mitochondrial superoxide radical have a shorter life span than species with a lower rate of formation of these radicals.
6. Studies that implicate free radical reactions in the pathogenesis of diseases such as atherosclerosis, Alzheimer's disease, and cancer which are more common in the elderly.

However, it is not known why free radical damage does not adversely affect certain cells such as gonadal germ cells. Although its appeal derives from a long-standing body of supporting correlative data, the free radical theory was more

rigorously tested only recently. Ongoing researches in the study of free radical biochemistry and the genetics of aging have been at the forefront of this work. Transgenic approaches in invertebrate models with candidate genes such as superoxide dismutase (SOD) involved in the detoxification of reactive oxygen species (ROS) have shown that the endogenous production of ROS due to normal physiologic processes is a major limiting factor for life span. Genes involved in ROS detoxification are highly conserved among eukaryotes; hence, the physiologic processes that limit life span in invertebrates are likely to be similar in higher eukaryotes.

The increased life span caused by certain mutations in the nematode *C. elegans* has been interpreted in terms of two metabolic theories of aging: the oxidative damage theory and the rate of living theory. New findings support the former, but not the latter interpretation. Some studies suggest that ROS generation is not the primary or initial cause of aging. ROS are closely associated with aging because they play a role in mediating a stress response to age-dependent damage, which suggests correlation between aging and ROS without implying that ROS damage is the earliest trigger or main cause of aging (Hekimi et al. 2011).

Hypoxia and Aging

Aging is also viewed as a manifestation of hypoxia. The acquisition and use of oxygen involve a series of steps, each subject to change with aging, as shown in Table 35.1.

The subject of hypoxia and aging has been discussed in detail by Jain (1989). Most studies of blood gas determinations have shown a linear regression of arterial pO_2 with aging. Blom et al. (1988) found that mean paO_2 was 95 mmHg (12.67 kPa) in those between the ages of 30 and 50. It dropped

Table 35.1 Effect of aging on the oxygen conductance system

Phase of the oxygen conductance system	Structure/functions reduced by aging
Ventilation of air	Thoracic compliance
	Lung compliance
	Vital capacity
	Maximum voluntary ventilation
	Closing volume
Diffusion of oxygen from bronchioles into alveolar sacs and across the alveolar membrane	Size of the alveolar sac
	Area of the alveolar membrane
Uptake of oxygen by blood flowing in the pulmonary capillaries	Pulmonary perfusion rate
	Ventilation/perfusion ratio
Delivery of oxygen to tissues	Tissue perfusion rate
	Tissue pO_2
Diffusion of the oxygen from the tissue capillary to the active cell	Decreased
Utilization/metabolism of oxygen in the cell	Intracellular enzyme systems

during successive decades until it was 77 mmHg (10.20 kPa) in those over the age of 70. The oxygen saturation, however, did not differ significantly in various age groups.

Changes in the Brain with Aging

A basic knowledge of changes in the brain structure and function with aging is important for understanding the neurological disorders of the elderly (Jain 2016). This is also important for designing strategies for management and rehabilitation.

Morphological Changes

The most striking change in the brain with age is a loss of volume and weight. The average weight of a newborn human brain is 350 g. It increases to 1400 g by the age of 20 years and declines to 1100 g by the age of 90. The reduction in brain weight occurs in the absence of disease and can be 5 % by the age of 70 years, 10 % by the age of 80 years, and 20 % by the age of 90 years. Most of the tissue loss takes place over the cerebral cortex, with more taking place over the frontal lobes and less over the parietal and temporal lobes and basal ganglia. The dentate nucleus shrinks by 29 %, whereas the brainstem has an insignificant loss of substance. With modern anatomical techniques, it is possible to determine the relative volume of gray and white matter of the brain. Atrophy involves mostly the gray matter, both cortical and subcortical. Cortical atrophy and ventricular enlargement indicating a loss of cerebral substance with advancing age have been shown on CT studies.

MRI studies show significant decreases in cross-sectional whole-brain, temporal lobe, and hippocampal volumes and a significant increase in ventricular volume with increasing age, with the most marked changes occurring after 70 years of age. Positive associations have been reported between general cognitive ability and estimated brain volume in youth and in measured brain volume in later life (Royle et al. 2013). These findings show that cognitive ability in youth is a strong predictor of estimated prior and measured current brain volume in old age.

The total number of neurons in the human cerebral cortex is ~10 billion, and it does not change with aging if pathologic processes are excluded. The decrease in brain size is counterbalanced by an increase in neuron density. Age-related loss of neurons is controversial. It is now generally accepted that there is widespread preservation of neuron numbers in the aging brain, and the changes that do occur are relatively specific to certain brain regions and types of neurons. Also, no proof exists that new neurons are added to the cerebral neocortex in the adult brain.

Cerebral Blood Flow and Metabolism in Aging

Using a Xenon-133 technique, several investigators have reported a decrease in the mean gray matter cerebral blood flow (CBF) with aging, whereas the white matter CBF remains stable with advancing age. Cerebral autoregulation is usually maintained in healthy adults below the age of 60 years but is frequently impaired in those above the age of 60 years. There is controversy regarding carbon dioxide reactivity of the cerebral blood vessels with aging. Reduction in cerebral vasoconstrictive response to hypercapnic carbon dioxide in the elderly has been attributed to a loss of elasticity due to atherosclerotic changes in the cerebral vessels. Carbon dioxide reactivity of the cerebral vessels has been shown to be unimpaired in those elderly subjects in whom cerebrovascular pathology has been ruled out.

Cerebral metabolism is not disturbed significantly with aging as far as glucose and oxygen utilization are concerned. It is difficult to define a healthy old person. Also, it is not possible to exclude occult disorders of the brain in the elderly. Psychosocial factors and the state of physical and mental activity can affect CBF and metabolism. Changes in cerebral metabolic rate for glucose are more clear-cut in dementias. The aging brain is more susceptible to metabolic insults. Other important metabolic changes in the aging brain are:

- An increase in metabolic waste in neurons
- An increase in cytosolic calcium concentration with activation of proteases and, hence, in the possibility of proteins or lipids intrinsic to the cell being degraded
- An increase in the extracellular concentration of glutamate and in glutamate binding
- An increased production of free radicals

A metabolic triad in the aging brain involves the coordination of mitochondrial function (energy transducing and redox regulation), insulin/insulin-like growth factor-1, and c-Jun N-terminal kinase (JNK) signaling (Yin et al. 2013). Disturbances in this triad may lead to neurodegenerative disorders.

Cumulative oxidative damage to mitochondrial DNA with subsequent defects in oxidative phosphorylation may reduce the capacity of the aging brain to cope with metabolic stress. Decrease of SOD, the primary defense against free radicals, may be a factor involved in aging of the brain.

Role of Hypoxia in the Decline of Mental Function with Aging

McFarland (1963) theorized that the aging process involves a diminished capacity of the central nervous system to use oxygen. He compared the decline of mental function resulting from aging with that resulting from hypoxia. Although there is impairment of functional activity with hypoxia in aging, the metabolic capacity of the brain is not totally exhausted.

Dysfunction of cerebral autoregulation with increasing age along with age-related structural and functional alterations in cerebral blood vessels starts a vicious circle, which includes accumulation of Aβ in the media of cortical arterioles, neurovascular uncoupling due to astrocyte end-feet retraction, and impairment of CBF and increases the neuronal degeneration and further susceptibility to hypoxia and ischemia (Popa-Wagner et al. 2015). A decreased cerebral glucose metabolism is an early event in Alzheimer's disease (AD) pathology and may precede the neuropathological Aβ deposition associated with AD. Aβ accumulation in turn leads to further decreases in the CBF closing the vicious cycle.

Applications of HBO in Geriatrics

Rationale

Although hypoxia accompanies the aging process and HBO can counteract hypoxia, there is no evidence that HBO can halt or reverse the aging process. If one accepts the free radical

theory of aging and also the free radical theory of the mechanism of oxygen toxicity, then HBO would be contraindicated, as it would aggravate the tissue damage by oxygen free radicals. There is no clinical or experimental evidence that this is so. In the first place, HBO is not used for the treatment of aging as such, and second, the pressures usually used (1.5–2 ATA) do not produce oxygen toxicity. Some degree of protection is afforded by the administration of antioxidants, such as vitamin E, to patients receiving HBO therapy.

The main object of HBO is to counteract tissue hypoxia and improve the metabolism. Both of these are important in disturbances of the brain, which constitute a major portion of the problems in geriatric patients treated by HBO.

Indications

Elderly patients may suffer from any of the conditions discussed in previous chapters where HBO has been found to be useful (with some obvious exceptions such as obstetrics and decompression sickness). The major indications are shown in Table 35.2. It should be noted that ischemia is a common factor in most of the indications listed in this table. Changes in mental function occur frequently in patients with cardiovascular disease over the age of 60. Decline of mental activity is also common in hospitalized patients.

Role of HBO in Rehabilitation of Elderly Patients

The role of HBO in rehabilitation is described in Chap. 36. Rehabilitation of elderly patients, particularly those with neurological disabilities, is a challenge. The capacity for physical exercise is reduced in these patients. HBO may not increase the physical performance in healthy adults, but it improves the physical performance capacity in those limited by pain and paralysis or spasticity. Physical therapy in such patients can be carried out in a hyperbaric chamber (see rehabilitation of stroke patients, Chap. 19).

HBO in the Management of Decline of Mental Function with Aging

HBO does not increase the mental performance in otherwise healthy and active elderly persons. Studies of Talton et al. (1970) showed that focused attention, alertness, motor coordination, and the facility to deal rapidly with symbolic material do not improve in the "normal" healthy elderly during HBO exposure at 2.8 ATA. HBO does not have any effect in primary degenerative dementias, but it improves mental function in patients with cerebrovascular insufficiency. HBO is part of a multidisciplinary approach to the patient with decline of mental function with aging. It is combined with brain jogging (mental exercises), physical exercise, and nootropic medications (to improve cerebral metabolism).

One technique of mental exercise (Jain 1988) was found very useful in counteracting mental decline with aging. Physical exercise has been known to reduce the age-related decline in aerobic

Table 35.2 Major Indications for HBO therapy in geriatric patients

1. Cerebrovascular insufficiency with neurological deficits such as hemiplegia
2. As an aid to physical therapy and rehabilitation
3. As prophylaxis against recurrence of acute episodes of stroke
4. Disorders of cognition, such as mild to major dementia secondary to vascular insufficiency
5. Peripheral vascular disease
6. Chronic myocardial ischemic disease
7. Photoaging of the skin

Fig. 35.2 The concept of hyperbaric oxygenation as an adjunct to mental training, nootropic drugs (cerebral metabolic enhancers), and physical exercise. The eventual benefit of life extension and improvement of quality of life is indirect

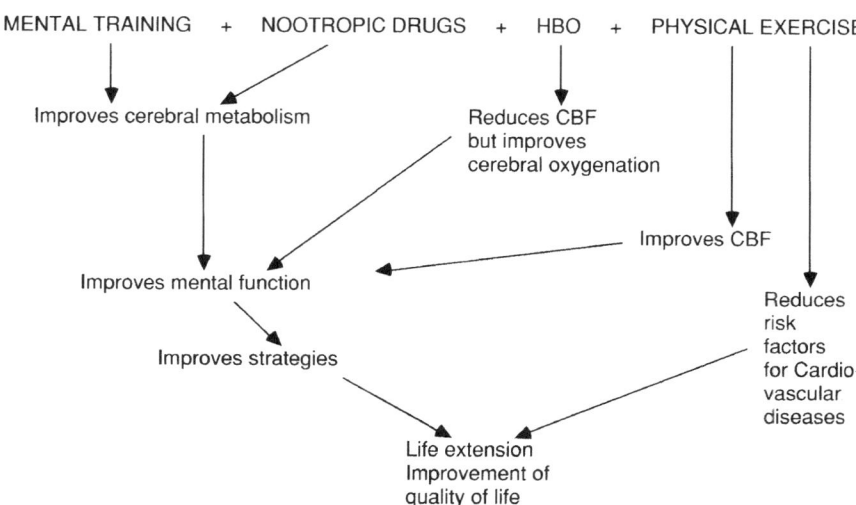

capacity and increase the life expectancy. It should also be stressed that physical exercise has an important role in improving cerebral circulation and function. Exercising skeletal muscles has been shown to release ATP in quantities sufficient to alter CBF and increase cerebral metabolism during exercise. It has been shown using the 131Xe method that exercise increases regional CBF in areas of the brain as specific as the prefrontal, somatosensory, and primary areas of the motor cortex.

Thus exercise may prevent or postpone a commonly existing cycle: disuse decreases metabolic demands in the motor and somatosensory brain tissue, which decreases the need for circulatory flow, which in turn may result in neuronal dysfunction, leading to disuse of brain tissue, and so on. The concept of mutually interacting beneficial effects of brain jogging, physical exercise, and nootropic drugs (cerebral metabolic enhancers) as adjuncts to HBO therapy in the elderly is shown in Fig. 35.2. Physical exercise improves mental function, increased mental activity, improves physical performance, and both together increase the life span. There is evidence that persons who are mentally active live longer. Mentally active persons develop better strategies for survival after myocardial infarction.

Whether the decline in the oxidative capacity of the human brain with aging can be postponed by chronic physical exercise is not established, but theoretical evidence indicates that it is possible. HBO improves the metabolic disturbances associated with hypoxia.

Role of HBO in Managing Photoaging of the Skin

Wrinkles occur in the skin with aging, which may be genetically programmed, but happens over time. There is a decrease production of fibroblast, collagen, and elastin, which results in skin wrinkling and elasticity loss. Extrinsic factors such as ultraviolet B (UVB) radiation during overexposure to the sun and smoking damage the skin. UVB induces matrix metalloproteinases (MMPs), which degrades basement membrane and rearranges the extracellular matrix and type I collagenase resulting in digestion of type I collagen that is important for supporting the skin and causes wrinkle formation.

A possible mechanism by which HBO therapy attenuates skin wrinkle formation from exposure to UVB radiation is shown in Fig. 35.3. UVB irradiation is shown to upregulate pathways that cause wrinkles. Hyperoxia is shown to inhibit the pathways activated by UVB such as HIF-1α, neutrophils, and angiogenesis pathways, which results in decreased wrinkles formation (Asadamongkol and Zhang 2014). Angiogenesis correlates with wrinkling of the skin and can be caused by not only through UVB radiation but also through hypoxic conditions by affecting and increasing HIF, which regulates the vascular networks. VEGF, a major angiogenesis factor, is a target gene of HIF protein and is upregulated in hypoxic areas.

Fig. 35.3 Possible mechanism by which HBO therapy attenuates skin wrinkle formation from exposure to UVB radiation. Abbreviations: HIF-1α, hypoxia inducible factor; MMPs, matrix metalloproteinases; VEGF, vascular endothelial growth factor. Reprinted with permission from Asadamongkol B, Zhang JH. The development of hyperbaric oxygen therapy for skin rejuvenation and treatment of photoaging. Med Gas Res 2014;4:7

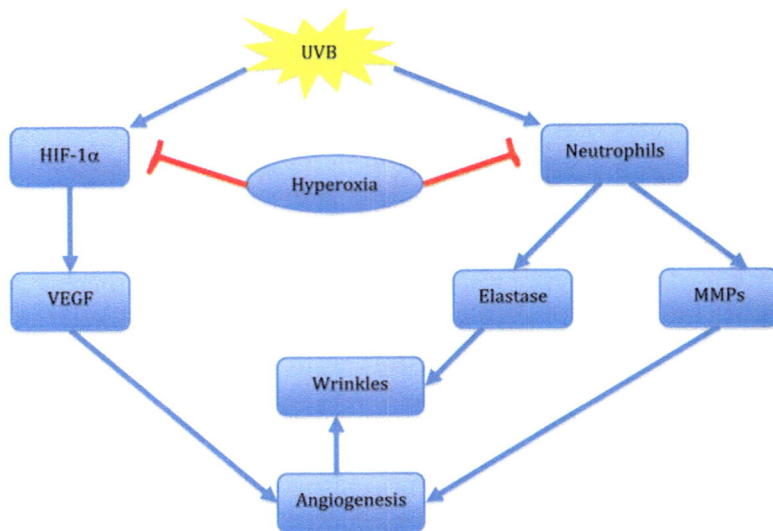

Safety of HBO Treatments in the Elderly

HBO is generally considered to be safe in the aged persons unless they have a medical contraindication. Some conditions such as cataracts occur more frequently in the elderly. Oxidation could account for the lipid compositional changes with loss of transparency that are observed to occur in the lens with age and in cataract. Animal experimental evidence indicates that increased lipid oxidation and hydrocarbon chain disorder correlate with increased lens nuclear opacity in the in vivo HBO model. HBO has been reported as a complication of very prolonged HBO therapy over a number of months and sometime years (see Chap. 32). Modern surgery is safe and effective for cataracts. Many elderly persons already have the lens removed for cataract developed as a result of aging or other causes.

Conclusion

HBO has proven to be helpful in geriatrics, and its most useful role is in vascular insufficiency syndromes. Since elderly inactive patients also suffer from mental decline in the absence of organic disease of the brain, a combination of HBO, nootropic drugs, brain jogging (mental exercises), and physical therapy is maximally effective for geriatric patients. If the genetic programming theory of aging is true, one cannot extend the life span, but one can help the patient achieve the maximal age determined for him or her at an optimal level of mental and physical functioning. There is no evidence that oxygen, whether normobaric or hyperbaric, given alone by any technique, can "rejuvenate" elderly people.

References

Asadamongkol B, Zhang JH. The development of hyperbaric oxygen therapy for skin rejuvenation and treatment of photoaging. Med Gas Res. 2014;4:7.

Blom H, Mulder M, Verweij W. Arterial oxygen tension and saturation in hospital patients: effect of age and activity. Br Med J. 1988;297:720.

Harman D. Free radical theory of aging: increasing the average life expectancy at birth and the maximum life span. J Anti Aging Med. 1999;2:199–208.

Hekimi S, Lapointe J, Wen Y. Taking a "good" look at free radicals in the aging process. Trends Cell Biol. 2011;21:569–76.

Jain KK. Mentaltraining: Grundlegende Prinzipien und Anwendungen. Natur Ganzheit Med. 1988;2:45–8.

Jain KK. Oxygen in physiology and medicine. Springfield: Charles C. Thomas; 1989.

Jain KK. Neurological disorders of aging. In: Greenamyre JT, editor. Medlink neurology. San Diego: Medlink; 2016.

McFarland RA. Experimental evidence of relationship between aging and oxygen want. Ergonomics. 1963;6:339–66.

Popa-Wagner A, Buga AM, Popescu B, Muresanu D. Vascular cognitive impairment, dementia, aging and energy demand. A vicious cycle. J Neural Transm (Vienna). 2015;122 Suppl 1:S47–54.

Royle NA, Booth T, Valdés Hernández MC, Penke L, Murray C, Gow AJ, et al. Estimated maximal and current brain volume predict cognitive ability in old age. Neurobiol Aging. 2013;34:2726–33.

Talton IH, Thompson LW, Dent SJ, Ferrari HA. Investigation of changes in blood gases, EEG and vigilance behavior during increased oxygen pressure in old and young community volunteers. Anaesthesist. 1970;19:241–4.

Yin F, Jiang T, Cadenas E. Metabolic triad in brain aging: mitochondria, insulin/IGF-1 signalling and JNK signalling. Biochem Soc Trans. 2013;41:101–5.

HBO as an Adjuvant in Rehabilitation and Sports Medicine

K.K. Jain

Abstract

This chapter deals with the role of HBO as an adjuvant to physical therapy. Physical exercise is facilitated under hyperoxia. HBO is particularly useful for rehabilitation of neurological disorders including stroke and trauma to the central nervous system. Other applications include rehabilitation after myocardial infarction and in peripheral vascular disease. Finally, the rationale and applications of HBO in sports injury, e.g., for rapid resolution of pain and swelling is discussed. There is no evidence that HBO enhances performance of healthy athletes.

Keywords

HBO and physical exercise • HBO and physiotherapy • HBO and sports injuries • Hyperbaric oxygen (HBO) • Myocardial infarction • Peripheral vascular disease • Rehabilitation • Sports medicine • Stroke

Introduction

Physical therapy is an essential part of rehabilitation in many chronic diseases and in dealing with the sequelae of cerebrovascular insufficiency and myocardial ischemia, as well as in many neurological disabilities. Physical exercise in various forms is an important component of physical therapy and preventive medicine programs. Hyperbaric oxygenation (HBO) has also proven useful in many medical problems, such as infections and gangrene. There has been very little work on the combination of HBO and physical exercise.

Exercise physiology—under normoxia, hypoxia, and hyperoxia—has been discussed in Chap. 4, which should be read in conjunction with this chapter. The role of HBO in the treatment of various disorders has been considered in the appropriate chapters. Important points that are relevant to rehabilitation are repeated here.

Rehabilitation is a multidisciplinary undertaking to aid the functional recovery of patients and their integration into society. It has an important role to play in all branches of medicine and particularly so in neurological disorders; rehabilitation is not only physical but psychological as well. Rehabilitation uses the techniques of physical medicine, and currently these include ultraviolet light, electrotherapy, and ultrasound. HBO can be added to these. Traditionally, rehabilitation therapy has followed recovery from an acute illness. In some cases, rehabilitation measures should already start during the acute phase of an illness and should also aim at preventing further recurrences of the disease process.

Role of HBO in Rehabilitation

Indications

The conditions in which HBO has been found to be a useful adjunct to rehabilitation are shown in Table 36.1.

K.K. Jain, MD, FRACS, FFPM (✉)
1 Blaesiring 7, Basel 4057, Switzerland
e-mail: jain@pharmabiotech.ch

© Springer International Publishing AG 2017
K.K. Jain, *Textbook of Hyperbaric Medicine*, DOI 10.1007/978-3-319-47140-2_36

Table 36.1 Conditions in which HBO is a useful adjunct to rehabilitation

- Stroke
- Peripheral vascular disease
- CNS injury: traumatic brain injury and spinal cord injury
- Toxic encephalopathy, e.g., CO poisoning
- Multiple sclerosis
- Paraplegia
- Sports injuries
- Coronary heart disease
- Limb amputees

Advantages

The combination of HBO (1.5 ATA) with physical therapy has the following advantages:

Biochemical improvement. Excess concentrations of lactate, pyruvate, and ammonia, particularly in older people, are detrimental to fitness and contribute to fatigue, and there is significant increase of these substances during exercise. HBO reduces this.

Increase of capacity for strenuous exercise. HBO allows more strenuous and prolonged exercise than is possible under normobaric conditions. This is of particular advantage in the rehabilitation of chronic ischemic heart disease patients, for treatment of mild hypertension, and for lowering blood lipids.

Applications of HBO in Rehabilitation of Neurological Disorders

The role of HBO in the rehabilitation of stroke patients is described in Chap. 18. The rationale for HBO in stroke rehabilitation is summarized in Table 36.2. HBO has been found useful in the rehabilitation of patients with postoperative neurological deficits. In many neurological conditions, where the effect of HBO on the course of the disease remains uncertain, rehabilitation is greatly facilitated by conducting physical therapy during an HBO session, for example, in cases of multiple sclerosis and muscular dystrophy. The physical performance capacity of neurologically disabled patients is thus improved.

Rehabilitation of patients with CNS injuries

HBO is beneficial in the acute stages of traumatic brain injury (TBI) with cerebral edema, and the evidence for HBO therapy in the rehabilitation of the TBI patient is summarized in Table 36.3. Rehabilitation should start as soon as the patient has regained consciousness and can be moved. The

usefulness of HBO in the management of spinal cord injury (SCI) is described in Chap. 21, and its role in intensive rehabilitation is summarized in Table 36.4.

Evidence supporting the usefulness of HBO in TBI has been provided in other chapters of the book. HBO is a useful adjunct in the rehabilitation of sequelae of TBI in US war veterans, e.g., persistent post-concussion symptoms of mild TBI. A claim that HBO is not effective in TBI has been made in a poorly conducted unscientific study, which is quite obvious from critical readers' open comments appended to the publication in PubMed Commons (Cifu et al. 2014).

Role of HBO in Rehabilitation after Myocardial Infarction

There is some controversy regarding the usefulness of HBO in acute myocardial infarction. Exercise therapy is popular for the rehabilitation of patients who have recovered from acute episodes. Most of the beneficial effects of HBO in cardiovascular disease are associated with increased capacity for physical exercise. This is particularly true in cases with hypertension, where exercise therapy has been shown to reduce blood pressure. The role of HBO in the rehabilitation of myocardial ischemia is shown in Table 36.5.

HBO as an Adjunct to Rehabilitation in Peripheral Vascular Disease

The role of HBO in the management of peripheral vascular disease has been described in Chap. 25. Exercise therapy for patients with ischemic leg pain is facilitated by the use of HBO in situations where it is possible to extend the limit of performance by the use of normobaric oxygen. A treadmill controlled by the patient can be installed in a hyperbaric chamber for training therapy for those suffering ischemic leg pain. The benefits of exercise under HBO conditions are summarized in Table 36.6.

Table 36.2 Rationale of use of HBO in stroke rehabilitation

- Activates dormant neurons in the penumbra zone
- Relieves spasticity
- Facilitates movements
- Improves motor power
- Reduces stroke recurrences
- Increases physical and mental exercise capacity

Table 36.3 Role of HBO in the rehabilitation of traumatic brain injury

- Decreases cerebral edema in acute stage
- Decreases spasticity
- Accelerates recovery
- Improves cognitive function recovery in combination with brain jogging
- Relieves post-traumatic headaches

Table 36.4 HBO in rehabilitation of paraplegia

- Relieves spasticity
- Improves vital capacity
- Increases exercise capacity
- Decreases hyperammonemia resulting from exhaustive exercise

Table 36.5 HBO in rehabilitation of myocardial ischemia

- Improves exercise capacity
- Prevents recurrence of ischemic episodes
- Decreases BP in hypertensives
- Long-term use reverses atherosclerosis

Table 36.6 Benefits of exercise under HBO in patients with ischemic leg pain

- Increases painless exercise capacity
- Relieves pain both at rest and on activity
- Reduces biochemical disturbances resulting from exercise of ischemic muscles
- Counteracts the vasoconstricting effect of HBO
- Improvement is maintained after cessation of HBO when the ceiling effect is reached

HBO as an Adjunct to Rehabilitation of Limb Amputees

A study has assessed the effects of HBO therapy on prosthetic rehabilitation of patients with unilateral lower limb amputation (Igor et al. 2013). The results show that HBO accelerates prosthetic rehabilitation of lower limb amputees so that the patients were discharged from the hospital faster than the controls. HBO-treated patients had improved arterial Hb saturation and pulse palpability, less complications of the amputation stump, greater healthy leg thigh girth, stronger amputation stump, and better functional abilities as measured by Narang's scale and locomotor capabilities index.

HBO for Treatment of Sports Injuries

HBO has an important role in the acute management of trauma (see Chap. 30). The rehabilitation of an injured athlete should start right after the injury. The benefits of HBO in the rehabilitation of sports injuries are summarized in Table 36.7. Since the use of HBO was recommended in the *Handbook of Hyperbaric Oxygen Therapy* (precursor of this textbook) 25 years ago, HBO has been applied widely in the treatment of sports injuries. Some of the experiences have been reported in scientific journals, and some studies have been carried out to evaluate the beneficial effect.

The potential benefits of HBO for sports injuries appear to be a blunting of initial injury, possibly by controlling the

Table 36.7 Benefits of HBO in sports injuries

- Reduces swelling and pain in acute stage
- Speeds up recovery and return to active training
- Improves fracture healing
- Aids recovery from exhaustion and collapse

neutrophil adhesion and release of oxygen free radicals as well as an enhancement of healing processes requiring oxygen-like collagen formation and phagocytosis.

Borromeo et al. (1997) conducted a randomized double-blind study of 32 subjects with acute ankle sprains to compare treatment with HBO at 2 ATA ($N=16$) (treatment group) with treatment using air at 1.1 ATA ($N=16$) (control group) in a hyperbaric chamber. Each group received three treatments at their respective pressures: one for 90 min and two for 60 min each. Mean age, severity grade, and time to treatment were similar in both groups. The change from initial to final evaluation was significantly greater in the treatment group. Subjective pain index fell significantly with HBO as compared to the fall with air treatment. No differences were noted in passive or active range of motion when comparing HBO treatment with air treatment. Time to recovery was the same in both groups. Regression analysis to determine the influence of time to treatment, initial severity of injury, HBO, and age showed no effect of HBO treatment on time to recovery. Although this study did not show any lessening of the time of recovery, there was a reduction of the pain index.

HBO treatment has been reported to reduce post-injury swelling in animals and in humans. Positive results have also been reported regarding tissue remodeling after injuries involving bones, muscles, and ligaments with improved recovery. However, a systematic review of randomized clinical trials of the use of HBO for delayed soft tissue soreness after sports injuries found that comparisons tested within randomized controlled trials provided insufficient evidence to establish the effects of HBO therapy on ankle sprain or acute knee ligament injury (Bennett et al. 2010). These findings may be the result of sample size being too small to be confident where the true result lies. Ankle function displayed improvement of 95% (confidence interval of 0.15–2.65) suggesting statistical significance, but the scale used has not been validated. Although HBO seems to be promising in the recovery of injuries for high-performance athletes, there is a need for larger samples, randomized, controlled, double-blinded clinical trials combined with studies using animal models so that its effects and mechanisms can be identified to confirm that it is a safe and effective therapy for the treatment of sports injuries.

HBO, in conjunction with platelet-rich plasma (PRP) injection therapy, serves as a valuable addition to established rehabilitation techniques and protocols for the healing of musculoskeletal or soft tissue injuries. In a retrospective analysis, combination of HBO and PRP with physical therapy decreased the recovery time after hamstring injury in rugby players with a 38% reduction in injury time in players with a grade I injury and 45.7% reduction in players with a grade II injury (Botha et al. 2015). In terms of recurrent injuries, 62% of players with grade I injuries remained uninjured after treatment, and the percentage of reinjured players with grade II injuries was 0% after HBO, PRP, and physical therapy treatment.

HBO as an Adjunct to Sports Training

The effect of HBO on physical performance has been discussed in Chap. 4. There is no evidence that HBO can extend the limits of physical performance in normal healthy adults. Recovery from exhausting physical exercise is, however, hastened in line with the faster recovery from biochemical disturbances.

The role of oxygen inhalation in physical exercise was examined by Jain (1989). There is no conclusive proof that oxygen inhalation can extend human physical performance. As well, oxygen is a drug, and its use may not be permitted by some sports organizations, particularly the International Olympic Committee. Exercise under HBO conditions may have its limits, as strenuous exercise with rise of body temperature may predispose to oxygen toxicity. I have used HBO to aid exercise in neurologically disabled patients without any complications although their exercise capacity is somewhat limited. In normal healthy volunteers, no problems have been seen in carrying out non-exhaustive physical exercise. Further investigations are needed to determine the effects of exhaustive exercise under HBO conditions by trained athletes.

HBO is not a panacea for all pains and aches associated with sports. Delayed onset of muscle soreness after intensive training is one of the commonest complaints, particularly among those not conditioned to heavy exercise. This can occur in the absence of any direct trauma or injury to bones and ligaments. Byrnes et al. (1998) tested 21 college students without a history of recent weight training who followed a strenuous program of eccentric weight lifting to establish muscle soreness on the dominant arm that was allowed to recover for 14 days. Subjects were then randomized to three groups:

1. Control ($n=8$).
2. Preventive treatment with one session of HBO at 2.4 ATA for 120 min administered within 2 h of the injury and followed by four subsequent sessions ($n=6$).

3. Regenerative treatment by four HBO treatments beginning 24 h after injury ($n = 7$).

All subjects were tested for creatine phosphate kinase as a marker of muscle injury and MRI for muscle imaging, before the exercise and at intervals throughout the study period. There were no significant differences between the three groups. The authors concluded that HBO started immediately postexercise or applied 24 h later did not significantly alter the course of delayed onset of muscle soreness.

Future Prospects

Several professional athletic teams, in the fields of hockey, football, basketball, and soccer, utilize and rely on HBO as an adjuvant therapy for numerous sports-related injuries acquired from playing competitive sports (Babul and Rhodes 2000; Dolezal 2002). HBO treatment has effectively increased recovery from fatigue. This was clearly seen at the Nagano Winter Olympics, where sports players experiencing fatigue were successfully treated, enabling the players to continue performing in the games (Ishii et al. 2005). However, there is still a paucity of publications on the value of HBO for sports injuries. With the expansion of the use of HBO in rehabilitation, the construction of special rehabilitation facilities with HBO capabilities is foreseen. The most convenient method would be to have the whole physical therapy room pressurized and 100 % oxygen administered during the exercises. Such a construction is technically possible and economically feasible.

The role of HBO in sports medicine should be investigated further. At present, HBO is a useful aid in the rehabilitation of sports injuries. Whether it can improve the training and performance of athletes remains to be proven.

References

Babul S, Rhodes EC. The role of hyperbaric oxygen therapy in sports medicine. Sports Med. 2000;30:395–403.

Bennett MH, Best TM, Babul-Wellar S, Taunton JE. Hyperbaric oxygen therapy for delayed onset muscle soreness and closed soft tissue injury. Cochrane Database Syst Rev. 2010;4, CD004713.

Borromeo CN, Ryan JL, Marchetto PA, Peterson R, Bove AA. Hyperbaric oxygen therapy for acute ankle sprains. Am J Sports Med. 1997;25:619–25.

Botha DM, Botha CY, Collins MK, et al. The effect of hyperbaric oxygen and blood platelet injection therapy on the healing of hamstring injuries in rugby players: a case series report. Afr J Phys Health Educ Recr Dance. 2015;Suppl 1:29–39.

Byrnes W, Robinson D, Stevens B, et al. The effect of hyperbaric oxygen on the delayed onset of muscle soreness as quantified by magnetic resonance imaging. Undersea Hyperbaric Med. 1998;25:10 (Abstract).

Cifu DX, Hart BB, West SL, Walker W, Carne W. The effect of hyperbaric oxygen on persistent postconcussion symptoms. J Head Trauma Rehabil. 2014;29:11–20.

Dolezal V. Hyperbaric oxygen therapy in athletic injuries. Cas Lek Cesk. 2002;141:304–6.

Igor S, Mirko T, Dalibor P, Milutin R, Dusica D, Vladimir Z, et al. Hyperbaric oxygenation accelerates prosthetic rehabilitation of lower limb amputees. Undersea Hyperb Med. 2013;40:289–97.

Ishii Y, Deie M, Adachi N, Yasunaga Y, Sharman P, Miyanaga Y, et al. Hyperbaric oxygen as an adjuvant for athletes. Sports Med. 2005;35:739–46.

Jain KK. Oxygen in physiology and medicine. Springfield: Charles C. Thomas; 1989.

Valerie A. Larson-Lohr

Abstract

The movement of nursing into the specialty of hyperbaric medicine is relatively new and has occurred within the last 47 years. During this time, a professional organization was formed, a certification examination created, and two textbooks dedicated to hyperbaric nursing were published. Nursing has defined its unique role in this specialty, impacted the education of the patient, developed nursing interventions specific for the patient undergoing treatment under hyperbaric conditions, and performed research to answer questions relevant to advancing the field. This chapter is the journey of hyperbaric nursing, an overview of the specialty with a focus on nursing interventions and patient education.

Keywords

Baromedical nursing organization • History • Hyperbaric medicine • Hyperbaric oxygen (HBO) therapy • Hyperbaric nursing • Hyperbaric nursing certification • Nursing plan of care • Nursing education • Nursing research • Nursing interventions • Patient education

History

The practice of nursing within the specialty of hyperbaric medicine is relatively new and in fact has only been defined as a nursing specialty in the last 47 years.

Nurses first set foot within a multiplace hyperbaric chamber not as hyperbaric nurses but as surgical nurses in the late 1950s. It was under the leadership of Ita Boerema of The Netherlands that the first Cardiovascular Hyperbaric Operating room was developed. The nurses that entered these first hyperbaric operating rooms were trained in procedures that were necessary to ensure their safety and the ability to function in this new environment. Their nursing function and role was to assist with the surgery and provide care for the patient during and after the procedure. While these were the first nurses to enter a hyperbaric environment, they were surgical nurses not nurses practicing in the specialty of hyperbaric nursing.

During the same time frame as Dr Boerema's success with the cardiovascular hyperbaric operating room, W. H. Brummelkamp discovered that HBO inhibited anaerobic bacteria. Dr. Brummelkamp went on to pioneer the use of the HBO treatments for patients with gas gangrene that limb amputation was not an option. The nurses working in the surgical intensive care units were required to go into the multiplace chambers to render care to their patients during the hyperbaric treatment. Once again, their role and function was as surgical ICU nurses, not hyperbaric nurses.

Closely observing the success in Europe of hyperbaric operating rooms for cardiovascular surgery, the United States and Canada established their own hyperbaric operating facilities in the mid-1960s. This started to ignite an interest in this new therapy within the nursing field. While the demand was for nurses to function as cardiovascular and surgical ICU nurses, there were those nurses that saw a different place and role for nursing within the emerging clinical specialty of hyperbaric medicine.

In 1969, two nurses, one in Australia and the other in the United States, became the first nurses trained as hyperbaric nurses. Toni Bishop, a member of the Royal Australia Navy,

V.A. Larson-Lohr, MSN, APRN (✉)
Wound Healing Associates, 3346 Carbine Road, San Antonio, TX 78247, USA
e-mail: wound_nurse@juno.com

© Springer International Publishing AG 2017
K.K. Jain, *Textbook of Hyperbaric Medicine*, DOI 10.1007/978-3-319-47140-2_37

became interested in hyperbaric medicine after caring for patients who had received treatment within a multiplace hyperbaric chamber. She requested training and attended the School of Underwater Medicine at HMAS Penguin.

Alice le Veille, a former US Navy nurse, established a training curriculum for the hyperbaric medicine department at the Long Beach Naval Shipyard. She went on to work with Dr. George Hart and establish the hyperbaric medicine department at Long Beach Memorial Hospital. She continued her educational efforts across the United States for a number of years.

There was also a technical change that had a direct impact on the movement of nurses into the specialty of hyperbaric medicine. In 1969 the acrylic-hulled monoplace hyperbaric chamber was introduced. This change from a highly technical environment filled with complex control systems, fire suppression systems, air compression systems, and gas storage containers, to a simpler system where the chamber could be operated by one person who was also able to manage the care of the patient. This was often the registered nurse. The introduction of a monoplace hyperbaric chamber was a key factor that triggered the registered nurses movement into this new specialty as well as a "cost" saving method to deliver HBO therapy within a clinical setting.

In 1970, a third nurse in Seattle, WA, with a background in critical care and a love of research saw enormous possibilities for professional growth in the specialty of hyperbaric nursing. This was Diane Norkool. Working at Virginia Mason Medical Center Hyperbaric Center, Ms. Norkool developed the nursing care aspects from the occasional scuba diver to the patient with problem wounds. Ms. Norkool went on to complete her Master's thesis on the Effects of Intermittent Hyperbaric Oxygen on Full Thickness Burns in the Rat.

Over the next 20 years, there was steady movement within the clinical hyperbaric medicine community and the nurses that were drawn to the specialty. Hyperbaric oxygen therapy was moving from primary focus on the diving medicine into the clinical arena. The Undersea Medical Society became the Undersea and Hyperbaric Medical Society (UHMS) and in 1985, 35 registered nurses established the Baromedical Nurses Association (BNA). The mission of the BNA is to work on an international basis to define and implement the standards of practice, promote education, and support clinical research for the hyperbaric nurse. Diana Norkool became the first elected President of the BNA and in 1 year the BNA had 176 members. This was the first step in defining the specialty of hyperbaric nursing. Today the BNA has members in Europe, Asia, South and Central America, and the South Pacific.

Nurses drawn to hyperbaric nursing frequently had a background or interest in research, critical care, or emergency nursing. This served the fledgling specialty very well in establishing the role of the nurse in partnering with medicine to define the application of HBO in the clinical setting.

Nursing research during this era focused both on the use of supportive medical equipment, such as IV pumps, ventilators, cardiac pacemakers, and defibrillators as well as dealing with emergent patient issues as hypotension, bronchospasm, and hemotympanum within and during the hyperbaric treatment.

Over the next 6 years, the BNA worked to incorporate nursing focused presentations into the Annual Scientific Meeting of the UHMS and the Society's Chapter meetings. Diane Norkool, Valerie Messina, and Diana De Jesus-Greenberg worked diligently during this time to advance hyperbaric nursing by holding offices in the Chapter Society, working on committees, developing and teaching educational programs, and doing research. In 1995, Valerie Messina and Diana Norkool authored a chapter on Hyperbaric Nursing in the first edition of Eric Kindwall's textbook on Hyperbaric Medicine Practice (Messina and Norkool 1995).

This interest and movement toward a hyperbaric nursing specialty was not in the United States alone, it was worldwide. Canada, France, Japan, Australia, Great Britain, and India all had nurses asking and seeking answers about this new clinical specialty. Questions such as different modalities of pain control during therapy, psychological aspects of confined environment anxiety, and the uniqueness of specific diagnosis demanded unique specific nursing management. The nurses need to be able to expertly address the needs of the patient with decompression sickness as wells as the patient with necrotizing fasciitis.

The importance of defining an agreed upon set of competencies for Hyperbaric Nursing was another key to defining the specialty. What was it that made this specialty unique from all other nursing specialties? Thus was born the Nationally Recognized Certification exam. The nurses that formed the BNA, worked long hours to define a nationally recognized process for a certifying exam, write pertinent test questions that would become part of the test bank of questions, and prepare nursing to successfully sit this brand new certifying exam.

Diane Norkool worked with Dick Clarke, then President of the National Board of Diving and Hyperbaric Technology, to finalize the process of testing, to ensure the certification exam met the nursing regulatory criteria of being 40 % nursing focused (remainder of exam was on operational, safety, and technical aspects), and to overall manage the process.

In 1995 the BNA Certification Board was established and the first certification exam occurred later that year. The first nurses to sit the exam were the Board of the BNA. From the first Certified Hyperbaric Registered Nurse (CHRN) designation the certification exam has grown to Advanced Certified Hyperbaric Registered Nurse (ACHRN) for those with management, teaching, and research interests and a CHRN-C for the registered nurse clinician with a Masters degree and 5 or more years experience in hyperbaric nursing. Currently, there are over 900 certified registered nurses practicing in the specialty of Hyperbaric Nursing.

The final step to defining the specialty of hyperbaric nursing came with the publication of the first hyperbaric nursing textbook co-edited by Valerie Larson-Lohr and Helen Norvell published in 2002 (Larson-Lohr and Garcia 2002). The textbook contained essential and practical information for the hyperbaric nurse. It provided the first reference text that the hyperbaric nurse could use that was entirely focused on the specialty of hyperbaric nursing.

Ms. Larson-Lohr and Ms. Norvell along with Laura Josefsen and James Wilcox published a second *Hyperbaric Nursing and Wound Care* textbook in 2010 (Josefsen 2010). This book expanded past the sole emphasis on HBO therapy to reflect the current practice locations, which included the use of HBO therapy in the treatment of chronic wounds.

To paraphrase the forward of this text, Dr. Robert Warner III wrote "The field of hyperbaric medicine, specifically the nursing care of patient undergoing HBO treatment has advanced significantly since the landmark publication of first Hyperbaric Nursing textbook, *Hyperbaric Nursing and Wound Care*, will provide the knowledge base for hyperbaric nursing into the next decade." The specialty of hyperbaric nursing, through the work of dedicated, visionary and sacrificing nurses was born, defined and placed on a solid path for sustainability for the generations of nurses that follow.

The Nursing Process

The nursing process is a holistic approach to patient centered, goal-oriented care that takes into consideration not only the physical needs but also the psychosocial needs as well. The nursing process follows a scientific process based on the theories of nursing and provides a framework to identify the needed nursing care and the goals appropriate for each individual patient.

The BNA in 1998 published a standard of care for the patient receiving HBO therapy. These guidelines included a nursing plan of care, desired outcomes, and interventions for the nursing problems reflected within the specialty of hyperbaric nursing. These guidelines have since been adopted as the Standard of Care for the hyperbaric nurse (Tables 37.1 and 37.2).

Hyperbaric Patient Education

Nursing learned long ago that by having an engaged patient, the patient is more compliant, the family is more supportive, and the outcomes are better. An integral part of the nursing process is the education of the patient and their support team.

In today's world with the internet and social media, patients and families worldwide can look up information on

Table 37.1 BNA guidelines for standards of care for the patient receiving HBO therapy

1.	Anxiety related to knowledge deficit of HBO and treatment procedures
2.	Potential for injury related to transferring patient in/out of chamber, and within hyperbaric facility
3.	Potential for barotrauma to ears, sinuses, teeth, and lungs or cerebral gas embolism related to changes in atmospheric pressure inside oxygen chamber
4.	Potential for oxygen toxicity seizures related to delivery of 100 % oxygen at an increased atmospheric pressure
5.	Potential for inadequate therapeutic gas delivery related to delivery system and patient's needs/limitations
6.	Anxiety related to feelings of confinement associated with the hyperbaric oxygen chamber
7.	Pain related to associated medical problems
8.	Discomfort related to temperature and humidity changes inside hyperbaric chamber
9.	Potential for ineffective individual coping related to stresses of illness and/or poor psychosocial support systems
10.	Potential for dysrhythmia related to disease to disease pathology
11.	Potential for fluid volume deficit related to dehydration or fluid shifts
12.	Altered cerebral tissue perfusion related to:
	• Carbon monoxide poisoning
	• Decompression sickness
	• Acute necrotizing infection
	• Gas embolism
	• Other conditions
2.	Potential for alteration in comfort, fluid, and electrolyte balance to nausea and vomiting
3.	Altered health maintenance related to knowledge deficit for:
	• Management of chronic wound
	• Restrictions following decompression sickness
	• Systems to report after carbon monoxide poisoning
4.	Potential for pulmonary oxygen toxicity related to 100 % oxygen at an increased atmospheric pressure
5.	Potential for injury related to fire within the hyperbaric chamber

Table 37.2 BNA guidelines for interventions for problems in hyperbaric nursing

Problem	Goal/rationale	Actions
1.Anxiety related to knowledge deficit of hyperbaric oxygen therapy and treatment procedures Definition: Anxiety is a practical risk with hyperbaric oxygen treatments. It can occur before, during, or after the treatment Identify signs and symptoms of anxiety • Patient verbal admission of anxiety • Clenching of fists • Flushed face • Complaint of nausea or diarrhea • Sudden complaint of pain or discomfort • Feelings of being smothered or suffocated • Urgency to empty bladder • Defensive attitude • Hyperventilation • Profuse diaphoresis • Flat Affect • Tachycardia Restlessness	**Patient and/or family will state:** 1.Rationale for hyperbaric oxygen therapy 2.Goals of therapy 3.Procedures involved with hyperbaric oxygen therapy 4.Potential hazards of hyperbaric oxygen therapy **Purpose:** Familiarize the patient with the procedure, potential beneficial effects and safety precautions relating to his/her treatments to ensure patient's emotional comfort	1.Assess and document patient and/or family's understanding of rationale for and goals of hyperbaric oxygen therapy, procedures involved with, and potential hazards of hyperbaric oxygen therapy 2.Identify barriers of learning 3.Include information on the following when identified as a learning need: • Involve Interpreter if indicated • Apply age-specific teaching • Consider cultural/religious factors • Assess readiness to learn • Purpose and expected outcomes of hyperbaric oxygen therapy • Sequence of treatment procedures and what to expect (e.g., pressure, temperature, noises, wound care) • Gas delivery systems; hands-on practice of applying mask or hood • Ear clearing techniques • Pulmonary barotrauma • Prevention of oxygen toxicity 4.Provide continued opportunities for discussion and instruction 5.Provide patient and/or family with information brochure on hyperbaric oxygen therapy 6.Keep patient and/or family informed of all procedures 7.Document patient/family instruction, using the confirmation of instruction form and the general patient instruction form 8.**Potential for injury related to transferring patient in/out of chamber and within hyperbaric facility**
Identification: Equipment located in the hyperbaric facility should only items necessary to provide patient care. Excess items like personal belongings or other medical equipment unrelated to the function of HBO treatment contribute to potential injury hazards and therefore should be removed All necessary equipment in the facility should be in good working order at all times Only those personnel trained to operate the equipment should do so	**Patient will not experience any injury** **Purpose:** The patient has the right to expect safe care delivery throughout the admission	1.It is the responsibility of all staff, lead by the Safely Director to inspect the facility and identify equipment with the potential of causing harm to a patient in any state 2.Comply with the local Fall Risk Policy; assess patient's potential risk for fall and apply precautions as appropriate 3.All equipment with the potential for injury will be secured to prevent harm 4.Assist patient in and out of the chamber appropriately • 1–2 person assist as necessary • Use of gait belt, as necessary • Use of foot stool and/ or lower gurney to load patient • Use of slide board, as necessary • Use side rails on stretcher, as appropriate 5. Communicate transfer plan with patient and staff involved prior to taking action 6.**Potential for barotraumas to ears, sinuses, teeth, and lungs or cerebral gas embolism related to changes in atmospheric pressure inside hyperbaric oxygen chamber**

(continued)

Table 37.2 (continued)

Problem	Goal/rationale	Actions

	Prevention of barotraumas during HBO	**Ear Barotrauma**
		• Administers decongestants, per physician orders, prior to HBO
		• Patient education prior to HBO therapy should include: methods to equalize pressure in middle ear during therapy; patient demonstration of equalization techniques and importance of notifying chamber operator immediately when pressure or fullness is felt in middle ear
		Nursing interventions include:
		• Assess tympanic membrane pre- and post-HBO treatment, recording level of barotrauma using TEED scoring system
		• Assess patient's ability to equalize pressure
		• \Have HOB elevated during HBO therapy to assist in equalization of middle ear
		• Ensure operator of chamber understands chamber descent should stop when patient is unable equalize pressure and should return to the point of no pain/pressure prior to asking patient to equalize ears
		Pneumothorax
		• Identify those patients at greater risk for development of a pneumothorax
		• Implement protocols to decrease risk of pneumothorax in high risk patients
		• Observe for:
		   –Sudden, sharp chest pain
		   –Difficult, rapid breathing
		• Abnormal chest movements on the affected side
		Nursing interventions include:
		• Notify physician, follow physician's orders for patient management
		• Chamber should not be decompressed until preparations are made for emergency decompression of pneumothorax
		Document assessments

4.Potential for oxygen toxicity seizures related to delivery of 100 % oxygen at an increased atmospheric pressure	**Signs and symptoms will be recognized and promptly addressed. Seizing patients will suffer no harm**	1.Report patient assessment outcome to hyperbaric physician of: 2.Monitor patient during HBO and document signs and symptoms of **central nervous system** oxygen toxicity including: • Elevated body temperature • History of steroid use • History of oxygen seizures • Other high risk factors as appropriate • Numbness and twitching • Ringing in the ears or other auditory hallucinations • Vertigo • Blurred vision • Restlessness and irritability • Nausea (Note: CNS oxygen toxicity can ultimately result in a seizure.) 3.Change 100 % oxygen source to air for patient if signs and symptoms appear and notify the hyperbaric physician 4.Protect patient during seizure 5.**Potential for inadequate therapeutic gas delivery related to delivery systems and patient's needs/limitations**

(continued)

Table 37.2 (continued)

Problem	Goal/rationale	Actions

	Signs and symptoms of inadequate oxygen delivery will be recognized and reported promptly	1. Assess the patient's condition, needs, and limitations for the best suited gas delivery systems:
		2. Monitor the patient's response to the oxygen delivery system, including their ability to tolerate chosen system
		3. Assist the hyperbaric technician with the delivery system, as appropriate
		    • Head hood for children with facial deformities, or per patient preference (customize neck dam when possible for best fit)
		    • Face mask
		    • "T" piece (Briggs adapter), for patients who are intubated or with tracheostomy/laryngectomy
		    • Ventilator for intubated patients who require ventilation assistance
		Head Hood
		1. Assist patient with application and removal of hood
		2. After assembly, check for leaks
		3. Observe patient for signs and symptoms of CO_2 buildup, including restlessness
		Face mask/Mouth Piece
		1. assist patient with mask, application and removal, and reposition mask/mouth piece as needed (i.e., monoplace)
		2. Check form leaks, continuity of seal against the patient's face, keep tight fit around mouth piece
		T-Piece (Briggs adapter)
		1. Setup process
		2. Monitor patient's rate and depth of respirations, listen to breath sounds
		3. Notify the hyperbaric physician if patient is experiencing difficulty breathing. Have IV access for medication Administration if needed
		4. Suction as needed
		Ventilator
		1. Document management of ET cuff with NS prior to descent
		2. Keep suction equipment nearby and ready to use. Suction PRN
		3. Monitor and document patient's tidal volume, respiratory rate and breath sounds prior to chamber pressurization, after chamber pressurization, then every 10–15 min, or as ordered
		4. Monitor patient for respiratory distress. Notify hyperbaric physician if apparent
		5. Manually oxygenate the patient if necessary (resuscitator bag)
		6. Monitor $PtcO_2$ levels, or pulse oximetry or ABG levels if possible and as ordered. Notify hyperbaric physician of abnormal readings

(continued)

Table 37.2 (continued)

Problem	Goal/rationale	Actions
6.**Anxiety related to feelings of confinement associated with the hyperbaric oxygen chamber** Definition: Confinement anxiety is a practical risk with hyperbaric oxygen treatments. It can occur before, during, or after the treatment Identify signs and symptoms of anxiety •Patient verbal admission of anxiety •Clenching of fists •Flushed face •Complaint of nausea or diarrhea •Sudden complaint of pain or discomfort •Feelings of being smothered or suffocated •Urgency to empty bladder •Defensive attitude •Hyperventilation •Profuse diaphoresis •Flat Affect •Tachycardia Restlessness	**Patient will tolerate the hyperbaric oxygen therapy treatment** **Purpose:** • To prevent confinement anxiety during treatment • To assess the degree of confinement anxiety when it may occur and manage it effectively Relieving or decreasing contributing or precipitating factors may reduce its incidence	1.Patient interaction: • Address patient calmly • Establish eye contact with the patient • Reassure patient that he/she is safe 2.Assess patient for any history of confinement anxiety 3.Engage patient in problem-solving his/her feelings of confinement anxiety 4.Identify barriers of learning • Involve Interpreter if indicated • Apply age-specific teaching • Consider cultural/religious factors • Assess readiness to learn 5.Implement preventative measures as appropriate: • Education • Chamber tour • Antianxiety medication • Eliminate preconceived notions • Empower patient; he or she is in charge and may request to end treatment at anytime • Offer diversional activities; TV, music, books on tape, family member chamber side • Assure patient of nurse presence throughout treatment 6.Prior to, during, and after the hyperbaric oxygen therapy treatment, monitor and assess for signs and symptoms of confinement anxiety 7.Notify hyperbaric physician of patient's response to the antianxiety measures and ability to tolerate confinement 8.Document results of interventions 9.**Pain related to associated medical problems**
	Patient will state satisfaction with pain management	1.Assess patient's experience of pain and whether pain is increased during HBO 2.Medicate patient for pain before HBO as needed. Document efficacy of analgesic 3.Have analgesic available during HBO 4.Reposition patient for comfort 5.Avoid IM medications immediately prior to treatment 6.**Discomfort related to temperature and humidity changes inside hyperbaric chamber**

(continued)

Table 37.2 (continued)

Problem	Goal/rationale	Actions

Definition:
According to Charles' law when gas volume is kept constant the temperature of the gas will vary with the absolute pressure. As pressure increases, so does temperature; the reverse is true during decompression
	Patient will tolerate the internal climate of the chamber
	Purpose:
	Slowing the rate of gas flow through the chamber increases the relative humidity
	This effect is the result of a greater accumulation of the patient's evaporative moisture loss within the chamber
	The Increased humidity in a monoplace chamber decreases the risk of static electricity
		1.Identify barriers of learning:
		  • Involve Interpreter if indicated
		  • Apply age-specific teaching
		  • Assess readiness to learn
		2.Discuss with patient prior to treatment how the pressure environment affects the temperature
		3.Discuss with the patient how their exhalation contributes to the relative humidity in the chamber
		4.Periodically assess patient's comfort with humidity and temperature
		5.Offer the patient comfort measures:
		  • If the patient complains of being cold, first decrease the purge flow of the monoplace chamber; slowing the flow, increases the temperature
		  • If the patient continues to be cold, next offer a blanket keeping in mind that should a fire occur within the chamber, more fuel is available
		  • If the patient complains of being warm; slow compression rate and increase the chamber purge flow; offer a cool moist cotton cloth to take into the chamber
		  • Ensure the chamber facility temperature is maintained according to manufacturer recommendations; usually 68–72 °F

9.Potential for ineffective individual coping related to stresses of illness and/ or poor psychosocial support systems	**Patient will be able to comply with HBO treatment procedures**	1.Provide support and encouragement without exceeding treatment outcome expectations 2.Discuss with patient ability to cope with other care givers. Stay informed of progress and helpful approaches 3.Facilitate communication between patient and/or family and other HBO staff members 4.Encourage patient, if able, to discuss concerns and feelings 5.Document pertinent discussions and assessments 6.**Potential for dysrhythmia related to disease pathology**
	Signs and symptoms of dysrhythmia will be recognized and promptly addressed	1.As ordered, monitor EKG readings while patient is inside the chamber (especially if IP on telemetry) 2.Monitor and document blood pressure as indicated (by invasive or noninvasive methods) 3.Assess and document any signs of hypokalemia in patients with acute necrotizing infections 4.Maintain IV infusions as ordered 5.Maintain invasive pressure monitoring and record values, as indicated (make sure infusion pumps are plugged into D/C) 6.Obtain lab samples as ordered 7.Notify hyperbaric physician as needed 8.**Potential for fluid deficit related to dehydration or fluid shifts**
	Signs and symptoms of fluid volume deficit will be recognized and promptly reported	1.Assess fluid and electrolyte balance. Maintain hydration and/or pressure support as per physician order 2.Monitor patient's I & O as indicated 3.Monitor patient's vital signs as indicated 4.**Altered cerebral tissue perfusion to:**

(continued)

Table 37.2 (continued)

Problem	Goal/rationale	Actions
1.**Carbon monoxide poisoning** 2.**Decompression sickness** 3.**Gas embolism** **Other**	**Signs and symptoms of changing neurologic functioning will be recognized and promptly addressed**	1.Perform baseline neurological assessment prior to treatment 2.Monitor neurological checks per established protocol 3.Use a common language such as Glasgow Coma Score to facilitate communication and determination of altered level of consciousness 4.Assess and document patient's motor and sensory functioning 5.Provide reorientation and emotional support as needed 6.Notify physician of changes as per facility protocol 7.**Potential for alteration in comfort, fluid, and electrolyte balance to nausea and vomiting**
	Patient will experience decreased symptoms of nausea and vomiting	1.Assess and document patient's complaints of nausea 2.Maintain airway integrity to prevent aspiration 3.Notify hyperbaric physician of patient's nausea and administer medication as ordered 4.Place NG tube if ordered 5.Monitor and document amount of emesis on Patient's I & O record 6.**Altered health management related to knowledge deficit**
	Patient and/or family will be able to state/discuss factors appropriate to the management of their disease process during treatment	1.Assess for knowledge deficits related to underlying pathology 2.Identify patient's expectations of treatment 3.Begin discharge planning with patient during first visit. Supply information in format to match patient's preferred learning method 4.Document patient/family teaching, their understanding of instructions and any return demonstrations 5.Provide orientation to the hyperbaric environment to include: chamber orientation; middle ear equalization, fire hazards; safety policies and procedures; and risk and benefits of hyperbaric oxygen therapy 6.Appropriate information specific to the patient's disease process should be provided 7.Upon discharge, written instructions should be provided to patient and /or family 8.**Potential for pulmonary oxygen toxicity related to delivery of 100 % oxygen at an increased atmospheric pressure**
	Signs and symptoms of pulmonary oxygen toxicity will be recognized and promptly addressed	Monitor the patient during HBO and document signs and symptoms of **pulmonary oxygen toxicity** including: • Substernal irritation or burning • tightness in the chest • Dry, hacking cough • Difficulty inhaling a full breath • Dyspnea on exertion • Monitor Units of Pulmonary Toxicity Dose (UTPDs) to max of 1425/ day • Notify the hyperbaric physician if signs and symptoms of pulmonary oxygen toxicity appear • Add humidity to oxygen as needed to reduce chest discomfort

(continued)

Table 37.2 (continued)

Problem	Goal/rationale	Actions
6. **Potential for injury related to fire within the hyperbaric chamber** **Problem:** Hyperbaric oxygen involves placing a patient (fuel) in 100 % oxygen (oxidizer) under pressure in a chamber To complete the fire triad, an ignition source is necessary and this can occur from a spark in the chamber	**Patient will not experience any injury related to fire** **Purpose:** The patient has the right to expect safe care delivery throughout the admission	1. Follow fire prevention procedure per established policy and procedure 2. Hyperbaric oxygen treatment teaching and consent of the patient will include the risks of fire in the hyperbaric environment 3. Provide the patient and family an educational pamphlet that discusses the fire risks with HBO and what materials to be avoided for treatment 4. Staff will conduct a safety inspection prior to each treatment to ensure fire safety precautions are met. Prohibited items will not enter the chamber 5. The Safety Director will: • Screen patients with special circumstances (prohibited items) • Collaborate with the Medical Director to determine medical necessity • Identify ways to reduce fire risk • Sign a Prohibited Items release form, if indicated, to allow certain materials to enter the chamber 6. The chamber and patient will be confirmed as grounded prior to treatment 7. Staff will participate in quarterly unit fire drills to ensure preparedness

their disease process and treatments. Not all information is accurate or sound and we, as nurses, must be prepared with the knowledge and research to answer the patients' questions as completely as possible. So how do we impart this knowledge? First is understand what the questions are that the patient and family are asking, how do they best learn and to continue to provide educational support during the course of HBO therapy.

Lets start with understanding what question is the patient really asking. This may not be as obvious as it sounds. The patient and their family may not be ready to hear or accept a complete answer to their question, what they maybe doing is simply looking for support and encouragement to continue. This can be uncovered by observing the body language of the patient and through the development of a relationship with the patient. Care should always be taken to not give false hope but remain supportive and positive.

Ask the patient how they like to learn new information. Adults will learn best when there is a perceived need to learn. For instance, in treating a patient with a nonhealing wound, the patient must understand why they need HBO therapy and how it will help their wound to heal.

Adults learn best moving from the known to the unknown. Assess what the patient's background and knowledge is and build from there. For instance, an engineer will have a good understanding of pressure and how to measure it. This will be a good starting point to discuss how pressure is increased in a hyperbaric chamber and the effects.

Adult learners like to learn from active participation. Tour the unit with them, showing the hyperbaric chamber and allowing them to see and ask questions. If there is an oppor-

tunity to have the new patient speak with another who is already receiving HBO therapy makes for an initial positive supportive experience from which to build.

Opportunity to practice any new "skill" is important to the adult learner. An example is equalizing their ears during compression. First I like to find out if they have any experiences that caused a change in pressure within their ears, such as flying or traveling in the mountains. So this starts with a reference point. Then through demonstration and return demonstration they are able to practice the skill of equalizing the pressure within their ears during descent.

Other recommendations for patient education that can be combined with Adult Learner techniques are as follows:

1. Involve the family or support system of the patient. If all hear the same information, then misunderstandings can be avoided. Group discussion can also stimulate other questions that can improve understanding of the plan of care and adherence to it.
2. Use common language and avoid the medical jargon that is our second language.
3. Use known methods to confirm understanding.
   (a) Open-ended questions, stay away from yes/no answers
   (b) Avoid asking if they understand. This will frequently be answered in the affirmative, because it is easier, not because there is understanding
   (c) Use words that mean something to the lay public. An example is the word "positive." In medicine it may not mean a good thing, ex test is positive for cancer. In the lay public positive conveys a good feeling.

4. Keep what you want to teach to one or two topics at a time. Most people who are dealing with an illness cannot absorb more than that information.
5. Written instructions need to be clear, at a language level the patient can understand and given in an organized manner.
6. Always reinforce your teaching with each encounter
    (a) Ask the patient to restate what you have just taught
    (b) If possible reinforce teaching with a video or visual aid, which will also help with visual learners
    (c) Always provide written instructions for the patient to take home so they can review and refresh their memory of what was taught.

Having a good patient education program has a direct impact on the outcomes of the patient being treated. The outcome of a patient that appears noncompliant due to lack of instruction is different from a patient who is engaged in nursing plan of care.

Hyperbaric Nursing Research

The specialty of hyperbaric nursing has attracted many nurses with an interest in research. This has led to a large body of work by nurses, either in collaboration with a physician, technician, or focused entirely within the domain of nursing. Nurses such as Diane Norkool, Valerie Larson-Lohr, Valerie Messina, Christy Pirone, Craig Boussard, Helen Norvell, Jim Wilcox, Laura Josefsen, Julio Garcia, Monica Skarban, Stacy Handley, and many others have contributed to the body of nursing knowledge.

To review all the nursing research would require a book by itself, but there is one person whose activities in nursing research and education deserves mention. Christy Pirone entered the specialty of hyperbaric nursing in 1984 with the development and opening of the first hyperbaric unit at Methodist Hospital in Indianapolis. Ms Pirone was also a founding member of the BNA. In 1987, Ms Pirone departed for Australia. Over the next several years, she developed formal University level courses in hyperbaric nurses that culminated in the University of Adelaide Graduate Certificate in Hyperbaric Nursing Science.

During this time frame, Ms. Pirone started asking the questions concerning safety of nurse attendants in multiplace chambers and how incidences were report. This question culminated in 1992 launch of the Hyperbaric Incident Monitoring Study (HIMS) by Ms. Pirone—an anonymous, voluntary reporting system of incidents that could or did affect the safety of hyperbaric staff. All reports are held in the strictest confidence and used to critically examine what went wrong and it could be prevented in the future. The reports are not used in medical/legal claims to assign blame. In 1996, HIMS went international. Within one year of the international launch, 500 reports had been submitted. The impact of the HIMS database on hyperbaric safety is tremendous and the success of this international project is due to the dedication and perseverance of a hyperbaric nurse, Christy Pirone.

This chapter is the journey of how the specialty of hyperbaric nursing developed. It is an overview of the origination, growth, and contribution of the specialty to the care of the hyperbaric patient and the story of the nurses who worked to bring the specialty into existence. Hyperbaric nursing is still a relatively young nursing specialty and there many professional opportunities to those nurses who enter this field to build on the foundation and look to ways to continually improve the safety and care delivered.

References

Josefsen L. Assessment and documentation of the nursing process. In: Larson-Lohr V, Norvell H, Josefsen L, Wilcox J, editors. Hyperbaric nursing and wound care. Flagstaff: Best Publishing; 2010.
Larson-Lohr V, Garcia J. Assessing the critically ill hyperbaric medicine patient. In: Larson-Lohr V, Norvell HC, editors. Textbook of hyperbaric nursing. Flagstaff: Best Publishing; 2002.
Messina V, Norkool D. Hyperbaric Nursing. In: Kindwall E, Goldman RW, editors. Hyperbaric medicine procedures. Milwaukee: St. Luke's Medical Center; 1995.

Recommended Further Readings

Handley S, Clarke D. Hyperbaric history and the nursing evolution. In: Larson-Lohr V, Norvell H, Josefsen L, Wilcox J, editors. Hyperbaric nursing and wound care. Flagstaff: Best Publishing Company; 2010.
McHowell W. Care of the patient receiving hyperbaric oxygen therapy. In: Larson-Lohr V, Norvell HC, editors. Textbook of hyperbaric nursing. Flagstaff: Best Publishing; 2002.
Norkool D. Care of the Patient Receiving Hyperbaric Oxygen Therapy. In: Reiner A, editor. Manual of patient care standards. Gaithersburg: Aspen Publishers; 1988.
Norvell HC, Josefsen L, Fabius S, Larson-Lohr V. Patient education. In: Workman WT, editor. Hyperbaric facility safety: a practical guide. Flagstaff: Best Publishing; 1999.
Skarban M. Patient education. In: Larson-Lohr V, Norvell H, Josefsen L, Wilcox J, editors. Hyperbaric nursing and wound care. Flagstaff: Best Publishing; 2010.
Weaver L, editor. Hyperbaric oxygen therapy indications. 13th ed. Flagstaff: Best Publishing; 2014.

K.K. Jain

Abstract

A major cause of resistance of cancer to radiotherapy or chemotherapy is tumor hypoxia. This chapter deals with the causes of hypoxia in tumors and rationale for use of HBO for radiosensitization of solid tumors. Experimental as well as clinical studies are reviewed. There is considerable evidence for the efficacy of HBO as an adjunct to radiotherapy in various cancers, e.g., cancer of the cervix, head and neck cancer, and malignant tumors of the brain such as glioblastoma multiforme. Alternative methods of enhancing radiosensitivity of tumors are described as well as their potential for combination with HBO. Advantages as well as limitations of HBO as an adjunct to radiotherapy are discussed.

Keywords

HBO and chemotherapy • HBO and radiotherapy • Hyperbaric oxygen (HBO) • Radiosensitization of cancer • Tumor hypoxia

Introduction

Studies concerned with the relationship between oxygen tension and the effect of radiation in humans can be traced back to 1910 (Dische 1983). It has long been recognized that hypoxia influences the response of cells and tissues to radiation. Biological evidence for this was gathered in the 1950s, and HBO was introduced into radiotherapy by Churchill-Davidson et al. (1955). The technique developed by this team required a special radiotherapy unit and general anesthesia. Reducing the pressure from 4 ATA to 3 ATA and the avoidance of general anesthesia have made the technique simpler.

Role of Hypoxia in Tumors

Hypoxia has been noted in malignant tumors. Anemia is common in the cancer population and is suspected to contribute to intratumoral hypoxia. Thomlinson and Gray (1955) showed that the corded structure of some tumors could be explained in

terms of diffusion gradients of oxygen. At a specific distance from individual blood vessels, the tumor cells die, leaving cords or cuffs of viable cells around the blood vessel, enclosed in pockets of tumor cells. The recently dead cells are adjacent to the outer edge of the viable cord, and the long dead cells at greater distances. The radius of the cord, as measured in histological sections, was shown to be similar to the calculated diffusion distance for oxygen. It was postulated that one or two cell layers adjacent to necrosis would contain hypoxic but viable cells and hence be radioresistant.

The oxygen tension inside the tumor has been reported to be as low as 8 mmHg. It drops to even lower figures as the tumor enlarges and may drop to zero in the necrotic center of the tumor. Hypoxia increases the resistance of cancer to radiotherapy. With oxygen tension at zero, the amount of radiation required to be effective is three times that required with normal oxygen tension. Various approaches to coping with hypoxia in cancer include:

- Fractionation of total radiation dose to shrink the tumor and to allow tumor cells to reoxygenate in the intervals between sessions of radiotherapy.
- Oxygenation. This is usually achieved by HBO at 2–3 ATA. It is questionable if breathing 100 % oxygen at

K.K. Jain, MD, FRACS, FFPM (✉)
1 Blaesiring 7, Basel 4057, Switzerland
e-mail: jain@pharmabiotech.ch

© Springer International Publishing AG 2017
K.K. Jain, *Textbook of Hyperbaric Medicine*, DOI 10.1007/978-3-319-47140-2_38

normobaric pressure can be effective. Oxygen carrying solutions have also been used to improve oxygenation of the tumors.

- Modification of oxygen unloading capacity of the hemoglobin.
- Hypoxic cell sensitizers: metronidazole and misonidazole. These substances substitute for oxygen and act similarly to oxygen to "fix" the radicals. They kill the hypoxic cells that survive irradiation.
- Correction of anemia may be a worthwhile strategy for radiation oncologists to improve tumor hypoxia and improve response to radiotherapy as well as survival.

Rationale of Use of HBO as Adjunct to Radiotherapy

The theoretical basis for the use of HBO as an adjunct to radiotherapy is as follows:

- A number of proliferating cells in many tumors are under severely hypoxic or anoxic conditions.
- The reproductive integrity of such cells is substantially more resistant to damage by radiation than that of cells oxygenated to normal physiological levels.
- The larger the number of cells that lose their reproductive capability, the greater the chance of cure or palliation.

Four decades ago, opinions on this topic were as follows. Glassburn et al. (1977) stated: "It has not been demonstrated unequivocally that radiation under hyperbaric oxygen is superior to well fractioned, well-conceived conventional radio-therapy … well controlled studies especially in early stage disease are still necessary. It would be worthwhile to undertake such trials especially with tumors of the head and the neck which constitute the most promising site of tumor for study. As others have noted, even 5–10 % improvement in survival would mean many lives saved." Russian investigators were more enthusiastic about the role of HBO in radiotherapy. Sergeev et al. (1977) concluded: "Hyperbaric oxygen employed in radiotherapy increases the rate of neoplasm damage and reduces the rate of recurrences … No rise in percentage of distant metastases was noted in cases irradiated under hyperbaric oxygenation."

To demonstrate the effectiveness of HBO in increasing the radiosensitivity of tumors, one must show that it improves either the therapeutic ratio or the therapeutic efficiency. The radiation therapeutic ratio is the relation between the damage caused in the tumor and the damage caused to normal tissues exposed to the same dose of radiation under the same physiological conditions. The therapeutic ratio for a specified dose of radiation will be increased by HBO if the oxygen enhancement ratio (OER) for the tumor exceeds that of the normal

tissues. This is easy to achieve in small tumors but is difficult in large tumors because of the vasoconstriction produced by HBO. The term "radiation therapeutic ratio" should be used in reporting data on treatment with HBO, systemic radiation sensitizers, and whole-body hyperthermia. The term "radiation efficiency" should be used if local hyperthermia is applied to the tumor to increase the local effectiveness of treatment with HBO.

Hypoxia within tumor may be due to rise of interstitial pressure, which is a fundamental feature of cancer biology, and limits the efficacy of cancer treatment by radiotherapy or drugs due to heterogeneous distribution. Tumor pressure is also associated with increased metastatic potential and poor prognosis in some tumors. Increased pressure in solid tumors is multifactorial, and known causes include hyperpermeable tortuous tumor vasculatures, lack of functional intratumoral lymphatic vessels, abnormal tumor microenvironment, and stress exerted by proliferating tumor cells (Ariffin et al. 2014). Reduction of this pressure can enhance the uptake and homogenous distribution of many therapies. Agents that have been shown to reduce tumor pressure include antiangiogenic therapy, vasodilatory agents, antilymphogenic therapy, and proteolytic enzymes. Physical agents that reduce tumor pressure include radiation, HBO, and hyper- or hypothermia.

Another factor to be considered is the increase in tissue perfusion following radiation. Radiation biologists and oncologists have disputed the importance of hypoxic cells in clinical radiotherapy. Hypoxic tumor cells in animals do impair the radiation response of animal tumors, but it is questionable whether hypoxic cells persist following reoxygenation that occurs with increased perfusion following each radiation fraction. The use of bioreducible markers to positively label zones of viable hypoxic cells within solid tumors and to predict for tumor radioresistance is now possible. Several biomarkers of hypoxia have been identified, and their selective binding within tumors has been measured by both invasive and noninvasive assays (Jain 2010).

The role of HBO in treating radiation necrosis of normal tissues surrounding a tumor during high-dose radiation therapy was described in Chap. 17. The focus of this chapter is on the role of HBO as adjunct to treatment of cancer based on counteracting tumor hypoxia and as an adjunct to radiation therapy.

Experimental Studies of the Radiosensitizing Effect of HBO

The radiosensitizing ability of 100 % normobaric oxygen has been investigated in mouse mammary carcinoma using a variety of fractionated regimens and indicates that oxygen can play an important role in the management of cancers where hypoxia may limit the effect of radiotherapy. Some experimental studies

Table 38.1 Experimental studies of the effect of HBO on tumor radiosensitivity

Authors and year	Experimental design	Results
Fujimura (1974)	Rabbits with implanted VX2 maxillary carcinoma Two groups – Experimental. Radiotherapy under HBO – Control. Radiotherapy without HBO	1. Tumor disappeared in 53 % of the experimental group as compared to 13 % in control group 2. DNA synthesis inhibited more markedly in the experimental than in the control group
Ihde et al. (1975)	Study of effects of various durations of exposure to air and HBO on incorporation of tritiated thymidine into DNA of B16 melanoma in mice	Depression of incorporation of thymidine into DNA under HBO indicating reduction of tumor growth
Wiernick and Perrins (1975)	Study of rectal biopsies of patients with rectal carcinoma undergoing radiotherapy under HBO	A more extensive depression of pericryptal fibroblasts under HBO with radiation than under air. No difference after recovery
Milas et al. (1985)	Study of sensitivity of 4-day-old, induced pulmonary micrometastases of murine fibrosarcoma to ionizing radiation	Radiation sensitivity increased 1.13 times under HBO exposure
McDonald et al. (1996)	Twenty golden Syrian hamster cheek pouch carcinomas were induced with an established chemical carcinogen. Half of these underwent 30 HBO sessions (2.81 ATA/1 h), while the other half served as controls	At necropsy, animals receiving HBO therapy had significantly smaller tumors and fewer metastases
Kalns et al. (1998)	Carcinoma prostate cell monolayers grown under normoxic conditions were exposed to cisplatin, taxol, or doxorubicin for 90 min under HBO (3 ATA 100 % oxygen) or normal pressure air	HBO decreased the rate of growth and increased sensitivity to anticancer agents, but the effects were cell line dependent

of the effects of HBO on radiosensitivity of cancer are listed in Table 38.1. Brizel et al. (1997) have assessed tumor growth after exposure to radiation plus either HBO, carbogen, or carbogen/nicotinamide and the relationship between pretreatment tumor oxygenation and growth time. R3230AC carcinomas were grown in the flanks of F344 rats. Animals were randomized to one of seven radiation treatment groups: sham irradiation or irradiation plus room air, HBO (100 % O$_2$/3 ATA), nicotinamide, carbogen, carbogen/nicotinamide, or HBO/nicotinamide. Tumors received 20 Gy in a single dose. Irradiation with HBO, HBO/nicotinamide, and carbogen/nicotinamide increased growth time relative to room air. HBO was significantly more effective than carbogen/nicotinamide. Growth times for all tumors exposed to HBO were longer than those of the most fully oxygenated tumors (no baseline pO$_2$ values <10 mmHg) not exposed to HBO. These results suggest that HBO may improve radiation response by additional mechanisms separate from overcoming the oxygen effect.

Clinical Studies of HBO as Radiation Sensitizer

Carcinoma of the Cervix

The first pilot study involving the use of HBO as an adjunct to the radiotherapy of carcinoma of the cervix (stages III and IV) was published in 1965, which suggested that HBO might improve the survival of patients treated without intracavitary radiation and that any difference might be small if intracavitary radiation were added to HBO (Johnson 1965).

Watson et al. (1978) reported the results of the British Medical Research Council (MRC) randomized clinical trial of

HBO in the radiotherapy of advanced cancer of the cervix. A total of 320 cases were contributed by four radiotherapy centers in the United Kingdom. The use of HBO resulted in improved local control of the tumor and extended survival. The benefit was greatest in patients under the age of 55 with stage II disease. There was a slight increase in radiation morbidity, but it seemed that the benefit of HBO outweighed this factor and that there was genuine improvement of the therapeutic ratio. A randomized controlled trial of HBO in the radiotherapy of stage IIb and III carcinoma of the cervix was performed between 1971 and 1980 (Dische et al. 1999). HBO gave no benefit in the treatment of patients with stage IIb and III carcinoma of the cervix treated with radiotherapy using two fractionation regimes. There was evidence for an increase in late radiation morbidity when treatment was given in hyperbaric oxygen rather than in air and when, using ten fractions, a total dose of 45 rather than 40 Gy was achieved. The issue remains controversial—randomized trials have not settled it. Currently though, the interest in HBO as an adjunct to radiotherapy of carcinoma of the cervix has declined. In a retrospective analysis of patients in MRC trials, anemic patients (hemoglobin less than 10 g%) treated with blood transfusion and HBO had a better local tumor control than those treated in air (Dische 1983).

Head and Neck Cancer

Lee et al. (1996) have reviewed the rationale and results of clinical trials that utilize hypoxic sensitizers or cytotoxins in the treatment of head and neck carcinoma. Since the mid-1970s, clinical research in overcoming tumor hypoxia was mainly centered on the use of nitroimidazoles as hypoxic cell sensitizers. However, the results from several major clinical trials remain inconclusive. Hypoxic cytotoxins, such as tira-pazamine, represent a novel approach in overcoming radio-resistant hypoxic cells. Tirapazamine is a bioreductive agent which, by undergoing one electron reduction in hypoxic conditions, forms cytotoxic free radicals that produce DNA strand breaks causing cell death. In vitro and in vivo laboratory studies demonstrate that tirapazamine is 40–150 times more toxic to cells under hypoxic conditions as compared to oxygenated conditions. However, HBO trials for head and neck cancer, conducted since the 1970s, have demonstrated that HBO improved local control and survival rates in patients with head and neck cancer receiving radiotherapy. Combination of HBO with radiotherapy is considered to be useful for the following reasons:

- It allows a more uniform kill by improving the oxygenation, and therefore the radiosensitivity, at the cellular level.
- It is useful as an adjunct to surgical repair after radiation.

Other studies to evaluate HBO as an adjunct to radiotherapy are listed in Table 38.2. The number of patients in these studies varied from 50 to 120.

It has been shown that HBO enables the reduction of pre-operative radiation. This makes no difference in the immediate postoperative results but has the following advantages:

- Reduction of period of preoperative radiation and the interval between its discontinuance and the operation
- Increase in the rate of primary wound healing because of fewer radiation effects on the skin and the soft tissues
- Less impairment of the lymphocyte function

In conclusion it may be stated that most of the studies show some advantage of using radiotherapy in combination with HBO.

Carcinoma of the Lung

Cade and McEwen (1978) concluded from the results of a controlled trial on the effect of HBO plus radiotherapy in 281 patients that in cases of squamous cell tumors treated by large fractions of radiotherapy (3600 rads in six fractions), the survival rate was 24.6 % in the HBO group compared with 12.4 % in the air group.

Carcinoma of the Bladder

Kirk et al. (1976) treated 27 patients suffering from carcinoma of the bladder with radiotherapy (4 MeV linear accelerator) and HBO (3 ATA). There was a high incidence of

rapid onset of high-dose effects. The authors felt that to achieve maximal effect, the maximum value of the cumulative radiation effect was required. It appears that this is difficult to achieve in such cases. Cade et al. (1978) carried out a randomized clinical trial sponsored by Medical Research Council (MRC, UK) of HBO in carcinoma of the bladder in 241 patients. No benefit from the use of HBO was seen, and this study was abandoned. In a more recent study, 61 patients with locally advanced bladder carcinoma were treated using a phase II trial delivering radiotherapy to the bladder with inhalation of carbogen alone in 30 patients and the addition of oral nicotinamide prior to radiotherapy with carbogen (normobaric 95 % oxygen, 5 % carbon dioxide) in 31 patients (Hoskin et al. 1999). The results from these 61 patients were compared with those from two earlier attempts at hypoxic sensitization: the second MRC HBO trial in patients with bladder carcinoma and a phase III trial of misonidazole with radiotherapy in patients with bladder carcinoma. Although there was no difference between the HBO and misonidazole trials, when compared with the two earlier series, there was a large, statistically significant difference in favor of those patients receiving carbogen with or without nicotinamide for local control, progression-free survival, and overall survival. Although the advantage for the carbogen group may be explained in part by changes in radiotherapy practice over the period of the three studies, the improvement in local control is sufficiently great to support the hypothesis that hypoxia is important in modifying the control of bladder carcinoma using radiation therapy. Further evaluation of accelerated radiotherapy, carbogen, and nicotinamide in patients with bladder carcinoma is needed in a phase III trial.

Malignant Melanoma

Sealy et al. (1974) treated 22 malignant melanoma patients with large fractions of cobalt and HBO. Half of the lesions responded favorably to the treatment, including metastases. The authors concluded that radiotherapy, probably in combination with HBO, should receive more consideration in the treatment of malignant melanoma.

Malignant Glioma

In a study on glioblastoma cells that were exposed to HBO at 1.3 ATA and then irradiated with 2 Gy photons showed that HBO reverses radiation-induced increase in the mobility of tumor cells (Bühler et al. 2015).

The results of radiotherapy combined with HBO in 9 patients with malignant glioma were compared with those of radiotherapy without HBO in 12 patients (Kohshi et al. 1996). This is the first report of a pilot study of irradiation immedi-

Table 38.2 Clinical studies of HBO as an adjunct to the radiotherapy of head and neck cancer

Authors and year	Diagnosis and type of study	Results		
Glanzmann et al. (1974)	Malignant tumors of the oropharynx and laryngopharynx. Combined radiation and HBO. Results compared with literature reports of treatment by radiation alone	Improvement observed in the healing quotient in advanced tumors particularly those of the oropharynx		
Sealy et al. (1977)	Head and neck cancer. Random allocation to treatment by radiotherapy alone or combined with HBO	Higher death rate in HBO group but less local recurrences and longer life span		
Nelson and Holt (1978)	Advanced head and neck cancer Three groups	Group resolution rate 3-year survival		
	1. Cobalt radiotherapy	1	36.5%	19%
	2. Cobalt radiotherapy plus HBO	2	62.5%	29%
	3. Radiotherapy + HBO + microwave hyperthermia	3	94.0%	54%
Sause and Plenk (1979)	Squamous cell carcinoma of the head and neck. Randomized	Better tolerance of radiotherapy in immediate results were not different		
	1. Treated in air: 250 rads, four times 2. Total 6250 rads			
	2. Treated under HBO: 480 rads × 13 sessions = 6250 rads			
Churchill-Davidson et al. (1973)	Squamous cell carcinoma of the head and neck with metastases in cervical lymph nodes. Treated by HBO and radiotherapy and compared with patients treated previously by conventional surgery and radiation	No improvement in survival rate		
Darialova et al. (1985)	Laryngeal cancer. Randomized. Method of mean fractionation to overcome tumor hypoxia and to raise selective radiosensitivity	In the group with HBO plus radiation		
		1. Less frequent radiation reactions		
		2. Less metastases		
Henk (1986)	Head and neck cancer. Prospective-controlled trial to compare effects of ten fractions of radiotherapy under HBO versus 30 fractions under air	No difference in tissue effects between the two groups but survival rate was higher and recurrences less in HBO group		
Denham et al. (1987)	Squamous cell carcinoma arising from anterior two-thirds of the tongue, oropharynx, hypopharynx, and supraglottic larynx. Radiotherapy under HBO versus air	5-year survival was higher in the HBO group than in the group treated in air, but the difference was not significant		
Whittle et al. (1990)	Glottic cancer. Retrospective analysis of 397 patients. 240 treated in air and 157 under HBO	Local tumor control rate showed significant improvement in favor of HBO: stage I, 10%; stage II, 37%; stage III, 73%		
Haffty et al. (1999)	Randomized trial on 48 patients evaluating HBO at 4 ATA in combination with hypofractionated radiation therapy in patients with locally advanced squamous cell carcinoma of the head and neck (SCCHN)	Long-term outcome from this study demonstrates substantial improvements in response rate with the use of HBO		

ately after exposure to HBO in humans. All patients receiving this treatment showed more than 50% regression of the tumor, and in 4 of them, the tumors disappeared completely. Only 4 out of 12 patients without HBO showed decreases in tumor size, and all 12 patients died within 36 months. This new regimen seemed to be a useful form of radiotherapy for malignant gliomas. Beppu et al. (2003) added HBO to interferon-beta, ACNU as nimustine hydrochloride, and radiotherapy (IAR therapy), which is a common therapy for malignant glioma in

Japan. Although there was a good initial response in patients with residual tumors, the addition of HBO did not increase the survival time, but this is a problem specific to malignant glioma. Because HBO/IAR therapy could be applied to patients with poor prognostic factors, short treatment period, and acceptable toxicity, the authors recommend a prospective randomized trial to assess the benefit of this therapy.

Several studies have reported that radiotherapy immediately after HBO therapy was safe and seemed to be effective in patients with high-grade gliomas. Also, this approach may protect normal tissues from radiation injury. To accurately estimate whether the delivery of radiotherapy immediately after HBO therapy can be beneficial in patients with high-grade gliomas and other cancers, further prospective studies are warranted. Several studies have already reported that radiotherapy immediately after HBO therapy is safe and seemed to be effective in patients with high-grade gliomas (Ogawa et al. 2013). Also, this approach may protect normal tissues from radiation injury.

Advantages of HBO as an Adjunct to Radiotherapy

HBO is considered to be the most effective method for counteracting tumor hypoxia for enhancing the effect of radiotherapy on cancer. This approach has been shown to be effective in only some types of cancer. Concern has been expressed about the danger to the normal tissues of the body from the excessive free radical generation with HBO. In fact, the damage to the normal tissues is reduced by oxidation of cofactors in the peroxidation process. In recent years, radiotherapy immediately after HBO therapy has been emerging as an attractive approach for overcoming hypoxia in cancer treatment. The advantages of HBO combined with radiotherapy are:

- HBO is also a useful therapy for radiation-induced necrosis of normal tissues. Preemptive treatment with HBO following radiation therapy for head and neck cancer may prevent the onset of late radiation tissue injury (Wood and Bennett 2016).
- In a controlled study of patients with head and neck cancer treated by radiation with or without HBO, the survival was shown to be higher in the HBO group. The greatest advantage was seen in the less advanced tumors.
- In experimental bladder tumor, tissue oxygen tension has been shown to be higher in the bladder trigone region. HBO was shown to enhance the effect of combined chemotherapy and radiotherapy in this model (Akiya et al. 1988).

Limitations of HBO as Adjunct to Radiotherapy of Cancer

Drawbacks of HBO as Adjunct to Radiotherapy of Cancer

- HBO is effective only if hypoxia is present.
- HBO is not effective in the presence of metastases. It is certain that small metastatic lesions are hypoxic. Concern has been expressed that HBO may enhance the growth of metastases.

- If tumor vessels are occluded either spontaneously or therapeutically in an attempt to produce necrosis of the tumor, oxygen cannot penetrate the surviving hypoxic cells.
- In the case of some tumors where the intercapillary distance is 125 μm, about 20 % of the tumor cells are hypoxic (Vaupel et al. 1988). Even if 1 % of these survive the treatment, the tumor would grow back again. To eradicate the tumor completely would require further therapy beyond the tolerance limits of the body.
- Oxygen toxicity may occur at high pressures of HBO, but protective agents such as vitamin E and magnesium can reduce it.
- HBO is contraindicated in patients with acute radiation sickness as it may aggravate the symptoms.
- Application of radiation therapy under HBO conditions is technically difficult in the clinical setting since it may be effective only if tumor pO_2 remains elevated for a certain period of time after decompression, but a study has shown that pO_2 reaches baseline values again within 5–10 min after decompression (Thews and Vaupel 2016).

Alternative Methods for Enhancing Radiosensitivity of Cancer

Methods other than HBO with potential usefulness as radiosensitizers are briefly described in this section. Some of these can be combined with HBO.

- As an alternative to radiation, antiangiogenic approaches are being developed to target tumor vasculature to prevent tumor growth. Although antiangiogenic therapy alone can suppress the growth of established tumors, it can also potentiate the effects of radiation and chemotherapy. Because the latter treatments depend on adequate blood flow to the tumor to deliver oxygen and drugs, respectively, antiangiogenic therapy to reduce the tumor blood supply would interfere with this delivery. It is recommended that the antiangiogenic treatment should follow rather than precede a combination of radiation or chemotherapy with HBO. There is no evidence that HBO stimulates tumor angiogenesis.
- Hypoxia-mediated gene therapy is another approach.
- Modified quinone-based bioreductive drugs retain their potent cytotoxic effects under hypoxic conditions and can be delivered, selectively, to hypoxic tumors.
- Downregulation of miR-18a, a microRNA, sensitizes non-small cell lung cancer to radiation treatment, and it may help to develop a new approach for sensitizing radioresistant lung cancer cells by targeting miR-18a (Shen et al. 2015).

Combination of Other Methods with HBO and Irradiation for Cancer

Hyperthermia

Tumors can be destroyed by raising the core temperature to 42–43 °C by various devices. The mechanism of this treatment is based on the fact that cancer cells are heated preferentially by heat application due to lower vascularity in the tumor compared with the surrounding normal tissue. When this method is used in conjunction with radiation therapy or chemotherapy, higher partial pressures of oxygen in the tumor result in increase in tumor cell damage. The more broadly based the thermal radiation, the greater is the tendency to a rise of oxygen tension in the tumor.

General warming of the body, which is sometimes referred to as hyperthermia, involves temperatures of only 38.5 °C. This causes vasodilatation and increases oxygen uptake in the body. Hyperthermia has been used either before or after HBO sessions. Thermal enhancement is greater by hyperthermia given before irradiation compared with the reverse sequence.

Hypothermia

Lowering of body temperature is associated with reduced metabolism of the tissues and reduced oxygen consumption by the tumors. If the blood supply to a hypothermic tumor can be maintained, then the hypoxic fraction of the cells should be reduced and the radiation response increased. This hypothesis has been tested with radiation under HBO, and increased tumor response has been demonstrated (Nias et al. 1988).

Sealy et al. (1986) have suggested a combined approach for radiosensitization using hypothermia and HBO. Hypothermia causes reduction of oxygen utilization and hence a better redistribution of oxygen. The authors treated 31 patients in whom radiosensitivity was achieved by the use of hypothermia and HBO (3 ATA). Of the 29 patients in whom the treatment was completed, 27 had full regression of the tumors. The major problems of this technique are the logistics of combining the three modalities and the complications of hypothermia.

Vasodilators

Vasodilators increase the blood flow to the tumor but may cause a steal phenomenon. The use of vasodilators to counteract the vasoconstricting effect of HBO has been suggested but has not been tried experimentally or clinically.

Induced Anemia and Red Cell Infusion

This procedure has been shown to increase the effectiveness of radiation therapy under HBO. Sealy et al. (1989) showed improved 21-month survival of patients with cervical cancer undergoing radiation therapy when anemia was induced by venesection. Mice with transplanted tumors and anemia induced by iron-deficient diet showed decreased radiosensitivity when treatment was given in air, whereas HBO was successful in overcoming increased resistance to radiation (McCormack et al. 1990).

Radiation Sensitizing Agents

Combination of HBO with nitroimidazoles improves the efficacy of radiation therapy, and its effectiveness may be enhanced further by combining with treatment of induced anemia (Sealy 1991).

Use of Perfluorochemicals as Oxygen Carriers

These are highly fluorinated organic compounds which can dissolve large volumes of oxygen, and this property can be enhanced under hyperbaric conditions. Fluosol-DA and HBO (3 ATA) combination has been shown to increase the radiation response of malignant cells in rat rhabdomyosarcoma. The proportion of the severely hypoxic cells in the tumor is reduced to less than 1.5 % of the original number (Martin et al. 1987). Treatment with Fluosol-DA combined with breathing 100 % oxygen has been shown to be an effective adjuvant to radiation therapy and chemotherapy in several animal tumor systems. Dowling et al. (1992) demonstrated the safety of combined use of Fluosol with HBO (3 ATA) in a pilot study on patients with malignant glioma of the brain. Adverse reactions have been reported, and the safety of currently available preparations of perfluorochemicals should be viewed with caution. Perfluorooctylbromide (Oxydent) has been shown to increase radiosensitivity of experimentally induced sarcoma of mice and warrants further study as an adjunct to cancer chemotherapy Rockwell et al. 1992.

HBO and Antineoplastic Agents

Combination of antineoplastic agents and HBO induces dual injury to the mitochondrial respiration and cell membranes. HBO can be added to regimes combining radiotherapy with chemotherapy. Concomitant HBO enhances the effects of 5-fluorouracil on malignant tumors, but no clinical trials have been done to evaluate this combination.

HBO and Photodynamic Therapy

The use of HBO in photodynamic therapy of tumors is feasible. Combination of hematoporphyrin derivatives and laser radiation has been used for treatment of cancer. Addition of HBO to this regimen speeds up the photodynamic reaction processes by raising the transmission efficiency of light energy, increasing the quantum amount of oxygen, and extending the effective distance radius of oxygen.

Conclusion

Machin et al. (1997) have reviewed the survival outcome from the randomized phase III trials in solid tumors published on behalf of, or in collaboration with, the Cancer Therapy Committee of the British Medical Research Council over a 30-year period to the end of 1995. In all, 32 trials, involving over 5000 deaths in >8000 patients, have been published. Tumor types have included the bladder, bone, brain, cervix, colon and rectum, head and neck, kidney, lung, ovary, prostate, and skin. The MRC trials have made an impact on both clinical practice and research activities. Trials of HBO have defined the biological activity of this approach, and the appropriate dose of radiotherapy in patients with brain tumors has been found.

There is considerable evidence for the presence of hypoxia in human tumors. Vascular insufficiency has been demonstrated on histopathology of the tumors, direct oxygen measurements, and mapping of hypoxic areas by imaging techniques. It appears that hypoxia is probably responsible for failure to cure some tumors such as squamous cell carcinoma, but, even within tumors of the same type and stage, hypoxia does not occur to the same extent. Response to modifying agents also depends upon whether hypoxia is acute or chronic. New methods to detect hypoxic tumor cells (hypoxic cell stains) are being developed. The future prospects for the control of those tumors where hypoxia is a problem appear to be good.

A systematic review of randomized trials provides some evidence that HBO therapy improves local tumor control and mortality for cancers of the head and neck, and local tumor recurrence in cancers of the head and neck, and uterine cervix (Bennett et al. 2012). These benefits may only occur with unusual fractionation schemes. HBO is associated with significant adverse effects including severe tissue radiation injury. The methodological and reporting inadequacies of the studies included a demand of cautious interpretation of the results.

Of the various adjuvants to radiotherapy, HBO appears to be the best. It can be combined with other radiation enhancers. The effect of HBO in enhancing radiosensitivity is most pronounced in head and neck tumors. The objectives of future research projects to assess the role of HBO in cancer radiotherapy should be:

- To determine the effect of increasing oxygen tension on the radiosensitivity of a tumor model in animal experiments, where variable factors such as tumor pathology, size, location, etc. are eliminated.
- To identify the mechanism of radiosensitivity-enhancing action of oxygen. The current hypothesis is that "HBO, by increasing oxygen tension in the hypoxic tumor, increases its susceptibility to free radicals, which are generated in excess by the combined HBO and radiation." To prove this would require monitoring of oxygen tension in the tumor as well as measurement of free radicals in the tissues.
- To determine the most effective and safest measures that combine HBO and radiotherapy.
- Comparison of HBO with carbogen (95% oxygen + 5% carbon dioxide) as an adjunct to radiation therapy.

References

Akiya T, Nakada T, Katayama T, Ota K, Chikenji M, Matsushita T, et al. Hyperbaric oxygenation for experimental bladder tumor. Eur Urol. 1988;14:150–5.

Ariffin AB, Forde PF, Jahangeer S, Soden DM, Hinchion J. Releasing pressure in tumors: what do we know so far and where do we go from here? A review. Cancer Res. 2014;74:2655–62.

Bennett MH, Feldmeier J, Smee R, Milross C. Hyperbaric oxygenation for tumour sensitization to radiotherapy. Cochrane Database Syst Rev. 2012;4, CD005007.

Beppu T, Kamada K, Nakamura R, Oikawa H, Takeda M, Fukuda T, et al. A phase II study of radiotherapy after hyperbaric oxygenation combined with interferon-beta and nimustine hydrochloride to treat supratentorial malignant gliomas. J Neurooncol. 2003;61:161–70.

Brizel DM, Hage WD, Dodge RK, Munley MT, Piantadosi CA, Dewhirst MW. Hyperbaric oxygen improves tumour radiation response significantly more than carbogen/nicotinamide. Radiat Res. 1997;147:715–20.

Bühler H, Strohm GL, Nguemgo-Kouam P, Lamm H, Fakhrian K, Adamietz IA. The therapeutic effect of photon irradiation on viable glioblastoma cells is reinforced by hyperbaric oxygen. Anticancer Res. 2015;35:1977–83.

Cade IS, McEwen JB, Dische S, Saunders MI, Watson ER, Halnan KE, et al. Hyperbaric oxygen and radiotherapy: a Medical Research Council trial in carcinoma of the bladder. Br J Radiol. 1978;51:876–8.

Cade IS, McEwen JB. Clinical trials of radiotherapy in hyperbaric oxygen at Portsmouth, 1964–76. Clin Radiol. 1978;29:333–8.

Churchill-Davidson I, Metters JS, Foster CA, Bates TD. The management of cervical lymph node metastases by hyperbaric oxygen and radiotherapy. Clin Radiol. 1973;24:498–501.

Churchill-Davidson I, Sanger C, Thomlinson RH. High pressure oxygenation and radiotherapy. Lancet. 1955;268(6874):1091–5.

Denham JW, Yeoh EK, Wittwer G, Ward GG, Ahmad AS, Harvey ND. Radiation therapy in hyperbaric oxygen for head and neck cancer at Royal Adelaide Hospital – 1964 to 1980. Int J Radiat Oncol Biol Phys. 1987;13:201–8.

Dische S, Saunders MI, Sealy R, Werner ID, Verma N, Foy C, et al. Carcinoma of the cervix and the use of hyperbaric oxygen with radiotherapy: a report of a randomised controlled trial. Radiother Oncol. 1999;53:93–8.

Dische ST. The clinical use of hyperbaric oxygen and chemical hypoxic cell sensitizers. In: Steel GG, Adams GE, Peckham M, editors. The biological basis of radiotherapy. Amsterdam: Elsevier Scientific; 1983. p. 225–37.

Dowling S, Fischer JJ, Rockwell S. Fluosol and hyperbaric oxygen as an adjunct to radiation therapy in the treatment of malignant gliomas: a pilot study. Biomater Artif Cells Immobilization Biotechnol. 1992;20:903–5.

Fujimura E. Experimental studies on radiation effects under high oxygen pressure. J Osaka Dent Univ. 1974;19:100–8.

Glanzmann C, Magdeburg W, Bash H, Horst W. The results of radiotherapy of malignant tumours in the oropharynx and hypopharynx under hyperbaric oxygenation. Strahlentherapie. 1974;148:16–23.

Glassburn JR, Brady LW, Plenk HP. Hyperbaric oxygen in radiation therapy. Ann Cancer. 1977;39:751–65.

Haffty BG, Hurley R, Peters LJ. Radiation therapy with hyperbaric oxygen at 4 atmospheres pressure in the management of squamous cell carcinoma of the head and neck: results of a randomized clinical trial. Cancer J Sci Am. 1999;5:341–7.

Henk JM. Late results of a trial of hyperbaric oxygen and radiotherapy in head and neck cancer: a rationale for hypoxic cell sensitizers? Int J Radiat Oncol Biol Phys. 1986;12:1339–41.

Hoskin PJ, Saunders MI, Dische S. Hypoxic radiosensitizers in radical radiotherapy for patients with bladder carcinoma: hyperbaric oxygen, misonidazole, and accelerated radiotherapy, carbogen, and nicotinamide. Cancer. 1999;86:1322–8.

Ihde DC, Bostick FW, Devite VT. Cytokinetic effect of hyperbaric oxygen in two murine tumors. Proc Am Assoc Cancer Res. 1975;16:183.

Jain KK. Handbook of biomarkers. New York: Springer; 2010.

Johnson R. Preliminary observations and results with the use of hyperbaric oxygen and cobalt teletherapy in the treatment of carcinoma of the cervix. NCI Monogr. 1965;24:83–91.

Kalns J, Krock L, Piepmeier Jr E. The effect of hyperbaric oxygen on growth and chemosensitivity of metastatic prostate cancer. Anticancer Res. 1998;18(1A):363–7.

Kirk J, Wingate GW, Watson ER. High-dose effects in the treatment of carcinoma of the bladder under air and hyperbaric oxygen conditions. Clin Radiol. 1976;27:137–44.

Kohshi K, Kinoshita Y, Terashima H, Konda N, Yokota A, Soejima T. Radiotherapy after hyperbaric oxygenation for malignant gliomas: a pilot study. J Cancer Res Clin Oncol. 1996;122:676–8.

Lee DJ, Moini M, Giuliano J, Westra WH. Hypoxic sensitizer and cytotoxin for head and neck cancer. Ann Acad Med Singapore. 1996;25:397–404.

Machin D, Stenning SP, Parmar MK. Thirty years of medical research council randomized trials in solid tumours. Clin Oncol (R Coll Radiol). 1997;9:100–14.

Martin DF, Porter EA, Rockwell S, Fischer JJ. Enhancement of tumor radiation response by the combination of a perfluorochemical emulsion and hyperbaric oxygen. Int J Radiat Oncol Biol Phys. 1987;13:747–51.

McCormack M, Nias AHW, Smith E. Chronic anemia, hyperbaric oxygen and tumor radiosensitivity. Brit J Radiol. 1990;63:752–9.

McDonald KR, Bradfield JJ, Kinsella JK, Kumar D, Mader JA, Hokanson JA, et al. Effect of hyperbaric oxygenation on existing oral mucosal carcinoma. Laryngoscope. 1996;106:957–9.

Milas L, Hunter NM, Ito H, Brock WA, Peters LJ. Increase in radiosensitivity of lung micrometastases by hyperbaric oxygen. Clin Exp Metastasis. 1985;3:21–7.

Nelson AJ, Holt JA. Combined microwave therapy. Med J Aust. 1978;2:88–90.

Nias AH, Perry PM, Photiou AR. Modulating the oxygen tension in tumors by hypothermia and hyperbaric oxygen. J R Soc Med. 1988;81:633–66.

Ogawa K, Kohshi K, Ishiuchi S, Matsushita M, Yoshimi N, Murayama S. Old but new methods in radiation oncology: hyperbaric oxygen therapy. Int J Clin Oncol. 2013;18:364–70.

Sause WT, Plenk HP. Radiation therapy of head and neck tumours: a randomized study of treatment in air vs. treatment in hyperbaric oxygen. Int J Radiat Oncol Biol Phys. 1979;5:1833–6.

Sealy R. Hyperbaric oxygen in the radiation treatment of head and neck cancers. Radiother Oncol. 1991;20 suppl 1:75–9.

Sealy R, Berry RJ, Ryall RDH, Mills EE, Sellars SL. The treatment of carcinoma of the nasopharynx in hyperbaric oxygen: an outside assessment. Int J Radiat Oncol Biol Phys. 1977;2:711–4.

Sealy R, Harrison GG, Morrell D, Korrubel J, Korrubel J, Gregory A, Barry L, et al. A feasibility study of a new approach to clinical radiosensitization: hypothermia and hyperbaric oxygen in combination with pharmacological vasodilatation. Br J Radiol. 1986;59:1093–8.

Sealy R, Hockly J, Shepstone B. The treatment of malignant melanoma with cobalt and hyperbaric oxygen. Clin Radiol. 1974;25:211–5.

Sealy R, Jacobs P, Wood L, Levin W, Barry L, Boniaszczuk J, et al. The treatment of tumors by induction of anemia and irradiation in hyperbaric oxygen. Cancer. 1989;64:646–52.

Sergeev SI, Darialova SL, Lavnikova GA. Hyperbaric oxygenation in the preoperative radiotherapy of soft tissue sarcomas. Copr Onkol. 1977;23:17–27.

Shen Z, Wu X, Wang Z, Li B, Zhu X. Effect of miR-18a overexpression on the radiosensitivity of non-small cell lung cancer. Int J Clin Exp Pathol. 2015;8:643–8.

Thews O, Vaupel P. Temporal changes in tumor oxygenation and perfusion upon normo- and hyperbaric inspiratory hyperoxia. Strahlenther Onkol. 2016;192:174–81.

Thomlinson KH, Gray LH. The histological structure of some human lung cancers and the possible implications for radiotherapy. Br J Cancer. 1955;9:539–49.

Vaupel P, Kallinowski F, Groebe K. Evaluation of oxygen diffusion distances in human breast cancer using cell line specific in vivo data: role of various pathogenetic mechanisms in the development of tumor hypoxia. Arch Exp Med Biol. 1988;222:719–26.

Watson ER, Halnan KE, Dische S, Saunders MI, Cade IS, McEwen JB, et al. Hyperbaric oxygen and radiotherapy: a Medical Research Council report. Br J Radiol. 1978;51:879–87.

Whittle RJ, Fuller AP, Foley RR. Glottic cancer: results of treatment with radiotherapy in air and hyperbaric oxygen. Clin Oncol Royal Coll Radiol. 1990;2:214–9.

Wiernick G, Perrins D. The radiosensitivity of a mesenchymal tissue. The pericryptal fibroblasts sheath in the human mucosa. Br J Radiol. 1975;48:382–9.

Wood D, Bennett M. Pre-emptive treatment with hyperbaric oxygen following radiation therapy for head and neck cancer may prevent the onset of late radiation tissue injury. Diving Hyperb Med. 2016;46:124.

HBO Therapy and Organ Transplants

39

H. Alan Wyatt

Abstract

The effectiveness of hyperbaric oxygen (HBO) in ameliorating ischemia-reperfusion, modulating immune function, decreasing edema and inflammation, and improving tissue oxygenation is well-known. The use of HBO in enhancing the viability of stored organs and improving the post-transplant functionality of organs has been studied. The use of HBO has been shown to improve outcomes in vitro and in animal models. Case reports of HBO in human organ transplant have had positive outcomes. Further clinical trials are warranted, but the benign nature of the therapy argues for inclusion of HBO in transplant protocols.

Keywords

Hyperbaric oxygen • Organ transplant • Ischemia-reperfusion • Delayed graft function • Organ storage

Background

Organ transplantation has, since the first successful kidney transplant in the 1950s, become a relatively standard medical procedure. In 2015, there were 30,973 organ transplants in the US alone. Despite this, there remains a significant shortfall of organs; in the US during the same year, there were over 120,000 candidates on waiting lists to receive a transplant. Sadly, around 8000 of these patients die every year while awaiting a donor organ. Yet, with around 2.5 million deaths in the US every year, there should be more than enough viable organs to cover the need, and the ability to transplant some organs from living donors should further reduce the shortage. Unfortunately, rates of organ donation remain low. Religious and cultural preferences underlie some of the reluctance to donate; however, it is likely that increased public education and awareness would improve donation rates. Another method for improving donation rates is the use of an opt-out model. The US currently operates on an opt-in model, wherein a person must make an active declaration of their intent to become a donor, whereas, in the opt-out model, an active declaration must be made if a person does not wish to be a donor. Again, cultural and ethical considerations play a role, but it is interesting to note that in Europe, countries with similar cultures often have opposing policies: Germany is opt-in while Austria is opt-out; Sweden and Finland are opt-out while Denmark is opt-in. A recent study comparing the opt-in vs. opt-out model with respect to donation rates showed that countries with the opt-out model had higher levels of overall donation, although at the cost of lower living-donor rates (Shepherd et al. 2014). Finally, the presence of a well-organized system for the coordination of transplantation, which ensures the rapid and efficient transfer of the organ from the donor to the recipient, minimizes the potential for organ discard. In fact, Spain, which has the highest organ donation rates in the world, employs a combination of increased public education, increased regional and national co-ordination mechanisms, and an opt-out system. The importance of a well-coordinated system cannot be understated: organs, especially those from deceased donors, degrade rapidly. This donor pool is especially important because of the potential for abuses involving live-organ donation, includ-

H.A. Wyatt, MD, PhD, CHT (✉)
Department of Hyperbaric Medicine, West Jefferson Medical Center, Marrero, LA, USA
e-mail: undersea.medicine@gmail.com

© Springer International Publishing AG 2017
K.K. Jain, *Textbook of Hyperbaric Medicine*, DOI 10.1007/978-3-319-47140-2_39

ing: human trafficking, financial coercion, or even theft of organs during unrelated surgical procedures: as a result, the World Health Organization's Guiding Principle 3 (WHO Guiding Principles on Human Cell, Tissue and Organ Transplantation, 2010) encourages developing "its maximum therapeutic potential" of organ donation from deceased persons.

Given the significant organ shortage, any mechanism that would improve the viability of transplanted organs, either by prolonging the available window between removal from the donor and transplant, or by decreasing the post-operative complication rate, would be a valuable addition to the transplant process.

Role of HBO

There are a number of good reasons to believe that hyperbaric oxygen (HBO) may have a role to play in transplant medicine outside of its current use in treating wound infections in heart and lung transplant patients. Several studies have explored the use of HBO to increase the length of time that recovered organs may be safely stored prior to implantation (Guimaraes et al. 2005). Current work on preservation of organs through the use of such techniques as "supercooling" or sub-normothermic machine perfusion, or oxygenated vs. non-oxygenated perfusates has shown that there are many factors that influence the viability of stored organs. The current standard remains static cold storage, in which the organ is perfused in situ with a chilled solution to wash out the blood before being removed, double-bagged in a sterile solution, and packed in melting ice. Unfortunately, it is known that the cold itself results in oxidative stress, inflammation, and structural changes to the cytoskeleton, which have detrimental effects on the later function of the transplanted organ (Guibert et al. 2011). The main benefit of the cold is to reduce the rate of cellular metabolism and thus oxygen consumption, limiting hypoxic injury. However, cold storage only limits the extent of such injury, and certain metabolic processes continue which lead to an accumulation of injuries to the tissue, even at 4 °C. The amount of such preservation injury has been directly related to the severity of post-transplant ischemia-reperfusion injury (IRI) (Hosgood et al. 2011).

While IRI occurs in all deceased organ donor transplants, it is worse in those from donations after cardiac death (DCD). This is a major reason that livers from non-heart beating donors (NHBD) are considered poorer quality and are used much less than those from donors who have a heart beat (HBD), either live or brain-dead. The well-documented effect of HBO on IRI is one of the main reasons to think that there is a potential role for HBO in transplant medicine.

Ischemia-Reperfusion Injury

Ischemia-reperfusion can occur any time the blood supply to a tissue or organ is interrupted or severely restricted. The disruption of blood flow to the organ during transplantation results in decreased nutrient and oxygen delivery, as well as decreased metabolic waste removal. Ischemia leads to the switching of cellular metabolism to the anaerobic pathway, which depletes cellular ATP. At the same time, build-up of lactic acid causes a worsening cellular acidosis. While these lead to derangements in cellular metabolism that may result in cell death from ischemia alone, the majority of the damage to transplanted organs comes during the reperfusion phase (Salvadori et al. 2015). During reperfusion following ischemia, normalization of pH and oxygen levels results in activation of Ca^{++}-dependent proteases and the creation of reactive oxygen species (ROS) which lead to cell damage and death. IRI has been linked to delayed graft function, increased graft rejection, and possibly even chronic graft dysfunction.

HBO has been shown to ameliorate the effects of IRI in various animal models. While the exact mechanism of the effects of HBO has yet to be fully elucidated, it is clear that these mechanisms include: nitric oxide synthase-dependent nitric oxide (NO) upregulation (Jones et al. 2010), superoxide dismutase (SOD) upregulation, blocking the CD11/18 (beta-2 integrin)-mediated neutrophil adhesion in post-capillary venules, inhibiting the formation of ROS, and blocking the formation of inflammatory cytokines and interleukins (Strauss et al. 1983; Nylander et al. 1985; Zamboni et al. 1998; Kaelin et al. 1990; Thom 1992) . These actions protect the vascular endothelium, prevent the disruption of the endothelial basement membrane, and protect against microcirculatory failure. The significance of IRI in transplant medicine has led to a great deal of research to develop methods to reduce or eliminate the problem. A number of studies have examined the effect of inhaled carbon monoxide to reduce chemokine activation resulting from IR (Kaizu et al. 2007; Kohmoto et al. 2007). The use of a known toxin to attempt to prevent injury—when a safe and convenient alternative with documented effectiveness exists—makes little clinical sense.

Inflammation

While IRI plays a major role in acute transplant problems, rejection issues arise from lymphoid tissue activation as well. The importance of immunosuppression in transplant recipients is well-known. There are a number of different immune mechanisms involved in transplant rejection. These include CD4 and macrophage activation, and MHC-1 expression. MHC-1-related chain A antibodies appear to be associated with an increased frequency of acute rejection and decreased donor graft survival (Morales-Buenrostro and Alberu 2008). HBO is known to decrease the number of circulating CD4 cells, inhibit expression of MHC-1, and inhibit cytokine production that would otherwise lead to an increase in macrophage activation (Al-Waili et al. 2006).

As with some other recently proposed uses of HBO, the idea of using HBO in transplant medicine is not a new one. Several studies investigating the possible use of HBO in transplant medicine were conducted in the early 1970s. However, despite promising results, these were not translated from the laboratory to the clinic. Recently, however, there has been a resurgence of interest in the use of HBO, especially as the organ shortage grows worse, and the use of expanded donor-criteria donors (ECD) means that organs that are less than optimal are now being considered for use. Anything that can, in a benign and cost-effective way, increase the availability of viable organs and/or reduce the post-operative functional complications would be a tremendous help.

Lung Transplants

Ischemia-reperfusion injury to the lung following transplant is a well-known complication. It has been demonstrated that transplant-induced IRI in the lung is the result of a biphasic process involving the leukocytes from both the donor and the recipient (Fiser et al. 2001). Currently, one method of decreasing IRI is to use a heart-lung bypass machine with a leukocyte-depleting filter to remove leukocytes from the recipient's blood prior to reperfusion (Kurusz et al. 2002). One HBO treatment can effectively inhibit leukocyte adhesion for up to 24 h. It would, therefore, be possible to treat the donor, once the decision had been made to remove the organ and a recipient identified, prior to removal. Given the short treatment time, the recipient could also receive a treatment pre-op, possibly while the donor lungs are being evaluated. This would have the effect of suppressing both donor and recipient leukocyte adhesion.

The use of HBO as part of a preservation process might make it possible to store lungs for a longer period of time. Currently, lungs are one of the least tolerant organs to cold ischemia, with a maximum of 8 h, more tolerant only than the heart, at 6 h (Guibert et al. 2011). As previously noted, the main reason for the use of cold is to minimize metabolism and reduce oxygen demand. Might HBO in combination with normothermic or subnormothermic mechanical perfusion increase the viability time of donor organs? In fact, early in the development of lung transplantation protocols, continuous perfusion at normal or near-normal body temperatures was investigated. However, there were high rates of early graft dysfunction as a result of IRI and edema (Genco et al. 1992).

HBO has been used to treat other complications arising from lung transplant surgery, as well. These include: sternal osteomyelitis (Mills and Bryson 2006), respiratory infection, acute peripheral embolism, and arterial gas embolism (Higuchi et al. 2006). In all cases, HBO was shown to be a safe and effective therapy for these complications.

A small pilot study examining the effects of HBO on pulmonary function in patients suffering from chronic transplant rejection was initiated in New Orleans in 2005, but was disrupted by a natural disaster. However, some of the initial findings in the small group of end-stage patients were promising. For this study, four patients in the terminal stages of chronic lung rejection were enrolled to receive daily HBO. All patients had regular follow-up by a lung transplant team at a local teaching hospital. Although the study was disrupted by Hurricane Katrina in 2005, 3 of the 4 patients reported subjective improvements in their pulmonary function. Two of the four patients also had documented improvement of their pulmonary function tests. Of the 4, only 1 had received the full course of 40 treatments at the time the study was interrupted. The only patient to complete the initial phase of the trial, this patient had achieved a 10 % increase in FVC, despite having experienced a continuous decline in lung function over the preceding year and experienced a near doubling of his exercise tolerance. It is worth noting that all of the patients in this study were in the end-stages of chronic rejection and had very poor prognoses.

The relative ease with which HBO therapy can be delivered, even to a patient on mechanical ventilation, the short treatment duration, and the duration of the treatment effect seem to indicate that this treatment could be easily integrated into the transplant surgery protocol. A further role for HBO in the post-transplant period may also exist, as evidenced by the New Orleans pilot study of late post-transplant patients. Additionally, Duke University is preparing to begin a clinical trial of HBO in early post-transplant patients suffering from reduced blood flow and oxygenation of their airway tissues.

Pancreas Transplants

Once again, IRI is a major contributor to post-transplant complications. One of the main complications of pancreas transplantation is graft pancreatitis. Studies using a porcine model have demonstrated the role of IRI lipid peroxidation in the development of pancreatitis (Albendea et al. 2007). Animal studies of islet cell transplantation have demonstrated a beneficial effect of peritransplant HBO on the survival and function of transplanted islet cells (Juang et al. 2002). This study also examined the effect of HBO treatment regimen on the functional outcome of the transplant. In all cases, it was found that HBO improved the observed functional measures; however, those rats that received twice-daily treatment beginning 14 days prior to transplant and continuing through post-op day 28 showed both improved function and a greater beta-cell mass. While this represents an intensive level of HBO therapy, it would be difficult to extrapolate from the rat model to a specific clinical treatment requirements. However, the results are promising and again suggest that the role of HBO in organ transplants may extend beyond the immediate peri-transplant period.

While there are no current studies evaluating the degree of donor vs. host leukocyte contribution to IRI in pancreas transplants, it is not unreasonable to assume that both play a role as they do in the lung model.

Renal Transplants

The kidney is currently the most commonly transplanted organ and was the first successfully transplanted solid organ. Consequently, there is a significant body of research on all aspects of renal transplantation. The role of IRI in renal transplant complications is well-documented and is the major cause of intrinsic acute renal failure and a main cause of early renal dysfunction in cadaveric transplants (Gandolfo and Rabb 2008). A number of methods have been tried to decrease the amount of IRI sustained by the kidneys. Machine perfusion has been used increasingly in renal transplant preservation, especially as ECD kidneys have increased in prevalence, and has been shown to be beneficial in reducing delayed graft function and increasing 1-year graft survival (Moers et al. 2009). HBO has been tested in conjunction with various perfusates in transportable chambers in an attempt to increase preservation time and decrease IRI (Inuzuka et al. 2007; Rubbini et al. 2007). The results have been promising, with organs demonstrating significant preservation of function for up to 48 h.

Liver Transplants

In much the same way that renal transplant is the definitive treatment for end-stage renal disease, so is liver transplant the only viable option for end-stage liver disease. As in all other transplant models, IRI is a major factor in poor transplant outcome. Both delayed graft function and primary graft failure have been attributed to IRI (Bejaoui et al. 2015). The damage to the transplanted organ has been shown to be mediated by neutrophils (Ramaiah and Jaeschke 2007), ROS (Muralidharan and Christophi 2007), and cytokines (Colletti et al. 1996; Zwacka et al. 1998). Unlike some of the other organs discussed, the use of HBO in liver transplants has been more extensively researched. In addition to using HBO

for its suppressive effects on IRI, it has also been considered as a possible adjunct treatment in post-transplant hepatic artery thrombosis and primary graft dysfunction (Castro e Silva O et al. 2006). In this case report, 2 patients were treated with HBO, 1 of whom had developed hepatic artery thrombosis, the other a primary graft dysfunction. In both cases, the patients' liver function tests began to normalize soon after HBO was initiated.

A curious aspect of liver transplant is the development of IRI in the lung after liver transplant. Chemokines released secondary to hepatic IRI are reported to be responsible for the development of this condition (Colletti et al. 1995). In theory, the use of HBO on both donor and recipient could act to reduce the development of IRI in the transplanted organ and disrupt this chemokine release, protecting both the transplanted organ and the recipient lungs.

The use of HBO prior to transplantation on both donor and recipient has been reported (Bayrakci 2008; Kreimer et al. 2011). In the first case report, the use of HBO improved the function of a donor liver in situ prior to transplant, which then demonstrated good function in the recipient after transplant. The second study examined the effect of HBO on the function of failing livers in patients awaiting transplant. While not finding any statistically significant improvement in laboratory values of liver function studies, a reduction in the number of instances of encephalopathy was noted in 30 % of patients. Unfortunately, none of these patients received HBO immediately prior to transplantation, so what, if any, effects recipient pre-transplant HBO might have had on post-transplant liver function cannot be assessed. Previous studies have found that HBO improves liver regeneration in cirrhosis (Ozdogan et al. 2005).

The use of HBO in the case of small-for-size liver grafts has also been examined. Because of the perennial shortage of organs, techniques that allow the donation of a portion of the organ from a living donor have been developed. Initially, this involved donation of the smaller, left lobe of the liver to the recipient. However, the left lobe is often significantly smaller that the right and had been found insufficient to meet the metabolic demands of some recipients. As a result, some teams began using the larger, right lobe. This technique, however, imposes more surgical stress on the donor and cannot be used if the remaining left lobe amounts to less than 30 % of the donor's total liver volume. Several groups have examined the effect of HBO on the subsequent regeneration and function of such liver grafts. One group examined the use of HBO pretreatment in rats, which then underwent either a 70 or 90 % hepatectomy (Nori et al. 2007). The rats pretreated with HBO had more graft growth and better graft function than controls. Similar results have been reported previously on liver regeneration in rats after undergoing 15 % hepatectomy (Kurir et al. 2004). Additionally, Kurir's group found that the liver lobules in the HBO-treated rats were more histologically normal by light microscopy than those of controls.

Taken together, these findings indicate that HBO may have a plethora of uses in liver transplant medicine: acting as a bridge to improve the function of the failing liver, improving the viability and function of the deceased-donor liver, improving regeneration and function of whole-liver and liver graft transplants, in addition to combating IRI to reduce delayed graft function, primary graft dysfunction, and as an adjunct therapy for post-transplant hepatic artery thrombosis.

Face Transplants

From the first facial replant surgery in 1994, the field has advanced rapidly; the first partial transplant occurred in 2005, the first full facial transplant in 2010 and, most recently, the first full face and scalp transplant in 2015. In almost all of these cases, the recipient had suffered severe facial trauma resulting in significant soft-tissue scarring and requiring multiple reconstructive surgeries. Mechanisms have included electrical and thermal burns, animal predation, and firearm trauma. While any transplanted tissue will have complications arising from IRI and rejection, and there is no reason to suppose face transplants are any different, there are additional considerations for which HBO may have an application. Most solid organs have the advantage of a discrete circulation that is relatively straightforward to reconnect to that of the recipient. However, in the case of a face transplant, surgeons are essentially performing a large, free-flap procedure. In common with these types of surgeries, face transplant does not involve the anastomosis of many of the smaller vessels, especially on the venous return side, with those of the recipient. As a result, significant edema often occurs. Previous studies looking at the effect of HBO on flaps and grafts have shown the benefit of HBO in these procedures (Baynosa and Zamboni 2012). Additionally, it has been shown that the use of HBO along with leech treatment results in improvements in flap outcomes greater than with either therapy alone (Lozano et al. 1999).

A further potential benefit involves the use of HBO in preparation of the recipient tissue bed. As mentioned, all of the transplants to date have occurred in the settings of severe soft tissue trauma followed by repeated surgical trauma. The resultant disruptions to the normal blood flow make for a suboptimal wound bed. HBO has frequently been used to improve the vascularity of the wound bed in areas of soft-tissue trauma, thermal, or radiation burns. It is understood that the resultant angiogenesis is durable, therefore a course of HBO for recipients would be possible at any time once they are on the waiting list (indeed, there is no reason HBO could not be incorporated into earlier rounds of the reconstructive process) with treatment immediately prior to transplant, as has been discussed above.

Hand Transplants

Another procedure that has recently been high-profile is the hand transplant. As with face transplants, there are issues outside of those discussed above for transplanted organs, which may benefit from HBO. The use of HBO as an adjunctive therapy in limb replantation is currently approved, and the case of hand transplantation is essentially a special case of replantation. Studies have been conducted using HBO both pre-replant, for limb storage (Edwards et al. 1991; Zemmel et al. 1998), and post-replant, in the setting of prior prolonged warm ischemia (Salgado et al. 2010), all of which showed a significant improvement in replant outcome with the addition of HBO. The ability to pretreat a brain-dead donor with HBO prior to recovery of the hand (and, simultaneously, any other organs being recovered) should confer an added benefit not normally seen in the setting of traumatic amputation/replantation.

Miscellaneous Organs and Tissues

While the first successful heart transplant did not occur until 1969, research into HBO as an adjunct to improve viability of preserved hearts was already underway. As early as 1965, researchers were looking at the contractility and long-term viability of hearts preserved using a combination of HBO and hypothermia (Lempert et al. 1968; Makin and Howard 1966; Ladaga et al. 1966; Bui-Mong-Hung et al. 1968). It was found that the combination of HBO and hypothermia could successfully maintain viability of hearts subjected to prolonged (up to 48 h) cold storage. Additionally, canine hearts in static cold storage at 4 atm absolute oxygen tension at 2 °C were shown to remain viable after 24 h. Biopsies taken before and after storage were assayed and showed a marked reduction in glucose consumption and lactic acid production compared to controls (Lyons et al. 1966).

Heart, in common with all transplanted organs, suffers from the effects of IRI, which is an important cause of primary graft dysfunction. The IRI results in, among other effects, mitochondrial oxidative damage that is potentiated by cold ischemia (Dare et al. 2015).

HBO has also been used in other aspects of heart transplant, such as in the treatment of sternal osteomyelitis (Yu et al. 2011).

Many additional animal studies have examined the role of HBO in transplantation of various organs and tissues: thyroid (Talmage and Dart 1978), small bowel (Inuzuka et al. 2007; Sasaki and Joh 2007; Guimaraes et al. 2005), and skin (Jacobs et al. 1979). In all cases, investigators found a beneficial effect of the use of HBO on graft survival and function. In these cases, improved outcomes appear to be related to the inhibition of chemokine formation by attenuation of IRI.

Clinical Applications

There are at least three distinct phases where it would appear that HBO can be beneficially employed as part of the transplant protocol: pre-op treatment of the donor, during the organ storage process, and in treatment of the recipient pre- and/or post-op. By inactivating leukocytes and thus attenuating the IRI in both the donor and recipient, HBO should reduce the incidence and severity of the complications arising from IRI such as delayed graft function or primary graft dysfunction to which IRI is known to contribute. The use of HBO during the storage process has been shown to be beneficial in static cold storage models and mechanical perfusion models. By decreasing metabolic demand and reducing lactic acid production, a further reduction in IRI can be anticipated, along with the potential for increased viability with prolonged storage or the use of marginal organs.

The optimal treatment protocol would need to be determined clinically; however, our understanding of the mechanisms by which HBO blocks IRI in its current applications would suggest that even a single treatment of both donor and recipient within 24 h of surgery might significantly attenuate IRI. Based on some of the reported studies, additional post-op treatments may offer additional functional benefits. It is worth noting that, in all but DCD donors, treatment with HBO would exert its benefit simultaneously on all potentially recoverable organs in the body.

Conclusion

In view of the results obtained in the many animal studies, the well-understood pathways by which IRI induces damage, and the mechanisms by which HBO is known to block this type of insult, it seems reasonable to conclude that HBO will be an effective adjunct in the transplant process. Some indication of the renewed interest in the use of HBO may be gleaned from the recent inclusion of HBO on the list of non-covered indications established by CMS (Medicare). Certainly, cost-effectiveness is an important consideration in these days of ever-decreasing resources. However, the extreme organ shortage, the fact that transplant is often the only definitive treatment available for advanced organ failure, and the already high cost of transplantation all argue in favor of a method that is (relatively) cheap, safe, and effective to increase the pool of organs, decrease the wastage of marginal organs, and decrease the incidence of post-op organ dysfunction. The ease with which HBO can be delivered and the short treatment times required should make it relatively easy to incorporate its use into any transplant protocol. It is anticipated that this will continue to be a fertile area for future clinical research.

References

Albendea CD, Miana-Mena FJ, Garcia-Gil A, Fuentes-Broto L, Martinez-Ballarin E, Berzosa C, Gonzalvo E, Garcia JJ. Ischemia-reperfusion induces lipid peroxidation in the transplant of the pancreas in pigs. In: XXXIV Congress of the Spanish Society for Physiological Sciences 2007; 190, Supplement 655: p113.

Al-Waili NS, Butler GJ, Petrillo RL, Carrey Z, Hamilton RW. Hyperbaric oxygen and lymphoid system function: a review supporting possible intervention in tissue transplantation. Technol Health Care. 2006;14(6):489–98.

Baynosa RC, Zamboni WA. The effect of hyperbaric oxygen on compromised grafts and flaps. Undersea Hyperb Med. 2012;39(4):857–65.

Bayrakci B. Preservation of organs from brain dead donors with hyperbaric oxygen. Pediatr Transplant. 2008;12(5):506–9.

Bejaoui M, Pantazi E, Folch-Puy E, Baptista PM, Garcia-Gil A, Adam R, Rosello-Catafau J. Emerging concepts in liver graft preservation. World J Gastroenterol. 2015;21(2):396–407.

Bui-Mong-Hung VM, Leandri J, Laurent D. Influence of decompression procedure on heart viability after long-term storage using hyperbaric oxygen and hypothermia. Nature. 1968;219:1175–7.

Castro e Silva O, Sankarankutty AK, Martinelli AL, Souza FF, Teixeira AC, Feres O, et al. Therapeutic effect of hyperbaric oxygen in hepatic artery thrombosis and functional cholestasis after orthotopic liver transplantation. Transplant Proc 2006; 38(6): 1913–1917.

Colletti LM, Kunkel SL, Walz A, Burdick MD, Kunkel RG, Wilke CA, et al. Chemokine expression during hepatic ischemia/reperfusion induced lung injury in the rat. J Clin Invest. 1995;95:134–41.

Colletti LM, Kunkel SL, Walz A, Burdick MD, Kunkel RG, Wilke CA, et al. The role of cytokine networks in the local liver injury following hepatic ischemia/reperfusion in the rat. Hepatology. 1996;23(3):506–14.

Dare AJ, Logan A, Prime TA, Rogatti S, Goddard M, Bolton EM, et al. The mitochondria-targeted anti-oxidant MitoQ decreases ischemia-reperfusion injury in a murine syngeneic heart transplant model. J Heart Lung Transplant. 2015;34(11):1471–80.

Edwards RJ, Im MJ, Hoopes JE. Effects of hyperbaric oxygen preservation on rat limb replantation: a preliminary report. Ann Plast Surg. 1991;27:1.

Fiser SM, Tribble CG, Long SM, Kaza AK, Cope JT, Laubach VE, et al. Lung transplant reperfusion injury involves pulmonary macrophages and circulating leukocytes in a biphasic response. J Thorac Cardiovasc Surg. 2001;121:1069–75.

Gandolfo MT, Rabb H. Ischemia-reperfusion injury: pathophysiology and clinical approach. In: Ashan N, editor. Chronic allograft failure: natural history, pathogenesis, diagnosis and management. Austin, TX: Landes Bioscience; 2008. p. 39–47.

Genco CM, Connolly RJ, Peterson MB, Bernstein EA, Ramberg K, Zhang X, et al. Granulocyte sequestration and early failure in the autoperfused heart-lung preparation. Ann Thorac Surg. 1992;53:217–25.

Guibert EE, Petrenko AY, Balaban CL, Somov AY, Rodriguez JV, Fuller BJ. Organ preservation: current concepts and new strategies for the next decade. Transfus Med Hemother. 2011;38:125–42.

Guimaraes FAG, Taha MO, Simoes MJ, Moino CAA, Santos IV, Amador JC, et al. Use of hyperbaric oxygenation in small bowel preservation for transplant. Transplant Proc. 2005;38(6):1796–9.

Higuchi T, Oto T, Millar IL, Levvey BJ, Williams TJ, Snell GI. Preliminary report of the safety and efficacy of hyperbaric oxygen therapy for specific complications of lung transplantation. J Heart Lung Transplant. 2006;25(11):1302–9.

Hosgood SA, Bagul A, Nicholson ML. Minimising cold ischaemic injury in an experimental model of kidney transplantation. Eur J Clin Invest. 2011;41(3):233–40.

Inuzuka K, Unno N, Yamamoto N, Sagara D, Suzuki M, Nishiyama M, et al. Effect of hyperbarically oxygenated-per-fluorochemical with University of Wisconsin solution on preservation of rat small intestine using an original pressure resistant portable apparatus. Surgery. 2007;142(1):57–66.

Jacobs BB, Thuning CA, Sacksteder MR, Warren J. Extended skin allograft survival in mice during prolonged exposure to hyperbaric oxygen. Transplantation. 1979;28:70–2.

Jones SR, Carpin KM, Woodward SM, Khiabani KT, Stephenson LL, Wang WZ, et al. Hyperbaric oxygen inhibits ischemia-reperfusion induced neutrophil CD18 polarization by a nitric oxide mechanism. Plast Reconstr Surg. 2010;126(2):403–11.

Juang JH, Hsu BR, Kuo CH, Uengt SW. Beneficial effects of hyperbaric oxygen therapy on islet transplantation. Cell Transplant. 2002;11:95–101.

Kaelin CM, Im MJ, Myers RAM, Manson PM, Hoopes JE. The effects of hyperbaric oxygen on free flaps in rats. Arch Surg. 1990;125:607–9.

Kaizu T, Ikeda A, Nakao A, Tsung A, Toyokawa H, Ueki S, et al. Protection of transplant-induced hepatic ischemia/reperfusion injury with carbon monoxide via MEK/ERK1/2 pathway downregulation. Am J Physiol Gastrointest Liver Physiol. 2007;294:G236–44.

Kohmoto J, Nakao A, Stolz DB, Kaizu T, Tsung A, Ikeda A, et al. Carbon monoxide protects rat lung transplants from ischemia-reperfusion injury via a mechanism involving p38 MAP kinase pathway. Am J Transplant. 2007;7:2279–90.

Kreimer F, Corrêa de Araújo-Jr G, Campos JM, Martins-Filho ED, Carneiro D'Albuquerque LA, Ferraz Álvaro AB. Preliminary results of hyperbaric oxygen therapy on patients on the waiting list for liver transplantation. ABCD. Arquivos Brasileiros de Cirurgia Digestiva (São Paulo), 2011; 24(1), 48-51. Retrieved January 13, 2016, from http://www.scielo.br/scielo.php?script=sci_arttext&pid=S0102-67202011000100010&lng=en&tlng=en.

Kurir TT, Markotic A, Katalinic V, Bozanic D, Cikes V, Zemunik T, et al. Effect of hyperbaric oxygenation on the regeneration of the liver after partial hepatectomy in rats. Braz J Med Biol Res. 2004;37(8):1231–7.

Kurusz M, Roach JD, Vertrees RA, Girouard MK, Lick SD. Leukocyte filtration in lung transplantation. Perfusion. 2002;17 Suppl 2:63–7.

Ladaga LG, Nabseth DC, Besznyak I, Hendry WF, McLeod G, Deterling Jr RA. Preservation of canine kidneys by hypothermia and hyperbaric oxygen: long term survival of autografts following 24-hour storage. Ann Surg. 1966;163(4):553–8.

Lempert N, Blumenstock DA, Carter RD. Hyperbaric hypothermic preservation of the dog kidney with and without immediate contralateral nephrectomy. Surg Forum. 1968;16:196.

Lozano DD, Stephenson LL, Zamboni WA. Effect of hyperbaric oxygen therapy and medicinal leeching on survival of axial skin flaps subjected to total venous occlusion. Plast Reconstr Surg. 1999;104(4):1029–32.

Lyons GW, Dietzman RH, Lillehei RC. On the mechanism of preservation with hypothermia and hyperbaric oxygen. Trans Am Soc Art Int Organ. 1966;12(1):236–8.

Makin JS, Howard JM. Hyperbaric oxygen and profound hypothermia to preserve canine kidneys. Transplantation. 1966;4(3):349.

Mills C, Bryson P. The role of hyperbaric oxygen therapy in the treatment of sternal infection. Eur J Cardiothorac Surg. 2006;30(1):153–9.

Moers C, Smits JM, Maathuis MH, Treckmann J, van Gelder J, Napieralski BP, et al. Machine perfusion or cold storage in deceased-donor kidney transplantation. N Engl J Med. 2009;360:7–19.

Morales-Buenrostro LE, Alberu J. Anti-major histocompatibility class 1-related chain A antibodies in organ transplantation. Transplant Rev (Orlando). 2008;22(1):27–38.

Muralidharan V, Christophi C. Hyperbaric oxygen therapy and liver transplantation. HPB (Oxford). 2007;9(3):174–82.

Nori H, Shinohara H, Arakawa Y, Kanemura H, Ikemoto T, Imura S, et al. Beneficial effects of hyperbaric oxygen pretreatment on massive hepatectomy model in rats. Transplantation. 2007;84(12):1656–61.

Nylander G, Lewis D, Nordstrom H, Larsson J. Reduction of post-ischemic edema with hyperbaric oxygen. Plast Reconstr Surg. 1985;76:596–603.

Ozdogan M, Ersoy E, Dundar K, Albayrak L, Devay S, Gundogdu H. Beneficial effect of hyperbaric oxygenation on liver regeneration in cirrhosis. J Surg Res. 2005;129(2):260–4.

Ramaiah SK, Jaeschke H. Role of neutrophils in the pathogenesis of acute inflammatory liver injury. Toxicol Pathol. 2007;35(6):757–66.

Rubbini M, Longobardi P, Rimessi A, Pinton P, Morri A, Semprini G, et al. [A new transportable machine for the preservation of livers to be transplanted by means of hyper-baric oxygenation perfusion]. Chir Ital. 2007;59(5):723–34.

Salgado CJ, Jamali AA, Ortiz JA, Cho JJ, Battista V, Mardini S, et al. Effects of hyperbaric oxygen on the replanted extremity subjected to prolonged warm ischaemia. J Plast Reconstr Aesthet Surg. 2010;63:532–7.

Salvadori M, Rosso G, Bertoni E. Update on ischemia-reperfusion injury in kidney transplantation: Pathogenesis and treatment. World J Transplant. 2015;5(2):52–67.

Sasaki M, Joh T. Oxidative stress and ischemia-reperfusion injury in the gastrointestinal tract and antioxidant, protective agents. J Clin Biochem Nutr. 2007;40(1):1–12.

Shepherd L, O'Carroll RE, Ferguson E. An international comparison of deceased and living organ donation/transplant rates in opt-in and opt-out systems: a panel study. BMC Med. 2014;12:131.

Strauss MB, Hargens AR, Gershuni DH, Greenberg DA, Crenshaw AG, Hart GB, et al. Reduction of skeletal muscle necrosis using intermittent hyperbaric oxygen in a model compartment syndrome. J Bone Joint Surg. 1983;65A:656.

Talmage DW, Dart GA. Effect of oxygen pressure during culture on the survival of mouse thyroid allografts. Science. 1978;200:1066–7.

Thom SR. Dehydrogenase conversion to oxidase and lipid per- oxidation in the brain after CO poisoning. J Appl Physiol. 1992;73:1584–9.

Yu WK, Chen YW, Shie HG, Lien TC, Kao HK, Wang JH. Hyperbaric oxygen therapy as an adjunctive treatment for sternal infection and osteomyelitis after sternotomy and cardiothoracic surgery. J Cardiothorac Surg. 2011;6(1):141–6.

Zamboni WA, Roth AC, Russell RC, Graham B, Suchy H, Kucan JO. Morphologic analysis of the microcirculation during reperfusion of ischemic skeletal muscle and the effect of hyperbaric oxygen. Plast Reconstr Surg. 1998;91:1111–21.

Zemmel NJ, Amis LR, Sheppard FR, Drake DB. A temporal analysis of the effects of pressurized oxygen (HBO) on the pH of amputated muscle tissue. Ann Plast Surg. 1998;40:6.

Zwacka RM, Zhou W, Zhang Y, Darby CJ, Dudus L, Halldorson J, et al. Redox gene therapy for ischemia/reperfusion injury of the liver reduces AP1 and NF-kB activation. Nat Med. 1998;4:698–704.

Gerardo Bosco and Enrico M. Camporesi

Abstract

It is widely accepted that O_2 pretreatment before diving can be used for tissue denitrogenation, may reduce decompression requirements, and allows for a quicker restoration of platelet function after a decompression episode. Previous studies presented that anti-oxidative enzymes and related genes in the central nervous system such as catalase (CAT), superoxide dismutase (SOD), and hemo-oxygenase-1 were induced in tissues by HBO pre-breathing. Many patients have been treated with hyperbaric oxygen (HBO) pre-breathing in clinical practice. Even though the mechanisms of action have not been assessed, encouraging results were obtained. Although the number of publications on this topic is increasing, research that focuses on HBO pretreatment in a clinical setting is still scant. Until now, only a small number of publications have explored the connection between HBO pre-oxygenation, the human brain, and myocardial pathology and obtained robust results.

Keywords

Hyperbaric oxygen (HBO) treatment • Diving medicine • Pre-procedure oxygenation • Preconditioning

Introduction

During the few last decades, 100 % oxygen pre-breathing has been used for many different reasons in many different fields, such as the denitrogenation of the lungs and other tissues to extend useful apnea time during breath-old diving and before flights to high altitudes or up to very low environmental pressures (i.e., in space exploration) for denitrogenation prior to extravehicular activities (EVA). Breathing-elevated concentrations of oxygen during preoxygenation have been shown to generate effects that reflect the therapeutic and physiologic applications seen both in extreme settings and in particular clinical situations. At a normal environmental pressure, a common use of pre-oxygenation is in anesthetized patients where the extension of safe apnea times for intubation is a proven safety maneuver after muscle paralysis and rapid induction of anesthesia: this practice is an important clinical application that allows protracted laryngoscopy exposure time for tracheal intubation, specifically in subjects disposed to a quick desaturation succeeding apnea, such as pregnant women, children, and the obese.

Hyperbaric Medicine Perspective

Short-term hyperbaric O2 exposure has generated favorable results after extensive surgical procedures entailing cardiopulmonary bypass or major pancreatic surgery (Bosco et al. 2013). Oxygenated blood augments activities and amount of oxidants agents produced through the perfusion of ischemic tissue. Liberation of cytokines and reactive oxygen species (ROS) such as hydroxyl radical ($\cdot$OH), superoxide radical

G. Bosco, MD, PhD
Department of Biomedical Sciences, University of Padova, Padova, Italy

E.M. Camporesi, MD (✉)
University of South Florida, Tampa, FL, USA

Tampa General Hospital,
1 Tampa General Circle, Suite A327, Tampa, FL 33606, USA
e-mail: ecampore@health.usf.edu

© Springer International Publishing AG 2017
K.K. Jain, *Textbook of Hyperbaric Medicine*, DOI 10.1007/978-3-319-47140-2_40

(O_2^-), hydrogen peroxide (H_2O_2), and the activation of the complement system are possible dangerous consequences of early ischemic injury. This event has been described as ischemia-reperfusion (I/R) injury. Furthermore, animal studies have shown variability of endurance and susceptibility between various organs that have been investigated. There are several scientific publications that examined I/R injury in tissues such as lung, liver, kidney, brain, heart muscle, testis, and skeletal muscle (Yu et al. 2005). Atherosclerotic occlusive disease, arterial thrombosis or arterial embolism, and cardiovascular surgery are some of the situations in which I/R injury may affect skeletal muscles and bone (Grisotto et al. 2000). Furthermore, ischemia-reperfusion may often arise in surgery, such as when a tourniquet is applied to a limb to ensure a bloodless operative field (Ozyurt et al. 2007). Significant postoperative difficulties and multiple-organ dysfunctions are sequelae of I/R injury. In spite of advances in anesthetic methods and in surgical procedures, I/R represents an expected event during cardiac surgery. Reduced cardiac output as an acute effect and heart failure as a chronic sequel are the results of myocardial stunning, necrosis, or apoptosis in I/R injury during cardiopulmonary bypass (Bolli et al. 2004). Brain injury following cardiac surgery is an issue that is widely discussed in literature. Aftermath if I/R injury may be relatively less serious such as postoperative cognitive dysfunction and delirium, or serious such as stroke (Gao et al. 2005).

The complex origins of cerebral adverse effects after cardiac bypass surgery must be sought in the mutual influence among cerebral micro-emboli, decreased global cerebral perfusion, inflammation processes, cerebral temperature regulation, and hereditary weakness and may be useful in identifying potential therapeutic targets for pharmacologic neuroprotection (Sato et al. 2002). Preconditioning might initiate endogenous protective procedures able to reduce the structural and practical after-effects following outcome of ischemia. The studies in the ischemic preconditioning field were initially performed using a heart model from a dog in which the IR injury was overt initially (Murry et al. 1986) and it was evident in the brain tissues afterwards (Kitagawa et al. 1990). Later on, the desire to replicate the defensive functions of preconditioning in cardiac surgery led the pharmacologists to conduct numerous studies in order to recognize mediators such as volatile anesthetic agents and ischemic preconditioning (Hausenloy et al. 2007; Wu et al. 2003; Yellon et al. 1993). Preceding works presented that antioxidative enzymes and related genes in the central nervous system, including catalase (CAT), superoxide dismutase, and hemeoxygenase-1, were initiated by HBO preconditioning (Li et al. 2007; Sterling et al. 1993; Wada et al. 1996). Even though the number of scientific publications on this topic is rising, works that treat HBO preconditioning in a clinical setting are still few. According to a report, three sessions of HBO at 2.4 ATA (243.18 kPa) prior to on-pump coronary artery bypass graft (CABG) decreased neuropsychometric dysfunction and favorably controlled the inflammatory response after CPB (Alex et al. 2005). More recently, Yogaratnam and colleagues (Yogaratnam et al. 2010) stated that preoxygenation with a single session of HBO at 2.5 ATA (253.32 kPa) for 90 min before on-pump CABG surgery improved left ventricular stroke post-CABG surgery while reducing intraoperative blood loss, ICU length of stay, and postoperative complications. Other authors have portrayed the effective use of HBO to prevent restenosis after percutaneous transluminal coronary intervention (PTCI) in acute myocardial infraction (Shari et al. 2004). Moreover, preoxygenation could reduce the levels of cerebral and myocardial biomarkers such as S100B protein, neuron-specific enolase (NSE), and troponin I (cTnI) in the peri-and post-CABG surgery period (Li et al. 2011). Considerable reduction of the liberation of S100B and NSE, due to the repeated HBO preconditioning treatments, represents the most important conclusion of this final wide-ranging research. Another interesting consideration of this work is referred to such elements as serum troponin I, intrope usage, ventilator hours, length of ICU stay, postoperative duration of hospital stay, hemodynamics parameters, and serum CAT activity, while evaluating the consequences of HBO preconditioning on them. Optimistic outcomes on the cardiac and neurological functions were shown among on-pump surgical sufferers, treated with reiterative HBO preconditioning sessions, but this was not observed for off-pump CABG surgical sufferers. These facts suggest that HBO preconditioning was able to offset more ischemic events arising during cardiopulmonary bypass. A new empirical study identified a significant procedure implicated in setting of the helpful effect of preoxygenation, as the intracellular initiation of heme-oxygenase-1 in hepatic I/R injury (Liu et al. 2011). Further research is needed in order to understand if modifications of the different parameters of a preoxygenation procedure, such as pressure, frequency, or lag time before surgery, can lead to a different conclusion.

Diving Medicine

Decompression sickness (DCS) is a standard treatment for one of the common problems in diving medicine, which is treatable with HBO (Vann et al. 2009). It has been widely demonstrated that a positive reduction of air bubble production and platelet activation after a given immersion, using HBO and normobaric oxygen (NBO) pre-breathing maneuvers, can prevent the development of DCS (Arieli et al. 2011; Bosco et al. 2010). In fact, oxygen exposure is used with success in various diving activities in leisure time, in military applications (Castagna et al. 2009), in sport, and in commercial diving

(Piepho et al. 2007). It was shown that bubble formation was lower in divers after a set dive exposure with an in-water pre-oxygenation at depth of 6 or 12 m of seawater (msw) than preoxygenation at surface of water in open sea (Bosco et al. 2010). Furthermore, the same study presented a difference between HBO and NBO prebreathing in reducing bubble formation and platelet activation, with a more effective treatment with HBO (Bosco et al. 2010). Other studies considered the oxidative status and intracellular calcium (Ca^{2+}_i) of peripheral blood lymphocytes during a brief dive at the depth of 30 msw after the in-water preoxygenation session (Morabito et al. 2011). The main findings of this study were that an improvement of lymphocyte antioxidant action and a decrease of ROS quantity were related to O_2 preconditioning. Other effects due to O_2 preconditioning in water are preservation of calcium balance, which hints at a defensive role in the physiological functions of lymphocyte cell. Remarkably, an increase of catalase, SOD, and glutathione peroxidase mRNA gene expression, found by the researchers, suggests an improved antioxidant protection. Furthermore, no signs of Ca^{2+}_i augmentation were witnessed, which is evidence of a reduced oxidative stress (Morabito et al. 2011). It was suggested that a N_2 washout effect by oxygen at ground levels was quickly neutralized at depth (Landolfi et al. 2006). This concept was demonstrated by analyzing the comparison between groups of tissues that were not exposed to HBO and those that were subjected to preoxygenation. It was observed that the partial pressure of dissolved nitrogen in fast tissues at 4 ATA (405.30 kPa) compression was similar. Furthermore, the authors stated that an O_2 prebreathing at 1.6 ATA (162.12 kPa) was able to reduce post-decompression bubble formation from 4 ATA (405.30 kPa). This outcome is in accord with the process of gas nuclei removal through O_2 preconditioning (Arieli et al. 2002). Certainly, other preceding empirical works have revealed that lag period for restoration of a washed-out gas nuclei population may range from a few hours up to 100 h (Younth 1982). Similarly, research has established that breathing normobaric O_2 for a period of 30 min before an open water air dive produces significant decrease in bubble formation, which was detected after the assessment of venous gas emboli (VGE), Doppler ultrasound, and bubble formation score (Castagna et al. 2009). The greater the number of dives, the higher is the VGE production with a greater danger of evolving DCS, subsequent to repeated dives in a single day (Dunford et al. 2002; Hamilton and Thalmann 2003). Three different theories describe how O_2 pretreatment can induce the decrease of VGE: denitrogenation, gas nuclei removal, and hemodynamic effects (Castagna et al. 2009). Therefore, tissue N_2 super saturation prevents bubble formation (Behnke 1967). Furthermore, it is known that exercise can provide additional defense against the onset of DCS because of increased metabolic levels, enhanced ventilation, improved blood perfusion, and diffusion during oxygen pretreatment before altitude decompression

(Webb and Pilmanis 1999). In gas nuclei elimination, oxygen has the ability to substitute nitrogen in the cell nucleus by diffusion, thus removing preformed gas micronuclei before bubble production (Landolfi et al. 2006; Butler et al. 2006; Katsenelson et al. 2007). In addition, it has been proposed that O_2 is responsible for the removal of protein-coated bubbles by the lymphatic bed (Balestra et al. 2004), suggesting a reduction of gas nuclei in both venous and lymphatic systems (Castagna et al. 2009). However, it was observed that this process generates a decrease in the dimension of bubbles, but not their density (Arieli et al. 2002). Regarding hemodynamic consequences, it has been recognized that a 1-h O_2 pretreatment session at sea level in a group of healthy individuals resulted in a lower heart rate and cardiac output in conjunction with an augmented vascular resistance (Waring et al. 2003). These changes persisted well over an hour and after that the environmental 21 % O_2 was reinstated (Thomson et al. 2006).

References

Alex J, Laden G, Cale A, Bennett S, Flowers K, Madden L, et al. Pretreatment with hyperbaric oxygen and its effect on neuropsychometric dysfunction and systemic inflammatory response after cardiopulmonary bypass: A prospective randomised double- blind trial. J Thorac Cardiovasc Surg. 2005;130(6):1623–30.

Arieli Y, Arieli R, Marx A. Hyperbaric oxygen may reduce gas bubbles in decompressed prawns by eliminating gas nuclei. J Appl Physiol. 2002;92:2596–9.

Arieli R, Boaron E, Arieli Y, Abramovich A, Katsenelson K. Oxygen pretreatment as protection against decompression sickness in rats: pressure and time necessary for hypothesized denucleation and renucleation. Eur J Appl Physiol. 2011;111:997–1005.

Balestra C, Germonpre P, Snoeck T, Ezquer M, Leduc O, Leduc A, et al. Normobaric oxygen can enhance protein captation by the lymphatic system in healthy humans. Undersea Hyperb Med. 2004;31:59–62.

Behnke AR. The isobaric (oxygen window) principle of decompression. In: The new thrust seaward. Transactions of the third annual conference of marine technology society. San Diego: Marine Technology Society; 1967.

Bolli R, Becker L, Gross G, Mentzer Jr R, Balshaw D, Lathrop DA. Myocardial protection at a crossroads: the need for translation into clinical therapy. Circ Res. 2004;95:125–34.

Bosco G, Yang ZJ, Di Tano G, Camporesi EM, Faralli F, Savini F, et al. Effect of in-water oxygen prebreathing at different depths on decompression- induced bubble formation and platelet activation. J Appl Physiol. 2010;108:1077–83.

Bosco G, Guizzon L, Yang Z, Camporesi E, Casarotto A, Bosio C, et al. Effect of hyperbaric oxygenation and gemcitabine on apoptosis of pancreatic ductal tumor cells in vitro. Anticancer Res. 2013;33(11):4827–32.

Butler BD, Little T, Cogan V, Powell M. Hyperbaric oxygen pre-breathe modifies the outcome of decompression sickness. Undersea Hyperb Med. 2006;33:407–17.

Castagna O, Gempp E, Blatteau JE. Pre-dive normobaric oxygen reduces bubble formation in scuba divers. Eur J Appl Physiol. 2009;106:167–72.

Dunford RG, Vann RD, Gerth WA, Pieper CF, Huggins K, Wacholtz C, et al. The incidence of venous gas emboli in recreational diving. Undersea Hyperb Med. 2002;29:247–59.

Gao L, Taha R, Gauvin D, Othmen LB, Wang Y, Blaise G. Postoperative cognitive dysfunction after cardiac surgery. Chest. 2005;128:3664–70.

Grisotto PC, dos Santos AC, Coutinho-Netto J, Cherri J, Piccinato CE. Indicators of oxidative injury and alterations of the cell membrane in the skeletal muscle of rats submitted to ischemia and reperfusion. J Surg Res. 2000;92:1–6.

Hamilton RW, Thalmann ED. Decompression practice. In: Brubakk AO, Neuman TS, editors. Bennett & Elliott's physiology and medicine of diving. 5th ed. New York: Elsevier Science; 2003. p. 455–500.

Hausenloy DJ, Mwamure PK, Venugopal V, Harris J, Barnard M, Grundy E, et al. Effect of remote ischaemic preconditioning on myocardial injury in patients undergoing coronary artery bypass graft surgery: a randomised controlled trial. Lancet. 2007;370:575–9.

Katsenelson K, Arieli Y, Abramovich A, Feinsod M, Arieli R. Hyperbaric oxygen pretreatment reduces the incidence of decompression sickness in rats. Eur J Appl Physiol. 2007;101:571–6.

Kitagawa K, Matsumoto M, Tagaya M, Hata R, Ueda H, Niinobe M, et al. 'Ischemic tolerance' phenomenon found in the brain. Brain Res. 1990;528:21–4.

Landolfi A, Yang Z, Savini F, Camporesi E, Faralli F, Bosco G. Pretreatment with hyperbaric oxygenation reduces bubble formation and platelet activation. Sport Sci Health. 2006;1:122–8.

Li Q, Li J, Zhang L, Wang B, Xiong L. Preconditioning with hyperbaric oxygen induces tolerance against oxidative injury via increased expression of hemeoxygenase-1 in primary cultured spinal cord neurons. Life Sci. 2007;80:1087–93.

Li Y, Dong H, Chen M, Liu J, Yang L, Chen S, et al. Preconditioning with repeated hyperbaric oxygen induces myocardial and cerebral protection in patients undergoing coronary artery bypass graft surgery: a prospective, randomized, controlled clinical trial. J Cardiothorac Vasc Anesth. 2011;25(6):908–16.

Liu Y, Sun XJ, Liu J, Kang ZM, Deng XM. Hemeoxygenase-1 could mediate the protective effects of hyperbaric oxygen preconditioning against hepatic ischemia-reperfusion injury in rats. Clin Exp Pharmacol Physiol. 2011;38:675–82.

Morabito C, Bosco G, Pilla R, Corona C, Mancinelli R, Yang Z, et al. Effect of pre-breathing oxygen at different depth on oxidative status and calcium concentration in lymphocytes of scuba divers. Acta Physiol (Oxf). 2011;202:69–78.

Murry CE, Jennings RB, Reimer KA. Preconditioning with ischemia: a delay of lethal cell injury in ischemic myocardium. Circulation. 1986;74:1124–36.

Ozyurt H, Ozyurt B, Koca K, Ozgocmen S. Caffeic acid phenethyl ester (CAPE) protects rat skeletal muscle against ischemia-reperfusion-induced oxidative stress. Vascul Pharmacol. 2007;47:108–12.

Piepho T, Ehrmann U, Werner C, Muth CM. Oxygen therapy in diving accidents. Anaesthesist. 2007;56:44–52.

Sato Y, Laskowitz DT, Bennett ER, Newman MF, Warner DS, Grocott HP. Differential cerebral gene expression during cardiopulmonary bypass in the rat: evidence for apoptosis? Anesth Analg. 2002;94:1389–94.

Shari M, Fares W, Abdel-Karim I, Koch JM, Sopko J, Adler D, Hyperbaric Oxygen Therapy in Percutaneous Coronary Interventions Investigators. Usefulness of hyperbaric oxygen therapy to inhibit restenosis after percutaneous coronary intervention for acute myocardial infarction or unstable angina pectoris. Am J Cardiol. 2004;93(12):1533–5.

Sterling DL, Thornton JD, Swafford A, Gottlieb SF, Bishop SP, Stanley AW, et al. Hyperbaric oxygen limits infarct size in ischemic rabbit myocardium in vivo. Circulation. 1993;88:1931–6.

Thomson AJ, Drummond GB, Waring WS, Webb DJ, Maxwell SR. Effects of short-term isocapnic hyperoxia and hypoxia on cardiovascular function. J Appl Physiol. 2006;101:809–16.

Vann RD, Denoble PJ, Howle LE, Weber PW, Freiberger JJ, Pieper CF. Resolution and severity in decompression illness. Aviat Space Environ Med. 2009;80:466–71.

Wada K, Ito M, Miyazawa T, Katoh H, Nawashiro H, Shima K, et al. Repeated hyperbaric oxygen induces ischemic tolerance in gerbil hippocampus. Brain Res. 1996;740:15–20.

Waring WS, Thomson AJ, Adwani SH, Rosseel AJ, Potter JF, Webb DJ, et al. Cardiovascular effects of acute oxygen administration in healthy adults. J Cardiovasc Pharmacol. 2003;42:245–50.

Webb JT, Pilmanis AA. Preoxygenation time versus decompression sickness incidence. SAFE J. 1999;29:75–8.

Wu ZK, Iivainen T, Pehkonen E, Laurikka J, Tarkka MR. Arrhythmias in off-pump coronary artery bypass grafting and the antiarrhythmic effect of regional ischemic preconditioning. J Cardiothorac Vasc Anesth. 2003;17:459–64.

Yellon DM, Alkhulai AM, Pugsley WB. Preconditioning the human myocardium. Lancet. 1993;342:276–7.

Yogaratnam JZ, Laden G, Guvendik L, Cowen M, Cale A, Griffin S. Hyperbaric oxygen preconditioning improves myocardial function, reduces length of intensive care stay, and limits complications post coronary artery by-pass graft surgery. Cardiovasc Revasc Med. 2010;11:8–19.

Younth DE. On the evolution, generation, and regeneration of gas cavitation nuclei. J Acoust Soc Am. 1982;71:1473–81.

Yu SY, Chiu JH, Yang SD, Yu HY, Hsieh CC, Chen PJ, et al. Preconditioned hyperbaric oxygenation protects the liver against ischemia-reperfusion injury in rats. J Surg Res. 2005;128:28–36.

Anesthesia in the Hyperbaric Environment

41

Enrico M. Camporesi

Abstract

Use of anesthesia in the HBO environment is unusual. This chapter gives a historical perspective and describes the physics of anesthetic gases under pressure as well as the relevant physiology. There are practical aspects of anesthesia in hyperbaric environment of the chamber and several clinical indications are mentioned that require especially diligent attention to technique. Potential complications of anesthesia in the hyperbaric chamber are mentioned. Prophylactic bilateral myringotomy is recommended to avoid middle ear equilibration problems in an unconscious patient. Intravenous anesthesia is preferred to gaseous inhalation.

Keywords

Anesthetic gas physics • Complications of hyperbaric oxygen • Hyperbaric chamber • Hyperbaric oxygen • Intravenous anesthesia • Myringotomy • Nitrous oxide anesthesia • Respiration in hyperbaric environment

Historical Perspective

The administration of general anesthesia in the hyperbaric environment was first described by Paul Bert in 1878. His aim was to use nitrous oxide in anesthetic doses and to be able to provide adequate oxygenation. Through the use of elevated pressure, he reported this successful endeavor. His results were confirmed by Tindal in 1941 and were reconfirmed by Smith et al. in 1974.

In the 1940s and 1950s, cardiac surgical techniques clearly outgrew life support technology. Interest in the surgical treatment of congenital heart malformations grew rapidly after Blalock performed the first successful procedure for tetralogy of Fallot in 1944. When surgical correction of the septal and valvular abnormalities was attempted, the intracardiac portions of the procedures had to be done under hypothermia and cardiopulmonary arrest, as this provided a motionless heart. Limitations to this technique were primarily the short times of total circulatory arrest (less than 10 min) without significant ischemic CNS sequelae. General anesthesia under hyperbaric oxygenation (HBO) provided an added degree of protection and increased the safe cardiac arrest time up to 30 min. Several groups have reported their experiences with anesthesia under hyperbaric conditions, including Smith at Massachusetts General Hospital, Boerema in Holland, and McDowell at the Royal Infirmary in Glasgow (Smith 1965; Boerema 1961; McDowell et al. 1966). Anesthesia was usually achieved and maintained through the use of nitrous oxide, halothane, or methoxyflurane.

In the mid-1960s, a practical cardiopulmonary bypass machine was perfected for wider use. With the introduction of safe cardiopulmonary bypass pumps, cardiac surgery no longer needed to be performed in the hyperbaric chamber. Carotid endarterectomy had also been performed under hyperbaric conditions, but this practice fell into disfavor, as it was never firmly demonstrated to be beneficial.

A landmark report from a committee headed by Severinghaus reviewed the practice of anesthesia under

E.M. Camporesi, MD (✉)
University of South Florida, Tampa, FL, USA

Tampa General Hospital, 1 Tampa General Circle, Suite A327, Tampa, FL 33606, USA
e-mail: ecampore@health.usf.edu

© Springer International Publishing AG 2017
K.K. Jain, *Textbook of Hyperbaric Medicine*, DOI 10.1007/978-3-319-47140-2_41

hyperbaric conditions (Severinghaus 1965). No recommendations on choice of anesthetic were made in this report; rather, the advantages and disadvantages of commonly used techniques were presented. However, it was stated that intravenous techniques could prove especially useful in the hyperbaric setting.

Current Indications

Anesthetic care may be required at increased pressure for the following indications:

- Anesthesia delivered for the treatment of various conditions that produce transient hypoxemia, such as whole lung lavage (usually performed at 2–4 ATA).
- Delivery of anesthesia as a result of emergency surgical procedures required on a patient involved in a diving accident, which might occur while at pressures of up to 35 ATA (depth of saturation in deepest commercial diving).

The phenomenon of pressure reversal of barbiturate anesthesia in mammals has been in rats at pressures of 103 ATA (Winter et al. 1976). However, the clinical relevance of these findings proved of limited value, since therapeutic pressures of HBO do not exceed 6ATA. A comprehensive review of this argument appeared later (Kendig and Cohen 1977). Continuing studies, however, in the areas of high pressure physiology have extended the range of pressures tolerated by humans. The deepest exposure recorded for a human is at 69 ATA and was achieved during a study of physiological responses to exercise at Duke University Hyperbaric Center (Salzano et al. 1984).

Physical Considerations Concerning Anesthetic

Modern vaporizers work by forcing a gas, usually oxygen, at a known flow rate through a sintered bronze disk at the bottom of a pool of liquid anesthetic. The amount of anesthetic agent delivered to the patient depends on four factors:

- The particular vapor pressure of the agent (a function of the polarity of the agent, i.e., Vander Waals forces)
- The temperature of the liquid
- The flow of gas through the liquid
- The dilution of the anesthetic vapor with by-pass oxygen flow to constitute the desired concentration for delivery

The key point in calculating the required flows at various ambient pressures is that the vapor pressure of a liquid remains constant with variations in ambient pressure (Morris

1952). For example, the vapor pressure of halothane at 20 °C is 243 mmHg. According to Dalton's law of partial pressures, saturated halothane vapor at 1 ATA (760 mmHg) will contain 32 % halothane (243/760), while at 4 ATA (3040 mmHg) the same halothane partial pressure will produce a concentration of 8 % (243/3040). The amount of carrier gas required to dilute the saturated vapor to the desired inspired concentration (0.5–1 %, at the clinically useful doses) remains constant with changing ambient pressure. If the desired inspired partial pressure is 7.6 mmHg (1 % halothane at 1 ATA), each volume of saturated vapor must be diluted with 32 volumes of carrier gas at 1 ATA, or with 8 volumes at 4 ATA (which represents the same number of molecules).

Few empirical observations in this area used the Fluotec vaporizer at pressure and measured actual concentrations of gas delivered at different dial settings (McDowell 1987). The Fluotec vaporizer works by directing a stream of gas over a surface of liquid anesthetic and diluting the total gas output. McDowell found that the particular vaporizer tested would deviate at low settings (0.5–1 %), by delivering nearly twice the anesthetic gas concentration while at 2 atm. Gas concentrations did not vary significantly from 1 ATA at higher settings (from 2 to 4 %).

Flowmeters/rotameters are also affected by pressure, as they measure the flow of a gas on the principle that flow past a resistance is proportional to the pressure gradient. Density is the key variable, especially at high flow rates. Viscosity is a more significant variable at low rates, when the shape of the resistance is tubular. At increased ambient pressure, the approximate correction factor is:

$$F_1 = F_0 \times \sqrt{d_0 / d_1}$$

where F_1 represents the flow at ambient pressure, F0 the indicated flow, d0 the density at 1 ATA, and d1 the density at present ATA.

For example, at 4 ATA:

$$F_1 = F_0 \times 1 / 4$$

Therefore,

$$F_1 = 0.5 F_0$$

This calculation is a good correction estimate if one assumes that the supply line pressure gradient between the chamber and the outside is kept constant.

Physiological Considerations

The major alterations of increased pressures are reflected in the respiratory, the cardiac, and the central nervous systems.

Exposure for 24 h to high levels of oxygen (90–100 %) at 1–2 ATA can result in rapid damage to the mucosa of the tracheobronchial tree, manifested by hyperemic mucosa, increased secretions, and atelectasis. This might be of special importance in the patient with reactive airway disease or chronic obstructive pulmonary disease. Airway irritation could complicate endotracheal intubations, because of increased tendency to laryngospasm.

In chronic obstructive pulmonary disease, and any other pulmonary process that narrows the caliber of the airways, increased secretions and increased work of breathing at increased ambient pressure may lead to severe ventilatory difficulties. In addition, pulmonary bullae and other slow exchange zones, as well as mucus plugging, may cause a disastrous problem during decompression as they can lead to parenchymal rupture, pneumothorax, or air embolism secondary to barotrauma.

A reduction in vital capacity has been measured as an index of atelectasis, which correlates with the length and pressure of oxygen exposure and is predicted by empirical units, i.e., units of pulmonary toxicity dose (UPTD) (Clark and Lambertsen 1971). Reductions of vital capacity reverse within hours after termination of oxygen exposure (Don et al. 1970; Hickey et al. 1973).

Loss of pulmonary surfactant has been described after exposure to HBO. It is not clear whether peroxidation of surfactant plays a significant role in its destruction, but it is clearly demonstrated that surfactant production is inhibited. There is evidence, especially in practice, that adequate humidification of inspired gases protects against some of these pulmonary problems, especially airway irritation (Miller et al. 1987). The work of breathing is increased at increased ambient pressures. This is a result of increased turbulent flow due to high gas density. These pressure-induced changes can be minimized by using the largest possible endotracheal tubes.

Cardiovascular Effects

It has been demonstrated that significant peripheral vasoconstriction occurs with the exposure to high blood oxygen tensions. It has been shown in humans that, although the peripheral vasoconstriction does occur, the pulmonary vascular resistance is decreased (Barratt-Boyes and Wood 1958). Because of the peripheral vasoconstriction, one should avoid giving medications through intramuscular or subcutaneous routes.

Vasoconstriction can also occur in coronary vessels. A number of studies have demonstrated that coronary blood flow is significantly decreased during exposure to HBO. Patients with significant obstructive coronary disease should be approached cautiously, especially in the delivery of a general anesthetic under HBO.

Some studies have demonstrated that cardiac output can be reduced by as much as 12 % during hyperbaric hyperoxia.

Probably as a result of increased afterload, no significant changes in contractility have been demonstrated, in a sophisticated dog model exposed to 3 ATA O_2 (Savitt et al. 1994).

Central Nervous System

Oxygen is also a potent cerebral vasoconstrictor that affects pial as well as cerebral arterioles. This principle becomes important when treating patients with closed head injuries, as one would expect a protective effect of oxygen on neural structures in patients with closed head injuries or intracranial masses. Although few data on this subject are available, it is possible that seizure threshold may be reduced during general anesthesia in patients who are already at higher risk for seizures. Such patients should have prophylactic anticonvulsant medications before exposures to HBO at high pressures (3 ATA or above) under anesthesia.

The ability of the attending personnel in the chamber to make sound clinical decisions may be impaired while exposed to breathing air at high pressure. Inert gas narcosis is a well-described phenomenon in humans breathing air at increased atmospheric pressure. Although not always a significant problem, inert gas narcosis can be observed at pressures of 2 ATA and greater. Nitrogen narcosis is not unpleasant and it has been compared to alcohol intoxication. The affected individual may also experience drowsiness and euphoria and judgment can be impaired. The severity of nitrogen narcosis is directly proportional to the pressure to which a patient is exposed. Patients are usually not at risk since they are breathing high oxygen levels.

Nitrous Oxide Anesthesia

Despite mainly the theoretical value of the research, the most extensive and precise human study of nitrous oxide (N_2O) as a sole anesthetic agent in the hyperbaric environment was published by Russell et al. (1990). He described the physiologic effects of induction and maintenance of N_2O general anesthesia under stable hyperbaric conditions at 2.0 ATA (1520 mmHg) in eight healthy ASA 1 male volunteers ranging in age from 20 to 31 years. A large hyperbaric chamber housed the volunteer and two anesthesiologists: the chamber was compressed with air to 2.0 ATA and induction of anesthesia by mask was initiated at depth with large vital capacity breaths of 75 % N_2O and 25 % O_2. Unconsciousness was reached in a few breaths and intubation was facilitated by succinylcholine. Duration of anesthesia ranged from 2 to 4 h with spontaneous ventilation and extensive monitoring of the EEG and of respiratory gases via mass spectrometry.

Hypertension, tachycardia, tachypnea, bursts of increased sympathetic nervous system activity, and occasional clonus and opisthotonus were noted as characteristic of general anesthesia with hyperbaric N₂O. Further, no prolonged residual effects have been noted. Still, it appears that this anesthesia technique is not practical in a clinical setting. This important publication also established a more precise level of MAC for N₂O, closer to 1.2 ATA, refining the previously published value of 1.04 ATA (Hornbein et al. 1982).

Intravenous Anesthesia

Ross et al. (1977) were one of the first groups to advocate intravenous anesthesia for use in the hyperbaric chamber. This was a result of considering the problem of anesthetic gas pollution while delivering gaseous anesthetics at pressures of up to 35 ATA. Li (1987) reported the successful use of ketamine anesthesia in 48 patients undergoing open heart surgery while having oxygen administered at 3 ATA. Ketamine and benzodiazepines have been used along with muscle relaxants in the delivery of anesthesia to patients undergoing therapeutic lung lavages (Moon and Camporesi 1987). Approximately 20 patients have been treated with this anesthetic regimen without complications.

Pharmacokinetics in the Hyperbaric Environment

There is only a small volume of data concerning the pharmacokinetics of i.v. anesthetics in the literature. A few studies have been performed with specific agents using animal models. Drugs studied include meperidine and pentobarbital. No significant differences were observed in the half-life, volume of distribution, or plasma clearance of the drugs when pentobarbital and meperidine were measured at 2.8 or 6 ATA. Despite the fact that absolute pharmacokinetic values for the dog differ considerably from those of humans, these observations support the concept that intravenous anesthetic agents commonly used at 1 ATA can be judiciously administered at pressures of 2–6 ATA (Table 41.1).

Pressure reversal has been investigated and no significant differences were detected in the pharmacokinetics of pentobarbital

when given at 1, 2.8, or 6 ATA (Kramer et al. 1983a, b). In addition, one does not observe this phenomenon in practice, especially at 2.8 ATA. Pressure reversal could play a role if anesthesia is being delivered at much greater depths (e.g., >50 ATA).

Practical Aspects of Anesthesia in the Pressure Chamber

Noise

During decompression and compression, the air entering or escaping the chamber generates a significant level of noise, which can interfere with auscultation or the ability to hear equipment alarms. These traveling times are precisely when the anesthetist must be especially alert of the condition of the patient. Most complications in anesthetic management occur during these chamber pressure changes.

Airway Equipment

Laryngoscopes are not greatly affected by pressure as long as the battery handle is vented and can exchange gas at pressure. Sealed batteries have been shown to function adequately up to 35 ATA. Endotracheal tubes should be of the largest size appropriate for the patient, as when pressure rises, turbulent flow increases and will cause an increase in airway resistance and increasing ventilatory work. Tracheal tube cuffs should be filled with saline rather than air, since water is incompressible and the danger of volume variations in the cuff with changing ambient pressure is avoided.

Ventilators

It is imperative to minimize the amount of electrical equipment in the hyperbaric chamber where oxygen partial pressures are high and the danger of fire and explosion are very real.

Ventilators driven by compressed air are desirable. One must keep in mind that these ventilators function through a

Table 41.1 Pharmacokinetic parameters for meperidine (M) and pentobarbital (P) under normal and hyperbaric conditions (Mean ± SD)

Parameter/Drug	1 ATA	2.8 ATA	6 ATA
$t_{1/2}$ (min)/M	60.40 ± 43.6	44.90 ± 22.7	55.70 ± 17.5
$t_{1/2}$ (h)/P	4.49 ± 1.11	4.88 ± 1.89	6.08 ± 2.29
CLT (mL/(min/kg))/M	75.20 ± 49.8	84.40 ± 37.4	75.40 ± 40.0
CLT (mL/(min/kg))/P	2.82 ± 0.32	3.69 ± 1.23	2.67 ± 0.85
V (L/kg)/M	4.56 ± 2.06	5.18 ± 2.77	5.54 ± 1.63
V (L/kg)/P	1.11 ± 0.37	1.44 ± 0.42	1.29 ± 0.24

No statistically significant differences between different pressures were noted (Kramer et al. 1983 a, b)

pressure differential of about 50 psi. Therefore, as long as the supply line is adjusted to maintain this differential gradient above ambient pressure, the ventilators should work well at pressure, although they will exhibit somewhat lower peak flow rates.

Another consideration is the rate of oxygen leakage from the ventilator. This must be kept to a minimum, as standard operating procedure for multiplace hyperbaric units dictates that the ambient concentration of oxygen should not exceed 23 %. This can be achieved by choosing a ventilator with an inherently low oxygen leak and by scavenging and venting outside the chamber. Oil lubrication presents a high risk of fire. Lubrication used for the ventilator should be compatible with high oxygen tensions (e.g., tetrafluorethylene polymer-based lubricants).

Moon and colleagues reported the use of the Monaghan 225 ventilator under hyperbaric conditions (Moon et al. 1986). They found that this ventilator, after minor modifications, provided adequate ventilatory support at pressures of up to 6 ATA.

Monitoring

Because anesthesia is not commonly practiced under hyperbaric conditions, it is not administered according to set rules or special dosage tables that correct for pressure. Rather, the anesthesiologist must titrate the agents used to effect. This makes the importance of good monitoring paramount. Monitoring should include the usual monitors for vital signs. The need for accurate blood pressure readings and access for arterial blood sampling would suggest that an arterial line should be in place prior to any procedure that will require prolonged anesthesia under hyperbaric conditions.

Arterial oxygen measurements present a problem in the chamber. When a sample is drawn and passed through a lock to the surface, gas bubbling may occur during decompression, and the time that the sample remains in transit is also critical. Most blood gas analyzers used in clinical practice are not calibrated to measure oxygen tensions as high as those observed during hyperbaric therapy, therefore oxygen content is only an approximation when it is measured outside the chamber. A direct solution to the problem is to maintain blood gas measuring equipment in the chamber or in a lock pressurized to the same pressure as the therapeutic chamber. The disadvantage of this approach is that, although accurate blood gas measurements can be performed at pressure, trained personnel must remain available in the chamber to carry out the measurements. Pulse oximetry can also be monitored by splicing cables through chamber walls. Its use has been of value when treating patients with high pulmonary shunts, in order to increase ambient partial pressure of O_2 until there is restoration of high SO_2 levels. A respiratory mass spectrometer can be set up outside the chamber with a sampling line traversing the wall of the chamber in order to monitor the actual concentrations of O_2, CO_2, N_2, or N_2O inhalation agent continuously.

At usual therapeutic pressures (2.8 ATA), CNS oxygen toxicity is rarely a problem. If prolonged exposure to high oxygen tension or unusual depths is to be used, EEG should be monitored, especially when muscle paralysis impedes the visual recognition of seizures. Since convulsions are often the first signs of CNS toxicity, the EEG would be the only way to detect a seizure in an adequately paralyzed patient. Electrical activity from the ECG must be monitored as usual, but the monitor itself will usually remain outside the chamber, since it most often uses a CRT-based display. The monitor must remain visible to the attendants inside the chamber through a porthole window. The leads are passed through a pressure tight access to the outside of the chamber. Recently, a variety of flat-screen display monitors have been used to record digital and analog signals during the pressure phase.

Defibrillation is possible during the phase of pressure in the hyperbaric chamber and the use of an R2 defibrillator adaptor on a Life Pak 6S unit has been reported (Martindale et al. 1987). Self-adhering pads were used in order to reduce the danger of fire caused by sparking between defibrillator paddles. As with ECG monitors, the defibrillator unit must be kept outside the chamber and wires passed through the chamber wall and attached to the patient. Standard defibrillator paddles can be used if care is taken to make good paddle-skin contact through the use of a low resistance gel, and the paddles are positioned far enough from each other to prevent arcing across the paddles.

A neuromuscular transmission monitor can be used in the chamber without fear of fire or explosion as the amperage delivered is quite low. Any electrical equipment to be used inside the hyperbaric chamber must be flushed with nitrogen (N2) in order to provide an inert gas atmosphere in case of spark generation.

Prophylactic Myringotomy to Prevent Middle Ear Barotrauma

It is best to induce anesthesia while the patient is at 1 ATA and, after adequate anesthesia is obtained, perform bilateral myringotomy to avoid middle ear equilibration problems. This has been proven to be better than induction of anesthesia at depth, because the patient is more comfortable if the compression phase is avoided. As an alternative, tympanostomy tube may be inserted under local anesthesia beforehand, as it is being commonly used and has been shown to be a safe procedure (Lamprell et al. 2014). Prevention of middle ear barotrauma is described in more detail in Chapter 8.

Conclusion

Anesthesia is not usually performed in the hyperbaric chamber, but there are a few indications for its use in lifesaving hyperbaric therapy. Attention to detail is paramount while delivering anesthesia under hyperbaric conditions. I recommend that, where possible, i.v. anesthesia should be used. Ketamine and benzodiazepine, along with a muscle relaxant, have been proven to be very useful for induction and maintenance of anesthesia under hyperbaric conditions. Inhalation agents almost always leak into the operating environment and are avoided because of their possible effects on the operating team. An anesthetic should be delivered to be effective at pressure and not with any preconceived formulations. At pressures up to 6 ATA, pressure reversal of anesthesia should induce only minor changes from surface treatment.

Prophylactic myringotomy should be done to prevent middle ear barotrauma during anesthesia. A nasogastric tube should be used in every instance in order to drain expanding gastrointestinal air, which is introduced by masking at depth. It will expand to several times the original volume and cause a number of mechanical problems, including ventilatory difficulty and desaturation. If a gas is used, a volatile agent would be preferable to nitrous oxide, especially for prolonged anesthesia, as there is risk of the development of decompression sickness. An anesthetist may be involved in the transfer of patients requiring HBO treatment. The problems of low-altitude helicopter transfer or transport to a hyperbaric facility of patients with decompression sickness via fixed wing in a pressurized aircraft cabin, risk of dehydration, and the use of sedation are reviewed in a book chapter (Bratteboe and Camporesi 2001).

Finally, the anesthetist is an important member of the interdisciplinary team for acute hyperbaric oxygen therapy in a medical center where the other members are emergency room physicians and surgeons and where intensive care therapy is required. Some of the hyperbaric emergencies such as air embolism may arise during surgical procedures and require monitoring by the anesthetist as well as participation in the treatment if such an event should occur.

References

Barratt-Boyes BG, Wood EH. Cardiac output and related measurements and pressure values in the right heart and associated vessels, together with the analysis of the hemodynamic responses to inhalation of high oxygen mixtures in healthy subjects. J Lab Clin Med. 1958;51:72–90.

Boerema I. An operating room for high oxygen pressure. Surgery. 1961;47:291–8.

Bratteboe G, Camporesi EM. Diving injuries and hyperbaric medicine. In: Søreide E, Grande CM, editors. Prehospital trauma care. New York: Marcel Dekker; 2001. p. 639–56.

Clark JM, Lambertsen CJ. Pulmonary oxygen toxicity: a review. Pharmacol Rev. 1971;23:37–133.

Don HF, Wahba M, Cuadrado L, Kelkar K. The effect of anesthesia and 100% oxygen on the functional residual capacity of lungs. Anesthesiology. 1970;32:521–9.

Hickey RF, Visick WD, Fairley HB, Fourcade HE. Effects of halothane anesthesia on functional residual capacity and alveolar-arterial oxygen tension difference. Anesthesiology. 1973;38:20–4.

Hornbein TF, Egger II EI, Winter PM, Smith G, Wetstone D, Smith KH. The minimum alveolar concentration of nitrous oxide in man. Anesth Analg. 1982;61:553–6.

Kendig JJ, Cohen EN. Pressure antagonism to nerve conduction block by anesthetic agents. Anesthesiology. 1977;228:6–10.

Kramer WG, Welch DW, Fife WP, Chaikin BN, Gross DR. Salicylate pharmacokinetics in the dog at 6 ATA in air and at 2.8 ATA in 100% oxygen. Aviat Space Environ Med. 1983a;54:682–4.

Kramer WG, Welch DW, Fife WP, Chaikin BN, Medlock C, Gross DR. Pharmacokinetics of pentobarbital under hyperbaric and hyperoxic conditions in the dog. Aviat Space Environ Med. 1983b;54:1005–8.

Lamprell L, Young D, Vangaveti V, Orton J, Suruliraj A. Retrospective review of grommet procedures under general versus local anaesthesia among patients undergoing hyperbaric oxygen therapy. Diving Hyperb Med. 2014;44(3):137–40.

Li W. Myasthenia gravis treated by hyperbaric oxygenation. A report of 40 cases. Presented at the 9th international congress on hyperbaric medicine. Sydney, Australia, March 1–4, 1987.

Martindale LG, Milligan M, Fries P. Test of an R-2 defibrillation adapter in hyperbaric chamber. J Hyperbaric Med. 1987;2:15–25.

McDowell DG. Anesthesia in the pressure chamber. Anesthesia. 1987;19:321–36.

McDowell DG, Jennett WB, Bloor K, Ledingham IM. The effect of hyperbaric oxygen on oxygen tension of the brain during chloroform anesthesia. Surg Gynecol Obstet. 1966;122:545–9.

Miller WC, Suich DM, Unger KM. Hyperbaric environment for chronic hypoxemia. J Hyperbaric Med. 1987;2:211–4.

Moon RE, Camporesi EM. Pulmonary edema in a young, healthy woman. Chest. 1987;92(2):385–6.

Moon RE, Bergquist LV, Conklin B, Miller JN. Monaghan 225 ventilator under hyperbaric conditions. Chest. 1986;89:846–51.

Morris LE. A new vaporizer for liquid anesthetic agents. Anesthesiology. 1952;13:587–93.

Ross JAS, Manson HJ, Shearer A et al. Some aspects of anesthesia in high pressure environments. In: Proceedings International Congress on Hyperbaric Medicine. Aberdeen: Aberdeen University Press; 1977. p. 449–52.

Russell GB, Snider MT, Richard RB, Loomis JL. Hyperbaric Nitrous Oxide as a Sole Anesthetic Agent in Humans. Anesth Analg. 1990;70:289–95.

Salzano JV, Camporesi EM, Stolp BW, Moon RE. Physiological responses to exercise at 47 and 66 ATA. J Appl Physiol. 1984;57:1055–68.

Savitt MA, Elbeery JR, Owen CH, Rankin JS, Camporesi EM. Mechanism of decreased coronary and systemic blood flow during hyperbaric oxygenation. Undersea Hyperbaric Med 1994; 21 [abstract].

Severinghaus J. Hyperbaric oxygenation: anesthesia and drug effects. A committee report. Anesthesiology. 1965;26:812–24.

Smith RM. Anesthesia during hyperbaric oxygenation. Ann N Y Acad Sci. 1965;117:768–73.

Smith WDA, Mapleson WW, Siebold K, Hargreaves MD, Clarke GM. Nitrous oxide anesthesia induced at atmospheric and hyperbaric pressures. Parts I and II. Br J Anaesth. 1974;46:3–28.

Winter PM, Smith RA, Smith M, Eger 3rd EI. Pressure antagonism of barbiturate anesthesia. Anesthesiology. 1976;44:416–9.

Keith Van Meter

Abstract

For resuscitative effort in advanced cardiopulmonary life support (ACLS) or advanced trauma life support (ATLS) to be successful, one of the contributory therapeutic efforts must be to keep the mitochondrial intermembrane space (IMS), of especially the cells of the heart and brain, supplied with an oxygen tension of approximately one mmHg. This must be so before hypoxia itself degrades the inner mitochondrial membrane respiratory complexes I–V (or electron transport system, otherwise ETS). The ETS supplies the intramitochondrial membrane space with a reservoir of hydrogen ions to power adenosine triphosphate (ATP) synthase to couple adenosine diphosphate (ADP) with inorganic phosphate (Pi) to produce ATP. All of this is enabled by the flow of electron energy to oxygen docked at cytochrome aa3 (respiratory complex IV). ATP is essential to power most of all cellular function and certainly the success of resuscitation in ACLS or ATLS.

While conventional ACLS drugs have been tried over the years, the main American Heart Association (AHA) Class I interventions which have withstood the test time have been crystalloid intravenous fluid loading, chest compressions, defibrillation/cardioversion, and oxygen. The dose–response curve for oxygen use above a fraction inhaled oxygen of 100 % (FIO$_2$ 100 %) by the use of hyperbaric oxygen treatment has had encouraging results and is indicated in certain instances.

Keywords

Hyperbaric oxygen • ATLS • ACLS • Resuscitation • Mitochondria • ATP synthase • Electron transport system • Cytochrome aa3

Introduction

The success of prompt resuscitation from acute severe injury or illness (ASII) requires an adequate supply of high energy phosphates. Adenine triphosphate (ATP) is predominantly needed. Chains of respiratory enzymes are embedded in the inner membrane of the intermembrane space (IMS) of mitochondria.

K. Van Meter, MD (✉)
Section of Emergency Medicine, LSU Health Sciences Center, University Medical Center, LCMC Health, New Orleans, LA, USA

Tulane School of Medicine, New Orleans, LA, USA
e-mail: kwvanmeter@gmail.com

The electron transportation system (ETS) taps Kreb's cycle for a supply of electron's energy for ATP production. In effect, the ETS is an insulated conduit for conducting a flow of electron's energy to paramagnetic molecules of diatomic oxygen docked at the end of each ETS. The ETS is composed of four linked respiratory, enzymatic complexes I–IV. Specifically, oxygen docks at cytochrome aa3, last of the ETS complexes (complex IV). Sequentially the electron's energy on its way to oxygen through the ETS, power the chain of respiratory enzymes to transport hydrogen ions (H+) across the inner membrane to the IMS to enrich the IMS with a supply of H+. This reservoir of H+ powers the stator/rotor micromachine enzyme, ATP synthase (Complex V), after the ETS and separate from it (Dimroth et al. 2000). Figure 42.1 is a diagram of this process. Both the

Fig. 42.1 The ETS
(respiratory complexes I.IV)
fill the intermitochondrial
space with H+ to drive the
respiratory complex IV (ATP
synthase) to churn out
ATP. This ETS function is
powered by the docking of
molecular oxygen on
cytochrome a33 (complex IV)
where, in effect, the
paramagnetic oxygen atoms
draw electrons down the ETC
to place H+ in the
intramitochondrial membrane
space

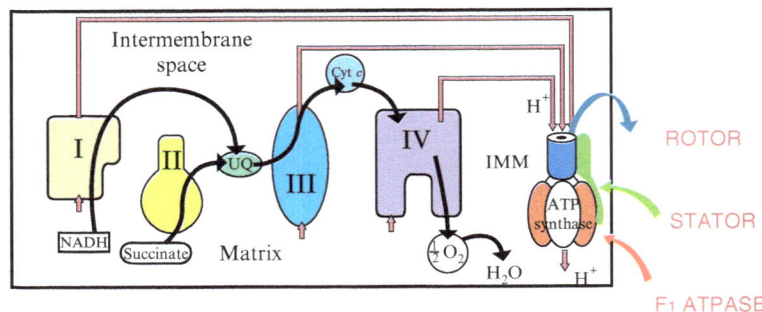

Fig. 42.2 Transverse section
of the portion of ATP synthase
which protrudes from the
inner membrane of the
mitochondrial space into the
mitochondrial matrix. This
part of the enzyme grabs onto
ADP and Pi to fuse them
chemically together with each
third rotation. Reprinted from
https://users.soe.ucsc.
edu/~hongwang/ATP_
synthase.html

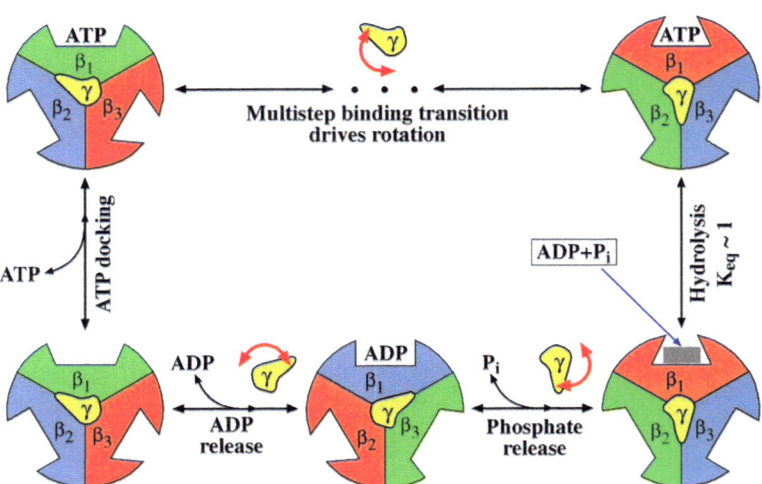

ETS and ATP synthase are embedded in the inner mitochondrial membrane, thereby the ETS is in good position to harvest H+ from the mitochondrial matrix and ATP synthase is in a good position to accept the harvest of H+ to power the ATP synthase micromachine itself.

The stream of H+ channeling through ATP synthase causes the stator/rotor component of the enzyme to rotate and thereby open the enzyme's conformational attachment sites for adenosine diphosphate (ADP) and inorganic phosphate (Pi) to join to form ATP. ATP synthase allows this otherwise improbable reaction to be fast and efficient as shown in Fig. 42.2. With a sufficient reservoir of H+ in the IMS, the enzymatic rotor of ATP synthase makes tertiary segmental turns on continuous, one-directional spin causing Pi and ADP to chemically mate to release a vital supply of ATP (Rich 2003).

An intact mitochondrial ETS straightforwardly behaves as a powerful antioxidant. Degradation of the respiratory chain occurs in hypoxia and allows an electron leak from the chain to nonenzymatically docked diatomic oxygen. This allows formation of reactive oxygen species (ROS). Intact enzymatic respiratory chains conduct electron energy efficiently for ATP production instead of ROS formation. In effect oxygen as it is attached to cytochrome aa3 accepts the "insulated" electron energy flow through an intact ETS. With the help of ATP synthase, cytochrome aa3, oxygen unites with H+ to form innocuous water (Michel 1999).

Figure 42.3 serves as a reminder of how central ATP is to basic biologic process (Knowles 1980; Hardie and Hawley 2001; McBride et al. 2006).

The energy requirements in ASII are often more than a magnitude higher than subject's baseline energy needs in health. In ASII, an inflammatory state ensues, highly consumptive of ATP. In systemic repair and recovery from ASII, cellular processes consume prodigious amounts of ATP. ATP is needed to power membrane cationic ionophores to transport cations to the correct sides of cellular membranes after cationic dyshomeostasis disruptively occurs in illness or injury (Burnstock 1990).

ATP's main chemical energy supply for cellular function:

1. Cell signaling
2. Cell differentiation (i.e., meuronal, myocyte, immune cell function)
3. Cell death
4. Cell cycles
5. Cell growth
6. Control of cellular membrane ionophors
7. Cellular genomic function
8. Cellular proteonomic function

Fig. 42.3 ATP is central to providing essential power for biologic processes

Indications

In the strictly regulated medical systems of most industrialized nations, the use of hyperbaric oxygen (HBO) in cardiopulmonary resuscitation (CPR) has special caveats. This is especially true in the United States where HBO has not been considered as a drug of potential use in ACLS/ATLS by the AHA, by the American College of Surgeons (ACS), or by the Centers for Medicare and Medicaid Services (CMS).

At this time, HBO can only be used in cases of cardiac resuscitation if the arrest occurred while the patient was concurrently being treated for acute comorbidities. The conditions include the following:

- Cases of decompression illness (DCI) in an aviator or diver
- Cases of carbon monoxide or cyanide intoxication
- Cases of acute crush injury
- Cases of iatrogenic, intraarterial, or venous gas embolism
- Cases where cardiopulmonary arrest occurs in any patient being treated in a hyperbaric chamber for any otherwise UHMS-approved HBO indication (Weaver 2014)

At present the only justifiable setting for use of HBO for CPR in the United States would be in a multiplace hyperbaric chamber, in a critical care area of a hospital (intensive care unit, operating room, anesthesiology recovery unit, cardiology procedural suite, or emergency department). The chamber would need to have all of the patient monitoring equipment and medications advised by AHA/ACS standards currently for patient care. Further, it would be most desirable that the unit have a 24/7 availability with technician, physician, and nurse staffing.

If this capability could be arranged, the lives potentially saved would shortly justify its use at first in large regional medical centers (Van Meter 2012a, b, 2014).

Cardiopulmonary Resuscitation

Oxygen must be present for ATP to form, but oxygen can be toxic. Recent literature addressing ACLS resuscitation management of acute myocardial ischemia comes with cautionary advisements about the use of supplemental oxygen administration at 1 atm of pressure. Advisement by the AHA 2015 guidelines is to not use supplemental oxygen in the specific instance of myocardial ischemia in a patient with a pulse oximetry determination of >94 % while breathing room air (AHA 2015; Stub et al. 2015).

Even with this restriction, oxygen has been considered a class I therapeutic agent by the AHA. With the exception of defibrillation, very few of the therapeutic agents in ACLS have withstood the test of time for all of their first-intended applications. This is reflected by the current AHA 2015 Guidelines update on both efficacy classification and guidelines for use of sodium bicarbonate, calcium chloride, vasopressin, and even to a partial extent, atropine, epinephrine, and hypothermia (Dumas et al. 2014; Patel et al. 2016; Vajkoczy et al. 2000).

The very pointed purpose of ACLS is to get oxygen to its cytochrome aa3 receptor in the ETS before the enzymatic chains themselves degrade from the ravages of hypoxia. In ACLS, the two most hypoxia-sensitive organs traditionally focused upon have been the heart and the brain. Oxygenated blood flow at 1 atm of ambient pressure has been quantified for predictive effect on outcome. This is best summarized in Fig. 42.4 (Van Meter et al. 2008).

Suboptimal delivery of oxygen to the intact mitochondrial respiratory enzymatic chains allows oxygen itself to be a source of ROS for reasons described.

The dissolved oxygen at 1 atm when one is breathing 100 % oxygen (fraction of inhaled oxygen 100 % or FIO_2 100 %) in plasma reaches 2.3 vol.%. In low flow states or by low levels of hemoglobin or by functionally impaired hemoglobin, the 2.3 vol.% of dissolved oxygen may provide substrate enough for the degrading mitochondrial enzymatic respiratory chains' to have an electron leak to form abundant ROS.

It may be that the potential antioxidant power of mitochondrial respiratory chains best exists in properly oxygenated mitochondria at 1 mmHg oxygen and not at some point below this level or above. Suboptimal 100 % oxygen in ACLS might therefore become an issue in myocardial ischemia as AHA suggests in the 2015 guidelines. Oxygen, as any drug, has a dose–response curve. There is a beneficial dose–response curve for oxygen for resuscitation of divers stricken with DCI. The necessary arrival of oxygen for cytochrome aa3 in ischemic nervous system tissue in DCI may require hyperbarically administered oxygen up to surface equivalent fraction of inhaled oxygen ($SEFIO_2$) levels of 200–300 % to resolve the ischemic injury (Van Meter 1999).

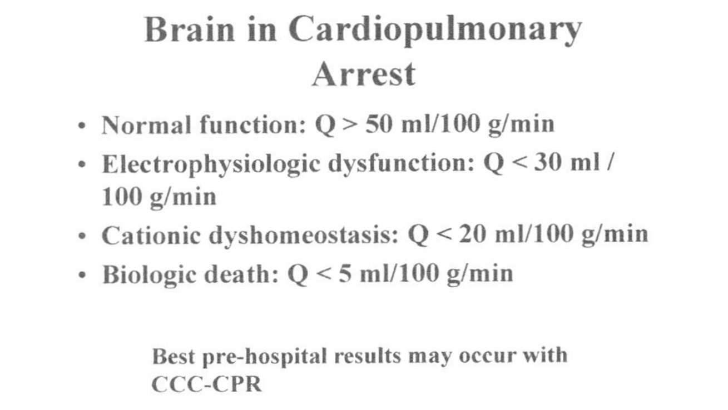

Brain in Cardiopulmonary
Arrest

- Normal function: Q > 50 ml/100 g/min
- Electrophysiologic dysfunction: Q < 30 ml / 100 g/min
- Cationic dyshomeostasis: Q < 20 ml/100 g/min
- Biologic death: Q < 5 ml/100 g/min

Best pre-hospital results may occur with
CCC-CPR

Fig. 42.4 The brain's function is dependent upon blood flow for purpose of oxygen delivery to the mitochondrial inner space to keep the oxygen tension at 1 mmHg oxygen. Short of this, the brain becomes dysfunctional

The use of HBO in ACLS has focused on the dose–response in $SEFIO_2$s and has been reported in published case reports and reproduced in controlled animal studies (Van Meter 2012a, 2012b; Van Meter et al. 1988; Van Meter and Harch 2009). Unimpaired survival has occurred with 23 min prolonged, non-intervened-upon normothermic cardiopulmonary arrest, $SEFIO_2$'s of 400–600 % achievable by systemic HBO in both humans and swine. In these instances, the subjects have not had the benefit of any intervention other than basic CPR begun only after 23 min of non-intervened-upon cardiopulmonary arrest (Fig. 42.5). The use of HBO has resulted in return of spontaneous circulation (ROSC) and consciousness as shown in Figs. 42.6 and 42.7.

It seems easier to explain rather than refute the 2015 AHA ACLS contention that in some instances FIO_2 100 % administered to a patient may be harmful. The suggestion has been made that results from ACLS provided to a patient in cardiopulmonary arrest might well be served with 21 % FIO_2 and worse with 100 % FIO_2 and best of all with $SEFIO_2$ 400 % afforded by HBO (Van Meter and Harch 2009).

Gas diffusion chemistry alone can explain how it is possible with low blood flow through parenchyma, for microvasculature to deliver dissolved oxygen to supply the mitochondria with physiologic amounts of oxygen. Even in badly damaged microvasculature, it has been demonstrated that a plasma flow through parenchyma exists (Bigelow 1964). In fact, over 50 years ago, Boerema demonstrated in both animals and humans the use of HBO to sustain "life without blood" (Boerema et al. 1959).

Experimentally HBO as opposed to normoxic oxygen has been demonstrated to confer the following effects:

1. Truncation of membrane lipid peroxidation in reperfusion of hypoxically insulted tissue (Thom and Elbuken 1991).
2. Lessening of leukocyte endothelial adherence in reperfusion injury (Thom et al. 1997).

3. Induction of at least 8101 genes to express half of which oversee reparative function and half of which oversee anti-inflammatory function (Godman et al. 2010).
4. Improve leukocyte microbe killing (both for aerobic and anaerobic microbes) (Knighton et al. 1984).
5. Expungement of adult medullary stem cells into the central circulation (Thom et al. 2006).
6. Lessing of impact of intravascular microparticles after ischemic insult (Thom et al. 2011).

Possible areas of future investigation may be to determine if: (1) increased cytosolic oxygen tension afforded by HBO may place cytochrome c (released into the cytosol by injured mitochondria) in an oxidized state to prevent induction of apoptotic caspase cascades, (2) if netosis of polymorphonuclear leukocytes might be made more effective in countering bacterial biofilm formation in bacterial sepsis (Zawrotniak and Rapala-Kozik 2013), (3) if glymphatic flow in the central nervous system is improved (Iliff et al. 2012), and (4) to see the effect of HBO on neuroglobin (Brunori and Vallone 2006) and cytoglobin (Schmidt et al. 2004).

Case Studies

Two clinical cases are presented, more to demonstrate the safety and simplicity of providing high-dose $SEFIO_2$ afforded by the availability of HBO for adjunctive use in ACLS in an otherwise medically primitive field setting. The presented cases occurred at offshore oil and gas field commercial diving accident sites. At these sites, as a part of the operational standard, HBO was available approximately a half-hour after the onset of the ASII insult (one half-hour was consumed to get the diver out of the water and under pressure for administration of an elevated $SEFIO_2$ in a hyperbaric chamber environment). What was key for the success in both presented cases was the availability of HBO administered within one half-hour of the insult. A hyperbaric chamber is the standard on all commercial offshore diving site either by way of deck decompression chambers for bounce diving or larger storage chambers for saturation diving (Van Meter 2012a, b).

Case 1

On a hot August day in 1983, a 35-year-old male commercial diver was attempting to break the suction imposed by river silt against the hull of a newly sunken tugboat in the Mississippi River. His task incorporated the use of an air lift which is a suction dredge that incorporated the injection of compressed air into the mouth of a large diameter pipe (Fig. 42.8). As the air rose on its way to the surface inside the pipe, a strong vacuum developed to suck sand and debris in

Fig. 42.5 Porcine non-intervened-upon 23-min normothermic cardiopulmonary arrest. Reprinted from Resuscitation, 78(2), Van Meter KW, Sheps S, Kriedt F, Moises J, Barratt D, Murphy-Lavoie H, et al., Hyperbaric oxygen improves rate of return of spontaneous circulation after prolonged normothermic porcine cardiopulmonary arrest, 200-214, Copyright 2008, with permission from Elsevier

	Initial ROSC after ACLS at 30 min	Sustained ROSC at 2 ½ hour
SEFIO$_2$ 100% (n=6)	0/6	0/6
SEFIO$_2$ 190% (n=6)	0/6	0/6
SEFIO$_2$	5/6	4/6

$$(p \leq 0.001)$$

K Van Meter
Resuscitation
2008;78(2):200-214

Fig. 42.6 At the BRI hyperbaric chamber laboratory, ACLS is augmented by hyperbaric oxygen use in swine study after prolonged normothermic, non-intervened-upon, 23-min cardiopulmonary arrest

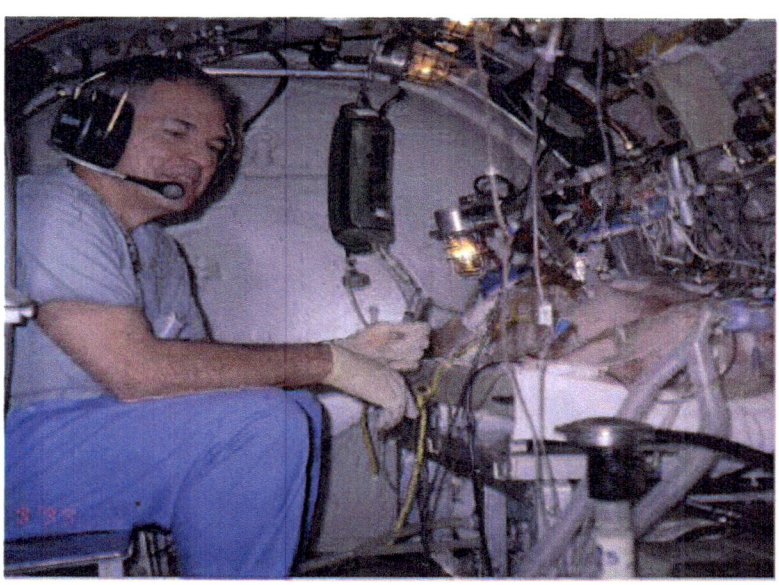

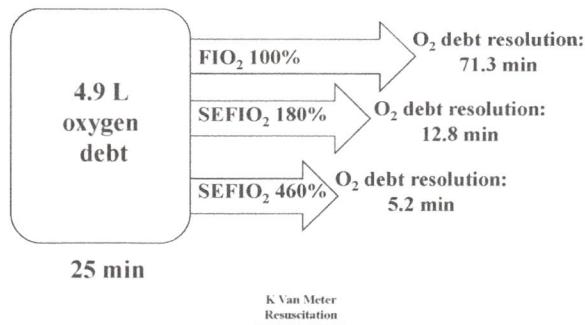

Fig. 42.7 Twenty-three minute, non-intervened-upon normothermic cardiopulmonary arrest in swine. Reprinted from Resuscitation, 78(2), Van Meter KW, Sheps S, Kriedt F, Moises J, Barratt D, Murphy-Lavoie H, et al., Hyperbaric oxygen improves rate of return of spontaneous circulation after prolonged normothermic porcine cardiopulmonary arrest, 200-214, Copyright 2008, with permission from Elsevier

ascent up the pipe, or "air lift," to dump material away from the work site (Fig. 42.9). In the course of his task, the diver became sucked up into the intake of an air lift in the Mississippi River at 89 ft of fresh water (ffw). The diver's head and helmet were drawn into the air lift. With his head and helmet now blocking the intake of the tube, a strong vacuum was drawn on his helmet neck dam, essentially suctioning his helmet to his head or more accurately, his lead to the larger space of the helmet's interior. His head and neck ecchymosed and the skin envelope separated from the face and cranium to produce a large, distorting head and neck space filling hematoma. In effect he had a severe head and neck Morel–Lavallee lesion (Shen et al. 2013; Tseng and Tornetta 2006). The stoma of his mouth narrowed with swelling and he lost consciousness. The air lift was shut down, and standby divers found him on the river bottom, out of his helmet in lifeless form. He was brought to the surface. No breathing or pulse was

Fig. 42.8 Drawing completed by patient to detail his workplace setting where he had undergone a surface-supplied air dive to attempt salvage of a sunken tugboat in the Mississippi River

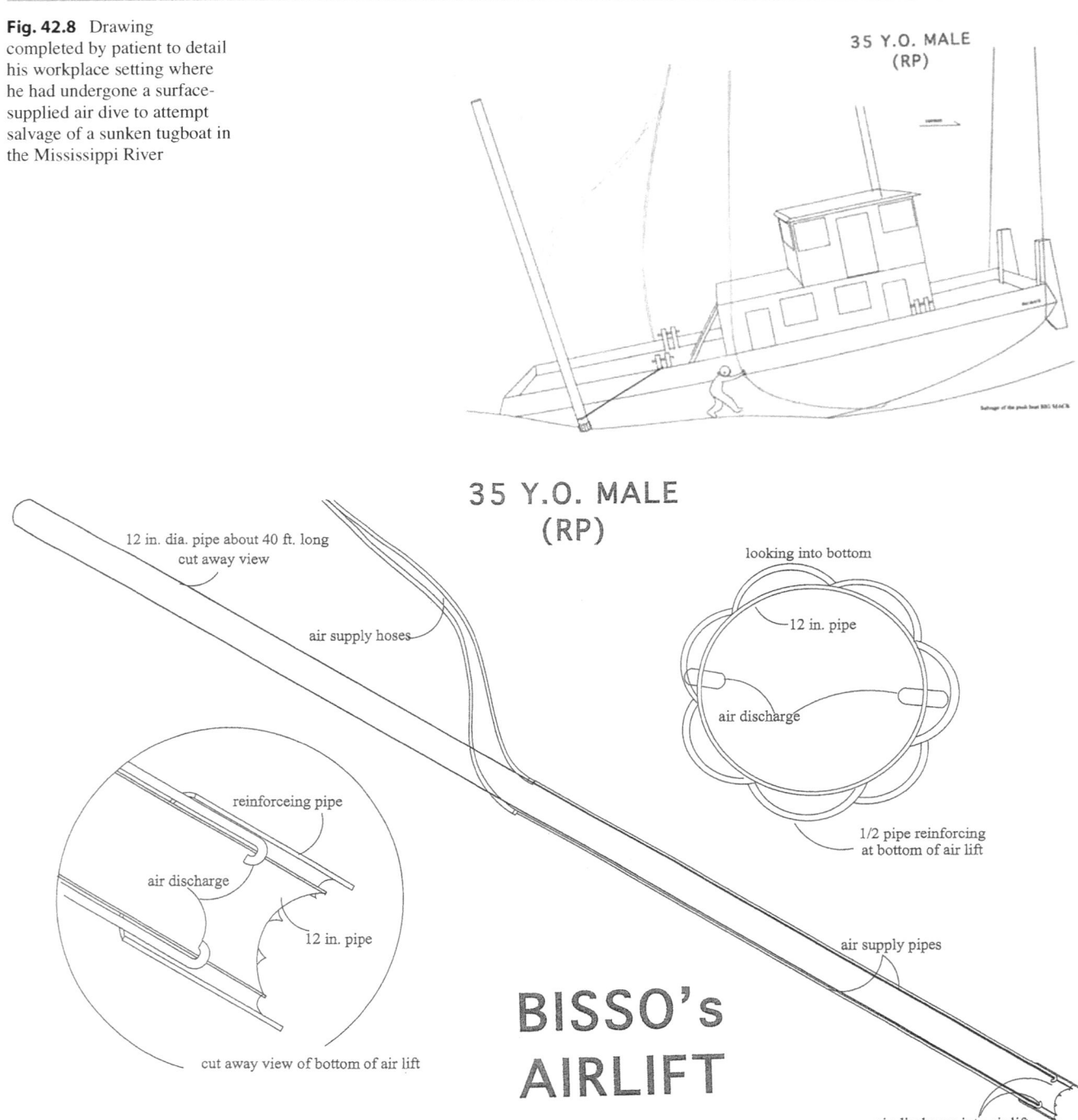

35 Y.O. MALE
(RP)

35 Y.O. MALE
(RP)

12 in. dia. pipe about 40 ft. long
cut away view

air supply hoses

looking into bottom

12 in. pipe

air discharge

reinforceing pipe

air discharge

12 in. pipe

1/2 pipe reinforcing
at bottom of air lift

air supply pipes

cut away view of bottom of air lift

BISSO's
AIRLIFT

air discharge into air lift

Fig. 42.9 Orifice of airlift into which the diver's helmeted head had been sucked

apparent in survey of his flaccid body. Twenty-three minutes had elapsed, before chest compressions (hands-only-CPR) were begun in the hot sun without use of mouth-to-mouth ventilations. His mouth and face were so grossly disfigured that his resuscitators admitted in a later debriefing that they could not bring themselves to ventilate him. There was no ambu-bag-valve-mask on-site. The patient was then compressed to 6 atm in a deck decompression chamber. He was stretched out into a supine position on the inner curve of a 56-in.-diameter chamber. His resuscitator straddled his body to give continuous, firm chest compressions to an essentially upright patient torso. The $SEFIO_2$ conducted to the nonoxygen scavenging mask on the actively unventilated patient at 165 fsw (6 ATA) was 600 % (an otherwise extreme breathing mix in normal circumstances). The diver awoke, shrugged off his mask, and resisted the attempts of his resuscitator who was a bit persistent at his efforts of chest compression. Shortly afterward, the resuscitator had a seizure from oxygen toxicity and was consoled by the now-resuscitated diver. The injured diver went on to receive pulsed HBO breathing treatments utilizing a downwardly adjusted oxygen mix ($SEFIO_2$ of 300 %). The swelling of head and neck markedly reduced over the next 3 days on his slow decompression to surface in the chamber. Notably during this time, his facial skin and scalp were dark and ecchymotic, while he breathed compressed air in the chamber, but when he was placed by mask on enriched HBO mix ($SEFIO_2$ of 280 %), his face lit to a bright tomato-red, as extravasated hemoglobin in the tissue became oxygenated. Slowly over the next 60 h, he decompressed to surface. In this 56-in.-diameter chamber, in the hot summer sun, aboard the deck of a barge on the Mississippi River, the diver recovered with the inside attendance of a fellow diver resuscitator and a physician who had locked-in to provide added assistance. In tight confines, all were captives of compressed air saturation and had to oblige slow decompression to surface (Fig. 42.10). By the time the injured diver reached surface, he had recognizable facial features (Fig. 42.11). He was completely oriented to person, place, time, and situation. After exhaustive examination, no neurologic abnormality was found aside from auditory diminution, which turned out to be an air conduction problem due to perforated tympanic membranes. His head CT evidenced no detectable abnormality to the brain, but did reveal pansinusitis with extensively fluid-filled sinus spaces from barotrauma. A day-long psychometric testing battery was normal and a 29-year follow-up brain SPECT scan and repeated daylong

psychometric testing battery were normal. In fact, he maintained his IQ of over 120 throughout the years. He remains in completely good mental health and has become a fine cabinet and furniture maker (Figs. 42.12, 42.13, 42.14, and 42.15).

As previously discussed, subsequent simulation of this normothermic cardiopulmonary arrest was carried on in randomized, controlled trials. First guinea pigs were used in a closed chest compression model (Van Meter et al. 1988). This model was followed by another randomized, controlled trial utilizing an open chest cardiac ventricular assist device for cardiac compressions (Van Meter 1999). Both studies yielded encouraging ROSC in the high-dose HBO ($SEFIO_2$ 400 % or greater) groups only. All animals were in persisting asystole at the beginning of attempts to resuscitate them. Universally, the normobaric (FIO_2 100 %) and conventional dose HBO ventilation groups ($SEFIO_2$ 180 %) could not be resuscitated to the endpoint of enduring ROSC. In fact, all of the animals ventilated with normobaric oxygen had only EKG flat lines during their attempted resuscitation.

Could it have been that in both studies, better oxygenation of the myocardium and suppression of the cardiac dysrhythmias by "narcotization" by hyperbaric inert gas or oxygen itself contributed to ROSC? In canine controlled studies, Rosenthal (Rosenthal et al. 2003) and more recently Huang (Huang et al. 2012) have demonstrated that HBO applied postresuscitation, successfully ameliorated neurologic sequelae which otherwise persisted in groups treated as normobaric oxygen controls. Likewise, Mathieu demonstrated similar successful neurologic outcomes by applying prompt HBO treatment to depressed French farmers who had attempted suicide by hanging (Mathieu et al. 1987). Recently, Yogaratnam has successfully shown in a randomized,

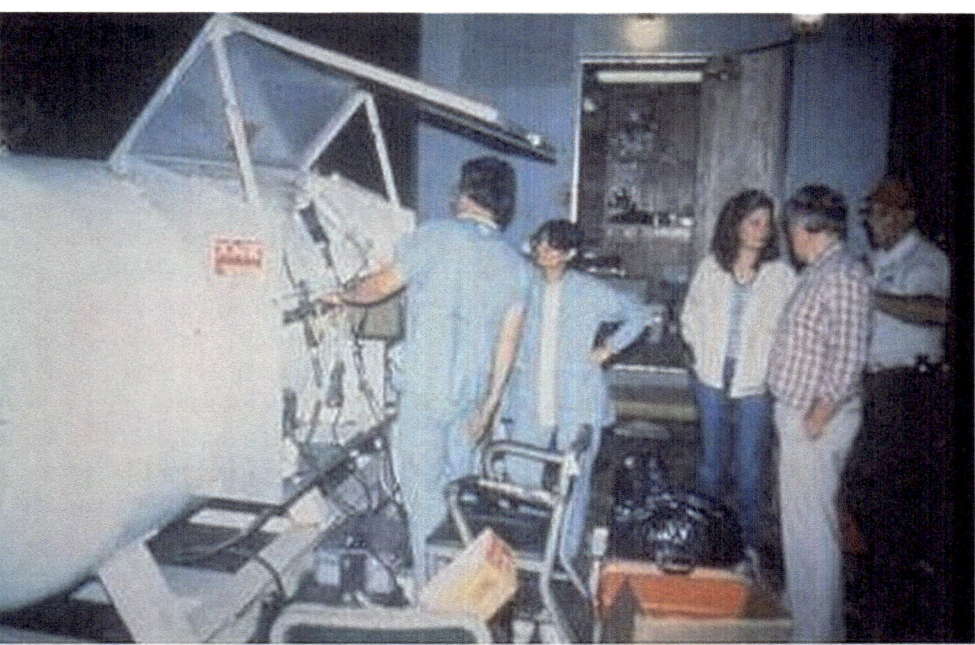

Fig. 42.10 Topside physician and technician tending to DDC in which the injured diver was entrapped during a 3-day decompression to surface

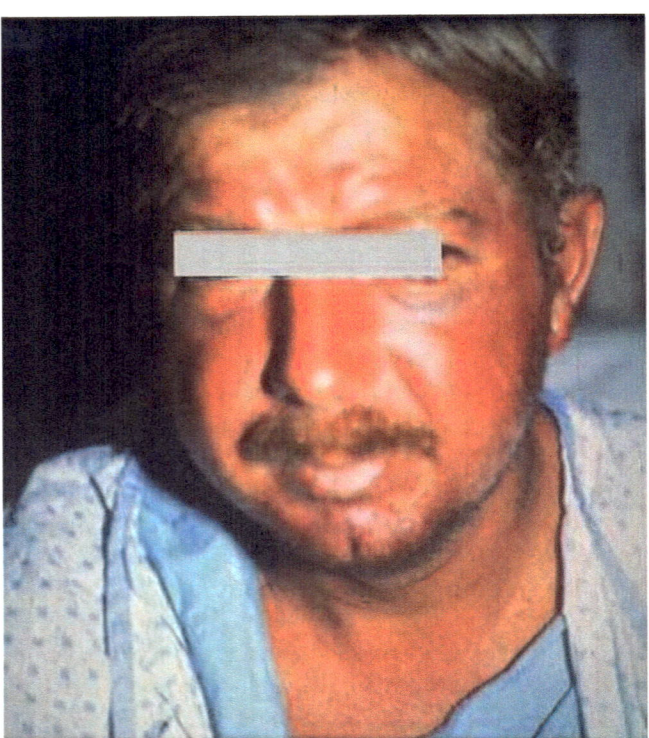

Fig. 42.11 Diver with markedly reduced facial injury after ascending in chamber to surface

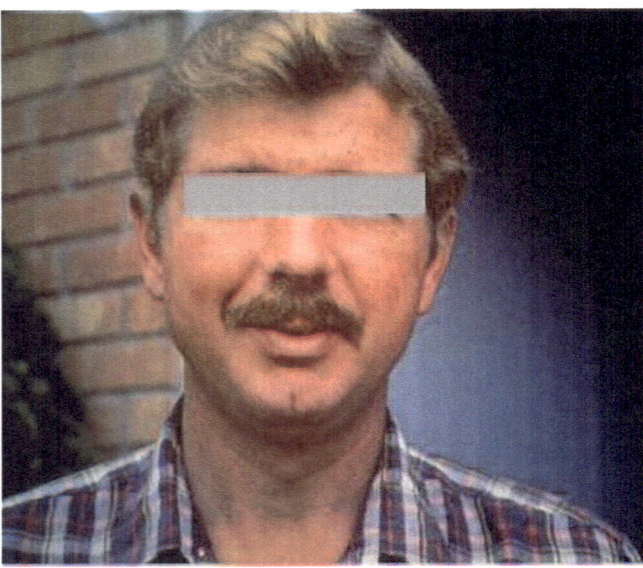

Fig. 42.12 At 1 month after accident, the patient's face resumed pre-injury appearance

controlled human trial that HBO ameliorated neurologic abnormalities in patients following coronary artery bypass grafting (Yogaratnam et al. 2010; Alex et al. 2005).

Again simple application of HBO acutely in a remote resuscitation site followed by short-interval HBO therapy was practical and most probably resulted in favorable treatment results.

Case 2

A 42-year-old, male commercial diver working in the Gulf of Mexico had a long history of intermittent, gnawing epigastric discomfort. The discomfort sometimes awoke him at night and would not relieve with ingestion of food. He was working in a 300 fsw heliox saturation chamber system storage depth aboard a diving vessel. He made downward 60 fsw excursions from the storage depth by way of transfer to the gulf floor by personal transfer chamber (PTC). On one excursion to the floor of the Gulf, he vomited coffee ground emesis, had a melanotic accidental loose stool, and become unconscious. He was fetched by the PTC bellman, who helmeted and dragged him back to the PTC. The PTC was brought to the surface and mated with the saturation deck storage chamber system. He was pushed into the saturation deck chamber and placed in a lateral decubitus position on the deck (Fig. 42.16). He was breathing shallowly at a rate of 40 breaths per minute. He was cold, diaphoretic, unconscious, and extremely pale. A diver medic locked-in to place a peripheral IV line but was unsuccessful in 32 separate attempts. Intraosseous access catheters were not available. Placement of a BIBS mask for enriched oxygen helium breathing (SEFIO$_2$ of 300 %) improved the diver's initial Glasgow Coma Scale (GCS) score of 3 to a GCS of 10 (eye = 2, verbal = 2, motor = 4). The patient would not comply with ingestion of oral fluids. Slow decompression to surface over 3 days was started (Fig. 42.17). The medic was instructed to use hypodermoclysis for parenteral administration of crystalloid fluids. Three liters of normal saline was slowly infused in several subdermal IV lines attached to subdermal needles placed in his extremities. The chamber SEFIO$_2$ was kept at 40 % and the mask SEFIO$_2$ was kept at 250 %. His fellow divers noted that his iatrogenically edematous extremities "made him look like a Michelin man." He became alert with total return of consciousness (GCS 15) and climbed into an upper bunk under his own power. Without the benefit of a packed red blood cell (PRBC) transfusion, he remained at a GCS of 15 over the 3-day decompression to surface. Attempts at getting blood for type and cross-match as well as for transfusion were unsuccessful. The blood hemolyzed badly on descent and ascent from the heliox storage depths at which the divers resided and could not be used. Type O or matched PRBCs were therefore unavailable to the diver. During decompression to surface the vessel made its way to port.

An initial HBO treatment was embedded into his saturation decompression profile. Then pulsed, intermittent, tailing breathing HBO treatments of short interval followed and were also embedded into his decompression profile during his slow ascent to surface. He had EKG leads placed on his chest wall shortly after his initial profuse diaphoresis abated and he stabilized. The intervals between HBO treatments

Fig. 42.13 Here is the patient several years later with his granddaughter; patient was high functioning and in good health

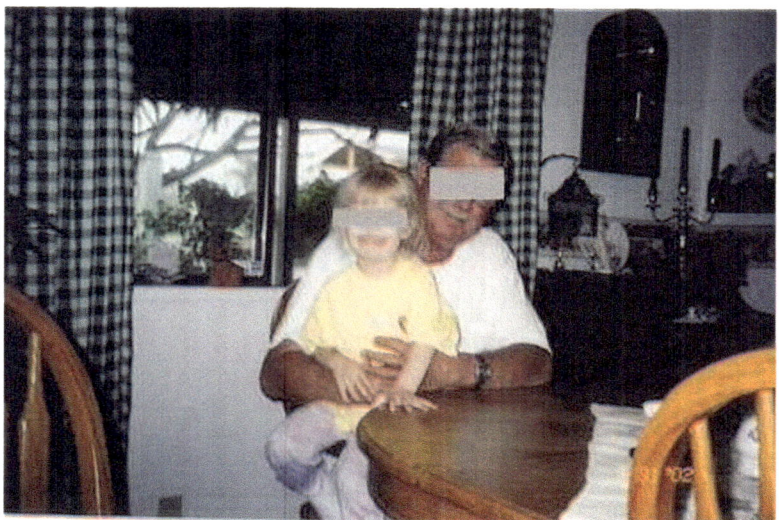

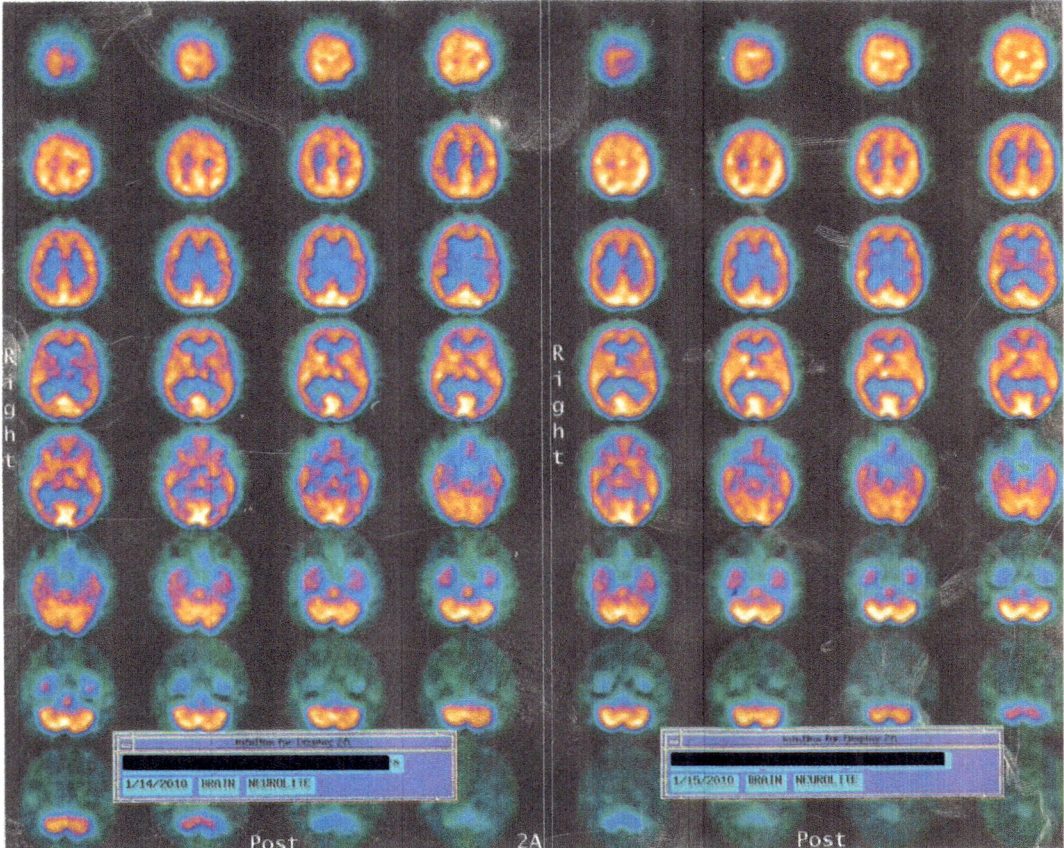

Fig. 42.14 Twenty-seven years later, the patient had an essentially normal SPECT brain scan before HBO challenge and an unchanged scan afterward

were gradually lengthened as long as his ST segments remained unelevated. When the ST segments on the cardiac monitor elevated, he was put back on HBO-enriched helium breathing mix (SEFIO$_2$ 300%). His measured hemoglobin (Hbg) on the hemolyzed, locked-out samples of blood was 2 g/dL by this time. Soon peripheral veins could be found and accessed for established IV lines. He tolerated oral chicken and beef broth, oral hematinics (folic acid and multivitamins), intramuscular iron injections, and subcutaneous erythropoietin.

Fig. 42.15 The patient, almost 30 years later, very coherently is being interviewed on a local New Orleans TV station about his accident

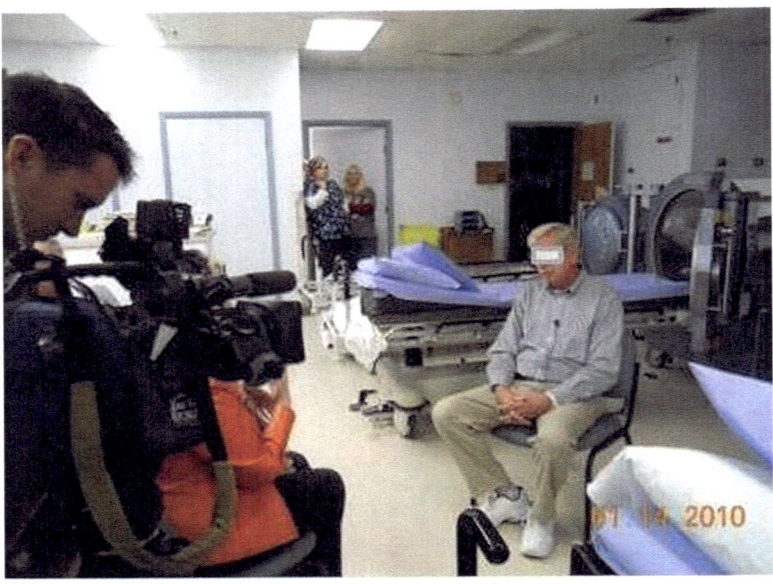

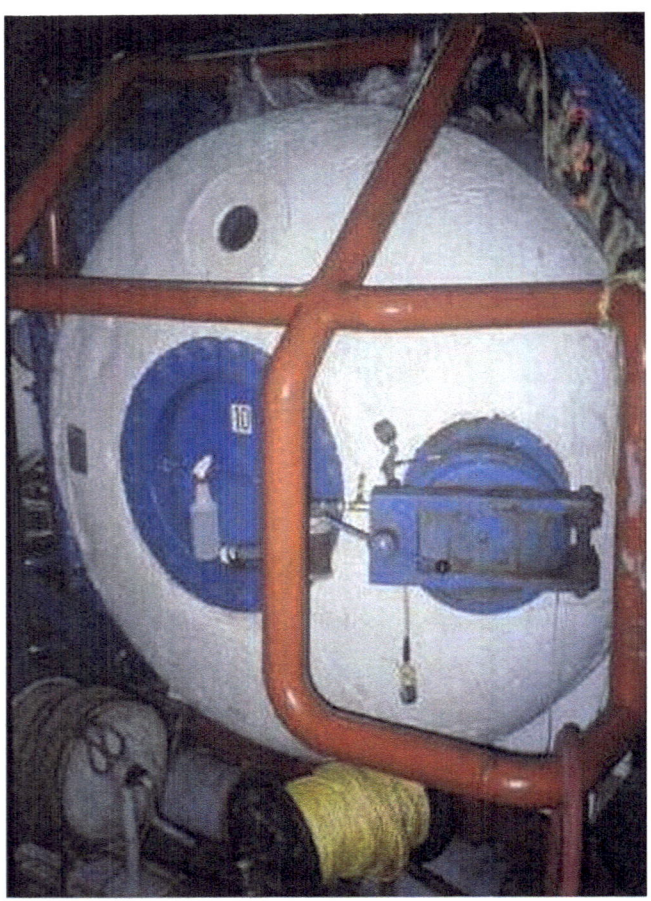

Fig. 42.16 Heliox saturation diving chamber at site of offshore operation where patient sustained a severe blood loss insult when a duodenal ulcer eroded a duodenal artery while he was on a diving work excursion on the sea floor

When he arrived at surface 3 days later, he was transfused with type O PRBCs brought by a transport ambulance awaiting the vessel at dockside. He was promptly transferred to the hospital (Fig. 42.18). His pretransfusion Hbg drawn by transport paramedics was 4 g/dL, and his Hbg after 6 units of PRBC transfusion was 10 g/dL. Endoscopy revealed a mature clot over a duodenal ulcer, which had eroded a duodenal artery. As a precaution, the vessel was endoscopically cauterized without complication. He went on to have an uneventful recovery. He had no evidence of injury to kidneys (creatinine and BUN and urinalysis were normal), heart (EKG and cardiac enzymes were normal), liver (liver profile was normal), or musculoskeletal (CPK levels were not elevated). An injury shock state, which may have resulted in multiorgan failure or death in a remove field site 3 days away from hospital-based intensive care, resolved well (Fig. 42.19).

Shoemaker described accumulated and unresolved oxygen debt after the onset of a shock state as a prognosticator of patient outcome. He contended that if oxygen consumption exceeded oxygen delivery by 8 L during the first 4 h of insult but was afterward promptly resolved, the patient would feel the effects of a bad flu-like syndrome or a mild systemic inflammatory response syndrome. If the accumulated oxygen debt was more than 22 L over the first 4 h before correction, the patient would suffer multiorgan failure. If the uncorrected oxygen debt were in excess of 32 L in the first 4 h, the patient would not survive given conventional attempts at resuscitation to follow (Shoemaker et al. 1988). The diver described in this case report suffered an accumulated estimated oxygen debt of 45 L in the first 4 h following his exsanguination before parenteral fluid and oxygen resuscitation could be fully implemented.

Fig. 42.17 Diver is shown by a topside TV monitor to be on the top bunk in the saturation diving system chamber; the diver is on a SEFIO$_2$ 260 % equivalent heliox mix while having a hemoglobin of 2 g/dL. The diver is alert, not short of breath, nondiaphoretic, and normotensive

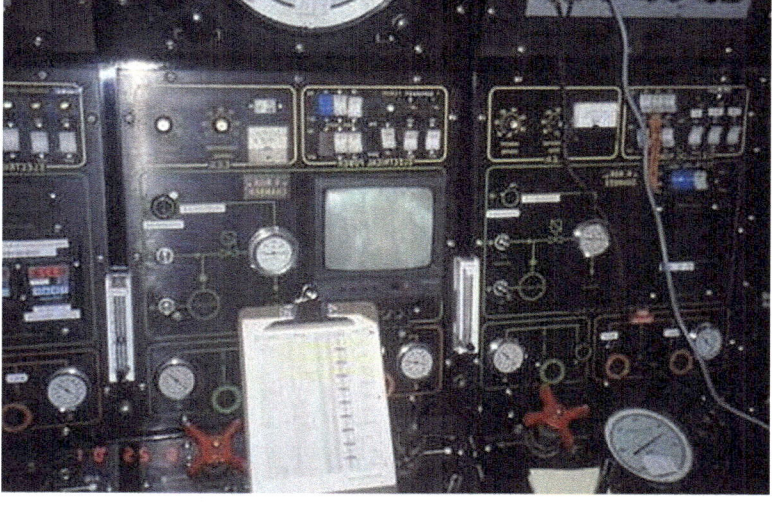

Fig. 42.18 Patient after transfusion of PRBCs and after hospital-based endoscopy; endoscopy discovered the duodenal ulcer, which was hemostatic. Patient was comfortable and was discharged home after a 3-day hospital stay

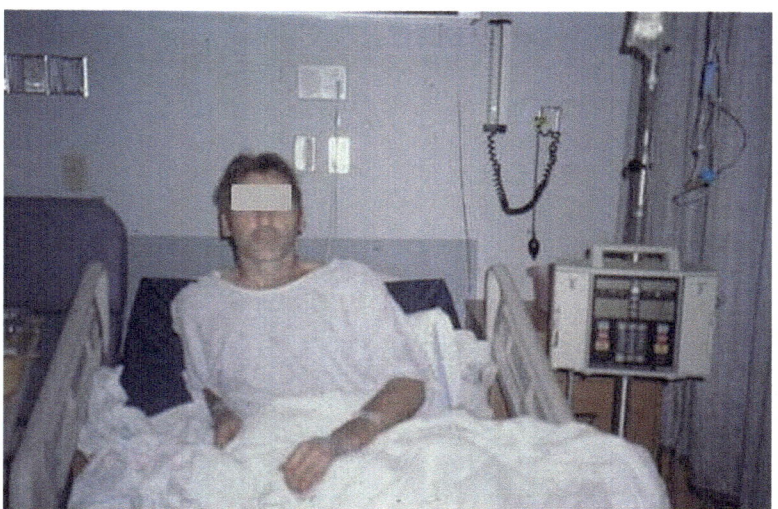

Fig. 42.19 Same diver 10 years later with family in good health celebrating the FIFA World Cup as a spectator in South Africa, 2010

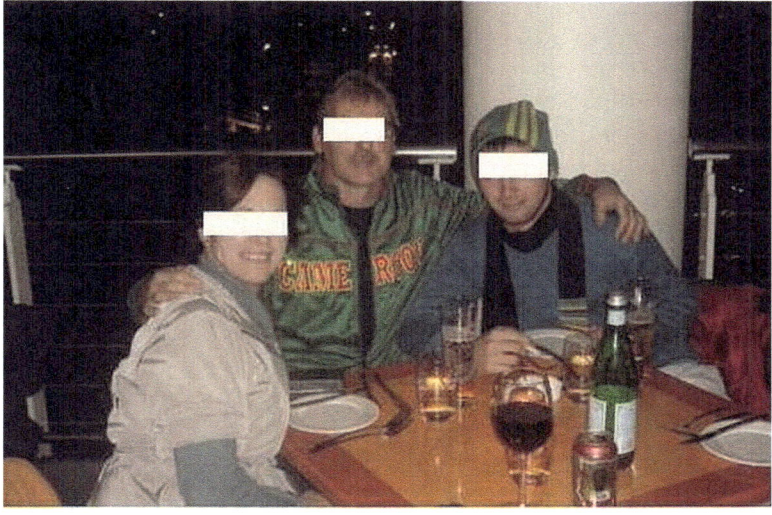

A systematic, evidence-based review of the published scientific literature reveals that use of HBO in severe blood loss anemia scored well in evaluation of efficacy (Van Meter 2012b). In the 1960 inaugural volume of the *Journal of Cardiovascular Surgery*, Ite Boerema published the results of an experiment in which normothermic swine sustained an acute removal of 40 % of their blood volume. After exsanguination, the animals were fluid loaded with crystalloid and colloid solution, then ventilated in a hyperbaric chamber on oxygen at 3 atm (SEFIO$_2$ of 300 %). The swine were attached to EKG leads for continuous cardiac monitoring. The researchers noted that when ventilated by 3 atm of air (SEFIO$_2$ 63 %), the animals had uniformly elevated ST segments and had dysrhythmias on their cardiograms. If they were ventilated by at least 3 atm of oxygen, the dysrhythmias and ST segments elevations normalized (Boerema et al. 1959).

Our laboratory has subjected 30 kg swine to an ACS Class IV hemorrhage (40 % removal of blood volume). After 20 min, each cc of blood shed by the animal was replaced by 3 cm^3 IV normal saline. The animals were kept normothermic, and then were taken to 5 atm for 5 min and ventilated with 100 % oxygen (SEFIO$_2$ of 500 %). They were then brought to 60 fsw and ventilated on oxygen (SEFIO$_2$ of 280 %) for 55 min. Then the shed blood was returned by IV infusion and then the animals were brought to surface with usual decompression stops. They recovered completely and have had a currently 3-year survival with no discoverable impairment. It is noteworthy that the HBO-treated animals with an acute hemoglobin of 2 g remained with normal vital signs. Likewise, brain tissue pO$_2$ monitored by a polarographic oxygen-sensing electrode (placed through a burr hole in the animal's cranium) returned to a normal 40 mmHg oxygen level in HBO-treated animals. Control animals kept on surface and fluid resuscitated while being ventilated with 100 % normobaric oxygen had brain tissue pO$_2$ of 0 mmHg (Van Meter 2014). This observation may have far-reaching implication for modification of the resuscitation methods used for patients suffering from severe blood loss in the military far-forward, in prehospital domestic locations, or even in the trauma center itself.

In the duodenal ulcer patient presented and in the experimental swine, the use of HBO allowed the plasma fraction of dissolved oxygen to bridge the subjects with crystalloid IV solutions until the subjects could be transfused with blood. The implication is that patients may be bridged with crystalloid solutions until damage control surgery effects hemostasis so that the patient can have retransfusion of shed blood or low-volume transfusion of matched units of PRBCs. Again, far-forward medical interventions may profit by the rather simple low-technology use of HBO-enriched breathing mix in the future as is already happening in commercial diving operations.

Discussion

Oxygen debt is not elusive in concept. By definition it is the estimated consumption of oxygen over and above the available delivered oxygen over time needed by the mitochondrial respiratory enzymatic chains to make ATP. The predicament in resuscitation medicine is that in ASII, the consumption of oxygen often increases while the delivery of oxygen diminishes. In ASII the rub is that the need systemically for ATP is high and is dependent on a maintained IMS oxygen partial pressure of 1 mmHg.

While there is not yet an accurate way at bedside to measure oxygen debt imposed by ASII, the debt must nevertheless be rapidly resolved if the resuscitative effort is to be successful and multiorgan failure prevented as a sequelae. Much as in the 2015 iterations of the "surviving sepsis" treatment guidelines, intravascular volume must be replenished to assist oxygen delivery to mitochondria (Delinger et al. 2008).

Sufficient oxygen delivery to mitochondria at 1 atm ambient pressure can be problematic. Provision of supplemental oxygen to the patient that does not diffuse a sufficient supply to cytochrome aa3 and can increase ROS as the AHA literature backed 2015 guidelines for ACLS suggest. Intravenous fluorocarbon delivery of oxygen has been fraught with side effects of the carrier itself (Cohn and Cushing 2009). The use of formulations of stroma-free hemoglobin has likewise had untoward side effects precluding their use (Winslow 2002). Coated oxygen micelles given intravenously have to-date ultimately been damaging to microvasculature (Kheir et al. 2012). Mechanical interventions like emergency room resuscitative endovascular balloon occlusion of the aorta (ER-REBOA) (Saito et al. 2015), extracorporeal life support (ECLS) (Dworschak 2013), and mechanical chest compression (Steen et al. 2005) still face reperfusion injury which could be ameliorated by concurrent HBO.

Over the past 33 years, New Orleans has had two emergency department-based multiplace chambers engineered to lock onto ambulance delivered hyperbaric transfer chambers to address prehospital cardiopulmonary arrest. One site was Jo Ellen Smith Memorial Hospital, opened in 1983, and the other was Charity Hospital, opened in 2005 (Fig. 42.20). Unfortunately, both hospitals suffered political closures before human ACLS-HBO trials could be started (Van Meter 2006). Still the future may once again hold for a multiplace hyperbaric chamber to be set up similarly for HBO life support (HBOLS) for resuscitation from ASII (Figs. 42.21 and 42.22).

The average healthy 70 kg adult at any one time has approximately 8.8 oz of ATP. During a 24 h period, the expended and regenerated ATP amounts to a total ATP amount of one's own body weight (Törnroth-Horsefield and

Fig. 42.20 Shown is a multiplace hyperbaric chamber with SICU/ICU capability in the Emergency Department at Charity Hospital's Trauma Center in 2005 in New Orleans, Louisiana

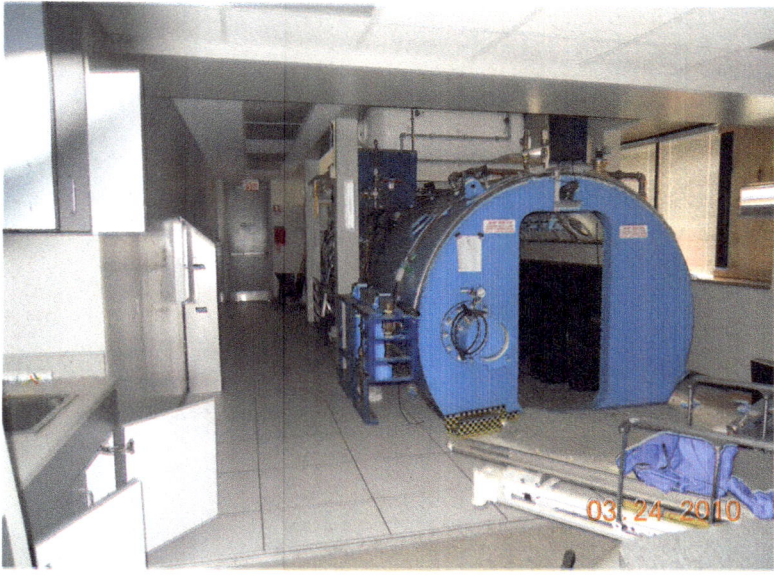

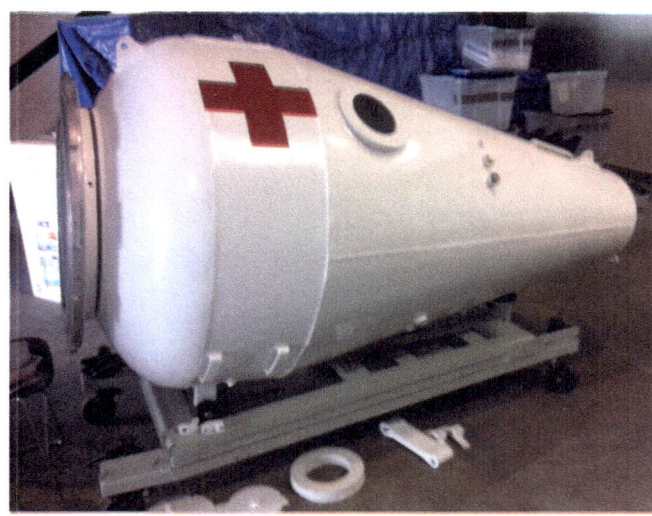

Fig. 42.21 An example of an EMS transport chamber which would admit the patient and paramedic in transport to a hospital-based unit from an event on the street; the ambulance would need no modification. Chamber would be powered by high-pressure D cylinders of compressed oxygen and air. The chamber would fit in the unmodified aisleway of a standard box compartment ambulance

Neutze 2008). By far the majority of this ATP is generated by the event of nascent diatomic oxygen docking on cytochrome aa3 to pull electron's energy to put H+ into the IMS to run the ATPase micromachine enzymatic turbine's end of shaft conformation to allow ADP + Pi to bind at an extraordinary rate. In ASII, acute inflammation initially steps up ATP consumption and regeneration until no longer can the supply keep up with the demand as the mitochondrial oxygen tension gets dragged below one mmHg pO_2. Cellular and interstitial edema and flagging circulatory perfusion combine to allow suboptimal dangerously low levels of oxygen to comingle with leaking respiratory enzymatic chains. The chains themselves cannot be repaired by reason of insufficient supply energy from ATP. In effect as mounting ATP debt occurs, ATP consumption outstrips supply paralleling a mounting oxygen debt by consumption of oxygen outstripping supply to cytochrome aa3 necessary under an optimal tissue oxygen tension of 1 mmHg. An inaccurate time lagging measurement of oxygen debt clinically has been by determination of serum lactate levels. More recently a polarographic-based needle probe which can be inserted in vivo into tissue can produce real-time continuous tissue quantitative levels of tissue ATP (Llaudet et al. 2005). With this probe, cooperative laboratories in New Orleans have demonstrated that after prolonged limb tourniqueting, a drop in ATP occurs. After tourniquet release, the muscle ATP levels deplete even more when the subject breathes 1 atm 100 % oxygen (FIO_2 100 %) and ATP levels increase threefold if the subject breathes oxygen at 2.4 atm ($SEFIO_2$ 240 %).

Future Applications

In the future, computerized tomography of near-infrared imaging may be able to track the total body cytochrome aa3 redox state to correlate it with total body ATP levels in ASII to give guidance for necessary $SEFIO_2$ to reduce effectively the patient' oxygen debt (or ATP debt) (Kriedt et al. 2010).

In concluding comment, oxygen is a drug and as a drug it has a dose–response curve which may be generalized for patients, but is certainly different to some extent in all subjects even over the span of each life. As a drug, oxygen,

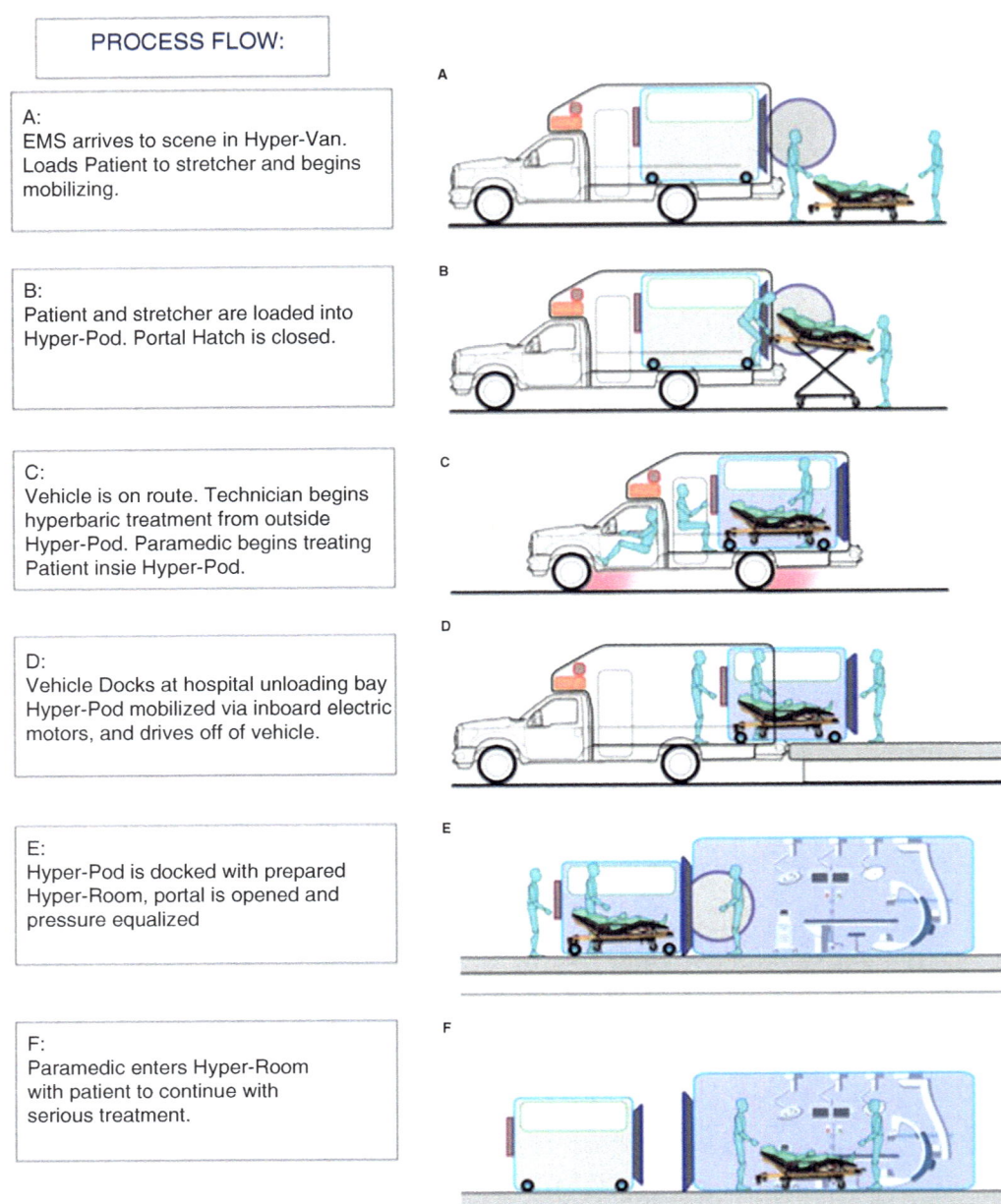

PROCESS FLOW:

A:
EMS arrives to scene in Hyper-Van. Loads Patient to stretcher and begins mobilizing.

B:
Patient and stretcher are loaded into Hyper-Pod. Portal Hatch is closed.

C:
Vehicle is on route. Technician begins hyperbaric treatment from outside Hyper-Pod. Paramedic begins treating Patient insie Hyper-Pod.

D:
Vehicle Docks at hospital unloading bay Hyper-Pod mobilized via inboard electric motors, and drives off of vehicle.

E:
Hyper-Pod is docked with prepared Hyper-Room, portal is opened and pressure equalized

F:
Paramedic enters Hyper-Room with patient to continue with serious treatment.

Design by Delise Design works, Los Angeles, California, 2016

Fig. 42.22 Design by Delisle Design Works, Los Angeles, California, 2016. Design patent pending/Illustrations Copyright 2016 Delise Design Works, LLC.

with its varying doses, may have productive as well as deleterious interaction with other drugs and therapies. HBO along with systemically applied pressure allows a yet not fully explored dosing potential for oxygen and for pressure. It is possible that many of the discarded or efficacy downgraded ACLS drugs and therapies may work better or worse in hyperbarically oxygenated patients during resuscitation. Perhaps some of the deleterious efforts produced by norepinephrine-induced ischemia may be ameliorated HBO during resuscitation of the ASII patients.

Conclusion

Without a constantly renewed oxygen supply, we would cease to have a constantly renewed ATP supply and without both, resuscitation fundamentally would be lackluster to impossible. Again HBO therapy is a low technology, easily applied therapy. Existing medical technology could easily throw together a chain of survival to begin with a code cart drawer replacement with a monoplace chamber managed with robotic arms (with cardiac and blood pressure cuff monitoring. Hayek Curiass (Lockart et al. 1992) negative ventilator vest with recess for a Lucas (Steen et al. 2005) cardiac chest compressor, and intraosseous venous access and fiber optic guided endotracheal intubation). With ambient air compression for the patient safe defibrillation through chest paste on electrodes has been tested after 1250 times on endotracheal intubated subject's ventilation with oxygen in hyperbaric environment (Van Meter et al. 1996).

It is up to the political winds of the medical world to allow this avenue of intervention in resuscitation to be pursued or not.

References

Alex J, Laden G, Cale AR, Bennett S, Flowers K, Madden L, et al. Pretreatment with hyperbaric oxygen and its effect on neuropsychometric dysfunction and systemic inflammatory response after cardiopulmonary bypass: a prospective randomized double blind trial. J Thorac Cardiovasc Surg. 2005;130(6):1623–30.

American Heart Association Guidelines and Update for CPR and ECC. Circulation 2015;132(18 suppl 2):469.

Bigelow WG. The microcirculation: some physiological and philosophical observation concerning the peripheral vascular system. Can J Surg. 1964;7:237–60.

Boerema I, Meyne NG, Brummelkamp WK, et al. Life without blood: a study of the influence of high atmospheric pressure and hypothermia on dilution of the blood. J Cardiovasc Surg. 1959;13:133–46.

Brunori M, Vallone B. A globin for the brain. FASEB J. 2006;20(13):2192–7.

Burnstock G. Overview: purinergic mechanisms. Ann N Y Acad Sci. 1990;603:1–17; discussion 18.

Cohn CS, Cushing MM. Oxygen therapeutics: perfluorocarbons and blood substitute safey. Crit Care Med. 2009;25:399–414.

Delinger RP, Levy MM, Carlet JM, Bion J, Parker MM, Jaeschke R, et al. Surviving Sepsis Campaign: international guidelines for management of severe sepsis and shock. Intensive Care Med. 2008;34(1):17–60.

Dimroth P, Kaim G, Matthey U. Crucial role of membrane potential for ATP synthesis by $F(1)F(o)$ syntheses. J Exp Biol. 2000;203(Pt 1):51–9.

Dumas F, Bougouin W, Geri G, Lamhaut L, Bougle A, Daviaud F, et al. Is epinephrine during cardiac arrest associated with worse outcomes in resuscitated patients? J Am Coll Cardiol. 2014;64(22):2360–7.

Dworschak M. Is extracorporal cardiopulmonary resuscitation for out-of-hospital cardiac arrest superior compared with conventional resuscitation. Crit Care Med. 2013;41(5):1365–6.

Godman CA, Chheda KP, Hightower LE, Perdrizet G, Shin DG, Giardina C. Hyperbaric oxygen induces a cytoprotective and angiogenic response in human microvascular endothelial cells. Cell Stress Chaperones. 2010;15(4):431–42.

Hardie DG, Hawley SA. AMP-activated protein kinase: the energy charge hypothesis revisited. Bioessays. 2001;23(12):1112–9.

Huang SF, Shen CH, Peng CK, et al. Successful treatment of post-ACLS hypoxic encephalopathy by hyperbaric oxygen—report of 2 cases. J Med Sci. 2012;32(2):93–6.

Iliff JJ, Wang M, Liao Y, Plogg BA, Peng W, Gundersen GA, et al. A paravascular pathway facilitates CSF flow through the brain parenchyma and the clearance of interstitial solutes, including amyloid B. Sci Transl Med 2012;4(147):147ra111.

Kheir JN, Scharp LA, Borden MA, Swanson EJ, Loxley A, Reese JH, et al. Oxygen gas-filled microparticles provide intervenous oxygen delivery. Sci Transl Med. 2012;4(140):1–10.

Knighton DR, Halliday B, Hunt TK. Oxygen as an antibiotic: the effect of inspired oxygen on infection. Arch Surg. 1984;119(2):199–204.

Knowles JR. Enzyme-catalyzed phosphoryl transfer reactions. Annu Rev Biochem. 1980;49:877–919.

Kriedt FA, Kriedt C, Patterson C, Van Meter KW. Determination of oxygen dosage effects on cytochrome oxidase after anoxia in brain. Adv Exp Med Biol. 2010;662:191–7.

Llaudet E, Hatz S, Droniou M, Dale N. Microelectrode biosensor for real-time measurement of ATP in biological tissue. Anal Chem. 2005;77(10):3267–73.

Lockart D, Langleben D, Zidulka A. Hemodynamic differences between continual positive and two types of negative pressure ventilation. Am Rev Respir Dis. 1992;146(3):677–80.

Mathieu D, Wattel F, Gosselin B, et al. Hyperbaric oxygen in treatment of posthanging cerebral anoxia. J Hyperbar Med. 1987;2(2):63–7.

McBride HM, Neuspiel M, Wasiak S. Mitochondria: more than just a powerhouse. Curr Biol. 2006;16(14):R551–60.

Michel H. Cytochrome c oxidase: catalytic cycle and mechanisms of proton pumping—a discussion. Biochemistry. 1999;38(46):15129–40.

Patel JK, Parikh PB. Association between therapeutic hypothermia and long-term quality of life in survivors of cardiac arrest: a systematic review. Resuscitation. 2016;103:54–9.

Rich PR. The molecular machinery of Keilin's respiratory chain. Biochem Soc Trans. 2003;31(Pt 6):1095–105.

Rosenthal RE, Silbergleit R, Hof PR, Haywood Y, Fiskum G. Hyperbaric oxygen reduces neuronal death and improves neurological outcome after canine cardiac arrest. Stroke. 2003;34(5):1311–6.

Saito N, Matsumoto H, Yagi T, Hara Y, Hayashida K, Motomura T, et al. Evaluation of the safety and feasibility of resuscitative endovascular balloon occlusion of the aorta. J Trauma Acute Care Surg. 2015;78(5):897–904.

Schmidt M, Gerlach F, Avivi A, Laufs T, Wystub S, Simpson JC, et al. Cytoglobin is a respiratory protein in connective tissue and neurons which is up-regulated by hypoxia. J Biol Chem. 2004;279(9):8063–9.

Shen C, Peng JP, Chen XD. Efficacy of treatment in per-pelvic Morel-Levallee lesion: a systematic review of the literature. Arch Orthoped Trauma Surg 2013;133(5)"635-640.

Shoemaker WC, Appel PL, Kram HB. Tissue oxygen debt as a determinant of lethal and nonlethal postoperative organ failure. Crit Care Med. 1988;16(11):1117–220.

Steen S, Slöberg T, Olssen P, Young M. Treatment of out-of-hospital cardiac arrest with LUCAS, a new device for automatic mechanical compression and active decompression resuscitation. Resuscitation. 2005;67(1):25–30.

Stub D, Smith K, Bernard S, Nehme Z, Stephenson M, Bray JE, et al. Air versus oxygen ST-segment-elevation myocardial infarction. Circulation. 2015;131(24):2143–50.

Thom SR, Elbuken ME. Oxygen-dependent antagonism of lipid peroxidation. Free Radic Biol Med. 1991;10(6):413–26.

Thom SR, Mendiguren I, Hardy K, Bolotin T, Fisher D, Nebolon M, et al. Inhibition of human neutrophil B2-integrin-dependent adherence by hyperbaric oxygen. Am J Physiol 1997;272(3 part 1):C770-C777.

Thom SR, Bhopale VM, Velazquez OC, Goldstein LJ, Thom LH, Buerk DG. Stem cell mobilization by hyperbaric oxygen. Am J Physiol Heart Circ Physiol. 2006;290(4):H1378–86.

Thom SR, Yang M, Bhopale VM, Huang S, Milovanova TN. Microparticles initiate decompression-induced neutrophil activation and subsequent vascular injuries. J Appl Physiol. 2011;110(2):340–51.

Törnroth-Horsefield S, Neutze R. Opening and closing the metabolite gate. Proc Natl Acad Sci U S A. 2008;105(50):19565–6.

Tseng S, Tornetta P. Percutaneous management of Morel-Levallee lesions" J Bone Joint Surg AM 2006;88(1):92-96.

Weaver LK (ed.). Undersea Hyperbaric Medical Society. Hyperbaric Oxygen Therapy Indications, 13th Ed. North Palm Beach, FL: Best Publishing; 2014.

Vajkoczy P, Roth H, Horn P, Lucke T, Thomé C, Hubner U, et al. Continuous monitoring of regional blood flow: experimental and clinical validation of a novel thermal diffusion microprobe. J Neurosurg. 2000;93(2):265–74.

Van Meter KW, Gottlieb SF, Whidden SJ. Hyperbaric oxygen as an adjunct in ACLS in guinea pigs after 15 minutes of cardiopulmonary arrest. Undersea Hyperb Med. 1988;15(suppl):55.

Van Meter KW, Swanson S, Sheps S, et al. Electrical defibrillation to treat ventricular fibrillation in a controlled, non-randomized pilot in swine. Presented at the Undersea and Hyperbaric Medical Society Gulf Coast Chapter Scientific Assembly, May 1996.

Van Meter KW. Medical field management of the injured diver. Respir Care Clin N Am. 1999;5(1):137–77. vi.

Van Meter KW. Katrina at Charity Hospital: much ado about something. Am J Med Sci. 2006;332(5):251–4.

Van Meter KW, Sheps S, Kriedt F, Moises J, Barratt D, Murphy-Lavoie H, et al. Hyperbaric oxygen improves rate of return of spontaneous circulation after prolonged normothermic porcine cardiopulmonary arrest. Resuscitation. 2008;78(2):200–14.

Van Meter KW, Harch PG. HBO$_2$ in emergency medicine. In: Jain KK, editor. Textbook of hyperbaric medicine. 5th ed. Göttingen, Germany: Hogrefe; 2009. p. 453–83.

Van Meter KW. Hyperbaric oxygen therapy as an adjunct to pre-hospital advanced trauma life support. Surg Technol Int. 2012a;21:61–73.

Van Meter KW. The effect of hyperbaric oxygen on severe anemia. Undersea Hyperb Med. 2012b;39(5):937–42.

Van Meter K. Hyperbaric oxygen clinical application in resuscitation from insult of acute severe anemia. Wound Care Hyperbar Med. 2014;5(4):29–34.

Weaver LK, editor. Indications for hyperbaric oxygen therapy. 13th ed. North Palm Beach: Undersea & Hyperbaric Medical Society (UHMS)/Best Publishing Company; 2014.

Winslow RM. Blood substitutes. Curr Opin Hematol. 2002;9(2):146–51.

Yogaratnam JZ, Laden G, Guvendik L, Cowen M, Cale A, Griffin S. Hyperbaric oxygen preconditioning improves myocardial function, reduces length of intensive care stay, and limits complications post coronary artery bypass graft surgery. Cardiovasc Revasc Med. 2010;11(1):8–19.

Zawrotniak M, Rapala-Kozik M. Neutrophil extracellular traps (NETS)—formation and implications. Acta Biochim Pol. 2013;60(3):277–84.

Fabio Faralli, Alberto Fiorito, and Gerardo Bosco

Abstract

The potential role of hyperbaric oxygen therapy (HBOT) in military medicine for treatment of combat casualties has raised interest and focused attention on aspects that are different from the usual and historic role associated with decompression illness (DCI) and diving medicine. The key sections of this chapter are HBOT and combat medicine, hyperbaric activities in military environment, diving medicine in military diving operations, and submarine medicine

Keywords

Military medicine • Hyperbaric oxygen therapy • Diving medicine • Submarine medicine • Decompression illness • Traumatic brain injury

Hyperbaric Oxygen Therapy and Combat Medicine

The potential role of hyperbaric oxygen therapy (HBOT) in military medicine for combat casualties treatment has raised interest and focused attention on assets different from the usual and historic role associated with decompression illness (DCI) and diving medicine. The use of HBOT therapy for the management of combat-related injuries has been suggested by several authors (Cramer 1985; Workman and Calcote 1989; Fitzpatrick 1997, 2000; Wright 2000; Hart 2004).

It was pointed out that HBOT, when properly and safely used, can be a powerful and valuable adjunct in acute surgical and trauma conditions, and military surgeons can utilize this useful adjunct to surgical practice, in conjunction with hyperbaric therapy specialists (MacFarlane et al. 2000).

F. Faralli, MD, Surg Rear Admiral (Ret) (✉)
Italian Navy, Arcola, Italy
e-mail: fabio.faralli1958@gmail.com

A. Fiorito, MD, LtC (Ret) • G. Bosco, MD, PhD
Department of Biomedical Sciences, University of Padova,
Lerici, Italy

Van Meter (2011) proposed an increasing role as an adjunct to prehospital advanced trauma life support for HBOT.

HBOT has been used for a variety of indications. Undersea & Hyperbaric Medical Society (UHMS) in the US and European Committee for Hyperbaric Medicine (ECHM) in the EU have a constantly updated list of indications based on scientific evidence and many of them can be typical consequences of war injuries (Kot and Mathieu 2011; Weaver 2014). It is important to note that HBOT is only an adjunctive treatment for majority of these indications. HBOT can prove to be an important factor in improving the prognosis in these patients in whom the standard care is proving to be inadequate (Verghese et al. 2013).

However, the lack of treatment facilities available for combat casualty care and management in a theater of operations may reduce the impact that HBOT can provide for an injured soldier and the number of patients that can be treated. Then a change in the HBOT technology has been postulated to maximize the effect of the hyperbaric treatment. HBOT mono place chambers can have a role in the treatment of battle casualties. Transportable recompression chambers can be an option for field hospital next to the battlefield. Latson and Zinszer (1999) evaluated for the US Navy two portable and collapsible one-man hyperbaric chambers, as Emergency Evacuation Hyperbaric Stretchers

(EEHS); they prospected, as indications for use of these systems, smoke inhalation, carbon monoxide poisoning, thermal burns, and crush injury, other than the classical DCI and arterial gas embolism. Unconsciousness or airway compromise is the most significant contraindication to the use of these systems, and the risk of fire is the prominent hazard when using oxygen.

The use of hyperbaric stretchers for aeromedical evacuation of scenario casualties to a definitive medical hyperbaric treatment facility was proposed (Krock et al. 2000).

Among the accepted and the experimental indications of HBOT, some of them may be typical of combat and military medicine.

Gas Gangrene: Crush Injuries and Traumatic Wounds

There are early reports of use of HBOT in gas gangrene from war wounds (Johnson et al. 1969; Shupak et al. 1984). HBOT therapy enhanced the survival rate of patients with gas gangrene, lowered the anesthetic risk, allowed for maximal tissue preservation, and helped avoid radical mutilating surgery.

The indication of HBOT in severe limb trauma is supported by its effect on peripheral oxygen transport, muscular ischemic necrosis, compartment syndrome, and infection prevention (Camporesi and Bosco 2014). A randomized double-blind placebo-controlled clinical trial made by Bouachour et al. (1996) showed the effectiveness of HBO in improving wound healing and reducing repetitive surgery. The authors proposed HBOT as a useful adjunct in the management of severe (grade III) crush injuries of the limbs especially in patients more than 40 years old. The involvement of Nitric Oxide System in experimental muscle crush injury may give further support to the use of hyperbaric oxygen (Rubinstein et al. 1998). MacFarlane et al. (2000) prospected the use of HBOT by military surgeons as an adjunct to the surgical therapy in various conditions with the aim to reduce morbidity and mortality.

A review on war extremity injures, including combat-related Type III fractures, and describing the impact of HBOT on wound healing and infectious complications, showed a reduction of the infectious complications when patient management included HBOT. This effect was more common among non-NATO patients than in NATO patients, who received the standard NATO wound management and antimicrobials; more cases of osteomyelitis were reported in the group of patients treated with HBOT (Roje et al. 2008).

More recent reviews with the aim to determine the effects of HBOT on the healing of acute surgical and traumatic wounds concluded that there is a lack of high quality randomized controlled trials and pointed out the need of further evaluation (Goldman 2009; Eskes et al. 2010; Murray et al. 2011)

Exceptional Loss of Blood

In the 1960s, the Dutch thoracic surgeon Boerema demonstrated that removing blood from the blood vessels of pigs and replacing it with a substitute liquid made of Ringer's Lactate solution, dextrose, and dextran, then pressurizing the pigs in a hyperbaric chamber while the animals breathed 100 % oxygen, enough oxygen could be dissolved in the simulated plasma and the animals survived (Boerema et al. 1960). Hart et al. (1987, Hart 1974) utilized an empirical- and symptom-based approach to treat exceptional blood loss with HBOT. A systematic review of the application of HBOT in the treatment of severe anemia concluded that the use of HBOT to treat severe anemia, especially when blood products are not available in a combat scenario, is an established and effective option (Van Meter 2005) made. A physiological approach has been described and an exhaustive guide to the management of an anemic patient using HBOT is available (Bartlett 2008).

Burns

There are several reports showing the effect of adjunctive HBOT in the treatment of severe burns (Wada et al. 1966; Ketchum et al. 1967; Winter and Perrins 1970). The use of HBOT in serious burns in a combat theater may reduce the need for surgery and length of hospital stay (Cianci et al. 1988, 1989) and, probably, may decrease mortality (Niu et al. 1987). The theoretical beneficial effect of HBOT on burn wounds is in bactericidal effects on possible infections, in the reduction of edema and of the systemic inflammatory response, in delimiting the size of burned tissue and increasing collagen formation. The best results seem to be obtained when the hyperbaric therapy is started in the first hours from the injury. Nevertheless, there are studies showing a marginal and not clear role of HBOT in the management of severe burns. A randomized study to evaluate possible positive effects of HBOT on the experimental burn wound healing supports the use of HBOT (Bilic et al. 2005). In this study, the authors demonstrated a beneficial effect on the burn wound healing by HBOT, and they postulated that such an effect was determined by a reduction of edema and a preservation of the microcirculation.

Even if the quantity and quality of the evidence-based studies on the potential benefits of HBOT in patients with burns is poor, its potential use in combat medicine deserves further research. It is recommended a careful selection and screening of the patients to achieve the best results (Cianci 2008).

Postconcussion Syndrome, Traumatic Brain Injuries, Posttraumatic Stress Disorders

The current military engagements in Afghanistan and Iraq and recent wars have resulted in a number of military personnel returning from deployments with traumatic brain injury (TBI)/postconcussion syndrome (PCS) and posttraumatic stress disorder (PTSD).

The symptoms of PCS are nonspecific and they include somatic symptoms (headaches, dizziness, fatigue, ringing in the ears, seizures, sensitivity to light), cognitive symptoms (memory and concentration problems), and affective symptoms (irritability, emotional lability, depression, anxiety, trouble sleeping). Usually there is negativity of the clinical examination and complementary explorations and often pain killers and sleeping aids are prescribed.

PTSD is a psychiatric disorder that may affect patients with traumatic brain injuries but an anatomy and clinical correlation between the symptoms of postconcussion syndrome and objectivable brain damage is still to be discovered (Auxéméry 2012).

HBOT seemed to be one of those treatments showing promising results easing the effects of those injuries. Some anecdotal evidence suggested HBOT treatment can improve TBI/PCS. The military medical community concluded that enough positive evidence exists in both military and nonmilitary case studies to more closely examine HBOT as a standard treatment for soldiers suffering from traumatic brain injuries. The rationale for the use of HBOT in TBI/PCS may be in the fact that elevated levels of dissolved oxygen by HBOT can have several reparative effects on damaged brain tissues (Boussi-Gross et al. 2013).

Harch et al. (2012) tested the safety and efficacy of 1.5 ATA HBOT in military subjects with chronic blast-induced mild to moderate TBI/PCS and PTSD. Sixteen military subjects received 40 1.5 ATA/60 min HBO sessions in 30 days. Symptoms, physical and neurological exams, SPECT brain imaging, and neuropsychological and psychological testing were completed before and within 1 week after treatment. Significant improvements occurred in symptoms, abnormal physical exam findings, cognitive testing, and quality-of-life measurements, with concomitant significant improvements in SPECT.

A single centre, double blind, randomized, sham controlled, prospective trial at the U.S. Air Force School of Aerospace Medicine, examined the effects of 2.4 atm absolute (ATA) HBOT on postconcussion symptoms in 50 military service members with at least one combat related, mild TBI. The results showed no effect on postconcussive symptoms after mild TBI using HBOT at 2.4 ATA (Wolf et al. 2012).

Bennett et al. (2012b) made a review of seven studies, involving 571 people (285 receiving HBOT and 286 in the control group). Given the modest number of patients, meth-

odological shortcomings of the trials and poor reporting, the results should be interpreted cautiously. The results showed that while the addition of HBOT may reduce the risk of death and improve the final Glasgow Coma Scale (GCS), there was little evidence that the survivors have a good outcome. The authors concluded that the routine application of HBOT to these patients cannot be justified from this review.

A collaborative study between the Department of Defense and the Department of Veterans Affairs looking at the use of hyperbaric oxygen on 60 military service members and its effect on persistent postconcussion symptoms concluded that there were no significant effects from using HBOT to manage symptoms of TBIs (Cifu et al. 2014).

Miller et al. (2015) made a randomized clinical trial to estimate the safety and the efficacy for symptomatic outcomes from standard PCS care alone, care supplemented with HBOT, or a sham procedure. HBOT showed no benefits over sham compressions but these two groups demonstrated improved outcomes compared with PCS care alone. This may suggest some placebo effect. Wang et al. (2016) recently performed a meta-analysis to evaluate the outcomes of HBOT in patients with TBI. The results showed a significant improvement in the GCS and Glasgow Outcome Scale (GOS).

In conclusion at the present, there are no clear evidence that HBOT can be an effective treatment for PCS and related disorders, but there are sign of its utility in TBI.

High Altitude Cerebral Edema and High Altitude Pulmonary Edema

In a case of deployment of soldiers in a high altitude combat theater, high altitude cerebral edema (HACO) and high altitude pulmonary edema (HAPO) can be an emergency to face up to. A portable, lightweight hyperbaric bag was developed to treat HACO and HAPO when immediate evacuation from high altitude was impossible (Kasic et al. 1989).

In a report on 9 HAPO and 7 HACO patients, observation time frames of 4 h and 6 h, respectively, were required to achieve resolution of the symptoms with no subsequent complications or deterioration (Taber 1990). The author considers the hyperbaric bag an effective adjunctive measure for the treatment of HAPO and HACO. A case of HAPO and HACO was reported occurring at moderate altitude that was successfully treated with the Gamow Bag (Freeman et al. 2004).

In the Wilderness Medical Society Consensus Guidelines for the Prevention and Treatment of Acute Altitude Illness, a 1B Recommendation Grade is given to the use of a portable hyperbaric chamber, but it is stressed that descent should not be delayed when it is feasible (Luks et al. 2010).

Gamow Bag has been used for the treatment of Altitude Mountain Sickness (AMS) with a series of hyperbaric treatment profiles developed by Life Support Technologies group for US military and NASA, which make use of vasoconstrictive effects of oxygen under 1.25 ATA pressure

(Butler et al. 2011). These profiles virtually eliminate AMS rebound after the initial treatment often seen in conventional AMS treatment, when the patient returns, after the treatment, directly to the same altitude where AMS symptoms first manifested reported the case of A patient with moderate acute mountain sickness at 3700 m above sea level was successfully treated by a transportable hyperbaric chamber that could be pressurized up to 15 psi of pressure (Saito et al. 2000).

Two cases of HAPO have been reported, where immediate descent was not possible in one of them, and the patient was treated with a hyperbaric chamber in view of life-threatening hypoxemia (Singhal et al. 2014). He showed some response inside the hyperbaric chamber, but when he was taken out of the chamber, he had cardiorespiratory arrest and died. The suggested cause of death was HAPO.

Despite these reports on hyperbaric treatment of high altitude illness, descent seems to remain the definitive treatment and the use of portable chambers can be an option when an immediate evacuation from altitude is impossible, as in a combat situation.

Hearing Loss and Tinnitus

Hearing loss and tinnitus are two of the most frequent service-connected disabilities in the military veterans. Reports indicate an alarming increase in the military population (Baldwin 2009). The recent war theaters have seen soldiers exposed to multiple hazards associated with these conditions, such as blasts/explosions, ototoxic chemicals, and high levels of noise (Theodoroff et al. 2015).

A MEDLINE search on this topic was conducted from 1960 to 2007 yielding 22 publications that revealed no demonstrable significant effect in four prospective studies (Desloovere 2007). On the other hand, retrospective studies indicate a better effect in acute cases (Lamm et al. 1998) and there is a study showing a psychological component in the improvement (Stiegler et al. 2006). A review showed no evidence of a beneficial effect of HBOT on chronic presentation of idiopathic sudden sensorineural hearing loss and/or tinnitus (Bennett et al. 2012a).

Spinal Cord Injury

A literature review has been made on the incidence, epidemiology, and management of combat-related spinal trauma with the aim to discuss the Clinical Practice Guidelines given by the USA Department of Defense in light of the published military experience (Schoenfeld et al. 2012). This review pointed out the dramatic increase of the incidence of spinal cord injuries (SCI) in the military involved in the Global War on Terror, in comparison with the conventional wars and recommend a reexam of the care procedure. The mRNA and protein expression of inducible nitric oxide synthase (iNOS) in the spinal cord and the serum nitric oxide (NO) content in a rat SCI model following HBOT have been studied (Huang et al. 2013). The results showed that the SCI was related to the excessive production of NO, and early HBOT could effectively protect the neurons in the spinal cord and promote the recovery of neurofunction, by the regulation of iNOS mRNA-iNOS-NO signaling pathway and the subsequent reduction of NO production in the spinal cord.

The mechanisms of action of HBOT in SCI have been investigated using an animal experimental model (Liu et al. 2014). The authors measured the expression levels of vascular endothelial growth factor (VEGF) and Connexin43 (CX43) in the injured spinal cord tissue. They found an improvement in neurological recovery when HBOT was applied after SCI and believed that the expression level changes of VEGF and CX43 could contribute to understand the molecular mechanisms of HBOT in these conditions.

Other studies on animal seemed to demonstrate a promising protective effect of HBOT in SCI (Zhou et al. 2013; Tan et al. 2014; Yaman et al. 2014)

A more recent study, again on an animal model, suggested that HBOT after SCI modified the inflammatory environment by modulating the macrophage populations. This, in authors' view, may promote the axonal extension and functional recovery (Geng et al. 2015).

Hyperbaric Oxygen Therapy and Military Response to Natural Catastrophes

At the present military response is worldwide accepted for assistance to civil communities in natural disasters. Most of the time, military support is activated only in large-scale disasters since small-scale disasters can be handled with the capacity of local resources. Many recent natural catastrophic events have shown the role the military can play, in different sectors, re-enforcing and integrating the civilian capabilities, including the possibility to offer HBOT for civilian casualties. The Italian Navy, after the Molise (Italy) Earthquake in 2002, sent a hyperbaric chamber to the Campobasso hospital, to treat patients with crush syndrome and risk of amputation (Fig. 43.1).

The Haiti Earthquake, in 2010, demonstrated the utility of HBOT: the hyperbaric chamber on-board of the Italian Navy aircraft carrier Cavour (Figs. 43.2 and 43.3) with a staff of surgeons and hyperbaric medicine specialists was effective in saving several limbs from amputation, especially in children with infected wounds. A retrospective analysis on the patients treated in that occasion, HBOT seemed to reduce both pain and Paracetamol consumption. In author's opinion, vasoconstriction caused by hyperbaric treatment, reducing posttraumatic edema of tissues and determining low releasing of acute inflammatory agents, could have analgesic effect on acute pain (Bosco et al. 2007; Lauretta 2012).

Fig. 43.1 Italian Navy hyperbaric chamber in the Campobasso Hospital

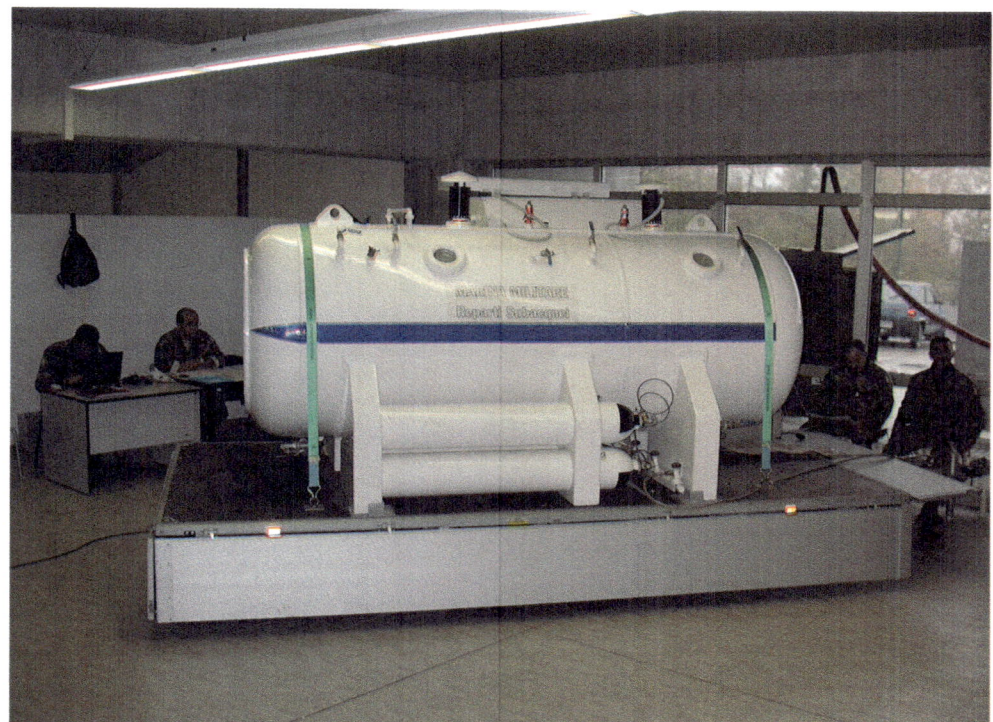

Fig. 43.2 Hyperbaric chamber and related equipment onboard the Italian Navy aircraft carrier Cavour

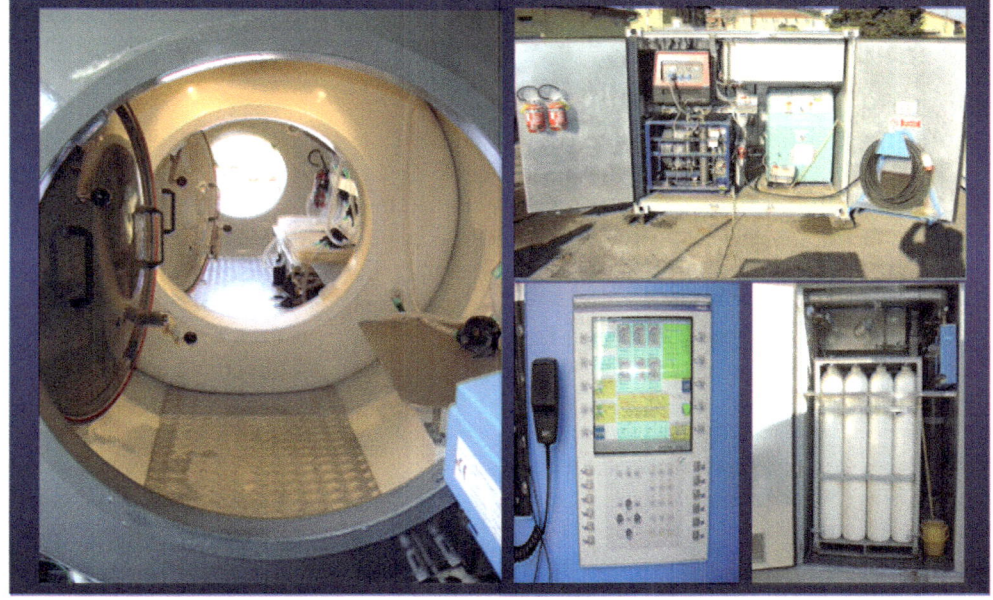

Hyperbaric Activities in Military Environment

Offensive Activities or Activities Carried out During Wartime

Around the fourth century, according to the sources of Plinio and Erodoto's tales, the figure of the "urinatores" appeared for the first time in the history. These were the first underwater workers whose interests ranged from research to war activities. With regard to the war field they were regularly paid and they even created a real corporation in the waters overlooking Rome. This seems to be one of the most ancient references related to underwater activity with military purpose in the history (Rossi et al. 2009). We had to wait until the Second World War to see the specific use of underwater equipment during raid activities, which began with the Deep-Sea Divers Corps of the Italian Navy, later called "raiders" (Bussoni 2013). This selected corps developed an underwater

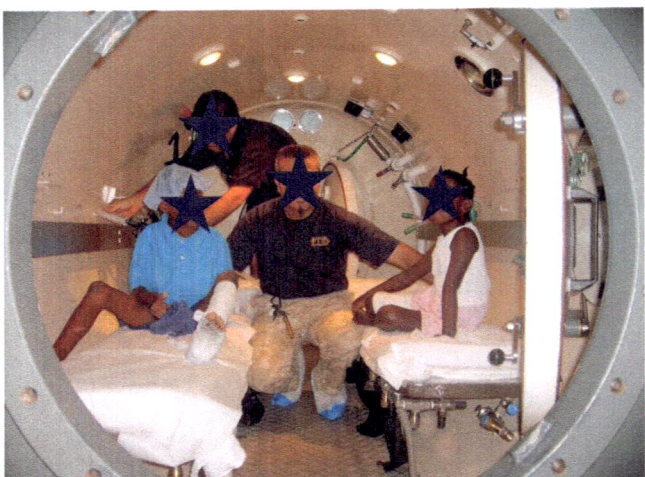

Fig. 43.3 Patients under treatment in the hyperbaric chamber onboard the Italian Navy aircraft carrier Cavour

breathing system with oxygen that had the peculiarity of being based on a closed circuit, meaning that it did not release any air bubble and for this reason they are not visible from the surface. The experiences of these men helped detecting the neurologic toxicity of oxygen from a clinical point of view and its limits of use. However, Paul Bert had already theoretically identified these limits during the second half of the nineteenth century (Bert 1943).

After that experience, the use of oxygen for military purposes spread out in most of the navies. In contrast to the two unquestionable advantages represented by invisibility from the surface and the endurance of a closed circuit breathing apparatus, which is superior to any other independent diving apparatus, there is the depth limitation in its use, which changes depending on the country but has a maximum of 12 m for short periods (Italy), around 10–15 min.

Defensive Activities or Activities Carried out During Peacetime

During peacetime, the military divers' corps are mainly employed to carry out research, rescue, inspection, and reclamation activities.

Research and Rescue Activities

The research of objects and wreckages on the sea bottom can either have an historical aspect, if the object is an evidence of ancient times, or can be linked to security and forensic medicine if it is carried out with the aim of finding wreckages of recent accidents. In this second and most frequent case, the procedure is a complicated one and requires an organization that involves the use of several surface means of transportation.

After signaling the event and the possible generic localization realized by the surface means, the ideal unit suitable for the research and the specific identification of the wreckage position is represented by the mine hunters. These ships are provided with a sophisticated equipment which is able to detect even extremely small objects on the bottom of the sea. International navies have mine hunters that are often provided with ready operation diver units and surface hyperbaric systems which are adequate for security tasks and potential first intervention in case of accidents. So the potential action of the mine hunter's personnel is limited to the free diving intervention equipment provided and without diving bell.

If the depth is higher than the limits prescribed by the equipment given to the operational crew or if the operation on the sea bottom is too long, the intervention of a surface unit with a kind of equipment which is suitable for more demanding diving operations is necessary, until reaching the saturation level. It is obvious that it is impossible to predict this kind of operation regarding the potential rescue of the personnel that is trapped inside the wreckage because the duration in this case is necessarily long.

Seabed Inspection Activities

An immersion in order to inspect an area of the seabed could be necessary. Among the most sensible objectives of that kind of research there could be pipelines or oil pipelines with the aim of evaluating the risks that could threaten the population or the marine life. Underwater installations assigned to research or to military use or ordinary training could be other objectives of the inspection activities.

Reclamation Activities

Because of conflicts or accidents of the surface transit units, there is the possibility of leaving potentially explosive devices that can be dangerous for the population. In this case the navy divers units are called in order to identify, rescue, and clear the area by removing explosive devices or material.

This kind of underwater activity requires two specific considerations. The first one is related to the diving equipment. In fact, there is the possibility that war scraps are activated by magnetic mechanisms. Considering this risk, it is essential that the personnel that is assigned to this kind of operation be provided with not-magnetic equipment in order to avoid the activation of the explosive. Another explosive activation system could be connected to vibrations. Vibrations produced by divers' breathing should not be able to stimulate activation of the explosives. The diving equipment used in this kind of operation should include devices to divide the bubbles, which act on exhaled breath and further reduce sounds and vibrations. The second consideration is about a particular kind of barotrauma that could affect divers who handle with this type of operations. There are some precise safety standards in order to regulate the charges explosion modality and the safety distance that must be kept. In any case, we should take into consideration that sometimes the personnel undergo explosion risks at short distance from the event, due to accident, mistake, or intention. The organs which are the most threatened by trauma risk are those that have air spaces and in particular lung and middle ear. Because of the possible trauma these organs can be affected in their soft tissues which can be lacerated and suffer from other serious damage.

Field of HBO Application in Military Diving Medicine

Military Diving Operations

The diving component within the military field is relevant in almost every nation, whether a country has access to the sea or the operations are limited to its internal waters. Apart from the offensive use in the strict sense, the component's scopes of work are harbors and ship canals' security, defensive systems installation and control, mine clearance activities, research and rescue of human beings, objects, and sunk boats.

Diving Methods

In order to fulfill the institutional tasks these units have essentially three diving methods: immersion with independent breathing apparatus, using different equipment and gas depending on the diving demands, bounce dive or saturation dive from a diving facility.

Technical and pathophysiological characteristics of these diving methods have been examined in the respective chapters. Following we will deal with some peculiarities in the military field in which a doctor could be interested.

Employee's Safety

The military field has an important difference if compared to the civil one. The personnel that is employed in diving operations act following orders and guidelines established in specific legislations where the safety value, even if taken into consideration in every organization, is in this case particularly emphasized due to a higher and more complex hierarchy of responsibilities. For this reason, it is frequently possible to notice an excess of regulations in security systems until reaching the point of having an abundance of employees. Bounce diving is a typical example of this case. In the commercial field, two divers carry out these operations. One has the task of tender and remains in the diving bell and the other one handles with the prescribed task. In the military field three divers usually carry out this kind of operation. Apart from the tender, who always remains in the diving bell, two other divers both handle with the task and at the same time look after the security of the buddy.

Personnel Training

Personnel training represents an essential moment in both civil and military field. Due to its importance, there are no particular differences. The only real advantage that can have diving operations within military field is that, apart from extremely rare cases, the personnel speak the same language. In an off shore environment, the staff involved have different backgrounds and in case of emergency there might be the possibility of not being fluent in the language during emergencies. In this case a situation, that is already an emergency, could get worse.

Personnel Recruitment

The recruitment process is considerably different too. Even if the characteristics of the evaluation parameters are mostly standard, due to the earlier said responsibility issue, within the military field it is possible to expect more restrictive measures and a stricter selection, most of all at the beginning.

Submarine Medicine

Submarines' Rescue

Among the tasks of the navies' divers units a particular aspect is the personnel on damaged submarines rescue. In this case we suppose that a submarine cannot go back to the surface due to an accident, that the crew on board is still alive and manage to send messages which let them give information about the event and the precise location.

When the danger signal is activated, the rescue system starts and it can be carried out in two ways. The American and soviet navies have airborne submarines able to be carried on surface units, to be brought where the accident took place and to carry out the rescue. Other navies in the Mediterranean area, especially the Italian navy, have surface units available which are already equipped with small submarines and systems of fixed rescue, diving bell McCann, that can be ready in 24–48 h and with the aim of quickly reaching the accident area only by sea.

Technical Aspects of Rescue Operations

From the procedural point of view both the small submarine and the diving bell work in the same way, this means that these devices need to reach the exit hatch of the submarine and

Table 43.1 Possibility of transfer under pressure according to maximum rescue depth in various navies around the world

Country	Maximum rescue depth	Transfer under pressure
Australia	525	Yes
Bulgaria	120	No
Canada	300	Yes
India	200	No
Italy	300	Yes up to 5 bar
Norway	610	Yes
Singapore	500	Yes
Sweden	450	Yes up to 6 bar
Turkey	207	No
USA	600	Yes

firmly anchor to it. At this point, there are three different compartments: the submarine, the rescue system, and the space between these two, which at the beginning is full of water and which is called "skirt." With a system that allows the introduction of pressurized gas in this space the water is eliminated and a valve that drains to the rescue system is used in order to create the same pressure in both the "skirt" and the rescue system area. The next passage will be the creation of the same pressure in both the submarine and the rescue system, always through a drain valve. At this point the submarine crew is collected depending on the rescue means' capacity and brought on the surface. The operation will be repeated until the whole crew has been evacuated.

The operative substantial difference between small submarine and diving bell is that the last one requires the employment of divers who have the task of connecting an iron cable at the height of the exit hatch of the damaged submarine. This cable will have the function of guiding the diving bell in order to reach the precise position for the rescue operation. The important limit of this operation is the limit of the divers with their diving tools. On the contrary, the small submarine moves independently, it doesn't require the intervention of deep-sea divers and can reach higher operative depths, currently ranging from 250 to 600 m.

Transfer Under Pressure

The main problem that the rescue team will have to deal with is the fact that there is a high probability that the atmosphere inside the damaged submarine is higher than the normal level, which is of one atmosphere. This fact could be a consequence of the entrance of water in a compartment or could be the result of the use of emergency gas inside the submarine or of technical accidents.

Depending on the length of the stay with this new pressure, hypothesizing it in several hours, the damaged crew should be considered saturated with a new pressure. Because of this situation, the crew cannot be transferred directly to the surface. Once collected from the damaged mean, the survivors will need to be brought to a suitable hyperbaric facility in order to accomplish the progressive decompression depending on the depth at which they had been saturated. This possibility, theoretically more frequent, has as a consequence the need for a surface unit to have a suitable hyperbaric environment. Possibility of transfer under pressure, which varies according to maximum rescue depth in various navies, is shown in Table 43.1.

References

Auxéméry Y. Mild traumatic brain injury and postconcussive syndrome: a re-emergent questioning [Article in French]. Encéphale. 2012;38(4):329–35.

Baldwin D. Tinnitus, a military epidemic: is hyperbaric oxygen therapy the answer? J Spec Oper Med. 2009;9(3):33–43.

Bartlett B. HBO and exceptional blood-loss anemia. In: Kindwall EP, Whalen HT, editors. Hyperbaric medicine practice. 3rd ed. Flagstaff, AZ: Best Publishing; 2008. p. 793–834.

Bennett MH, Kertesz T, Perleth M, Yeung P, Lehm JP. Hyperbaric oxygen for idiopathic sudden sensorineural hearing loss and tinnitus. Cochrane Database Syst Rev. 2012a;10, CD004739.

Bennett MH, Trytko B, Jonker B. Hyperbaric oxygen therapy for the adjunctive treatment of traumatic brain injury. Cochrane Database Syst Rev. 2012b;12:CD004609.

Bert P. Barometric pressure. Researches in experimental physiology. Translated by Hitchock MA and Hitchcock FA. Columbus: College Book; 1943.

Bilic I, Petri NM, Bezic J, Alfirevic D, Modun D, Capkun V, Bota B. Effects of hyperbaric oxygen therapy on experimental burn wound healing in rats: a randomized controlled study. UHM. 2005;32:1–9.

Boerema I, Meijne NG, Brummelkamp WH, Bouma S, Mensch MH, Kamermans F, et al. Life without blood. J Cardiovasc Surg. 1960;182:133–46.

Bosco G, Yang ZJ, Nandi J, Wang J, Chen C, Camporesi EM. Effects of hyperbaric oxygen on glucose, lactate, glycerol and anti-oxidant enzymes in the skeletal muscle of rats during ischaemia and reperfusion. Clin Exp Pharmacol Physiol. 2007;34(1-2):70–6.

Bouachour G, Cronier P, Gouello JP, Toulemonde JL, Talha A, Alquier P. Hyperbaric oxygen therapy in the management of crush injuries; a randomized double-blind placebo-controlled clinical trial. J Trauma. 1996;41(2):333–9.

Boussi-Gross R, Golan H, Fishlev G, Bechor Y, Volkov O, et al. Hyperbaric oxygen therapy can improve post concussion syndrome years after mild traumatic brain injury—randomized prospective trial. PLoS ONE. 2013;8(11):e79995.

Bussoni M. Incursori, oltre la leggenda. Un secolo di storia delle forze speciali della Marina Militare Italiana, Mattioli 1885, 2013.

Butler GJ, Al-Waili N, Passano DV, Ramos J, Chavarri J, Beale J, et al. Altitude mountain sickness among tourist populations: a review and pathophysiology supporting management with hyperbaric oxygen. J Med Eng Technol. 2011;35(3-4):197–207.

Camporesi EM, Bosco G. Mechanisms of action of hyperbaric oxygen therapy. Undersea Hyperb Med. 2014;41(3):247–52.

Cianci P. Ajunctive hyperbaric oxygen therapy in the treatment of thermal burns. In: Kindwall EP, Whalen HT, editors. Hyperbaric medicine practice. 3rd ed. Flagstaff, AZ: Best Publishing; 2008. p. 921–38.

Cianci P, Leuders H, Lee H, et al. Adjunctive hyperbaric oxygen reduces the need for surgery in 40-80% burns. J Hyper Med. 1988;3:97–104.

Cianci P, Leuders H, Lee H, Shapiro RL, Sexton J, Williams C, et al. Adjunctive hyperbaric oxygen therapy reduces length of hospitalization in thermal burns. J Burn Care Rehabil. 1989;10:342–5.

Cifu DX, Hart BB, West SL, Walker W, Carne W. The effect of hyperbaric oxygen on persistent post concussion symptoms. J Head Trauma Rehabil. 2014;29(1):1120.

Cramer FS. Care of the injured soldier: a medical readiness role for clinical hyperbaric oxygen therapy. Mil Med. 1985;150:372–5.

Desloovere C. Hyperbaric oxygen therapy for tinnitus. B-ENT. 2007;3 Suppl 7:71–4.

Eskes A, Ubbink DT, Lubbers M, Lucas C, Vermeulen H. Hyperbaric oxygen therapy for treating acute surgical and traumatic wounds. Cochrane Database Syst Rev. 2010;10, CD008059.

Fitzpatrick DT. Applications of HBO therapy in army medicine. US Army Med Dept J. 1997;17–22.

Fitzpatrick DT. Role of HBO therapy in combat casualty care. US Army Med Dept J. 2000;4–9.

Freeman K, Shalit M, Stroh G. Use of the Gamow Bag by EMT-basic park rangers for treatment of high-altitude pulmonary edema and high-altitude cerebral edema. Wilderness Environ Med. 2004;15:198–201.

Geng CK, Cao HH, Ying X, Zhang HT, Yu HL. The effects of hyperbaric oxygen on macrophage polarization after rat spinal cord injury. Brain Res. 2015;1606:68–76.

Goldman RJ. Hyperbaric oxygen therapy for wound healing and limb salvage: a systematic review. PM R. 2009;1:471–89.

Harch PG, Andrew SR, Fogarty E, Amen D, Pezzullo JC, Lucarini J, et al. A Phase I study of low-pressure hyperbaric oxygen therapy for blast-induced post-concussion syndrome and post-traumatic stress disorder. J Neurotrauma. 2012;29:168–85.

Hart GB. Exceptional blood loss anemia. JAMA. 1974;228:1028–9.

Hart BB. Hyperbaric oxygen therapy: an adjunct to optimal combat trauma management. In: Proceedings of the NATO Research and Technology Office (Human Factors and Medicine) Symposium on Combat Casualty Care in Ground Based Tactical Situations: Trauma Technology and Emergency Medical Procedures 2004 August 16-18. St Peach Beach, USA. NATO Scientific Report No: RTO-MP-HFM-109.

Hart GB, Lennon PA, Strauss MB. Hyperbaric oxygen in exceptional acute blood-loss anaemia. J Hyper Med. 1987;2:205–10.

Huang H, Xue L, Zhang X, Weng Q, Chen H, Gu J, et al. Hyperbaric oxygen therapy provides neuroprotection following spinal cord injury in a rat model. Int J Clin Exp Pathol. 2013;6(7):1337–42.

Johnson JT, Gillespie TE, Cole JR, Markowitz HA. Hyperbaric oxygen therapy for gas gangrene in war wounds. Am J Surg. 1969;118(6):839–43.

Kasic JF, Smith HM, Gamow RI. A self-contained life support system designed for use with a portable hyperbaric chamber. Biomed Sci Instrum. 1989;25:79–81.

Ketchum SA, Zubrin JR, Thomas AN, Hall AD. Effect of hyperbaric oxygen on small first, second and third degree burns. Surg Forum. 1967;18:65–7.

Kot J, Mathieu D. Controversial issues in hyperbaric oxygen therapy: a European Committee for Hyperbaric Medicine Workshop. Diving Hyperb Med. 2011;41(2):101–4.

Krock LP, Galloway TR, Sylvester J, Latson GW, Wolf EG Jr. Into the Theater of Operations: Hyperbaric Oxygen on the Move. RTO HFM Symposium on "Operational Medical Issues in Hypo- and Hyperbaric Conditions," Toronto, Canada, 16-19 October 2000.

Lamm K, Lamm H, Arnold W. Effect of hyperbaric oxygen therapy in comparison to conventional or placebo therapy or no treatment in idiopathic sudden hearing loss, acoustic trauma, noise-induced hearing loss and tinnitus. A literature survey. Adv Otorhinolaryngol. 1998;54:86–99.

Latson GW, Zinszer MA. Evaluation of Emergency Evacuation Hyperbaric Stretchers (EEHS) Navy Experimental Diving Unit Technical Report No. 5-99, September 1999

Lauretta F. The analgesic effect of the hyperbaric oxygen therapy. WebmedCentral Disaster Medicine. 2012;3(2), WMC002954.

Liu X, Zhou Y, Wang Z, Yang J, Gao C, Su Q. Effect of VEGF and CX43 on the promotion of neurological recovery by hyperbaric oxygen treatment in spinal cord-injured rats. Spine J. 2014;14(1):119–27.

Luks AM, McIntosh SE, Grissom CK, Auerbach PS, Rodway GW, Schoene RB, et al. Wilderness Medical Society consensus guidelines for the prevention and treatment of acute altitude illness. Wilderness Environ Med. 2010;21:146–55.

MacFarlane C, Cronje FJ, Benn CA. Hyperbaric oxygen in trauma and surgical emergencies. J R Army Med Corps. 2000;146:185–90.

Miller RS, Weaver LK, Bahraini N, Churchill S, Price RC, Skiba V, et al. Effects of hyperbaric oxygen on symptoms and quality of life among service members with persistent postconcussion symptoms: a randomized clinical trial. JAMA Intern Med. 2015;175(1):43–52.

Murray CK, Obremskey WT, Hsu JR, Andersen RC, Calhoun JH, Clasper JC, et al; Prevention of Combat-Related Infections Guidelines Panel. Prevention of infections associated with combat-related extremity injuries. J Trauma. 2011;71(2 Suppl 2): S235–57.

Niu AKC, Yang C, Lee HC, Chen SH, Chang LP. Burns treated with adjunctive HBO_2 therapy—a comparative study in humans. J Hyper Med. 1987;2:75–82.

Roje Z, Roje Z, Eterović D, Druzijanić N, Petričević A, Roje T, Capkun V. Influence of adjuvant hyperbaric oxygen therapy on short-term complications during surgical reconstruction of upper and lower extremity war injuries: retrospective cohort study. Croat Med J. 2008;49(2):224–32.

Rossi C, Russo F, Russo F. History of mechanism and machine science, Ancient engineers & inventions, vol. 8. New York: Springer; 2009.

Rubinstein I, Abassi Z, Coleman R, Milman F, Winaver J, Better OS. Involvement of nitric oxide system in experimental muscle crush injury. J Clin Invest. 1998;101(6):1325–33.

Saito S, Aso C, Kanai M, Takazawa T, Shiga T, Shimada H. Experimental use of a transportable hyperbaric chamber durable for 15 psi at 3700 meters above sea level. Wilderness Environ Med. 2000;11(1):21–4.

Schoenfeld AJ, Lehman Jr RA, Hsu JR. Evaluation and management of combat-related spinal injuries: a review based on recent experiences. Spine J. 2012;12(9):817–23.

Shupak A, Halpern P, Ziser A, Melamed Y. Hyperbaric oxygen therapy for gas gangrene casualties in the Lebanon War, 1982. Isr J Med Sci. 1984;20(4):32–6.

Singhal S, Bhattachar SA, Paliwal V, Pathak K. Delayed-onset high-altitude pulmonary edema. Int J Adv Med Health Res. 2014;1:96–8.

Stiegler P, Matzi V, Lipp C, Kontaxis A, Klemen H, Walch C, Smolle-Jüttner F. Hyperbaric oxygen (HBO_2) in tinnitus: influence of psychological factors on treatment results? Undersea Hyperb Med. 2006;33(6):429–37.

Taber RL. Protocols for the use of a portable hyperbaric chamber for the treatment of high altitude disorders. J Wilderness Med. 1990;1:181–92.

Tan J, Zhang F, Liang F, Wang Y, Li Z, Yang J, Liu X. Protective effects of hyperbaric oxygen treatment against spinal cord injury in rats via toll-like receptor 2/nuclear factor-kB signaling. Int J Clin Exp Pathol. 2014;7(5):1911–9.

Theodoroff SM, Lewis MS, Folmer RL, Henry JA, Carlson KF. Hearing impairment and tinnitus: prevalence, risk factors, and outcomes in US service members and veterans deployed to the Iraq and Afghanistan wars. Epidemiol Rev. 2015;37:71–85.

Van Meter KW. A systematic review of the application of hyperbaric oxygen in the treatment of severe anemia: an evidence-based approach. Undersea Hyperb Med. 2005;32:61–83.

Van Meter K. Hyperbaric oxygen therapy as an adjunct to prehospital advanced trauma life support. Surg Technol Int. 2011;21:61–73.

Verghese G, Verma R, Bhutani S. Hyperbaric oxygen therapy in the battlefield. Med J Armed Forces India. 2013;69:94–6.

Wada J, Ikeda K, Kegaya H, Ajibi H. Oxygen hyperbaric treatment and severe burn. Jap Med J. 1966;13:2203–6.

Wang F, Wang Y, Sun T, Yu HL. Hyperbaric oxygen therapy for the treatment of traumatic brain injury: a meta-analysis. Neurol Sci. 2016;37(5):693–701.

Weaver LK. Hyperbaric oxygen therapy. 13th ed. Flagstaff, AZ: Best Publishing; 2014.

Winter G, Perrins DJD. Effects of HBO$_2$ treatment on epidermal regeneration. In: Wada J, Iwa T, editors. Book of proceedings of the fourth international congress on hyperbaric medicine. Baltimore, MD: Williams & Wilkins; 1970. p. 370–80.

Wolf G, Cifu D, Baugh L, Carne W, Profenna L. The effect of hyperbaric oxygen on symptoms after mild traumatic brain injury. J Neurotrauma. 2012;29(17):2606–12.

Workman WT, Calcote RD. Hyperbaric oxygen therapy and combat casualty care: a viable potential. Mil Med. 1989;154(3):111–5.

Wright JK. Relevance of hyperbaric oxygen to combat medicine. In: Proceedings of the NATO Research and Technology Office (Human Factors and Medicine) Symposium on Operational Medical Issues in Hypo- and Hyperbaric Conditions 2000 October 16-19. Toronto, Canada. NATO Scientific Report No: RTO-MP-062.

Yaman O, Yaman B, Aydın F, Var A, Temiz C. Hyperbaric oxygen treatment in the experimental spinal cord injury model. Spine J. 2014;14(9):2184–94.

Zhou Y, Liu XH, Qu SD, Yang J, Wang ZW, Gao CJ, Su QJ. Hyperbaric oxygen intervention on expression of hypoxia-inducible factor-1α and vascular endothelial growth factor in spinal cord injury models in rats. Chin Med J (Engl). 2013; 126(20):3897–903.

Hyperbaric Medicine as a Specialty

K.K. Jain

Abstract

This chapter outlines relation of hyperbaric medicine to other specialties and describes training for hyperbaric medicine for physicians as well as technicians. Courses and examinations are outlined. Finally, suggestions are made to set up a program for practice of hyperbaric medicine.

Keywords

Hyperbaric medicine • Hyperbaric oxygen (HBO) • Diving medicine • Undersea and hyperbaric medicine • Medical economics • Hyperbaric physicians

Introduction

Hyperbaric medicine is not universally recognized as a full specialty although the American Board of Hyperbaric Medicine (ACHM) is the first pathway to clinical certification in hyperbaric medicine when it launched the Physician Certification in Hyperbaric Medicine in 2003. The ACHM endorses the certification examinations offered by the American Board of Wound Healing, which offers certification for physicians, and allied healthcare professionals, in wound care and hyperbaric medicine. These set the gold standard for certification; it is the only organization that is endorsed by several professional societies. Physicians in the USA can obtain board certification in Undersea and Hyperbaric Medicine through the American Board of Emergency Medicine and the American Board of Preventive Medicine, with a current certification from one of the 24 primary member boards of the American Board of Medical Specialties.

Most of the contemporary experts in hyperbaric medicine have another primary medical specialty. Only a small number of physicians devote their full time to hyperbaric medicine, and there are only a handful of professors of hyperbaric medicine around the world (none in the USA). Some hyperbaric physicians are qualified in diving medicine, also called undersea and hyperbaric medicine, which is the diagnosis, treatment, and prevention of conditions caused by humans entering the undersea environment. The time has now come for hyperbaric medicine to be recognized as a full medical specialty. Further development and research can best be carried out by dedicated, full-time physicians.

Because new techniques in medicine come in and go out of fashion with the passage of time, medical specialties should not be created on the basis of techniques alone. Hyperbaric medicine is more than a technique for administering oxygen under pressure. It is total care of the patient with emphasis on the pathology that can be corrected by hyperbaric oxygenation (HBO). Normobaric oxygen therapy can be prescribed by any physician, anywhere, and sometimes by nonphysicians as well, but HBO is restricted to use by those who have special training and experience with this method of treatment. This therapy requires the use of a hyperbaric chamber.

Hyperbaric medicine is better recognized as a specialty of medicine in some countries such as Russia, Japan, and China. These countries have the largest number of hyperbaric facilities in academic centers with chairs in hyperbaric medicine.

K.K. Jain, MD, FRACS, FFPM (✉)
1 Blaesiring 7, Basel 4057, Switzerland
e-mail: jain@pharmabiotech.ch

© Springer International Publishing AG 2017
K.K. Jain, *Textbook of Hyperbaric Medicine*, DOI 10.1007/978-3-319-47140-2_44

Relation of Hyperbaric Medicine to Other Medical Specialties

Hyperbaric Medicine and Diving Medicine

Historically, hyperbaric medicine is an offshoot of diving medicine, which itself is not recognized as a full medical specialty. The American Medical Association recognizes the subspecialty training in "undersea and hyperbaric medicine" held by someone who is already board certified in some other specialty. Diving medicine has assumed importance due to the large navies, increasing recreational diving and offshore oil drilling. Some of the physicians involved in diving medicine have background training in environmental and occupational medicine, but they have developed an interest in hyperbaric medicine because the treatment of decompression sickness involves use of HBO and they use hyperbaric chambers.

The primary specialties of physicians who are currently active in hyperbaric medicine vary greatly and do not necessarily correlate with their clinical interests within hyperbaric medicine. The primary specialties of these physicians are internal medicine (with its subspecialties), general surgery (with subspecialties such as orthopedics, neurosurgery, plastic surgery, and chest surgery), anesthesia, and emergency medicine. Locating the hyperbaric facility within some other restricted specialty in a general hospital has some disadvantages such as the following:

• There may not be enough work load within the specialty to keep the hyperbaric facility in full use.
• Some departments may be reluctant to send their patients to another department.

Ideally, the hyperbaric medicine service should be an independent department available for service to patients and their physicians from other departments in the hospital as well as referred by elsewhere.

Training in Hyperbaric Medicine

Most of the present generation of hyperbaric physicians are self-taught or have some training by preceptorship. There are few residency training programs in hyperbaric medicine as such, but there are 4-year programs in diving medicine in Europe that include training in hyperbaric medicine. Fellowships in hyperbaric medicine have been available in some hyperbaric centers in the USA. If hyperbaric medicine is recognized as a specialty, the following should be the requirements of a training program in the discipline.

Admission Requirements

Graduation in medicine followed by 2 years of graduate training in medicine or surgery. Special cases would be those with training in a specialty or those who have been in general medical practice for some years.

Training Program

The training program should be at least 3 years. The first year should be devoted to study of basic subjects and research followed by 2 years of clinical work. Guidelines for making up the training schedule for the first year are:

• A research project involving HBO; animal experiments or clinical investigation.
• Instruction in physiology relevant to hyperbaric medicine.
• Hyperbaric technology; study of function of various chambers and ancillary equipment.

Those with previous research experience in hyperbaric medicine can be exempted from this year and receive their basic instruction during the following year of clinical work. Two years of clinical work should be residency in a recognized hyperbaric center. The training may be divided between two training centers affiliated with a training program. Private practice clinics may be used to supplement university hospital-based training. There should be balanced exposure to acute as well as chronic conditions with a good mix of clinical material.

Optional extra training or fellowship for 1 year should be used for advanced training in a special area such as neurological rehabilitation, treatment of burns, or management of decompression sickness, in an institution that specializes in such activities. An advanced research project may be carried out during this year. This fellowship would be suitable for those planning academic careers in hyperbaric medicine.

Examinations

These should be conducted by specialty boards in hyperbaric medicine at the end of the training period. The examination should have written, and additional oral or practical parts. The written examination should be designed to test the knowledge of basic subjects relevant to hyperbaric medicine as well as of the theory of hyperbaric medicine. An oral examination would be the most important factor in deciding on certification of the candidate.

For those who are certified in internal medicine or general surgery, the training program should be reduced to 2 years—1 year of basic studies and 1 year of clinical training. Those with some experience in hyperbaric medicine may be allowed to take their examinations after 1 year of fellowship.

The training should be conducted in approved centers and the number of trainees should be limited. The aim should be to produce specialists of a high caliber who will advance hyperbaric medicine.

Proposal for a Curriculum for a Diploma Course in Hyperbaric and Diving Medicine

In accordance with some of the concepts discussed in the preceding text, a proposal is made for a curriculum for a diploma course in hyperbaric and diving medicine. This edition of *Textbook of Hyperbaric Medicine* can be used as source for developing the curriculum. This proposal consists of many modules shown in Tables 44.1 and 44.2, the duration of which can be adjusted as well as duration of the whole course. Modules can be selected for courses varying from 6 months (minimum) to 3 years. 1 hour = 1 lecture. Optional courses can be designed for economics and ethical aspects of hyperbaric medicine.

Table 44.1 Modules in basic sciences for HBO course

1. History of diving and hyperbaric medicine	2 h
2. Oxygen: physics, biochemistry, physiology	20 h
3. Molecular biology	20 h
4. Physiology: hyperbaric, hypobaric, high altitude	20 h
5. Hypoxia: pathomechanismcourse	6 h
6. Oxygen toxicity and free radicals	10 h
7. Diving physiology	20 h
8. Compression and decompression	12 h
9. Exercise under hyperbaric conditions	8 h
10. Basics and rationale of hyperbaric oxygen therapy	12 h
11. Training in research methods	20 h
12. Bioinformatics/statisticscourse	10 h
Total	150 h

Table 44.2 Modules in hyperbaric technologies

1. Basis construction of hyperbaric chambers	10 h
2. Operation of various hyperbaric chambers (practical)	30 h
3. Monitoring equipment/devices in hyperbaric chambers (practical)	10 h
4. Anesthesia in hyperbaric environments	10 h
5. Safety in hyperbaric chambers	10 h
6. Diving equipments	10 h
7. Technologies relevant to diving medicine	20 h
Total	100 h

Training of Nonphysician Healthcare Personnel for Hyperbaric Medicine

Bulk of the daily work of running hyperbaric chambers and taking care of patients requires paramedical personnel—nurses and technicians. Chapter 37 covers the role of the nurse and training for hyperbaric medicine. Apart from running the hyperbaric chambers, they also have to be educated in the fundamentals of hyperbaric medicine with knowledge of relevant physiology. There are a number of courses available for hyperbaric technicians. The National Board of Diving and Hyperbaric Medical Technology has an approval process for these courses in the USA. Those who successfully complete formal training in hyperbaric technology become eligible to take an examination, upon completion of a defined preceptorship period.

Practice of Hyperbaric Medicine

This should be hospital based or at least affiliated with a hospital. Several methods of developing a hyperbaric medical service have been described. A sample development plan for a hyperbaric medical program is shown in Table 44.3.

Key referral specialties for the hyperbaric program include orthopedic surgery, oral and maxillofacial surgery, radiation oncology, plastic surgery, infectious diseases, and emergency medicine. The pattern of practice in each country is guided by local socioeconomic factors. The indications for

Table 44.3 Sample plan outline for developing a hyperbaric medicine program

1. Preliminary meeting of interested parties, e.g., local practicing hyperbaric physicians, heads of clinical departments of the hospital(s) interested in using hyperbaric facilities, facility administrators, insurance carriers, and invited outside expert in hyperbaric medicine
2. Finalization of the program and setting up of a starting date
3. Start with formal announcement, a half day series of lectures by hyperbaric experts, followed by open house for medical staff of host institution
4. Media coverage is important with local newspaper as well as TV coverage of the facility and spreading information about hyperbaric medicine in the community
5. Publication and distribution of good quality brochures describing the program as well as periodic newsletters describing interesting new developments with contributions by the staff
6. Periodic tour of the facility should be provided for small interested groups
7. Physicians working at the facility should actively participate and present relevant material on hyperbaric medicine at various medical meetings in the region in addition to publishing in medical journals
8. The program should provide courses for training nurses and technicians in hyperbaric medicine

HBO vary in each country (see Chap. 8). The most stringent list of indications is that of the Undersea and Hyperbaric Medical Society in the USA.

Economic Aspects

Economic aspects of the practice of medicine are important in some countries. The cost-effectiveness of HBO for a disease has become a criterion for approval of this treatment in the USA. Many of the clinical studies using HBO deal with this aspect and HBO has been shown to be a cost-effective treatment for the following conditions:

- Nonhealing wounds
- Chronic osteomyelitis
- Osteoradionecrosis
- Burns
- Gas gangrene
- Diabetic foot

Some of the reasons for this cost-effectiveness are:

- HBO reduces the length of hospitalization.
- HBO obviates the need for surgical procedures in many cases.

Although the initial cost of equipment for hyperbaric medicine is high, the operational costs can be kept low in a multiplace chamber that is run to full capacity with non-acute cases.

Most of the medical care in the USA is provided by physicians in private practice, and the insurance companies may refuse payment for methods of treatment that are not yet recognized in conventional medicine, or where the cost is much higher than any benefit obtained.

Conclusion

HBO has become a recognized treatment for a number of disorders although its role in many other conditions remains experimental, controversial, or simply unknown to the medical profession at large. The main indications for HBO as the primary therapy are decompression sickness, air embolism, and CO poisoning. In all other disorders where it has been used, it remains an adjunctive therapy. There is a rational basis for HBO therapy in disorders, where hypoxia plays an important role in the pathophysiology. Clinical results in many of these indications have been excellent although controlled studies are lacking.

As a drug, HBO has a specific effect on the structure and the function of the human body both in health and disease. It has a defined range of effectiveness that varies according to the disorder under treatment. It is the drug with the longest list of indications, but it is not a panacea. Like other drugs, it has certain contraindications, as well as toxic and overdose effects.

In contrast to the restricted list of indications recommended by the Undersea and Hyperbaric Medical Society, application of HBO in various disorders that span most systems of the body have been described in this book. Less than half of these indications are recognized—the others are experimental or speculative. Evidence has been provided from the literature with brief comments at the end of each chapter. The central nervous system disorders and their rehabilitation constitute the most important indications and therefore proportionately more space has been allocated to these problems.

K.K. Jain

Abstract

This chapter deals with the role of research in hyperbaric medicine. It is discussed under the topics of animal experiments and clinical trials. Application of biotechnology to research in combination with HBO is described. Biomarkers can be used to monitor the effects of HBO. Controlled clinical trials are important as most of the evidence for efficacy or lack of it is obtained in clinical treatment of thousands of patients. Clinical trials are difficult to design, conduct, and finance as there are no profitable products for marketing as in the case of pharmaceutical companies developing new drugs.

Keywords

Hyperbaric oxygen (HBO) • Trials HBO • Animal experimental research • Hyperbaric medicine • Biotechnology and HBO • Biomarkers

Introduction

A considerable amount of research has been carried out on the effect of HBO on experimental animals, and further investigations continue. Many of the effects of hypoxia/ischemia and the responses to various therapeutic measures have been studied in laboratory animals. Although there are no ideal animal models of human diseases, the information gained from such studies is useful in understanding the pathophysiology of hypoxia/ischemia and response to oxygen therapy at various pressures. Eventually, the effects of HBO are studied during treatment of diseases.

Most of the current indications for HBO are based on evidence obtained from uncontrolled clinical trials. There are few of the randomized, double-blind, and controlled studies that are emphasized these days before recognition of any new therapeutic method or for reevaluation of older well-established methods.

Basic Research in HBO

There is a need for research in the following areas:

1. Study of basic molecular and chemical biology of oxygen and understanding the physiology of oxygen transport
2. More precise tools for measuring detailed organ function and cellular pO_2 in particular
3. Understanding cellular responses and cell–cell interactions in both hypoxia and hyperoxia, especially in the injured state
4. Need for controlled clinical research based on basic research

Perhaps there should be a study of the variable response of different species to HBO, which could then serve as a guide to researchers as well as to readers who want to compare the result of different studies. Important areas where research is required are identified in various chapters of this book. Some important topics are listed in Table 45.1.

K.K. Jain, MD, FRACS, FFPM (✉)
1 Blaesiring 7, Basel 4057, Switzerland
e-mail: jain@pharmabiotech.ch

© Springer International Publishing AG 2017
K.K. Jain, *Textbook of Hyperbaric Medicine*, DOI 10.1007/978-3-319-47140-2_45

Table 45.1 Important areas for research in hyperbaric medicine

Basic research

- Monitoring of the level of free radicals in normal as well as hypoxic conditions and determining the effect of HBO on both
- Determination of mitochondrial oxygen tension and the effect of HBO on it
- Use of biotechnologies in HBO research

Animal experiments

- Toxic encephalopathies

Studies on human volunteers

- Effect of physical exercise under HBO
- Pharmacokinetics of commonly used drugs under hyperbaric conditions

Studies on human patients

- Superior mesenteric artery thrombosis
- Treatment of adverse effects of drugs
  - Hepatotoxicity
  - Toxic epidermal necrolysis
- Treatment of acute mountain sickness
- Combination of HBO with approved biotechnology-based therapies
- Personalized hyperbaric medicine

Longitudinal studies (long-term follow-up)

- Rehabilitation of patients in chronic post-stroke stage as an adjunct to physical therapy
- Multiple sclerosis
- Cerebral palsy
- Anoxic encephalopathies
- Ischemic leg pain as an adjunct to exercise

Controlled clinical trials

- Acute stroke
- Spinal cord injury
- Traumatic brain injury and its sequelae
- Diabetes mellitus

Table 45.2 Biotechnologies relevant to human health

Antisense therapy
Biomarkers
Biochips/microarrays
Cell therapy
DNA vaccines
Gene therapy
Genetic engineering
Genomics
Molecular diagnostics
Monoclonal antibodies
Nanobiotechnology
Proteomics
Recombinant DNA technology
RNA interference (RNAi)
Sequencing
Synthetic biology
Systems biology

Application of Biotechnologies in Hyperbaric Medicine

Biotechnology, which implies processing of materials by biological agents to provide goods and services, has been used since World War I, and one example was brewing of beer. In the pharmaceutical industry, biotechnology has been used for application of biological organisms in industrial manufacture of defined products which are mostly proteins. Introduction of the term genetic engineering in 1932 opened the way for application of biotechnology in life sciences although practical tools used in modern molecular biology had been developed at that time. Synthesis of human insulin in 1978 started the field of biotechnology-based drugs as part of biopharmaceutical industry. Recombinant DNA is an important method that is used to make alterations to an organism's genome, usually causing it to over- or under-express a certain gene of interest or express a mutated form of it. The results of these experiments can provide information on that gene's role in the organism's body.

Biotechnologies relevant to human health are shown in Table 45.2. Those relevant to hyperbaric medicine include biomarkers, gene expression, stem cell therapy/regenerative medicine, nanobiotechnology, etc. The role of biotechnologies in the development of personalized hyperbaric medicine will be described in Chap. 46.

Biomarkers of Effect of HBO

A biomarker is a characteristic that can be objectively measured and evaluated as an indicator of a physiological as well as a pathological process or pharmacological response to a thera-

Animal Experimental Studies

Animal experimental studies require laboratories that are difficult to organize outside an academic center. Proper care of animals, compliance with regulations for ethical treatment of animals, etc. are better managed in larger laboratories with well-trained staff. Research in hyperbaric medicine requires the use of special small animal chambers mentioned in Chap. 7. Limiting factors for research in hyperbaric medicine are as follows:

- Basic pathophysiology of several disorders treated with HBO is not well understood.
- Animal models of some diseases do not adequately represent human illnesses. There are species differences in response to HBO so that the animal results cannot always be extrapolated to humans.

peutic intervention. Classical biomarkers are measurable alterations in blood pressure, blood lactate levels following exercise, and blood glucose in diabetes mellitus. Any specific molecular alteration of a cell on DNA, RNA, metabolite, or protein level can be referred to as a molecular biomarker. In the era of molecular biology, biomarkers usually mean molecular biomarkers (Jain 2010). Characteristic findings of some diseases on molecular imaging are biomarkers as well. Biomarkers can be used to monitor the effect of HBO. For example, initial and posttreatment levels of serum neuron-specific enolase and S-100β levels, which are biomarkers of neuronal cell injury, can be compared in patients with carbon monoxide poisoning, who received normobaric oxygen or HBO therapy (Yildirim et al. 2015).

Overexpression of the enzyme matrix metalloproteinase-9 (MMP-9) has been implicated as a contributory factor to some of the sequelae associated with cerebral ischemia, cell death, nonhealing wounds, traumatic brain injury, aneurysms, and plaque instability in atherosclerosis. A study showed that MMP-9 levels were raised in urine after surgery but reduced after HBO therapy at 2.5 ATA for 1 h/day×5 (Cummins and Gentene 2010). This indicated that MMP-9 can be used as a biomarker of effect of HBO. The understanding of how HBO therapy modulates MMP-9 may provide an additional insight into mechanisms and future potential therapies.

A prospective clinical trial is evaluating inflammatory and vasoactive biomarkers as prognostic markers of severity and mortality in patients with necrotizing soft tissue infections and investigating whether HBO therapy is able to modulate these biomarkers (Hansen et al. 2015).

Action of HBO on Gene Expression

Gene expression is the process by which information from a gene is used in the synthesis of a functional gene product, usually a protein. However, in nonprotein-coding genes such as rRNA genes or tRNA genes, the product is a functional RNA. Chronic diseases are usually caused by a synergistic action of genetic and environmental factors. The molecular events are caused or paralleled by specific gene expression changes. Analysis of these changes provides an understanding of the disease at the molecular level.

An example is given of the human brain, which has a more complex pattern of gene expression than any other region of the body. Several technological advances enable the analysis of thousands of expressed genes in a small brain sample. These techniques include sequencing of cDNA libraries, serial analysis of gene expression (SAGE), and the high density DNA microarrays. Gene expression measurements may be used to identify genes that are abnormally regulated as a secondary consequence of a disease state or to identify the response of brain cells to treatments.

Microarray analysis of gene expression in rat neurons after exposure to varying levels of oxygen pressures (2, 4, and 6 ATA) identified 183 genes significantly altered (increased or decreased) in response to pressure and/or oxidative stress (Chen et al. 2009). Among them, 17 genes changed in response to all exposure conditions. More genes were altered in response to hyperbaric air than HBO. Altered genes included factors associated with stress responses, transport/neurotransmission, signal transduction, and transcription factors. The results may serve as guidance for selection of biomarkers of hyperoxia and HBO response and provide a starting point for further studies to investigate the global molecular mechanisms underlying hyperbaric oxidative stress.

Induction of antioxidant gene expression. Global gene expression changes in human endothelial cells in vitro following a HBO, comparable to a clinical treatment, reveal an upregulation of antioxidant, cytoprotective, and immediate early genes, which coincides with an increased resistance to a lethal oxidative stress (Godman et al. 2010). Repeated exposure to increasing pressures and durations of HBO might have useful applications in promoting wound healing in the aged and preventing against disorders associated with aging where oxidative stress plays a role.

Gene Expression in Stroke

Over 5000 differentially expressed genes can be identified in stroke-affected tissue by microarray analysis. The expression pattern is altered by HBO treatment and correlates with beneficial effects seen on other parameters. For example, in animal stroke models, HBO limits leukocyte accumulation to the infarct site by attenuation of stroke-inducible proinflammatory chemokine response and reduces stroke lesion volume (Rink et al. 2010). These findings provide key information relevant to understanding oxygen-dependent molecular mechanisms in the brain affected by acute ischemic stroke.

Gene Expression in Decompression

The use of HBO to expedite decompression from saturation has not been proven and may increase risk of toxicity to the pulmonary system. To evaluate any benefit of HBO during decompression, a study used a 70-kg swine model of saturation and examined lung tissue by microarray analysis for evidence of RNA regulation (Malkevich et al. 2010). Swine were compressed to 5 ATA for 22 h to achieve saturation and then underwent decompression on air (AirD) or HBO (HBOD) starting at 2.36 ATA. Animals were evaluated for type I and type II decompression sickness (DCS) for 24 h. Control animals were placed in the chamber for the same duration, but were not compressed. Animals were sacrificed 24 h after exposure, and total RNA was isolated from lung samples for microarray hybridizations on the Affymetrix platform.

Table 45.3 Combined effects of stem cells and HBO in experimental models of various diseases

Type of stem cell	Experimental model/reference	Effect and mechanism
Neural stem cells (NSCs)	NSCs, isolated from rat cortex, exposed to HBO at 2 ATA for 60 min (Chen et al. 2010)	HBO promotes differentiation of NSCs into neurons
Endogenous NSCs	Neonatal rat with hypoxic–ischemic brain damage given HBO at 2 ATA once daily for 1 W (Wang et al. 2009)	NSCs migrate to the cortex and differentiate into mature neurocytes
Amniotic fluid mesenchymal stem cells (MSCs)	Rat sciatic nerve injury model treated with local application of MSCs in combination with HBO at 2 ATA once daily for 1 h (Pan et al. 2009)	Peripheral nerve regeneration was enhanced by suppression of apoptosis in implanted cells and the attenuation of an inflammatory response
Circulating stem cells	In vivo exposure to HBO 2.8 ATA for 90 min combined with lactate as an oxidative stressor (Milovanova et al. 2009)	HBO plus lactate activates a physiological redox-active autocrine loop in stem cell, which stimulates vasculogenic growth and differentiation of SCs in vivo
Rat NSCs	Proliferation after HBO therapy in vitro (Zhang et al. 2011)	HBO therapy promotes neurogenesis by β-catenin-induced activated Ngn1 gene and represses astrocytogenesis by β-catenin-induced downregulated BMP-4 gene
Umbilical cord MSCs	Rat models of severe traumatic brain injury treated with HBO in combination with stem cells (Zhou et al. 2016)	Growth-associated protein-43 expression and calaxon-like structures increased along with neurological improvement in rats treated with combination

There was no evidence of type I DCS or severe cardiopulmonary DCS in any of the animals. Three genes (nidogen 2, calcitonin-like receptor, and pentaxin-related gene) were significantly upregulated in both the AirD and HBOD groups compared to controls. Three other genes (TN3, platelet basic protein, and cytochrome P450) were significantly downregulated in both groups. It is concluded that HBO during decompression from saturation does not reduce the incidence of DCS. Gene expression is similar in both the AirD and HBOD groups, particularly in genes related to immune function and cell signaling.

HBO as Adjunct to Cell therapy and Regenerative Medicine

Cell therapy is the prevention or treatment of human disease by the administration of cells that have been selected, multiplied, and pharmacologically treated or altered outside the body (ex vivo). Cell therapy is described in detail in a special report on this topic (Jain 2016). The aim of cell therapy is to replace, repair, or enhance the function of damaged tissues or organs. The scope of cell therapy can be broadened to include methods to modify the function of cells of the body in vivo for therapeutic purposes. Various types of cells are used in cell therapy, but currently the focus is on stem cells.

Although the bone marrow is the best-known reservoir of stem cells, only one of 100,000 cells in the marrow is a stem cell. Therefore, methods for stem cell engraftment, mobilization, expansion, and proliferation are important for cell transplantation and stem cell-mediated applications. Several methods including pharmaceuticals are used for mobilization and expansion of stem cells in vivo/in vitro. Mobilization of stem cells by HBO is more effective and safer than pharmaceutical strategies. A typical course of HBO increases the number of stem cells circulating in a patient's body eightfold. By causing an oxidative stress, HBO activates a physiological redox-active autocrine loop in circulating stem cells in the mouse model that stimulates vasculogenesis (Milovanova et al. 2009). Thioredoxin system activation leads to elevations in HIF-1 and HIF-2, followed by synthesis of HIF-dependent growth factors.

Effects of HBO combined with various types of stem cells in experimental models of diseases and mechanisms of action are shown in Table 45.3. Most of the examples are in neurological disorders. Clinical relevance is seen in some clinical studies of HBO. One example is that of a prospective case series where HBO therapy was shown to stimulate colonic stem cells and induce mucosal healing in patients with refractory ulcerative colitis (Bekheit et al. 2016).

Nanobiotechnology and HBO

Nanotechnology is the creation and utilization of materials, devices, and systems through the control of matter on the nanometer-length scale (10–9 m). Nanomedicine is the application of nanobiotechnology in healthcare ranging from nanoscale studies of molecular basis of disease to diagnostics and therapeutics (Jain 2012). Nanomedicine is contributing to advances in healthcare by refining molecular diagnostics and drug delivery and providing innovative therapeutics. Some examples of use in relation to HBO therapy are:

- MRI contrast agent using manganese oxide nanoparticles produces images of the anatomic structures of the brain, which are as clear as those obtained by histological examination.
- MRI with superparamagnetic iron oxide nanoparticle can visualize and track stem cells transplanted into the body for therapeutic purposes.
- Phosphorescent nanosensors using dendrimers have a high selectivity for oxygen and can be used for in vivo measurement of pO_2 (Lebedev et al. 2009).

Clinical Trials of HBO Therapy

A clinical trial is defined as any research project that prospectively assigns people or a group of people to an intervention, with or without concurrent comparison or control groups, to study the cause and effect relationship between a health-related intervention and a health outcome. Potential bias in allocating patients to active and control treatment is one of the main problems with uncontrolled studies, which led to need for randomized trials. The general methods of conducting controlled studies are well known to clinical investigators. There are basically three types of clinical trials with HBO:

1. Patients receive HBO as a primary treatment and controls do not receive HBO.
2. HBO is an add-on therapy to conventional medical treatment and controls receive no HBO.
3. HBO treatment is compared with sham treatment in a hyperbaric chamber.

All three methods may be combined in a trial which has several groups.

Problems with Clinical Trials of HBO

Although randomized controlled trials have become the standard technique for changing diagnostic or therapeutic methods, the use of this method poses several problems:

- Blinding is difficult in controlled trials with HBO.
- In life-threatening illnesses such as air embolism and DCS, it would be unethical to deny a patient HBO treatment in a controlled trial. Clinical trials would essentially be limited to conditions which are not a threat to the patient's life or those where HBO is an adjuvant treatment.
- Financial support for clinical trials in hyperbaric medicine is very slim. Although HBO is a drug, it does not have a commercial sponsor. For new pharmaceuticals, the manufacturers support the high cost of clinical trials which are necessary to get the drugs approved for general use.
- Shortage of patients for trials in any individual medical center. This limitation can be overcome by multicenter studies, but it is more difficult to implement a uniform HBO protocol than it is in the case of pharmaceuticals.

Another problem in carrying out these studies is that in the usual setting of a hyperbaric chamber, the control patient and the investigator would not be blind to the nature of the experiment. To overcome this difficulty, one technique for randomized controlled studies uses a protocol respirator unit, which allows the patient to breathe a specific mixture of gases known only to an umpire, but not known to the patient or the investigator. All the control patients breathe a mixture of 8.9 % oxygen and 91.1 % nitrogen on the assumption that at a pressure of 2.4 ATA, it is equivalent to breathing air. Those in the experimental group breathe 100 % oxygen at the same pressure. The drawbacks of this method are:

- Possible undesirable side effects of nitrogen under pressure
- Possible DCS in the control group
- Errors in gas mixture; if 100 % nitrogen is breathed, the consequences can be disastrous

In the past 40 years, the use of an air sham (21 % oxygen, 1.14–1.5 ATA) in clinical and animal studies, instead of observational or crossover controls, has led to false acceptance of the null hypothesis (declaring no effect when one is present), due to the biological activity of these "sham" controls (Figueroa and Wright 2015). In the clinical trials sponsored by the US Department of Defense/Veterans Administration, previously published reports on the use of HBO therapy on stroke and mild TBI have helped to highlight the biological activity of pressurized air, validate the development of a convincing control for future studies, and demonstrate the effectiveness of a hyperbaric intervention.

Equipment for double-blind studies is commercially available (Dräger AG, Lübeck, FRG).

There are some situations in which controlled studies on a large number of patients cannot be done. Even when such studies are done, they do not necessarily resolve the issues. Careful documentation in a small patient population with longitudinal studies may prove more useful.

Ethical Aspects of Clinical Trials with HBO

It would be unethical to deprive a patient of HBO in a life-threatening situation where HBO has shown to be effective in uncontrolled studies. There are ethical objections to double-blind studies in the case of patients for whom HBO therapy has been shown to be nearly 100 % effective in well-conducted uncontrolled clinical trials. An example of this is the physical therapy for chronic post-stroke patients under simultaneous HBO. The difference between the patients treated with HBO and those treated outside is so great that any controlled study on these patients may have to be called off. The response to HBO in these patients is reproducible on multiple applications, and the benefit persists with prolonged therapy. Another situation where a controlled study would be unethical is in life-threatening situations such as CO poisoning and gas gangrene. Extensive clinical trials in several countries over the past several years have established the superiority of results in these illnesses when HBO is added to the conventional therapy. Apart from the decreased mortality, there is improvement of quality of life in patients treated with HBO. If controls were to be deprived of this, they cannot be compensated for it by crossing over at a subsequent date to the HBO group, for then it may be too late.

Ideally, clinical trials should be based on solid basic experimental research in animals. In conditions where there is no suitable animal model, it may be ethical to conduct controlled clinical trials without previous animal data.

Clinical trials should be designed with professional statistical input, and the results whether positive or negative should be considered valuable information. To ignore these principles would be considered unethical.

Conclusion

Research, both experimental in animals as well as clinical in humans, is important for further development of hyperbaric medicine. Application of biotechnology to research in combination with HBO is important. HBO enhances the effect of stem cell therapy and is important for development of regenerative medicine. Biomarkers can be used to monitor the effects of HBO. Controlled clinical trials are important as most of the evidence for efficacy or lack of it is obtained in clinical treatment of thousands of patients. Clinical trials are difficult to design, conduct, and finance as there are no profitable products for marketing as in the case of pharmaceutical companies that are developing new drugs.

References

Bekheit M, Baddour N, Katri K, Taher Y, El Tobgy K, Mousa E. Hyperbaric oxygen therapy stimulates colonic stem cells and induces mucosal healing in patients with refractory ulcerative colitis: a prospective case series. BMJ Open Gastroenterol. 2016;3(1), e000082.

Chen Y, Nadi NS, Chavko M, Auker CR, McCarron RM. Microarray analysis of gene expression in rat cortical neurons exposed to hyperbaric air and oxygen. Neurochem Res. 2009;34:1047–56.

Chen CF, Yang YJ, Wang QH, Yao Y, Li M. Effect of hyperbaric oxygen administered at different pressures and different exposure time on differentiation of neural stem cells in vitro. Zhongguo Dang Dai Er Ke Za Zhi. 2010;12:368–72.

Cummins Jr FJ, Gentene LJ. Hyperbaric oxygen effect on MMP-9 after a vascular insult. J Cardiovasc Transl Res. 2010;3:683–7.

Figueroa XA, Wright JK. Clinical results in brain injury trials using HBO$_2$ therapy: another perspective. Undersea Hyperb Med. 2015;42:333–51.

Godman CA, Joshi R, Giardina C, Perdrizet G, Hightower LE. Hyperbaric oxygen treatment induces antioxidant gene expression. Ann N Y Acad Sci. 2010;1197:178–83.

Hansen MB, Simonsen U, Garred P, Hyldegaard O. Biomarkers of necrotising soft tissue infections: aspects of the innate immune response and effects of hyperbaric oxygenation-the protocol of the prospective cohort BIONEC study. BMJ Open. 2015;5(5), e006995.

Jain KK. Handbook of biomarkers. New York: Springer; 2010.

Jain KK. Handbook of nanomedicine. 2nd ed. New York: Springer; 2012.

Jain KK. Cell therapy. Basel: Jain PharmaBiotech; 2016.

Lebedev AY, Cheprakov AV, Sakadzić S, Boas DA, Wilson DF, Vinogradov SA. Dendritic phosphorescent probes for oxygen imaging in biological systems. ACS Appl Mater Interfaces. 2009;1:1292–304.

Malkevich N, McCarron RM, Mahon RT. Decompression from saturation using oxygen: its effect on DCS and RNA in large swine. Aviat Space Environ Med. 2010;81:15–21.

Milovanova TN, Bhopale VM, Sorokina EM, Moore JS, Hunt TK, Hauer-Jensen M, et al. Hyperbaric oxygen stimulates vasculogenic stem cell growth and differentiation in vivo. J Appl Physiol. 2009;106:711–28.

Pan HC, Chin CS, Yang DY, Ho SP, Chen CJ, Hwang SM, et al. Human amniotic fluid mesenchymal stem cells in combination with hyperbaric oxygen augment peripheral nerve regeneration. Neurochem Res. 2009;34:1304–16.

Rink C, Roy S, Khan M, Ananth P, Kuppusamy P, Sen CK, et al. Oxygen-sensitive outcomes and gene expression in acute ischemic stroke. J Cereb Blood Flow Metab. 2010;30:1275–87.

Wang XL, Yang YJ, Xie M, Yu XH, Wang QH. Hyperbaric oxygen promotes the migration and differentiation of endogenous neural stem cells in neonatal rats with hypoxic-ischemic brain damage. Zhongguo Dang Dai Er Ke Za Zhi. 2009;11:749–52.

Yildirim AO, Eroglu M, Kaldirim U, Eyi YE, Simsek K, Durusu M, et al. Serum neuron-specific enolase and S-100β levels as prognostic follow-up markers for oxygen administered carbon monoxide intoxication cases. Indian J Biochem Biophys. 2015;52:29–33.

Zhang XY, Yang YJ, Xu PR, Zheng XR, Wang QH, Chen CF, et al. The role of β-catenin signaling pathway on proliferation of rats neural stem cells after hyperbaric oxygen therapy in vitro. Cell Mol Neurobiol. 2011;31:101–9.

Zhou HX, Liu ZG, Liu XJ, Chen QX. Umbilical cord-derived mesenchymal stem cell transplantation combined with hyperbaric oxygen treatment for repair of traumatic brain injury. Neural Regen Res. 2016;11:107–13.

K.K. Jain

Abstract

This chapter deals with personalization of HBO therapy in keeping with the current trends in hyperbaric medicine. Decision whether to use HBO or not and selection of appropriate schedule of HBO treatment can be guided by measurable characteristics of an individual including genotype rather than following a routine applicable to all patients with the same diagnosis. Efficacy and safety of HBO can be improved by personalized approaches. Although initially expensive, personalized hyperbaric medicine would result in cost saving in the long run.

Keywords

Personalized medicine • Precision medicine • Molecular hyperbaric medicine • Biomarkers • Molecular imaging • Genes and oxygen toxicity • Personalized hyperbaric medicine • Pharmacogenetics of HBO

Introduction

Personalized medicine simply means the prescription of specific therapeutics best suited for an individual. It is usually based on pharmacogenetic, pharmacogenomic, pharmacoproteomic, and pharmacometabolomic information, but other individual variations among patients and environmental factors are also taken into consideration (Jain 2015).

The concept of personalized medicine is not new. The ancient medical systems were personalized. In the Ayurvedic practices of India, therapy is customized to the individual's constitution (Prakruti)—ancient counterpart of genotype. The traditional Chinese medicine with acupuncture and herbs takes individual variations into consideration, and this system is still practiced in modern China as well as in Western countries. In homeopathic medicine, founded in the eighteenth century in Germany, prescribing is highly individualized to a person's "constitutional picture" rather than to specific diseases. Some of the older therapies are now lumped under alternative medicine, and some skeptics place HBO therapy in the same category.

Although pharmacogenetics is known in pharmacology since 1959 and the term pharmacogenomics was coined in 1997, their applications for personalized medicine were not advocated until the publication of the first monograph with the title *Personalized Medicine* in 1998; and this term started to be indexed in MEDLINE in 1999 in relation to its modern application. Even after the human genome was sequenced in 2000, its potential applications were referred to as genomic medicine. The term "personalized medicine" is now widely accepted as it has a broader scope than genomic medicine although some prefer to call it "precision medicine," which uses one of the several adjectives used earlier to describe the superiority of personalized medicine over conventional medicine. Personalized approaches are used in the treatment of most of the diseases, and the most frequent application is in oncology.

Personalized hyperbaric medicine started in the 1980s when Dr. Richard Neubauer started to assess response of individual stroke patients to HBO by SPECT before making decisions for further treatment. This is similar to the use of diagnostics biomarkers to monitor pharmaceutical therapy for verifying its efficacy, which is an important part of personalized management of diseases. In the post-genomic age,

K.K. Jain, MD, FRACS, FFPM (✉)
1 Blaesiring 7, Basel 4057, Switzerland
e-mail: jain@pharmabiotech.ch

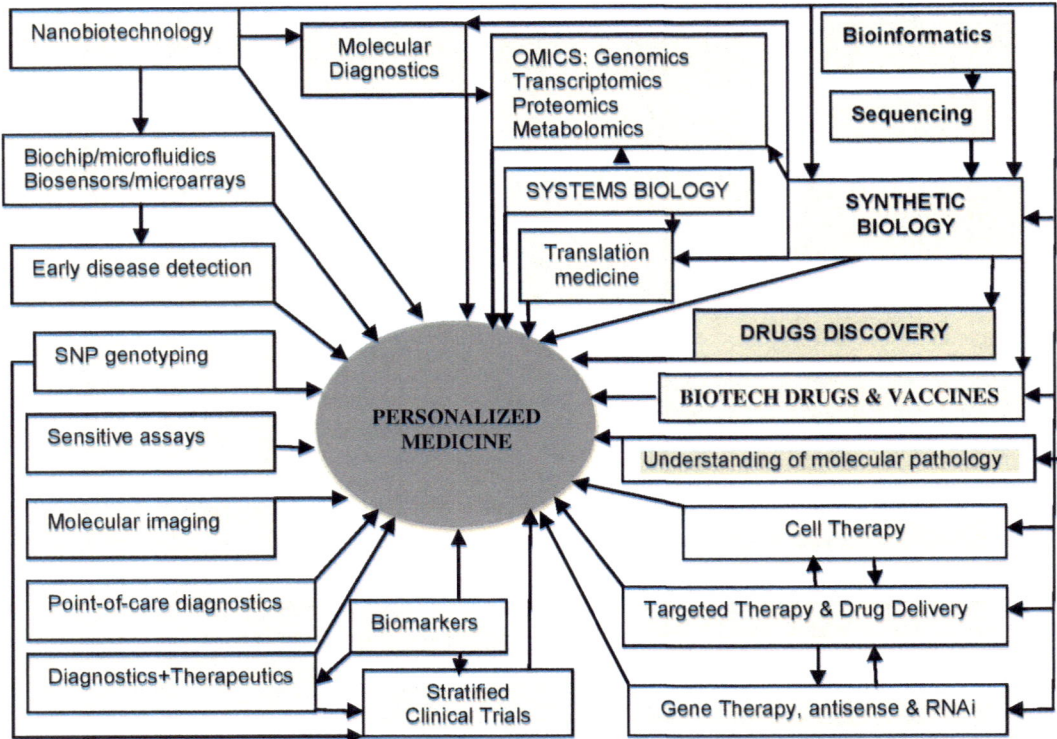

Fig. 46.1 Relation of personalized medicine to other technologies (© Jain PharmaBiotech)

genes could be viewed as biomarkers of response to HBO as well as predictors of oxygen toxicity. This will enable determination of suitability of HBO and dose and duration of treatment for individual patients.

Concept of personalized medicine as "systems medicine" is the best way of integrating new technologies and translating them into clinical application for improving healthcare. A schematic view of interrelationship of various technologies is shown in Fig. 46.1.

Molecular Diagnostics as Guide to HBO Therapy

Molecular diagnostics, the use of diagnostic testing to understand the molecular mechanisms of an individual patient's disease, will be pivotal in the delivery of safe and effective therapy for many diseases in the future. Diagnostics influence as much as 70 % of healthcare decision-making, and a new generation of diagnostics tests that provide insights at the molecular level is delivering on the promise of personalized medicine. The role of molecular diagnostics in personalized medicine covers the following aspects:

- Early detection and selection of appropriate treatment determined to be safe and effective on the basis of molecular diagnostics (Jain 1916a)
- Monitoring therapy as well as determining prognosis

Various molecular diagnostic technologies are described in a special report on this topic (Jain 2016b). Important among these are technologies used for detection of biomarkers, DNA sequencing, and imaging. Nanobiotechnology has made significant contribution to refinement of these technologies.

Genotyping for determination of single nucleotide polymorphisms (SNPs) in clinical trials is important for the design and interpretation of clinical studies. Advantages of molecular genetic profiling in clinical studies are:

- Contribution to molecular definition of the disease
- Correlation of drug response to the genetic background of the patient
- Prediction of dose-response and adverse effects
- SNP mapping data can be used to pinpoint, a common set of variant nucleotides shared by people who do not respond to a therapeutic.

Role of Sequencing in Personalized Medicine

The genome sequence is an organism's blueprint: the set of instructions dictating its biological traits. The term DNA sequencing refers to methods for determining the exact order of the three billion nucleotide bases—adenine, guanine, cytosine, and thymine—that make up the DNA of the 23 pairs of human chromosomes. In de novo sequencing, short DNA fragments purified from individual bacterial colonies are individually sequenced and assembled electronically into one long, contiguous sequence. This method does not require any preexisting information about the sequence of the DNA. Resequencing using next-generation technologies means determination of variations of DNA sequence in an organism where the nominal sequence is already known. It is often performed using PCR to amplify the region of interest (preexisting DNA sequence is required to design the PCR primers). Resequencing is more relevant for translation into diagnostics and clinical applications. Sequencing technologies are described in more detail in a special report on this topic.

DNA sequencing has now become a routine tool in molecular diagnostics. Among various technologies, sequencing will play an important role in the development of personalized medicine. The detailed map of human genetic variation promised by the 1000 Genomes Project will allow a more in-depth analysis of the contribution of genetic variation in responses to therapeutic interventions. Future studies utilizing this new resource may greatly enhance our understanding of the genetic basis of therapeutic response and other complex traits, which will help to advance personalized medicine (Zhang and Dolan 2010). By the end of the second decade of the twenty-first century, it is anticipated that the general population will have the opportunity to carry a chip card, like a credit card, with all the genetic information of the person coded on it. Such a database can be constructed by taking a blood sample of the individual, resequencing the functional DNA, and identifying the genetic variations in functional genes.

Biomarkers for Personalized HBO Therapy

A biological marker (biomarker) is simply a molecule that indicates an alteration in physiology from normal. For example, any specific molecular alteration of a cancer cell either on DNA, RNA, or protein level can be referred to as a molecular marker. A biomarker is defined as a characteristic that is objectively measured and evaluated as an indicator of normal biologic processes, pathogenic processes, or pharmacologic responses to a therapeutic intervention. The topic of biomarkers has been discussed in a book (Jain 2010). The expression of a distinct gene can enable its identification in a tissue with none of the surrounding cells expressing the specific marker. Potential applications of biomarkers relevant to personalized medicine are:

- The biomarker would specifically and sensitively reflect a disease state and could be used for diagnosis, for predicting response to therapy as well as for disease monitoring during and following therapy.

- A dramatic increase in the identification of potential molecular targets for therapy and reduction in the cost of high-throughput genomic sequencing have enabled biomarker tests for molecularly targeted therapies to help selection of the most effective therapy for a patient's condition and avoid treatments that could be ineffective or harmful.

Imaging for Personalized HBO Therapy

Molecular imaging provides in vivo information in contrast to the in vitro diagnostics. PET is the most sensitive and specific technique for imaging molecular pathways in vivo in humans (see Chap. 10). Because of cost and logistical difficulties, SPECT is more practical for use in conjunction with HBO therapy.

Brain Imaging as Guide to Therapy of Multiple Sclerosis

MRI has been useful for guiding treatment of multiple sclerosis (MS) with HBO (see Chap. 22). Resolution of MRI lesions is evidence for efficacy of HBO treatment and its continuation for a longer duration. Resolution of edema surrounding an acute lesion may be an indicator of the mode of action of HBO.

A study has shown decreased cerebral perfusion in secondary progressive-MS patients with a moderate to severe disability score and its association with clinical parameters (Taghizadeh Asl et al. 2016). Because of its accessibility, rather low price, practical ease, and providing objective quantitative information, brain perfusion SPECT can be complementary to MRI in disease surveillance and monitoring.

Imaging Tumor Hypoxia for Personalized Cancer Therapy

The role of HBO in treating tumor hypoxia for overcoming resistance to anticancer therapy was described in Chap. 38. Tumor oxygenation is difficult to measure. Fluoromisonidazole (FMISO) is the lead radiopharmaceutical in PET imaging for the evaluation, prognosis, and quantification of tumor hypoxia, as it is less affected by blood flow, and although the images have less contrast than FDG-PET, its uptake after 2 h is an accurate reflection of inadequate regional oxygen partial pressure at the time of radiopharmaceutical administration (Rajendran and Krohn 2015). Tumor hypoxia imaging, pre-treatment or intra-treatment, will likely become an important in vivo imaging biomarker of the future to personalize anticancer therapies for hypoxic tumors including HBO as an adjunct.

Pharmacogenomics and Pharmacogenetics of HBO

Oxygen Toxicity and Genes

If oxygen is considered to be a drug, there should be individual variations in susceptibility to high-dose oxygen toxicity. This is parallel to the well-known individual variations in adverse drug reactions that have been documented in pharmacogenetics for several years. However, the role of genetic susceptibility in oxygen toxicity has not be studied, although there are studies linking some gene mutations to susceptibility to oxidative damage and diseases known to be caused by oxidative stress.

Rodent models of oxygen-induced retinopathy (OIR) provide important insights into the pathogenesis of human retinopathy of prematurity. An overview of work with rat OIR has identified marked and consistent variations in susceptibility to OIR among different inbred rat strains and provides strong evidence for a genetic determinant of susceptibility to OIR (van Wijngaarden et al. 2010). Furthermore, differences in retinal angiogenic factor gene expression among different inbred rat strains exposed to cyclic hyperoxia have been characterized. A key determinant of susceptibility to OIR appears to be the extent to which proangiogenic factor genes, such as vascular endothelial growth factor and erythropoietin, are expressed during the period of hyperoxic exposure. Those strains in which expression is relatively well maintained are less susceptible to retinopathy than are those in which expression is reduced.

Susceptibility to HBO-Induced Cataract Formation

Methionine sulfoxide reductase A (MsrA) in lens cells provides resistance to oxidative stress by maintenance of mitochondrial function that is important for the lens transparency. Correspondingly, increased protein methionine sulfoxide (PMSO) is associated with lens aging and human cataract formation, suggesting that loss of MsrA activity is associated with this disease. MsrA gene deletion in mice exposed to HBO leads to oxidization of cyt c in the lenses. Introduction of wild-type MsrA gene can restore the in vitro activity of cyt c through its repair of PMSO. These results provide evidence that repair of mitochondrial cyt c by MsrA could play an important role in defense of the lens against cataract formation (Brennan et al. 2009).

Economical Aspects of Personalized HBO Therapy

Biotechnology-based therapies are expensive reflecting the long development and approval process. Molecular diagnostics are relatively cheaper reflecting the shorter development process and less regulatory hurdles. Nevertheless, these are still more expensive than HBO therapies. The cost of sequencing the human genome is coming down to below $1000 and some companies are aiming to bring it down eventually to less than $100. It is possible to integrate the diagnostics with HBO, considering that expensive brain imaging is already being used in practice.

One of the economic reasons given for combining the use of molecular diagnostics with expensive biotechnology treatments is to spare the unnecessary use in patients who are not responders or might suffer adverse effects. This argument may not hold in case of HBO because it does not have the same problems as biotechnology-based therapeutics, which are approved by authorities who do not cover the relatively inexpensive HBO treatments.

Conclusion

With the trend toward personalization of medical care, HBO should adapt to approaches already established for individualizing treatment to improve the efficacy. Further molecular studies relevant to HBO are needed in the following areas:

- Basic studies on molecular mechanisms of action of HBO
- Genotyping of patients to obtain information for correlating certain genotypes with response or lack of response to HBO and for identifying patients who are likely to develop adverse effects from hyperoxygenation
- Increasing use of HBO for stratifying patients in clinical trials as well as in practice as adjunct to new biotechnology-based therapies such as cell therapy

References

Brennan LA, Lee W, Cowell T, Giblin F, Kantorow M. Deletion of mouse MsrA results in HBO-induced cataract: MsrA repairs mitochondrial cytochrome c. Mol Vis. 2009;15:985–99.

Jain KK. Handbook of biomarkers. New York: Springer; 2010.

Jain KK. Textbook of hyperbaric medicine. 2nd ed. New York: Springer; 2015.

Jain KK. Molecular diagnostics. Basel: Jain PharmaBiotech; 2016a.

Jain KK. DNA sequencing. Basel: Jain PharmaBiotech; 2016b.

Rajendran JG, Krohn KA. F-18 fluoromisonidazole for imaging tumor hypoxia: imaging the microenvironment for personalized cancer therapy. Semin Nucl Med. 2015;45:151–62.

Taghizadeh Asl M, Nemati R, Chabi N, Salimipour H, Nabipour I, Assadi M. Brain perfusion imaging with voxel-based analysis in secondary progressive multiple sclerosis patients with a moderate to severe stage of disease: a boon for the workforce. BMC Neurol. 2016;16:79.

van Wijngaarden P, Brereton HM, Coster DJ, Williams KA. Hereditary influences in oxygen-induced retinopathy in the rat. Doc Ophthalmol. 2010;120:87–97.

Zhang W, Dolan ME. Impact of the 1000 genomes project on the next wave of pharmacogenomic discovery. Pharmacogenomics. 2010;11:249–56.

The Future of Hyperbaric Medicine

47

K.K. Jain

Abstract

This chapter outlines advances in medicine in the next decade as a background for the role of hyperbaric medicine in multidisciplinary care. Futuristic medicine will be personalized. HBO needs to be combined with biotechnologies for further progress. Suggestions are made for hyperbaric medicine to keep up with advances in other disciples of medicine.

Keywords

Hyperbaric medicine • Futuristic medicine • Hyperbaric oxygen (HBO) • Multidisciplinary healthcare • HBO and personalized medicine

Introduction to Future Medicine

Anticipated advances in healthcare in the next decade are outline here as a background for discussion of future of hyperbaric medicine. Some of these advances are as follows:

Important Medical Advances in the Next Decade

Molecular Diagnostics

Refinements, particularly with use of nanobiotechnology, will extend the present limit to detect traces of biochemical in the body and single microorganisms. Biochips/biosensors and point-of-care diagnostics will expand the use of diagnosis to select proper treatment at an early stage (Jain 2016a). Genotyping will become routine.

Sequencing

Advances in next-generation sequencing will have a considerable impact on molecular diagnostics and personalized medicine (Jain 2016b). Portable sequencers will be available in small laboratories at point of care.

Molecular Imaging

Refinements of contrast materials and introductions of new technologies will enable in vivo visualization of pathology various organs, particularly the brain with detail matching histological examination. Therapy may be combined with imaging, e.g., nanoparticle-based imaging may be followed by therapy based on the same nanoparticles.

Biomarkers

Discovery and validation of new biomarkers will increase with refinements in molecular diagnostics (Jain 2010). In addition to use in clinical trials, biomarkers will be applied more often in clinical practice to guide treatment and serve as basis of molecular diagnostics.

Pharmaceuticals

Marked improvement in drug discovery and development with the use of cells rather than animal models. Development of personalized medicines to start with to replace some of the repositioned drugs. Increase in the discovery of new viable drugs with less failures and improved translation from preclinical to clinical stage. Development of nanomedicines with targeted delivery that are more effective and less toxic than conventional drugs. The use of drugs with companion diagnostics, particularly for the treatment of cancer, will increase.

K.K. Jain, MD, FRACS, FFPM (✉)
1 Blaesiring 7, Basel 4057, Switzerland
e-mail: jain@pharmabiotech.ch

Remote Monitoring of Vital Signs

Remote monitoring of human body functions and disease diagnosis by electronic devices, conducted on a limited scale now, will become more widespread.

Drug Delivery

Marked improvement in drug delivery technologies for targeted delivery (Jain 2014b). Increase in use of nanobiotechnology and methods for controlled passage of drugs through barriers such as blood-brain barrier. Increase in use of transdermal patches for controlled delivery of drugs as an alternative to injection for systemic administration. Further development of alternative routes such as transnasal for drug delivery to the brain.

Synthetic Biology

There will be an increase in applications for improving diagnostics and drug development. Synthetic biology will also contribute to the development of personalized medicine (Jain 2013a).

Nanomedicine

Nanobiotechnologies play an important role in advancing areas already mentioned and will play an important role in the development personalized medicine (Jain 2017). Nanobots, navigating to various parts of the body via circulation, will be able to detect disease and deliver treatment.

Robotics

There will be an increase and further refinements in the use of robotics in healthcare for surgical procedures, assisting medical personnel and in rehabilitation.

Cell Therapy

The use of stem cells in treatment of various diseases will increase (Jain 2016c). Cell therapy will be used in combination with other regenerative therapies.

Gene Therapy

More gene therapy approvals are expected in the next decade. Gene-editing technologies such as CRISPR (clustered regularly interspaced short palindromic repeats) will be approved for limited applications within ethical restrictions (Jain 2016d).

Regenerative Medicine

Cell-based regenerative therapies using nanofiber scaffolds for repair of damaged organs. Printing of organs to overcome organ donor shortage, e.g., by use of liver cells.

Geriatric Medicine

Advances in understanding of the aging process will enable strategies to slow down the aging process and promote healthy aging. Life span will increase also due to improvement in management of diseases common in the elderly.

Virtual Medicine

Application of virtual reality for therapeutic purposes in neuropsychiatric disorders

Advances in Bioinformatics

These will accompany advances in medical research for analysis of immense new data and to facilitate translation of research into clinical practice. This will also be important for the development of personalized medicine.

Advances in Surgery

Success of some biotechnology-based innovative approaches will obviate the need for some classical operations. The trend toward minimally invasive surgery will continue. Some procedures will be miniaturized beyond microsurgery to nanosurgery, e.g., by use of nanolasers.

Personalized Medicine

Many of the advances mentioned in this section are linked to advances in personalized medicine (Jain 2015).

Social Media and Future Medicine

With proliferation in the use of social media and wide availability of healthcare and scientific information on the Internet, there will be greater dissemination of new discoveries to general audiences. Interaction between the scientists and the public will influence the development of medicine.

Important Areas for Future Development

Advances in healthcare will impact all therapeutic areas, but the following will be most notable.

Cancer

This is the most active area for research and applications of new technologies (Jain 2014a). The most promising developments will be in immunotherapies for cancer, bringing us closer to cure of cancer. As a multifactorial disease, cancer will require combination of various approaches.

Neurological Disorders

New biotechnologies have already made a significant contribution to understanding and management of neurological disorders (Jain 2013b). Cell/gene therapies and nanotechnologies are among promising technologies. Significant advances are expected in the next decade particularly in the ongoing projects on brain mapping or connectomics. This knowledge will form the basis of rational therapies for some of the disorders that are challenging for management. Significant advances are expected in the management of Alzheimer disease and stroke.

Cardiovascular Disorders

In addition to advances in biomedical engineering, biotechnology will have considerable impact on prevention and management of cardiovascular disorders (Jain 2011). Cell therapy and nanobiotechnology will be among important technologies.

Tropical Diseases and Emerging Viral Infections

Tuberculosis and malaria are old problems that plague most of the developing world. New biotechnology-based measures for prevention and eradication of these diseases are foreseen in the next decade. Emerging viral epidemics is another challenge where biotechnology-based solutions are being applied.

Diabetes

Further development of bionic pancreas for closed-loop insulin delivery adjusted to constant measurement of blood glucose levels. Stem cell and gene therapies for diabetes are in development.

Role of HBO in Future Medicine

HBO will play a greater part in the practice of medicine in the future. Availability of hyperbaric chambers in every major medical facility in the developed countries is foreseen by the end of the first decade of the twenty-first century. Already, there is greater awareness of this form of therapy among physicians and patients. A considerable amount of research work still needs to be done to place hyperbaric medicine on a sound scientific basis. There will be increasing use of new biotechnologies in hyperbaric medicine in keeping with trends in other areas of medicine.

Role of Hyperbaric Oxygen in the Multidisciplinary Healthcare Systems of the Future

Modern medicine is increasing in complexity. In spite of advances in new biotechnologies, the pathophysiology of most of the diseases is not fully understood. Several established treatments are still empirical. Increasing activity in molecular biological approach to diseases is indicating that only a minority of the disease genes discovered fit in with the concept of one gene the one disease phenomenon. Several of the common diseases are polygenic and multifactorial in origin. Increasing numbers of risk factors are being identified.

This has implications for treatment. Even if a single cause of the disease is identified (e.g., mutation in a gene), correction of this defect, even if possible, is usually not enough. The patient may need to control risk factors and therapies to give relief and aid recovery from the damage done by the disease process. As more methods of treatment become available, medicine is assuming a multidisciplinary form. It is a rare patient who receives only one medicine. The increasing number of options requires a discussion of the choice of treatments and integration of treatments in the best interests of the patients. A simplified concept of the relationship of some forms of treatment to HBO is shown in Fig. 47.1. Mainstream medicine and those who practice it have contact with practitioners of other forms of therapy.

Alternative/complementary medicine is gaining increasing popularity. Acupuncture has been combined with HBO. Most physicians have no objection to their patients receiving this form for minor self-limiting diseases or for those where no treatment is available. Cell therapy, particularly involving the use of stem cells, can be combined with HBO. New technologies to facilitate regeneration can be combined with HBO for repair of fractures and wound healing. Gene therapy, on the other hand, is being developed for some serious and previously incurable diseases. The role of physical therapy and rehabilitation in patient care is increasingly recognized, and it can be enhanced by HBO, e.g., in chronic poststroke patients.

Basis of HBO use in multidisciplinary approach to disease management is shown in Fig. 47.2. The level of importance for HBO depends upon the level of evidence available. Only examples are given, with no effort to compile an exhaustive list of diseases for which HBO has a rational basis. Simply because no other treatment is available for a condition is no argument for giving priority to HBO for any condition.

Future Needs in Hyperbaric Medicine

Some of the suggested measures for hyperbaric medicine to keep up with advances in other areas of healthcare and further improve the results are as follows:

- Hyperbaric physicians need to familiarize themselves with new biotechnologies and their potential applications in combination with HBO.
- There should be a greater effort toward integration of HBO with other methods of treatment.
- Personalized approaches to management of diseases should be adopted wherever possible.
- For optimal instruction and research, chairs should be established for hyperbaric medicine at the university level.
- Politicians and funding agencies should be lobbied for increased funding for research.

Fig. 47.1 Important
components of the
multidisciplinary approach to
disease management and
relation to hyperbaric oxygen

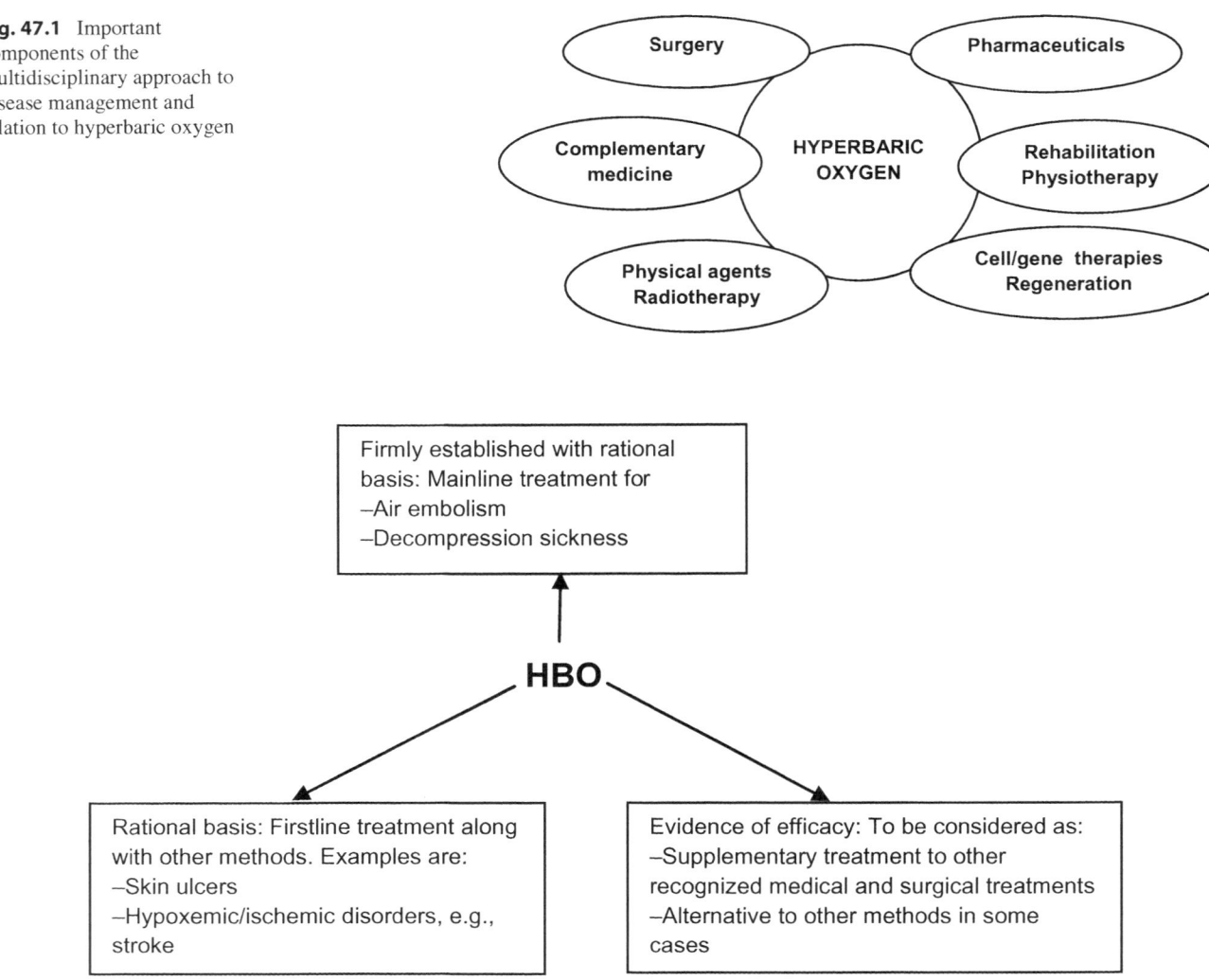

Fig. 47.2 Basis of HBO use in multidisciplinary approach to disease management

References

Jain KK. Textbook of personalized medicine. 2nd ed. New York: Springer; 2015.
Jain KK. Molecular diagnostics. Basel: Jain PharmaBiotech; 2016a.
Jain KK. DNA sequencing. Basel: Jain PharmaBiotech; 2016b.
Jain KK. Cell therapy. Basel: Jain PharmaBiotech; 2016c.
Jain KK. Gene therapy. Basel: Jain PharmaBiotech; 2016d.
Jain KK. Handbook of biomarkers. New York: Springer; 2010.

Jain KK. Applications of biotechnology in cardiovascular therapeutics. New York: Springer; 2011.
Jain KK. A handbook of nanomedicine. 3rd ed. New York: Springer; 2017.
Jain KK. Synthetic biology and personalized medicine. Med Princ Pract. 2013a;22:209–19.
Jain KK. Applications of biotechnology in neurology. New York: Springer; 2013b.
Jain KK. Applications of biotechnology in oncology. New York: Springer; 2014a.
Jain KK, editor. Drug delivery systems. 2nd ed. New York: Springer; 2014b.

Ethical Issues, Standards, and Quality Control in the Practice of Hyperbaric Medicine

48

Caroline E. Fife, Kristen A. Eckert, and Wilbur Thomas Workman

Abstract

We will discuss the safety and ethics of hyperbaric oxygen therapy (HBOT) amidst a boom in public demand and usage. Although there are 14 indications recognized by the Undersea and Hyperbaric Medical Society (UHMS) in the United States, there are dozens of off-label indications (most unsupported by scientific evidence) for which HBOT is utilized in clinics, medical spas, and the home. In many cases, "hyperbaric oxygen therapy" is being provided with compressed air in inflatable chambers at 1.3 ATA. These "mild hyperbaric" treatments do not meet the definition of HBOT according to the UHMS. Furthermore, clinical trials have been published that evaluate the efficacy of these "mild hyperbaric" treatments, using oxygen partial pressures so low that they could have been achieved breathing oxygen with a simple face mask at sea level atmospheric conditions. Thus, some studies purporting to demonstrate the effectiveness of HBOT did not even employ HBOT. Despite the excellent safety record of HBOT in general, when pure oxygen *is* provided to patients under hyperbaric conditions, there is a risk of side effects and adverse events including deaths from hyperbaric chamber fires, gas mishandling, and poor decompression practices, all of which might have been prevented by adherence to safety regulations and proper training. The risk of HBOT must be weighed against the potential benefit, and this is difficult to do when the benefit is unknown. The economic implications of the rise in HBOT use are significant. Fraudulent use of HBOT can occur with approved as well as off-label indications. Consumers may pay out of pocket for unproven treatments without a clear understanding of the scientific evidence for its use, or third party payers may pay for the improper use of HBOT in patients who do not meet coverage criteria and maybe unlikely to benefit. A more clear definition of what constitutes "hyperbaric oxygen therapy" would improve publication standards for clinical trials involving HBOT. The creation of a national registry to make outcome data available and more federal resources directed at the enforcement of safety standards would reduce patient risk.

C.E. Fife, MD (✉)
CHI St. Luke's Wound Clinic, The Woodlands, TX, USA

Baylor College of Medicine, Houston, TX, USA

Intellicure, Inc., The Woodlands, TX, USA
e-mail: cfife@intellicure.com

K.A. Eckert, MPhil
Strategic Solutions, Inc., Cody, WY, USA

W.T. Workman, BS, MS
Quality Assurance and Regulatory Affairs, Undersea and
Hyperbaric Medical Society, San Antonio, TX, USA

© Springer International Publishing AG 2017
K.K. Jain, *Textbook of Hyperbaric Medicine*, DOI 10.1007/978-3-319-47140-2_48

Keywords
Hyperbaric oxygen therapy • Off-label use • Ethics • Safety • Fire hazard • HBOT • Registry • UHMS • FDA

Alternative Medical Treatments and Off-Label Use of Hyperbaric Oxygen

For many years, the United States (US) Food and Drug Administration (FDA) has deferred to the Undersea and Hyperbaric Medical Society (UHMS) to establish the list of indications for which hyperbaric oxygen (HBOT) has sufficient evidence to support its use (UHMS 2015; Fife and Fife 2009). Hyperbaric oxygen chambers are Class II medical devices and are cleared for marketing and use by the FDA for 13 indications (Fife and Fife 2009; FDA 2013). These are air or gas embolism, carbon monoxide poisoning and carbon monoxide poisoning complicated by cyanide poisoning, clostridial myositis and myonecrosis, crush injury, compartment syndrome and other acute traumatic ischemias, decompression sickness, enhanced of selected problem wounds, exceptional blood loss anemia, necrotizing soft tissue infections, osteomyelitis (refractory), delayed radiation injury (soft tissue and bony necrosis), skin grafts and flaps (compromised), thermal burns, and intracranial abscess. Recently, the UHMS has added idiopathic sudden sensorineural hearing loss to its list of approved indications (UHMS 2015), but the FDA does not recognize this indication. It should be noted that the list of indications for which HBOT is considered proven differs from country to country outside of the US (Hyperbaric Chambers 2011), and within some countries like Canada, there are even differences between the provinces regarding the conditions for which HBOT is considered a proven therapy. In the US, while the FDA does not regulate the practice of medicine, it does regulate the safety and effectiveness of medical devices and claims made with regard to the use of medical devices (US FDA 2015). Hyperbaric chamber manufacturers and purveyors of HBOT are considered to be making "false claims" if they advertise the use of HBOT and/or a hyperbaric chamber for any indication outside of the 13 conditions listed earlier. Such instances of "false claims" are subject to FDA oversight and censure. Nevertheless, HBOT is promoted on the Internet for dozens of other conditions by independent clinics, hospitals, and patient advocacy groups. As of 2008, a patient advocacy website lists 59 centers in the US that treat patients with HBOT for off-label indications, such as autism, Lyme disease, mitochondrial disease, cerebral palsy, Ménière's disease, migraine, multiple sclerosis, Parkinson's disease, chronic fatigue syndrome, and stroke, among others (Healing-arts.org 2008). There are at least 106 HBOT clinics in the US that advertise the use of HBOT for Lyme disease alone (see Chap. 15).

The increase in off-label use of HBOT has led the FDA to release a statement strongly cautioning healthcare consumers that HBOT is not clinically proven to be an effective treatment of cancer, autism spectrum disorder (ASD), heart disease, multiple sclerosis, and other diseases and conditions (US FDA 2013). Nearly 30 complaints were filed by the FDA against centers using HBOT for off-label conditions, and the agency fears that misinformed consumers may endanger their health. This consumer warning was supplemented by five warning letters issued to the manufacturers of inflatable, low pressure hyperbaric chambers for misbranding their devices (Gaffney 2013). As payers increasingly restrict coverage for the approved indications of HBOT (e.g., diabetic foot ulcers), there has been a dramatic increase in the use of off-label HBOT.

Today, there are hyperbaric chambers in hospitals, independent clinics, medical spas, and private homes. Portable chambers are marketed for family use at home (Portable Hyperbaric Chambers Australia 2014; Cronin 2012) and include a quick step-by-step user video, the purpose of which is to obviate the need for the formal technical safety training that professional HBOT operators undergo (Portable Hyperbaric Chambers Australia 2014). This chapter will review the challenges associated with the shift in the use of HBOT away from approved indications to off-label indications and away from traditional medical settings.

The Risks of the Public Information Gap

The new consumer trend in hyperbaric medicine poses ethical and safety challenges on multiple fronts. Even if the scientific data were available to resolve questions of efficacy, limited marketing regulations (Chan and Brody 2001), lack of enforcement recourses, and the desperation of many patients and family members have aligned to create the perfect storm of potentially high-risk behaviors with maximum opportunity for disaster from a safety standpoint.

The Wall Street Journal reports that a single HBOT treatment can cost the consumer $150–250 at medical spas and alternative medicine centers where reimbursement by insurers is highly unlikely (Walker 2015). While this per treatment cost may be considered economical compared to the charges at a local hospital, mandated safety standards for equipment and properly trained personnel are far less likely to be in place. Thus, vulnerable people may pay relatively large amounts of money for an unproven treatment administered in a potentially unsafe environment. Individuals are enticed to undergo off-label HBOT treatment by the myriad of anecdotal reports readily available online touting the benefits of HBOT for conditions such as autism, without the necessary scientific background to weigh the strength of evidence. Balanced information may be difficult to obtain. One mother whose child had failed to improve after a lengthy course of HBOT for cerebral palsy posted a comment about the child's lack of progress in an Internet chat room, and several angry parents berated the mother for her "negativity" (Caroline Fife, personal communication, October 26, 2015).

The first ethical issue that must be addressed is that of the financial burden that patients or their family members may incur (which can approach many thousands of dollars) for the off-label use of HBOT when the potential benefit may be unknown. Furthermore, HBOT, while a relatively safe treatment overall, is not without side effects. Otic barotrauma occurs in 0.5–10 % of patients and 1:10,000–1:50,000 suffer from treatment-related oxygen toxicity seizures (Fife and Fife 2009). A relative contraindication to HBOT is chronic obstructive pulmonary disease or emphysema, air trapping from which can predispose to pulmonary over-pressurization, pneumothorax, arterial gas embolism, and even death.

The off-label use of HBOT is ethical only when the potential benefits are greater than the risks to the patient. For most of the approved indications, the likelihood of benefit can be easily estimated from published data. Thus, the risk-to-benefit ratio can be determined. However, when the likelihood of benefit is unknown or perhaps nonexistent, any risk of complication or side effect would seem to be unacceptable. It is not clear whether patients treated for off-label indications undergo an appropriate consent process. A recent news article reported the success of HBOT for a stroke patient at a local hyperbaric center (Libov 2014). The radiologist, who provided patient treatments at the facility, is quoted in the news article as saying that HBOT has been "proven effective" in treating chronic obstructive pulmonary disease and emphysema, in addition to rheumatoid arthritis, multiple sclerosis, cerebral palsy, and autism. Thus, it is hard to imagine that patients treated at this facility undergo adequate informed consent regarding the risks of HBOT in the presence of certain preexisting conditions (e.g., chronic obstructive pulmonary disease and emphysema which might predispose to pulmonary barotrauma), prior to HBOT if conditions considered relative contraindications are considered indications for treatment. Some disturbing cases have been reported in the literature, including a case of "medical child abuse" (Heild 2014), in which a malnourished boy in Santa Fe, New Mexico was treated with HBOT at an independent clinic for nonexisting conditions at the insistence of his

mother, who was suspected to suffer from Munchausen by proxy syndrome. The pediatrician involved was also accused of lying about his professional qualifications and has since then closed his practice. Another disturbing news report from Tennessee (RAYCOM 2013) revealed that two individuals posing as ministers and falsely claiming to be doctors of natural medicine and certified in hyperbaric medicine used two inflatable hyperbaric chambers for a variety of unproven indications, including hair loss. They had taken a physicians' hyperbaric training course using false medical credentials. The Tennessee Health Department confirmed that they did not have medical licenses (RAYCOM 2013).

Is There an Alternative to HBOT?

The next issue from an ethical standpoint is whether there currently exists a proven medical treatment for the off-label indication. HBOT is aggressively marketed for some conditions that may have less costly and overall more accessible therapeutic treatment options available. For example, the off-label use of HBOT is often promoted for mental health illness such as anxiety disorders or depression, conditions which may be successfully managed with more evidence-based treatments at much lower cost (Garakani and Mitton 2015). There is currently great interest in the use of HBOT for traumatic brain injury with several clinical trials currently underway, as well as possible beneficial effect on post-traumatic stress disorder in military patients (Harch et al. 2009, 2012). For many conditions, HBOT is attractive because there are no alternative therapies available.

Safety and Fire Hazard Issues from Misuse of Hyperbaric Chambers

Poor fire safety practices may pose the greatest risk of patient endangerment with regard to HBOT. As of the end of 2015, there have been 90 fatalities reported worldwide since 1923 caused by fires in hyperbaric chambers (Hyperbaric Chambers 2011; Walker 2015; Sheffield and Sheffield 2008; Sheffield and Desautels 1997; Zimlich 2012). There have been at least six fatalities due to unsafe gas handling (e.g., the patient receiving the wrong gas) (Hyperbaric Chambers 2011; Sheffield and Sheffield 2008), and one fatality due to decompression sickness as a result of inadequate decompression (Sheffield and Sheffield 2008). In total, at least 98 people have died in accidents related to the use of pressurized chambers. On the one hand, given the hundreds of thousands of hyperbaric treatments that have been administered, this is an extraordinary safety record. On the other hand, this safety record was achieved as a result of increasingly stringent safety requirements, and each fatality was possibly avoidable had proper safety practices been followed. Sheffield and Sheffield highlight five basic safety issues which must be considered when properly handling a hyperbaric chamber: fire safety, gas handling, and decompression, integrity of the pressure vessel, and staff training (Sheffield and Sheffield 2008).

There were no national fire safety standards in place for clinical hyperbaric chambers in the US prior until the late 1960s (Sheffield and Desautels 1997). Strict fire safety codes were created by the National Fire Protection Association (NFPA) following fatal fires in oxygen-enriched environments in the 1960s (Sheffield and Desautels 1997). These comprehensive guidelines are updated every 3 years in response to the general increased level of knowledge and expertise on the use of hyperbaric chambers (NFPA 2015). A summary of the current NFPA Health Care Facilities Safety Codes in Table 48.1 are the minimum safeguards that should be in place to protect patients and personnel from HBOT fires (NFPA 2015). This code not only applies to health care facilities as noted earlier, but also to any facility that falls under the NFPA's Life Safety Code and operates a hyperbaric chamber. Beginning with the 2000 edition of NFPA 101, compliance to the hyperbaric safety requirements of NFPA 99 was invoked by reference therefore making adherence to these well-established safety requirements mandatory is just about any location including strip shopping malls, business occupancies, etc. (NFPA 2015).

A chamber fire is caused by three components: ignition, oxygen, and fuel (flammable material) (Sheffield and Desautels 1997). Therefore, fire prevention focuses on limiting and/or eliminating these risk components. Over the past few decades, most chamber fires were caused by prohibited ignition sources such as electronics that were brought inside the chamber by the occupant (Sheffield and Desautels 1997). It is, therefore, particularly distressing to see Internet advertisements for off-label use of HBOT featuring children inside of hyperbaric chambers using laptop computers or other prohibited electronic devices. Advertisements like this send a clear and unambiguous message that chamber operators do not understand either hyperbaric safety regulations or the risks associated with oxygen use (Ibuki Health and Wellness 2015). Even more distressing, the manufacturer of a portable hyperbaric chamber for home use advertises on their website that their customers may use laptops, tablets, and portable music devices in the chamber (again with accompanying photographs of children using electronic devices), because the chamber uses pressurized air with an oxygen concentrator (1.3 ATA/4.3 psi), instead of pure oxygen (Cronin 2012). It is clear that even the manufacturer does not understand the simple math of the hyperbaric environment, the safety codes that govern the use of any hyperbaric chamber, or the FDA labeling requirements for inflatable hyperbaric chambers. It is important to note that the FDA labeling requirements for inflatable hyperbaric chambers prohibit the use of enriched air in any of the inflatable chambers that have been cleared for marketing through their PreMarket Notification Clearance Program (510[k]) (US FDA 2015). Enriched air is achieved when oxygen concentrators are used to provide the "treatment gas" which is exhaled directly in to the interior of the chamber, thus raising the oxygen partial pressure beyond 27%. At 1.3 ATA of air, the oxygen partial pressure is equivalent to 27% at sea level. According to the NFPA, when the oxygen concentration is >23.5% by volume, an oxygen enriched atmosphere is present (Sheffield and Desautels 1997). The conditions of every fatal chamber since 1980 involved >28% oxygen and the presence of flammable material (Sheffield and Desautels 1997). Additional factors that were involved in the fatal chamber fires were faulty electrical components (e.g., light bulbs, motors, and temporary electrical extension cords), inadequate extinguishments, and lack of vigilance to prevent the use of ignition sources (including spark-generating toys) in the chamber. A chamber pressurized with room air at 1.3 ATA has achieved an oxygen partial pressure which the NFPA would consider to be an oxygen-enriched atmosphere and one which certainly poses an increased risk of fire, particularly when combined with an ignition source. A mobile phone ignited the fire that killed a hyperbaric patient in China (Sheffield and Desautels 1997).

The most recent HBOT fatality in the international hyperbaric community was in China in 2014 when a 65-year-old male died resulting from a hyperbaric chamber fire caused by the patient smoking (Newton 2014).

The most recent HBOT-related fatality in the US occurred in 2012, when a female chamber operator was killed in conjunction with a chamber fire and explosion at an equine hyperbaric facility (Zimlich 2012). The ignition source was a spark from the horse's metal shoe against the metallic chamber wall. This case was a great shock to the veterinary community, which has had no formal certification or regulations on the use of HBOT on animals. A similar equine hyperbaric chamber fire occurred in the United Kingdom in 2008 which was fatal to a promising 3-year-old thoroughbred (W.T. Workman, personal communication, November 27, 2015). Human chambers have been adapted for animal use, or homemade chambers have been used for HBOT on animals, a practice which increases the risk to both the animals and the human chamber operators (Rech et al. 2008). A homemade chamber exploded killing two people in South Africa in 2004 (Sheffield and Sheffield 2008). For patient care in the US, clinical hyperbaric chambers must be constructed in accordance with the American Society of Mechanical Engineers Standards for Pressure Vessels (Boiler and Pressure Vessel Code and Pressure Vessels for Human Occupancy (Sheffield and Sheffield 2008; ASME 2013). While the FDA has cleared several inflatable hyperbaric chambers for marketing, they did so without requiring the manufacturer to comply with this well-established industry

Table 48.1 National Fire Protection Association fire safety code requirements for hyperbaric chambers (NFPA 2015)

Category	Code focus
Construction and equipment requirements	• Construction
	• Wall and door fire rating
	• Fire sprinkler protection
	• Piping
	• Medical oxygen and air
	• Gas storage
	• Hyperbaric chamber fabrication
	• Must comply with the design, fabrication, testing, and installation requirements of ASME Boiler and Pressure Vessel Code, Section VIII, Division 1 (22) and ASME PVHO-1-2012, Safety Standard for Pressure Vessels for Human Occupancy (23).
	• Illumination
	• Chamber ventilation
	• Sources of air for chamber atmospheres
	• Temperature and humidity control
	• Emergency depressurization and facility evacuation capability
	• Fire protection
	• Electrical systems and service
	• Chamber grounding
	• Communications and monitoring
	• Oxygen monitoring
	• Chamber gas supply monitoring
	• Other equipment and fixtures
Administration and maintenance	• Recognition of hazards
	• Responsibility
	• Establishes requirement for a designated Safety Director
	• Rules and regulations
	• Emergency procedures
	• Potential ignition sources: hot objects, cell phones, pager, spark-generating toys, personal entertainment devices such as laptops, smart phones, and tablets
	• Potential ignition sources: flammable, burnable materials
	• Potential ignition sources: silk, wool, synthetic textiles/materials, flammable hairsprays, hair oils, skin oils, cosmetics, lotions, oils, etc.
	• Potential ignition sources: battery-operated devices (in particular lithium and lithium ion batteries)
	• Personnel
	• Patient grounding
	• Textiles
	• Mattresses
	• Equipment
	• Handling of gases
	• Maintenance and maintenance documentation
	• Routine and major
	• Electrical safeguards
	• Housekeeping

ASME The American Society of Medical Engineers

standard. Many hyperbaric practitioners do not realize that criminal manslaughter charges have been filed against the physicians and chamber operators involved in recent hyperbaric fire deaths. Malpractice insurance does not protect a clinician against criminal charges, and the likelihood of prevailing in court is low when there is an obvious lack of adherence to fire safety standards.

With the surge in the number of centers offering HBOT and increased usage of HBOT among the general public, patient safety may be at risk worldwide due to the lack of experienced, formally trained staff (Sheffield and Sheffield 2008; Alcantara et al. 2010). Sheffield and Sheffield recommend that physicians should take at least 40 h of a UHMS Designated Introductory Course in Hyperbaric Medicine and that nurses and technologists also take at least 40 h of a National Board of Diving & Hyperbaric Medical Technology-approved introductory course (Sheffield and Sheffield 2008). Advanced practitioners practicing hyperbaric medicine are recommended to have either subspecialty board certification in Undersea and Hyperbaric Medicine (UHM) or a Certificate of Added Qualification in UHM. Given the relatively cavalier way in which the use of electronics is promoted and depicted inside inflatable hyperbaric chambers, it may be that the primary reason more safety problems have not been reported in conjunction with off-label use is that patients are being treated with concentrations of oxygen that are very nearly the same as that of sea level air. In other words, the great irony may be that the reason more fires have not occurred in association with inflatable hyperbaric chambers, in particular, is that they are not delivering HBOT.

The Controversy of Low Pressure Oxygen

HBOT is defined by the UHMS as the administration of oxygen at pressures ≥ 1.4 ATM (UHMS 2015). Breathing 100 % oxygen at the equivalent of 1 atm of pressure ("sea level") is not hyperbaric oxygen.

Inflatable chambers can achieve atmospheric pressures of 1.3 ATA. These light, portable devices were originally designed for the treatment of acute mountain sickness. Acute mountain sickness is the only indication for which the FDA has cleared the inflatable chambers. However, they are now heavily marketed for home use and are often found in health spas. This trend is clearly outside the boundaries of the FDA's intended clearance action. As discussed earlier, breathing air at 1.3 ATA pressure is equivalent to breathing 27 % oxygen at sea level. This means that the same amount of oxygen a patient obtains by breathing air inside an inflatable chamber at 1.3 ATA can be provided without the chamber—simply by giving a little extra oxygen to a patient in a regular room with a face mask. Proponents of "low pressure or mild oxygen therapy" insist that the additional 0.3 ATA of pressure achieved with the inflatable chamber is somehow beneficial in its own right, a theory that has no scientific grounds (Mitchell and Bennett 2014). In essence, inflatable chambers are merely providing their users with sea level oxygen concentrations, falsely advertised as hyperbaric oxygen, raising multiple ethical concerns for a public unable to understand the physics involved. There are risks with inflatable chambers, including sudden depressurization and the fact that small plastic

pieces have been observed to come loose from them and be propelled at very high velocities due to the differential rate of pressure between the chamber and the environment (not unlike the injuries that have been sustained from ruptured tires). There has been at least one fatality attributed to the failure of a chamber component of an inflatable chamber. In 2011, a 19-year-old male with ASD died while sleeping inside a home use inflatable chamber (Walker 2015). During the night, the quick disconnect supply valve somehow became disconnected, thus preventing a continuous air supply to the chamber, and the boy suffocated (Oxy-Health et al. 2014). One has to wonder if this fatality would have occurred if the inflatable chamber was designed to meet ASME design requirements (American Society of Medical Engineers 2012).

The use of low pressure oxygen is not limited to inflatable chambers. Regrettably, the inability to properly define what constitutes HBOT has led to misleading publications regarding HBOT (Rossignol et al. 2009). In a randomized controlled trial (RCT) widely cited by advocates of HBOT for autism, 62 young children with ASD were treated with HBOT at 1.3 ATM in a traditional hyperbaric chamber with 24 % oxygen or with a sham involving pressurized air at 1.03 ATM and 21 % oxygen (Rossignol et al. 2009). The authors found that the "HBOT group" significantly improved in their overall functioning, language and social skills, eye contact, and cognitive behavior compared to the control group. The HBOT group treated with 1.3 ATA pressure and 24 % oxygen received 237 mmHg PO_2, which is equivalent to 31 % O_2 at sea level. In other words, the children who were touted as receiving "hyperbaric oxygen therapy," got a lower partial pressure of oxygen than they would have received if they had been treated with a nonrebreather face mask and 100 % oxygen at sea level. The experimental group did not, in fact, receive "hyperbaric oxygen therapy" according to the definition of HBOT. A similar problem occurred with a study evaluating neurologically impaired adults and children treated with 1.3 ATA and 24 % oxygen (Heuser et al. 2015). Using common sense, a cheaper and safer (and therefore more ethical therapy) would have been the use of an oxygen mask therapy in both studies (Rossignol et al. 2009; Hu et al. 2015). Oxygen breathing at sea level could provide a higher partial pressure of oxygen at a lower risk of side effects and at much lower cost. This easier alternative to "low pressure HBOT" with face mask oxygen has not been discussed in the autism community.

The "Chamber" Effect

In his analysis of the placebo effect in HBOT, Bennett (2014) prefers the placebo definition used by Moerman and Jonas (2002): "a substance or procedure … that is objectively without specific activity for the condition being treated." The increasing use of low pressure oxygen therapy under the guise of HBOT seems to be partly driven by a placebo effect that may be linked to placing the patients inside a hyperbaric chamber (Mitchell and Bennett 2014; Bennett 2014). Patients enter what they feel is a highly technical device. The pressure changes require them to equalize their ears, and they undergo an experience which they are convinced is likely to result in benefit (Bennett 2014). In fact, none of the blinded, sham-controlled RCTs that evaluated HBOT in cerebral palsy and mild traumatic brain injury demonstrated a HBOT benefit compared to the control, although both treatment and control groups reported improvements, no doubt an influence of a placebo effect (Bennett 2014).

Evidence supports the effect of a placebo in producing endorphins that can lead to measurable, physiological changes in a patient (Bennett 2014). If the placebo sham has a therapeutic effect, then it is not a placebo, but rather a form of treatment. Advocates of low pressure oxygen believe that the 131 kPa of air that is commonly used as the sham control in RCTs is actually beneficial in its own right (Hu et al. 2015; Bennett 2014). The therapeutic effect observed when breathing air at 131 kPa may be a result of exposure to pressure or small increases in nitrogen concentration or the inspired partial pressure of oxygen (Bennett 2014). The traumatic brain injury trial by Wolf et al. (2012) showed that the sham (ambient air at 1.3 ATA) had higher efficacy than 100 % oxygen at 2.4 ATA although both groups improved. They argued that HBOT was less effective than the sham and the sham's greater efficacy resulted from the placebo effect (Wolf et al. 2012; Boussi-Gross et al. 2013). Indeed, other skeptics of low pressure oxygen therapy argue that the lack of differences between treatment and sham groups is evidence that the HBOT and the sham work the same, which is to say, HBOT is not more effective than the placebo effect on that particular condition being tested (Bennett 2014; Boussi-Gross et al. 2013; Collet et al. 2001). Moreover, in an RCT that evaluated low pressure oxygen therapy (24–28 % oxygen at 1.3 ATM) versus a placebo (simulated pressurization of ambient air using airflow noise) on children with ASD, the authors found no significant improvement in the use of "mild" HBOT (Bennett 2014; Granpeesheh et al. 2010). To summarize thus far, for all of the earlier studies, there has been no significant benefit of the treatment arm over the sham group. Either this is due to the placebo effect, or oxygen partial pressures as little as 205 mmHg (equivalent to 27 % at sea level) can have a salutary effect on some neurological conditions. If that is so, given that an oxygen mask could provide the same therapeutic effect as either the sham or the "low pressure HBOT" groups in these studies, to insist on a more expensive therapy that has greater potential risk to the patient is hard to argue from an ethical standpoint. There is evidence that simply entering the hyperbaric chamber is a powerful contributor to the placebo effect. While patients

may have imbued the chamber with almost shamanistic properties, the very real physics of the hyperbaric environment put constraints on the design of controlled trials, as discussed in the following section.

Ethical Challenges with HBOT Clinical Trial Design

The optimal way to design a controlled trial of HBOT remains controversial. Since there is ample evidence that patients perceive "going in the chamber" to have a salutary effect, some exposure to the hyperbaric environment appears necessary for control subjects. Sham treatments have been used with success whereby the chamber is compressed only enough to give subjects the sensation of pressure on the tympanic membranes and create the audible "noise" of the hyperbaric experience. Interviews with patients at the conclusion of trials have shown that subjects were unable to identify that they were receiving a sham treatment. This approach requires considerable coordination and monitoring of hyperbaric chamber operators who might inadvertently indicate to a subject that they are not in the active treatment group. Another option is to compress the chamber but have the patient breathe a gas other than oxygen. It must be remembered that if the patient is allowed to breathe compressed air, the partial pressure of oxygen continues to increase as pressure increases, even though the oxygen percentage is unchanged. Therefore, at 2.0 ATA, the partial pressure of oxygen when breathing compressed air is equivalent to the respiration of 42 % oxygen at sea level. Because previous work has suggested a possible therapeutic effect of oxygen in this range, another option is to breathe a gas mixture in which the percentage of oxygen is reduced in order to maintain a partial pressure of oxygen equivalent to sea level. At 2.0 ATA, this would mean providing the subject with a gas mixture of approximately 11 % oxygen, with the balance nitrogen (89 % nitrogen rather than the 79 % nitrogen in air). Although the oxygen *percentage* is reduced by half, since the atmospheric pressure is twice that of sea level, the subject would still be respiring approximately 160 mmHg of oxygen, exactly the same as sea level. Therefore, the subjects would not be hypoxic while in the chamber. However, they would be breathing a greatly increased amount of nitrogen and thus be at increased risk of developing decompression sickness (more commonly referred to as "the bends"). Even control subjects respiring compressed *air* may be placed at risk of decompression sickness depending on the atmospheric pressure and duration of the treatment to which the subjects are exposed.

The risk to control subjects may have gone unrecognized in one important hyperbaric clinical trial. Löndahl et al. (2010) performed a RCT of HBOT in diabetic foot ulcers which demonstrated that Wagner grade ulcers of 2, 3 or 4 were more likely to completely heal if treated with HBOT than with air (52% vs. 29% healed, $p = 0.03$). The HBOT group received 100% oxygen at 2.5 ATA for 85 min, and the control group received 21% oxygen at 2.5 ATA for 85 min. Both groups required 10 additional minutes of compression and decompression breathing air. This brought the total "dive time" of the control group to 95 min. Using standard diving decompression tables, a compressed air exposure to 2.5 ATA (15.0 m) over 70 min requires a decompression stop which was not provided in the protocol (NAUI Worldwide 2015). Thus, the control subjects were exposed to a "dive profile" which was in excess of the "no decompression limit" for most sport diving tables. Alarmingly, in the control group, one patient was hospitalized for 24 h after "temporarily losing consciousness after a treatment session." It is possible that this represented a case of unrecognized decompression illness. This possibility was not discussed in the paper, nor was the serious risk to the control group mentioned in the publication. It must be remembered that, despite the increased risk of decompression sickness, the subjects in the control group were still respiring an *increased* partial pressure of oxygen above that found at sea level and perhaps sufficient to have some therapeutic effect. This study is important for several reasons. The study demonstrated clear benefit from HBOT despite the fact that the controls received enough additional oxygen to have had some therapeutic effect. However, while the trial design could be viewed as ideal from an "evidence-based" standpoint, the controls were exposed to enough compressed nitrogen to risk a serious adverse event such as decompression illness. More troubling is that the possible risk to control subjects may not have been identified by the investigators themselves, their institutional review board, or the reviewers of the manuscript. If the unique physics of the hyperbaric environment are not clearly understood by the investigators performing hyperbaric clinical trials, it is understandable why the general public may be unable to interpret the information about studies with low pressure oxygen published under the title of "hyperbaric oxygen therapy."

Despite the challenges imposed by the laws of physics, the biggest impediment to HBOT research has been the lack of adequate funding. Oxygen is not made by a pharmaceutical company. Most conditions for which HBOT is promoted for off-label use are unlikely to garner major research funding. Until there is medical consensus on the off-label use of HBOT, the principles of autonomy, beneficence, and nonmaleficence should guide the physician's decision concerning the off-label use of HBOT (Fife and Fife 2009; Chan and Brody 2001).

Informed Consent

The informed consent process between physician and patient provides an opportunity for the patient to understand the potential risks and benefits of any treatment. Although practitioners view obtaining informed consent as a necessary part of any procedure, the process of informed consent takes on even greater importance when it involves the off-label use of a medical device or drug and is the primary way we acknowledge patient autonomy. Off-label use of drugs is commonplace. Many pharmaceuticals originally marketed for one purpose have since been found to be even better suited for another purpose, e.g., the common use of antidepressant amitriptyline in management of neuropathic pain rather than depression. Off-label use of HBOT is not unethical per se, assuming certain standards are followed as part of the informed consent process. Indeed, HBOT can be used unethically for *approved* conditions, if patients are provided treatment for reasons other than its potential clinical benefit. In order for the patient to make an informed decision regarding the off-label use of HBOT, the physician must disclose the following information to the patient: the existence of alternative medical treatments for the condition, the level and type of scientific data (i.e., animal studies vs. RCTs) that support the use of HBOT, the risks of HBOT specific to the patient, exactly how much the treatment will cost the patient, and any financial incentive that the physician might have in recommending HBOT (e.g., if the physician owns the hyperbaric facility and stands to gain financially by recommending that the patient undergo treatment) (Fife and Fife 2009; Chan and Brody 2001). While informed consent does not have to be written, since the physician needs to document the details of the consent process, it makes sense for this to take the form of a written document.

Physicians can make case-by-case decisions to use HBOT for off-label indications. This is part of the practice of medicine. However, when the off-label use of HBOT is repeatedly performed with the intent to apply potential findings to the care of other patients, the clinician is now engaged in research. To perform research in an ethical manner, a protocol must be approved by an IRB and patients must be informed that they are subjects in a research study in which they have the right to consent or decline to participate (Fife and Fife 2009; Paris 2003).

Desperate Measures

Decisions surrounding the off-label use of HBOT can be particularly difficult when indications with insufficient data are encountered in patients with desperate medical situations. For example, online advocacy groups target the parents of children with ASD and cerebral palsy, encouraging them to seek treatment with HBOT (Healing-arts.org. 2008). A parent's love for their sick child can be a powerful advocacy tool for off-label HBOT. One would assume that the best interest of the pediatric patient is the sole determinant of physician's treatment decision (Paris et al. 2001), but questions about this have been raised in court (Le 2015). In Florida, a distressed and desperate father pleaded with pediatric intensive care physicians to provide HBOT to his 20-month-old son who suffered anoxic damage to the brain following a near drowning accident in his backyard pool (Le 2015). While the father believed HBOT represented the last hope for his son's recovery, the physicians refused on the grounds that there was insufficient evidence to support its use in such cases, and out of concern for the possibility of HBOT-associated risks in a critically ill child. A legal battle ensued resulting in a circuit court judge issuing an order that the hospital install a hyperbaric chamber, given that the parents had agreed to pay for all the associated costs and waive any potential treatment liability. However, in the interim, the patient's condition had worsened to a persistent vegetative condition so there was no possible expectation of benefit from HBOT. This case has interesting ethical implications. Paris et al. suggest that if the parents' perceived "last chance of recovery" maintains the patient's dignity and is not a burden on the community at large, then the off-label use of HBOT is considered ethical because the family will know that every possible treatment was attempted for their child (Paris 2003). What is not addressed with regard to this case are the unique implications of a court demanding that a hyperbaric chamber be installed where one is not currently available, with no apparent understanding of the planning needed to ensure compliance with fire codes and to train personnel to ensure the safe operation of such a facility, and whether this would in fact, have represented a "burden on the community".

HBOT Fraud

In medical practice, it is unethical to provide HBOT for an off-label use by disguising the reason for treatment as an approved indication in order to obtain coverage by a third-party payer (Fife and Fife 2009). With regard to approved uses, when physicians, hospitals, or management companies misrepresent medical information in order to provide HBOT to a Medicare beneficiary, then they are committing Medicare fraud. Fraudulently billed HBOT services have been the target of government investigation since 2000, with the release of a report on the use and appropriateness of HBOT by the US Department of Health and Human Services Office the Inspector General (OIG) (Le 2015; USDHHS 2000). The

OIG report concluded that, of the US$49.9 million paid in hyperbaric-related charges to hospitals and physicians, $16 million (32%) were "inappropriately billed" as a result of failure to support claims with proper medical documentation (e.g., medical records did not describe adequately the procedures reported on the claim), $14.2 million (28%) were paid in error, and another $4.9 million (10%) were paid for services that did not meet Medicare's medical necessity criteria (e.g., therapy sessions that were excessive). Furthermore, the OIG suspected that 74% of inappropriate payments did not have an attending physician present during the HBOT session, a requirement for payment (Le 2015; USDHHS 2000).

Since its launch in 2007, the Medicare Fraud Strike Force comprised of federal, state, and local investigators in nine US cities has specifically targeted hyperbaric fraud, which is prosecuted by the Department of Justice (Le 2015). These cases begin in the court system as a civil case, but can become criminal cases, depending on the severity. A guilty verdict results in very serious consequences, which have thus far included 5 years imprisonment, up to $2.6 million in restitution, 50 h of community service, and $3.6 million to resolve the liability of overpaid HBOT services. The alarming findings of the US investigation on HBOT and the ongoing, increased activities of the Strike Force could have dire consequences on HBOT coverage in the US. Le suggests that it is not unlikely that CMS could eliminate Medicare coverage for HBOT in the future (Le 2015). Sadly, unethical standards in the delivery of hyperbaric medicine for *approved* indications may have done more harm to the field than unsubstantiated claims over off-label indications. The increasingly Draconian measures the US healthcare system is employing to limit overuse and improper use of HBOT could create a scenario in which the "approved" indications are no longer covered by payers, and HBOT is primarily available on a cash basis for off-label use.

HBOT Market Regulations

Food, Drug, and Cosmetic Act (FDC) 510(k) Clearance

In the US, the FDA, which regulates the marketing of both medical devices and drugs, classifies hyperbaric chambers as "Class II medical devices," because they do not support or sustain human life (Class III), but are not as innocuous as, for example, a tongue depressor (Class I). The Food, Drug and Cosmetic Act requires medical device manufacturers to notify FDA of their intent to market a new medical device at least 90 days in advance using a process known as Premarket Notification, often referred to by the name of the subsection of the act in which it is found, "510(k)" (US FDA 2015).

This process allows the FDA to determine whether a new device (not in commercial distribution prior to May 28, 1976) is substantially equivalent to a device which has already been classified. The 510(k) clearance process is relatively uncomplicated for hyperbaric chambers that have not undergone substantial changes in design or composition when compared to predecessor chambers. In the 510(k) process, manufacturers must also stipulate that there are no substantial changes to the *intended use* of the chamber. This means that since 1978, all hyperbaric chambers cleared by the FDA can only be promoted for those conditions that are listed as approved in the UHMS Hyperbaric Oxygen Therapy Committee report (UHMS 2015; Fife and Fife 2009). In order for a chamber to be approved to treat an indication that is not listed by the UHMS, the manufacturer would have to provide the FDA with compelling evidence to support the use of HBOT for that condition. Advertising and promotion of off-label use of HBOT places the healthcare entity in breach of FDA regulations (US FDA 2015), even if the clinician is promoting an IRB approved research protocol (Fife and Fife 2009), and the FDA is within it purview to seize assets including the hyperbaric chamber. Warning letters have been issued by the FDA in the past for off-label advertisement of HBOT (US FDA 2013). If research is to be performed using HBOT on an unapproved indication, then an investigational device exemption has to first be requested from the FDA. However, as explained in Chap. 7, updated guidelines regarding the promotion of off-label uses are pending from the FDA in the wake of several lawsuits which successfully argued that off-label promotion is protected free speech and thus, allowable as long as the information provided is "truthful and nonmisleading" (Boumil 2013; Inside Health Policy 2015).

In addition to the requirements noted earlier, the FDA also defines a hyperbaric chamber as a prescriptive device meaning that the chamber can only be sold or used under prescriptive authority of a licensed practitioner. This requirement is believed to be widely ignored in many facilities that are using inflatable chambers. Frequently the rational for not requiring a prescription for use is that inflatable chambers are being used for alternative medicine and the FDA does not regulate alternative medicine. While this may be true, the FDA does regulate the device (hyperbaric chamber) (W.T. Workman, personal communication, November 27, 2015).

National Hyperbaric Oxygen Therapy Registry

The off-label use of HBOT is increasing without a commensurate increase in funding for HBOT research. The ethical use of HBOT necessitates access to data, the only likely source of which may be the individuals who are currently providing off-label treatments or even the patients themselves. A medical registry was initially proposed by Chan and Brody (2001) as a potential tool to assess the potential effectiveness of HBOT on certain, unapproved indications. As discussed in Chap. 15, a national HBOT registry could generate data to analyze the effect of HBOT on off-label uses; it would also help the public identify HBOT providers with good safety and ethical practices for off-label uses.

Chan and Brody provided a framework by which off-label indications could be evaluated for their suitability in a national registry (Fife and Fife 2009; Chan and Brody 2001). Factors included whether alternative treatments to HBOT are costly and have suboptimal outcomes, whether human and animal data support the rationale for using HBOT, whether the benefits outweigh the risks to both the patient and clinic staff, whether there is a significant burden of disease, whether a high public demand exists, and whether there are defined outcome measures. Patients participating in such a national registry would need to undergo informed consent, and there would need to be local IRB approval (Chan and Brody 2001). It is unfortunate, given the large number of patients being treated with HBOT for chronic lyme disease, for example (see Chap. 15), that a national registry has not been created for this purpose. While such a registry might not be able to prove that HBOT is effective for the disease, a registry could define a group of patients who do not appear to benefit, identify the patient factors associated with improvement (which might inform a subsequent controlled trial), and perhaps suggest the ideal treatment protocol.

Conclusion

HBOT is a very safe medical treatment, but side effects (e.g., otic barotrauma, oxygen toxicity seizures) do occur and catastrophic events (e.g., deaths from fire) are possible. The ethical use of HBOT necessitates a risk vs. benefit assessment which may be impossible for some off-label indications when the likelihood of benefit is unknown. HBOT has been provided in an unethical manner even for "approved" indications as evidenced by recent Medicare fraud settlements. HBOT can be provided for off-label use in an ethical manner if there is a scientific rationale for its use, if the patient is informed of alternative treatments and the risks of HBOT, if the cost of therapy is clearly understood by the patient, and if the clinician discloses any financial incentives that might affect patient decision making. Case-by-case medical decisions to use HBOT for off-label indications do not require approval by Institutional Review Board (IRB), but if data are being collected with the intention of using that information to direct the care of future patients, then the activity should be considered research and IRB approval should be sought. The promotion of the off-label use of HBOT can be considered a breach of FDA regulations, but this issue is under FDA review.

The desperation of many patients and family members, and the many conditions for which there are few currently accepted satisfactory treatments (e.g., autism), combined with the ease of dissemination of information on the Internet and Social Media has produced enormous pressure to use HBOT off-label. Some studies claiming to involve "hyperbaric oxygen therapy" used oxygen pressures that could easily have been achieved or exceeded with an oxygen mask at sea level without the need for a hyperbaric chamber at all. No mechanism exists by which information about HBOT can be vetted for accuracy, and unsafe practices from a fire safety standpoint have occurred, particularly using inflatable chambers, based on easily viewed Internet advertisements. Cutbacks on insurance coverage for approved indications (as a result of healthcare austerity measures) could pressure even the most conservative hospitals and clinicians to offer HBOT for off-label indications, particularly if the FDA loosens restrictions on the marketing of the off-label use of medical devices.

Improved market regulations and oversight, better emphasis on the use of real HBOT as opposed to "low pressure oxygen/mild "HBOT" (sic), and the creation of a national registry to make available more and better patient outcome and side effects data are all urgently needed to protect patients and strengthen the code of ethics in hyperbaric medicine.

References

Alcantara LM, Leite JL, Trevizan MA, Mendes IA, Uggeri CJ, Stipp MA, et al. Legal issues of Brazilian hyperbaric nursing: why regulate? Rev Bras Enferm. 2010;63:312–6. Article in Portuguese.

The American Society of Medical Engineers (ASME). ASME Boiler and Pressure Vessel Code. An International Code. ASME, 2013. http://files.asme.org/Catalog/Codes/PrintBook/34011.pdf. Accessed 30 November 2015.

The American Society of Medical Engineers (ASME). ASME PVHO-1-2012. Safety Standard for Pressure Vessels for Human Occupancy. ASME, 2012. http://files.asme.org/Catalog/Codes/PrintBook/32398.pdf. Accessed 30 November 2015.

Bennett MH. Hyperbaric medicine and the placebo effect. Diving Hyperb Med. 2014;44:235–40.

Boumil MM. Off-label marketing and the first amendment. N Engl J Med. 2013;368:103–5.

Boussi-Gross R, Golan H, Fishlev G, Bechor Y, Volkov O, Bergan J, et al. Hyperbaric oxygen therapy can improve post concussion syndrome years after mild traumatic brain injury—randomized prospective trial. PLoS One. 2013;8, e79995.

Chan EC, Brody B. Ethical dilemmas in hyperbaric medicine. Undersea Hyperb Med. 2001;28:123–30.

Collet JP, Vanasse M, Marois P, Amar M, Goldberg J, Lambert J, et al. Hyperbaric oxygen for children with cerebral palsy: a randomised multicentre trial. HBO-CP Res Group. Lancet. 2001;357:582–6.

Cronin S. Mild hyperbaric oxygen chambers. 12 May 2012, Om Life. http://www.omlifeme.com/hyperbaric/. Accessed 20 July 2015.

Fife WP, Fife CE. Textbook of hyperbaric medicine. In: Jain KK, editor. Hyperbaric oxygen therapy in chronic Lyme disease. 5th ed. Göttingen Germany: Hogrefe; 2009. p. 149–55.

Gaffney A. FDA says medical device popular with elite athletes regularly misbranded. Regulatory Affairs Professionals Society. 22

August 2013. http://www.raps.org/focus-online/news/news-article-view/article/3980/. Accessed 30 November 2015.

Garakani A, Mitton AG. New-onset panic, depression with suicidal thoughts, and somatic symptoms in a patient with a history of Lyme disease. Case Rep Psychiatry. 2015;2015:457947.

Granpeesheh D, Tarbox J, Dixon DR, Wilke AE, Allen MS, Bradstreet JJ. Randomized trial of hyperbaric oxygen therapy for children with autism. Res Autism Spectr Disord. 2010;4:268–75.

Harch PG, Fogarty EF, Staab PK, Van Meter K. Low pressure hyperbaric oxygen therapy and SPECT brain imaging in the treatment of blast-induced chronic traumatic brain injury (post-concussion syndrome) and posttraumatic stress disorder: a case report. Cases J. 2009;2:6538.

Harch PG, Andrews SR, Fogarty EF, Amen D, Pezzullo JC, Lucarini J, et al. A phase I study of low-pressure hyperbaric oxygen therapy for blast-induced post-concussion syndrome and post-traumatic stress disorder. J Neurotrauma. 2012;29:168–85.

Healing-arts.org. Hyperbaric Oxygen Therapy Providers and Treatment Centers in the United States Treating Autism, Cerebral Palsy and Other Neurological Disorders. 2008. http://www.healing-arts.org/children/hyperbaricoxygen therapy_hbot.htm. Accessed 15 August 2015.

Heild C. Doctor accused of treating child who wasn't sick. Albuquerque Journal. 14 December 2014. http://www.abqjournal.com/512358/news/doctor-accused-of-treating-child-who-wasnt-sick.html. Accessed 20 July 2015.

Heuser G, Heuser SA, Rodelander D, Aguilera O, Uszler M. Treatment of Neurologically Impaired Adults and Children with "Mild" Hyperbaric Oxygen (1.3 ATA and 24% Oxygen). The Proceedings of the 2nd International Symposium of Hyperbaric Oxygenation for Cerebral Palsy and the Brain Injured Child. http://hyperbaricstudies.com/wp-content/uploads/Treatment-of-Neurologically-Impaired-Adults-and-Children-with-Mild-Hyperbaric-Oxygen.pdf. Accessed 11 September 2015.

Hu Q, Manaenko A, Guo Z, Huang L, Tang J, Zhang JH. Hyperbaric oxygen therapy for post concussion symptoms: issues may affect the results. Med Gas Res. 2015;5:10.

Hyperbaric Chambers, life-saving devices or killer machines? International Business Times. 24 January 2011. http://www.ibtimes.com/hyperbaric-chambers-life-saving-devices-or-killer-machines-258533. Accessed 20 July 2015.

Ibuki Health and Wellness. Hyperbaric oxygen therapy. http://ibuki-health.com/hyperbaric-oxygen-therapy/. Accessed 20 July 2015.

Inside Health Policy. Federal Judge Lets Amarin Promote Vascepa Off-Label, Says FDA Policies Violate 1st Amendment. August 7, 2015. http://insidehealthpolicy.com/login-redirect-no-cookie?n=84883&destination=node/84883. Accessed 10 August 2015.

Le PJ. Lessons to learn from federal convictions of HBOT fraud. Today's Wound Clinic. http://www.todayswoundclinic.com/articles/lessons-learn-federal-convictions-hbot-fraud. Accessed 20 July 2015.

Libov C. Oxygen therapy heals stroke damage. Newsmax. 25 March 2014. http://www.newsmax.com/Health/Headline/stroke-treatment-hyperbaric-oxygen-therapy-HBOT-COPD-Valerie-Green/2014/03/25/id/561674/. Accessed 30 October 2015.

Löndahl M, Katzman P, Nilsson A, Hammarlund C. Hyperbaric oxygen therapy facilitates healing of chronic foot ulcers in patients with diabetes. Diabetes Care. 2010;33:998–1003.

Mitchell SJ, Bennett MH. Unestablished indications for hyperbaric oxygen therapy. Diving Hyperb Med. 2014;44:228–34.

Moerman DE, Jonas WB. Deconstructing the placebo effect and finding the meaning response. Ann Intern Med. 2002;136:471–6.

National Fire Protection Association (NFPA). NFPA 99. In: NFPA: Health Care Facilities Code 2015 Edition. http://www.nfpa.org/codes-and-standards/document-information-pages?mode=code&code=99&tab=about. Accessed 21 July 2015.

National Fire Protection Association (NFPA). NFPA Online Catalog. NFPA 101: Life Safety Code, Prior Years. http://catalog.nfpa.org/NFPA-101-Life-Safety-Code-Prior-Years-P4160.aspx. Accessed 30 November 2015.

NAUI Worldwide. NAUI Dive Tables. NAUI Worldwide, 2015. http://naui.org/tables.aspx. Accessed 28 October 2015

Newton J. Patient killed after blowing up hospital ward when he decided to smoke a cigarette while undergoing treatment in high pressure oxygen chamber. Daily Mail.com. Updated July 31, 2014. http://www.daily-mail.co.uk/news/article-2711646/Patient-killed-blowing-hospital-ward-decided-smoke-cigarette-undergoing-treatment-high-pressure-oxygen-chamber.html#ixzz3szv6pHqM. Accessed 30 November 2015.

Sparks vs Oxy-Health, LLC/Oxy-Health Corporation, Civil Action 5:13-cv-00649-FL, 2014.

Paris JJ, Ferranti J, Reardon F. From the Johns Hopkins Baby to Baby Miller: what have we learned from four decades of reflection on neonatal cases? J Clin Ethics. 2001;12:207–14.

Paris JJ, Schreiber MD, Reardon FE. Hyperbaric oxygen therapy for a neurologically devastated child: whose decision is it? J Perinatol. 2003;23:250–3.

Portable Hyperbaric Chambers Australia. The Salus 36. Portable Hyperbaric Holdings Pty Ltd, 2014. http://02hyperbaricchambers.com/salus36-chamber/. Accessed July 20, 2015.

RAYCOM. World Now. Pastors use hyperbaric chambers as alternative medicine. 31 October 2013. Updated May 1, 2014. http://raycom-group.worldnow.com/story/23847706/pastors-use-hyperbaric-chambers-as-alternative-medicine. Accessed 20 July 2015.

Rech FV, Fagundes DJ, Hermanson R, Rivoire HC, Fagundes AL. A proposal of multiplace hyperbaric chamber for animal experimentation and veterinary use. Acta Cir Bras. 2008;23:384–90.

Rossignol DA, Rossignol LW, Smith S, Schneider C, Logerquist S, Usman A, et al. Hyperbaric treatment for children with autism: a multicenter, randomized, double-blind, controlled trial. BMC Pediatr. 2009;9:21.

Sheffield PJ, Desautels DA. Hyperbaric and hypobaric chamber fires: a 73-year analysis. Undersea Hyperb Med. 1997;24:153–64.

Sheffield PJ, Sheffield RB. Safety first: In the hyperbaric environment. Today's Wound Clinic. 2008;2(4). http://www.todayswoundclinic.com/articles/safety-first-hyperbaric-environment. Accessed 22 July 2015.

U.S. Department of Health and Human Services. Office of Inspector General. Hyperbaric Oxygen Therapy. Its Use and Its Appropriateness. October 2000; OEI 06-99-00090. http://oig.hhs.gov/oei/reports/oei-06-99-00090.pdf. Accessed 30 September 2015.

U.S. Food and Drug Administration (FDA). Hyperbaric oxygen therapy: don't be misled. FDA, 2013. Updated 15 May 2015. http://www.fda.gov/ForConsumers/ConsumerUpdates/ucm364687.htm. Accessed 20 July 2015.

U.S. Food and Drug Administration. Medical devices. 510(k) Clearances. Updated January 13, 2015. http://www.fda.gov/MedicalDevices/ProductsandMedicalProcedures/DeviceApprovalsandClearances/510kClearances/default.htm. Accessed 30 September 2015.

U.S. Food and Drug Administration. Regulatory information. FD&C Act Chapter V: Drugs and Devices. Updated September 25, 2015. http://www.fda.gov/RegulatoryInformation/Legislation/FederalFoodDrugandCosmeticActFDCAct/FDCActChapterVDrugsandDevices/default.htm. Accessed 30 September 2015.

Undersea & Hyperbaric Medical Society (UHMS). Indications for hyperbaric oxygen therapy. UHMS, 2015. https://www.uhms.org/resources/hbo-indications.html. Accessed 23 July 2015.

Walker J. Hyperbaric oxygen therapy gets more popular as unapproved treatment. The Wall Street Journal. 5 January 2015. http://www.wsj.com/articles/hyperbaric-oxygen-therapy-gets-more-popular-as-unapproved-autism-treatment-1420496506. Accessed 20 July 2015.

Wolf G, Cifu D, Baugh L, Carne W, Profenna L. The effect of hyperbaric oxygen on symptoms after mild traumatic brain injury. J Neurotrauma. 2012;29:2606–12.

Zimlich R. Equine hyperbaric oxygen chamber explosion in Florida kills woman and horse. Investigation could lead to new oversight on hyperbaric therapies. DVM360 Magazine. February 22, 2012. http://veterinarynews.dvm360.com/equine-hyperbaric-oxygen-chamber-explosion-florida-kills-woman-and-horse?rel=canonical. Accessed 20 July 2015.

K.K. Jain

Abstract

Hyperbaric medicine is practiced throughout the world, but the indications vary from one country to another. As examples, HBO developments in various countries are described here as well as the worldwide distribution of hyperbaric facilities. Since the USA is covered in Chap. 50 and Latin America in Chap. 51, the rest of the countries are included in this chapter with examples limited to Germany, China, Japan, and Russia.

Keywords

Hyperbaric oxygen (HBO) • Hyperbaric medicine • Indications for HBO • Hyperbaric chambers • Hyperbaric medicine in China • Hyperbaric medicine in Russia • Hyperbaric medicine in Japan • Hyperbaric medicine in Germany

Introduction

The practice of medicine varies around the world and so does hyperbaric medicine. It was considered appropriate to include a brief description of trends in the practice of hyperbaric medicine around the world. It was not possible to include all the countries. Only those countries outside of the USA where hyperbaric medicine is practiced on a significant scale are included. A brief description of hyperbaric medicine in the USA is given in Chap. 50 and Latin America in Chap. 51. This chapter will briefly describe the current state of hyperbaric medicine in China, Japan, Russia, and Germany. The European hyperbaric centers are list on the Oxynet website: http://www.oxynet.org/03HBOCenters/Index03.php. Within Europe, Italy, and Germany, each has the largest number of hyperbaric centers, i.e., ~30 in each. Turkey is next with ~28 hyperbaric centers, and France is in the third place with 20 hyperbaric centers. There are 13 hyperbaric centers in the UK. Hyperbaric medicine is not covered in the National Health Service of the UK. Most of the monoplace chambers are privately owned and used by multiple sclerosis patients.

Hyperbaric Medicine in China

The first Chinese hyperbaric chamber was built in 1964 by Dr. Wen-ren Li at Fujian Medical University Union Hospital; hyperbaric medicine developed rapidly in China after the cultural revolution, and there are now >5000 hyperbaric chambers in the country (Yan et al. 2015). The total staff including physicians, nurses, technicians, and research scientists is over 35,000. The number of patients treated yearly with HBO exceeds 2.5 million. Apart from the routine practice, research is being carried out on the mechanisms of action of HBO and its role in the management of the following conditions:

- Stroke
- Persistent vegetative state
- Autoimmune diseases
- Cancer
- Rejection in transplants

The Chinese Professional Committee of Hyperbaric Oxygen drafted the indication and contraindication stan-

K.K. Jain, MD, FRACS, FFPM (✉)
1 Blaesiring 7, Basel 4057, Switzerland
e-mail: jain@pharmabiotech.ch

© Springer International Publishing AG 2017
K.K. Jain, *Textbook of Hyperbaric Medicine*, DOI 10.1007/978-3-319-47140-2_49

dards of practice in 1982 in an effort to reduce the number of patients experiencing toxic side effects of HBO therapy. The Chinese Medical Association revised the indication and contraindication standards in 2004 and 2013; the 2004 version is widely used in clinical practice, followed by the indications and contraindications of 2004. Indications and contraindications for hyperbaric oxygen in China are shown in Table 49.1.

There is considerable research activity in hyperbaric medicine in China. By mid-2016, there are ~15,000 articles that can be retrieved from various databases using "hyperbaric oxygen" and "China" as keywords, of which 395 articles appeared in PubMed. This amount of hyperbaric oxygen research suggests that HBO therapy in China is still in the development stage. The amount of published HBO research has been increasing every year during the past decade.

Hyperbaric Medicine in Japan

This account is partially based on the chapter on this topic in the 5th edition of this textbook written by late Prof. Hideo Takahashi from University of Nagoya and has been updated by the current author. Before World War I, research on hyperbaric medicine in Japan was focused mainly on the environmental physiology of Ama diving or the industrial hygiene of caisson workers. Hyperbaric air was used for stroke rehabilitation in the late 1050s. Clinical work in hyperbaric medicine started in 1960s with the construction of a hyperbaric surgical theater and a hyperbaric recovery room at Tokyo University. Around the same time, a series of clinical investigations of hyperbaric oxygen therapy were initiated at Nagoya University, which led to the installation

Table 49.1 Indications for HBO approved by the Chinese Medical Association 2013

Emergency indications, first line
1. Acute carbon monoxide poisoning and other harmful gas poisoning
2. Gas gangrene, tetanus, and other anaerobic bacteria infections
3. Decompression sickness
4. Air embolism syndrome
5. A variety of risks for acute brain dysfunction after cardiopulmonary resuscitation (CPR)
6. Aid in the treatment of shock
7. Brain edema
8. Pulmonary edema (except cardiac pulmonary edema
9. Crush syndrome
10. Compromised blood supply after skin transplantation of limbs (finger, toe)
11. Drug and chemical poisoning
12. Acute ischemia anoxic encephalopathy
Second-line indications, nonemergency, adjunctive
1. Carbon monoxide poisoning or other toxic encephalopathy
2. Sudden deafness
3. Ischemic cerebrovascular disease (cerebral arteriosclerosis, transient ischemic attack, cerebral thrombosis, cerebral infarction)
4. Craniocerebral injury (concussion, cerebral contusion of intracranial hematoma removal surgery, brain stem injury)
5. Cerebral hemorrhage recovery
6. Poor healing fractures
7. Central serous retinal inflammation
8. Vegetative state
9. Plateau adaptation insufficiency syndrome
10. Peripheral nerve injury
11. Intracranial benign tumor surgery
12. Periodontal disease
13. Viral encephalitis
14. Facial paralysis
15. Osteomyelitis
16. Aseptic osteonecrosis
17. Cerebral palsy
18. Fetal developmental delays
19. Diabetes and diabetic foot
20. Coronary atherosclerotic heart disease (angina and myocardial infarction)
21. Rapidity arrhythmia (atrial fibrillation, premature beat, tachycardia)
22. Myocarditis

(continued)

Table 49.1 (continued)

23. Peripheral vascular disease; vasculitis, e.g., Raynaud's disease; deep vein thrombosis; etc.
24. Vertigo
25. Chronic skin ulcer (arterial blood supply obstacles, venous congestion, bedsore)
26. Spinal cord injury
27. Peptic ulcer
28. Ulcerative colitis
29. Infectious hepatitis (use the special chamber of infectious disease)
30. Burns
31. Frostbite
32. Plastic surgery
33. Skin grafting
34. Sports injuries
35. Radioactive damage (bone and soft tissue, cystitis, etc.)
36. Malignant tumors (with radiotherapy or chemotherapy)
37. Otic nerve injury
38. Fatigue syndrome
39. Angioneurotic headache
40. Pustular
41. Psoriasis
42. Pityriasis rosea
43. Multiple sclerosis
44. Acute Guillain-Barre syndrome
45. Recurrent oral ulcer
46. Paralytic ileus
47. Bronchial asthma
48. Acute respiratory distress syndrome
Absolute contraindication
Untreated tension pneumothorax
Relative contraindications
1. Intraventricular external drainage
2. Fracture of the skull base with cerebrospinal fluid leakage
3. Birth weight < 2000 g in premature and low birth weight infants
4. Serious infection of the upper respiratory tract
5. High blood pressure (syst BP > 180 mmHg, diast BP > 110 mmHg)
6. Patients with chronic obstructive pulmonary disease with CO_2 retention

of the world's largest hyperbaric chamber there (see Chap. 7). Many new indications for HBO were developed there. This was followed by installation of multiplace chambers at Osaka and Kyoto Universities. The Japanese Society for Hyperbaric Medicine (JSHM) was formed in 1969. In 1982, JSHM launched the Educational Course in Hyperbaric Medicine for hyperbaric nurses and engineers. In 1981, the *Japanese Journal of Hyperbaric Medicine*, the official journal of JSHM started to publish quarterly. Currently accepted indications for HBO by JSHM are listed in Table 49.2.

At the end of year 2015, the total number of hyperbaric chambers in Japan was ~820, of which 760 were monoplace (93%) and 60 multiplace (7%). These chambers are located at 620 medical facilities. The total number of clinical chambers is still growing and at least one university hospital introduces a new multiplace chamber every year.

Historically, Japanese hyperbaric medicine has emphasized clinical applications, and fundamental research to provide a scientific background for clinical indications has tended to be delayed. By conducting more basic investigations, many new indications will be established in the future. One of the most important goals of HBO therapy is to participate in cancer therapy; the combination of hyperbaric medicine and oncology is considered to be an attractive new horizon.

Hyperbaric Medicine in Russia

Russia has extensive hyperbaric facilities. There are >60 centers with hyperbaric facilities and ~1400 hyperbaric chambers are currently in use. HBO therapy indications in Russia do not resemble those recommended by the Undersea and Hyperbaric Medical Society in the USA. HBO is used in the following areas of medicine in Russia: cardiology, pulmonology, gastroenterology, hepatology, nephrology, hematology, oncology, endocrinology, rheumatology, allergology

Table 49.2 Currently accepted indications for hyperbaric oxygen therapy in Japan as recommended by the Japanese Society for Hyperbaric Medicine

Emergency (acute) indications

1. Acute carbon monoxide and other gas-induced intoxications, including delayed intoxications
2. Gas gangrene
3. Air embolism and decompression sickness
4. Acute peripheral vascular disorders:
    (a) Severe burn injury and frostbite
    (b) Combined with large crush injury or massive vascular damage
5. Shock
6. Myocardial infarction and other coronary insufficiencies
7. Consciousness disorders and brain edema after brain embolism or severe cranial injury
8. Acute and severe hypoxic disorder of the brain
9. Paralytic ileus
10. Acute obstructive disorders of the retinal artery
11. Sudden deafness
12. Severe spinal cord disorders

Nonemergency (chronic) indications

1. Malignant neoplasms, combined with radiation or chemotherapy
2. Peripheral circulatory disorders with refractory ulcers
3. Skin grafts
4. Subacute myelo-opticoneuropathy (SMON)
5. Motor paresis, as the later sequelae of cerebrovascular attack, severe cranial injury, or craniotomy
6. Delayed syndromes in carbon monoxide intoxication
7. Spinal cord neuropathy
8. Osteomyelitis and radiation necrosis

and immunology, infectious disease, emergency medicine, diving medicine, general surgery, orthopedic surgery, thermal injuries, neurology, neurosurgery, obstetrics and gynecology, neonatology and pediatrics, otolaryngology, clinical toxicology, ophthalmology, urology, and psychiatry. There are >60 approved indications for HBO therapy in Russia, and some of these are shown in Table 49.3.

Hyperbaric Medicine in Germany

Germany is chosen as an example in Europe as it has played an important part in the development of modern hyperbaric medicine, particularly in the applications for neurological disorders. Important work in this area was done in the late 1960s and early 1970s at the University Neurosurgical Clinic, Bonn, by Professor K.H. Holbach and colleagues, of whom Prof. Wassmann continued this work. The author (K.K.J.) had an opportunity to work with this team. HBO was applied to patients with head injuries and stroke, and the important contribution was the response to HBO for selecting patients for extra-intracranial bypass operation. This application of HBO did not spread in clinical practice for the next decade when the group in Bonn moved to other centers and followed other interests in neurosurgery. In 1980s, research was done into the applications of HBO for inner ear disorders, particularly

sudden deafness. In 1986, the author returned to Germany and during the following 3 years had a chance to work on the clinical applications of HBO in a rehabilitation clinic. This is where the work on treatment of chronic stroke patients was carried out.

In Germany, the professional scientific association for hyperbaric oxygen therapy is the "Gesellschaft für Tauch- und Überdruckmedizin e.V." This professional association evaluates possible applications of HBO therapy from a medical perspective. On its websites (https://www.gtuem.org/), there is a directory with contact details of pressure chambers in Germany, Austria, and Switzerland.

In 1989, there were only four active hyperbaric chambers for clinical HBO therapy in Germany. In recent years, there has been a rapid expansion of hyperbaric facilities in Germany, and as of mid-2016, there are 30 hyperbaric centers in Germany. The breakdown according to availability and scope of service is as follows:

Centers for emergency use of HBO and for diving accidents	6
Centers with 24 h service for HBO therapy and availability of intensive care beds	5
Centers with 24 h availability of outpatient HBO therapy but no hospital beds	4
Centers with limited hours of service for HBO therapy	15

Table 49.3 Indications for hyperbaric oxygen in Russia

Vascular diseases
Arterial obstructions in the limbs before and after surgery (embolism, trauma, thrombosis)
Arteriosclerosis
Gas embolism in the blood vessels
Ulcers caused by defective blood circulation
Cardiac disorders
Heart strain
Heart rhythm disturbances
Irregular heartbeat
Paroxysmal extrasystole
Cardiac insufficiency
Cardiosclerosis decompensation
Cardiac insufficiency after heart surgery
Heart contraction disturbances
Cardiopulmonary insufficiency
Pulmonary disorders
Lung abscess before and after surgery
Nonspecific chronic lung affections with cardiopulmonary insufficiency signs
Gastrointestinal disorders
Stomach and duodenal ulcers
Intestinal obstruction
Liver diseases
Acute viral hepatitis
Hepatic encephalitis
Liver cirrhosis
Obstructive jaundice
Hepatic insufficiency after resuscitation
Toxic hepatitis

Germany has only multiplace chambers (monoplace chambers are not approved in Germany currently), and >60,000 patients were treated in the year 2015. Most of these patients (about 85%) are treated on an ambulatory basis. Some of these chambers are in university centers where research is done, and others are private business enterprises with little research activity.

Germany has the usual indications accepted in most Western countries. Most HBO therapies are conducted for the following indications:

- Tinnitus
- Acute hearing loss with or without tinnitus
- Noise-induced hearing loss, acoustic trauma
- Chronic wound(s)
- Diabetic foot: nonhealing wound(s)
- Bone marrow necrosis
- Radiation cystitis
- Radiation proctitis
- Borreliosis/lyme arthritis

Use for tinnitus and hearing loss is more common in Germany than in other countries.

World Distribution of Hyperbaric Facilities

Some idea of the quantity of hyperbaric medical facilities in the world can be obtained by a review of the statistics regarding the distribution of hyperbaric chambers in various countries. Accurate information on this subject is difficult to obtain, but the available figures are shown in Fig. 49.1. The largest number of chambers is located in China (>5000) and the USA with 2400 chambers is next. Russia has ~1800, Japan has ~820, and Europe has ~480 hyperbaric chambers.

The total number of hyperbaric chambers in the world is not known. The number of chambers does not necessarily correlate with the number of patients or the number of treatments given. There is no separation of multiplace and monoplace chambers in the statistics for most countries.

Worldwide Distribution of Hyperbaric Chambers

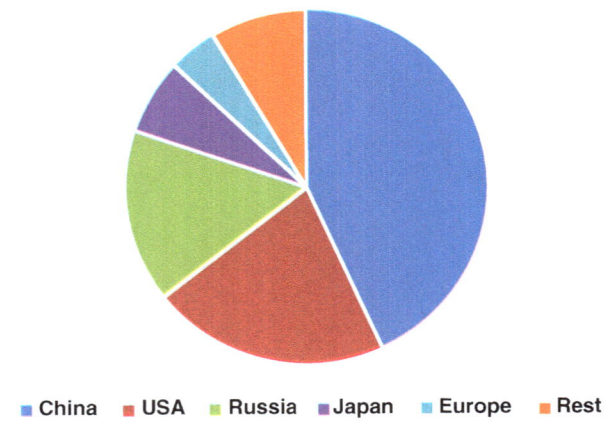

■ China ■ USA ■ Russia ■ Japan ■ Europe ■ Rest

Fig. 49.1 World distribution of hyperbaric chambers

Conclusion

Hyperbaric medicine is practiced worldwide with the greatest activity in China, Russia, and the USA. The USA has the most regulated applications of HBO with the most restrictive list of applications. Japan is also active in hyperbaric medicine in clinical applications as well as in research. China has the largest number of hyperbaric chambers and is most active in basic as well as clinical research in HBO therapy. Within Europe, Germany and Italy are most active in hyperbaric medicine and have the largest number of hyperbaric centers.

Reference

Yan L, Liang T, Cheng O. Hyperbaric oxygen therapy in China. Med Gas Res. 2015;5:3.

Hyperbaric Medicine in the United States

50

Thomas M. Bozzuto

Abstract

This chapter discusses the practice of hyperbaric medicine in the United States, the various organizations involved in the practice, certifying agencies for practitioners, the status of certification, and the current legislative and reimbursement issues.

Keywords

Hyperbaric medicine • American College of Hyperbaric Medicine • Undersea and Hyperbaric Medical Society • Baromedical Nurses Association • National Board of Diving and Hyperbaric Medical Technology

Introduction

The early history of hyperbaric medicine in the United States has been partially covered in Chap. 1. The first organization formed to encompass this specialty was the Undersea Medical Society (UMS), which was primarily devoted to diving medicine, as the original name indicated prior to addition of the word hyperbaric. Later, in order to include the practice of clinical hyperbaric medicine, the name of the society was changed to Undersea and Hyperbaric Medical Society (UHMS). As of 2015, there are now seven chapters of the parent organization including one in Canada and one in Brazil. A chapter is currently forming in Saudi Arabia. There are 2,303 UHMS members as of 2016 and approximately 17 % of its membership is international. In 1992, the first board certification examination in the sub-specialty of Undersea Medicine was offered by the American Board of Preventive Medicine (ABPM). Ten physicians took the examination. It then went dormant until 1998. The name of the examination was then changed to Undersea and Hyperbaric Medicine to reflect the increase in clinical hyper-

baric medicine practice, and in 2000, the American Board of Emergency Medicine (ABEM) began offering the same sub-specialty board certification. Later, the American Osteopathic Board of Preventive Medicine (AOBPM) started offering the Certificate of Added Qualification (equivalent to the ABEM Sub-Specialty Board Certification). Since the last edition of this textbook, all three examining bodies have retired the "grandfathering clause" and now a one-year fellowship is required in order to take the examination. There are currently approximately 533 physicians who are sub-specialty certified in Undersea and Hyperbaric Medicine through either ABEM or ABPM, and 28 through AOBPM. In 2012, the UHMS initiated a category of Fellowship in Undersea and Hyperbaric Medicine which is awarded to members who have shown dedication and excellence in the field by recommendation of current fellows. As of this writing there are 58 fellows, one of whom has passed away. The UHMS will celebrate its 50th anniversary with an Annual Scientific Meeting at the Wyndam Rio Mar Beach Resort and Spa in Puerto Rico from 22 to 24 June 2017 (www.uhms.org).

The first organization of physicians devoted to hyperbaric medicine was the American College of Hyperbaric Medicine (ACHM) which was founded in 1983 by Drs. Richard Neubauer, Charles Shilling, William Maxfield, and J.R. Maxfield. A key figure in the development of hyperbaric medicine in the United States was Dr. Edger End. He carried out the earlier trials of HBO in CO poisoning. He is also the

T.M. Bozzuto, DO, FACEP, FFACHM, UHM/ABEM (✉)
Phoebe Putney Memorial Hospital, Wound Care and Hyperbaric Center, 803 N Jefferson St., Suite A, Albany, GA 31701, USA
e-mail: tbozzuto@ppmh.org

© Springer International Publishing AG 2017
K.K. Jain, *Textbook of Hyperbaric Medicine*, DOI 10.1007/978-3-319-47140-2_50

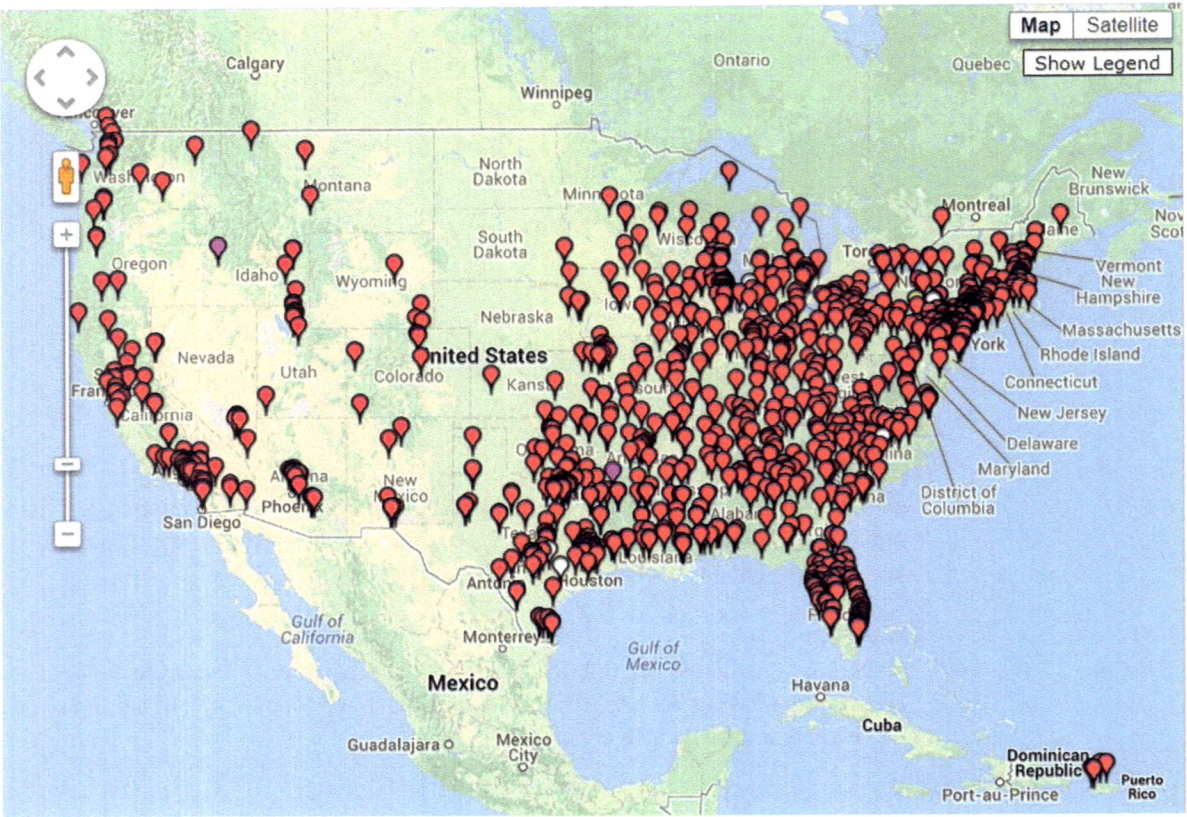

Fig. 50.1 Hospital-based hyperbaric programs in the United States

inventor of SCUBA gear and the use of liquids as an oxygen substitute for respiration while diving, among numerous other innovations. He was a visionary who predicted that the use of HBO would extend beyond treatment of wounds into other clinical applications, particularly in diseases of the nervous system. Drs. End and Neubauer published a paper on the use of HBO in stroke in 1980. Dr. Neubauer applied and investigated the use of HBO in neurological disorders such as stroke, multiple sclerosis, and hypoxic encephalopathies. He also pioneered the use of SPECT scan in evaluating the effect of HBO in stroke. Other applications of SPECT are in reassessing the late effects of decompression sickness on the brain.

Distribution of hospital-based hyperbaric programs in the United States is shown in Fig. 50.1.

In the year 2014, the number of hyperbaric facilities had increased to approximately 1200, with approximately 50 to 70 multiplace chambers and about 2300 to 2400 monoplace chambers, but the figures for the breakdown into various categories are not available. Because of the growth of contract management companies who contract with hospitals to run the hyperbaric units, and the increasing cost of staffing, with many emergency patients being uninsured, the number of 24/7 hyperbaric facilities in the United States has decreased

dramatically. The number of freestanding "hyperbaric" centers in spas, chiropractors' offices, homes, etc., using "low pressure" chambers (Gamow Bags) promoting off-label uses for hyperbaric oxygen therapy has increased dramatically.

In an effort to raise the quality of care provided to the hyperbaric patient, the Undersea & Hyperbaric Medical Society (UHMS) established a clinical hyperbaric facility accreditation program in 2001. The objective of the program is to ensure that clinical hyperbaric facilities are:

- Staffed with the proper specialists who are well-trained
- Using quality equipment that has been properly installed and maintained, and being operated with the highest level of safety possible
- Providing high quality of patient care
- Maintaining the appropriate documentation of informed consent, patient treatment procedures, physician involvement, etc.

Since the first survey in September 2002, the UHMS has accredited 235 centers, with 197 being active. Fifty-eight surveys are scheduled for 2016. At the present time, accreditation is voluntary in all states except for Utah. The Utah Medicaid Program Office requires UHMS-specific accreditation to be reimbursed for hyperbaric oxygen therapy by that program.

There is a growing international interest in hyperbaric facility accreditation. The UHMS is working with representatives from Brazil, Mexico, Australia, New Zealand, Singapore, Sweden and others to establish accreditation programs in these respective countries.

American College of Hyperbaric Medicine

The American College of Hyperbaric Medicine (ACHM) continues to serve as a medical specialty society for physicians practicing hyperbaric medicine. In the US, ACHM works to deliver support and services to nearly 200 physicians in 40 states, many of whom practice clinical hyperbaric medicine. A small number of physicians from outside the United States also belong to the organization. One of the most important roles of the College involves responding to events impacting the field. Advocacy efforts help create a cohesive group of clinical hyperbaric physicians. Functions and goals of the ACHM are:

Development of Hyperbaric Medicine as a Specialty. A goal of the College is to develop an image of hyperbaric medicine as a distinct medical specialty. In support of that goal, it represents hyperbaric physicians before organized medicine bodies, supports certification of experienced hyperbaric physicians, sponsors special events for hyperbaric fellows, and maintains an active publications program. Among other things, the College publishes hyperbaric protocols and a directory of clinical hyperbaric physicians. There is an examination for certifying specialists in hyperbaric Medicine in the United States and in other countries. There is also Fellowship recognition for certified hyperbaric physicians who are members of the College and have made significant contributions to the field.

Specialist Certification. The ACHM has joined with the American Professional Wound Care Association to offer certification examinations for hyperbaric medicine and wound care (these examinations are not recognized by the American Board of Medical Specialties). A certification program, which includes an examination, helps to create an identifiable group of expert hyperbaric physicians. Fifty-seven physicians have taken the hyperbaric examination and 12 have taken both. Both the UHMS and ACHM have promulgated position papers on physician credentialing and they can be found on their respective websites.

A New Examination. The American Professional Wound Care Association (APWCA) was contacted about two years ago by members of the American College of Hyperbaric Medicine (ACHM) who expressed their opinion that there was a need for a certification process in wound care available to their members that was physician oriented. After reviewing options, they concluded that the APWCA was the most appropriate organization for them to work. An ad hoc committee was established with key members of both organizations which investigated the concept further and found that there is a growing need for some formal process to distinguish those who are skilled in the art and science of wound care. An examination construction committee was established with members from the two professional societies. This gave a tremendous jump start to the creation of a physician certifying examination. While the APWCA has supported this initiative at many levels and will endorse the examination, a separate testing organization will administer the certification process. The development of this physician examination is a first step toward the long-term goal of achieving specialty recognition of wound care by the American Board of Medical Specialties, American Osteopathic Association, and the Council of Podiatric Medical Education.

Reimbursement for Hyperbaric Treatments. In recent years, the ACHM successfully worked together with a consortium of hyperbaric groups (including the UHMS) to resolve a serious funding crisis that threatened to close as many as 80% of the hyperbaric chambers in the US. In the end, hospital-based facilities received increased Medicare fees for their services. College officers often work to assure adequate reimbursement for hyperbaric treatments and represent hyperbaric physicians before bodies that determine reimbursement policies for hyperbaric medicine. They provide information at the request of such bodies. College officials are now working to increase Medicare payment rates to hyperbaric physicians.

In early 2003, ACHM was pressing the Centers for Medicare and Medicaid Services (CMS) to appropriately adjust the overhead expensive RVU (relative value unit) of the CPT Code 99183 (physician attendance and supervision of hyperbaric oxygen therapy) to accurately reflect the high overhead of availability of hyperbaric medical services and high physician costs of providing this service, and to appropriately adjust the total RVU of CPT 99183 to accurately reflect the requirement for constant attendance and supervision during the hyperbaric oxygen therapy session as mandated by Medicare guidelines.

The ACHM asked CMS to increase reimbursement rates to physicians because of the significant overhead involved in on call duties, treating indigent patients and emergency treatments.

After a reimbursement battle lasting more than 4 years, CMS recently increased payments for facility fees to hospitals with hyperbaric centers. Hopefully the move will stop closures of US hyperbaric centers. Over a dozen ceased operations while the new policy was being developed.

The crisis arose over the proposal by CMS predecessor, the Health Care Financing Administration (HCFA) to stop paying for an important hyperbaric indication. Effective the spring of 2000, HCFA had announced plans to end payments for using hyperbaric oxygen therapies to prepare compromised wound beds for skin grafts. To resolve the crisis, a delay was requested, and another hyperbaric organization, the Undersea and Hyperbaric Medical Association (UHMS) proposed that HCFA create a new indication, ischemic wound. ACHM supported this proposal.

While CMS refused to create an indication for ischemic wound, officials said they would reconsider this policy if more evidence were presented. A final Medicare policy on payments for diabetic wounds of the lower extremities (DWLE) was published in December 2002 and took effect April 1, 2003. The preparation of scientific data by hyperbaric physicians and submission to CMS helped produce the favorable final DWLE policy.

Medicare officials agreed to pay for treatment of DWLE for patients at hospital facilities who meet strict guidelines. Criteria include (1) patients who have Type I or Type II diabetes and have a lower extremity wound due to diabetes, (2) patients who have a wound classified as a Wagner Grade II or higher, and (3) patients who have failed an adequate course of standard wound therapy. It will not pay for treating DWLE with hyperbaric oxygen as an initial treatment. The benefit category for HBO therapy (DWLE) was hospital outpatient services, physician services, or incident to physician services. In practice this means freestanding centers are paid no technical fees for DWLE or other CMS-approved indications. Freestanding centers only receive physician fees for services provided; however, freestanding centers' physician fees are slightly higher to compensate for the loss of technical fees.

Another crisis arose in 2015 when Blue Cross/Blue Shield circulated an (internal) assessment of hyperbaric treatments, leading to some historically well documented treatments being labeled as investigational, and therefore not reimbursed. One of the most significant of these is radiation injury, which accounts for approximately 40–60% of all hyperbaric treatments rendered in the United States. For most hyperbaric programs, loss of the revenue generated from this therapy will lead to program closure, as they will no longer be self-supporting. The ACHM has already seen a "chilling" effect as hospitals are postponing entry into the field of hyperbaric medicine until the full impact of the BCBS decision is assessed. The College initiated a Radionecrosis Registry whereby facilities could enroll and electronically submit their data which will be collected, de-identified and submitted to third-party payors. This Radionecrosis Registry will serve as the basis for reporting outcomes, success rates, and cost savings when compared with historical controls and the natural course of the disease in patients without hyperbaric therapy. At the present time, three states (Idaho, Pennsylvania, and Hawaii) are affected by the BCBS central office recommendation for non-payment of these services. So far, the registry as reached over 1000 cases making it the largest study ever conducted in hyperbaric medicine.

Medicare has published Quality Measures for Hyperbaric Medicine and Wound care which are linked to physician reimbursement (Figs. 50.2 and 50.3).

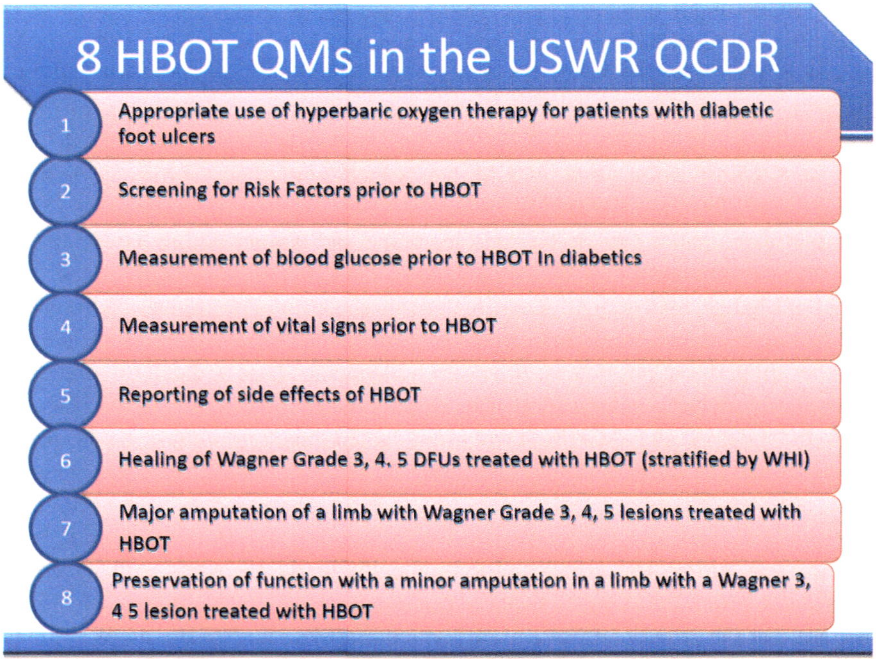

Fig. 50.2 Quality measures for hyperbaric oxygen therapy

8 HBOT QMs in the USWR QCDR

1. Appropriate use of hyperbaric oxygen therapy for patients with diabetic foot ulcers
2. Screening for Risk Factors prior to HBOT
3. Measurement of blood glucose prior to HBOT In diabetics
4. Measurement of vital signs prior to HBOT
5. Reporting of side effects of HBOT
6. Healing of Wagner Grade 3, 4, 5 DFUs treated with HBOT (stratified by WHI)
7. Major amputation of a limb with Wagner Grade 3, 4, 5 lesions treated with HBOT
8. Preservation of function with a minor amputation in a limb with a Wagner 3, 4 5 lesion treated with HBOT

Fig. 50.3 Quality measures
for wound care

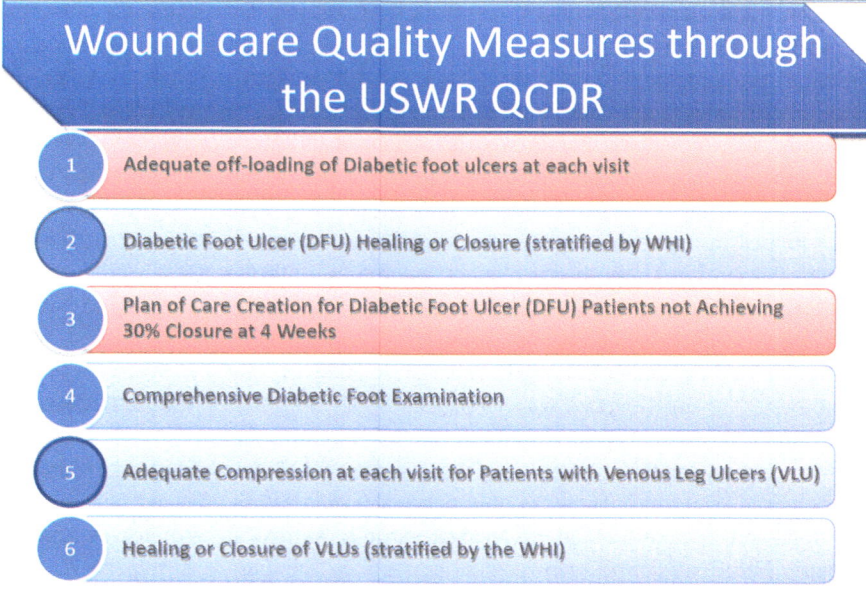

Despite a strong scientific rationale and compelling basic science data, the field of hyperbaric medicine faces existential threats in the US from changes in Medicare coverage policy, a perceived lack of sufficient high quality evidence to satisfy some payers, increasing regulatory burdens, and reductions in reimbursement rates, to name only a few issues. The majority of hyperbaric treatments are provided in hospital-based outpatient clinics which bill for services under "provider-based" rules. These clinics can charge a hospital facility fee for providing the hyperbaric service as long as a properly credentialed advanced practitioner provides direct supervision. Both the Centers for Medicare and Medicaid Services (CMS) and some regional Medicare Administrative Carriers (MACs) have established criteria which practitioners must meet in order to bill Medicare for hyperbaric chamber supervision, the Current Procedural Terminology (CPT®)[1] code for which is 99183, "physician attendance and supervision of hyperbaric oxygen therapy, per session." The UHMS has created training and credentialing recommendations for physicians who would supervise hyperbaric treatments (https://www.uhms.org/resources/news-announcements/108-uhms-credentialing-and-privileging-guidelines-for-hyperbaric-medicine-physicians-in-the-u-s-a.html) and has also detailed the responsibilities and activities which comprise the supervision of a patient undergoing a hyperbaric oxygen therapy treatment.

National Board of Diving and Hyperbaric Medical Technology

National Board of Diving and Hyperbaric Medical Technology (NBDHMT) is the long-established and respected certification organization for those who support the delivery of undersea medicine and hyperbaric oxygen therapy. The Board was introduced in 1985 and first called the National Association of Diver Medic Technicians (DMTs). Its dual purpose was the formalization of DMT training standards and introduction of DMT certification. DMT training had first occurred in 1975 as a method to enhance on-site medical presence at geographically remote commercial oilfield installations. Previous efforts to incorporate training and certification into existing organization had been unsuccessful.

In 1991, the name was changed to reflect growing certification interest by hospital-based hyperbaric technicians and hyperbaric nurses. Certification in hyperbaric technology was introduced in that same year. Hyperbaric nursing certification became available in 1995. This was followed by certification in veterinary hyperbaric technology in 2011.

Baromedical Nurses Association

Hyperbaric nursing had its origins in the 1950s, in Europe. Nurses were called upon to support multiplace chambers as the practice of hyperbaric medicine evolved from the treatment of divers (undersea medicine) to those illnesses and diseases suffered by more traditional patient populations.

---

[1] Personal communication, Dr. Caroline Fife.

Initially, nurses learnt their roles via on-the-job training. By the 1960s, formal training became available and was soon an essential prerequisite. This period coincided with the introduction of monoplace hyperbaric chambers.

Many such hyperbaric nurses were experienced in critical care, emergency room, and medical-surgical areas, which reflected the nature of the early referable indications. They were cross-trained in hyperbaric oxygen therapy. Nurses eventually became involved and published in clinical research. In 1978, the first US hyperbaric conference included workshops specifically for nurses. It was sponsored by the Baromedical Department at Memorial Medical Center in Long Beach, CA. In 2002, the first Hyperbaric Nursing Textbook was published.

In 1985, the specialty of hyperbaric nursing became formally recognized with the founding of the Baromedical Nurses Association. The BNA, now an international organization, develops and maintains standards of practice in baromedical nursing. The BNA defines baromedical nursing as "the diagnosis and treatment of human response to actual or potential health problems in the altered environment of the hyperbaric chamber." The role of the hyperbaric nurse is multifunctional and includes the clinician, educator, research, and manager. The goal of hyperbaric nursing is to provide safe, cost-effective, quality patient care, according to established standards.

In the early 1990s, a BNA committee chaired by Diane Norkool wrote the first set of nursing certification questions with the goal to provide an added competency to hyperbaric nursing. Dick Clarke, President of the NBDHMT, invited the BNA to be a part of the NBDHMT certification process. This occurred and established according to nursing regulatory guidelines in that 40 % of the examination would directly relate to nursing activities, the balance of the examination being technical, safety, and operational. The Baromedical Nurses Association Certification Board (BNACB) was established in 1995. The first nursing certification was given in 1995 and was taken by the Board members of the BNA. There are currently over 900 hyperbaric certified nurses. The nurse may achieve the level of CHRN (Certified Hyperbaric Registered Nurse), ACHRN (Advanced Certified Hyperbaric Registered Nurse), or CHRNC (Certified Hyperbaric Registered Nurse Clinician).

Indications for Use of Hyperbaric Oxygen

Hyperbaric medicine represents an emerging medical specialty whose scientific basis, while supported by over 6,000 studies, continues to be explored. The UHMS supports use of hyperbaric therapy for the 14 indications published in the Undersea and Hyperbaric Medical Society Hyperbaric Oxygen Committee Report (Table 51.1). The 13th Edition was published in April 2014. It also supports research into investigational uses of hyperbaric oxygen therapy.

Resources

Undersea and Hyperbaric Medical Society (www.uhms.org)
American College of Hyperbaric Medicine (www.achm.org)
American Board of Wound Healing (www.abwh.net)
American Professional Wound Care Association (www.apwca.org)

Table 51.1 UHMS approved indications for hyperbaric oxygen therapy (2014)

1. Carbon monoxide poisoning
2. Cyanide poisoning
3. Air or gas embolism
4. Clostridial myositis and myonecrosis (gas gangrene)
5. Crush injury, compartment syndrome and other acute traumatic ischemias
6. Decompression sickness
7. Arterial insufficiencies
   (a) Central retinal artery occlusion[a,c]
   (b) Enhancement of healing in selected problem wounds[b]
8. Severe anemia[c]
9. Intracranial abscess[c]
10. Necrotizing soft tissue infections
11. Osteomyelitis (refractory)
12. Delayed radiation injury (soft tissue or bone)
13. Compromised skin grafts or flaps
14. Acute thermal burn injury[c]
15. Idiopathic sudden sensorineural hearing loss[a,c]

[a]Conditions added since last edition of textbook
[b]Includes diabetic wounds
[c]Conditions approved by UHMS but not approved by Medicare (some third-party insurance companies will cover these conditions)

Baromedical Nurses Association (www.bna.org)

National Board of Diving and Hyperbaric Medical Technology (www.NBDHMT.org)

Organizations for Subspecialty Certification

American Board of Emergency Medicine (www.abem.org)

American Board of Preventive Medicine (www.theabpm.org)

American Osteopathic Board of Preventive Medicine (www. abopm.org)

Currently Offered Fellowship Training Locations in Undersea and Hyperbaric Medicine

CRESE at the University of Buffalo

Buffalo, NY

Contact: Dr. David R. Pendergast

716-829-3830

Postdoctoral Fellowship

The Center for Research and Education in Special Environments in the School of Medicine and Biomedical Sciences at the University at Buffalo is recruiting for a Postdoctoral Fellow with interest in one or more of the following fields: undersea and hyperbaric medicine, environmental physiology, gravity, or exercise physiology. This is a 3-year Office of Naval Research-funded fellowship. The successful candidate must have a Medical Degree or Ph.D. or equivalent. CRESE is a grant-supported multidisciplinary, officially recognized University Organized Research Center. The major facilities include a human-rated hyperbaric/hypobaric chamber, animal/cell hyperbaric chambers, human centrifuge, climatic chamber, and annular swimming pool. Additionally, there are exercise, biochemistry, animal surgery, and open laboratories and offices. Applications will be considered until the position is filled.

Duke University Medical Center

Durham, NC

Contact: Jake Freiberger, MD, MPH

Email: john.freiberger@duke.edu

(919) 684-6726

Home Page: dukedivemedicine.org

Hyperbaric fellows work in the Center for Hyperbaric Medicine and Environmental Physiology, an integral part of Duke University Medical Center. Four slots are available each year, 2 of which are associated thru Intermountain Healthcare. Applicants must be eligible for licensure as a trainee in the state of North Carolina and they must have completed an ACGME certified residency program and be board eligible in their specialty. The fellowship is highly

competitive and the training is designed to prepare the fellow to become a leader in the field of Undersea and Hyperbaric Medicine through the development of clinical competence and research expertise.

Hennepin County Medical Center

Minneapolis, MN

Contact: Stephen Hendriksen, MD

Email: Stephen.Hendriksen@hcmed.org

612-873-7420

Home Page: http://www.hcmc.org/education/fellowships/ hyperbaric-fellowship/index.htm

Undersea and Hyperbaric Medicine Fellowship

Since opening our first hyperbaric chamber in 1964, Hennepin County Medical Center has pioneered the field of undersea and hyperbaric medicine. Our fellowship is an ACGME accredited one year program whose graduates fulfill the requirements to sit for the American Board of Medical Specialists' certification examination for special competency in Undersea and Hyperbaric Medicine. The Primary Hospital: Hennepin County Medical Center, Minneapolis, MN is a Level I Trauma Center and referral center for all hyperbaric emergencies for western Wisconsin, the eastern Dakotas, Iowa and all of Minnesota. Fellows practice in our new state-of-the art Center for Hyperbaric Medicine, which opened in 2012. More information can be found at our website:

Please contact us if interested in applying and for more details:

Stephen Hendriksen, MD

Center for Hyperbaric Medicine

Division of Undersea and Hyperbaric Medicine

Department of Emergency Medicine

Hennepin County Medical Center

612-873-7420

Kent Hospital

15 Health Lane, Bldg. 2D

Warwick, RI 02886

Contact: Mary Beth Hanley, DO

Email: mhanley@KentRI.org

Tel (401)-736-4646

*Currently approved for DO's only

Home Page: http://www.kentri.org/graduateeducation/ hyperbaric/

Louisiana State University

New Orleans, LA

Contact: Tracy LeGros, MD

Email: tlegros1@cox.net

(504) 366-7638

Home Page: www.medschool.lsuhsc.edu/emergency_medicine/fellowship_hyperbarics.aspx

Fellowship in Diving and Hyperbaric Medicine

Louisiana, LSU Health Sciences Center/Charity Hospital, New Orleans. One year fellowship includes extensive opportunities in clinical and animal research, publishing, and teaching experiences. Divers Alert Network and Gulf Coast Commercial Diving Referral Center. Clinical teaching locations includemultiplace and monoplace units. Program directors: Dr. Tracy L LeGros.

Accredited Program: effective July 1, 2008

SUNY Upstate Medical University

Syracuse, NY
Contact: Marvin Heyboer III, MD, FACEP, FUHM and
    William Santiago, MD
E-Mails: Heyboerm@upstate.edu; santiagw@upstate.edu
Phone: (315) 464-4363
Home Page: http://www.upstate.edu/emergency/education/fellowships/hyperbaric.php

Fellowship in Undersea and Hyperbaric Medicine

This ACGME accredited fellowship program at SUNY Upstate Medical University offers comprehensive training for a physician who is board-eligible in any ABMS or Osteopathic specialty. The program provides intensive training in clinical hyperbaric medicine while including all aspects of wound care and diving medicine. There are didactic lectures based on core curriculum and participation in research within hyperbaric medicine. Opportunities also exist for clinical activity to maintain skills in trainees' primary specialty. Program Director: Marvin Heyboer III, MD, FACEP, CWS, FACCWS.

United States Air Force School Of Aerospace Medicine

Lackland, TX
Contact: Devin Beckstrand, MD
E-Mails: devin.beckstrand@us.af.mil
Phone: (210) 292-3483
Home Page: https://kx.afms.mil/kj/kx2/HyperbaricMedicine/Pages/fellowship_requirements-31may12[1].aspx

University of California San Diego

Contact: Peter Witucki, MD, FACEP
E-Mail: pwitucki@ucsd.edu
Phone: (619) 543-6463 or (619) 543-6218

Home Page: http://emergencymed.ucsd.edu/education/fellowships/hyperbaric
University of Pennsylvania
Philadelphia, PA
Contact: Kevin Hardy, MD and Wendy Kelly
E-Mail: whermann@mail.med.upenn.edu
Phone: (215) 898-9095
Home Page: http://www.uphs.upenn.edu/ifem/hbofellowshipoutline.pdf

Fellowship in Undersea and Hyperbaric Medicine

The ACGME accredited fellowship program at The University of Pennsylvania offers comprehensive training for two physicians who are board-eligible in any ABMS specialty. Our program provides intensive training in diving and hyperbaric medicine, including all aspects of wound care and elective opportunities in critical care. A series of didactic lectures occurs weekly, and there are opportunities for research and clinical activity to maintain skills in trainees' primary specialty.

On-line information is found at http://www.uphs.upenn.edu/emergency-medicine/education/fellowships/hyperbaric-medicine/
Interested candidates should contact:
Wendy Kelly at 215-898-9095
or
e-mail: wherrman@mail.med.upenn.edu

Two Postdoctoral Positions:

Two Postdoctoral Positions are offered to study fundamental mechanisms of oxygen in angiogenesis, cell-to-cell adhesion or free radical production/pathogenesis as well as the clinical effects of hyperbaric oxygen. Individuals with clinical experience who are interested in obtaining research training will receive special consideration. An exceptional opportunity exists for collaborative basic and clinical research as part of a NIH-funded Specialized Center of Research in Hyperbaric Oxygen Therapy.

Clinical Hyperbaric Medicine Fellowship:

One position is offered to a board-eligible, licensed physician for intensive training in undersea and hyperbaric medicine. Fellows are actively involved with the clinical program of Penn's Institute for Environmental Medicine, and are provided opportunities for involvement in basic and clinical research as a part of the training.

Cuauhtémoc Sánchez-Rodríguez

Abstract

This chapter deals with the history and general organization of hyperbaric medicine in 39 countries of Latin America. There is considerable activity in this field, but no regulatory standards have been set. Most of the regulations are similar to those in the USA and indications for use of HBO are similar.

Keywords

Hyperbaric medicine • Hyperbaric oxygen • Latin America • Hyperbaric chambers • Regulation of hyperbaric medicine

History

Hyperbaric chambers have been used in Latin America from the early 1990s during the construction of the Panama Canal. The first written report of clinical hyperbaric oxygen was by Osorio de Almeida (Brazil) for the treatment of Lepromatous leprae in 1936. The early development happened mainly in the national navies, one exception was Cuba that had the development of clinical and undersea medicine almost simultaneously. The civilian clinical units started in the 1960 and 1970s and slowly became the most important centers in hyperbaric medicine.

Introduction

Thirty-nine different countries form Latin America with a great diversity of cultures and languages. Although Spanish is the most common, it is still not the official language. Mexico has 56 different languages and dialects; 10% of the total population does not speak Spanish. This great diversity also stands for design, fabrication, operation, and safety measures for hyperbaric chambers. It also extends to the diversity of treatment protocols and accepted conditions for hyperbaric oxygen therapy.

The Latin American Chapter of the UHMS was formed in 1993 and worked as a center of information for the newly formed units in the area. It also had a meeting in a different county every 2 years. The meeting covered the areas of diving, hyperbaric oxygen, and safety. It made efforts to standardize the development of the field in the area. It set the minimum standards for safety, guidelines for training, staffing of hyperbaric, construction and operation of hyperbaric chambers, and accepted and investigative conditions. Unfortunately, it was dissolved in the early 2000s. Never the less, Latin America is the fastest growing area in diving and hyperbaric medicine in the world.

The majority of the hyperbaric chambers in Latin America are multiplace. The introduction of monoplace chambers has been slow in the area, due to lack of experience with this type of chambers (most of the people working on chambers come with a naval background and used to work with multiplace chambers) and for economical reasons; oxygen is very expensive in South America.

Unfortunately, in the last 5 years we have experienced a rise of non-medical freestanding clinics that would use cheap chambers produced without any type of certification, to provide treatment to more than 150 conditions without any ethical or medical guidelines. You can see clinics in beauty

C. Sánchez-Rodríguez, MD, MSc, MPH (✉)
Department of Hyperbaric Medicine, Agustín O'Horan,
SSY, Av. Iztaes s/n x Canek, Col. Centro, Mérida,
Yucatán 97000, Mexico
e-mail: cuau57@hotmail.com

© Springer International Publishing AG 2017
K.K. Jain, *Textbook of Hyperbaric Medicine*, DOI 10.1007/978-3-319-47140-2_51

parlors or in the backyard of lay people giving treatment to not-accepted conditions. Also, the locally produced chambers do not follow any code of pressure vessels for their construction. Not only the chambers are unsafe, but they also use an oxygen cylinder to exchange the inside atmosphere for 10 min and pressurize the chamber, but once they are at pressure, they will not exchange again the inside atmosphere until the end of the treatment (usually 1 h).

Due to the lack of adequate information and knowledge in the field, physicians are taken by surprise by charlatans and buy one of these chambers and start using strange protocols. This same group has introduced the concept of ultra-low pressures, so they start treating the patient at 2 fsw and raise slowly the pressure until by the end of several days they get to a real treatment pressure, above 1.5 ATA. They call this the acclimatization to pressure. The scientific ethical units are starting to produce important contributions for the development of diving and hyperbaric medicine.

Existing General Standards

There are great differences between the different countries in the area. Most have regulations for pressure vessels (PV), but there is still none for pressure vessels for human occupancy (PVHO). Different organisms are the certifying agencies for PV (local navies, engineering institutions, labor department, etc.). Nevertheless, there are still no regulations for monoplace chambers. Although there are different organisms that certify PV, most of the area has American Society for Mechanical Engineers (ASME) certifying engineers, and ASME PVHO standards could be easily established. One of the major restrains to standardized ASME in the area is monetary; it is 30–40 % more expensive than to follow local certifications. The gas bottles and liquid oxygen systems follow the international certifications used in the USA (Compressed Gas Association—CGA). The fire suppression regulations are nonexisting in most countries, although there are local regulations for clinics and hospitals; hyperbaric chambers have not yet been addressed in most of the countries.

Responsible Existing Authorities

In Latin America, there are authorities similar to those in the USA that regulate most of our activity.

Industry

The industry follows the international regulations in gas handling and containers of gas under pressure. There are codes for pressure vessels, tanks, and other containers. Hospitals follow the strict regulations similar or equivalent to those in the USA. Chambers for the commercial diving industry follow international regulations (ASME, CGA, ADC, etc.). Nevertheless, our main problem is with freestanding units that do not meet or do not follow any regulation.

Labor

The Department of Labor regulates certain activities related to pressure vessels, specially related to integrity of the PV, and safety related to those working under abnormal environments. In some countries, they regulate all PV for the industry and for hospitals, including hyperbaric chambers.

Health

Health departments are starting to regulate all medical activities, although in some countries there are no real regulations for hyperbaric oxygen health providers. In others, you must have a medical degree to practice medicine, but now you will need to be board-certified to practice in hospitals.

Insurance

The insurance carriers are slowly gaining power in Latin America and are starting to regulate or request minimum standards to accredit a hyperbaric unit or reimburse the treatments. They are trying to have similar regulations as those in the USA.

Latin American Consensus

There is a great need to have a consensus meeting that addresses the following issues:

- Minimum standards for fabrication, inspection, installation, and operation of hyperbaric chambers (in and outside hospitals).
- Minimum standards for training of personnel working in a hyperbaric unit (technicians, nurses, respiratory therapist, physicians, etc.).
- Minimum staffing for hospital and freestanding hyperbaric units.
- Treatment protocols, accepted and investigative conditions. Minimum ethical standards for the treatment of investigative conditions, and basic and clinical research protocols.

The whole purpose of the consensus meeting is to standardize all of the hyperbaric activity in the area and avoid the unsafe, unethical, and non-scientific use of chambers. It is also needed to standardize the treatment protocols which would allow us to produce multinational multicenter research protocols that could reach statistical significance sooner. It is a real challenge to put together so many different countries and come to an agreement on minimum standards for the issues listed above, but it is need for hyperbaric medicine to be accepted and take its place in modern medicine in Latin America.

In diving medicine, Divers Alert Network (DAN) of Latin America, a branch of IDAN at that moment, set a precedent where it was divided in five areas (Mexico and the Caribbean, Central America, northern part of South America, southern part of South America, and Brazil) and created courses and documents for safety, training, and standardized the management of diving-related accidents. The area directors and subdirectors and attending physicians worked as volunteers. Many silent heroes gave a lot of their time and knowledge to make this happen.

Implementation of Minimum Standards and Regulations

Although we have standards in the area for multiplace chambers (at least PV), there is a need to extend the existing standard to PVHO and for monoplace chambers. A Latin American master document that contains the minimum standards for multiplace and monoplace chambers is very much needed. This document would serve as a foundation. Currently, most of the existing regulations in the USA are applied in our countries, although we need PVHO and National Fire Protection Association (NFPA), or their equivalent, in the area.

Hyperbaric chambers in accredited hospitals and clinics have no problems (except for PVHO and NFPA) because they, by law, have to meet certain standards that are generally similar to those in the USA. Our real problems are the freestanding chambers that do not follow any code or regulation. There is not an entity that investigates or regulates this type of freestanding chambers. In some countries, the Navy, Labor Department, or other institution regulates all the PV and the activity around them, but this codes or rules are not presently being enforced.

Our real challenge is to create a document that has the minimum requirements and that states where to get all the related information to upgrade these requirements. The second phase would be to try to enforce locally this minimum requirement to standardize the activity in the area. The ultimate goal would be that all the area followed the same codes and guidelines, so we can guarantee the safe and ethical use of diving and hyperbaric medicine in Latin America.

Index

A

ABEM. *See* American Board of Emergency Medicine (ABEM)
ABPM. *See* American Board of Preventive Medicine (ABPM)
Acetazolamide therapy, 478
Acetylcholinergic neurons, 140
ACGME accredited fellowship program, 628
ACHM. *See* American College of Hyperbaric Medicine (ACHM)
Acute acoustic trauma, 448–453, 458
Acute anemia, 403–404
Acute mountain sickness (AMS), 110
Acute myocardial infarction (MI)
    cardiac arrhythmias, 381
    cardiac resuscitation, 381
    chronic ischemic heart disease, 380
    diagnostic procedures, 379
    HBO and thrombolysis, 379, 380
    heart failure, 381
    normobaric oxygen, 379
    PTCA, 379
Acute obstructive bowel symptoms, 411
Acute pancreatitis
    animal study, 415
    causes, 415
    HBO applications, 415
Acute peripheral vascular ischemia, 436
Acute pulmonary oxygen toxicity, 84
Acute severe injury/illness (ASII), 555
Acute stroke, HBO role, 258–266
    animal models
        advantage, 258
        hyperglycemia, 261
        ischemia/hypoxia, 258–261
        MCAO, 258, 261, 262
    cerebral ischemia and free radicals, 258
    controlled clinical studies, 266
    neuroprotective effect, 262
    RBC, 257
    uncontrolled clinical studies
        cerebrovascular disease, 262–264
        clinical trials, 265
        EfHBOT, 266
        thrombosis, 264
Acute vision loss, 469
Adenine triphosphate (ATP), 555
Adhesive intestinal obstruction
    adhesions, 410
    clinical trial, 411
    decompression therapy, 411
    HBO, 411

Adjunctive therapy, 167
Adrenocortical function, 421–422
Advanced Certified Hyperbaric Registered Nurse (ACHRN), 516
Adynamic ileus, 410
Aging
    brain changes, 505–506
    free radicals, 503–504
    hypoxia, 504–505
    mental function, 506
    metabolism, 505–506
    morphological changes, 505
    oxygen conductance system, 505
    theories, 503–505
Air bubbles, 126
Air cysts, 81
Air embolism
    AGE and VGE, 123
    alveolar-capillary disruption, 123
    causes, 123, 124
    cerebral metabolism, 128
    delayed treatment, 131
    HBO application, 126–127
    hydrogen peroxide poisoning, 130
    invasive medical procedures, 129
    mechanisms, 124
    neurological deficits, 123
    obstetrical procedures, 129
    spontaneous recovery, 130
    treatment, 125, 126
Altitude Mountain Sickness (AMS), 573
Altitude sickness, 103
American Board of Emergency Medicine (ABEM), 621
American Board of Preventive Medicine (ABPM), 621
American College of Hyperbaric Medicine (ACHM), 583, 621
    APWCA, 623
    CMS, 623
    DWLE, 624
    functions and goals, 623
    Radionecrosis Registry, 624
    UHMS, 624, 625
American Diabetes Association, 194
American Osteopathic Board of Preventive Medicine (AOBPM), 621
American Professional Wound Care Association (APWCA), 623
American Society for Mechanical Engineers (ASME), 632
Amino acids, 58–59
Ammonia, 58–59
Ammonia metabolism, 21
Amphotericin B (AMB), 167
Anaerobic cellulitis, 162

Anaerobic glycolysis, 134
Ancillary equipment, 72
Anemia, 533
Anesthesia, 552, 553
    cardiovascular effects, 551
    central nervous system, 551
    historical perspective, 549–550
    indications, 550
    intravenous anesthesia, 552
    middle ear barotrauma, prevention, 553
    nitrous oxide (N₂O), 551, 552
    pharmacokinetics, 552
    physiological considerations, 550–552
    in pressure chamber
        airway equipment, 552
        monitoring, 553
        noise, 552
        ventilators, 552, 553
Angiogenesis, 188
Animal experimental studies, 588
Anoxia, 159
Anoxic brain injury, 359
Anterior ciliary arteries, 472
Anterior segment ischemia (ASI), 472, 473
Anticancer agents, 88
Antineoplastic agents, 533
Antioxidants, 90, 91
Antiplatelet drugs, 128
Anxiety reactions, 85
Apligraf (Organogenesis Inc.), 194
APWCA. See American Professional Wound Care Association (APWCA)
Arterial gas embolism (AGE), 465
Arterial insufficiency, 193
Arteriovenous malformations, 217
Arteritic ischemic optic neuropathy (AION), 474
Ascorbic acid, 60
Asymmetric dimethylarginine (ADMA), 190
Autism spectrum disorder (ASD), 372

B
Bacterial gangrene, 162
Bacteriology, 164
Baromedical Nurses Association (BNA), 516, 626
Barotraumatic lesions, 83
Barthel index, 252
Basic fibroblast growth factor (bFGF), 214
Battle casualties, 441
Benign intracranial hypertension (BIH), 369
Biochemical effects of HBO
    acid-base balance, 20
    biomarkers, 20
Bioinformatics, 600
Biological signals, 234
Biomarkers, 588–589, 597, 599
Birth injury, 357
Blood loss, 403–404
Blood volume, 402
Blood–brain barrier (BBB), 45, 124, 228, 346, 347
Bone mineral density (BMD), 440
Brain abscess, 335–336
Brain dysfunction, 235
Brain edema, 229
Brain fibroblastic growth factor (bFGF), 303
Brain imaging, 597
Brain injury, 355, 359, 362
Brain tumors, 334

Branch retinal artery occlusion (BRAO), 470, 476, 481
Bronchial asthma, 430
Bronchitis, 430
Brown-Séquard syndrome, 117

C
Canadian Neurological Scale (CNS), 253
Cancer, 600
Carbon monoxide poisoning, 133, 135–154, 491
Carbon tetrachloride (CCl₄) poisoning, 154, 155
Carboxyhemoglobin (COHb), 134–137, 139–144, 146–153
Carboxymyoglobin (COMb), 134
Carcinoma, 529
    bladder, 530
    lung, 530
Cardiac arrhythmias, 381
Cardiac pacemakers, 86
Cardiac surgery
    advantages, HBO, 381, 383
    CNS complications, 383–384
    HBO preconditioning, 383
    IRI, 382
    LDH, 382
    open-heart surgery, 382
    retransfusion, 382
Cardiology, 377–380
    HBO clinical application (see Acute myocardial infarction (MI))
Cardioprotection, 383
Cardiopulmonary resuscitation, 557–558
Cardiovascular diseases
    hyperoxia and atherosclerosis, 375, 376
    hypoxia, 375, 376
    NBO, 375
    risk factors, 375
Cardiovascular disorders, 601
Cardiovascular system, 19–20
Carotid bodies (CBs), 424
Carotid endarterectomy, 337
    EC/IC bypass operation, 336
    HBO, 336, 337
Cataract, 464–465
Catecholamines, 422
Ceiling effect, 393
Cell therapy, 255, 590, 600
Centers for Medicare and Medicaid Services (CMS), 623, 625
Central nervous system (CNS), 49, 495
Central retinal artery, 465
    occlusion, 466–469
Central retinal vein, 466, 472
    occlusion, 474–476
Cerebral anoxia, 300
Cerebral blood flow (CBF), 227, 235–236, 326–328, 330, 340, 505–506
Cerebral edema, 45–46, 229–230, 232
    control of, 326
    HBO, 336
    HBO therapy, 338
    and intracranial pressure, 341
    neurosurgery, 341
    postoperative, 342
    vascular occlusion, 337
Cerebral embolism
    clinical features, 125
    diagnosis, 125
    pathophysiology, 124–125
Cerebral glucose metabolism, 226

Cerebral hemodynamic, 217
Cerebral hypoxia, 46, 47, 229, 292
Cerebral infarction, 241, 248, 257, 258, 265
Cerebral ischemia, 228, 230
    DNA damage and repair, 248
    gene expression, 248
    oxygen free radicals, 246–247
Cerebral malaria, 371
Cerebral metabolism, 21, 56
Cerebral oxygenation, 230
Cerebral palsy (CP)
    causes of, 355
    children with cerebral anoxic injury, 359–360
    clinical trials, 358–360
    Cornell study, 360
    effectiveness studies, 360–361
    in HBO, 357–358
    in HBOT, 360
    hyperbaric oxygen therapy, 365
    molecular diagnostic procedures, 366
    oxygen therapy in neonatal period, 355–357
    postneonatal onset, 361
    side effects, 361–362
    spastic diplegia, 363, 364
    SPECT brain imaging study, 361
    TOVA, 361
    in utero, 362
Cerebral vasomotor paresis, 229
Cerebrospinal fluid (CSF), 228
Cerebrovascular diseases, 404
Cerebrovascular surgery
    HBO, 336–341
Certified Hyperbaric Registered Nurse (CHRN), 516
Cervical myelopathy, 334
Chamber claustrophobia, 85
Chandler's grading system, 218
Chemoradiotherapy (CRT), 219
Chinese hyperbaric chamber, 615
Chronic brain injury, 362
Chronic idiopathic intestinal pseudo-obstruction, 411
Chronic ischemic heart disease, 380–381
Chronic laryngitis, 458
Chronic lyme disease (CLD), 177, 178
Chronic myocardial insufficiency, 384
Chronic obstructive pulmonary disease (COPD), 429
Chronic osteomyelitis, 171, 172
Chronic poststroke stage
    depression, 257
    spasticity management, 256, 257
    vascular Dementia, 257
Chronic stable disease, 346
Cilioretinal arteries, 466, 469
Claustrophobia, 85
Clinical trial, HBO
    defined, 591
    ethical aspects, 592
    problems, 591, 592
    types, 591
Clinically isolated syndrome (CIS), 346
Clinicopathological correlation, 212
Clostridial infections, 165
CMS. See Centers for Medicare and Medicaid Services (CMS)
CNS drugs
    anesthetics, 89
    ethanol, 89
    injuries, 510

narcotic analgesics, 89
pentobarbital, 89
scopolamine, 89
stimulants, 89
CNS cochlear microphonics (CM), 450
Coma, 275, 276, 305
Comatose Patients, 233
Comex 30, 113
Compartment syndromes, 437
Compound action potentials (CAP), 450
Compressed air, 72, 74, 76, 77
Computerized tomography (CT), 96
    advantages and disadvantages, 236
    principles, 236
Congenital malformations, 489–490
Congenital spherocytosis, 404–405
Continuous bladder irrigation (CBI), 74
Controlled trials vs. observational studies, 274
Coronary artery bypass graft (CABG), 382
Coronary artery disease, 384
Corticosteroids, 203
Critical limb ischemia (CLI), 386
Crush injuries, 435
    compartment syndromes, 437
    diagnosis, 434
    late complications, 433
    pathophysiology, 434
    traumatic ischemia, 435, 436
    treatment, role of HBO
        BPI, 435
        PtcO$_2$, 435
Cutaneous ulcers, 188
Cyanide poisoning, 147, 153–154
Cystoid macular edema (CME), 476–478
Cytochrome aa3, 555–557, 566, 567
Cytochrome c oxidase, 134
Cytotoxic brain edema, 230

D
Decompression illness (DCI), 557, 571
Decompression sickness (DCS), 26, 28–30, 85, 104–108, 546
    2 ATA, 104
    altitude, 109–110
    blood examination, 112
    bone scanning, 112
    decompression illness, 104
    delayed treatment, 119–120
    diagnosis, 111–112
    in diving, 108–109
    drugs, 118–119
    dysbarism, 103
    early treatment, 119
    electrophysiological studies, 112
    emergency management and evaluation, 113
    extravehicular activity, 103
    facial baroparesis, 117
    gas formation, 104
    helium and oxygen environment (heliox), 104
    imaging, 112
    late sequelae, 118
    management, altitude, 117
    monoplace vs. multiplace chambers, 118
    neurological, 121
    neuropsychological assessment, 113
    ocular complications, 111

Decompression sickness (DCS) (*cont.*)
    oxygen *vs.* gas mixtures, 118
    pathophysiology
        bubble-induced CNS injury, 106–107
        changes in blood, 107
        DON, 108
        free radicals, 108
        gas formation, 104–105
        pulmonary changes, 106
    preventive measurement, 120–121
    prognosis, 121
    recompression and HBO treatment, 113–116
    retinal angiography, 112
    risk factors, 120
    spinal cord, 117
    steady-state conditions, 104
    type II, 120
    ultrasonic detection, bubbles, 111, 112
    X-rays, 112
Decompression syndrome (DCS), 431
Decubitus ulcers
    HBO role, 199
    pathophysiology, 199
Delayed neuropsychiatric sequelae (DNS), 235
Delayed radiation injuries, 218, 219
Dementia
    causes, 372
    defined, 372
Demyelination, 346
Department of Defense (DoD), 329
Department of Veterans Affairs (DVA), 329
Dermatology
    necrobiosis lipoidica diabeticorum, 206
    pyoderma gangrenosum, 206–207
Descemet's membrane, 465
Diabetes mellitus, 423–424, 491, 601
Diabetic foot infection (DFI), 161, 195
Diabetic macular edema (DME), 479
Diabetic retinopathy (DR), 479, 480
Diabetic ulcer
    adjuncts to HBO, 194–195
    barotrauma rate, 197
    clinical use of HBO, 195–196
    critical evaluation of HBO, 196
    division, 197
    HBO role, 194
    hyperglycemia, 194
    leg amputation rate, 194
    treatment, 194, 196–197
Diagnostic equipment
    ECG and EEG, 73
    glucose-monitoring devices, 73
    $tcpO_2$, 73
Dichlormethane, 151
Dimethyl sulfoxide (DMSO), 332
Diphosphoglycerate, 134
Diploma course, 585
Disseminated sclerosis, 346
Distal airway epithelial cells, 54
Diver's headache, 28
Diver's vertigo, 30
Divers Alert Network (DAN), 633
Diving chambers, 68
Diving medicine, 3–4, 23, 31, 546, 583, 584
    gas nuclei elimination, 547
    O_2 preconditioning, 547
    preoxygenation, 547

Diving, high-pressure effects
    central nervous system lesions, 28
    headache, 28
    hearing and vestibular impairment, 28, 29
    microbubble damage in BBB, 28
    middle ear damage, 29, 30
    peripheral nerve conduction velocity, 28
    taste sensation, 30
    vertigo, 30
DNA damage, 21
Drug delivery, 600
Drug interactions, 87
Dysbaric osteonecrosis (DON), 25, 108
Dysbarism, 103
Dyspnea, 219

E
Ear surgery, 81
ECD SPECT brain imaging, 315
Economic analysis, 196–197
Electron transport system (ETS)
    ATP, 556
        mitochondrial matrix, 556
        paramagnetic molecules, 555
Electrophysiological studies, 234–235
Embryonic stem cells (ESCs), 400
Emphysema, 431
Endoscopic retrograde cholangiopancreatography, 130
Endothelial progenitor cells (EPCs), 194
Entrapped intestinal balloons, 415
Enzyme inhibition, 50
Epilepsy, 59
Epinephrine/norepinephrine, 422
Erythropoiesis, 400
Euglobulin fibrinolytic activity (EFA), 19
European Stroke Scale, 253
Eustachian tube, 83
Exercise, 35–38
    ammonia metabolism, 37
    brain function, 33
    effect of HBO
        blood flow, muscles, 37
        skeletal muscle, 37
        toxic effects, 38
    effects on human body, 34
    hyperbaric conditions
        general effects, 35, 36
        lactate production and clearance, 36
    hyperbaric environments, 34, 35
    hyperoxia, 35
    hypoxia, 34
    oxygen, 33
Experimental allergic encephalomyelitis
        (EAE), 347
Extracellular SOD (EC-SOD), 60
Extracranial carotid occlusive disease, 337
Extracranial/intracranial (EC/IC) arterial bypass,
        338–341
    HBO, 338–339
    patients selection, 339–341
Eye diseases
    central retinal artery occlusion, 466–469
    decompression sickness, 465
    hyperoxic conditions, 462–463
    radiation retinopathy, 469–472
    recurrent pterygium/scleral necrosis, 472

F

Face transplants, 541
Facial palsy, 457
Fetal hypoxia, 490–491
Fibromyalgia syndrome (FMS), 181
Fire safety
    clinical monoplace chamber, 77
    fatal hyperbaric fires, 77
    monoplace chamber, 77
    multiplace hyperbaric chambers, 77
Flap survival
    and grafts, 204
    animal experiments, 204
    clinical applications, 203–204
    drugs and biological preparations, 203
Focal hypoxia signals, 346
Food and Drug Administration (FDA), 611–613
Forced vital capacities (FVC), 20
Fournier's gangrene, 163
Fractures
    arterial injuries, 440
    BMD study, 440
    cartilage, 439
    HBO treatments, 439
    hyperoxia, 439
    pseudoarthrosis, 440
Free radical scavengers, 88, 91
Frenzel's maneuver, 83
Frost bite
    clinical features, 199
    laboratory studies, 199
    management, 200
    pathogenesis, 199
Future medicine, 600, 601

G

GABA shunt, 44
Gas gangrene
    diagnosis, 164
    gangrene treatment, 164–165
    gas-forming anaerobic organisms, 163
    HBO, 165–166
    necrotic condition, 163
Gastroenterology, 407–413
    acute pancreatitis, 415
    entrapped intestinal balloons, 415
    IBD (*see* Inflammatory bowel disease (IBD))
    infections (*see* Gastrointestinal tract infections)
    intestinal obstruction
        adhesive intestinal obstruction, 410, 411
        adynamic ileus, 410
        animals studies, 409, 410
        categories, 408
        intestinal gas origin, 409
    ischemic disorders, 414, 415
    PCI (*see* Pneumatosis cystoides intestinalis (PCI))
    peptic ulceration
        antibacterial effect, 408
        clinical assessment, 408
        experimental studies in animals, 408
        gastric mucosal ischemia, 407
    radiation enterocolitis, 413
Gastrointestinal tract infections
    necrotizing enterocolitis, 413
    pseudomembranous colitis, 413
    TM, 412

Gene expression
    antioxidant induction, 589
    in decompression, 590
    human brain, 589
    microarray analysis, 589
    in stroke, 590
Gene therapy, 255, 256, 600
Genes, 597–598
Geriatrics
    medical specialty, 503
Glasgow coma scale (GCS), 275, 573
Glasgow outcome scale (GOS), 573
Glaucoma, 481
Global ischemia/anoxia, 274–308
    animal studies
        antiapoptotic effect/neurons preservation, 303
        bFGF, 303
        gene-signaling trophic effects, 302
        HBO therapy, 277–286
        microcirculation, 302
        neonatal ischemic/hypoxic birth injury, 302
        normobaric oxygen (NBO), 304
        pregnant uterine harvest/global ischemia model, 302
        stem cells, 303
        swine study, 302
        Van Meter dose–response study, 302
    HBO therapy
        carbon monoxide rat model, 276
        characterization, 275
        chronic traumatic brain injury rat model, 275
        microcirculation, 276
        trophic effect, 276
        WBCs, 276
    human clinical studies
        acute, 290–295
        categories, 304
        chronic, 298–301, 307
        coma, 305
        CSF pressure, 305
        HBO, 304, 305
        HBOT, 308
        heat stroke, 306
        hyperacute period, 287–290
        intravascular gas, 305
        subacute global ischemia/coma cases, 296, 297, 306, 307
        TBI patients, 305, 306
Glucocorticoid, 421
Glucose metabolism, 21
Glucose oxidation quotient (GOQ), 225
Glycolysis, 225
Grading of Recommendations Assessment, Development, and Evaluation (GRADE), 196
Gross Motor Function Measure (GMFM), 358, 359, 361
Growth and differentiation factor 15 (GDF15), 54
Gynecology
    animal experimental studies, 492
    clinical applications, 492

H

H+ channeling, 556
Haldane effect, 16
Hand transplants, 541
Hansen's disease, 168–169
HBO life support (HBOLS), 566
HBO preconditioning (HBO-PC), 229

HBO therapy, 355–366, 369, 373–374, 591–592
  anxiety reactions, 85
  ASD, 372
  BIH (see Benign intracranial hypertension (BIH))
  BNA guidelines, 517
  claustrophobia, 85
  clinical trials HBO (see Clinical trials HBO)
  cognitive impairment, 373
  contraindications, 81–83, 86
  decompression sickness, 85
  drug-induced neuropathy, 370
  genetic effects, 85
  hyperbaric chamber, 86
  indications, 81, 82
  inflammatory necrotic tissue, 187
  intervention, 305, 317
  management of neuromuscular disorders
      muscular dystrophies, 373–374
      myasthenia gravis, 374
  mental dysfunction, 373
  Middle Ear Barotrauma, 83–84
  in nonhealing wounds, 193
  neurotoxicity, 59
  ophthalmological complications, 84
  oxygen seizures, 84
  patients selection, 86
  peripheral neuropathic pain, 370
  peripheral neuropathy, 370
  plastic surgery, 187
  pulmonary complications, 84
  surgical procedures, 187
  Susac's syndrome, 371
  trigeminal neuralgia, 371
  ulcers, 193
  vascular headaches, 371, 372
HBO-induced DNA damage, 85
HBO-induced wound healing, 189–190
Head and neck cancer, 529–530
Heart disease, 491
Heart failure, 381
Heat shock protein (HSP), 40, 248
Helium-oxygen mixtures, 119
Hematocrit, 398
Hematuria, 219
Hemiplegics, 234
Hemodialysis, 469, 474
Hemodilution, 128
Hemoglobin, 13, 399
Hemolytic anemia, 404
Hemorheology, 397, 400
Hemorrhagic cystitis and proctitis, 220
Hepatic encephalopathy
  HBO, 417
  MRI diagnosis, 416
  treatment, 416
Hepatocellular carcinoma (HCC), 88
Hexamethylpropyleneamine oxime (HM-PAO), 238
High altitude cerebral edema (HACO), 573
High altitude pulmonary edema (HAPO), 573, 574
High pressure water gun injection injury, 437
High-pressure neurological syndrome (HPNS)
  clinical features, 26
  neurotransmitters, 27
  pathophysiology, 26, 27
  prevention and management, 27, 28

HMPAO SPECT brain imaging
  post near drowning, 312, 313
  postinjury, 309
  single HBO treatment, 311, 314
HMPAO–SPECT brain imaging, 120
Hospital-based hyperbaric programs, 622
Host defense mechanisms
  oxygen tension, 159
  phagocytic leukocytes, 159
Hydrogen cyanide (HCN), 153
Hydrogen peroxide (H_2O_2), 50
Hydrogen peroxide poisoning, 130
Hydrogen sulfide (H2S) poisoning, 154
Hydroxocobalamin, 146
Hydroxyethyl starch (HES), 452
Hydroxyl radicals (OH·), 50
Hyperacute and acute studies, 318
Hyperbaric air therapy
  compressed air, 4
  history, 4
  hyperbaric chamber, 5, 8
Hyperbaric chambers, 7, 53, 64, 74–78, 110, 117, 120, 553, 575, 615,
      617, 619, 620, 631, 633
  ancillary equipment, 72
  animal experiments, 68–70
  cardiopulmonary resuscitation, 73–74
  care of tracheotomy, 74
  CBI (see Continuous bladder irrigation (CBI))
  combined treatment and diver testing, 69
  contaminant and value, 76
  defibrillators usage, 74
  diving medicine, 68
  endotracheal tubes, 74
  hyperlite 1-man portable, 65
  mobile multiplace chamber, 67, 68
  model 500A, specifications, 73
  monoplace chambers, 63, 64
  multiplace chambers (see Multiplace chambers)
  oxygen masks, 72
  patient monitoring devices, 75
  pleural suction drainage, 74
  portable chamber, 78
  pressure usage, 71
  regulatory issues
      FDA classes, 78
      GMP regulations, 78
      labeling, 78
  risk-benefit analysis, 75
  safety
      atmospheric control, 76
      breathing control system, 76
      fire, 76, 77
      operational safety, 75
  safety and fire hazard, 605–608
  selection, 70
  transdermal patches, 74
  types, 63, 64
Hyperbaric medicine practice, 79, 187, 516, 584–585
  ACHM, 583
  air therapy, 4, 5
  application of biotechnologies, 588, 589
  in bioinformatics, 600
  cell therapy, 600
  cerebral adverse effects, 546
  in China, 615–616

diploma course, 585
and diving medicine, 3–4, 584
drug delivery, 600
economic aspects, 586
future needs, 601
in Germany, 618, 619
I/R injury, 546
in Japan, 617, 618
in Latin America, 631
molecular diagnostics, 599
molecular imaging, 599
nanomedicine, 600
nonphysician healthcare personnel, 585
preoxygenation, 546
program outline, 586
remote monitoring, 600
in Russia, 617, 619
sequencing, 599
standards and regulations, 633
training
    admission requirements, 584–585
    examinations, 584–585
    training program, 584
Hyperbaric Nursing and Wound Care, 517
Hyperbaric nursing research, 525
Hyperbaric oxygen therapy (HBOT), 133–135, 141, 144–155, 461,
        463–470, 472–482, 571, 572, 609, 610
adjuvant to antibiotics, 161
in AIDS, 167–168
case study
    battered child syndrome, 313, 314
    coma treatment, 308, 309
    drowning, chronic phase, 311, 312
cell DNA, 212
cerebrovascular diseases, 404
chronic laryngitis, 458
chronic noise exposure, 455
clinicopathological correlation, 212
congenital malformations, 489–490
decompression sickness, 7
dephlogisticated air, 7–9
diving medicine, 3
effectiveness, 347
ethical issue, 605
Facial Palsy, 457
gas gangrene, 572
hearing loss, 453–455
hemoglobin molecule, 399
hemorheology, 400
history, 8
hyperbaric chamber, 5
hyperbaric oxygenation, 348
hypoxia, 348
immune system treatment, 401–402
indications, 616–617
infections treatment, 161–169
inner ear, 455
intravenous high-dosage methylprednisolone, 346
ionizing radiation, 212
leprosy, 168–169
leukocytes, 400
loss of blood, 572
low pressure oxygen, 608
malignant otitis externa, 447, 457–458
mechanism, 178–181
medical registry, 183

medicare fraud, 611
Meniere's disease, 456
military response, 574
Multidisciplinary Healthcare Systems, 601
nanotechnology, 590
neonatology, 491–492
neurological disorders, 401
Neuro-otological Vascular Disturbances, 455–457
off-label use, 604, 605
osteomyelitis, 170–171, 447
otological complications, 457
oxygen carriers, 403
perinatal disturbances, 421
plasma oxygen tension, 347
platelets and coagulation, 400
postconcussive symptoms, 573
pregnancy, 489
radiation physics and biology, 211
RBCs, 397
sham treatment, desperate measures, 609–611
skin and mucous membranes, 213
soft tissue infections treatment, 162
stem cells, 400–401
tank treatment, 5
TBI/PCS, 573
tinnitus, 447–449
toxic effects, 7
UHMS, 604
unit of radiation, endocrine organs, 211–212, 421
VHL, 347
viscosity, 398
Hyperbaric oxygenation (HBO), 20, 70–71,
        88–90, 109, 110, 113–117, 119–121,
        376–378, 583
aging process, 506
alveolar oxygen pressures, 17
ammonia metabolism, 21
anticancer agents, 88
antimicrobials
    aminoglycoside antibiotics, 88
    carbapenem antibiotics, 88
    sulfonamides, 88
arterial O_2, 18
blood flow effect, 15
cardiovascular drugs
    adrenomimetic and adrenolytic blockers, 88
    antianginal drugs, 89
    digitalis/digoxin, 89
    heparin, 89
    hypoxia and hyperoxia, 376
CNS
    anesthetics, 89
    ethanol, 89
    insulin, 90
    Losartan, 90
    narcotic analgesics, 89
    pentobarbital, 89
    practical considerations, 90
    reserpine and guanethidine, 90
    salicylates, 90
    scopolamine, 89
    stimulants, 89
    theophylline, 90
biochemical effects
    acid-base balance, 20
    biomarkers, 20

Hyperbaric oxygenation (HBO) (*cont.*)
    capillary level, 14
    capillary oxygen pressure drop, 18
    cardiovascular system, 19–20
    cerebral metabolism, 21
    density, 17
    enzymes
        Cyclooxygenase inactivation, 20
        Cytochrome Oxidase (CCO), 20
        Heme oxygenase (HO), 20
        Succinic Dehydrogenase (SDH), 20
        Tyrosine hydroxylase, 20
    in geriatric patients, 507
    glucose metabolism, 21
    healthy human body, 19–20
    hyperoxia, 19
    indications, 506
    intracellular pO_2, 16
    mental function, 506–507
    metabolic effects on heart, 376, 377
    metabolism, 506
    microcirculation, 20
    molecular level, 21
    myocardial infarction, 377, 378
    nervous system, 20–21
    oxidative stress, 20
    oxygen
        delivery, 14, 15
        pathway, 12
        solubility, 17
        transport and utilization, 14–15
        uptake curve, 18
        utilization in cell, 15
    oxygen-hemoglobin dissociation curve, 13, 14
    oxygen-hemoglobin reaction, 15–16
    partial pressures, 17
    photoaging, 507–508
    physical basics, 11–12
    pressure comparison, 17
    rehabilitation, 506
    respiratory system, 20
    retention of CO_2, 18
    temperature, 17
    theoretical considerations, 16–19
    tissue oxygen tension, 18–19
    transport phase, 12–13
    treatments, 508
    ventilation phase, 12
Hyperbaric patient education, 517–525
Hyperbaric physicians, 583, 584
Hyperbaric technologies, 585
Hyperbaric treatment
    cardiovascular surgery, 128–129
    cerebral edema, 128
Hyperglycemia, 261
Hyperoxia, 19, 327, 428, 439
Hyperoxic acute lung injury (HALI), 428
Hyperoxic conditions, 462
Hyperoxic myopia, 464
Hyperoxygenated choriocapillaris, 463
Hyperoxygenated choroid, 463
Hyperperfusion, 96, 97
Hyperthermia, 533
Hypothalamo-hypophysio-adrenal system (HHAS), 490
Hypothermia, 60, 129, 498, 533
Hypovolemia, 403–404

Hypoxemia, 229
Hypoxia, 42–46, 48, 133–135, 137–141, 146, 147, 151–155, 274, 348, 504–505, 527–528, 597
    brain, 42
        BBB, 45
        brain damage, 46
        CBF regulation, 45
        cerebral edema, 45, 46
        cerebral metabolism, 42–44
        electrical activity, 46
        GABA Shunt, 44
        ischemic–hypoxic disturbances, 45
        mental function disturbances, 46
        microcirculation disturbances, 45
        neurotransmitter metabolism, 44, 45
        pyruvate and citric acid cycle, 44
        structural changes, 46
    cardiovascular system, 41
    causes, 41
    cellular metabolism, 40
    general metabolic effects, 41–42
    HBO, 46, 47
        carotid body, 48
        free radicals, 48
        hypoxic states, 48
        nitric oxide synthase, 48
    HIF, 40
    Hsps, 40
    oxidative stress, 40
    pathophysiology, 39–41
    respiratory function, 41
Hypoxia-inducible factor (HIF), 40
Hypoxic brain damage, 46
Hypoxic–ischaemic encephalopathy (HIE)
    necrotizing enterocolitis, 496–497
    newborn, 496

I
Idiopathic sudden sensorineural hearing loss (ISSHL), 181, 449
Impairment of consciousness, 304, 307
Inducible nitric oxide synthase (iNOS), 190, 231
Infected wounds, 199
Infertility treatment, 492
Inflammation, 538–539
Inflammatory bowel disease (IBD), 201
    Crohn's disease, 412
    oxidative stress biomarkers, 412
    ulcerative colitis, 412
Inflammatory processes, 430
Interleukin-10 (IL-10), 232
Intermembrane space (IMS), 555
International Federation of Multiple Sclerosis Societies, 349
Intestinal obstruction
    adhesive intestinal obstruction, 410, 411
    adynamic ileus, 410
    animals studies, 409, 410
    categories, 408, 409
    intestinal gas origin, 409
Intracellular adhesion molecules (ICAM-1), 497
Intracerebral hemorrhage (ICH), 262
Intracranial aneurysms, 337–338
Intraocular pressure (IOP), 463
Intravenous anesthesia, 552
Intravenous perfluorocarbon emulsions, 55
Intrinsic inflammatory disorders, 477–478

Ionizing radiation, 212
Ischemia/hypoxia, 275
Ischemia–reperfusion injury (IRI) injury, 382, 546
Ischemic central retinal vein occlusion, 474–476
Ischemic cerebrovascular disease, 249
Ischemic disorders, 414, 415
Ischemic leg pain, 391–393
Ischemic neuropraxia, 117
Ischemic optic neuropathy, 473–474
Ischemic penumbra, 276
Ischemic tissue, 467

J
Japanese Society for Hyperbaric Medicine, 618

K
Keratometry, 464
Klausenbach Study
    HBO sessions, 267
    outcome, 267, 269
Kreb's cycle, 555
Kurtzke disability score (KDS), 349

L
Lactic dehydrogenase (LDH), 382
Laryngeal cancer, 218
Laser Doppler flowmetry (LDF), 213
Latin America
    consensus, 632–633
    cultures and languages, 631
    hyperbaric chambers, 631
    meeting, 631
    oxygen cylinder, 632
LDH. See Lactic dehydrogenase (LDH)
Leprosy, 168–169
Leukocytes, 400
Limb reimplantation, 440–441
Lipase sphingomyelinase D, 200
Lipoperoxides, 50
Lipopolysaccharide, 348
Liver disease, 416, 417
    effect of HBO
        animal study, 416
        applications, 416
        hepatic encephalopathy, 416, 417
        normal liver, 416
Liver transplants, 540
Lung injury, 54
Lung mechanics, 428
Lung transplants, 539
Lyme disease
    vs. chronic lyme disease, 175–178
    HBOT, 178–183
    statistics, 179–180
    treatment, 181–183

M
Macular hole surgery, 479
Magnetic resonance angiography (MRA), 236
Magnetic resonance imaging (MRI), 20, 94, 96, 345
    advantages and disadvantages, 236–237
    diffusion-weighted imaging, 237
    principle, 236

Magnetic resonance spectroscopy (MRS), 145, 346
Malignant disease, 82
Malignant glioma, 530–532
Malignant melanoma, 530
Malignant otitis externa, 172
Mandibular osteoradionecrosis, 215
Market regulations
    FDC, 611, 612
    National Hyperbaric Oxygen Therapy Registry, 612
Matrix metalloproteinases (MMPs), 192
MCAO. See Middle cerebral artery occlusion (MCAO)
Medicare Administrative Carriers (MACs), 625
MEDLINE, 448
Meniere's disease, 456
Methemoglobinemias, 134, 154–155
Methionine sulfoxide reductase A (MsrA), 598
Methylene chloride, 151
Metronidazole, 528
Microcirculation, 20
Microembolism, 107, 346
Microvascular occlusion, 212
Middle cerebral arterial blood flow velocity (MCV), 228
Middle cerebral artery occlusion (MCAO), 258
Middle ear barotrauma, 83–84
Middle ear damage in diving, 29–30
Military diving medicine
    methods, 577
    operations, 577
    employee's safety, 577
    personnel training, 577
    recruitment process, 577
Military medicine, 573 (see also Hyperbaric oxygen therapy (HBOT))
    hearing loss and tinnitus, 574
    oxygen, 576
    spinal cord injury, 574
Military, hyperbaric activities
    defensive, 576–577
    offensive, 575–576
    reclamation, 576, 577
    research and rescue, 576
    seabed inspection, 576
Miscellaneous arteriopathies, 393
Misonidazole, 528
Molecular diagnostics, 596
Mono sclerosis, 346
Monoplace chambers
    advantages, 63, 64
    disadvantages, 64
    Gamow bag, 64
    oxygen flow mechanisms, 63
MS Therapy Centres, 350
Mucormycosis
    fungal disease, 167
Multidisciplinary Healthcare Systems, 601, 602
Multiplace chambers
    advantages, 64
    for ICU, 66, 67
    mobile multiplace chamber, 67, 68
    surgical procedures, 67
Multiple sclerosis (MS), 597
    definition, 345
    oxygen treatment, 349
    patients' assessment, 351
    specific abilities, 351
    urinary frequency, 351
Muscular dystrophy, 373–374
Myasthenia gravis, 374

Myocardial infarction, 510
Myonecrosis, 163
Myringotomy, 553

N
N-acetylcysteine (NAC), 203
Nanobiotechnology, 590
Nanomedicine, 600
National Board of Diving and Hyperbaric Medical Technology
    (NBDHMT), 516, 625
National Fire Protection Association (NFPA)
    fire safety code, 607, 633
National Hyperbaric Oxygen Therapy Registry, 612
Necrobiosis lipoidica diabeticorum, 206
Necrotizing enterocolitis, 413, 496–497
Necrotizing fasciitis (NF), 162
Neonatal brain injury, 355
Neonatal ischemic/hypoxic birth injury, 302
Neonatal patients
    hyperbaric chamber, 499
    hypothermia and oxygen toxicity, 499
    ischemia–reperfusion injuries, 499
    lesions, 499
Nervous system, 20–21, 26
    HPNS (see High-pressure neurological syndrome (HPNS))
    neuropsychological effects, 25–26
    nitrogen narcosis, 26
Neurological disorders, 510, 600–601
    BBB, 228
    CBF, 226–228
    cerebral metabolism, 225
    GOQ, 226
    HBO treatment, 228
    HBO-PC, 229
    hyperbaric chamber, 233
    hypoxia and ischemia, 225
    neuroprotection, 230
    OHCob, 226
Neurological indications, 233
Neuronal nitric oxide synthase (nNOS), 50, 56
Neuropathology, 59
Neuroprotection, 230–232
    cell therapy, 255
    gene therapy, 255, 256
    oxygen carriers, 255
Neuroprotective agents, 230
Neurosurgery, 129
Neurotransmitters, 56
Neurotrophic factors (NTFs), 248
Neutrophils, 106, 108, 346
New York University Medical Center, 349
Nicotinamide, 203
Nitric oxide synthase (NOS), 55, 189–190
Nitrogen dioxide poisoning, 431
Nitrogen narcosis, 26
Nocardia asteroides, 167
Nonarteritic ischemic optic neuropathy (NAION), 473, 474
Noncardiac pulmonary edema, 106
Non-Hb hemoproteins, 134
Nonhealing wounds, 188–189, 213
Nonischemic CRVO, 476
Nonsteroidal anti-inflammatory agents (NSAIDs), 477
Normobaric oxygen (NBO) therapy, 146–154, 191, 375, 583
Normobaric vs. hyperbaric oxygen, 55
Nosocomial infections, 169

NTFs. See Neurotrophic factors (NTFs)
Nuclear transcription factor kappa B (NFkB), 496
Nursing plan of care
    BNA Certification Board, 516
    HBO application, 515, 516
    hyperbaric medicine, 515, 516
    ICU nurses, 515
    Nationally Recognized Certification exam, 516
    nursing textbook, 517
    process, 517

O
Obstetrics
    experimental studies, 490
    fetal hypoxia, 490–491
    threatened abortion, 490
Ocular blood flow occlusion, 462
Ocular contraindications, 465
Ocular injury, 469
Ocular oxygen tension, 462
Oedema, 345, 347, 348
Ophthalmological complications, HBO, 84
Ophthalmology, 466
Optic neuritis, 82, 346, 347
Opt-out model, 537
Organ storage process, 542
Organ transplantation
    clinical applications, HBO, 542
    delayed graft function, 540
    face transplants, 541
    hand transplants, 541
    HBO, 538
    inflammation, 538–539
    ischemia-reperfusion injury, 538
    kidney transplant, 537
    liver transplants, 540
    lung transplants, 539
    opt-out model, 537
    organs and tissues, 541
    pancreas transplants, 539
    renal transplants, 540
Osteomyelitis, 169, 170
    jaw, 172
    sternum, 172
Osteonecrosis
    causes, 441, 442
    chest wall, 216
    diagnosis, 442
    HBO, 443, 444
    surgical procedures, 442
    temporal bone, 216
Osteopontin (OPN), 341
Osteoradionecrosis, 214–221
    basic studies, 214–215
    mandible, 215–216
    vertebrae, 216
Outer surface protein A (OspA), 176
Oxidative stress, 20
Oxygen
    as antibiotic, 159–160
    carriers, 255, 403, 533
    conductance system, 505
    inhalation, 512
    masks, 72
    seizures, 84

Oxygen toxicity, 90, 91, 597–598
  aerosol therapy, 60
  ammonia and amino acids, 58–59
  antioxidative defense mechanisms, 62
  ascorbic acid, 60
  brain and seizures, 59
  cerebral metabolism, 56
  chemiluminescence index, 61
  clinical monitoring, 59–60
  CNS, 49
  cytochrome c, 60
  distal airway epithelial cells, 60
  factors, 55–56
  free radical mechanisms, 50
  free radical scavengers, 61
  HBO neurotoxicity, 59
  hyperbaric oxygen (HBO), 49
  hyperoxic injury, 60
  hypothermia, 60
  magnesium sulfate suppresses, 60
  mammalian cell lines, 62
  medicine, 49
  molecular basis, 62
  neuropathology, 59
  neurotransmitters, 56
  normobaric vs. hyperbaric oxygen, 55
  oxygen-induced retinopathy, 55
  pathology, 50, 53, 54
  prevention/treatment, 60
  pulmonary, 54–61
  ROS, 50
  signs and symptoms, CNS toxicity, 52, 59
  vitamin E (tocopherol), 60
Oxygen transport and utilization, 14–15
Oxygen utilization in cell, 15
Oxygen-Hemoglobin Dissociation Curve, 13–14
Oxygen-induced retinopathy, 55
Oxygen-induced seizures, 59

P
Painless vision loss, 466, 469, 481
Panama Canal, 631
Pancreas transplants, 539
Paraplegics, 233–234
Paraquat poisoning, 431
Pars plana vitrectomy (PPV), 476, 477
Pathogenesis, 164
Patient monitoring devices, 75
Pattern shift visual evoked potential (PSVEP), 144
Penicillin, 165
Penicillin-G, 166
Penile amputation, 441
Penumbra zone, 246
Peptic ulceration
  antibacterial effect, 408
  clinical assessment, 408
  experimental studies in animals, 408
  gastric mucosal ischemia, 407
Perfluorochemicals, 533
Perinatal brain injury, 355
Perineal Crohn's disease (CD), 201
Peripheral blood mononuclear cells (PBMCs), 85

Peripheral nerve injuries, 438, 439
  HBO
    applications, 439
    edema, 438
    gait analysis, 438
    nerve regeneration, 438
    pinch-reflex test, 438
Peripheral neuropathy, 370
Peripheral vascular disease (PVD), 388, 510–511
  causes, 385
  clinical and laboratory assessment, 387
  clinical applications, HBO, 390, 391
  HBO, 389
  hyperbaric therapy, 390
  ischemia causes, 386
  limb ischemia, 386
  management, 388
    drug therapy, 388
    exercise therapy, 388
    surgery, 388
    surgical procedures, 388
  NBO, 389
  skeletal muscles, biochemical changes, 386, 387
  surgery, 393
  symptom, 386
Perivenous syndrome (PS), 108
Personal transfer chamber (PTC), 562
Personalized hyperbaric medicine
  Ayurvedic practices, 595
  clinical application, 596
  constitutional picture, 595
  economical aspects, 598
  hypoxia, 597
  imaging, 597
  molecular diagnostics, 596
  pharmacogenomics, 595
  prescription, 595
  sequencing, 596–597
  SPECT, 595
Pharmacogenomics, 595
Photoaging, 507–508
Photodynamic therapy, 534
Phycomycotic fungal infections, 167
Physical therapy, 509
Placental growth factor (PlGF), 401
Plasma, 402
Platelets and coagulation, 400
Pneumatosis cystoides intestinalis (PCI), 413–414
Pneumatosis intestinalis
  clinical study, 414
  normobaric oxygen therapy, 414
  PCI, 413
Pneumothorax (PTX), 84, 431
Positron Emission Tomography (PET), 145, 237
Post-concussion syndrome (PCS), 327, 329, 573
Postoperative anterior segment ischemia, 472–473
Postoperative complications
  cerebrovascular surgery, 336
  intracranial aneurysms, 337–338
Posttraumatic stress disorder (PTSD), 327, 573
Precision medicine, 595
Preconditioning, 546
PregnancyHBO therapy, 491

PregnancyMEDLINE, 491
Pregnant uterine harvest/global ischemia model, 302
Pre-HBOT ocular examination, 465
Preoxygenation, 545–547
Pressure and action of drugs, 30–31
Pressure effect on human body, 25–29
    ammonia metabolism, 24
    blood cells and platelets, 24
    cardiovascular system, 25
    endocrine system, 25
    hematological and biochemical effects, 23–24
    nervous system effects (*see* Nervous system)
    physical effects, 23
    respiratory system and blood gases, 24
    skeletal system, 25
Pressure ulcers, 199
Pressure vessels (PV), 632
Pressure vessels for human occupancy (PVHO), 632
Priapism, 404
Primary percutaneous transluminal coronary angioplasty
        (PTCA), 379
Proctitis, 220
Proliferative vitreoretinopathy, 480
Prostaglandins, 422
Protein methionine sulfoxide (PMSO), 598
Protoporphyrin IX-triplet state lifetime technique
        (PpIX-TSLT), 16
Pseudoarthrosis, 440
Pseudomembranous colitis, 413
Pseudomonas aeruginosa, 172
Psoriasis, 207
Psychological stress, 190
PTCA. *See* Primary percutaneous transluminal coronary angioplasty
        (PTCA)
Pulmonary barotrauma, 84, 106, 129
Pulmonary complications, HBO, 84
Pulmonary disorders
    arterial hemodynamics, 427
    respiratory insufficiency, 429
Pulmonary edema, 430–431
Pulmonary embolism, 430
Pulmonary gas exchange, 428
Pulmonary oxygen toxicity, 428
Pulmonary symptoms, 103
Purpura fulminans, 207
Pyoderma gangrenosum, 206–207, 478

Q
Quality measures, 624, 625

R
Radiation Biology, 212
Radiation effects
    bone, 213
    nervous system, 212
Radiation encephalopathy, 217
Radiation enterocolitis, 413
Radiation injuries, 214
Radiation myelitis, 216
Radiation retinopathy (RR), 469, 471, 472
Radiation sensitizing agents, 533
Radiation therapy, 218
Radiation-Induced Hemorrhagic Cystitis, 219–220
Radiation-induced necrosis (RIN), 217

Radiation-induced optic neuropathy (RION), 217
Radionecrosis, 211–214
    larynx, 218–219
Radiopharmaceutical, 93, 94
Radiosensitivity, 212, 528–529, 532
Radiotherapy, 528, 532
Rankin scale, 252
Reactive oxygen species (ROS), 50, 556
Recompression, 107–113, 116–119, 121
Red blood cells (RBCs)
    CO_2 and H_2O, 397
    deformability, 397–398
    erythropoiesis, 400
    hemoglobin, 399
    oxygen exchange, 398–399
    stored blood, 399
    structure and biochemistry, 399
Red cell infusion, 533
Refractory pseudomonas keratitis, 478
Regenerative medicine, 590, 600
Regional cerebral blood flow (rCBF), 56
Regulation of hyperbaric medicine
    codes, 632
    health, 632
    insurance, 632
    labor, 632
Rehabilitation, HBO role
    acute myocardial infarction, 510
    advantages, 510
    CNS injuries, 510
    indications, 509, 510
    ischemic leg pain, 511
    limb amputees, 511
    myocardial ischemia, 511
    neurological disorders, 510
    paraplegia, 511
    peripheral vascular disease, 510
    physical therapy, 509
    stroke, 511
    traumatic brain injury, 511
Renal transplants, 540
Reperfusion injury, 247–248, 274
Repetitive transcranial magnetic stimulation (rTMS) therapy, 449
Research
    animal experimental studies, 588
    application of biotechnologies, 588, 589
    in hyperbaric medicine, 587, 588
Respirators and ventilators, 72
Respiratory insufficiency, 429
Respiratory system, 20
Retina, 462
Retinal artery occlusions, 470–471
Retinal blood supply, 462
Retinal injury, 467
Retinal oxygen toxicity, 463–464
Retinitis pigmentosa (RP), 479
Retinopathy, 464
Retinopathy of prematurity (ROP), 356, 357
Retrolental fibroplasia, 55, 355–357, 464
Reversible ischemic neurological deficit (RIND), 338
Rheumatoid arthritis
    clinical applications, 445
    HBO therapy, 444
    inflammatory process, 444
Rhinocerebral mucormycosis, 167
Robotics, 600

S

Safety and fire hazard
    clinical hyperbaric chambers, 606
    FDA labeling requirements, 606
    fire causes, 606
    NFPA, 606
    UHM, 608
Salmonella abortus, 348
Scleroderma, 207, 208
Sechrist monoplace hyperbaric chamber, 64, 65
Secondary keratoendotheliosis, 480
Seizure disorders, 82
Seizures control, 128
Self-contained breathing apparatus (SCUBA), 106
Sequencing, 596–597
Shock
    cardiogenic shock, 385
    oxygen delivery , blood, 384–385
    pathophysiology, 384
    traumatic and hypovolemic, 385
Shock lung, 431
Sickle cell disease, 480
Single photon emission computerized tomography
        (SPECT), 145, 237–238, 359–367
Sinus Pain, 84
Skin flaps
    animal experimental studies, 202–203
    ischemic injury, 201
    myocutaneous flap, 202
    pedicle graft, 201
    split skin grafting, 201
    tissue hypoxia, 202
Social media, 600
Soft tissue gas, 165
Soft tissue infections, 162, 163
Soft tissue necrosis, 218
Somatosensory-evoked potentials
        (SSEPs), 331, 334
Spasticity, 357–360, 362
SPECT brain function imaging, 94, 95
    case studies, 95
        HBOT, 95
        hyperbaric oxygen therapy, 95
        stroke, 94, 95
    clinical utilization, 94
    heads imaging, 95
    image comparison, 94
    radioisotope, 96
SPECT brain imaging, 318
Spider bite
    animal experimental studies, 200
    antivenom, 200
    Loxosceles reclusa, 200
    treatment, 200–201
    vesicle formation, 200
Spinal cord injury (SCI), 231, 330–334, 342, 348, 574
Spinal cord symptoms, 103
Spinal epidural abscess, 334
Sports injuries, 511–512
Sports training, 512–513
Squamous cell carcinoma, 221
Standard cortisone treatment (SCT), 449
Stem cells, 400–401
Stem cells and HBO, 591
Stereotactic radiosurgery, 217
Steroids, 128

Stroke, 244–248, 252–255, 267, 336–341
    acute ischemic stroke, 253
        concomitant disorders, 254
        medical emergency, 254
        medical therapies, 253, 254
        rehabilitation, 253, 254
        surgical therapies, 254
    causes, 243, 244
    cerebral infarct, 244, 246
    cerebral ischemia, 246, 247
    complications, 250
    definition, 241
    diagnosis, 251, 252
    effects of HBO, 269, 270
    epidemiology, 242
    glutamate, 246
    ischemia
        brain changes, 244, 245
        cerebral metabolism, 246, 247
    neuroprotective agent (*see* Neuroprotection)
    pathogenesis
        cytokines and adhesion molecules, 248
        DNA damage, 248
        gene expression, 248
        HSP, 248
        NTFs, 248
    pathophysiology, 243
    recovery, 249, 250
    rehabilitation (*see* Klausenbach study)
    reperfusion injury, 247
    risk factors, 242–248
    scales
        Barthel index scores, 252
        CNS, 253
        European Stroke Scale, 253
        NIH, 252
        Rankin scale, 252
        UNSS, 252
    spasticity and dementia, 251
    stages, 244, 245
    symptoms, 244
    vascular dementia, 251
Stroke rehabilitation, 511
Subjects somatosensory evoked potentials (SSEP), 234
Submarine medicine
    rescue operations, 577
    submarines' rescue, 577
    transfer under pressure, 578
Sudden deafness
    acute acoustic trauma, 450
    causes, 449
    clinical studies, 452–453
    cortilymph pO_2, 449
    experimental studies, 450–452
    hair cells, 449
    HBO, 449
    treatment, 449
Superoxide dismutase (SOD), 54
Surface equivalent fraction of inhaled oxygen (SEFIO$_2$), 557
Susac's syndrome, 371
Synthetic biology, 600

T

Temporal bone, 216
Temporal visual field defects (TVFD), 479

Testosterone, 422
The MS National Therapy Centres, 349
The Undersea and Hyperbaric Medical Society (UHMS), 196
Thermal burns, 206
    cellular elements, 204
    clinical application, 205, 206
    experimental studies, 205
    pathophysiology, 204
    polymorphonuclear neutrophilic leukocytes, 204
    vascular permeability, 204
Thoracic surgery, 81
Thyroid disease, 423
Thyroid glands, 421
Tinnitus, 447–449
Tissue oxygen tensions, 190, 191
Tissue poisons, 133, 134
Tolerance to oxygen
    adaptation, 61
    drugs, 61
    interruption of exposure, 61
    newborn mammals, 61
Topical application by a small hyperbaric chamber (TOPOX), 191, 192
Toxemias, 491
Toxic amblyopia, 478, 479
Toxic brain injury, 359, 362
Toxic epidermal necrolysis, 207
Toxic megacolon (TM), 412, 413
Transcutaneous oximetry (TcPO$_2$), 213
Transcutaneous oxygen monitor (TCOM), 498
Transcutaneous oxygen pressure (tcpO$_2$), 73, 190
Transportable recompression rescue chamber (TRRC), 120
Transverse myelitis, 346
Traumatic brain injury, 355, 362
    HBO, 328
Traumatic brain injury (TBI), 226, 304, 325–331, 334, 341, 342, 573
Traumatic ischemia
    amputation, 436
    causes, 435
    HBO treatments, 436
    transcutaneous oxygen, 436
Traumatology
    definition, 433
Treatment of ulcers, 188
Tuberculosis, 169
Tumor radiosensitivity, 529, 531
Type I DCS, 108, 110, 112, 113
Type II DCS, 108–111, 113, 118, 120

U
Ulcers, 193
Undersea and Hyperbaric Medical Society (UHMS), 82, 495, 604, 621
Undersea and Hyperbaric Medicine (UHM), 583, 608, 628
Undersea Medical Society (UMS), 621
Unidentified bright objects (UBOs), 345

Unified neurological stroke scale (UNSS), 252
Unit pulmonary toxic dose (UPTD), 54
United States, hyperbaric medicine
    ABEM, 621
    ABPM, 621
    ACHM, 621
    hospital-based hyperbaric programs, 622
    UHMS, 621, 622
UNSS. *See* Unified neurological stroke scale (UNSS)
Urine methylguanidine (MG), 20
Uveitis, 480

V
Vacuum-assisted closure (VAC), 437
Vascular dementia, 251
Vascular endothelial growth factor (VEGF) expression, 192, 203, 356, 574
Vascular headaches, 371
Vascular pathologies, 391
Vasoconstriction, 126
Vasodilators, 533
Venous ulcers
    pathophysiology, 197
    treatment, 197–198
Vestibular symptoms, 103
Viral infections, 601
Vision
    factors, 462
    loss, 467–469, 473–476, 481, 482
    process, 462
Visual-evoked response (VER), 463
Vitreoretinopathy, 480
Von Hippel Landau protein (VHL), 347

W
White matter hyperintensities (WHMs), 345
Whole body irradiation, 212
Wound Care and Hyperbaric Medicine Program, 627
Wound healing
    adjuncts to HBO, 192–193
    angiogenesis, 188
    cell types, 188
    clinical applications, 191–193
    experimental studies, 189
    nitric oxide, 189–190
    nonhealing wounds, 188–189
    oxygen role, 188
    psychological stress, 190
    rationale of using oxygen, 189

X
Xanthine-oxidase-derived reactive oxygen species, 140

Printed by Printforce, the Netherlands